Haematology and Blood Transfusion
Hämatologie und Bluttransfusion 37

Springer
Berlin
Heidelberg
New York
Barcelona
Budapest
Hong Kong
London
Milan
Paris
Santa Clara
Singapore
Tokyo

W. Hiddemann T. Büchner
B. Wörmann J. Ritter U. Creutzig
W. Plunkett M. Keating (Eds.)

Acute Leukemias V

Experimental Approaches and Management of Refractory Disease

With 211 Figures and 202 Tables

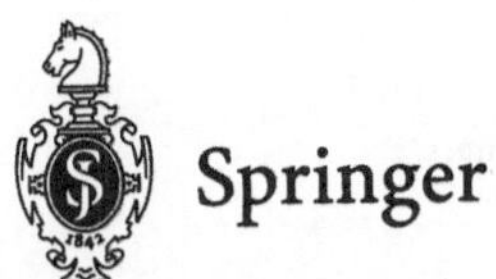

Springer

Prof. Dr. W. Hiddemann
Priv.-Doz. Dr. W. Plunkett
Department of Internal Medicine
University of Göttingen
Robert-Koch-Strasse 40
37075 Göttingen, Germany

B. Wörmann, M.D., Ph.D.
M.J. Keating, M.D., B.S.
Department of Internal Medicine
MD Anderson Cancer Center
1515 Holcombe Blvd.
Houston, TX 77030, USA

Prof. Dr. T. Büchner
Department of Internal Medicine
Prof. Dr. J. Ritter
Department of Pediatric Oncology
University of Münster
Albert-Schweitzer-Strasse 33
48145 Münster, Germany

Prof. Dr. U. Creutzig
Koordinierungsstelle
Deutsche Krebsgesellschaft e.V.
Thea-Bähnisch-Weg 12
30657 Hannover, Germany

ISBN 978-3-642-78909-0 ISBN 978-3-642-78907-6 (eBook)
DOI 10.1007/978-3-642-78907-6

Library of Congress Cataloging-in-Publication Data. Acute leukemias V: experimental approaches and management of refractory disease/W. Hiddemann... [et al.] (eds.). p. cm. – (Haematology and blood transfusion = Hämatologie und Bluttransfusion: 37) Includes bibliographical references and index.
ISBN 978-3-642-78909-0 1. Leukemia – Treatment – Congresses. I. Hiddemann, W. II. Series: Hämatologie und Bluttransfusion: 37. [DNLM: 1. Leukemia – therapy – congresses. 2. Acute Disease – congresses. 3. Antineoplastic Agents – pharmacokinetics – congresses. 4. Antineoplastic Agents – therapeutic use – congresses. 5. Drug Resistance – congresses. W1 HA1655 v.37 1996/WH 250 A1895 1996] RC643.A3172 1996 616.99'41906–dc20 DNLM/DLC for Library of Congress 96-41598

Softcover reprint of the hardcover 1st edition 1996

Cover design: Springer-Verlag, Design & Production

Typesetting: Thomson Press (India) Ltd., Madras

The text printed in this book was taken directly from data supplied by the editors.

SPIN: 10132922 23/3145/SPS – 5 4 3 2 1 0 – Printed on acid-free paper

Preface

150 years after the first description of the clinical picture of "white blood" and the introduction of the term "leukemia" by R.Virchow it appears, that the leukemias, and the acute leukemias in particular, serve as an impressive example for the major improvements that have been achieved in the treatment but also in the understanding of the biology of malignant disorders. The international symposia "Acute Leukemia" which are held at Münster since 1986 have developed into an international forum to review the current progress and the future perspectives of leukemia research and therapy at a high scientific and clinical level. Since the possibility for active participation in these symposia is somewhat restricted we are glad to have the opportunity to extend the information that was presented at the symposium "Acute Leukemias V - Experimental Approaches and Management of Refractory Disease" which was held from February 27 to March 2, 1994 to a broader audience of basic scientists and clinicians. This meeting was especially designed to discuss experimental approaches and the management of refractory disease which allows to evaluate new experimental therapies on the basis of preclinical studies. Hence, topics such as the pharmacokinetics of cytostatic agents, drug resistance, the application of growth factors for the modulation of cytotoxicity as well as clinical trials in both acute myeloid and lymphoblastic leukemias and the biology of residual disease were all addressed in different sessions and discussed by well recognized experts in the respective fields. The results summarized in these Proceedings are mostly new and previously unpublished and demonstrate the rapid transformation of basic research into clinical practice. This development will continue to translate into further improvements of therapy which will ultimately benefit patients with these disorders.

July 1995

W. Hiddemann · T. Büchner
B. Wörmann · J. Ritter
U. Creutzig · W. Plunkett
M. Keating

Table of Contents

Leukemia Cell Biology

Cell Differentiation and Programmed Cell Death: A New Approach to Leukemia Therapy
L. SACHS 3

CD34 and CD38 Expression on Blasts in Myelodysplastic Syndromes and Secondary AML
W. VERBEEK, C. RIES, D. GROVE, M. UNTERHALT, W. HIDDEMANN, and B. WÖRMANN 11

Heterogeneity of HRX-FEL Fusion Transcripts in Adult and Pediatric t(4;11) ALL
F. GRIESINGER, T. JAHN, H. ELFERS, W.-D. LUDWIG, M. FALK, H. RIEDER, J. HARBOTT, F. LAMPERT, B. HEINZE, D. HOELZER, E. THIEL, H. RIEHM, B. WÖRMANN, C. FONATSCH, and W. HIDDEMANN 15

Pharmacokinetics – Clinical Implications

Fludarabine and Ara-C Combination for Treatment of Adult Acute Myelogenous Leukemia: Pharmacokinetic and Pharmacodynamic Effects
V. GANDHI, M. DU, A.J. CHAPMAN, P. HUANG, E. ESTEY, M.J. KEATING, and W. PLUNKETT 25

Pharmacokinetics of Ara-CMP-Stearate (YNK01) – Phase I Study of the Oral Ara-C Derivative
J. BRAESS, E. SCHLEYER, B. RAMSAUER, M. UNTERHALT, C. KAUFMANN, S. WILDE, M. SCHÜSSLER, and W. HIDDEMANN 32

Differential Effect of GM-CSF on the Intracellular Ara-C Metabolism in Normal Bone Marrow Mononuclear Cells and Acute Myeloid Leukemia (AML) Blasts
C. REUTER, C. ROLF, E. SCHLEYER, M. UNTERHALT, B. WÖRMANN, T. BÜCHNER, and W. HIDDEMANN 41

Intracellular Retention of Cytosine-Arabinoside-Triphosphate in Leukemic Blast Cells from Children
J. Boos, M. Schiller, B. Pröbsting, U. Creutzig, and J. Ritter 50

The Pharmacokinetics of Epipodophyllotoxins – Clinical Relevance
K.B. Mross 53

Targeted Drug Therapy in Childhood Acute Lymphoblastic Leukemia
M.V. Relling, C.-H. Pui, and W.E. Evans 62

Asparagine Levels in Children on E. Coli- and Erwinia-Asparaginase Therapy
J. Boos, G. Werber, E. Verspohl, E. Ahlke, U. Nowak-Gött, and H. Jürgens 67

Chemo-Resistance

Pharmacologic Modulation of Multidrug Resistance in Acute Leukemia: Results and Challenges
A.F. List, B. Glinsmann-Gibson, and W.S. Dalton 73

Kinetic Resistance, Regrowth Resistance, and Multidrug Resistance in the Treatment of Acute Myelogenous Leukemia (AML)
H.D. Preisler and A. Raza 79

Topoisomerases – from Basic Research to Clinical Implications
F. Gieseler 89

Mechanisms of Acquired ARA-C and DAC-Resistance in Acute Myeloid Leukemia (AML): Development of a Model for the Study of Mutational Loss of Deoxycytidine Kinase (DCK) Activity
A.P.A. Stegmann, M.W. Honders, J.E. Landegent, and R. Willemze 94

Expression of P-Glycoprotein in Children and Adults with Leukemia – Correlation with Clinical Outcome
S. Kaczorowski, M. Ochocka, R. Aleksandrowicz, M. Kaczorowska, M. Matysiak, and M. Karwacki 101

Multidrug Resistance in Acute Myelogenous Leukemia: Relevance to Clinical and Laboratory Data
A. Zaritskey, I. Stuf, T. Bykova, K. Titov, N. Medvedeva, N. Anikina, and B. Afanasiev 108

Mitoxantrone/Cytarabine with or without Quinine as a Potential MDR-Reserving Agent for the Treatment of Acute Leukemias
E. Solary, D. Caillot, F. Witz, P. Moreau, P. Genne, B. Desablens, J.Y. Cahn, A. Sadoun, B. Pignon, J.F. Abgrall, F. Maloisel, D. Guyotat, P. Casassus, N. Ifrah, P. Lamy, B. Audhuy, P. Colombat, and J.L. Harousseau 112

In Vitro Modulation of Multidrug Resistance by BIBW22BS in Blasts of De Novo or Relapsed or Persistent AML
J. Schröder, M. Esteban, S. Kasimir-Bauer, U. Bamberger, A. Heckel, M.E. Scheulen, and S. Seeber 118

In Vitro Drug Resistance Profiles in Childhood Acute Lymphoblastic Leukemia
R. Pieters, G.J.L. Kaspers, E. Klumper, E.R. van Wering, A. van der Does-van den Berg, and A.J.P. Veerman 124

Growth Factors – Modulation

The Expression and Regulation of G-CSF and GM-CSF
E. Vellenga 131

In Situ Nick Translation as a Measure of Cell Death. Application to the Study of Growth Factors and Drug Sensitivity
M. Minden, C.W. Wang, and E.A. McCulloch 134

Molecular Mechanisms of Ara-C Signalling: Synergy and Antagonism with Interleukin-3
C. Belka, C. Sott, F. Herrmann, and M.A. Brach 139

Hematopoietic Recovery and Priming – Therapeutic Effects of GM-CSF in the Treatment of AML
T. Büchner, W. Hiddemann, B. Wörmann, R. Rottmann, G. Maschmeyer, W.-D. Ludwig, M. Zühlsdorf, K. Buntkirchen, A. Sander, J. Aswald, I. Binder, S. Prisett, and M.C. Sauerland 145

Improved Antileukemic Activity of the Combination of Ara-C with GM-CSF and IL-3 Fusion Protein (PIXY321)
K. Bhalla, A.M. Ibrado, G. Bullock, C. Tang, S. Ray, Y. Huang, and V. Ponnathpur 149

A Double-blind Controlled Study of G-CSF Started Two Days Before Induction Chemotheraphy in Refractory Acute Myeloid Leukemia
R. Ohno, T. Naoe, A. Kanamaru, M. Yoshida, A. Hiraoka, T. Kobayashi, T. Ueda, S. Minami, Y. Morishima, Y. Saito, S. Furusawa, K. Imai, Y. Takemoto, Y. Miura, H. Teshima, and N. Hamajima 156

Effects of Growth Factors In Vitro on Acute Lymphoblastic Leukemia Cells
G.J.L. Kaspers, R. Pieters, C.H. Van Zantwijk, G.H. Broekema, K. Hählen, and A.J.P. Veerman 163

The Experience of Polish Children's Leukemia Lymphoma Study Group on G-CSF and GM-CSF Interventional Use in Neutropenia Associated with Chemotheraphy of Childhood Acute Lymphoblastic Leukemia (ALL)
A. Chybicka, J. Boguslawska-Jaworska, J. Armata, W. Balwierz, K. Boruczkowski, J. Kowalczyk, M. Matysiak, M. Ochocka, U. Radwańska, and D. Sonta-Jakimczyk 167

Induction Therapy with Idarubicin, Ara-C, and VP-16 Followed by G-CSF and Maintenance Immunotherapy with Interleukin-2 for High-Risk AML
A. GANSER, G. HEIL, G. SEIPELT, J.TH. FISCHER, W. LANGER, W. BROCKHAUS, K. KOLBE, T.H. ITTEL, N. BRACK, H.G. FUHR, L. BERGMANN, and D. HOELZER 175

Incidence of Infections in Adult Patients (>55 Years) with Acute Myeloid Leukemia Treated with Yeast-Derived GM-CSF (Sargramostim): Results of a Double-Blind Prospective Study by the Eastern Cooperative Oncology Group
J.M. ROWE, A. RUBIN, J.J. MAZZA, J.M. BENNETT, E. PAIETTA, J.W. ANDERSON, R. GHALIE, and P.H. WIERNICK 178

Chemotheraphy in AML

New Approaches in the Treatment of AML and MDS
M.J. KEATING 187

S-HAM Salvage Therapy of Relapsed and Refractory AML Followed by Interleukin 2 Postremission Therapy
W. HIDDEMANN, M. UNTERHALT, M. KEMPER, E. SCHLEYER, P. SCHÖNROCK-NABULSI, L. UHAREK, M. FROMM, D. BRAUMANN, M. PLANKER, U. KUBICKA, J. KAROW, S. LANGE, C. TIRIER, B. WÖRMANN, C. SAUERLAND, A. HEINECKE, and TH. BÜCHNER for the German AML Cooperative Group . . . 195

Mitoxantrone-Etoposide or HD-ARA-C/Mitoxantrone for Remission Induction in Children with First Relapse of AML
K. STAHNKE, J. RITTER, J. BOOS, and U. CREUTZIG 200

Sequential Mitoxantrone, Ara-C and VP-16 (s-MAV) Followed by Immuno-Maintenance-Therapy with Interleukin-2 (IL-2) in the Treatment of Refractory and Relapsed Acute Myelogenous Leukemia
G. HÜBNER, J. WENDLER, B. OTREMBA, I. FACKLER-SCHWALBE, and H. LINK 203

Mitoxantrone, Etoposide and Cyclosporine A Therapy for Relapsed and Refractory Acute Myelogenous Leukemia, A Pediatric Oncology Group Phase II Trial
G.V. DAHL, N. BROPHY, H. GRIER, H. WEINSTEIN, B. SIKIC, and R. ARCECI 206

Sequential Chemotherapy with Mitoxantrone, Etoposide and Cytarabine for Previously Treated Acute Myeloid Leukemia. EMA 886 Regimen
E. ARCHIMBAUD, X. THOMAS, V. LEBLOND, M. MICHALLET, P. FENAUX, F. DREYFUS, X. TROUSSARD, C. CORDONNIER, J. JAUBERT, P. TRAVADE, J. TRONCY, D. ASSOULINE, and D. FIÈRE 210

Treatment of Childhood Acute Nonlymphoblastic Leukemia – Final Results of the Austrian-Hungarian Study AML-IGCI-84
F.M. FINK, G. MANN, P. MASÁT, E.R. PANZER-GRÜMAYER, P. KAJTAR, G. KARDOS, CH. URBAN, D. SCHULER, and H. GADNER for the IGCI Pediatric Study Group 213

TAD Double Induction, HDAra C Consolidation, Rotation Maintenance in ANLL: the Results and Prophylaxis of Hepatitis and Fungal Infection
S. Pushkareva, N. Gorbounova, E. Oboukhova, A. Davtian, M. Kontchalovski, G. Selidovkin, and A. Baranov 217

Chemotherapy in ALL

Salvage Therapy of Childhood ALL: Prognosis of Marrow Relapse After Intensive Front-line Therapy
G. Henze, R. Hartmann, and R. Fengler on behalf of the BFM Relapse Study Group 223

Salvage Therapy of Adult ALL
M. Freund, G. Heil, K. Pompe, R. Arnold, C. Bartram, Th. Büchner, H. Diedrich, C. Fonatsch, A. Ganser, W. Hiddemann, P. Koch, K. Kolbe, H. Link, H. Löffler, W.D. Ludwig, G. Maschmeyer, N. Schmitz, M. Schwonzen, E. Thiel, and D. Hoelzer on behalf of the German Relapsing Acute Lymphocytic Leukemia Study Group (GRALLSG) 229

Protocol RACOP in the Treatment of Resistant and Relapsed ALL
R.A. Kutcher, V.G. Isaev, V.G. Savchenko, E.N. Parovitchnikova, L.S. Lubimova, and L.P. Mendeleeva 235

Treatment of Philadelphia Chromosome Positive ALL with Interferon Alpha
J.L. Harousseau, F. Guilhot, P. Casassus, and D. Fière 239

Six Years' Experience with Treatment of Recurrent Childhood Lymphoblastic Leukemia. Report of the Polish Children's Leukemia/Lymphoma Study Group
J. Boguslawska-Jaworska, A. Chybicka, J. Armata, W. Balwierz, H. Bubala, B. Filiks-Litwin, J. Kowalczyk, D. Lukowska, M. Ochocka, U. Radwanska, R. Rokicka-Milewska, D. Sonta-Jaikimczyk, W. Strojny, and E. Zelenay . . . 243

Interim Results of a Phase II Study with Idarubicin in Relapsed Childhood Acute Lymphoblastic Leukemia
A. Neuendank, R. Hartmann, R. Fengler, R. Erttmann, R. Dopfer, F. Zintl, E. Koscielniak, and G. Henze 254

Leukemia-Lymphoma in Children with Primary Nodal Peripheral and Mediastinal Involvement
M. Matysiak and M. Ochocka 258

Immunotherapy of Acute Leukemias

Induction of Immunity Against Leukemia
S. de Vos, D.B. Kohn, W.H. McBride, and H.P. Koeffler 265

IL2 in Acute Leukemia
D. Blaise, A.M. Stoppa, M. Attal, J. Reiffers, J. Fleury, M. Michallet, E. Archimbaud, R. Bouabdallah, J.A. Gastaut, and D. Maraninchi 274

Is There a Role for Interleukin-2 Gene Transfer in the Management of Acute Leukemia?
R. Foa, A. Cignetti, A. Giillio Tos, A. Carbone, P.F. do Celle, and A. Guarini 279

Use of Roquinimex in the Myeloid Leukemias
J.M. Rowe, B.I. Nilsson, and B. Simonsson 285

The Inhibition of Lymphokine Activated Killer Cell Activation Mediated by AML Culture Supernatants Might Be Due to Transforming Growth Factor Beta 1
D.K. Schui, J. Brieger, E. Weidmann, P.S. Mitrou, D. Hoelzer, and L. Bergmann 294

Natural Killer Cell Alloreactivity Against Acute Leukemia Blasts: The Level of Activity Depends on the Individual Target-Effector Pair
B. Glass, L. Uharek, H. Ullerich, T. Gaska, H. Löffler, W.M. Müller-Ruchholtz, and W. Gassmann 298

Cellular Immunotherapy of Acute Leukemias After High Dose Chemotherapy with Cytarabin (ARA-C) and Cyclophosphamide (CY) in a Murine Model
L. Uharek, B. Glass, T. Gaska, M. Zeis, H. Löffler, W.M. Müller-Ruchholtz, and W. Gassmann 306

Interleukin-2 Bolus Infusion as Consolidation Therapy in 2nd Remission of Acute Myelocytic Leukemia
L. Bergmann, G. Heil, K. Kolbe, E. Lengfelder, E. Puzicha, H. Martin, J. Lohmeyer, P.S. Mitrou, and D. Hoelzer 312

Interleukin-2 Postremission Therapy in Acute Myeloid Leukemia (AML): In Vitro and In Vivo Effects of a Five Day Continuous Infusion of IL-2 on Phenotype and Function of Peripheral Lymphocytes
H.S.P. Garritsen, C. Constantin, F. Griesinger, A. Kolkmeyer, R. Doornbos, B.G. de Grooth, J. Greve, B. Wörmann, and W. Hiddemann . . 317

Comparison of Immunological and Molecular Markers When Using Interleukin-2 (IL-2) Alone or in Combination with γ-Interferon (IFN-γ) in the Maintenance Therapy of Acute Myeloid Leukemia (AML)
A. Neubauer, O. Knigge, R. Zimmermann, D. Krahl, C.A. Schmidt, J. Oertel, and D. Huhn 324

Immunological Response to IL-2 AND α-IFN-Treatment After Autologous BMT in Patients with BCR-ABL-positive ALL
H. Martin, L. Bergmann, J. Bruecher, S. Christ, B. Schneider, B. Wassmann, and D. Hoelzer 329

Bone Marrow Transplantation

Conditioning Regimens for Bone Marrow and Peripheral Blood Stem Cell Transplantation
A.M. Carella 337

Influence of Different Conditioning Regimens on Stroma Precursors
K. Momotjuk, L. Gerasimova, V. Savchenko, S. Kulikov,
L. Mendeleeva, and L. Lubimova 345

Autologous Bone Marrow Transplantation in Relapsing Acute Leukemias
C. Annaloro, A. Della Volpe, R. Mozzana, A. Oriani, E. Pozzoli, D. Soigo,
E. Tagliaferri, and G. Lambertenghi Deliliers 350

Autologous Vs. Unrelated Donor Bone Marrow Transplantation
for Acute Lymphoblastic Leukemia Considerations and Logistics
D. Weisdorf 356

Comparison Between Allogeneic and Autologous Bone Marrow
Transplantation for Childhood Acute Lymphoblastic Leukemia
in Second Remission
P. Bordigoni, G. Leverger, A. Baruchel, H. Espérou-Bourdeau, Y. Perel,
G. Michel, F. Bernaudin, C. Bergeron, G. Cornu, B. Lacour, G. Couillaud,
B. Pautard, J.P. dommergues, and J.L. Stephan for the Société
d'Hématologie et d'Immunologie Pédiatrique (SHIP) France 360

Comparison of Allogeneic and Autologous Bone Marrow Transplantation
for Treatment of Childhood Acute Myeloblastic Leukemia (AML)
in First Complete Remission
F. Zintl, J. Hermann, D. Fuchs, A. Müller, J. Füller, and H. Vogelsang . . . 369

Long-Term Results in Adult AML: Comparison of Postremission
Chemotherapy vs. Autologous BMT vs. Allogeneic BMT
W. Helbig, R. Krahl, M. Kubel, H. Schwenke, M. Herold, F. Fiedler,
A. Franke, V. Lakner, R. Rohrberg, D. Kämpfe, F. Strohbach, G. Schott,
U.V. Grünhagen, N. Grobe, R. Pasold, M. Stauch, J. Fleischer,
C. Klinkenstein, C. Boewer, J. Steglich, P. Richter, R. Pillkahn,
R. Schubert, I. Rudorf, K. Eisengarten, and D. Morgenstern
for the East German Study Group (EGSG) 373

Allogeneic BMT in Patients with AML Influence of the Prior Response
to Induction Chemotherapy on Outcome After BMT
R. Arnold, D. Bunjes, B. Hertenstein, C. Duncker, J. Novotny,
M. Stefanic, M. Theobald, G. Heil, M. Wiesneth, and H. Heimpel 380

Donor Leukocyte Infusions (DLI) in the Treatment of AML Patients
Relapsed After Allogeneic Bone Marrow Transplantation
V. Savchenko, L. Mendeleeva, L. Lubimova, H. Parovitchnikova,
H. Gribanova, L.P. Poreshina, and M. Petrov 383

Recombinant Human Erythropoietin After Bone Marrow Transplantation –
A Placebo Controlled Trial
H. Link, M.A. Boogaerts, A. Fauser, R. Or, J. Reiffers, N.C. Gorin,
A. Carella, F. Mandelli, S. Burdach, A. Ferrant, W. Linkesch, S. Tura,
A. Bacigalupo, F. Schindel, and H. Heinrichs 386

Novel Therapeutic Approaches

Combination of rhSCF + rhG-SCF, But Not rhG-CSF Alone Potentiate the Moblization of Hematopoietic Stem Cells with Increased Repopulating Ability into Peripheral Blood of Mice
N.J. DRIZE, J.L. CHERTKOV, and A.R. ZANDER 391

High-dose Therapy and Autografting with Mobilized Peripheral Blood Progenitor Cells in Patients with Malignant Lymphoma
R. HAAS, H. GOLDSCHMIDT, R. MÖHLE, S. FRÜHAUF, S. HOHAUS, B. WITT, U. MENDE, M. FLENTJE, M. WANNENMACHER, and W. HUNSTEIN 398

Cord Blood Banking for Hematopoietic Stem Cell Transplantation
E. GLUCKMAN 405

Molecular Basis for Retinoic Acid Effects in Acute Promyelocytic Leukemia
C. CHOMIENNE 409

Acute Promyelocytic Leukemia: Advantage of A-Trans Retinoic Acid (ATRA) over Conventional Chemotherapy
E. LENGFELDER, M. SIMON, D. HAASE, F. HILD, and R. HEHLMANN 415

Studies of 2-Chlorodeoxyadenosine (Cladribine) at St. Jude Children's Research Hospital
V.M. SANTANA, W.R. CROM, and R.L. BLAKLEY 420

The Role of 2-Chlorodeoxyadenosine (2-CDA) in the Treatment of Lymphoid Malignancies: Preliminary Observations
T. URASIŃSKI, I. JANKOWSKA-KUREK, and E. ZUK 425

Cytarabine Ocfosfate, a New Oral Ara-C Analogue, in the Treatment of Acute Leukemia and Myelodysplastic Syndromes
R. OHNO and YNK-01 Study Group 428

Tumor Immunotherapy by IL-2 and IL-2 Gene Transfected Cells
A. LINDEMANN, F.M. ROSENTHAL, A. MACKENSEN, H. VEELKEN, P. KULMBURG, M. LAHN, and R. MERTELSMANN 432

Myeloid Differentiation Mediated Through New Potent Retinoids and Vitamin D_3 Analogs
E. ELSTNER, M.I. DAWSON, S. DE VOS, S. PAKKALA, L. BINDERUP, W. OKAMURA, M. USKOKOVIC, and H.P. KOEFFLER 439

Residual Disease

Functional Assays for Human AML Cells by Transplantation into SCID Mice
T. LAPIDOT, C. SIRARD, J. VORMOOR, T. HOANG, J. CACERES-CORTES, M. MINDEN, B. PATERSON, M.A. CALIGIURI, and J.E. DICK 453

Cytogenetics and Clonal Evolution in Childhood Acute Lymphoblastic Leukemia (ALL)
J. HARBOTT, I. REINISCH-BECKER, J. RITTERBACH, W.-D. LUDWIG, A. REITER, and F. LAMPERT 456

Molecular Biology of Acute Lymphoblastic Leukemia: Implications for Detection of Minimal Residual Disease
A. Beishuizen, E.R. van Wering, T.M. Breit, K. Hählen, H. Hooijkaas, and J.J.M. van Dongen 460

Detection of AML1/ETO-Rearrangements in Acute Myeloid Leukemia with a Translocation t(8;21)
U. Jaeger, R. Kusec, and O.A. Hass 475

Mastocytosis in AML-M2 with t(8;21) – a New Characteristic Association
D. Kämpfe, W. Helbig, R. Rohrberg, J. Boguslawska-Jaworska, and O.A. Haas 478

Acute Myeloid Leukemia with Translocation (8;21). Cytomorphology, Dysplasia and Prognostic Factors in 41 Cases
T. Haferlach, J.M. Bennett, H. Löffler, W. Gassmann, J. Andersen, N. Tuzuner, P.A. Cassileth, C. Fonatsch, B. Schlegelberger, E. Thiel, W.-D. Ludwig, M.C. Sauerland, A. Heinecke, and T. Büchner for AML Cooperative Group and ECOG 481

Simultaneous Occurrence of t(8;21) and del(5q) in Myeloid Neoplasms
K. Clodi, A. Gaiger, C. Peters, J. Boguslawska-Jaworska, U. Jäger, and O.A. Hass 486

Detection of MLL/AF4 Recombination by PCR Technique
R. Repp, A. Borkhardt, J. Hammermann, S. Brettreich, R. Gossen, E. Haupt, J. Harbott, and F. Lampert 490

Detection of Different 11q23 Chromosomal Abnormalities by Multiplex-PCR Using Automatic Fluorescence-Based DNA-Fragment Analysis
R. Repp, A. Borkhardt, E. Haupt, R. Gossen, S. Schlieben, I. Reinisch-Becker, J. Harbott, and F. Lampert 493

Designing Probe Sets for the Detection of Chromosome Abnormalities in Acute Myeloid Leukemia Using Fluorescence In Situ Hybridization
K. Fischer, C. Scholl, G. Cabot, M. Moos, R. Schlenk, P. Theobald, R. Haas, M. Bentz, P. Lichter, and H. Döhner 497

The Amplification of the Wilms Tumor Gene (wt-1) mRNA Using the Polymerase Chain Reaction Technique (PCR) May Enable Sensitive Detection of Small Blast Populations in AML
J. Brieger, E. Weidmann, K. Fenchel, P.S. Mitrou, L. Bergmann, and D. Hoelzer 501

Distribution of Cells with a "Stem Cell Like" Immunophenotype in Acute Leukemia
B. Wörmann, D. Grove, M. Falk, S. Könemann, Y. Markloff, S. Toepker, A. Heyll, C. Aul, J. Ritter, T. Büchner, W. Hiddemann, L.W.M.M. Terstappen, and F. Griesinger 506

Expression of Human Endogenous Retroviral (HERV) Sequences in Hematological Disorders
M. Simon, P. Kister, C. Leib-Mösch, G. Papakonstantinou, M. Schenk, W. Seifarth, and R. Hehlmann 514

DNA-Analysis by Flow-Cytometry
of up to Nine Year Old Methanol/Acetic Acid Fixed Samples
of Childhood Acute Lymphoblastic Leukemia (ALL)
K. Romanakis, A. Argyriou-Tirita, H. Zankl, and O.A. Hass 520

Biological Entities in Acute Myelogenous Leukemia According
to Morphological, Cytogenetic and Immunological Criteria:
Data of Study AML-BFM-87
U. Creutzig, J. Ritter, J. Harbott, M. Zimmermann, H. Löffler,
S. Schwartz, F. Lampert, and W.D. Ludwig 524

Expression of CD7 and CD15 on Leukemic Blasts Are Prognostic Parameters
in Patients with Acute Myelocytic Leukemia – Irrelevance of CD34
K. Fenchel, C. Heller, E. Weidmann, B. Wörmann, J. Brieger, A. Ganser,
P.S. Mitrou, L. Bergmann, and D. Hoelzer 536

IL-2 Receptor (IL-2R) Alpha, Beta, and Gamma Chains Expressed
on Blasts of Acute Mylelocytic Leukemia May Not Be Functional
E. Weidmann, J. Brieger, K. Fenchel, D. Hoelzer, L. Bergmann,
and P.S. Mitrou 542

Stromal Function in Long Term Bone Marrow Culture of Patients
with Acute Myeloid Leukemia
M.Y. Lisovsky and V.G. Savchenko 547

Fluorescence In Situ Hybridization for the Diagnosis and Follow-up
of BCR-ABL Positive ALL
G.P. Cabot, M. Bentz, K. Fischer, A. Ganser, M. Moos, C. Scholl,
P. Lichter, and H. Döhner 552

Supportive Care

Incidence and Severity of Amphotericin B-induced Acute Toxicity
in Leukemic Patients After Treatment with Three Different Formulations
(Amphotericin B, AmBisome and Amphotericin B/Intralipid) – A Pilot Study
M. Arning, K.O. Kliche, A. Wehmeier, A.H. Heer-Sonderhoff,
and W. Schneider 559

Pulmonary Infiltrates in Patients with Hematologic Malignancies:
Clinical Usefulness of Non-bioptic Bronchoscopic Techniques
M. von Eiff, N. Roos, M. Zühlsdorf, M. Thomas, and J. van de Loo 562

Fludarabine in Chronic Lymphocytic Leukemia and Maligant Lymphomas

New Aspects in the Treatment of Chronic Lymphocytic Leukemia
J.L. Binet and the French Cooperative Group on CLL 569

The Use of Fludarabine in Chronic Lymphocytic Leukemia
and Malignant Lymphomas
M.J. Keating 572

Response to Fludarabine in Patients with Low Grade Lymphoma
A. PIGADITOU, A.Z.S. ROHATINER, J.S. WHELAN, P.W.M. JOHNSON,
R.K. GANJOO, A. ROSSI, A.J. NORTON, J. AMESS, J. LIM, and T.A. LISTER 578

Fludarabine in Combination with Mitoxantrone and Dexamethasone
in Relapsed and Refractory Low-Grade Non-Hodgkin's Lymphoma
C. POTT, M. UNTERHALT, D.S. SANDFORD, H. MARKERT, M. FREUND,
A. ENGERT, W. GASSMANN, W. HOLTKAMP, M. SEUFERT, K. HELLRIEGEL, B. KNAUF,
R. NIEBERDING, B. EMMERICH, P. KOCH, B. WÖRMANN, and W. HIDDEMANN . . . 581

Novantrone – Current Status and Future Perspectives

New Anthracyclines – A Comparative Analysis of Efficacy and Toxicity
A.D. HO 591

Hematologic and Therapeutic Effects
of High-Dose AraC/Mitoxantrone (HAM) in the Induction Treatment
of Patients with Newly Diagnosed AML. A Trial by AML Cooperative Group
T. BÜCHNER, W. HIDDEMANN, B. WÖRMANN, A. BOECKMANN, H. LÖFFLER,
W. GASSMANN, G. MASCHMEYER, W.-D. LUDWIG, E. LENGFELDER, A. HEYLL,
B. LATHAN, G. INNIG, E. AUGION FREIRE-INNIG, K. BUNTKIRCHEN,
M.C. SAUERLAND, and A. HEINECKE 595

Comparison of Front-Line Chemotherapy for Intermediate Grade
and Follicular Non-Hodgkin's Lymphoma Using the CAP-BOP Regimens
J.M. VOSE, J.R. ANDERSON, P.J. BIERMANN, and J.O. ARMITAGE
for the Nebraska Lymphoma Study Group 599

Prednimustine and Mitoxantrone in the Treatment
of Low-Grade Non-Hodgkin Lymphomas
M. UNTERHALT, P. KOCH, C. POTT-HOECK, R. HERRMANN, and W. HIDDEMANN
for the German Low-Grade Lymphoma Study Group 604

Mono- Versus Combination-Chemotherapy in Metastatic Breast Cancer
E. HEIDEMANN 609

Authors and Institutions

ANNALORO, C.
University of Milano, Hospital Maggiore di Milano, Istituto di Scienze Medicine, Centro Trapianti di Midollo, Via F. Sforza 35, 20122 Milano, Italy

ARCHIMBAUD, E.
Hospital Edouard Herriot, Dept. of Hematology, 69437 Lyon Cedex 03, France

ARNING, M.
University Hospital, Dept. of Hematology and Oncology, Moorenstr. 5, 40225 Düsseldorf, Germany

ARNOLD, R.
University Hospital, Dept. of Internal Medicine III, Steinhövelstr. 9, 89075 Ulm, Germany

BERGMANN, L.
University Hospital, Dept. of Hematology, Theodor-Stern-Kai 7, 60596 Frankfurt, Germany

BHALLA, KAPIL N.
Medical Univ. of South Carolina, 903 CSB, Hematology/Oncology, 171 Ashley Avenue, Charleston, SC 29425, USA

BINET, J.-L.
Départment d'Hematologie, Groupe Hospitalier Pitié-Salpètrière, 47, Boulevard de l'Hôpital, 75651 Paris Cedex 13, France

BLAISE, D.
Bone Marrow Transplant Unit, Institut Paoli Calmettes, 232 Boulevard Saint Marguerite, 13274 Marseille Cedex 09, France

BOGUSLAWSKA-JAWORSKA, J.
Medical Academy Wroclaw, Dept. of Childrens Hematology, ul. Smoluchowskiego 32/4, 55-209 Wroclaw, Poland

BOOS, J.
University Hospital, Dept. of Pediatrics, Albert-Schweitzer-Str. 33, 48149 Münster, Germany

Bordigoni, P.
Hôpital d'Enfants, Unité de Transplantation Medullaire de Pédiatrie 2, Rue du Morvan, 54511 Vandoeuvre-les-Nancy, France

Borkhardt, A.
University Hospital, Dept. of Pediatrics, Feulgenstr. 12, 35392 Giessen, Germany

Brach, Marion A.
Max-Delbrück-Center of Molecular Medicine, Robert-Rössle-Str. 10, 13125 Berlin, Germany

Braess, J.
University Hospital, Dept. of Hematology and Oncology, Robert-Koch-Str. 40, 37075 Göttingen, Germany

Brieger, J.
University Hospital, Dept. of Hematology, Theodor-Stern-Kai 7, 60590 Frankfurt, Germany

Büchner, T.
University Hospital, Dept. of Internal Medicine, Albert-Schweitzer-Str. 33, 48129 Münster, Germany

Cabot, G.-P.
University Hospital, Dept. Hematology and Oncology, Hospitalstr. 3, 69115 Heidelberg, Germany

Carella, A.M.
Hospital S. Martino, Div. of Hematology, Via Acerba 10/22, 16148 Genova-Quarto, Italy

Chomienne, C.
Hôspital St. Louis, Institut Universitaire Hématologie, 1 Avenue Claude Vellefaux, 75475 Paris Cedex 10, France

Chybicka, A.
Medical Academy, Pediatric Haematologic Clinic, A.M. Wroclaw, ul. Bujwida 44, 50-345 Wroclaw, Poland

Clodi, K.
St. Anna Kinderspital, CCRI, Kinderspitalgasse 6, 1090 Wien, Austria

Creutzig, U.
Deutsche Krebsgesellschaft e.V., Koordinierungsstelle, Thea-Bähnisch-Weg 12, 30657 Hannover, Germany

Dahl, G.
Lucile Packard Childrens Hospital, Stanford University, Dept. of Pediatrics, 725 Welch Road, Palo Alto, CA 94305, USA

de Vos, S.
Cedars-Sinai Medical Center, UCLA, Hematology and Oncology Division, 8700 Beverly Boulevard, Los Angeles, CA 90048-1865, USA

DRIZE, N.
Russian Research Center for Hematology, Dept. of Hematology and BMT, Novozykovski pr. 4a, 125167 Moscow, Russia

ELSTNER, E.
Cedars-Sinai Medical Center UCLA, Hematology and Oncology Division, 8700 Beverly Boulevard, Los Angeles, CA 90048-1865, USA

FENCHEL, K.
University Hospital, Dept. of Hematology, Theodor-Stern-Kai 7, 60590 Frankfurt, Germany

FINK, F.M.
University Hospital, Dept. of Pediatrics, Anichstr. 35, 6020 Innsbruck, Austria

FISCHER, K.
University Hospital, Dept. of Hematology and Oncology, Hospitalstr. 3, 69115 Heidelberg, Germany

FOA, R.
Sezione Clinical Dipartimento di Scienze, Biomediche e Oncologia Umana, Via Genova 3, 10126 Torino, Italy

FREUND, M.
University Hospital, Dept. of Hematology and Oncology, Postfach 10 08 88, 18055 Rostock, Germany

GANDHI, V.
M.D. Anderson Cancer Center, University of Texas, Dept. of Medical Oncology, 1515 Holcombe, Houston, TX 77030, USA

GANSER, A.
University Hospital, Dept. of Internal Medicine, Theodor-Stern-Kai 7, 60596 Frankfurt, Germany

GARRITSEN, H.
University Hospital, Institut Transfusionsmedizin/Transplantationsimmunologie, Domagkstr. 11, 48149 Münster, Germany

GIESELER, F.
University Hospital, Dept. of Internal Medicine, Klinikstr. 8, 97070 Würzburg, Germany

GLASS, B.
University Hospital II, Chemnitzstr. 33, 24116 Kiel, Germany

GLUCKMAN, E.
Hospital St. Louis, Dept. of Bone Marrow Transplantation, 1, Avenue Claude Vellefaux, 75475 Paris Cedex, France

GRIESINGER, F.
University Hospital, Dept. of Hematology and Oncology, Robert-Koch-Str. 40, 37075 Göttingen, Germany

Haas, R.
University Hospital V, Hospitalstr. 3, 69115 Heidelberg, Germany

Haferlach, T.
University Hospital II, Chemnitzstr. 33, 24116 Kiel, Germany

Harbott, J.
University Hospital, Dept. of General Pediatrics, Hematology and Oncology, Feulgenstr. 12, 35392 Giessen, Germany

Harousseau, J.-L.
Centre Hospitalier Regional et Universitaire de Nantes, Service d'Hématologie Clinique, Place Alexis Ricordeau, B.P. 1005, 44035 Nantes Cedex 01, France

Heidemann, E.
Diakonissenkrankenhaus, Dept. of Internal Medicine II, Rosenbergstr. 38, 70176 Stuttgart, Germany

Helbig, W.
University Hospital, Dept. of Hematology and Oncology, Johannesallee 32, 04103 Leipzig, Germany

Henze, G.
University Hospital Rudolf Virchow, Dept. of Pediatrics, Div. of Hematology and Oncology, Reinickendorfer Str. 61, 13347 Berlin, Germany

Hiddemann, W.
University Hospital, Dept. of Hematology and Oncology, Robert-Koch-Str. 40, 37075 Göttingen, Germany

Ho, A.D.
UCSD Cancer Center, University of California, Division of Hematology and Oncology, 200 West Arbor Drive, San Diego, CA 92103-8421, USA

Hübner, G.
Medical School of Hannover, Dept. of Hematology and Oncology, Konstanty-Gutschow Str. 8, 30625 Hannover, Germany

Jäger, U.
University Hospital I, Lazarettgasse 14, 1090 Wien, Austria

Kaczorowski, S.
Rozrostowych Akademii Medycznej, Klinika Hematologii i Chorob, ul. Dzialdowska 1, 01-184 Warszawa, Poland

Kämpfe, D.
University Hospital, Dept. of Internal Medicine, Ernst-Grube-Str. 40, 06120 Halle/Saale, Germany

Kaspers, G.-J.J.L.
Free University Hospital, Dept. of Pediatrics, De Boelelaan 1117, 1081 HV Amsterdam, The Netherlands

KEATING, M.J.
M.D. Anderson Cancer Center, Dept. of Internal Medicine, 1515 Holcombe Blvd., Houston, TX 77030, USA

KUTCHER, R.
Russian Research Center for Hematology, Dept. of Hematology and Bone Marrow Transplantation, Novozykovski pr. 4a 125167 Moscow, Russia

LAPIDOT, T.
Hospital for Sick Children, Dept. of Genetics, 555 University Avenue, Toronto, Ontario M5G 1X8, Canada

LENGFELDER, E.
University Hospital, Dept. of Internal Medicine III, Wiesbadener Str. 7–11, 68305 Mannheim, Germany

LINDEMANN, A.
University Hospital, Dept. of Internal Medicine I, Hugstetter Str. 55, 79106 Freiburg, Germany

LINK, H.
Medical School of Hannover, Dept. of Hematology and Oncology, Konstanty-Gutschow-Str. 8,30625 Hannover, Germany

LISOVSKY, M.Y.
Russian Research Center, Dept. of Hematology and BMT, Novozykovski pr. 4a, 125167 Moscow, Russia

LIST, A.
University of Arizona, Dept. of Medicine, College of Medicine, Tucson, AZ 85724, USA

LISTER, T.A.
St. Bartholomew's Hospital, Dept. of Clinical Oncology, West Smithfield, EC1 A7BE London, Great Britain

MARTIN, H.
University Hospital III, Dept. of Hematology, Theodor-Stern-Kai 7, 60596 Frankfurt, Germany

MATYSIAK, M.
Medical Academy, Dept. of Pediatric Hematology, ul. Dzialdowska 1, 01-184 Warszawa, Poland

MINDEN, M.D.
Princess Margaret Hospital, Ontario Cancer Institute, 500 Sherbourne Street, Toronto, Ontario M4X 1K9, Canada

MOMOTJUK, K.
Russian Research Center, Dept. of Hematology and BMT, Novozykovski pr. 4a, 125167 Moscow, Russia

MROSS, K.B.
University Hospital Eppendorf, Dept. of Hematology and Oncology, Martinistr. 52, 20251 Hamburg, Germany

Neubauer, A.
University Hospital Rudolf Virchow, Dept. of Hematology and Oncology, Spandauer Damm 130, 14050 Berlin, Germany

Neuendank, A.
University Hospital Rudolf Virchow, Dept. of Pediatric Hematology and Oncology, Reinickendorfer Str. 61, 13347 Berlin, Germany

Ohno, R.
Hamamatsu University, School of Medicine, Dept. of Medicine II, 3600 Handacho, 431-31 Hamamatsu, Japan

Pieters, R.
Free University Hospital, Dept. of Pediatrics, Academish Ziekenhuis, P.O. Box 7057, 1007 MB Amsterdam, The Netherlands

Pott, C.
University Hospital, Dept. of Hematology and Oncology, Robert-Koch-Str. 40, 37075 Göttingen, Germany

Preisler, H.D.
St. Luke's Medical Center, Rush-Presbyterian Cancer Institute, Dept. of Med. Oncology, 1725, W. Harrison Street, Chicago, IL 60612, USA

Pushkareva, S.
Clinic and Institute of Biophysics, Dept. of Hematology, Marshal Novikov St. 23, 123098 Moscow, Russia

Relling, M.
St. Jude Children's Research Hospital, Pharmacokinetics and Pharmacodynamics Section, Pharmaceutical Department, 332 North Lauderdale, P.O. Box 318, Memphis, TN 38101-0318, USA

Repp, R.
University Hospital, Dept. of General Pediatrics, Hematology and Oncology, Feulgenstraße 12, 35392 Giessen, Germany

Reuter, C.
University of Virginia, Health Sciences Center, School of Medicine, Box 441, Dept. of Microbiology, Charlottesville, 22908 VA USA

Romanakis, K.
University Hospital, Dept. of Biology and Genetics, Erwin-Schrödinger-Str., 67663 Kaiserslautern, Germany

Rowe, J.M.
University of Rochester Medical C, Dept. of Hematology and Oncology, 601 Elmwood Avenue, Box 610, Rochester, NY 14642, USA

Sachs, L.
The Weizmann Institute of Science, Dept. of Molecular Genetics and Virology, 76100 Rehovot, Israel

SANTANA, V.M.
St. Jude Children's Research Hospital, 332 North Lauderdale, P.O. Box 318, Memphis, TN 38101, USA

SAVCHENKO, V.
Dept. of Hematology and BMT, Russian Research Center for Hematology, Novozykovski pr. 4a, 126167 Moscow, Russia

SCHRÖDER, J.
University Hospital, Westdeutsches Tumorzentrum (Tumorforschung), Dept. of Internal Medicine, Hufelandstr. 55, 45122 Essen, Germany

SHUI, D.K.
University Hospital, Dept. of Hematology, Theodor-Stern-Kai 7, 60590 Frankfurt, Germany

SIMON, M.
University Hospital, Dept. of Internal Medicine III, Wiesbadener Str. 7-11, 68305 Mannheim, Germany

SOLARY, E.
Centre Hospitalier Régional et Universitaire de Dijon, Le Bocage, Service d'Hématologie Clinique, B.P. 1542, 21034 Dijon Cedex, France

STAHNKE, K.
University Hospital, Dept. of Pediatrics II, Prittwitzstr. 43, 89075 Ulm, Germany

UHAREK, L.
University Hospital II, Chemnitzstr. 53, 24116 Kiel, Germany

UNTERHALT, M.
University Hospital, Dept. of Hematology and Oncology, Robert-Koch-Str. 40, 37075 Göttingen, Germany

URASINSKI, T.
Pomeranian Med. Academy, I Pediatric Dept., ul. Unii Lubelskiej 1, 71-344 Szczecin, Poland

VAN DONGEN, J.J.M.
University Hospital, Dept. of Immunology, Postbus 1738, 3000 DR Rotterdam, The Netherlands

VELLENGA, E.
University Hospital Groningen, Dept. of Hematology, Oostersingel 59, 9700 RB Groningen, The Netherlands

VERBEEK, W.
University Hospital, Dept. of Hematology and Oncology, Robert-Koch-Str. 40, 37075 Göttingen, Germany

VON EIFF, M.
University Hospital, Dept. of Internal Medicine A, Albert-Schweitzer-Str. 33, 48129 Münster, Germany

VOSE, J.
University of Nebraska, Medical Center, Dept. of Internal Medicine, 600 South 42nd Street, Omaha, NE 69198-3330, USA

WEIDMANN, E.
University Hospital, Dept. of Hematology, Theodor-Stern-Kai 7, 60590 Frankfurt, Germany

WEISDORF, D.
University of Minnesota, Box 480, UMHC, Hematology, 420 Delaware Street S.E., Minneapolis, MN 55455, USA

WILLEMZE, R.
Academisch Ziekenhuis, Dept. of Hematology, Postbox 9600, 2300 RC Leiden, The Netherlands

WÖRMANN, B.
University Hospital, Dept. of Hematology and Oncolgy, Robert-Koch-Str. 44, 37075 Göttingen, Germany

ZARITSKEY, A.
Clinical Center for Advanced Technologies, Bone Marrow Transplantation Center, pr. Dynamos, 197042 St. Petersburg, Russia

ZINTL, F.
University Hospital, Dept. of Pediatrics, Hematology and Oncology, Kochstr. 2, 07745 Jena, Germany

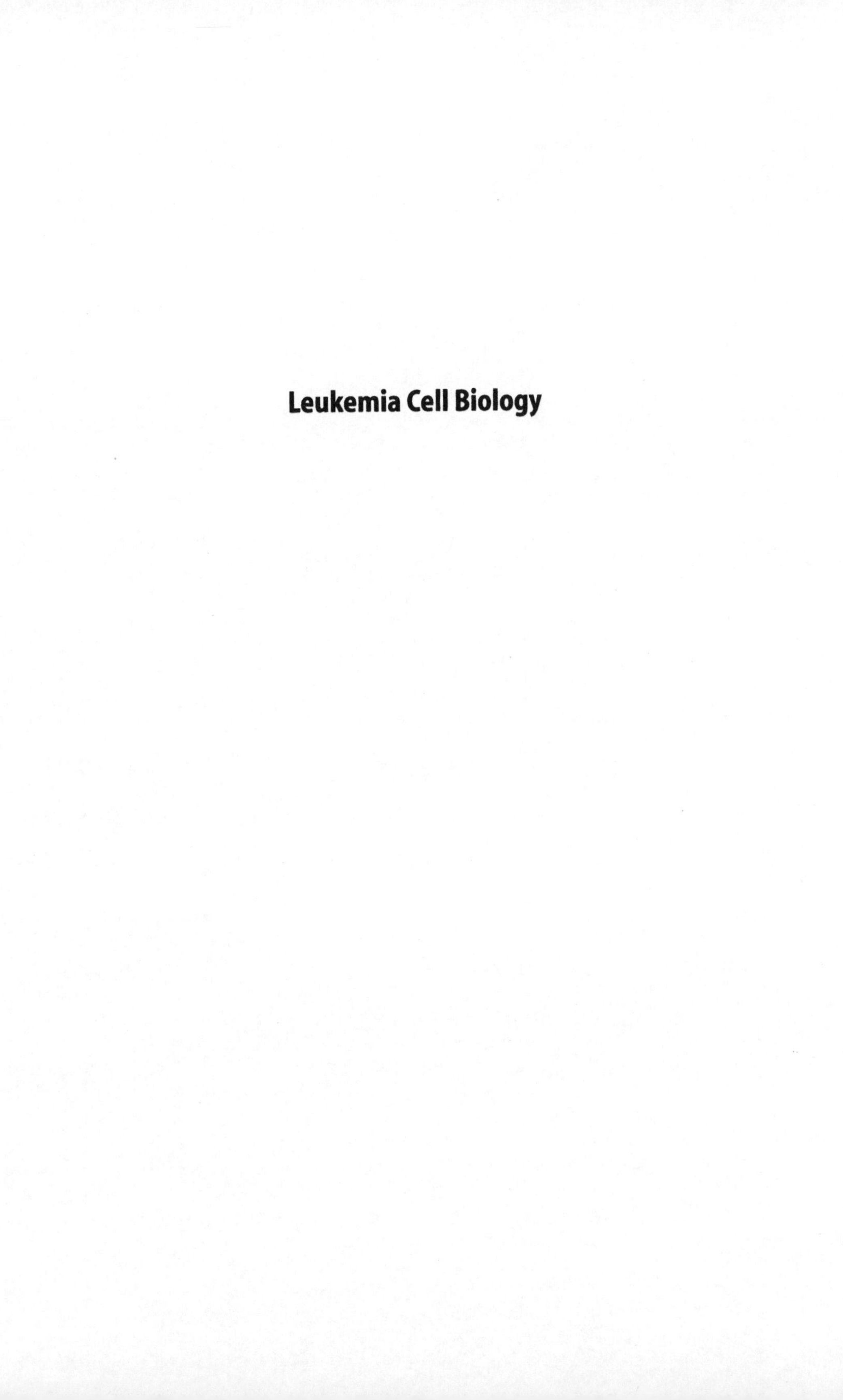

Leukemia Cell Biology

Acute Leukemias V
Experimental Approaches
and Management of Refractory Diseases
Hiddemann et al. (Eds.)

Cell Differentiation and Programmed Cell Death: A New Approach to Leukemia Therapy

Leo Sachs

Abstract. The establishment of a cell culture system for the clonal development of hematopoietic cells has made it possible to discover the proteins that regulate cell viability, growth and differentiation of different hematopoietic cell lineages and the molecular basis of normal and abnormal cell development in blood forming tissues. These regulators include cytokines now called colony stimulating factors and interleukins. Different cytokines can induce cell viability, multiplication and differentiation, and hematopoiesis is controlled by a network of cytokine interactions. Cytokines induce viability by inhibiting programmed cell death (apoptosis) including inhibition of apoptosis in leukemic cells treated with cytotoxic chemotherapy and irradiation therapy. Apoptosis and development of hematopoietic cells are also controlled by different genes including the tumor suppressor gene wild-type p53 and the oncogenes mutant p53, deregulated c-myc and bcl-2. Identification of the molecular controls of normal cell viability, growth and differentiation have made it possible to identify changes in the developmental program that result in leukemia. When normal cells have been changed into leukemic cells, the malignant phenotype can again be suppressed by inducing differentiation and apoptosis. Results on the suppression of malignancy in myeloid leukemia have shown that suppression of malignancy does not have to restore all the normal controls, and that genetic abnormalities which give rise to malignancy can be bypassed and their effects nullified by inducing differentiation and apoptosis. The results provide a new approach to therapy.

"The described cultures thus seem to offer a useful system for a quantitative kinetic approach to hematopoietic cell formation and for experimental studies on the mechanism and regulation of hematopoietic cell differentiation" [1].

In order to analyze the controls that regulate viability, multiplication and differentiation of normal hematopoietic cells to different cell lineages and the changes in these controls in disease, it is desirable and convenient to study the entire process in cell culture starting from single cells. Analysis of the molecular control of different types of hematopoietic cells therefore began with the development of a cell culture system for the cloning and clonal differentiation of different types of normal hematopoietic cells. This cell culture system was then used to discover a family of cytokines that regulate cell viability, multiplication and differentiation of different hematopoietic cell lineages, to analyze the origin of some hematological diseases, and to identify ways of treating these diseases with normal cytokines. I will mainly discuss cells of the myeloid cell lineages which have been used as a model system.

The discovery of colony stimulating factors: cytokines that control development of different cell lineages. Hematopoiesis cannot be maintained in cultures containing only hematopoietic cells suggesting that these cells require specific factors to maintain viability, growth and differentiation [2–6]. The culture system that was initially developed to study normal hematopoiesis, thus included in addition to normal cells from blood forming

Department of Molecular Genetics and Virology, the Weizmann Institute of Science, Rehovot 76100, Israel tissues of mice also feeder layers of other cell types such as normal embryo fibroblasts. These other cell types were chosen as possible candidates for cells that produce the regulatory molecules required for the cloning and differentiation of different hematopoietic cell lineages. The first such system [1], using cells cultured in liquid medium (Table 1), showed that it was possible to obtain by this procedure clones containing mast cells or granulocytes in various stages of differentiation. To make it simpler to distinguish and isolate separate clones, this system was then applied to the cloning of different cell lineages in semi-solid medium containing agar or methylcellulose [7–9]. Analysis of the first types of clones obtained in agar with these feeder layers showed clones containing macrophages, granulocytes, or both macrophages and granulocytes, in various stages of differentiation.The experiments also showed that these clones could originate from single cells [7–10]. This assay in agar or methylcellulose was then applied to cloning and clonal differentiation of normal human macrophages and granulocytes [11,12] and to the cloning of all the other blood cell lineages including erythroid cells [13], B lymphocytes [14], T lymphocytes [15] and megakaryocytes [16,17].

When blood forming cells were cloned in a semi-solid substrate such as agar, another more solid agar layer was placed between the feeder layer cells and the cells seeded for cloning. This showed that the inducer(s) required for the formation of macrophage and granulocyte clones were secreted by the feeder layer cells and can diffuse through agar [7]. This finding led to the discovery (Table 1) that the inducers required for the formation of macrophage and granulocyte clones are present in conditioned medium produced by the feeder cells [8,10]. These inducers were found in the conditioned medium from different types of normal and malignant cells (reviewed in [18,19]). These media were then used to purify the inducers [20–24]. A similar approach was later used to identify the protein inducers for cloning of T lymphocytes [25] and B lymphocytes (reviewed in [26]). When cells were washed at various times after initiating the induction of clones, there was no further development of either macrophage or granulocyte clones unless the inducer was added again [27]. The development of clones with differentiated cells thus requires both an initial and continued supply of inducer.

In cells belonging to the myeloid cell lineages, four different proteins that induce cell multiplication and can thus induce the formation of clones (colony inducing proteins) have been identified (reviewed in [3–6]). The same proteins have been given different names. After they were first discovered in cell culture supernatant fluids [8–10], the first inducer identified was called mashran gm from the Hebrew word meaning to send forth with the initials for granulocytes and macrophages [28]. This and other growth-inducing proteins were then re-named including macrophage and granulocyte inducers (MGI) [20]-type 1, (MGI-1), are now called colony stimulating factors (CSF) [29], and one protein is called interleukin-3 (IL-3) [24] (Table 2). Of these four CSFs, one (M-CSF), induces the development of clones with macrophages, another (G-CSF), clones with granulocytes, the third (GM-CSF), clones with granulocytes, macrophages, or both macrophages and granulocytes, and the fourth, (IL-3), clones with macrophages, granulocytes, eosinophils, mast cells, erythroid cells, or megakaryocytes (Table 2). The CSFs induce cell viability and cell multiplication (reviewed in [3–6,30,31]) and enhance the functional activity of mature cells (reviewed in [29]). Cloning of genes from mice and humans for IL-3, GM-CSF, M-CSF and G-CSF has shown that these proteins are coded for by different

Table 1. Establishment of the cell culture system for cloning and clonal differentiation of normal hematopoietic cells and discovery of the molecular regulators of this clonal development in cell culture supernatants

Cloning and differentiation in liquid medium (mast cells and granulocytes) [1]
Cloning and differentiation in agar (macrophages and granulocytes) [7–9]
Cloning and differentiation in methylcellulose (macrophages and granulocytes) [8]
Inducers for cloning and differentiation secreted by cells [7]
Inducers for cloning and differentiation in cell culture supernatants (macrophages and granulocytes) [8,10]

Table 2. Induction of growth and differentiation of normal myeloid precursor cells by different hematopoietic cytokines

Nomenclature	Location on chromosome		Induction of colonies*	Induction of differentiation	
	Mouse	Human		Direct	Indirect**
MGI-1M = CSF-1 = M-CSF	3	5	+(M)	-	+
MGI-1G = G-CSF	11	17	+(G)	-	+
MGI-1GM = GM-CSF	11	5	+(G, M)		
IL-3	11	5	+(G, M, others)	-	+
MGI-2 = IL-6	5	7	-	+(G, M, Meg)	-
IL-1	2	2	-	-	+(G, M, Meg)
D-factor = HILDA = LIF	11	22	-	CD	CD
DIF = TNF	17	6	-	CD	CD

*Colonies with macrophages (M), granulocytes (G), granulocytes and macrophages (G, M) and granulocytes, macrophages, eosinophils, mast cells, megakaryocytes or erythroid cells (G, M, others), megakaryocytes (Meg)
** The four CSFs, including IL-3 and IL-1, induce production of IL-6. CD = cell death. References in [5]

genes (reviewed in [32]). Since the discovery of CSFs, other cytokines have been found including various ILs and stem cell factor.

It appeared unlikely that a CSF that induces cell multiplication is also a differentiation inducer whose action includes stopping cell multiplication in mature cells. Indeed, a protein that acts as a myeloid cell differentiation inducer and does not have colony stimulating activity was identified and called macrophage and granulocyte inducer-type 2 (MGI-2), (reviewed in [3–6]). Studies on amino acid sequence of the purified protein, neutralization by monoclonal antibody and myeloid cell differentiation-inducing activity of recombinant protein have shown that MGI-2 is interleukin 6 (IL-6) [5] and there are presumably other normal hematopoietic cell differentiation inducers. Studies on myeloid leukemic cells have identified other differentiation inducing proteins called D-factor and differentiation-inducing factor (DIF) (reviewed in [5]). D-factor was identified as a protein that has also been called LIF and HILDA, and DIF was found to be a form of tumor necrosis factor (TNF). IL-6 can induce viability and differentiation of normal myeloid precursors, but LIF and TNF which induce differentiation in certain clones of myeloid leukemic cells do not induce viability or differentiation of normal myeloid cells (reviewed in [5]) (Table 2).

Network of Hematopoietic Cytokines

Production of specific cell types has to be induced when new cells are required and has to stop when sufficient cells have been produced. This requires an appropriate balance between inducers and inhibitors of development. The development of normal hematopoietic cells is positively regulated by several CSFs and ILs and can be negatively regulated by TNF and by a cytokine called transforming growth-factor b1 (TGF-b1). TGF-b1 can selectively inhibit the activity of some CSFs and ILs and can also inhibit the production of these cytokines [33]). The control of the hematopoietic system thus shows considerable flexibility. A good way to obtain such flexibility would be for the different factors to function within a network of interactions and this is indeed how the hematopoietic cytokines act [5,34,35] (Fig. 1). An important function of the network is to selectively control programmed cell death.

Parts of this network function not only within the hematopoietic cell system but also for some non-hematopoietic cell types. For example, in endothelial cells that make blood vessels there is an induction of IL-6 when new blood vessels are being formed and the production of IL-6 is switched off when angiogenesis has been completed [36]. The transient expression of IL-6 in the endothelial cells indicates a role for IL-6 in angiogenesis in addition to its role in regulating the development of myeloid and lymphoid hematopoietic cells. IL-6 can also induce the production of acute phase proteins in liver cells [26]. The pleiotropic effects of a cytokine such as IL-6 raises the question whether these effects on different cell types are direct, or are indirect by IL-6 switching on production of other regulators that vary in the different cell types. Interpretation of experimental data on the effect of

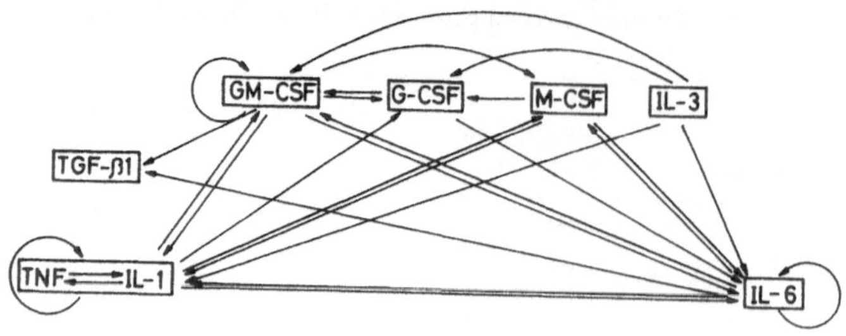

Fig. 1. Network of interactions between hematopoietic regulatory proteins

each cytokine therefore has to take into account that the regulator functions in a network of interactions, so as to avoid an incorrect assignment of a specific effect to a direct action of a particular cytokine. This network has also to be taken into account in the clinical use of these cytokines. What can be therapeutically useful may be due to the direct action of an injected cytokine, or to an indirect effect due to other cytokines that are switched on in vivo.

A network of interactions allows considerable flexibility depending on which part of the network is activated. It also allows a ready amplification of response to a particular stimulus such as bacterial lipopolysaccharide (LPS) [5,35]. This amplification can occur by autoregulation and by transregulation of genes for the hematopoietic cytokines [5]. There is also a transregulation by these cytokines of receptors for other cytokines [37,38]. In addition to the flexibility of this network both for the response to present-day infections and to infections that may develop in the future, a network may also be necessary to stabilise the whole system. Hematopoietic cytokines induce during differentiation sustained levels of transcription factors that can regulate and maintain gene expression in the differentiation program [39]. Interactions between the network of hematopoietic cytokines and transcription factors can thus ensure the production of specific cell types and stability of the differentiated state.

Differentiation of Leukemia Cells by Normal Regulators of Hematopoiesis. In normal hematopoietic cells induction of growth by a cytokine is coupled to induction of cell differentiation (reviewed in [40]). One mechanism for such coupling is the induction of a differentiation inducer such as IL-6 by the different CSF's [40]. In contrast, myeloid leukemic cells show an uncoupling between induction of growth and differentiation and it was therefore questioned whether myeloid leukemic cells can still be induced to differentiate to mature non-dividing cells by cytokines that induce differentiation in normal myeloid cells? This question has been answered by showing that there are clones of myeloid leukemic cells that can be induced to differentiate to mature macrophages or granulocytes through the normal sequence of gene expression by incubation with the normal myeloid differentiation-inducing protein IL-6. These are called D+ clones (D for differentiation). The mature cells, which can be formed from all the cells of a leukemic clone, then stop multiplying like normal mature cells and are no longer malignant in vivo. In addition to D+ clones that can be induced to differentiate by IL-6, there are other D+ clones from other myeloid leukemias that can be induced to differentiate by incubation with GM-CSF, IL-3, or G-CSF (reviewed in [2-6,40]). In these clones the growth inducers presumably induce production of an appropriate differentiation inducer. D+ leukemic cells that respond to IL-6 can also be induced to differentiate by IL-1a and IL-1b, and this is mediated by the endogenous production of IL-6 [5].

Studies in animals and humans have shown that normal differentiation of D+ myeloid leukemic cells to mature nondividing cells can be induced not only in culture but also in vivo [41]. These leukemias, therefore, grow progressively when there are too many leukemic cells for the normal amount of differentiation inducer in the body. The development of leukemia can be inhibited in mice with these D+ leukemic cells by increasing the amount of differentiation inducing protein, either by injecting it or by injecting a compound that increases its production by cells in the body [42,43]. Induction of differentiation in vivo like in vitro can occur directly, or by an indirect mechanism that involves induction of the appropriate differentiation inducing protein either by the same cells or by other cells in the body. After injection of myeloid leukemic cells into fetuses, D+ leukemic cells can participate in hematopoietic cell differentiation in apparently healthy adult animals [44,45].

The D+ myeloid leukemic cells have an abnormal chromosome composition, and suppression of malignancy in these cells was not associated with chromosome changes. It was obtained by induction of the normal sequence of cell differentiation by a normal myeloid regulatory protein. In this suppression, the stopping of cell multiplication by inducing differentiation to mature cells bypasses genetic changes that produced the malignant phenotype [46].

The study of different clones of myeloid leukemic cells has also shown that in addition to D+ clones there are differentiation defective clones called D− clones. Some D− clones are induced by a normal myeloid cytokine to an intermediate stage of differentiation which then slows down the growth of the cells, and others could not be induced to differentiate even to this intermediate stage. But even these D− cells can be induced to differentiate by other compounds, either singly or in combination, that can induce the differentiation program by alternative pathways. The stopping of cell multiplication by inducing differentiation by these alternative pathways bypasses the genetic changes that inhibit response to the normal differentiation inducer (reviewed in [4,5,40]). Studies on the genetic changes in D− clones of myeloid leukemias have shown that differentiation defectiveness may be due to changes in homeobox genes. These include re-arrangement of the Hox-2.4 homeobox gene which results in abnormal expression of this gene in the leukemic cells [47]. This abnormal expression inhibits specific pathways of myeloid cell differentiation [48]. In other leukemias with a deletion in one chromosome 2 [49] there is a deletion of one copy of Hox-4.1 [50].

Studies with a variety of chemicals other than normal hematopoietic cytokines have shown that many compounds can induce differentiation in D+ clones of myeloid leukemic cells. These include certain steroid hormones, chemicals such as cytosine arabinoside, adriamycin, methotrexate and other chemicals that are used today in cancer chemotherapy, and irradiation. At high doses these compounds used in cancer chemotherapy and irradiation kill cells by inducing programmed cell death, whereas at low doses they can induce differentiation. Not all these compounds are equally active on the same leukemic clone [2,51]. A variety of chemicals can also induce differentiation in clones that are not induced to differentiate by a normal hematopoietic cytokine, and in some D− clones induction of differentiation requires combined treatment with different compounds [51]. In addition to certain steroids and chemicals used today in chemotherapy and radiation therapy, other compounds that can induce differentiation in myeloid leukemic cells include insulin, bacterial lipopolysaccharide, certain plant lectins, tumor promoting phorbol esters and retinoic acid [2,40,51,52]. In addition to the normal myeloid cytokines, the steroid hormones, insulin and retinoic acid are physiological compounds that can induce differentiation. It is possible that all myeloid leukemic cells no longer susceptible to the normal hematopoietic cytokines by themselves can be induced to differentiate by the appropriate combination of compounds. The therapeutic potential of this differentiation-directed approach to leukemia treatment has already proved useful in acute promyelocytic leukemic patients treated with retinoic acid [52].

Regulation of Programmed Cell Death

Normal myeloid precursor cells depend on hematopoietic cytokines for viability, multiplication and differentiation (reviewed in 3–5, 31, 40]). Withdrawal of these cytokines leads to death by programmed cell death [53] (apoptosis) [54]. Although viability factors such as the CSFs are also growth factors, viability and growth are separately regulated (reviewed in [31]). Certain myeloid leukemic cells are growth factor independent and do not require an exogenously added cytokine for cell viability and growth. Induction of differentiation in these leukemic cells with IL-6 induces in the differentiating cells a growth factor dependent state so that the cells lose viability by apoptosis following withdrawal of IL-6 [30,38,55–57]. This induction of the program for cell death occurs before terminal differentiation, and the differentiating cells can be rescued from apoptosis and continue to multiply by re-adding IL-6, or by adding IL-3, M-CSF, G-CSF, or IL-1 [38]. The differentiating leukemic cells can also be rescued from apoptosis by the tumor promoting phorbol ester

12-o-tetradecanoylphorbol-13-acetate (TPA) but not by the non-promoting isomer 4-a-TPA [30]. TPA rescued the differentiating cells from apoptosis by a different pathway than rescue with these cytokines. TPA can thus act as a tumor promoter by inhibiting programmed cell death [30]. The program for cell death is present in normal myeloid precursor cells and in more differentiated cells including mature granulocytes and macrophages. Induction of programmed cell death in myeloid leukemic cells is a physiological process that can be used to suppress leukemia.

Programmed cell death can also be induced in myeloid leukemic cells without inducing differentiation (reviewed in [31]). Wild-type p53 protein is a product of a tumor suppressor gene which is no longer expressed in many types of tumors including myeloid leukemias (reviewed in [58]). There is a clone of myeloid leukemic cells that completely lacks expression of p53 protein and mRNA [59]. This p53 negative clone of myeloid leukemic cells was transfected with DNA encoding a temperature sensitive p53 mutant (Ala to Val change at position 135). The Val 135 mutant behaves like other p53 mutants at 37.5¡C but like wild-type p53 at 32.5¡C. There was no change in the behavior of the transfected cells at 37.5¡C but activation of the wild-type p53 protein at 32.5¡C resulted in apoptotic cell death. This induction of apoptosis was not associated with differentiation [59]. Apoptosis can, therefore, be induced in myeloid leukemic cells not only by a differentiation-associated process, but also by expression of wild-type p53 (Table 3) in undifferentiated leukemic cells. This induction of apoptosis by wild-type p53 was inhibited by IL-6 [59]. These results show that wild-type p53 mediated apoptosis in these myeloid leukemic cells is a physiological process. Experiments with p53 knock-out mice have shown that wild-type p53 is also involved in mediating apoptosis in normal myeloid precursors deprived of the appropriate cytokine concentration required for cell viability [60]. The induction of apoptosis in myeloid leukemic cells by various cytotoxic agents can be enhanced by deregulated expression of c-myc [61]. The oncogene mutant p53 [61] and bcl-2 ([62,63] and reviewed in [64]) (Table 3) can suppress the enhancing effect on cell death of deregulated c-myc, and thus allow induction of cell proliferation and inhibition of differentiation which are other functions of deregulated c-myc. The suppression of cell death by mutant p53 and bcl-2 increases the probability of developing tumors. Experiments with p53 knock-out mice have also shown that there are wild-type p53 dependent and p53 independent pathways of inducing apoptosis [60,65,66]. These and other experiments have shown that there are alternative pathways to apoptotic cell death [31]. Alternative pathways to regulate apoptosis can be useful to control selective cell viability. Treatments that downregulate the expression or activity of mutant p53 or bcl-2 in tumor cells should be useful for cancer therapy [31]. Indeed, induction of differentiation by IL-6 or G-CSF downregulated bcl-2 expression and increased the susceptibility of the cells to induction of apoptosis [67].

Table 3. Control of apoptosis by a tumor suppressor gene and oncogenes

Deregulated expression of	Apoptosis		
	Induction	Enhancement	Suppression
Wild-type p53	+	–	–
c-myc	–	+	–
Mutant p53	–	–	+*
bcl-2	–	–	+

*Mutant p53 suppresses the enhancement of apoptosis by deregulated c-myc [61]. Other references in [31]

References

1. Ginsburg H., Sachs L. 1963. Formation of pure suspensions of mast cells in tissue culture by differentiation of lymphoid cells from the mouse thymus. J. Natl. Cancer Inst. 31: 1–40.
2. Sachs, L. 1978. Control of normal cell differentiation and the phenotypic reversion of malignancy in myeloid leukaemia. Nature, 274: 535–539.
3. Sachs, L. 1986. Growth, differentiation and the reversal of malignancy. Scientific American, 254: 40–47.
4. Sachs, L. 1987. The molecular control of blood cell development. Science, 238: 1374–1379.
5. Sachs, L. 1990. The control of growth and differentiation in normal and leukemic blood cells. The 1989 Alfred P. Sloan Prize of the General Motors Cancer Research Foundation. Cancer, 65: 2196–2206.
6. Sachs, L. 1993. The molecular control of hemopoiesis and leukemia. C.R. Acad. Sci. Paris, Sciences de la vie, 316: 882–891.
7. Pluznik D.H., Sachs L. 1965. The cloning of normal "mast" cells in tissue culture. J. Cell Comp. Physiol. 66: 319–324.

8. Ichikawa Y., Pluznik D.H., Sachs L. 1966. In vitro control of the development of macrophage and granulocytes colonies. Proc. Natl. Acad. Sci. USA 56: 488–495.
9. Bradley T.R., Metcalf D. 1966. The growth of mouse bone marrow cells in vitro. Aust. J. Exp. Biol. Med. Sci. 44: 287–300.
10. Pluznik D.H., Sachs L. 1966. The induction of clones of normal "mast" cells by a substance from conditioned medium. Exp. Cell Res. 43: 553–563.
11. Paran M., Sachs L., Barak Y., Resnitzky P. 1970. In vitro induction of granulocyte differentiation in hematopoietic cells from leukemic and non-leukemic patients. Proc. Natl. Acad. Sci. USA 67: 1542–1549.
12. Pike B., Robinson W.A. 1970. Human bone marrow growth in agar gel. J. Cell Physiol. 76: 77–84.
13. Stephenson J.R., Axelrad A.A., McLeod D.L., Shreeve M.M. 1971. Induction of colonies of hemoglobin-synthesizing cells by erythropoietin in vitro. Proc. Natl. Acad. Sci. USA 68: 1542–1546.
14. Metcalf D., Nossal G.J.V., Warner N.L., Miller J.F.A.P., Mandel T.E., Layton J.E., Gutman G.A. 1975. Growth of B lymphocyte colonies in vitro. J. Exp. Med. 142: 1534–1549.
15. Gerassi E., Sachs L. 1976. Regulation of the induction of colonies in vitro by normal human lymphocytes. Proc. Natl. Acad. Sci. USA 73: 4546–4550.
16. Metcalf D., McDonald H.R., Odartchenko N., Sordat B. 1975. Growth of mouse megakaryocyte colonies in vitro. Proc. Natl. Acad. Sci. USA 72: 1744–1748.
17. Lotem J., Sachs L. 1989. Regulation of meagakaryocyte development by interleukin-6. Blood 74: 1545–1551.
18. Sachs L. 1970. In vitro control of growth and development of hematopoietic cell clones. In: Regulation of Hematopoiesis, Vol. 1, A.S. Gordon, ed. New York: Appleton-Century-Crofts, 217–233.
19. Sachs L. 1974. Regulation of membrane changes, differentiation and malignancy in carcinogenesis. Harvey Lectures, Vol. 68, New York: Academic Press, 1–35.
20. Landau T., Sachs L. 1971. Characterization of the inducer required for the development of macrophage and granulocyte colonies. Proc. Natl. Acad. Sci. USA 68: 2540–2544.
21. Burgess A.W., Camakaris J., Metcalf D. 1977. Purification and properties of colony-stimulating factor from mouse lung conditioned medium. J. Biol. Chem. 252: 1998–2003.
22. Stanley E.R., Heard P.M. 1977. Factors regulating macrophage production and growth. Purification and some properties of the colony stimulating factor from medium conditioned by mouse cells. J. Biol. Chem. 252: 4305–4312.
23. Lipton J., Sachs L. 1981. Characterization of macrophage and granulocyte inducing proteins for normal and leukemic myeloid cells produced by the Krebs ascites tumor. Biochim. Biophys. Acta. 673: 552–569.
24. Ihle J.N., Keller J., Henderson L., Klein F., Palaszinski E. 1982. Procedures for the purification of interleukin-3 to homogeneity. J. Immunol. 129: 2431–2436.
25. Mier J.W., Gallo R.C. 1980. Purification and some characterisitics of human T-cell growth factor from phytohemagglutinin-stimulated lymphocyte-conditioned media. Proc. Natl. Acad. Sci. USA 77: 6134–6138.
26. Hirano T., Akira S., Taga T., Kishimoto T. 1990. Biological and clinical aspects of interleukin 6. Immunol. Today 11: 443–449.
27. Paran M., Sachs L. 1968. The continued requirement for inducer for development of macrophage and granulocyte colonies. J. Cell. Physiol. 72: 247–250.
28. Ichikawa Y., Pluznik D.H., Sachs L. 1967. Feedback inhibition of the development of macrophage and granulocyte colonies. I. Inhibition by macrophages. Proc. Natl. Acad. Sci. USA 58: 1480–1486.
29. Metcalf D. 1985. The granulocyte-macrophage colony-stimulating factors. Science 199: 16–22.
30. Lotem J., Cragoe E.J., Sachs L. 1991. Rescue from programmed cell death in leukemic and normal myeloid cells. Blood 78: 953–960.
31. Sachs L., Lotem J. 1993. Control of programmed cell death in normal and leukemic cells: New implications for therapy. Blood 82: 15–21.
32. Clark S.C., Kamen R. 1987. The human hematopoietic colony-stimulating factors. Science 236: 1129–1237.
33. Lotem J., Sachs L. 1990. Selective regulation of the activity of different hematopoietic regulatory proteins by transforming growth factor b1 in normal and leukemic myeloid cells. Blood 76: 1315–1322.
34. Lotem J., Shabo Y., Sachs L. 1991. The network of hematopoietic regulatory proteins in myeloid cell differentiation. Cell Growth Differ. 2: 421–427.
35. Sachs L. 1991. Keynote Address for Symposium on: A Visionary Assessment of the Scientific, Clinical and Economic Implications of Hematopoietic Growth Factors. Cancer (May 15 Supplement) 67: 2681–2683.
36. Motro B., Itin A., Sachs L., Keshet E. 1990. Pattern of interleukin 6 gene expression in vivo suggests a role for this cytokine in angiogenesis. Proc. Natl. Acad. Sci. USA 87: 3092–3096.
37. Lotem J., Sachs L. 1986. Regulation of cell surface receptors for different hematopoietic growth factors on myeloid leukemic cells. EMBO J. 5: 2163–2170.
38. Lotem J., Sachs, L. 1989. Induction of dependence on hematopoietic proteins for viability and receptor upregulation in differentiating myeloid leukemic cells. Blood 74: 579–585.
39. Shabo Y., Lotem J., Sachs L. 1990. Induction of genes for transcription factors by normal hematopoietic regulatory proteins in the differentiation of myeloid leukemic cells. Leukemia 4: 797–801.
40. Sachs L. 1987. The molecular regulators of normal and leukaemic blood cells. The Wellcome Foundation Lecture 1986. Proc. Roy. Soc. Lond. B 231: 289–312.

41. Lotem J., Sachs L. 1978. In vivo induction of normal differentiation in myeloid leukemic cells. Proc. Natl. Acad. Sci. USA 75: 3781–3785.
42. Lotem J., Sachs L. 1981. In vivo inhibition of the development of myeloid leukemia by injection of macrophage and granulocyte inducing protein. Int. J. Cancer 28: 375–386
43. Lotem J., Sachs L. 1984. Control of in vivo differentiation of myeloid leukemic cells. IV. Inhibition of leukemia development by myeloid differentiation-inducing protein. Int. J. Cancer 33: 147–154.
44. Gootwine E., Webb C.G., Sachs, L. 1982. Participation of myeloid leukaemic cells injected into embryos in haematopoietic differentiation in adult mice. Nature, 299: 63–65.
45. Webb C.G., Gootwine E., Sachs, L. 1984. Developmental potential of myeloid leukemia cells injected into mid-gestation embryos. Develop. Biol. 101: 221–224.
46. Sachs L. 1987. Cell differentiation and by-passing of genetic defects in the suppression of malignancy. Cancer Res., 47: 1981–1986.
47. Blatt C., Aberdam D., Schwartz R., Sachs, L. 1988. DNA rearrangement of a homeobox gene in myeloid leukaemic cells. EMBO J., 7: 4283–4290.
48. Blatt C., Lotem J., Sachs, L. 1992. Inhibition of specific pathways of myeloid cell differentiation by an activated Hox-2.4 homeobox gene. Cell Growth Differ., 3: 671–676.
49. Azumi J., Sachs, L. 1977. Chromosome mapping of the genes that control differentiation and malignancy in myeloid leukemic cells. Proc. Natl. Acad. Sci. USA, 74: 253–257.
50. Blatt C., Sachs, L. 1988. Deletion of a homeobox gene in myeloid leukemias with a deletion in chromosome 2. Biochem. Biophys. Res. Commun., 156: 1265–1270.
51. Sachs L. 1982. Normal development programmes in myeloid leukaemia. Regulatory proteins in the control of growth and differentiation. Cancer Surveys 1: 321–342.
52. Degos L. 1992. All-trans-retinoic acid treatment and retinoic acid receptor alpha gene rearrangement in acute promyelocytic leukemia: a model for differentiation therapy. Int. J. Cell Cloning 10: 63–69.
53. Williams G.T., Smith C.A., Spooncer E., Dexter T.M., Taylor D.R. 1990. Haemopoietic colony stimulating factors promote cell survival by suppressing apoptosis. Nature 343: 76–79.
54. Arends M.J., Wyllie A.H. 1991. Apoptosis: Mechanisms and roles in pathology. Int. Rev. Exp. Pathol. 32: 223–254.
55. Fibach E., Sachs L. 1976. Control of normal differentiation of myeloid leukemic cells. XI. Induction of a specific requirement for cell viability and growth during the differentiation of myeloid leukemic cells. J. Cell. Physiol. 89: 259–266.
56. Lotem J., Sachs L. 1982. Mechanisms that uncouple growth and differentiation in myeloid leukemia cells. Restoration of requirement for normal growth-inducing protein without restoring induction of differentiation-inducing protein. Proc. Natl. Acad. Sci. USA 79: 4347–4351.
57. Lotem J., Sachs L. 1983. Coupling of growth and differentiation in normal myeloid precursors and the breakdown of this coupling in leukemia. Int. J. Cancer 32: 127–134.
58. Levine A.J., Momand J., Finlay C.A. 1991. The p53 tumor suppressor gene. Nature 351: 453–456.
59. Yonish-Rouach E, Resnitzky D., Lotem J., Sachs L., Kimchi A., Oren M. 1991. Wild type p53 induces apoptosis of myeloid leukaemic cells that is inhibited by interleukin 6. Nature 352: 345–347.
60. Lotem J., Sachs, L. 1993. Hematopoietic cells from mice deficient in wild-type p53 are more resistant to induction of apoptosis by some agents. Blood 82:1092–1096.
61. Lotem J., Sachs, L. 1993. Regulation by bcl-2, c-myc and p53 of susceptibility to induction of apoptosis by heat shock and cancer chemotherapy compounds in differentiation competent and defective myeloid leukemic cells. Cell Growth Differ., 4: 41–47.
62. Bissonnette R.P., Echeverri F., Mahboudi A., Green D.R. 1992. Apoptotic cell death induced by c-myc is inhibited by bcl-2. Nature 359: 552–554.
63. Fanidi A., Harrington E.A., Evan, G.I. 1992. Cooperative interaction between c-myc and bcl-2 proto-oncogenes. Nature 359: 554–556.
64. Korsmeyer S.J. 1992. Bcl-2 initiates a new category of oncogenes: Regulators of cell death. Blood 80: 879–886.
65. Lowe S.W., Schmitt E.M., Smith S.W., Osborne B.A., Jacks T. 1993. p53 is required for radiation-induced apoptosis in mouse thymocytes. Nature 362: 847–849.
66. Clarke A.R., Purdie C.A., Harrison D.J., Morris R.G., Bird C.C., Hooper M.L., Wylie A.H. 1993. Thymocyte apoptosis induced by p53-dependant and independant pathways. Nature 362: 849–852.
67. Lotem J., Sachs L. 1994. Control of sensitivity to induction of apoptosis in myeloid leukemic cells by differentiation and bcl-2 dependent and independent pathways. Cell Growth Differ. 5: 321–327.

Acute Leukemias V
Experimental Approaches
and Management of Refractory Diseases
Hiddemann et al. (Eds.)

CD34 and CD38 Expression on Blasts in Myelodysplastic Syndromes and Secondary AML

W. Verbeek, C. Ries, D. Grove, M. Unterhalt, W. Hiddemann, and B. Wörmann

Abstract. The expression of a "stem cell like" blast immunophenotype (CD34+/CD38−) has been associated with a poor prognosis in AML. Advanced myelodysplastic syndromes and secondary AML's are another patient population with an inferior prognosis. We hypothesized that a stem cell origin of these disorders results in a higher incidence of a CD34+/CD38− blast immunophenotype. This could be biologically related to a higher chemoresistence. The data presented here shows that a "stem cell like" blast immunophenotype is rare in RAEB. In addition there is no significant difference between primary AML and secondary AML or RAEB-T.

Introduction

Pluripotent hematopoietic progenitor cells are characterized by the expression of CD34 (Civin et al. 1984). Based on the acquisition of further antigens such as the lineage non restricted CD38 and HLA-DR and lineage restricted antigens such as CD19, CD33 and CD5, this pool of progenitor cells can be divided into further subpopulations. The most immature hematopoietic progenitor cell has been characterized as CD34+/CD38−/HLA-DR- and has a frequency of approximatly 0.01 % in normal bone marrow (Huang et al. 1992). Their capacity to differentiate into the different hematopoietic cell lineages as well as fibroblasts has been elegantly demonstrated by single cell sorting in combination with subsequent colony assay (Huang et al. 1992). CD34 is also expressed in 50–80% of the leukemic blasts from patients with newly diagnosed acute myeloid leukemia. Expression of CD34 has been associated with a higher proportion of clonogenicity (Löwenberg et al. 1985). In a study on 235 patients with newly diagnosed acute myeloid leukemia we have recently demonstrated that the early differentiation pathway of pluripotent progenitor cells is well conserved on myeloid leukemic blasts (Terstappen et al. 1992). About 1/3 of AML samples expressed the "stem cell like" immunophenotype of CD34+/CD38−/HLA-DR-. The subgroup had an inferior prognosis with a lower remission rate and shorter remission duration than patients with a more mature immunophenotype (Wörmann et al. 1993). In this study we have analyzed the immunophenotype of leukemic blasts in patients with advanced stages of myelodysplastic syndromes (MDS) and secondary AML. In MDS multilineage involvement of hematopoiesis has been demonstrated by the detection of cytogenetic changes in different lineages, which is in good agreement with the hematological picture (Nylund et al. 1994). We hypothesize that the frequency of CD34+/CD38− blasts is higher in patients with MDS and secondary AML than in primary AML. This "stem cell like" immunophenotype might also explain the higher degree of chemoresistance in these entities.

Patients, Material and Methods

Diagnosis. Diagnosis of MDS and classification was performed according to the morphological criteria defined by the FAB group (Bennett et al.

Department of Hematology and Oncology, University of Göttingen, Göttingen, Germany

1982). Secondary leukemia was defined by a previous history of myelodysplasia or another form of antecedent hematological disorder for at least 6 months or previous chemo- or radiotherapy.

Cell preparation. Nucleated cells were isolated from bone marrow samples by NH_4Cl erythrocyte lysis. 2 × 105 – 1 × 106 cells were stained with 15 µl of CD34 FITC conjugated monoclonal antibody (Becton Dickinson, San José, California, USA) and a Phycoerythrin conjugated anti CD38 antibody (BDIS) and a PerCP conjugated anti HLA-DR antibody (BDS) for 15–30 minutes on ice. Unspecific binding was removed by two 3-minute washes with Phosphate Buffered Saling (PBS).

Data acquisition and analysis. Dual (FITC and PE) or three color immunofluorescence was quantitated in a BD FACS can equipped with an argon laser. Antibody conjugates of the same murine isotypes specificity were used as negative controls. For each sample 10–20.000 events were recorded. Data were stored in list mode and analyzed with the BD Lysis, consort 30 software and the Paint a gate program. Immunofluorescence was analyzed within the characteristic light scatter gate region for blast cell morphology. Four populations of cells were distinguished based on differential expression of CD34 and CD38 as previously described (Terstappen et al. 1992).

Definition of CD34 subpopulations. Population I includes the most immature cells with high CD34 expression and lack of CD38 ("stem cell like" immunophenotype). Cells in population III are characterized by coexpression of CD34 and CD38, population II has an intermediate expression of CD38. Population IV is charaterized by a negativity for CD34 and expression of CD38. The number of cells in each population was determined as percentage of all cells within the blast gate. Five novel bone marrows were analyzed as controls for the MDS samples.

Results

CD34/CD38 antigen expression of the blast populations of 10 RAEB, 8 RAEB-T and 49 sAML patients were investigated by dual colour immunophenotyping.

In RAEB blast populations were characterised by a relatively mature CD34 positive/ CD38 positive immunophenotype (population III and IV).

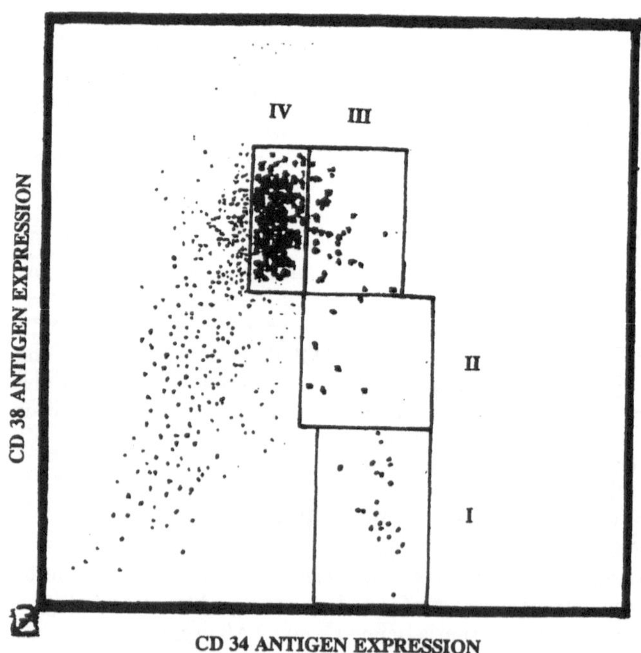

Fig. 1

Only in one out of 10 cases the CD34+/CD38− population was significantly increased when compared to normal controls. This case showed a clearly separated population of stem cell like blasts. In RAEB-T an expansion of population I was demonstrated in 3 out of 8 cases. In AML secondary to myelodysplasia 20 of 49 patients showed a significant percentage of stem cell like blasts. Immature blasts in RAEB-T and s-AML showed a continuous acquisition of the CD38 antigen. However, the relative distribution of blasts in the different steps of maturation differed considerably. The broad variations between cases were similar to primary AML.

In one patient with RAEB we repeated immunophenotyping after one year without clinical progression. The individual immunophenotype remained stable over this time period. Another case progressing from RAEB to sAML developed a new stem cell like blast population at the time of transformation. Statistical evaluation demonstrated a tendency towards an increased number of stem cell like blasts in the blast populations of secondary AML compared to RAEB. In addition we compared the incidence of stem cell like blasts between the group of secondary AML's analyzed in this study and a large population of 178 de novo AML's investigated previously. The incidence was 41% and 36% respectively. This marginal difference did not reach a statistical significance (p= 0,6476).

Conclusions

The main populations of blasts accumulating in RAEB does not exhibit a stem cell like immunophenotype (CD34+/CD38−). This finding is in accordance to data by Oertel et al. who investigated CD34 expression in RAEB by immunohistochemistry. The stem cell origin of RAEB is not reflected by the phenotype of the mayor blast population. Cells with blast morphology are most likely derived from a CD 34+/CD38− progenitor cell which retained the capacity for limited phenotypic maturation. A tendency towards a higher frequency of immature blast populations in the group of sAML compared to RAEB may be explained by the expansion of an immature clone at the time of transformation. This event could be demonstrated in one case. Patient 10, the only RAEB case with a separated CD 34+/CD38− blast population received intensive chemotherapy after progression to sAML. At the time of immunophenotyping his bone marrow was again classified as RAEB. The separated PI blasts could belong to residual sAML blast population incompletely eliminated by chemotherapy. Concerning the incidence of CD34+/CD38− blast populations no difference has been found between primary and secondary AML. The poor prognosis of AML following MDS is not related to the immaturity of its mayor blast population.

References

1. Bennett JM, Catovsky D, Daniel M-T: Proposals for the classification of the myelodysplastic syndromes. Br.J. of Haematol 33: 329–331, 1982
2. Civin CI, Strauss LC, Brovall C, Fackler MJ, Schwartz JF, Shaper JH: Antigenic analysis of hematopoiesis: A hematopoietic progenitor cell surface antigen defined by a monoclonal antibody raised against KG1a cells J. Immunol. 133: 157, 1984
3. Campos L, Guyotat D, Archimbaud E, Devaux Y Treille D, Larese A, Maupas J, Gentilhomme O.,Ehrsam A, Fiere D: Surface marker expression in adult acute myeloid leukemia: correlation with initial characteristics, morphology and response to therapy. Br. J. Haematol 72: 161–166, 1989
4. Huang S, Terstappen LWMM: Formation of haematopoietic microenvironment and haematopoietic stem cells from single human bone marrow stem cells. Nature 360: 745–749, 1992
5. Huang S, Terstappen LWMM: Lymphoid and myeloid differentiation of single human CD34+, HLA-DR- ,CD38- hematopoietic stem cells. Blood 83: 1515–1526, 1993
6. Kristensen J.S. Hokland P: Monoclonal antibody ratios in malignant myeloid diseases: diagnostic and prognostic use in myelodysplastic syndromes. Br. J. Haematol 74, 270–276, 1990
7. Delwel R, Löwenberg B: Variable differentiation of human acute myeloid leukemia during colony formation in vitro: A membrane marker analysis with monoclonal antibodies. Brit J Haematol 59: 37 1985
8. Masuya M, Kita K, Shimizu N, Ohishi K, Katayama N, Sekine T. Otsuji A, Miwa H. Shirakawa S: Biologic characteristics of acute leukemia after myelodysplastic syndrome. Blood 81: 3388–3394, 1993
9. Nylund S, Verbeek W, Larramendy ML, Ruutu T, Heinonen K, Hallman H, Knuutila S: Cell lineage involvement in four patients with myelodysplastic syndrome an t(1;7) or trisomy 8 studied by simultaneous immunophenotyping and fluorescence in situ hybrisation. Cancer Genet Cytogenet 70: 120–124, 1993

10. Oertel J., Kleiner S., Huhn D: Immunotyping of blasts in refractory anaemia with excess of blasts. Br. J Haematol. 84, 305–309, 1993
11. San Miguel J.F. Gonzalez M., Canizo M.C., Anta J.P., Hernandez J., Ortega F., Borrasca L: The nature of blast cell in myelodysplastic syndromes evolving to acute leukemia. Blut 22: 357–363, 1986
12. Wörmann B., D.Grove D., Unterhalt M.; Toepker S., Aul C. Heyll A. Büchner TH., Hiddemann W., Terstappen LW.M.M: Characterisation of CD 34+/CD38− acute myeloid leukemia. ASH Abstract, 1993

Acute Leukemias V
Experimental Approaches
and Management of Refractory Diseases
Hiddemann et al. (Eds.)

Heterogeneity of HRX-FEL Fusion Transcripts in Adult and Pediatric t(4;11) ALL

F. Griesinger[1], T. Jahn[1], H. Elfers[1], W.-D. Ludwig[2], M. Falk[1], H. Rieder[3], J. Harbott[4], F. Lampert[4], B. Heinze[5], D. Hoelzer[6], E. Thiel[7], H. Riehm[8], B. Wörmann[1], C. Fonatsch[3], and W. Hiddemann[1]

Abstract. The t(4;11) is the cytogenetic hallmark of a subgroup of pre-pre-B-ALL characterized by coexpression of myeloid differentiation antigens, a high prevalence in infants and an incidence of 5–7% in children and adults. Prognosis is very poor in infants, and may be somewhat better in children and adults. The molecular correlate of t(4;11) is a fusion gene composed of HRX (ALL-1, MLL) on 11q23 and FEL (AF-4) on 4q21. HRX shows homology to Drosophila trithorax, and to murine ALL-1 and most likely represents a DNA-binding transactivating factor of unknown function in human hematopoiesis and/or embryogenesis. Replacement of 3′ zinc finger domains of HRX by 3′ protein domains of the FEL fusion partner may alter protein-DNA interaction specificity and thereby confer transforming potential to HRX fusion proteins. The aims of the study were i) to analyze the incidence of HRX-FEL fusion genes in adult pre-pre-B-ALL coexpressing CD15 and/or CDw65 by RT-pcr. ii) to characterize HRX-FEL fusion genes by sequence determination in different age groups. Twenty-three pre-pre-B-ALL (7 infants, 14 adults and two cell lines) were selected either based on cytogenetic demonstration of t(4;11) (n = 12, group A) or on a CD15/CDw65+ pre-pre-B-ALL phenotype, highly suggestive of a t(4;11) (n = 10, group B). HRX-FEL-fusion gene transcripts were detected in 13 of 13 pre-pre-B-ALL in group A and in 9 of 10 adult pre-pre-B-ALL in group B. More than one HRX-FEL-fusion gene amplification product was detected in 4 of 22 pre-pre-B-ALL, suggesting differential splicing of fusion genes. All 16 HRX-FEL positive samples coexpressed CDw65, while only 12 of 15 coexpressed CD15. The most common fusion genes join HRX exons 6 (4 adults) or 7 (6 adults, 3 infants) to FEL exon "a". The third fusion product represents a join between HRX exon 6 and FELnt 1458 (3 adults, 1 infant). Additional types of fusion genes with breakpoints more 3′ on FEL and/or more 5′ of exon 6 on HRX are suspected in 2 infants and 2 adults. In conclusion, i) HRX-FEL fusion transcripts may be detected in the vast majority of immunophenotypically suspected t(4;11). Coexpression of CDw65 may show a better correlation with t(4;11) than CD15. ii) HRX-FEL fusion genes are heterogeneous, and there is a tendency for a lower incidence of HRX exon 6 fusions in infants. Whether these differences will hold true and correlate with prognosis will have to be studied in a larger number of patients in a prospective study.

Introduction

Acute leukemias represent clonal expansions of malignant transformed lymphohematopoietic

[1]Division of Hematology and Oncology, Department of Internal Medicine, University of Göttingen, FRG
[2]Division of Hematology and Oncology, Department of Internal Medicine, Rössle Clinic, Berlin-Buch, FRG
[3]Institute of Human Genetics, University of Lübeck, FRG
[4]Department of Pediatric Hematology and Oncology, University of Gießen, FRG
[5]Institute of Occupational and Social Medicine, University of Ulm, FRG
[6]Division of Hematology, Department of Internal Medicine, University of Frankfurt, FRG
[7]Division of Hematology and Oncology, Department of Internal Medicine, Free University of Berlin, FRG
[8]Department of Pediatric Hematology and Oncology, University of Hannover, FRG

precursor cells. A variety of genetic alterations resulting in a malignant phenotype have been identified. In acuteleukemias, "master genes" which physiologically play a role in differentiation and presumably lineage commitment have been implicated in leukemia associated chromosomal translocations [1]. A new such candidate gene, HRX (ALL-1, MLL), is located on chromosome 11q23 [2, 3, 4] and forms fusion genes with a number of genes located most frequently on chromosomes 4, 6, 9, and 19 [5]. HRX is homologous to Drosophila trithorax, involved in Drosophila morphogenesis, and homologous to murine ALL-1 which may be associated with murine skeletal malformation [6]. Based on the protein structure of HRX (AT-hooks, zinc fingers, prolin-rich domain) it most likely represents a DNA-binding transactivating factor. However its function in human hematopoiesis is unclear.

Replacement of 3′ zinc finger domains of HRX by 3′ protein domains of the respective fusion partner may alter protein-DNA interaction specificity and thereby confer transforming potential to HRX fusion proteins. HRX fusion proteins are associated with ANLL (M5) [5], and pre-pre-B-ALL with coexpression of myeloid differentiation antigens. CD15 and CDw65 [7,8] are frequently associated with a t(4;11) (q21;q23) and formation of a HRX-FEL fusion gene product. This leukemia may constitutes up to 50% of infant and 5–7% of childhood and adult ALL [5]. Prognosis in infants is dismal with chemotherapy alone [9,10,11], and it may be somewhat better in children and adults. The presence of a t(4;11) is a stratification criterion in most adult and childhood ALL protocols for intensive therapeutic approaches.

In order to learn more about genetic alterations of the HRX gene in ALL, a total of 23 (16 adult, 7 infant) pre-pre-B-ALL, selected either by cytogenetic demonstration of t(4;11) or by a CD15/CDw65+pre-pre-B-ALL phenotype, highly suggestive of a t(4;11), were studied by RT-pcr for the presence of a HRX-FEL fusion transcript and sequences of HRX-FEL fusion genes were analyzed.

Material and Methods

Patients and cell lines. Five adult pre-pre-B-ALL, 6 infant pre-pre-B-ALL and two cell lines (RS 4;11, MV 4;11, the latter kindly provided by Dr. John H. Kersey, University of Minnesota) had a cytogenetically proven t(4;11) (q21;q23). Pre-pre-B-ALL was defined by a CD10-, CD19+, CD20±, CD22±, CD24−, CD34±, CD38+ phenotype.

Nine adult pre-pre-B-ALL and 1 infant ALL were selected solely because of coexpression of CD15 and/or CDw65, but t(4;11) had not been demonstrated by karyotype in these cases (see Table 1).

RNA-extraction and RT-pcr. mRNA was extracted using a cellulose based RNA-extraction-kit (Fast Track and Micro Fast-Track, Invitrogen, San Diego, CA). First strand cDNA synthesis was performed with an AMV-based reverse transcription kit (cDNA cycle kit, Invitrogen, San Diego, CA) according to the manufacturer's instructions by random priming. Primers used for amplification of HRX-FEL-fusion genes were primer 1 (HRX 5′): GAA AGCCCG TCG AGG AAA AGA, primer 2 (FEL 3′): TGC TTT CTG ACT CTG CACTGC, primer 3 (HRX 5′5′): GAG AAA ATG TCA GAA TCT ACA ATG, primer 4(FEL 3′3′): CGC TGC TGC CCT TAC TCT CT. PCR was performed for 30 cycles at a stringent annealing temperature of 63 °C. "Nested" pcr was performed with primers 5 and 6; primer 5 (ALL-1 5′5′): ATC AGG TCCAGA GCA GAG C; primer 6 (AF-4 3′): GGG AAA GGA AAC TTG GAT GG. Pcr was performed for 25 cycles at a stringent annealing temperature of 58 °C. As a positive control for the quality of mRNA, β-actin RT-pcr was performed for 25 cycles at a stringent annealing temperature of 58 °C using primer β-actin 5′: ACT CCA TGC CCA GGA AGG A, and primer β-actin 3′: GAC CCA GAT CAT GTT TGA GA.

Sequence analysis. Primary amplification products – generated with primers 1 and 2 – were asymmetrically amplified and sequenced using primers 5 and 6 with a T7-polymerase based sequencing kit (Sequenase 2.0, USB, Cleveland, OH) or alternatively were sequenced on an automated sequencer (ABI) by cycle sequencing.

Immunophenotyping. Three color immunophenotyping was performed on a FACScan using FITC-conjugated anti-CDw65 monoclonal antibody (BMA0210-FITC,Behring, Marburg, FRG) and FITC-conjugated anti-CD15 monoclonalantibody (Leu-M1-FITC, Becton and Dickinson, San Josá□á, CA) in combination with PE-conju-

Table 1. List of patients. All patients were β-actin positive. nd: not done

Pt#	Phenotype	% CD15+	% CDw65+	Karyotype	HPX/FEL
Adult pre-pre-B-ALL with cytogenetic detection of t(4;11)					
14	prepreB	10	49	46, XY[6]/46, XY, t(4;11)(q21;q23) [16]	pos
20	prepreB	89	45	46, XX, t(4;11) (q21;q23) [2]	pos
27	prepreB	10	45	46, XY[1]/46, XY, t(4;11) (q21;q23) [15]	pos
32	prepreB	57	77	46, XY [9]/46, XY, t(4;11) (q21;q23) [5]	pos
33	prepreB	43	61	46, XY, t(4;11) (q21;q23) [13]	pos
MV 4;11	prepreB	nd	nd	Chen et al. Blood 1993	pos
RS 4;11	prepreB	nd	nd	Stong et al. Blood 1985	pos
Infant pre-pre-B-ALL with cytogenetic detection of t(4;11)					
17	prepreB	31	50	46, XX, t(4;11) (q21;q23) [5]	pos
29	prepreB	39	49	46, XX, t(4;11) (q21;q23) [3]	pos
31	prepreB	19	75	46, XX, t(4;11) (q21;q23), i(7q10), del (11) (q23) [5]	pos
1.1	prepreB	30	nd	46, XX, t(4;11) (q21;q23)	pos
1.2	prepreB	33	nd	46, XX, t(4;11) (q21;q23)	pos
1.3	prepreB	66	nd	46, XX, t(4;11)(q21;q23)	pos
Adult pre-pre-B-ALL without cytogenetic detection of t(4;11)					
1	prepreB	59	30	46, XY [33]	pos
7	prepreB	5	15	46, XX [6]	pos
8	prepreB	90	83	46, XY [14]	pos
10	prepreB	nd	55	46, XX [18]/47, XX+C [2]	pos
12	prepreB	52	8	46, XY [13]/52–55, XY, +X, dup(1) (q32q21), +4, +6, +8, +10, −13, +14, +15, +21, +mar [30]	pos
18	prepreB	84	89	46, XX [14]	pos
22	prepreB	58	52	nd	pos
24	prepreB	17	30	nd	pos
28	prepreB	28	15	nd	pos
Infant pre-pre-B-ALL without cytogenetic detection of t(4;11)					
1.4	prepreB	45	15	nd	pos

gated anti-CD19 and PerCP conjugated anti-CD20 monoclonal antibodies.

Results and Discussion

HRX-FEL-fusion gene transcripts were detected by RT-pcr in all (13 of 13) pre-pre-B-ALL with cytogenetically proven t(4;11). Thus, with our selection of primers, all HRX-FEL fusion sites are readily detectable with a single step RT-pcr without the necessity to perform a "nested" pcr.

HRX-FEL-fusion gene transcripts were detected in 9 of 10 (89%) adult pre-pre-B-ALL without cytogenetic demonstration of t(4;11). One pre-pre-B-ALL (pt #12), coexpressing CD15, but not CDw65, was negative. These results are considerably higher than those of other groups, indicating that in the order of 30% 11q23 abnormalities will be detected by molecular genetic approaches which are missed by conventional cytogenetics [9,12]. The discrepancy is most likely due to a highly selected population of immunologically characterized pre-pre-B-ALL, as well as differences in the quality of cytogenetic analysis, as concordance rates between karyotype and molecular analysis varied considerably between cytogenetic reference laboratories.

Table 2. Summary or results of cytogenetic demonstration of t(4;11) and detection of HRX-FEL fusion transcripts by RT-pcr. *2 patients with ⩾20,2 with 10–19, 1 with ⩽10 metaphases, 3 patients no karyotype done, 1 patient not available

	HRX-FEL+	HRX-FEL−	n
t(4;11)+	13	0	13
t(4;11)−	9*	1	10
n	22	1	23

Table 3. Association of CDw65 (A) and CD15 (B) coexpression with presence of t(4;11). pre-pre-B-ALL were scored positive, if > 10% of leukemic blasts expressed the respective differentiation antigen by three color immunophenotyping

A	HRX-FEL+	HRX-FEL−	n
CDw65+	17	0	17
CDw65−	0	1	1
n	17	1	18
B	**HRX-FEL+**	**HRX-FEL−**	**n**
CD 15+	16	1	17
CD 15−	3	0	3
n	19	1	20

CDw65 coexpression showed a better correlation with t(4;11)/HRX-FEL fusion gene than CD15 coexpression. This was also true for those pre-pre-B-ALL which were selected based on presence of t(4;11) by cytogenetics, irrespective of their phenotype. These results may warrant inclusion of CDw65 rather than CD15 for the selection of pre-pre-B-ALL for routine screening of t(4;11)/HRX-FEL fusion transcripts.

More than one HRX-FEL-fusion amplification product was detected in 4 of 22 pre-pre-B-ALL, suggesting differential splicing of fusion genes as t(4;11) was cytogenetically demonstrated only on one allele in all cases in which cytogenetic analysis was available. Furthermore,

Table 4. Sequences of HRX-FEL fusion genes. Assignment of nucleotides to the HRX and FEL genes was based on the published intron/exonboundaries, FEL exons "a" and "b" according to Downing et al. Blood 1994. The numbering of nucleotides is according to Morrisey et al., Blood, 1993, and Tkachuk et al. Cell 1992. *samples with ⩾2 fusion transcripts

Pt#10, #24, #27, #32			
	EXON 6	**EXON 7**	
HRX-Germline	AAAACCAAAAGAAAAG	GAAAAACCACCT...	
FUSION GENE	AAAACCAAAAGAAAAG		*CAGACCTACTCCAATGAAGTCC*
FEL Germline			*CAGACCTACTCCAATGAAGTCC*
			FEL(exon "a") nt:1413
MV 4;11, Pt#1, #20			
	EXON 6	**EXON 7**	
HRX-Germline	AAAACCAAAAGAAAAG	GAAAAACCACCT...	
FUSION GENE	AAAACCAAAAGAAAAG		*GAAATGACCCATTCATG*
FEL Germline			*TCGAAGGAAATGACCCATTCATG*
			FEL (exon "b") nt:1458
RS 4;11, Pt's #8, #14, #22, #28, #33,#1.2*, #1.4*			
	EXON 7	**EXON 8**	
HRX-Germline	ATCAGAGTGGACTTTAAG	GAGGATTGTGAA...	
FUSION GENE	ATCAGAGTGGACTTTAAG		*ACCTACTCCAATGAAGTCC*
FEL Germline			*CAGACCTACTCCAATGAAGTCC*
			FEL(exon"a") nt:1416
RS 4;11, #17*, #1.2*, #1.3*,#1.4*			
	EXON 7	**EXON 8**	
HRX-Germline	ATCAGAGTGGACTTTAAG	GAGGATTGTGAA...	
FUSION GENE	ATCAGAGTGGACTTTAAG		*CAGACCTACTCCAATGAAGTCC*
FEL Germline			*CAGACCTACTCCAATGAAGTCC*
			FEL(exon"a") nt:1413
Pt#17*, #1.2*			
	EXON 8	**EXON 9**	
HRX-Germline	AGTGGGCATGTAGAG	GTTTGTGTATTG...	
FUSION GENE	AGTGGGCATGTAGAG		*CAGACCTACTCCAATGAAGTCC*
FEL Germline			*CAGACCTACTCCAATGAAGTCC*
			FEL(exon "a") nt:1413

both splice variants of FEL exon "a" [13] were demonstrated by sequence analysis in 2 infants (1.2 and 1.4) as well as in the cell line RS4;11 (see Table 4), which were not separated on agarose or PAGE gel electrophoresis. Five different fusion gene products were identified with three breakpoints on FEL and two on HRX . The most common fusion genes join HRX exons 6 or 7 with the two splice variants of FEL exon "a", demonstrated in 17 of 22 sequenced fusion products. The fourth fusion product represents a join between HRX exon 6 and FEL exon "b",

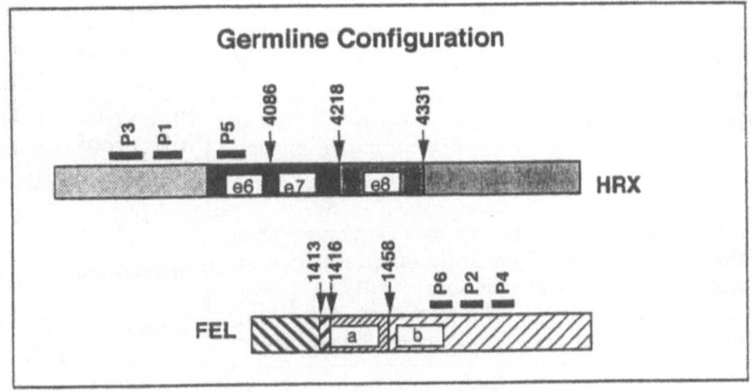

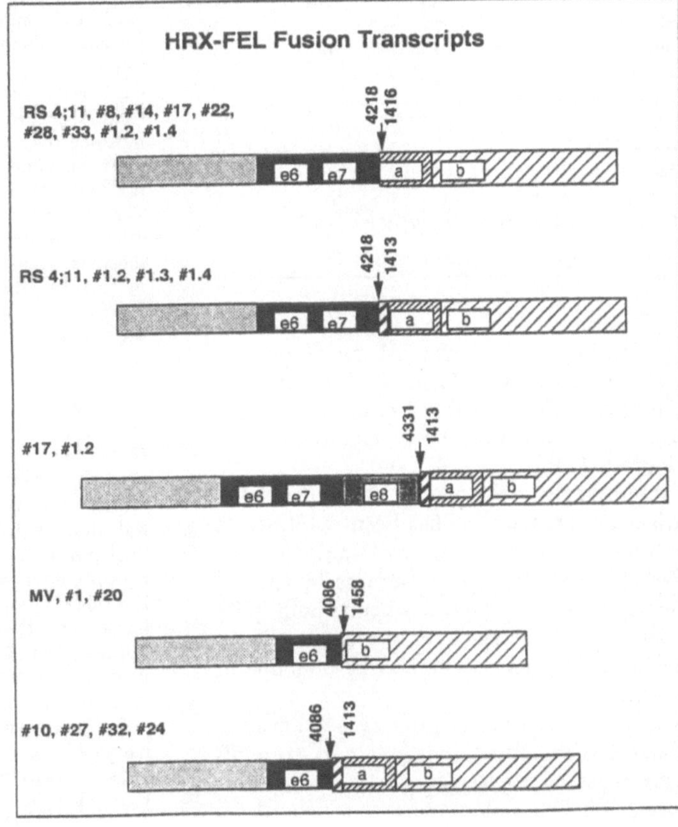

Fig. 1. Schematic representation of heterogeneous fusion transcripts in pre-pre- B-ALL. e = exon. Exon assignment as in Table 4

Table 5. HRX (A) and FEL (B) exon assignment as in Table 4

A	e6	e7	e8	n
infant	0	4	2	6
adult	7	6	0	13
n	7	10	2	19
B	a	b	c	n
infant	6	0	0	6
adult	10	3	0	13
n	16	3	0	19

Table 6. HRX (A) and FEL (B) exon assignment as in Table 4. Data are from Borkhardt et al. Leukemia 1994, Griesinger et al. Leukemia 1994, and this poster, Biondi et al. Blood 1993, Morrisey et al. Blood 1993, Hilden et al. Cancer Res 1993, Cotter et al. PNAS 1993

A	e6	e7	e8	n
infant	7(23%)	11(37%)	12(40%)	30
pediatric	1	3	1	5
adult	11(52%)	10(48%)	0	21
n	19	24	11	55
B	a	b	c	n
infant	25(83%)	5(17%)	0	30
pediatric	5(100%)	0	0	5
adult	16(76.5%)	2(9.5%)	3(14%)	21
n	45	7	3	55

observed in 3 samples, the fifth fusion product between exon 8 and FEL exon"a" shown in 2 infant pre-pre-B-ALL. These results are consistent with published results in infant and adults pre-pre-B-ALL.

Interestingly, only one or the other splice variant of FEL exon "a" has been published to form the fusion gene in RS4;11 [13,14], while we have observed both splice variants in our cell line sample. It is not known, whether both splice variants are transcribed in the same cell, or whether individual cells transcribe only one or the other.

Based on the sizes of primary amplification products of samples #7, #18, #29 and #31 additional types of fusion genes with breakpoints more 3′ on FEL and/or more 5′ of exon 5 on HRX may be suspected.

With a low number of fusion genes studied, there seems to be a lower incidence of usage of exon 7 in infants. In our small series, none of the infants had a HRX exon 6 fusion gene product, while 7 of 13 fusion genes in adult pre-pre-B-ALL "used" this exon. A review of the literature listing all published and sequenced HRX-FEL fusion genes also shows a lower incidence of HRX exon 6 as being the fusion site in infants as compared to both adults and childhood pre-pre-B-ALL [15–20].

It is tempting to speculate that differences of fusion genes are associated with a different prognosis in infants and adults. However, definitive proof will await a prospective study with a homogeneously treated patient population.

References

1. Rabbitts TH. Translocations, master genes, and differences between the origins of acute and chronic leukemias. Cell, 1991,67: 641–644.
2. Cimino G, Lo Coco F, Biondi A, Elia L, Luciano A, Croce CM, Masera G, Mandelli F, Canaani E. ALL-1 gene at chromosome 11q23 is consistently altered in acute leukemia of early infancy. Blood 1993; 82: 544–546.
3. Gu Y, Nakamura T, Alder H, Prasad R, Canaani O, Cimino G, Croce CM, Canaani E. The t(4;11) chromosome translocation of human acute leukemias fuses the ALL-1 gene, related to drosophila trithorax, to the AF-4 gene. Cell 1992; 71: 701–708.
4. Tkachuk DC, Kohler S, Cleary ML. Involvement of a homolog of drosophila trithorax by 11q23 chromosomal translocations in acute leukemias. Cell 1992; 71: 691–700.
5. Thirman MJ, Gill HJ, Burnett RC, Mbangkollo D, McCabe NR, Kobayashi H, Ziemin van der Peil S, Kaneko Y, Morgan R, Sandberg AA, Chaganti RSK, Larson RA, Le Beau MM, Diaz MO, Rowley JD. Rearrangement of the MLL gene in acute lymphoblastic and acute myeloid leukemias with 11q23 chromosomal translocations. N Engl J Med 1993;329: 909–914.‰
6. Ma Q, Alder H, Nelson KK, Chatterjee D, Gu Y, Nakamura T, Canaani E, Croce CM, Siracusa LD, Buchberg AM. Analysis of the murine ALL-1 gene reveals conserved domains with human ALL-1 and identifies a motif shared with DNA methyltransferases. Proc Natl Acad Sci USA 1993; 90: 6350–6354
7. Borowitz MJ, Carroll AJ, Shuster JJ, Look AT, Behm FG, Pullen DJ, Land VJ, Steuber P, Crist WM. Use of clinical and laboratory features to define prognostic subgroups in B-precursor acute lymphoblastic leukemia: Experience of the Pediatric Oncology Group. In Ludwig W-D, Thiel E, eds. Recent Results in Cancer Research. Recent Advances in Cell Biology of Acute Leukemia. Berlin, Springer, 1993; pp. 257–267.
8. Ludwig W-D, Harbott J, Bartram CR, Komischke B, Sperling C, Teichmann JV, Seibt-Jung H, Notter

M, Odenwald E, Nehmer A, Thiel E, Riehm H. Incidence and prognostic significance of immunophenotypic subgroups in childhood acute lymphoblastic leukemia: Experience of the BFM Study 86. In Ludwig W-D, Thiel E, eds. Recent Results in Cancer Research. Recent Advances in Cell Biology of Acute Leukemia. Berlin, Springer, 1993; pp. 269–282.

9. Rubnitz JE, Link MP, Shuster JJ, Carroll AJ, Hakami N, Frankel L, Pullen DJ, Cleary ML. Frequency and significance of HRX rearrangements in infant acute lymphoblastic leukemia. Blood 1993; 82: 190a (Abstract 744)

10. Riehm H, Gadner H, Henze G, Kornhuber B, Lampert F, Niethammer D, Reiter A, Schellong G. Results and significance of six randomized trials in four consecutive ALL-BFM studies. In Büchner Th, Schellong G, Hiddemann W, Ritter J, eds. Acute Leukemias: II. Prognostic factors and treatment strategies. Berlin, Springer. 1990; pp. 439–450.

11. Chen C-S, Hilden JM, Frestedt J, Domer PH, Moore R, Korsmeyer SJ, Kersey JH. The chromosome 4q21 gene (AF-4/FEL) is widely expressed in normal tissues and shows breakpoint diversity in t(4;11)(q21;q23) acute leukemia. Blood 1993b; 82: 1080–1085.

12. Chen C-S, Sorensen PHB, Domer PH, Reaman GH, Korsmeyer SJ, Heerema NA, Hammond FD, Kersey JH. Molecular rearrangements on chromosome 11q23 predominate in infant acute lymphoblastic leukemia and are associated with specific biologic variables and poor outcome. Blood 1993; 81: 2386–2393.

13. Nakamura T, Alder H, Gu Y, Prasad R, Canaani P, Kamada N, Gale RP, Lange B, Crist WM, Nowell PC, Croce CM, Canaani E. Genes on chromosomes 4, 9, and 19 involved in 11q23 abnormalities in acute leukemia share sequence homology and/or common motifs. Proc Natl Acad Sci USA, 1993;90: 4631–4635.

14. Hilden JM, Chen C-S, Moore R, Frestedt J, Kersey JH. Heterogeneity in MLL/AF-4 fusion messenger RNA detected by the polymerase chain reaction in t(4;11) acute leukemia. Cancer Res 1993; 53: 3853–3856.

15. Corral J, Forster A, Thompson S, Lampert F, Kaneko Y, Slater R, Kroes WG, van der Schoot CE, Ludwig W-D, Karpas A, Pocock C, Cotter F, Rabbitts TH. Acute leukemias of different lineages have similar MLL gene fusions encoding related chimeric proteins resulting from chromosomal translocations. PNAS 1993; 90: 8538–8542.

16. Borkhardt A, Repp R, Haupt E, Brettreich S, Buchen U, Gossen R, Lampert F. Molecular analysis of MLL-1/AF4 recombination in infant acute lymphoblastic leukemia. Leukemia 1994; 8: 549–553.

17. Biondi A, Rambaldi A, Rossi V, Elia L, Caslini C, Basso G, Battista R, Barbui T, Mandelli F, Masera G, Croce C, Canaani E, Cimino G. Detection of ALL-1/AF4 fusion transcript by reverse transcription pcr for diagnosis and monitoring of acute leukemias with the t(4;11) translocation. Blood, 1993; 82: 2943.

18. Morrissey J, Tkachuk DC, Milatovich A, Francke U, Link M, Cleary ML. A serine/proline-rich protein is fused to HRX in t(4;11) acute leukemias. Blood 1993; 81: 1124–1131.

19. Downing JR, Head DR, Raimondi SC, Carroll AJ, Curcio-Brint AM, Motroni TA, Hushof MG, Pullen DJ, Domer PH. The der (11) encoded MLL/AF-4 fusion transcript is consistently detected in t(4;11)(q21;q23) containing acute lymphoblastic leukemia. Blood 1994; 83: 330–335.

20. Griesinger F, Elfers H, Ludwig W-D, Falk M, Rieder H, Harbott J, Lampert F, Heinze B, Hoelzer D, Thiel E, Riehm H, Wášármann B, Fonatsch C, Hiddemann W. Detection of HRX-FEL fusion transcripts in pre-pre-B-ALL with and without cytogenetic demonstration of t(4;11). Leukemia 1994;8: 542–548.

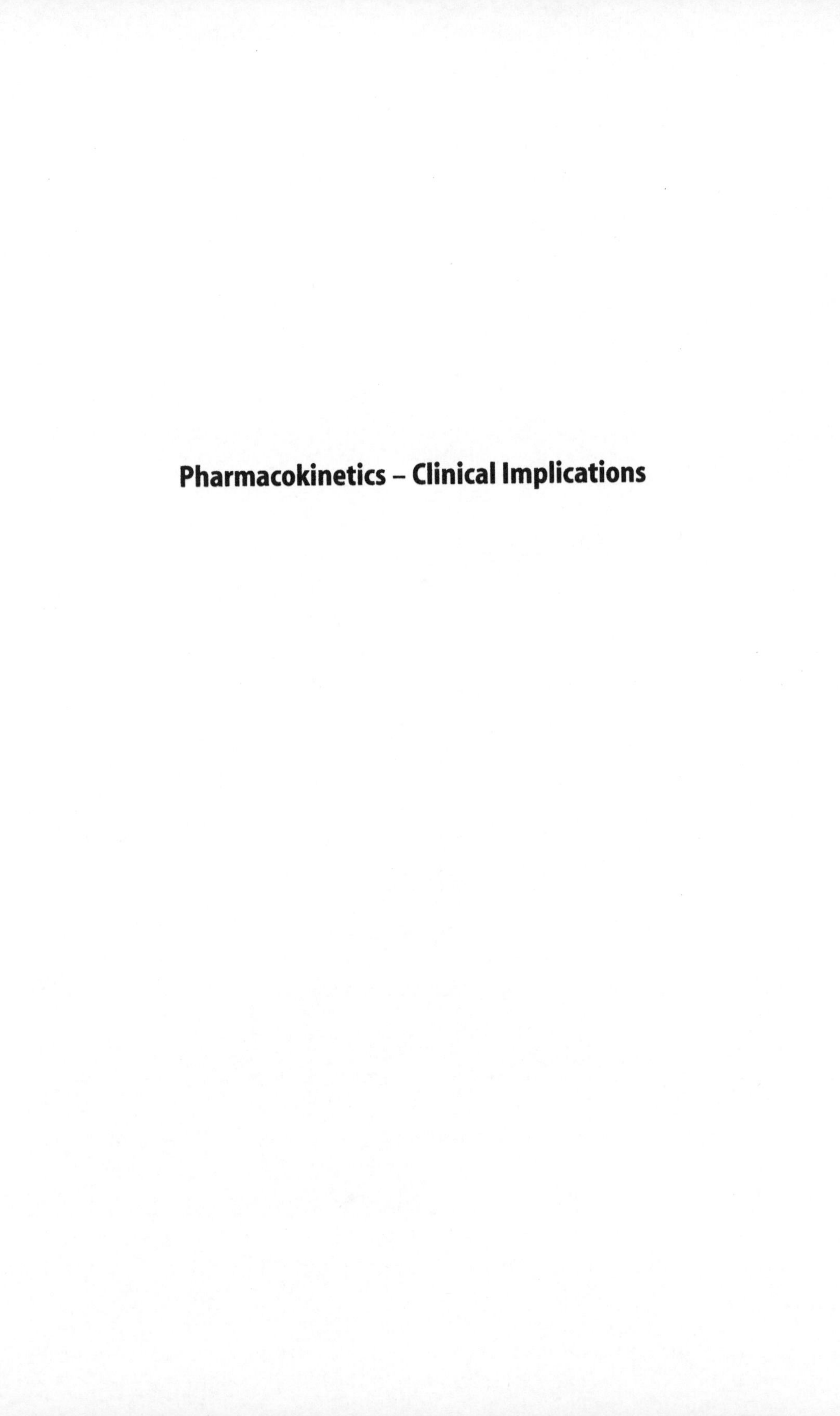

Pharmacokinetics – Clinical Implications

Acute Leukemias V
Experimental Approaches
and Management of Refractory Diseases
Hiddemann et al. (Eds.)

Fludarabine and Ara-C Combination for Treatment of Adult Acute Myelogenous Leukemia: Pharmacokinetic and Pharmacodynamic Effects

Varsha Gandhi, Min Du, Amy J. Chapman, Peng Huang, Elihu Estey, Michael J. Keating, and William Plunkett

Abstract. Based on pharmacologic, clinical, and biochemical investigations, fludarabine and arabinosylcytosine (ara-C) were combined to treat patients with acute myelogenous leukemia. Fludarabine's effect in this combination therapy was multifaceted, both on the pharmacokinetics and pharmacodynamics of ara-C triphosphate (ara-CTP) in the circulating leukemia cells. Pharmacokinetically, fludarabine infusion increased the rate of ara-CTP accumulation by a median of two-fold (P = 0.001), hence enhancing ara-CTP peak levels and the area under the concentration times time curve of ara-CTP during therapy. In addition, fludarabine infusion added fludarabine triphosphate (F-ara-ATP), a new cytotoxic metabolite, to the leukemia cells (peak, 38 % 16 μM). Pharmacodynamically, fludarabine affected DNA synthesis by perturbing deoxynucleotide pools and incorporating F-ara-ATP into the growing DNA chain. The limited data available on the deoxynucleotide pools after fludarabine infusion suggested a decrease in the dATP pool in the circulating blasts. Finally, an in vitro model system which used primer extension as an assay for DNA synthesis suggested that both ara-CTP and F-ara-ATP are recognized as substrates by polymerase a. DNA polymerase a was able to incorporate these analogs consecutively on the extending primer. When present together during DNA synthesis, these analogs, resulted in synergistic (at low concentrations) or additive (above the 10 μM level of each analog) inhibition of DNA primer elongation. These studies demonstrated that the effects of fludarabine are multifaceted on both the pharmacokinetic and pharmacodynamic aspects of the drugs actions.

Fludarabine was used in combination with arabinosylcytosine (ara-C) to treat patients with acute myelogenous leukemia (AML). The rationales for this combination therapy were obtained from several different studies. Clinical and pharmacological results obtained in patients who received ara-C as a major therapeutic agent demonstrated that the pharmacokinetics of ara-C triphosphate (ara-CTP) in leukemia blasts are directly related to response to ara-C therapy [1–3] and that the dose rate of 0.5 g/m2/h (intermediate dose) of ara-C saturates the ability of leukemia cells to accumulate ara-CTP [4–6]. Our previous biochemical experience with the combination of fludarabine and ara-C in K562 human leukemia cells [7] and in leukemic lymphocytes in vitro and ex vivo [8] provided a compelling rationale for combining fludarabine with ara-C because fludarabine as its triphosphate (F-ara-ATP) potentiated the rate of ara-CTP accumulation. Hence, the area under concentration times time curve (AUC) of ara-CTP could be enhanced in leukemia cells by infusing intermediate dose ara-C in combination with fludarabine. This postulate was tested and confirmed in several clinical studies in which these two agents were combined to treat patients with chronic lymphocytic leukemia [9,10], acute lymphocytic leukemia [11], and acute myelogenous leukemia [12–14]. In this present paper we review these data in the circulating blasts from patients with AML and focus on the multifaceted influence of fludarabine on

Department of Clinical Investigation and Hematology, The University of Texas M. D. Anderson Cancer Center, Houston, Texas

the pharmacokinetics of ara-CTP and pharmacodynamics of this combination.

Pharmacokinetic Modulation

All pharmacologic studies were done with patients who had relapsed AML and had given their informed consent to receive this combination therapy. Patients received a dose of 1.0 g/m^2 of ara-C infused over 2 h. Twenty h later, a 30-min infusion of fludarabine (30 mg/m^2), and 4 h later (24 h after the start of first ara-C dose) a second and identical dose of ara-C were infused. On each subsequent day, patients were infused with one dose of fludarabine and one dose of ara-C for the 6-day course of therapy. Pharmacokinetic studies were done during the first two days of therapy when ara-C was given alone or 4 h after fludarabine (designated as ara-C alone or fludarabine + ara-C, respectively), to permit comparison of the ara-CTP accumulation rates in the same patient. For pharmacokinetic investigations, four patients were studied on this combination protocol. The first patient was studied twice, and was designated as patient 1 during the first course and as patient 5 during his second course of therapy. Patient characteristics and their clinical response to these treatments have been published [15].

Plasma Pharmacology and Effect of Fludarabine

The ara-C dose (intermediate dose) rate (0.5 g/m^2/h) was chosen as one that would produce plasma ara-C concentrations at 10 μM or above, a level that would maximize the rate of ara-CTP accumulation in leukemia blasts. This dose rate gives values for ara-CTP AUC equal to those of high-dose ara-C rates (3 g/m^2 over 1–3 h) [4,5] which result in equal response rates, yet has less toxicity [6,16]. When ara-C was infused alone or 4 h after fludarabine, plasma ara-C levels were generally 10 μM or above (Table 1). Comparison of plasma levels at 1 and 2 h of both ara-C and its deaminated metabolite arabinosyluracil (ara U) demonstrated that mean values were similar when ara-C was given alone or 4 h after fludarabine (Table 1). These studies suggested that fludarabine infusion does not affect the plasma pharmacokinetics of ara-C or its deamination to ara-U.

Table 1. Effect of fludarabine on plasma pharmacokinetics

Nucleoside	Mean concentration ± SD, μM		P
	ara-C alone	fludarabine +ara-C*	
ara-C, 1 h	18 ± 12	20 ± 7	0.925
ara-C, 2 h	23 ± 8	26 ± 9	0.441
ara-U, 1 h	51 ± 15	55 ± 23	0.497
ara-U, 2 h	130 ± 36	112 ± 43	0.238

*ara-C infusion 4 h after fludarabine infusion
Ara-C and ara-U levels were determined at the indicated times in plasma by reverse-phase high-pressure liquid chromatography. Data are presented as mean% SD of values obtained from 5 individuals. P values were obtained by comparing values from each patient with or without fludarabine by paired two-tailed t test

Cellular Pharmacology and Effect of Fludarabine

The accumulation of ara-CTP was generally linear up to 3 h after the beginning of the ara-C infusion. Thereafter, ara-CTP was eliminated in a monophasic pattern. Using a pharmacokinetic approach, we characterized the action of fludarabine on ara-CTP concentrations by comparing the peak cellular ara-CTP, the intracellular AUC of ara-CTP, and the rates of ara-CTP accumulation and elimination during and after each ara-C infusion in five patients. The peak ara-CTP during the first dose ranged from 332 to 939 μM, whereas during the second dose of ara-C peaks were higher, ranging from 625 μM to 1386 μM. The peak ara-CTP concentration was elevated by a median of 1.7-fold after fludarabine infusion (P = < 0.001, Table 2). AUC values for ara-CTP accumulation and elimination during the first dose varied among patients between 1560 μM-h and 6930 μM-h. Similarly, during the second dose, the AUC of ara-CTP was heterogeneous among patients. Comparison of the ara-CTP AUC during the first and second doses of ara-C (Table 2) indicated a significant 1.9-fold increase during the second dose. Because the AUC is a sum of accumulation and elimination rates of ara-CTP, we determined whether the increased intracellular exposure to ara-CTP resulted from a decrease in the rate of ara-CTP elimination by comparing the half-time ($t^{1/2}$) of ara-CTP retention before and after fludarabine infusion (Table 2). These values ranged from 1.8 to 4.0 h among the 5 patients during the first

Table 2. Effect of fludarabine on cellular pharmacokinetics

	Mean values ± SD			
	ara-C alone	fludarabine+ara-C*	Ratio#	P
Peak ara-CTP, μM	568 ± 224	965 ± 281	1.7	<0.001
AUC ara-CTP, μM-h	3284 ± 2162	5736 ± 3023	1.9	0.004
ara-CTP elimination rate, t1/2 h	2.8 ± 1.0	3.0 ± 0.9	1.1	0.426
ara-CTP accumulation rate μM/h	230 ± 62	463 ± 19	2.0	0.001
Peak F-ara-ATP, μM	-	38 ± 16	-	

*ara-C infusion 4 h after fludarabine infusion
#mean fludarabine + ara-C values
mean ara-C alone values
Intracellular levels of ara-CTP were determined in circulating AML blasts by highpressure liquid chromatography. Data are presented as mean % SD of values obtained from 5 individuals. *P* values were obtained by comparing values from each patient with or without fludarabine by paired two-tailed *t* test

course of ara-C and from 2.0 to 4.3 h during the second course (Table 2), with a ratio of 1.1, indicating that fludarabine infusion did not affect the rate of ara-CTP elimination (P = 0.426). The last parameter, the rates of ara-CTP accumulation before and after fludarabine infusion (Table 2) demonstrated a significant increase during the second ara-C infusion (P = 0.001). The mean increase following fludarabine infusion was twofold. Taken together, these results demonstrated that the increase in ara-CTP AUC was caused by a higher rate of anabolism of ara-C rather than by a slower rate of catabolism of ara-CTP. Finally, combining fludarabine with ara-C added a new cytotoxic metabolite, F-ara-ATP. The F-ara-ATP peak occurred 4 h after the start of fludarabine infusion (24 h after the start of therapy). The mean F-ara-ATP peak level was 38 μM, with a range among these patients between 20 and 60 μM. Even the lowest peak level was sufficient to modulate ara-C, which was infused at this time. Unlike ara-CTP, F-ara-ATP was eliminated at a slower rate ($t^{1/2}$, 5–10 h). With these pharmacological characteristics, leukemia cells retain both ara-CTP and F-ara-ATP for a long time after infusion of each drug to affect cytotoxicity.

Pharmacodynamic Modulation

Effect of fludarabine on deoxynucleotides. Because F-ara-ATP inhibits ribonucleotide reductase [17–19], the sole enzyme responsible for the de novo pathway for maintaining deoxynucleotides [20], the deoxynucleotide (dNTP) pools are expected to be affected by fludarabine infusion [7]. Furthermore, leukemia blasts accumulated F-ara-ATP to levels (15–60 μM) sufficient to inhibit this important enzyme: $IC_{50} = 1$ μM for ADP reduction and $IC_{50} = 9$ μM for CDP reduction [17]. To compare the effect of fludarabine infusion on the dNTP pool in circulating leukemia blasts before and after fludarabine infusion, the blasts were isolated before therapy and 4 h after fludarabine infusion. Nucleotides were extracted by methanol, and dNTPs were quantitated as described [21]. The data from three patients (Table 3) indicated that the dATP

Table 3. Effect of fludarabine on deoxynucleotide pools

	Deoxynucleotides, μM				
Patient	Time	dATP	dCTP	dGTP	dTTP
1	#before	9.6	5.5	2.4	1.6
	#after	5.2	4.2	3.7	5.7
2	before	12.4	ND*	12.2	2.4
	after	9.9	1.6	2.9	3.2
3	before	7.3	2.8	10.4	4.0
	after	5.1	3.3	1.4	5.5

* Below limit of detection
\# Before, before fludarabine infusion; after, 4 h after fludarabine infusion
Leukemia blasts were isolated from peripheral blood obtained from patients before and 4 h after fludarabine infusion. Intracellular levels of dNTP were measured as described in the text

pool was consistently lowered after fludarabine infusion. This is in keeping with the data from K562 cells [7] and the fact that the IC_{50} for ADP reduction was quite low [17]. There was minimal or no effect on dCTP and dGTP pools, and the dTTP pool was increased.

The effect on dNTPs result in a two-pronged potentiation. First, because the activity of deoxycytidine kinase is regulated by deoxynucleotides, lowering of dNTPs activates this enzyme [7]. Ara-C is phosphorylated by deoxycytidine kinase and this potentiates ara-CTP accumulation. The second action is targeted toward DNA synthesis. F-ara-ATP competes with dATP, and ara-CTP competes with dCTP for incorporation into DNA. The lowered dNTP pool enhances incorporation of ara-nucleotides [22–24].

Effect of fludarabine on DNA synthesis. The principal mechanism by which these analog triphosphates exert cytotoxicity is by incorporation into DNA and inhibition of DNA synthesis [22–27]. To determine the combined effect of these two ara-nucleotides on the DNA synthesizing machinery, an in vitro model system of DNA primer extension assay was employed. A DNA primer was elongated by DNA polymerase α purified from human leukemia cells over a synthetic template as shown in Figure 1. A 17-nucleotide primer labeled at the 5'-end with ^{32}P was annealed to a defined-sequence template of 31 nucleotides in length. With this custom sequence of the template, DNA polymerase a gets a "running start" [28] of 6 nucleotides by incorporating dGTP and dTTP until it comes to the critical sites. At these sites, F-ara-ATP or dATP and ara-CTP or dCTP would be incorporated in specified sequence. Polymerase α then completes the elongation by adding 6 more nucleotides. The elongation of the radiolabeled primer to the final product, near the end of the template, was analyzed on a DNA sequencing gel. A profile of a gel using this assay is shown in Figure 2.

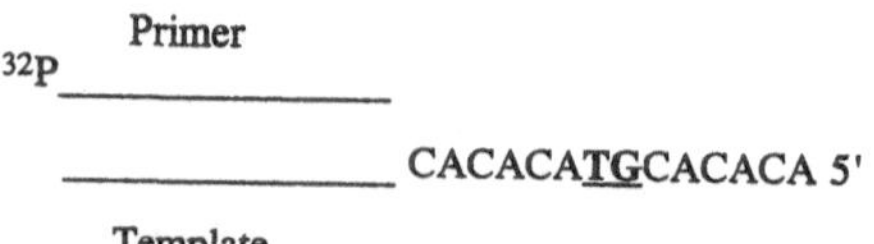

Fig. 1. Template-primer complex used as an in vitro model system to study DNA elongation. Sites on the template designated as critical sites are underlined and bold

As is apparent in the control reaction in the first lane of Figure 2, the primer was elongated by polymerase a to a final product when all 4 deoxynucleotides were present at 5 μM. This was the lowest concentration of deoxynucleotides that supported linear kinetics of the uninhibited reaction. Addition of either F- ara-ATP or ara-CTP in lanes 2 or 3, resulted in termination of DNA primer elongation at the A or C site, consequently decreasing the radioactivity in the final product. Addition of both arabinosylnucleotides resulted in bands at both A and C positions and a major reduction in the final product. The radioactivity in the product in each lane was quantitated by a betascope and was expressed as a percentage of the radioactivity in the control reaction (Table 4). When ara-CTP was used alone, there was a dose dependent increase in the inhibition of DNA elongation. When F-ara-ATP was used at 10 μM, primer extension was inhibited by 37 percent. The combination of a fixed concentration of 10 μM F-ara-ATP with ara-CTP at increasing concentrations indicated

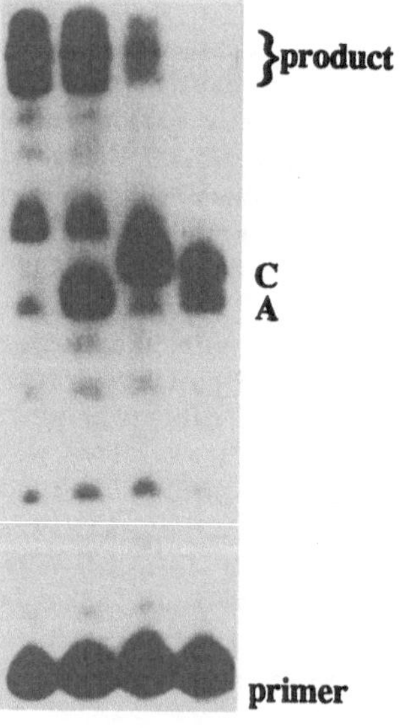

Fig. 2. Incorporation of single analog versus two analog molecules in DNA primer by DNA polymerase a. Lane 1 is a complete reaction containing 5 μM of dNTPs. Lane 2 is the same as lane 1 but with 10 μM F-ara-ATP. Lane 3 is the same as lane 1 but with 10 μM ara-CTP. Lane 4 contains both F-ara-ATP (10 μM) and ara-CTP (10 μM) in addition to 5 μM dNTPs

a greater decrease in primer extension compared to that of a single drug. The expected percentage inhibition values from these combinations, tabulated in the last column of Table 4, are the product of inhibition by F-ara-ATP at 10 µlM and of ara-CTP alone at the indicated concentrations. A comparison of the observed values with those expected suggested that, at 1 and 3 µM ara-CTP the combination of ara-CTP and F-ara-ATP resulted in greater than additive inhibition. At higher concentrations, however, the result was additive. Similar results were obtained when the F-ara-ATP concentration was varied and ara-CTP was kept constant at 3 µM.

To further determine the consequences of incorporating these analogs alone or in combination, we deleted the competing deoxynucleotide from the reaction mixture, thus forcing the polymerase to incorporate an arabinosyl nucleotide. A single analog incorporation resulted in 89% to 95% inhibition of DNA synthesis, whereas incorporation of both in sequence inhibited DNA primer extension by 99%. These results demonstrated that both F-ara-ATP and ara-CTP can incorporate in tandem, and that incorporation of two arabinosyl nucleotides results in greater inhibition of DNA elongation than when a single analog was incorporated.

Additional effects of fludarabine. Both fludarabine and ara-C infusions have been shown to block cells in S-phase [29,30]. Because both drugs are S-phase-specific, alternate infusion of these analogs could selectively affect the partially synchronized population of leukemia blasts, when it proceeds into S-phase after the first drug. Finally, fludarabine is recognized as an effective agent for indolent leukemia and lymphomas in which a majority of cells are quiescent [31,32]. One can postulate that, aside from its effect on actively dividing cells, fludarabine may affect the AML cell population that is quiescent [33]. This may prove synergistic, because ara-C is active primarily in cycling cells.

Conclusion

Fludarabine, when combined with the ara-C therapy, affects both the pharmacokinetics of ara-CTP and the pharmacodynamics of drugs actions. The pharmacokinetic aspect brings on a new metabolite, F-ara-ATP, in the cells. Accumulation of F-ara-ATP decreases dNTP pools in leukemia cells and thus enhances deoxycytidine kinase activity. This results in increased rate of ara-C phosphorylation resulting in a higher peak of ara-CTP. The rate of ara-CTP elimination, however, remains similar to that of ara-C given alone, hence it stays longer in the circulating cells. When both metabolites are at less than 10 µM, they may work together and synergistically to maintain the inhibition of DNA synthesis. The lowered dATP or dCTP pool may, in addition, enhance the incorporation of these antimetabolites into growing DNA. Taken together, these multifaceted effects may prolong

Table 4. Inhibition of DNA primer extension by ara-CTP and ara-CTP with F-ara-ATP

	Percentage of Inhibition, mean % SD ara-CTP with		
ara-CTP, µM	only ara-CTP	10 µM F-ara-ATP	expected
0	0%0	37%6	37
1	19%10	69%6	49
3	29%18	69%10	55
10	74%3	87%4	84
30	89%2	88%1	93
60	90%4	94%2	93

The reaction mixture contained 5 µM of all four dNTPs without any ara-NTP (control) or with ara-CTP at different concentrations with or without 10 µM F-ara-ATP. The expected value is a product of values with F-ara-ATP at 10 µM and ara-CTP at the respective concentrations. DNA primer extension was measured as described under experimental procedures. The values are mean % SD from 3 to 7 different gels

the duration of inhibition of DNA synthesis and hence cytotoxicity.

Acknowledgements. Research from the authors' laboratory was supported in part by grants CA28596, CA32839, CA55164, and CA57629 from the National Cancer Institute, DHHS, and grant DHP-1 from the American Cancer Society.

References

1. Plunkett W, Iacoboni S, Estey E, Danhauser L, Liliemark JO, Keating MJ (1985) Pharmacologically directed ara-C therapy for refractory leukemia. Semin Oncol 12 (suppl): 20–30
2. Kantarjian HM, Estey EH, Plunkett W, Keating MJ, Walters RS, Iacoboni S, McCredie KB, Freireich EJ (1986) Phase I-II clinical and pharmacologic studies of high-dose cytosine arabinoside in refractory leukemia. Am J Med 81: 387–394
3. Estey E, Plunkett W, Dixon DO, Keating MJ, McCredie KB, Freireich EJ (1987) Variables predicting response to high dose cytosine arabinoside therapy with refractory acute leukemia. Leukemia 1: 580–583
4. Plunkett W, Liliemark JO, Adams TM, Nowak B, Estey E, Kantarjian H, Keating MJ (1987) Saturation of 1-b-D-arabinosylcytosine 5'-triphosphate accumulation in leukemia cells during high-dose 1-b-D-arabinosylcytosine therapy. Cancer Res 47: 3005–3011
5. Plunkett W, Liliemark JO, Estey E, Keating MJ (1987) Saturation of ara-CTP accumulation during high-dose ara-C therapy: Pharmacologic rationale for intermediate-dose ara-C. Semin Oncol 14: (suppl 1): 159–166
6. Estey EH, Plunkett W, Kantarjian H, Rios MB, Keating MJ (1993) Treatment of relapsed or refractory AML with intermediate-dose arabinosylcytosine (ara-C): Confirmation of the importance of ara-C triphosphate formation in mediating response to ara-C. Leukemia Lymphoma 10 (suppl) 115–121.
7. Gandhi V, Plunkett W (1988) Modulation of arabinosylnucleoside metabolism by arabinosylnucleotides in human leukemia cells. Cancer Res 48: 329–334
8. Gandhi V, Nowak B, Keating MJ, Plunkett W (1989) Modulation of arabinosylcytosine metabolism by arabinosyl-2-fluoroadenine in lymphocytes from patients with chronic lymphocytic leukemia: Implications for combination therapy. Blood 74: 2070–2075
9. Gandhi V, Kemena A, Keating MJ, Plunkett W (1992) Fludarabine infusion potentiates arabinosylcytosine metabolism in lymphocytes of patients with chronic lymphocytic leukemia. Cancer Res 52: 897–903
10. Gandhi V, Robertson LE, Keating MJ, Plunkett W (1994) Combination of fludarabine and arabinosylcytosine for treatment of chronic lymphocytic leukemia: Clinical efficacy and modulation of arabinosylcytosine pharmacology. Cancer Chemother Pharmacol (in press)
11. Suki S, Kantarjian H, Gandhi V, Estey E, O'Brien S, Beran M, Rios MB, Plunkett W, Keating M (1993) Fludarabine and cytosine arabinoside in the treatment of refractory or relapsed acute lymphocytic leukemia. Cancer 72: 2155–2160
12. Gandhi V, Estey E, Keating MJ, Plunkett W (1993) Fludarabine potentiates metabolism of cytarabine in patients with acute myelogenous leukemia during therapy. J Clin Oncol 11: 116–124
13. Gandhi V, Estey E, Keating MJ, Plunkett W (1993) Biochemical modulation of arabinosylcytosine for therapy of leukemias. Leukemia Lymphoma 10 (suppl): 109–114
14. Gandhi V (1993) Fludarabine for treatment of adult acute myelogenous leukemia. Leukemia Lymphoma 11 (suppl 2): 7–13
15. Estey E, Plunkett W, Gandhi V, Rios MB, Kantarjian H, Keating MJ (1993) Fludarabine and arabinosylcytosine therapy of refractory and relapsed acute myelogenous leukemia. Leukemia Lymphoma 9: 343–350
16. Hiddemann W (1991) Cytosine arabinoside in the treatment of acute myeloid leukemia: The role and place of high-dose regimens. Annals of Hematology 62: 119–128
17. Tseng W-C, Derse D, Cheng Y-C, Brockman RW, Bennett LL Jr (1982) In vitro biological activity of 9-b-D-arabinofuranosyl-2-fluoroadenine and the biochemical actions of its triphosphate on DNA polymerases and ribonucleotide reductase from HeLa cells. Mol Pharmacol 21: 474–477
18. White EL, Shaddix SD, Brockman RW, Bennett LL Jr (1982) Comparison of the action of 9-b-D-arabinofuranosyl-2-fluoroadenine on target enzymes from mouse tumor cells. Cancer Res 42:2260–2264
19. Parker WB, Shaddix SC, Chang C-H, White EL, Rose LM, Brockman RW, Shortnacy AT, Montgomery JA, Secrist III JA, Bennett LL (Jr) (1991) Effects of 2-chloro-9-(2-deoxy-2-fluoro-b-D-arabinofuranosyl)adenine on K562 cellular metabolism and the inhibition of human ribonucleotide reductase and DNA polymerase by its 5'-triphosphate. Cancer Res 51: 2386–2394
20. Reichard P (1988) Interactions between deoxyribonucleotides and DNA synthesis. Ann Rev Biochem 57: 349–374
21. Sherman PA, Fyfe JA (1989) Enzymatic assay for deoxynucleoside triphosphates using synthetic oligonucleotides as template primers. Anal Biochem 180: 222–226
22. Major PP, Egan EM, Beardsley GP, Minden MD, Kufe DW (1981) Lethality of human myeloblasts correlated with the incorporation of arabinofuranosylcytosine into DNA. Proc Nat Acad Sci USA 78: 3235–3239
23. Townsend AJ, Cheng Y-C (1987) Sequence specific effects of ara-5-aza-CTP and ara-CTP on DNA synthesis by purified human DNA polymerases in vitro: Visualization of chain elongation on a defined template. Mol Pharmacol 32: 330–339

24. Huang P, Chubb S, Plunkett W (1990) Termination of DNA synthesis by 9-b-D-arabinofuranosyl-2-fluoroadenine: A mechanism for cytotoxicity. J Biol Chem 265: 16617–16625
25. Ohno Y, Spriggs D, Matsukage A, Ohno T, Kufe D (1988) Effects of 1-b-D-arabinofuranosylcytosine incorporation on elongation of specific DNA polymerases, DNA primase, and ribonucleotide reductase. Mol Pharmacol 34: 485–491
26. Spriggs D, Robbins G, Mitchell T, Kufe D (1986) Incorporation of 9-b-D-arabinofuranosyl-2-fluoroadenine into HL-60 cellular RNA and DNA. Biochem Pharmacol 35: 247–252
27. Parker WB, Bapat AR, Shen J-X, Townsend AJ, Cheng Y-C (1988) Interaction of 2-halogenated dATP analogs (F, Cl, and Br) with human DNA polymerases, DNA primase, and ribonucleotide reductase. Mol Pharmacol 34: 485–491
28. Goodman MF, Creighton S, Bloom LB, Petruska J (1993) Biochemical basis of DNA replication fidelity. Crit Rev Biochem Mol Biol 28: 83–126
29. Smets LA, Homan BJ (1985) S1-phase cells of the leukemia cell cycle sensitive to 1-b-D-arabinofuranosylcytosine at a high-dose level. Cancer Res 45: 3113–3117
30. Dow LW, Bell DE, Poulakos L, Fridland A (1980) Differences in metabolism and cytotoxicity between 9-b-D-arabinofuranosyladenine and 9-b-D-arabinofuranosyl-2-fluoroadenine in human leukemic lymphoblasts. Cancer Res 40: 1405–1410
31. Keating MJ, Kantarjian H, O'Brien S, Koller C, Talpaz M, Schachner J, Childs CC, Freireich EJ, McCredie KB (1991) Fludarabine: A new agent with marked cytoreductive activity in untreated chronic lymphocytic leukemia. J Clin Oncol 9: 44–49
32. Hochster HS, Kim K, Green MD, Mann RB, Meiman RS, Oken MM, Cassileth PA, Statt P, Ritch P, O'Connell MJ (1992) Activity of fludarabine in previously treated non-Hodgkin's low-grade lymphoma: Results of an Eastern Cooperative Oncology Group study. J Clin Oncol 10: 28–32
33. Andreeff M (1986) Cell kinetics of leukemia. Semin Oncol 23: 300–314

Acute Leukemias V
Experimental Approaches
and Management of Refractory Diseases
Hiddemann et al. (Eds.)

Pharmacokinetics of Ara-CMP-Stearate (YNK01) – Phase I Study of the Oral Ara-C Derivative

Jan Braess[1], Eberhard Schleyer[1], Bernhard Ramsauer[1], Michael Unterhalt[1], Cornelia Kaufmann[1], Sabine Wilde[1], Martin Schüssller[2], and Wolfgang Hiddemann[1]

Abstract. Ara-CMP-Stearate (1-beta-D-Arabinofuranosylcytosine-5'-stearylphosphate, YNK 01, Fosteabine) is an the orally applicable prodrug of cytosine-arabinoside (Ara-C). During a recently started phase-I study in patients with advanced low-grade non-Hodgkin lymphomas or acute myeloid leukemia the pharmacokinetic parameters of Ara-CMP-Stearate (kindly provided by ASTA Medica, Frankfurt, FRG) were determined by HPLC analysis. 72 hours after a first starting dose which served for the determination of baseline pharmacokinetic parameters, Ara-CMP-Srearate was administered over 14 days by once daily oral application. Ara-CMP-Stearate was started at a dose of 100 mg/d and was escalated in subsequent patients to 200 mg/d, 300 mg/d and 600 mg/d. Plasma and urine concentratiions of Ara-CMP-Stearate, Ara-C and Ara-U were measured during the initial treatment phase and within 72 hours after the end of the 14 day treatment cycle. So far six patients have been treated with 100 mg/d, three with 200 mg/d and another six with 300mg/d. One patient was treated consecutively with 100 mg, 300 mg and 600 mg. Fitting the results of the plasma concentration measurements of Ara-CMP-Stearate to a one compartment model, the following pharmacokinetic parameters were obtained (average and variation coefficient VC). Ara-CMP-Stearate dose independent parameters: Lag time = 1.04 h (0.57), $t_{max=}$5.72 h (0.30), $t_{1/2}$ = 9.4 h (0.36). Dose dependent parameters: at 100 mg : AUC = 1099 ng·ml/h (0.31), concentration$_{max}$ = 53.8 ng/ml (0.28), at 200 mg: AUC = 2753 ng·h/ml (0.32), concentration$_{max}$ = 154.8 ng/ml (0.46), at 300 mg: AUC = 2940 ng·h/ml (0.66), concentration $_{max}$ = 160.0 ng/ml (0.59). The long lag time and late$_{max}$ can be explained by resorption in the distal part of the small intestine. No Ara-CMP-Stearate was detected in urine samples (limit of detection = 500pg/ml). Pharmacokinetcic parameters of ARA-C following Ara-CMP-Stearate application showed the following characteristics: $t_{1/2}$ = 24.3 h (0.39), AUC (100mg) = 262 ng·h/ml (0.93), AUC (200mg) = 502 ng·h/ml (0.87), AUC (300mg) = 898 ng·h/ml (1.07). Since Ara-CMP-Stearate causes intravascular hemolysis after i.v. administration, it was not possible to determine its bioavailability by comparing the AUC after oral and i.v. application. Instead, the renal elimination of ARA-U, as the main metabolite of ARA-C was measured during the first 72 h period and after the last application. This approach allowed to estimate that an average of 15.8% of Ara-CMP-Stearate (VC 0.82) had undergone resorption and final metabolism to ARA-U. The observed half lifes for ARA-C($t_{1/2}$ = 24,4h, VC = 0,39) and Ara-U ($t_{1/2}$ = 22,0 h, VC = 0,35) after Ara-CMP-Stearate administration were substantially longer than those after intravenous application of Ara-C suggesting a prolonged release of Ara-C from the prodrug due to a slow hepatic metabolism of Ara-CMP-Stearate. These data show that Ara-CMP-Stearate is able to maintain prolonged ARA-C plasma levels and suggest that ARA-C concentrations as in low dose and probably in standard dose ARA-C therapy can be achieved by oral application of Ara-CMP-Stearate.

[1]Department of Internal Medicine, Division Hematology and Oncology, University of Göttingen, Germany
[2]ASTA Medica, Frankfurt/M, Germany

Introduction

Because of its rapid deamination by cytidine deaminase the plasma half-live of Ara-C is short and is in the range of t1/2 10–40 min minutes, only [9,10]. Therefore, continous intravenous infusion or repeated s.c. injections are required to maintain prolonged cytotoxic drug levels. In an attempt to overcome this limitation and to develop an orally applicable compound a series of lipophilic Ara-C analogues were synthesized [11] in the early 1980. Among these substances 1-beta-D-arabinofuranosylcytosine-5'-stearyl-phosphate (Fosteabine, YNK01, Ara- CMP-Stearate) revealed the highest antileukemic activity in in vitro and animal models [12]. Ara-CMP-Stearate is metabolized by the liver and is converted to ara-C at a low rate [13, 14]. Hence, Ara-C is released into the circulation over a prolonged period of time. Ara-CMP-Stearate may therefore not only provide a more convenient way of drug application through the oral route but may also allow to maintain long-lasting Ara-C plasma levels by its slow and prolonged hepatic conversion. These perspectives and their clinical relevance need to be substantiated in controlled studies. In addition, more information is needed about the pharmacokinetics of Ara-CMP-Stearate and about potential interindividual differences in uptake and metabolism between individual patients. These questions were addressed by the current investigation as part of a clinical phase I study in patients with advanced low-grade lymphomas and acute myeloid leukemia.

Patients

The current study was open for patients suffering from advanced low grade non-Hodgkin-lymphomas or end stage acute myeloid leukemia. Six patients were treated with 100mg/day, three with 200mg/day and another six with 300mg/day. One patient was treated consecutively with 100mg/day, 300mg/day and 600mg/day in order to estimate intraindividual differences during dose-escalation. Patients with WHO grade 3 or better, Age > 18 years, normal liver and kidney function were admitted into the study. All patients provided their written informed consent after having been informed about the investigational nature of the current evaluation.

Treatment

Each course consisted of a single test dose followed three days later by a once daily oral administration of Ara-CMP-Stearate over 14 days. Ara-CMP-Stearate was applied as capsules of 100mg. A dose escalation was carried out in consecutive patients comprizing 100 mg/d, 200 mg/d, 300 mg/d and 600 mg/d after treatment of at least 3 patient at each dose level with tolerable toxicity. Prior to its initiation the study was approved by the local ethic commitee. It is also in accordance with the Helsinki declaration.

Pharmacokinetic Analysis

Blood samples were taken before the first application of the drug and at 1 h, 2 h, 4 h, 6 h, 8 h, 12 h, 16 h, 20 h, 24 h, 28 h, 32 h, 48 h, 62 h and 76 h after the initial test dose and after the last dose of the 14 days regimen in order to establish the half-lifes of Ara-CMP-Stearate, Ara-C and Ara-U. In addition, seven samples were taken on every second day in order to estimate the development of a pseudo steady state trough level of all three substances. Urine was collected during the first 72 hours and after the last dose of the 14 days regimen in order to determine the renal excretion of all three substances. On this basis the metabolic bioavailability of Ara-CMP-Stearate could be estimated by the proportion that is absorbed after oral application and metabolized to Ara-C or Ara-U of which more than 95% is excreted through the kidneys. This approach was chosen since a standard cross-over evaluation of drug concentrations after intravenous and oral administration was not possible due to the induction of hemolysis after intravenous application of Ara-CMP-Stearate. Blood samples were collected in heparinized vacutainers to which 250 µg of tetrahydrouridine (THU), was added for the inhibition of cytidine deaminase. The specimens were immediately centrifuged, plasma was removed and instantly frozen at −20 °C until analysis. Urine specimens were similary prepared. After measuring the total urine volume and stirring thoroughly an aliquot of 50 ml was obtained and frozen at −20 °C.

Plasma and urine concentrations of Ara-CMP-Stearate were determined by HPLC analysis [15]. In brief, this highly sensitive assay involves ion-pairing on a reversed-phase C_6H_5

phenyl column with a mobile phase of 50% acetonitril and 50% 0.04 M sodium phosphate buffer for isocratic elution. In order to reach a low limit of quantification in the range of 5 ng/ml (variation coefficient 6.8%) and of 500 pg/ml (variation coefficient 7.3) for plasma and urine respectively enrichment on C18 enrichment cartridges was performed prior to elution onto the analytical column. Prior to analysis sample clean-up was performed using tubes filled with C18 material. Signal detection was performed by an ultraviolet detector at 275 nm. Recovery following sample preparation was between 52–64%.

Ara-U concentrations were determined by a HPLC assay with a limit of detection of 20 ng/ml and 0.5 µg/ml for plasma and urine respectively. A 3µ C_{18} reversed phase column and a 5µ SA cation exchange column were used with 0.1 M sodium phosphate buffer as the mobile phase. Before the separation on the analytical columns, samples were eluted onto C_{18} cartridges for cleansing. Plasma samples were prepared by precipitation of proteins using $HClO_4$ and speed-vac drying of the supernatant.

Ara-C analaysis had to be performed by using a radio-immuno-assay first described by Enomoto et al. [16] in order to reach a sufficiently low limit of detection. Conditions were slightly changed in order to facilitate sample preparation by precipitating plasma samples with a low volume of acetonitril and speed-drying the supernatant. The limit of detection was 100 pg/ml and 1 ng/ml for plasma and urine respectively. The intra assay variation coefficient is 18% at the detection limit.

All data were analyzed by using the TOPFIT pharmacokinetic computer program which allows an optimized adaptation of variation coefficients between the observed and calculated data, respective [17]. The data of all three substances were fitted to a linear one compartment model as described by the extended Batemann equation. This equation originally describes a first order pharmacokinetic model following a single application of a drug that is in turn resorbed according to first order kinetics. It can be extended by adding cumulation factors to include multiple drug applications :

$$C_{pn} = [(f{\cdot}D{\cdot}k_a)/Vd{\cdot}(k_a - k_e))]{\cdot}[r_e{\cdot}e^{-ket} - r_a{\cdot}e^{-kat}]$$

where Cp = concentration at a given time point, n,re,ra = specific cumulation factors, D = given dose, f = percentage of dose absorbed, Vd = volume of distribution, ka = time constant of absorption, ke = time constant of elimination, t = time following last application. The plasma decay curve of Ara-CMP-Stearate, Ara-C and Ara-U and the cumulative renal elimination of the latter two substances were determined independently assuming a first order rate constant of conversion of Ara-CMP-Stearate to Ara-C.

Results

Pharmacokinetic analyses were performed in 16 patients during 18 cycles of Ara-CMP-Stearate therapy. In order to facilitate comparative evaluations drug doses were assessed on the basis of calculated square meter concentrations rather than on the absolute levels that were clinically administered. Tables 1–3 depict the pharmaco-

Table 1. Pharmacokinetic parameters of Ara-CMP-Stearate at three dose levels

Ara-CMP-Stearate dose	$t_{1/2}$ in h	AUC in ng.h/ml	$\text{concentration}_{max}$ in ng/ml	time of $\text{concentration}_{max}$ in h
average	11.9	1099	53.8	5.08
VC	0.27	0.31	0.28	0.41
(calculated for 50 mg/m²)				
average	7.2	2753	154.8	6.91
VC	0.17	0.32	0.46	0.33
(calculated for 100 mg/m²)				
average	9.1	2940	160.0	5.54
VC	0.34	0.66	0.59	0.24
(calculated for 150 mg/m²)				
average (total)	9.4	–	–	5.72
VC	0.36			0.30

Table 2. Pharmacokinetic parameters of Ara-C at three dose levels of Ara-CMP-Stearate

Ara-CMP-Stearate dose	$t_{1/2}$ in h	AUC in ng·h/ml	$concentration_{max}$ in ng/ml in h	time of $concentration_{max}$ in h	$elimination_{renal}$ in % of dose	$clearance_{renal}$ in ml/min
average	21.9	268	9.1	8.2	1.2	41.2
VC	0.38	0.89	1.16	0.50	0.91	0.62
(calculated for 50 mg/m²)						
average	21.8	502	6.7	30.6	0.6	30.9
VC	0.31	0.87	0.38	0.31	0.51	1.20
(calculated for 100 mg/m²)						
average	26.1	898	16.7	25.5	0.6	23.9
VC	0.47	1.07	1.29	0.55	0.85	1.49
(calculated for 150 mg/m²)						
average (total)	24.4	-	-	22.7	0.8	30.5
VC	0.39			0.67	0.98	1.00

Table 3. Pharmacokinetic parameters of Ara-U at three dose levels of Ara-CMP-Stearate

Ara-CMP-Stearate dose	$t_{1/2}$ in h	AUC in ng·h/ml	$concentration_{max}$ in ng/ml	time of $concentration_{max}$ in h	$clearance_{renal}$ in ml/min	renal elimination in % of dose
average	18.2	1800	31.7	24.1	89.3	21.3
VC	0.33	0.84	0.31	0.41	0.41	0.92
(calculated for 50 mg/m²)						
average	25.1	3197	78.2	15.3	94.1	20.1
VC	0.43	0.93	1.08	0.45	0.25	0.70
(calculated for 100 mg/m²)						
average	25.3	3460	71.9	13.5	72.2	9.2
VC	0.27	0.58	0.76	0.57	0.52	0.21
(calculated for 150 mg/m²)						
average (total)	22.0	-	-	18.5	84.4	15.8
VC	0.35			0.49	0.39	0.88

kinetic parameters of Ara-CMP-Stearate (Table 1), Ara-C (Table 2) and Ara-U (Table 3) after application of 50 mg/m², 100 mg/m² and 150 mg/m² Ara-CMP-Stearate calculated from the 0 h to 475 h blood and 0 to 76 h urine sample period, respectively. Lag-time and metabolic bioavailability of the mother drug and half-lifes and clearances of all three substances were shown to be dose independent parameters at the applied doses and are illustrated in Figure 1. Using a complex user defined compartment model this figure shows the pharmacokinetics of one typical case after the application of 150 mg/m² Ara-CMP-Stearate. As in all other patients optimum results with variation coefficients > 0.90. were obtained when fitting the experimental data to a linear one compartment model. Figures 2 and 3 show the plasma concentrations of Ara-CMP-Stearate and Ara-C at the 300 mg dose level. Absorption of the mother drug was rather slow resulting in a late t_{max} of approximately 6 hours. Similarly, Ara-CMP-Stearate is first detected in the plasma after a lag-time of 1.16 hours. Ara-C and Ara-U reach maximum concentrations after approximately 20 hours and are excreted into the urine with a half-life of 24.4 hours and 22.0 hours respectively.

Plasma AUCs are dose dependent parameters and show a linear increase with higher doses of Ara-CMP-Stearate (Tables 1–3). Until the 300 mg/day dose level no signs of any decreased resorption of Ara-CMP-Stearate could be detect-

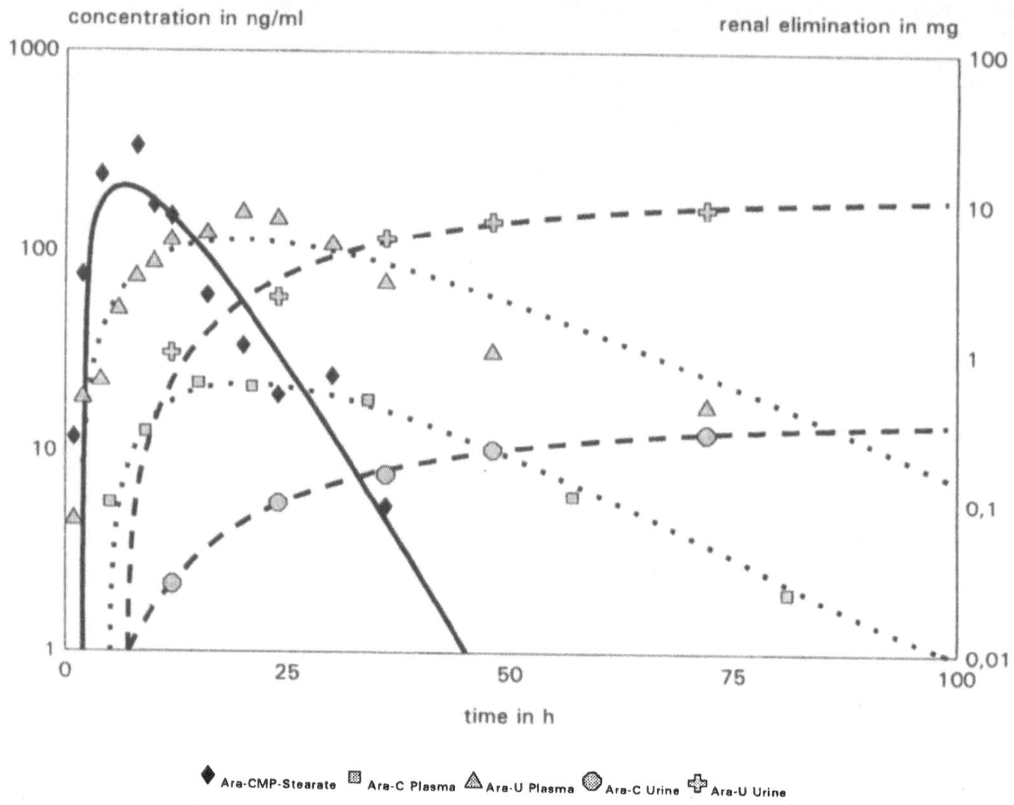

Fig. 1. Pharmakokinetics of Ara-CMP-Stearate, Ara-C and Ara-U following application of 300 mg Ara-CMP-Stearate

ed. Instead the plasma AUCs rose from an average of 1099 ng·h/ml in the 100 mg/day dose group to 2753 ng·h/ml in the 200 mg/day dose group and to 2940 ng·h/ml in the 300 mg/day dose group. A linear relation between oral drug dose and plasma AUC is also revealed by the results of a single patient receiving consecutively 100 mg/day (AUC = 646 ng·h/ml), 300 mg/day (AUC = 1690 ng·h/ml) and 600mg/day (AUC = 4635 ng·h/ml). A comparison of results between different patients indicates distinct interindividual differences in the absorption and in the subsequent metabolism of Ara-CMP-Stearate. This is demonstrated by the coefficients of variation for the AUCs of Ara-CMP Stearate, Ara-C and Ara-U (Table 1, 2, 3). When comparing the variation coefficients of renal excretion of Ara-C and of Ara-U which lie between 0.62 and 1.49 and between 0.21 and 0.92 respectively, variability in Ara-C metabolism seems to be slightly higher than in the case of Ara-U which is consistent with the results on plasma AUC variability.

Ara-CMP-Stearate, Ara-C and Ara-U plasma levels that are obtained after the application of 300 mg/d represent the formation and maintenance of a pseudo steady-state level (Fig. 2). These figure also show that there is no accumulation of either Ara-CMP-Stearate, Ara-C or Ara-U but that long lasting plasma levels of Ara-C and Ara-U are maintained as result from their long half-lifes.

Discussion

After the demonstration of a significant antileukemic activity of Ara-CMP-Stearate in experimental systems and patients with secondary leukemias and myelodysplastic syndroms [22,23], the current study provides for the first time more extensive information about the

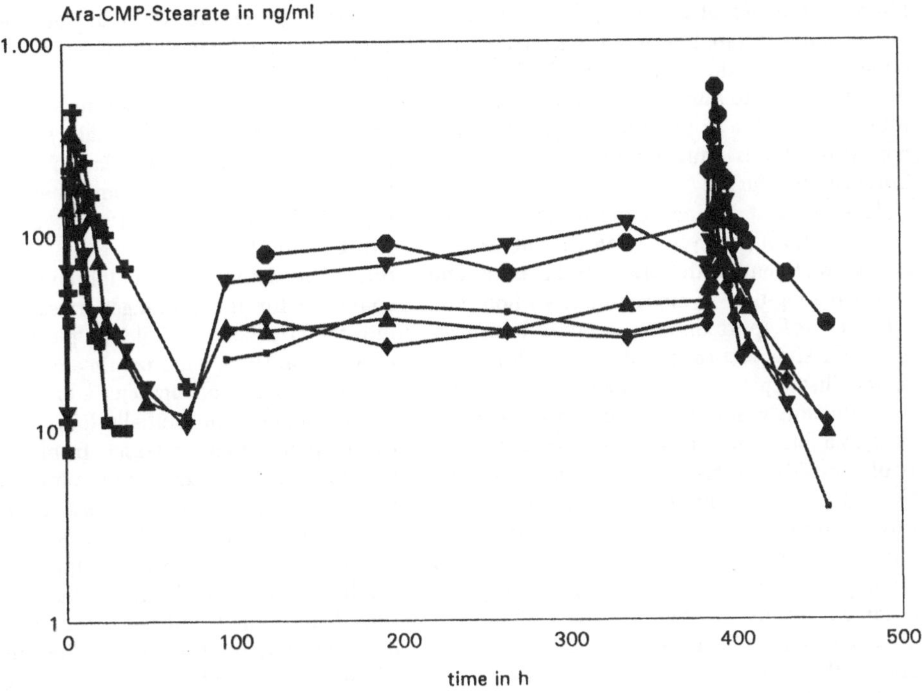

Fig. 2. Ara-CMP-Stearate plasma level under application of 300 mg/body/day Ara-CMP-Stearate

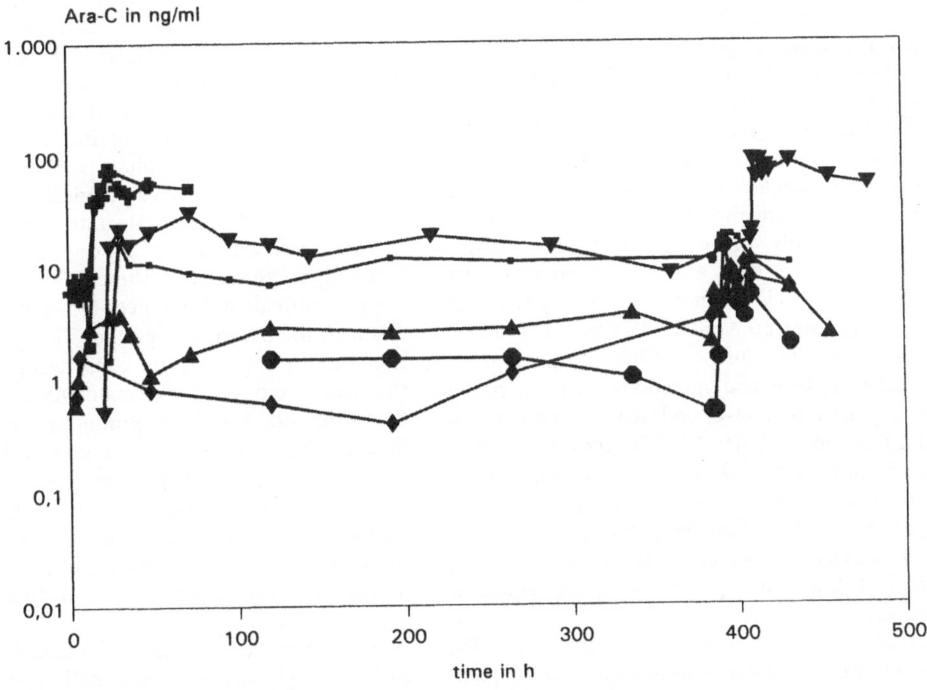

Fig. 3. Ara-C plasma level under application of 300 mg/body/day Ara-CMP-Stearate

pharmacokinetics of this promising new agent and its main metabolites Ara-C and Ara-U. The obtained data indicate that Ara-CMP-Stearate not only allows to administer Ara-C via the oral route but that it also provides long lasting plasma Ara-C levels thus mimicing a continous intravenous infusion.

Plasma and urine concentrations were analysed during 18 cycles in 16 patients undergoing treatment with Ara-CMP-Stearate and revealed a lag-time of approximately 1 hour and a late t_{max} of approximately 6 hours both suggesting a slow resorption of Ara-CMP-Stearate in the distal part of the small intestine. This behaviour fits well to the chemical nature of the drug as a fatty acid. The metabolic bioavailability of Ara-CMP-Stearate was calculated indirectly through the renal elimination of Ara-U since a direct comparison of intravenous and oral administration is prohibited by the induction of hemolysis after intravenous application. The obtained results indicate a bioavailability of approximately 15%. These data are in accordance with preceding experiments by Takayama et al. [18] that have shown that only a small percentage of 2.4% of the total given dose is excreted unchanged into the bile. This means that of the 80–85% of Ara-CMP-Stearate that is found unchanged in the faeces more than 95% has not been resorbed but has passed the gastrointestinal tract without systemic effects or metabolism.

So far there has been no indication that either absorption of the parent compound or its metabolism is reaching a steady state level. Further dose escalation with higher plasma levels seems therefore feasible. The plasma half-life of Ara-CMP-Stearate is around $t_{1/2} = 9$ hours and is highly reproducible in all analyzed patients. Since only a small percentage of the absorbed dose is eliminated via biliary excretion [18] and since no Ara-CMP-Stearate is found in the urine this long half-life mainly reflects hepatic uptake and metabolism of the parent compound to Ara-C and Ara-U. Increases of plasma levels of Ara-CMP-Stearate were linear to intraindividual dose escalation suggesting a constant absorption of the drug in a given patient. On the other hand interindividual differences in plasma levels of both the parent drug and of Ara-C at a given dose level require to assess Ara-C through levels in each case to ashure adequate plasma concentrations. The high intraindividual reproducibility of the pharmacokinetics of Ara-CMP-Stearate, Ara-C and Ara-U however indicate that such determinations must not be performed repeatedly in individual cases.

Following hepatic uptake the stearate moiety of Ara-CMP-Stearate is gradually shortened first by microsomal omega oxydation [19] which is then followed by peroxisomal beta oxydation [14]. The late $t_{max} = 20$ hours of both Ara-C and Ara-U indicate that these steps are relatively time consuming and are therefore partly responsible for the prolonged release of Ara-C into the circulation. While the plasma half lifes of Ara-C and Ara-U are 14 min and 4 hours after intravenous or subcutaneus administration of Ara-C they are substantially longer and nearly overlapping after release from Ara-CMP-Stearate with t_{max} of 22.7 and 18.5 hours and half-lifes of 24.4 and 22.0 hours, respectively [9,10]. The nearly identical half-lifes of Ara-C and Ara-U following Ara-CMP-Stearate application is the result of a typical flip-flop situation with the slow hepatic metabolism of the mother drug being the rate limiting factor. The processes of elimination of both Ara-C and Ara-U and of deamination of Ara-C to Ara-U [24] by far exceed hepatic metabolism of the mother drug to Ara-C. Accordingly the terminal half-life of both metabolites represents mainly the rate of metabolism and is therefore nearly identical for both substances. This observation is clearly represented by the parallel plasma decay curves of Ara-C and Ara-U in Figure 1. These long lasting plasma levels make Ara-CMP-Stearate not a mere prodrug of Ara-C but indicate that this drug possesses distinct pharmacokinetic properties which may well have a clinical impact.

Similarly to Ara-CMP-Stearate, plasma levels of Ara-C rise with increasing dose but are substantially more variable. These findings strongly suggest individual differences in hepatic metabolism of the parent compound. This phenomenon can be explained by considering the fact that Ara-C and Ara-U excretion will always add up to the total metabolic product of Ara-CMP-Stearate. Slight differences in metabolism that will eg lower the Ara-U percentage of this metabolic product from 90% to 80% will mean only a slight variation for Ara-U excretion whereas increasing the Ara-C percentage of the metabolic product from 10% to 20% will double total Ara-C excretion.

This estimation is supported by the fact that a similarly high variability in hepatic metabolism has been found also for other drugs that are mainly metabolized via the cytochrom P450 dependent peroxisomal oxydation system like barbiturates or mephenytoin [20]. Distinct pharmacogenetic polymorphisms has been demonstrated for this enzyme complex [21]. These metabolic effects emphasize the need to monitor Ara-C rather than Ara-CMP-Stearate plasma concentrations for an optimized adaption of treatment.

The current study shows that by oral application of Ara-CMP-Stearate Ara-C plasma levels can be achieved which are comparable to those obtained by subcutaneous administration of so called low dose therapy i.e. 20 mg/m²/d. Because of its more convenient way of application Ara-CMP-Stearate therefore may provide the means for a future development of this therapeutic approach.

Since no signs of saturation of either absorption or metabolism to Ara-C was observed further dose escalation can be expected to result in even higher plasma concentrations of Ara-C that are comparable to those during standard dose regimens. The unique ability of Ara-CMP-Stearate to produce long lasting plasma levels of Ara-C may even improve the prolonged exposure of leukemic cells to Ara-C.

Further studies are needed to establish the clinical relevance of this approach and to define the most appropriate indications for its use.

References

1. Büchner Th, Hiddemann W. Treatment strategies in acute myeloid leukemia (AML). First line chemotherapy. Blut 1990; 60: 61–67.
2. Champlin R, Gale RP. Acute myelogenous leukemia: recent advances in therapy. Blood 1987; 69: 1551–1562.
3. Bolwell BJ, Cassileth PA, Gale RP. High dose cytarabine: a review. Leukemia 1988; 2: 253–260
4. Bolwell BJ, Cassileth PA, Gale RP. Low dose cytosine arabinoside in myelodysplastic and acute myelogenous leukemia: a review. Leukemia 1987; 1: 575–579.
5. Cheson BD, Jasperse DM, Simon R, Friedmann MA,. A critical appraisal of low-dose cytosine arabinoside in patients with acute non lymphocytic leukemia and myelodysplastic syndromes. Journal of Clinical Oncology 1986; 4: 1857–1864.
6. Hiddemann W. Cytosine arabinoside in the treatment of acute myeloid leukemia: the role and place of high dose regimens. Annals of Hematology 1991; 62: 119–128.
7. Peters WG, Colly LP, Willemze R. High dose cytosine arabinoside: pharmacological and clinical aspects. Blut 1988; 56: 1–11.
8. Capizzi RL, White JC. Dose dependent cellular and systemic pharmacokinetics of cytosine arabinoside. Haematology and Blood Transfusion 1992; 34: 266–274.
9. Breithaupt H, Pralle H, Eckhardt T, von Hattingberg M, Schick J, Löffler H. Clinical results and pharmacokinetics of high dose cytosine arabinoside. Cancer 1982; 50: 1248–1257.
10. Hiddeman W, Schleyer E, Unterhalt M, Zühlsdorf M, Rolf C, Reuter C, Kewer U, Uhrmeister C, Wörmann B, Büchner T. Differences in the Intracellular Pharmacokinetics of Cytosine Arabinoside (AraC) between Circulating Leukemic Blasts and Normal Mononuclear Blood Cells. Leukemia 1992; 6: 1273–1280.
11. Saneyoshi M, Morozumi M, Kodama K, Machida H, Kuminaka A,Yoshino H. Synthetic nucleosides and nucleotides. XVI. Synthesis and biological evaluation of a series of 1-β-D-arabinofuranosylcytosine-5'-alkyl or arylphosphates. Chemical Pharm Bull (Tokyo) 1980; 28: 2915–2923.
12. Kodama K, Morozumi M, Saitoh K, Kuninaka A, Yoshino A, Saneyoshi M. Antitumor activity and pharmacology of 1-β-D-arabinofuranosylcytosine-5'-stearylphosphate: An orally active derivate of 1-β-D-arabinofuranosylcytosine. Japanese Journal of Cancer Research 1989; 80: 679–685.
13. Preiss B, Bloch K. Omega oxidation of long fatty acids in rat liver. Journal of Biological Chemistry 1964; 239: 85–88.
14. Yoshida Y, Yamada J, Watanabe T, Suga T, Takayama H. Participation of the peroxisomal β-oxidation system in the chain shortening of PCA_{16}, a metabolite of the cytosine arabinoside prodrug , YNK01, in rat liver. Biochemical Pharmacology 1990; 39: 1505–1512
15. Ramsauer B, Braess J, Unterhalt M, Kaufmann CC, Hiddemann W, Schleyer E. A highly sensitive HPLC assay for quantification of YNK01 – a lipophilic derivate of cytosine-arabinoside. Journal Chromatographia – Biomedical Applications; in press.
16. Enomoto K, Nakagawa Y, Yamashita K, Takayama K, Hashimoto Y. Quantification of Ara-C and Ara-U by radioimmunoassay. Research Laboratories, Pharmaceutical Group, Nippon Kayaku Co. LTD unpublished report.
17. Heinzel G. Topfit-Curve fitting programs. in Pharmacokinetics during drug development: Data analysis and evaluation techniques. Eds Bozler G and Van Rossum JM 1982; 207–208.
18. Takayama H, Esumi Y. Metabolic fate of YNK01 (I), absorption distribution metabolism and excretion after single administration to rats. Research Laboratories, Pharmaceutical Group, Nippon Kayaku Co. LTD 1990; unpublished report.
19. Takayama H. Metabolism of YNK01 in rat hepatocytes. Research Laboratories, Pharmaceutical Group, Nippon Kayaku Co. LTD 1990; unpublished report.
20. Guengerich FP. Characterization of human microsomal cytochrome P-450. Annual Review of Pharmacology and Toxicology 1989; 29: 241–264.

21. Idle JR, Smith RL. Polymorphism of odidation at carbon centers of drugs and their clinical significance. Drug Metabolism Review 1979; 9: 301–317.
22. Ryuzo Ohno, Noriyuki Tatsumi, Masami Hirano, Kuniyuki Imai, Kiyoji Kimura. Treatment of myelodysplastic syndromes with orally administered 1-β-D-Arabinofuranosylcytosine-5′-Stearylphosphate. Oncology 1991; 48: 451–455
23. Ueda T, Imamura S, Kawai Y, Wano Y, Kamiya K, Tsutani H, Nakamura T. Successful treatment of myelodysplastic syndrome with 1-β-D-arabinofuranosylcytosine-5′-stearylphosphate. Leukemia Research 1990; 14: 1067–1068.
24. Laliberte J, Marquez VE, Momparler RL. Potent inhibitors for the deamination of cytosine arabinoside and 5-aza-2′-deoxycytidine by human cytidine deaminase. Cancer Chemotherapy Pharmacology 1992; 30: 7–11.

Acute Leukemias V
Experimental Approaches
and Management of Refractory Diseases
Hiddemann et al. (Eds.)

Differential Effect of GM-CSF on the Intracellular Ara-C Metabolism in Normal Bone Marrow Mononuclear Cells and Acute Myeloid Leukemia (AML) Blasts

Christoph Reuter[1], Claus Rolf[2], Eberhard Schleyer[1], Michael Unterhalt[1], Bernhard Woermann[1], Thomas Buechner[2], and Wolfgang Hiddemann[1]

Abstract. This study examines the effect of recombinant human granulocyte-macrophage colony-stimulating factor (GM-CSF) on the intracellular metabolism of cytosine arabinoside (ara-C) in mononuclear bone marrow cells (NBMMC) from 8 healthy volunteers and leukemic blasts from 50 patients with acute myeloid leukemia (AML). Pretreatment with rh GM-CSF (100 U/ml) for 48 hrs significantly enhanced DNA synthesis: Median ^{3}H-TdR uptake into the DNA increased from 2.15 to 3.68 pmol/10^5 cells in AML blasts and from 3.09 to 7.4 pmol/10^5 cells in NBMMC ($p<0.05$). 14 AML cases did not respond to GM-CSF. Median ara-C mediated inhibition of DNA synthesis was significantly higher in AML blasts as compared to NBMMC (76.5 vs 55.0% and 99.0 vs 96.0% at 0.05 and 5.0 μM ara-C, respectively, $p<0.01$). Similarly, intracellular ara-CTP levels were higher in AML blasts as compared to NBMMC (46.5 vs 18.7, 167.8 vs 48.0 and 59.5 ng/10^7 cells at 1, 10, 100 μM extracellular ara-C, respectively, $p<0.01$). Overall DNA polymerase and DNA polymerase α activity increased from median 80.9 to 94.1 and from 3.1 to 5.7 pmol/min × mg in AML blasts as compared to median 96.7 to 189.8 and 1.2 to 2.2 pmol/min × mg in NBMMC ($p<0.05$). Median deoxycytidine and thymidine kinase activity were only slightly increased in the presence of GM-CSF. The GM-CSF induced increase of the ^{3}H-ara-C incorporation into the DNA was slightly higher in GM-CSF responding AML blasts as compared to NBMMC (median 2.0 vs 1.7 fold at 0.06 μM ara-C, $p<0.05$). The differential effect of GM-CSF on the metabolism of ara-C in normal versus leukemic cells may cause a selective increase in the antileukemic cytotoxicity of ara-C in the presence of GM-CSF.

Introduction

Cytosine arabinoside (ara-C) is one of the most active agents in the treatment of acute myeloid leukemia (AML) and provides the basis for the majority of currently applied treatment regimens [1]. Recent in vitro investigations [2–17] indicate that pretreatment of AML blasts with hematopoietic growth factors such as GM-CSF or IL-3 enhances the ara-C mediated cytotoxicity against leukemic cells. This increase might be due to an increase of the cell fraction in the S-phase of cell cycle, an increase of intracellular ara-CTP/dCTP pool ratios, and an enhanced ara-C incorporation into the blast cell DNA by activation of DNA polymerase α [2–16]. Furthermore, it has been reported that GM-CSF, IL-3 and a combination of both cytokines preferentially enhance the metabolism of ara-C in leukemic versus normal mononuclear bone marrow cells [9, 10, 12–14]. Enhanced ara-C cytotoxicity to normal bone marrow progenitors has only been reported for both G-CSF and GM-CSF at low extracellular ara-C concentrations (0.01 and 0.1 μM) [14]. The mechanisms underlying this phenomenon are still not fully understood.

The present study evaluates and compares the effect of GM-CSF on several parameters of the intracellular ara-C metabolism in leukemic

[1]Department of Hematology and Oncology, University of Göttingen, D-37075 Göttingen, Germany
[2]Department of Internal Medicine, University of Münster, D-48149 Münster, Germany

blasts of 50 AML cases and normal bone marrow mononuclear cells (NBMMC) (n = 8) such as deoxycytidine kinase (dCK), thymidine kinase (TK), overall DNA polymerase, DNA polymerase α, ara-C mediated inhibition of DNA synthesis, ara-C incorporation into blast cell DNA and intracellular ara-CTP levels. Our results indicate that GM-CSF increases ara-C mediated cytotoxicity against leukemic blasts and NBMMC through enhancement of DNA polymerase activity and ara-C incorporation into the DNA. In addition, our data suggest differences in the intracellular ara-C pharmacology in AML blasts and NBMMC which may allow a selective increase in the antileukemic cytotoxicity of ara-C.

Methods

Cells and incubation procedure. Bone marrow aspirates and peripheral blood (n = 6) were obtained from 50 patients (median age 50.5 years, range 12–81) with newly diagnosed AML and from 8 healthy volunteers. FAB subtypes included 2 M0, 7 M1, 8 M2, 1 M3, 14 M4, 7 M4eo, 9 M5, and two secondary AML after myelodysplastic syndrome (MDS). Leukemic cells comprized >70% of the total cell population. Cells were subjected to Ficoll-Hypaque density gradient (1.007 g/cm^3) separation before further processing. Blast cells and NBMMC were cultured for 48 hrs in the absence or presence of GM-CSF (100 U/ml) kindly provided by Behringwerke (Marburg, Germany) at a concentration of 1.5 × 10^6/ml in 30 ml of Iscove's modified Dulbecco's medium (IMDM) supplemented with 10% heat inactivated fetal calf serum (FCS), glutamine (292 μg/ml) and antibiotics (penicillin 60,2 μg/ml, streptomycine 133 μg/ml) at 370C in a 5% CO_2 atmosphere. Throughout this investigation a single lot of fetal calf serum was used.

Cell extract preparation. Cells were washed in 0.9% NaCl. For preparation of cell extracts, 10^7 cells were suspended in 100 μl 50 mM Tris-HCl pH 7.4. Cell were lysed by freeze thawing of the suspension for three times. Cellular debris and unsolved proteins were pelleted by centrifugation at 12,000 g for 15 min at 47 °C.The supernatant was assayed for enzyme activities and protein concentration [18].

^{3}H-thymidine and ^{3}H-ara-C incorporation into the DNA. ^{3}H-thymidine (TdR) (2 Ci/mmol) and ^{3}H-ara-C (30 Ci/mmol) were obtained from Amersham-Buchler, Braunschweig, Germany. After preincubation in the presence or absence of GM-CSF 400,000 (^{3}H-TdR) and 800,000 (^{3}H-ara-C) cells were plated in 24-well microtiter plates in a final volume of 2 ml IMDM. ^{3}H-TdR and ^{3}H-ara-C and increasing amounts of unlabeled ara-C (0.06–100 μM final concentration) were added for 4 and 24 hrs additional hours, respectively. Cells were harvested on DE81 filter paper (Whatman, England) as described [17].

Enzyme assays. Overall DNA polymerase, DNA polymerase α, deoxycytidine kinase and thymidine kinase activity were determined as previously described [17].

Determination of intracellular ara-CTP levels. The determination of the intracellular ara-CTP levels was performed as previously described [19].

Results

Effect of GM-CSF on DNA synthesis and on ara-C mediated inhibition of DNA synthesis. Figure 1 shows the effect of GM-CSF on the ^{3}H-TdR incorporation into the DNA of AML blasts and NBMMC. Median ^{3}H-TdR uptake into the DNA increased from 2.15 to 3.68 pmol/10^5 cells in AML cases (n = 35) and from 3.09 to 7.4 pmol/10^5 cells (n = 8) in NBMMC ($p < 0.05$). 14 AML cases did not respond to GM-CSF pretreatment. The median ara-C mediated inhibition of DNA synthesis was significantly higher in AML blasts as compared to NBMMC (76.5 vs 55.0% and 99.0 vs 96.0% at 0.05 and 5.0 μM ara-C, respectively). GM-CSF pretreatment had no influence on the ara-C mediated inhibition of DNA synthesis in AML blasts (median 82.0 vs 76.5% at 0.05 μM ara-C and 99 vs 99% at 5.0 μM ara-C). In contrast, GM-CSF pretreatment of NBMMC resulted in a slight increase of this inhibition (median 63.5 vs 55% at 0.05 μM and median 96 vs 94% at 5.0 μM extracellular ara-C concentration) (Table 1).

Effect of GM-CSF on the intracellular ara-CTP levels. Figure 2 depicts the effect of GM-CSF pretreatment on the intracellular ara-CTP levels in AML blasts and NBMMC. Following GM-CSF treatment both AML blasts and NBMMC revealed no effect on the intracellular ara-CTP levels as compared to control samples. Furthermore, intracellular ara-CTP levels were found to be 2–40 fold

Fig. 1. Effect of GM-CSF on the ³H-TdR incorporation into the DNA of AML blasts and NBMMC. After 48 hrs in vitro preincubation of the cells in the presence or absence of GM-CSF (100 U/ml) the DNA incorporation of tritiated thymidine was determined as described in "Methods". 3H-TdR uptake into the DNA is given in Pikomoles per 100,000 cells. AML cases are represented by empty squares, NBMMC by empty crosses

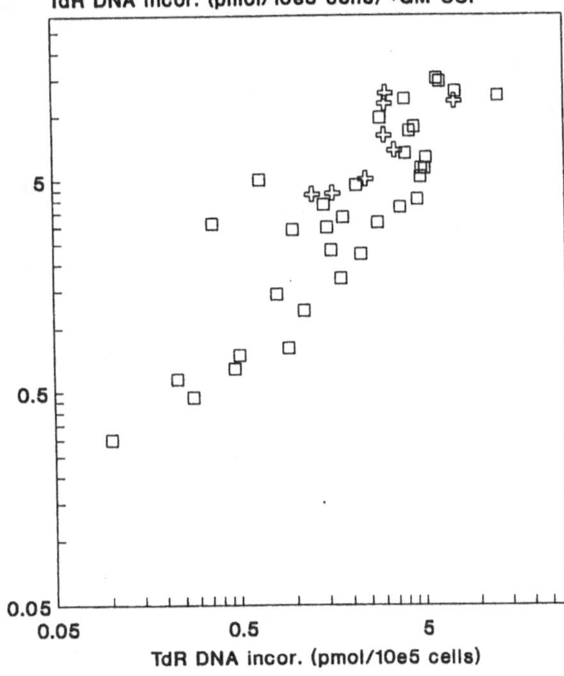

Table 1. Effect of GM-CSF on DNA synthesis and on ara-C mediated inhibition of DNA synthesis

	AML blasts	NBMMC
³H-TdR uptake (pmol/10⁵ cells)		
median	2.15(2.25+/3.2−)	3.09
range	0.1–13.0	1.25–7.5
n	35	8
+GM-CSF		
median	3.68(4.8+/3.1−)	7.4
range	0.3–14.9	4.25–12.7
Ara-C mediated inhibition of DNA synthesis (% of control)		
0.05 μM ara-C		
median	76.5	55.0
range	26–94	32–82
n	32	8
5.0 μM ara-C		
median	99	94
range	83–100	90–99
0.05 μM ara-C+GM-CSF		
median	82	63.5
range	41–94	41–77
n	29	8
5.0 μM ara-C+GM-CSF		
median	99	96
range	91–100	94–99

Values in parenthesis are for GM-CSF responsive (+) and non-responsive (–) AML blasts

lower in NBMMC as compared to AML blasts (median values: 18.7 vs 46.9, 48.0 vs 167.8 and 59.5 vs 337.5 ng/10^7 cells at 1, 10 and 100 μM extracellular ara-C, respectively, $p<0.01$).

Effect of GM-CSF on enzyme activity of DNA polymerase, thymidine kinase and deoxycytidine kinase. The effect of GM-CSF on the enzymes activities of overall DNA polymerase (POL), DNA polymerase α (POLA), thymidine kinase (TK) and deoxycytidine kinase (DCK) is shown in Figure 3 and Table 2. Overall DNA polymerase activity ranged from 12.9 to 210.4 pmol/min × mg (median 80.9) in AML blasts (n = 48) and from 20.6 to 301.5 pmol/min × mg (median 96.7) in NBMMC (n = 7). DNA polymerase α activity was slightly higher in AML blasts (n = 42) as compared to NBMMC (n = 5) (median 3.1 vs 1.2 pmol/ min × mg, range 0.04–28.9 vs 0.2–3.2 pmol/min × mg). In the presence of GM-CSF overall DNA polymerase α activity (POL) and DNA polymerase activity increased from median 80.9 to 94.1 and from 3.1 to 5.7 pmol/min × mg in AML blasts as compared to median 96.7 to 189.8 and 1.2 to 2.2 pmol/min × mg in NBMMC ($p<0.05$). GM-CSF pretreatment of AML blasts resulted in a slight

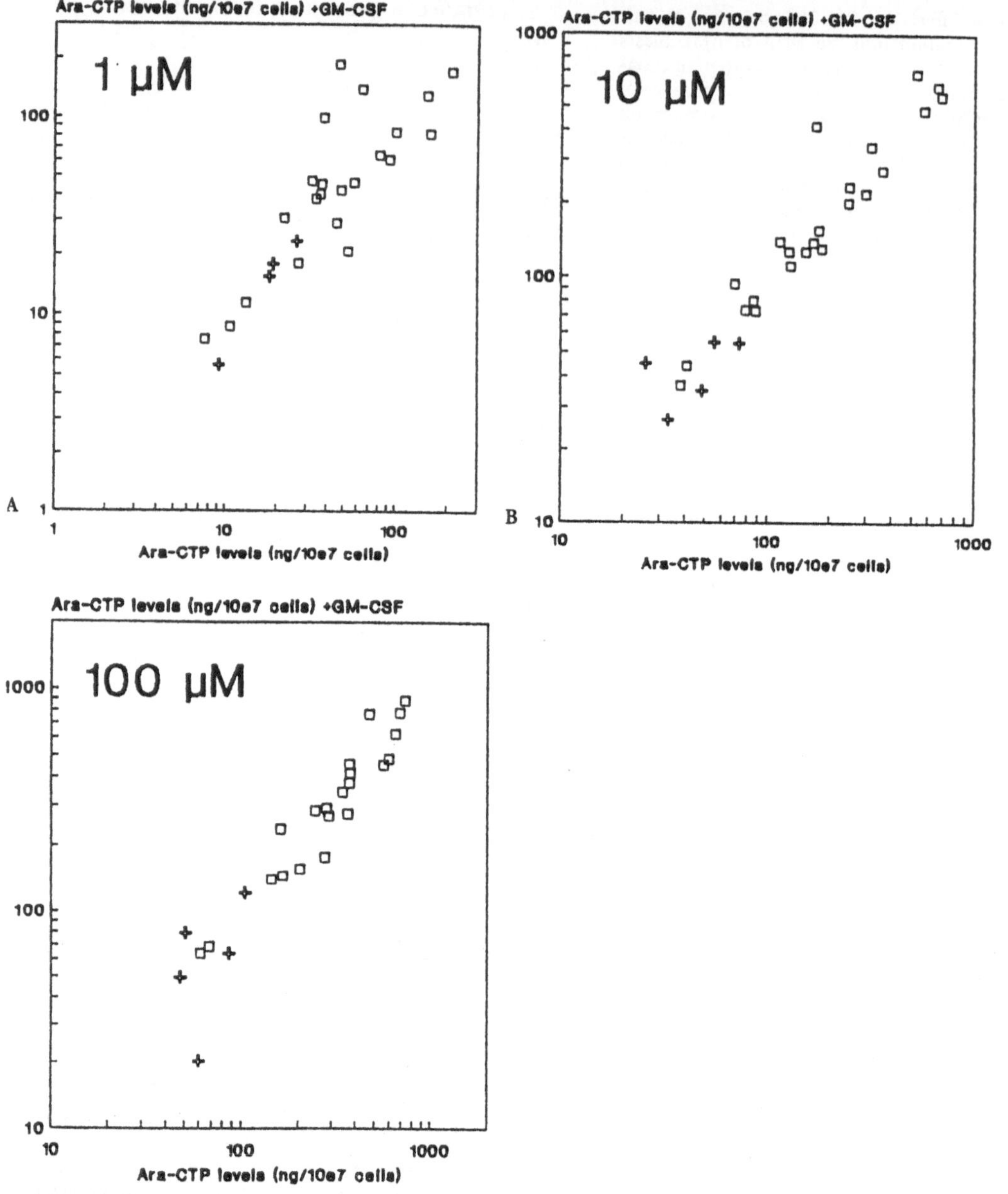

Fig. 2. Effect of GM-CSF on the intracellular ara-CTP levels in AML blasts and NBMMC. AML blasts (empty squares) and NBMMC (empty crosses) were preincubated for 48 hrs in the presence or absence of GM-CSF (100 U/ml). Ara-C was added for additional 12 hrs in increasing concentration (1, 10 100 μM, respectively). The determination of the intracellular ara-CTP levels was performed as previously described by Schleyer et al. [19]

increase of deoxycytidine kinase (dCK) activity (n = 40) (median 9.7 to 11.3 pmol/min × mg). In contrast, NBMMC (n = 6) showed no change in dCK activity in the presence of GM-CSF (19.5 vs 19.5 pmol/min × mg). Thymidine kinase activity was significantly higher in AML blasts (n = 39) as compared to NBMMC (n = 7) ($p < 0.05$) and was slightly increased in the presence of GM-CSF (median increase from 6.4 to 7.8 and from 1.9 to 3.6 pmol/min × mg, respectively).

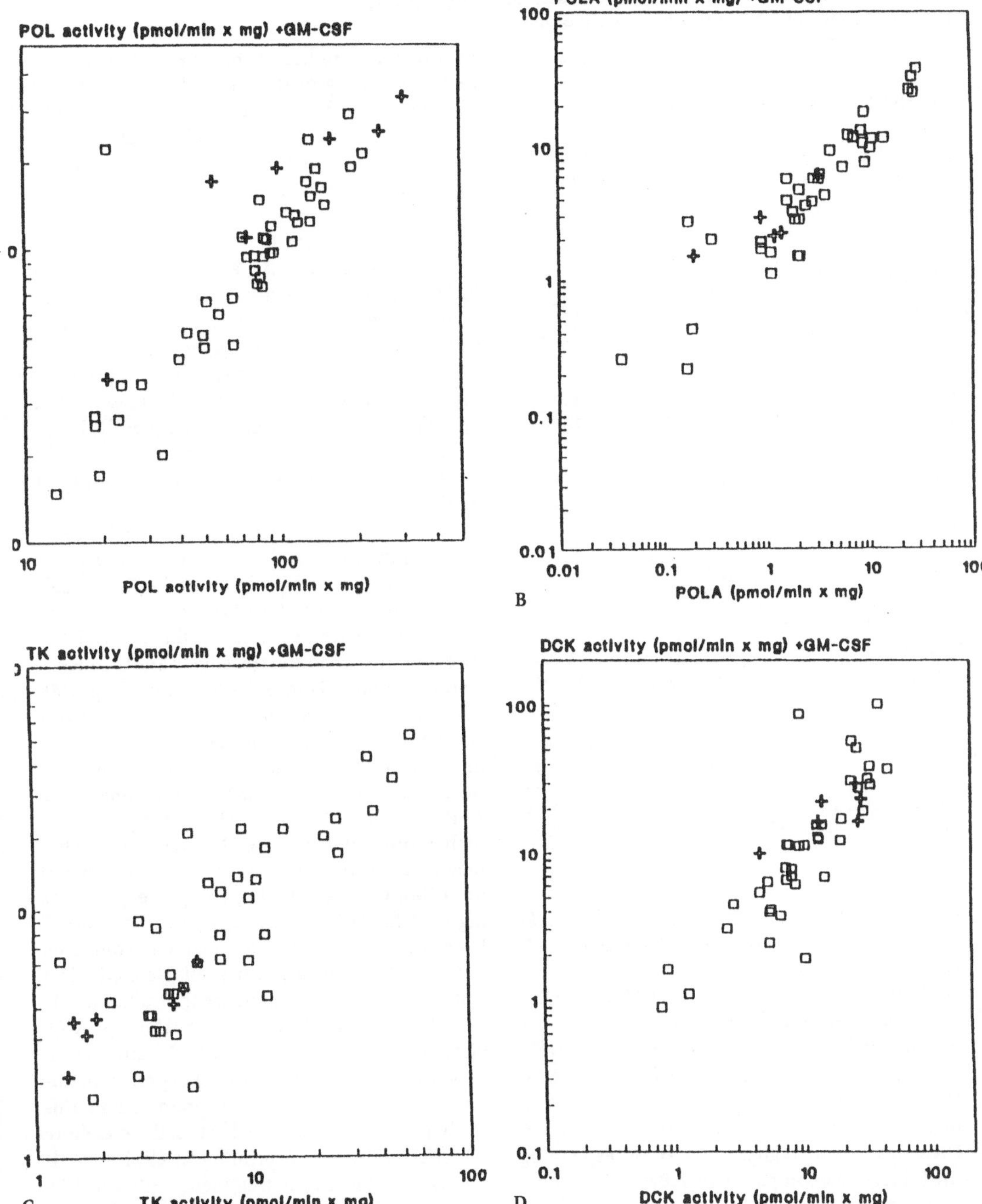

Fig. 3. Effect of GM-CSF on the enzyme activities of DNA polymerase, thymidine kinase and deoxycytidine kinase. AML blasts (empty squares) and NBMMC (empty crosses) were preincubated for 48 hrs in the presence or absence of GM-CSF (100 U/ml). Cells were harvested and enzyme activities were determined as described (see "Methods"). Enzyme activities of overall DNA polymerase (POL) and DNA polymerase α (POLA) are given in Pikomoles ^{3}H-dCTP incorporated into "activated" DNA per min per mg of protein, thymidine kinase (TK) and deoxycytidine kinase (DCK) activity is given in Pikomoles phosphorylated ^{3}H-TdR or ^{3}H-ara-C per min per mg of protein

Table 2. Effect of GM-CSF on enzyme activities of DNA polymerase, thymidine and deoxycytidine kinase

	AML blasts	NBMMC
Overall DNA polymerase		
median	80.9	96.7
range	12.9–210.4	20.6–301.5
n	46	7
+GM-CSF		
median	94.1	189.9*
range	14.7–289.6	36–331.7
DNA polymerase α		
median	3.1	1.2*
range	0.04–28.9	0.2–3.2
n	41	5
+GM-CSF		
median	5.7	2.2*
range	0.2–37.7	1.5–6.1
Thymidine kinase		
median	6.4	1.9*
range	1.3–56	1.4–5.6
n	39	7
+GM-CSF		
median	7.8	3.6*
range	1.7–51.3	2.1–6.1
Deoxycytidine kinase		
median	9.7	19.5
range	0.8–44.1	4.6–27.9
n	40	6
+GM-CSF		
median	11.3	19.5
range	0.9–102	9.9–29.7

Enzyme activities are given in pikomoles/min × mg of protein (see "Methods").* = $p < 0.05$ (Wilcoxon-test)

Effect of GM-CSF on ara-C incorporation into the DNA. Figure 4 depicts the differential effect of GM-CSF on the ^{3}H-ara-C incorporation into the DNA. ^{3}H-ara-C uptake into the DNA was determined in 31 AML cases and in samples from 8 healthy volunteers. Median ^{3}H-ara-C DNA incorporation increased 1.2–1.7 fold after GM-CSF pretreatment. The GM-CSF induced increase of the ara-C incorporation into the DNA was slightly higher in GM-CSF responding AML blasts as compared to NBMMC (median 2.0 vs 1.7 fold, $p < 0.05$).

Discussion

In previous studies it has been shown that hematopoietic growth factors like GM-CSF and IL-3 increase the percentage of cycling AML blasts in S-phase, favorably affect intracellular ara-CTP/dCTP pool ratios in AML blasts as compared to NBMMC, increase DNA polymerase α activity and thereby increase the incorporation of ara-C into the blast cell DNA [2–17]. These effects are associated with increased in vitro cytotoxicity against clonogenic leukemic cells but not against normal CFU-GM or CFU-GEMM [9, 10, 12–14]. In the present study, we report that GM-CSF pretreatment of NBMMC also results in increased DNA polymerase α activity and subsequently in an enhanced ara-C uptake into the DNA. Ara-CTP levels were not affected by GM-CSF priming in neither NBMMC and AML blasts. The incorporation of ara-C has been found to closely correlate with the cytotoxicity of ara-C on clonogenic leukemic cells and with its clinical efficacy [20]. Interestingly, GM-CSF pretreatment resulted in a slightly higher increase of the ara-C DNA incorporation at low extracellular ara-C concentrations (0.06 μM) in GM-CSF responding AML blasts versus NBMMC (median increase 2.0 versus 1.7 fold, $p < 0.05$). In contrast, the median increase of DNA synthesis after GMC-CSF treatment was higher in NBMMC as compared to AML blasts. AML blasts showed significantly higher intracellular ara-CTP levels and higher median DNA polymerase α values as compared to NBMMC. These findings might explain the higher GM-CSF induced increase of the ara-C DNA incorporation in AML blasts as compared to NBMMC. With currently available methods it is difficult to directly compare the values determined for AML blasts and NBMMC as AML blasts were not directly compared with normal bone marrow cells of equivalent degree of maturation. However, the results presented in this study provide an additional rationale to explore the effect of GM-CSF priming in clinical trials (21–24) of concurrent treatment with GM-CSF and ara-C in AML and suggest that GM-CSF

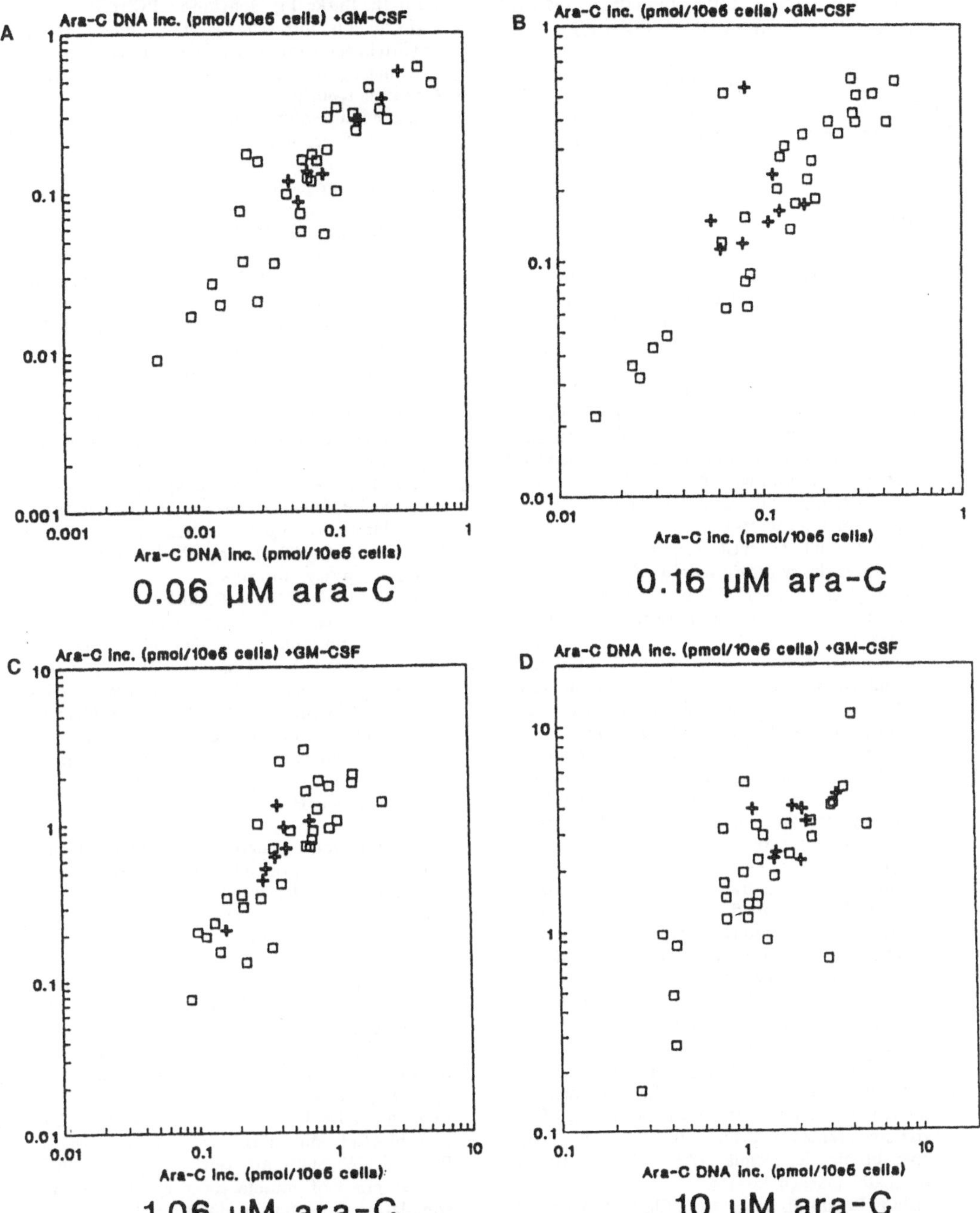

Fig. 4. Effect of GM-CSF on the incorporation of ara-C into the DNA of AML blasts and NBMMC. AML blasts (empty squares) and NBMMC (empty crosses) were pretreated in vitro for 48 hrs with or without GM-CSF (100 U/ml). Cells were incubated for additional 24 hrs with increasing concentrations of ^{3}H-ara-C (0.06, 0.16, 1.06 and 10 μM, respectively) in the presence or absence of GM-CSF. ^{3}H-Ara-C uptake into the DNA was measured as described in "Methods" and is given in Pikomoles ara-C incorporated into the DNA of 100,000 cells

responsive AML cases might benefit of GM-CSF pretreatment prior to induction therapy.

Acknowledgements. This study was supported by a grant from the Dr. Mildred-Scheel-Stiftung für Krebsforschung, Germany (W24/87/Hi 1).

References

1. Hiddemann W. Cytosine arabinoside in the treatment of acute myeloid leukemia: the role and place of high-dose regimens. Ann.Hematol. 1991; 62: 119–128.
2. Hiddemann W, Kiehl M, Zuehlsdorf M, Busemann C, Schleyer E, Woermann B, Buechner T. Granulocyte-macrophage colony-stimulating factor and interleukin-3 enhance the incorporation of cytosine arabinoside into the DNA of leukemic blasts and the cytotoxic effect on clonogenic cells from patients with acute myeloid leukemia. Sem.Oncol. 1992; 19: 31–37.
3. Lista P, Porcu P, Avazi GC, Pegoraro L. Interleukin-3 enhances the cytotoxic activity of 1-β D-arabinofuranosylcytosine (ara-C on acute myeloblastic leukemia (AML) cells. Br. J. Heamatol. 1988; 69: 121–123.
4. Miyauchi J, Kelleher CA, Wang C, Minkin S, McCulloch EA. Growth factors influence the sensitivity of leukemic stem cells to cytosine arabinoside in culture. Blood 1989; 73: 1271–1278.
5. Cannistra SA, Groshek P, Griffin JD. Granulocyte-macrophage colony-stimulating factor enhances the cytotoxic effects of cytosine arabinoside in acute myeloblastic leukemia and in the myeloid blast crisis phase of chronic myeloid leukemia. Leukemia 1989; 3: 328–334.
6. Butturini A, Alessandra MA, Gale RP, Perocco P, Tur S. GM-CSF incubation prior to treatment with cytarabine or doxorubicine enhances drug activity against AML cells in vitro: A model for leukemia chemotherapy. Leukemia Res. 1990; 14: 743–749.
7. Brach M, Klein H, Platzer E, Mertelsmann R, Hermann F. Effect of interleukin-3 on cytosine arabinoside-mediated cytotoxicity of leukemic myeloblasts. Exp. Hematol. 1990; 18: 748–753.
8. Lista P, Porcu P, Avanzi GC, Pegorarro L. Interleulin 3 enhances the cytotoxic activity of 1-β arabino-furanosyl-cytosine (ara-C) on acute myeloblastic leukaemia (AML) cells. Br. J. Haematol. 1988; 69: 121–123.
9. Lista P, Rossi BM, Resegotti L, Clark SC, Pegoraro L. Different sensitivity of normal and leukemic progenitor cells to ara-C and IL-3 treatment. Br. J. Heamatol. 1990; 76: 21–26.
10. Van Der Lely N, Witte T, Muus P, Raymakers R, Preijers F, Haanen C. Prolonged exposure to cytosine arabinoside in the presence of hematopoietic growth factors preferentially kills leukemic versus normal clonogenic cells. Exp. Hematol. 1991; 19: 267–272.
11. Karp JE, Burke PJ, Donehower RC. Effect of rh GM-CSF on intracellular ara-C pharmacology in vitro in acute myelocytic leukemia: comparability with drug-induced humoral stimulatory activity. Leukemia 1990; 4: 553–556.
12. Bhalla K, Birkhofer M, Arlin Z, Lutzky J, Graham G. Effect of recombinant GM-CSF on the metabolism of cytosine arabinoside in normal and leukemic human bone marrow cells. Leukemia 1988; 2: 810–813.
13. Bhalla K, Birkhofer M, Arlin Z, Grant S, Lutzky J, Safah H, Graham G. Differential effect of interleukin-3 on the metabolism of high dose cytosine arabinoside in normal versus leukemic human bone marrow cells. Exp. Hematol. 1991; 19: 669–673.
14. Bhalla K, Holladay C, Arlin Z, Grant S, Ibrado AM, Jasiok M. Treatment with interleukin-3 plus granulocyte-macrophage colony-stimulating factor improves the selectivity of ara-C in vitro against acute myeloid leukemia blasts. Blood 1991; 78: 2674–2679.
15. te Boekhorst PAW, Loewenberg B, Vlastuin M, Sonneveld P. Enhanced chemosensitivity of clonogenic blasts from patients with acute myeloid leukemia by G-CSF, IL-3 or GM-CSF stimulation. Leukemia 1993; 7: 1191–1198.
16. Yang GS, Minden MD, McCulloch EA. Influence of schedule on regulated sensitivity of AML blasts to cytosine arabinoside. Leukemia 1993; 7: 1012–1019.
17. Reuter C, Auf Der Landwehr U I, Auf Der Landwehr U II, Schleyer E, Zuehlsdorf M, Ameling C, Rolf C, Woermann B, Buechner T, Hiddemann W. Modulation of intracellular metabolism of cytosine arabinoside in acute myeloid leukemia by granulocyte macrophage colony stimulating factor. Leukemia 1994; 8: 217–225.
18. Bradford MM. A rapid and sensitive method for the quantitation of microgram quantities of proteins utilizing the prinziple of protein-dye binding. Anal. Biochem. 1976; 72: 248–254.
19. Schleyer E, Ehninger G, Zuehlsdorf M, Proksch B, Hiddemann W. Detection and separation of intracellular ara-CTP by ion-pair high performance liquid chromatography: a sensitive, isocratic, highly reproducible and rapid method. J. Chromatography 1989; 497: 109–120.
20. Kufe D, Spriggs D. Biochemical and cellular pharmacology of cytosine arabinoside. Sem. Oncol. 1985; 12(2): 34–48.
21. Aglietta M, De Felice L, Stacchini A, Petti MC, Bianchi ACM, Aloe Spiriti MA, Sanavio F, Apra F, Piacibello W, Stern AC, Gavosto F, Mandelli F. In vivo effect of granulocyte-macrophage colony stimulating factor on the kinetics of human acute myeloid leukemia cells. Leukemia 1991; 5: 979–984.
22. Bettelheim P, Valent P, Andreeff M, Tafuri A, Haimi J, Gorischek C, Muhm M, Sillaber Ch, Haas O, Vieder L, Maurer D, Schulz G, Speiser W, Geissler K, Kier P, Hinterberger W, Lechner K. Recombinant human granulocyte-macrophage colony-stimulating factor in combination with standard induction chemotherapy in de novo acute myeloid leukemia. Blood 1991; 77: 700–711.

23. Cannistra SA, Di Carlo J, Groshek P, Kanakura Y, Berg D, Mayer RJ, Griffen JD. Simultaneous administration of granulocyte-macrophage colony-stimulating factor and cytosine arabinoside for the treatment of relapsed acute myeloid leukemia. Leukemia 1991; 5: 230–238.
24. Estey E, Thall PF, Kantarjian H, O'Brien S, Koller CA, Beran M, Gutterman J, Deisseroth A, Keating M. Treatment of newly diagnosed acute myelogenous leukemia with granulocyte-macrophage colony-stimulating factor (GM-CSF) before and during continous-infusion high-dose ara-C + daunorubicin: comparison to patients treated without GM-CSF. Blood 1992; 79: 2236–2255.

Acute Leukemias V
Experimental Approaches
and Management of Refractory Diseases
Hiddemann et al. (Eds.)

Intracellular Retention of Cytosine-Arabinoside-Triphosphate in Leukemic Blast Cells from Children

J. Boos, M. Schiller, B. Pröbsting, U. Creutzig, and J. Ritter

Abstract. Pharmacokinetic parameters of intracellular Ara-CTP were investigated in 65 children with leukemia (50 ALL, 15 AML). Separated peripheral or bone marrow blast cells were incubated for one hour in Ara-C containing medium (1 or 3 μg/ml) followed by reincubation in Ara -C free medium for three hours to determine the intracellular formation and retention of Ara-CTP.

The Ara-CTP retention showed marked differences in the morphologically classified groups at the time of initial diagnosis: non-T-ALL 67±25% (x±SD, n=33), T-ALL 37±15% (n=8) and AML 34±18% (n=14). The difference between AML ($p<0.0006$) as well as T-ALL $p<0.002$ and non-T-ALL was significant.

The maximal accumulation of Ara-CTP (after 1h incub.), however, was not significantly different between AML, T-ALL, non-T-ALL and blast cells from children in relapse.

The similar cellular accumulation (C_{max}, 1h Ara-C incubation) of Ara-CTP in all groups with a significantly more rapid decrease (3h without Ara-C) in T-ALL and AML represents a pharmacokinetic rationale for continuous Ara-C infusion in these subgroups as an alternative to the intensification by HD-Ara-C schedules.

Introduction

Cytarabine (Ara-C) is one of the most important cytotoxic drugs in the treatment of childhood acute leukemia. Dosing and schedules vary widely (100 mg/m²/24h–3000 mg/m²/3h) and are still subjects of intense discussions.

Cellular uptake and intracellular phosphorylation to the nucleotide cytosine-arabinoside-triphosphate (Ara-CTP) is the precondition for the cytostatic effect of cytarabine. Several studies reported correlation of the leukemic cells' ability to build and retain the metabolite Ara-CTP intracellularly with clinical response to therapy in AML [1, 2]. Strategies were suggested to individualize Ara-C infusion regimens on the basis of intracellular Ara-CTP pharmacokinetics [1]. The prognostic relevance of intracellular Ara-CTP pharmacokinetics depends on the applied Ara-C schedule [3].

Observations in lymphoblastic leukemias are rare [4, 5] and especially in pediatric patients missing. Therefore, questions remain regarding to pharmacokinetic basis for the optimal dose and duration of Ara-C infusions in children with AML and ALL.

Methods

The intracellular Ara-CTP retention in 65 children with leukemia (50 ALL, 15 AML) was investigated.

Peripheral or bone marrow blast cells were separated from heparinized samples by Ficoll-Hypaque centrifugation and then incubated for one hour in Ara-C containing medium (RPMI, 10% fetal calf serum, 1 or 3 μg/ml Ara-C) followed by reincubation in Ara-C free medium for three hours to determine the intracellular formation and retention of Ara-CTP. Retention at the end of the second incubation period was

Department of Pediatric Hematology & Oncology, University of Münster, 48129 Münster, Germany

expressed in % of the 1h level. Under these conditions the Ara-CTP formation could be suppressed by coincubation of dipyridamol (5 μg/ml), an inhibitor of the nucleoside transport system [7], indicating that the cellular uptake was controlled by the carrier system.

Extraction of the cells following 1 and 1+3 hours of incubation and quantification by high performance liquid chromatography was described elsewhere [6].

Results

Ara-CTP-formation. The maximum Ara-CTP levels formed following one hour incubation with 1 μg/ml Ara-C resulted in a wide range of cellular Ara-CTP concentrations but did not show any significant difference between T-ALL, non-T-ALL, ALL in relapse or AML (see Fig.1 and Table 1).

Ara-CTP-retention. Intracellular Ara-CTP-retention was comparable in common-ALL (65±25%, n=30) and the pre-B-ALL subtype (62±24%, n=11, relapses included), both, therefore, were summarized as non-T-ALL.

Table 1. Ara-CTP-level following I hour incubation

	non-T-ALL	T-ALL	AML	ALL-Relapse
n	26	8	12	7
z	167	225	186	282
±s	169	144	97	117
Median	120	162	159	243

(pMol/10 mill cells)

The Ara-CTP-retention showed marked differences in the depicted morphologically and immunologically classified groups:

The differences between AML as well as T-ALL and non-T-ALL were significant (non-T-ALL/AML: $p<0.00006$, non-T/T-ALL: $p<0.002$). The difference between initially diagnosed non-T-ALL and non-T-ALL in relapse shows a trend with $p=0,07$.

Discussion

The cellular pharmacology of the cytotoxic Cytarabine-anabolite Ara-CTP differs between morphological and immunological subtypes in blast cells from children with acute leukemias.

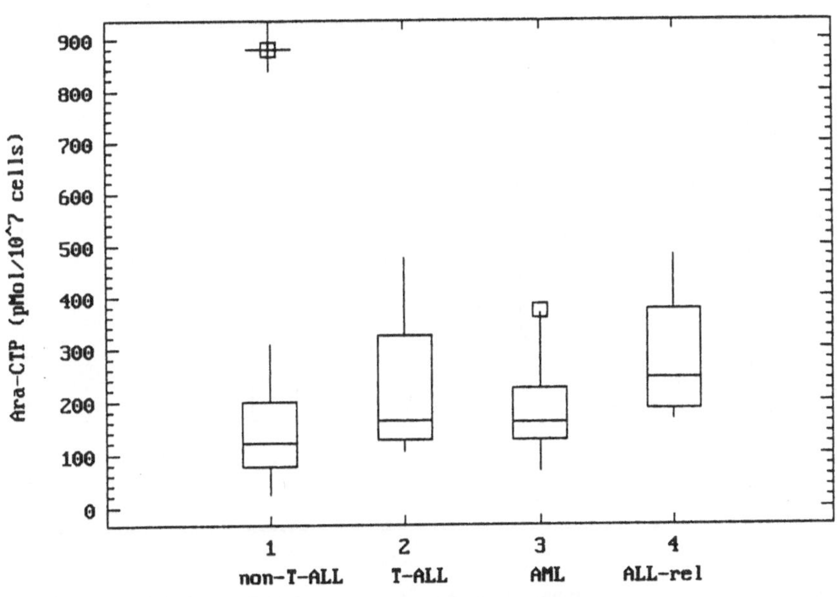

Fig. 1. Intracellular Ara-CTP concentration following 1 hour incubation with 1 μg/ml Ara-C

The Ara-CTP retention was found to be comparable in T-ALL and AML and in both groups significantly lower than in common-ALL.

The finding of a low Ara-CTP retention in T-ALL ist in contrast to results from a Japanese group [5] who even reported prolonged intracellular retention in T-ALL compared to other subtypes.

The cellular Ara-CTP decreased more rapidly in cells from normal bone marrow than in non-T-ALL (see Table 2, Fig. 2) but in the same order as in AML and T-ALL.

A specified amount of Ara-CTP once formed within the cells, therefore, will be removed from T-ALL and AML cells more rapidly than from non-T-ALL cells. Only in non-T-ALL the intracellular treatment intensity of a single dose of Ara-C will be higher compared to normal bone marrow.

These differences may provide the basis for a favorably tolerated treatment of acute lymphoblastic leukemias with bolus injections of Ara-C. In pediatric AML, however, there was a clinical benefit from the introduction of continuous infusion into the treatment protocol [8]. Continuous infusion theoretically should overcome the short intracellular half-life by continuous Ara-CTP formation.

Table 2. Ara-CTP-retention in leucemic blast cells

	x±s	median	range	n
non-T-ALL	67±25%	64%	26–130%	33
non-T-relapse	51±16%	52%	32–60%	11
T-ALL	37±15%	31%	20–60%	8
AML	34±18%	29%	9–64%	14
norm. BM	44±24%	37%	22–55%	7

The formation on the other hand was comparable in the different entities. Neither T-ALL nor AML showed a significantly lower formation of Ara-CTP. Even in relapse no reduction of Ara-CTP formation could be observed.

The present data give no supporting evidence that high Ara-C concentrations are needed to overcome resistance on the level of nucleoside transport or the phosphokinase activity.

The pharmacokinetic differences between the different entities always concerned the intracellular Ara-CTP-retention or the T½ of Ara-CTP. Therefore, the cellular AUC of Ara-CTP following bolus injection or short term infusion are expected to be significant lower in T-ALL, AML and ALL in relapse compared to non-T-ALL.

These data indicate, that first and foremost the time of exposure during Ara-C therapy might be important and might influence the therapeutic effect more than the height of Ara-C dosage.

While most therapeutic protocols tried to intensify Ara-C therapy by increasing the doses

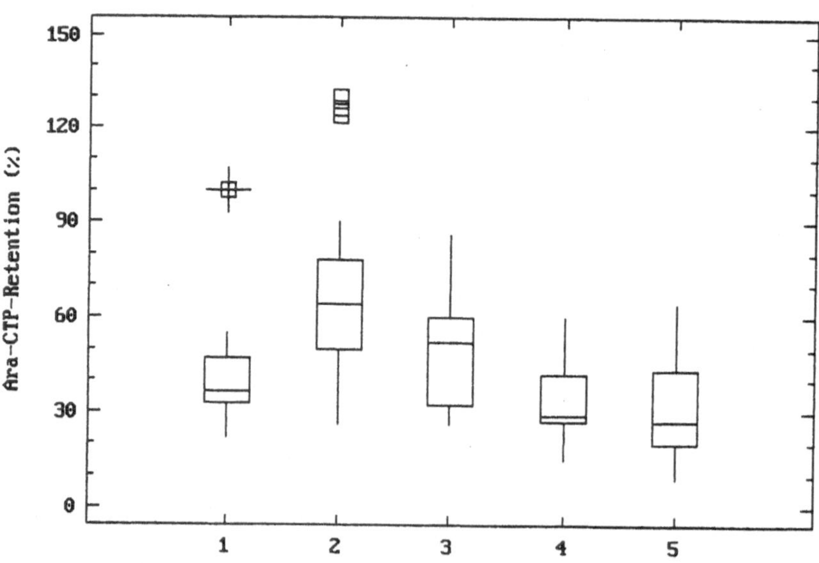

Fig. 2. Ara-CTP-retention in 1: normal bone marrow, 2: initial non-T-ALL, 3: relapsed non-T-ALL, 4: T-ALL and 5: AML. (4 and 5 initial, relapses excluded)

(HD-Ara-C regimens) during the last years, our data indicate, that prolonged duration of Ara-C infusions may be a superior intensification strategy to dose escalation especially in T-ALL and AML.

Acknowledgement. Supported by Deutsche Forschungsgemeinschaft.

References

1. Plunkett W, Iacoboni S, Estey E, Danhauser L, Liliemark JO, Keating MJ: Pharmacologically directed ara-C therapy for refractory leukemia. Semin Oncol 12 (Suppl 1): 20–30; 1985
2. Rustum YM, Preisler HD: Correlation between leukemic cell retention of 1-β-D-Arabinofuranosylcytosine 5'-Triphosphate and response to therapy. Cancer Res 39: 42–49; 1979
3. Preisler HD, Rustum YM, Azarnia N, Priore R: Abrogation of the prognostic significance of low leukemic cell retention of cytosine arabinoside triphosphate by intensification of therapy and by alteration in the dose and schedule of administration of cytosine arabinoside. Cancer Chemother Pharmacol 19: 69–74; 1987
4. Abe I, Saito S, Hori K, Suzuki M, Sato H: Role of dephosphorylation in accumulation of 1-β-D-Arabinofuranosylcytosine-5'-triphosphate in human lymphoblastic cell lines with reference to their drug sensitivity. Cancer Res 42: 2846–51; 1982
5. Tanaka M, Yoshida S: Efficient formation of cytosine arabinoside-5'-triphosphate in leukemic blasts of human T-cell acute lymphoblastic leukemia. Leukemia Research 13(10): 931–936; 1989
6. Boos J: A simple isocratic ion-pair high-performance liquid chromatographic determination of 1-β-D-arabinofuranosylcytosine 5'-triphosphate for intracellular drug-monitoring and in vitro incubation assays. Journal of Pharmaceutical & Biomedical Analysis 9: 47–52; 1991
7. Jarvis MS: Nitrobenzylthioinosine-sensitive nucleoside transport system: Mechanism of inhibition by Dipyridamole. Mol Pharmacol 30: 659–665; 1986
8. Creutzig U, Ritter J, Schellong G for the AML-BFM Study Group. Identification of two risk groups in childhood acute myelogenous leukemia after therapy intensification in study AML-BFM-83 as compared with study AML-BFM-78. Blood 75: 1932–1940; 1990

Acute Leukemias V
Experimental Approaches
and Management of Refractory Diseases
Hiddemann et al. (Eds.)

The Pharmacokinetics of Epipodopyllotoxins – Clinical Relevance

K. B. Mross

Introduction

Etoposide (VP-16) is a semisynthetic derivative of podophyllotoxin, an anticancer drug that has been used for more than 1000 years [1]. VP-16 is a phase-specific drug, acting in the late S or early G2 phases of the cell cycle [2]. The drug has been very active in germ cell tumors, small cell lung cancer, lymphomas and leucemias. For many cytotoxic drugs, an escalation of drug dosage usually leads to an increased antitumor effect. The limited toxicity, primarily myelosuppression, of VP-16 at the standard dose levels (300–500 mg/m²) makes it a suitable drug for much higher dosages. In fact the dosages administered for preparatory chemotherapy regimens in allogeneic and autologous bone marrow transplantation for hematologic malignancies are 6–10 times higher (60 mg/kg or 3000 mg/m²). Nevertheless, the optimal schedule for high-dose VP-16 chemotherapy has to be determined. In vitro studies have clearly demonstrated that the duration of cell exposure to etoposide dictates the drug's degree of tumorcell kill [3]. To achieve the same degree of cell kill in e.g. small cell lung cancer lines, 100 times the 24 hour incubation dose of VP-16 was required in a 1 hour exposure [4]. The results within clinical trials were similar. In case of five daily infusions of VP-16 in patients with small cell lung cancer this application mode (5 day split) was greatly superior to a 24 hour infusion [5]. In high dose regimens containing VP-16 it is a common procedure to administer the total VP-16 drug amount within a short infusion time (6–10 hours) [6]. The most fundamental question relates to the optimal schedule of etoposide in the high dose setting. It is possible that the optimal etoposide schedule and dose varies from patient to patient and tumor to tumor depending on the intra-individual capacities for clearance and metabolization and on the variable proportion of cycling cells open to attack by such a phase-specific action of VP-16. Within the bone marrow transplantation (BMT) project of the University Hospital in Hamburg the pharmacokinetic of three different schedules for high-dose VP-16 was studied in patients, receiving etoposide, cyclophosphamide and busulfan as conditioning chemotherapy regimen before BMT. Three sequential pharmacokinetic studies have been performed using different schedules for VP-16 administration for patients with hematological malignancies. The first study consisted of a 6 hour infusion schedule, the second investigation used a 34 hour infusion schedule and the third tested a 3-day regimen with 1 hour infusions every 24 hours.

Patients and Methods

Totally 23 patients have been entered into the three pharmacokinetic studies. 9 patients received a 6 hour infusion, 7 patients received a 34 hour infusion and 7 patients received three 1 hour infusion in daily intervalls. The patients had different diagnosis (AML, ALL, CML, NHL, HD and MDS). The mean age was 40 years ranging from 15 to 55 years. 15 patients received an allogeneic and 8 patients an autologous bone marrow. The supportive care was identical in all

Department Oncology and Hematology, University Hospital Eppendorf, D-20251 Hamburg, Germany patients, all were isolated in laminar air flow rooms, receiving the same drugs: ciprofloxacin, amphothericin B for gut decontamination, cotrimoxazole for pneumocstis carinii prophylaxis, metoclopramide and dexamethasone as antiemetics, phenytoin as seizure prophylaxis, and ceftazidime and vancomycin +/− tobramycin in case of fever; in case of persisting fever amphothericin B was administered if fungal infection was suspected. Red blood cells and platelet infusions were given when necessary. GVDH prophylaxis for allogeneic transplant recipients consisted of cyclosporin A and prednisone or methothrexate starting one day before BMT took place.

Treatment. VP-16 was administered at doses of 30–45 mg/kg at day −4 in case of a 6 hour infusion, at days −4 and −3 in case of a 34 hour infusion and at days −5, −4 and −3 in case of the daily 1 hour infusion on three consecutive days. Busulfan was given orally at a dose of 1 mg/kg every 6 hours on days −8 to −5. Cyclophosphamide was administered at a dose of 60 mg/kg as 1 hour infusion on days −4 and −3.

Blood samples. Blood sampling (10 ml heparinized) was performed before VP-16, during VP-16 administration and after the end of the infusion up to two days after the BMT resulting in total numbers of blood samples between 24 and 30. Samples were centrifuged on the ward and stored in the refrigerator until plasma samples were aliquotted and stored in the freezer until analysis was performed.

HPLC assay for the determination of VP-16. A solid-liquid extraction procedure with CN-material filled cartridges was used. VP-16 was separated by use of a CN-material filled analytical column and quantified by evaluations of signals from the electrochemical detector. The lowest amount of VP-16 detectable in a 1 ml plasma sample was 50 ng/ml. For a detailed assay characteristics see reference [7]. "Free" VP-16 levels (not bound to protein respectively albumine) were determined by use of ultrafiltrate samples. 1 ml plasma was centrifuged through a membrane filter integrated into a centrifuge tube (Centrisart, Sartorius, Göttingen, FRG). The assay procedure was validated according to good laboratory practice (GLP) rules.

Toxicity. The hematologic toxicity was monitored daily by complete blood counts. Toxicities were graded using a score system developed at the BMT center in Seattle.

Pharmacokinetic calculations. All concentration versus time curves were analyzed with a pharmacokinetic data analysis system named TopFIT [8]. All c(t)-curves were fitted according to a three-compartment model because of the results of the inbuilt statistics (F-ratio test, Akaike Information Criterion (AIC) and analysis of the residuals) which gave best results by use of this model type. All grafic and statistical evaluations (t-test: grouped data) were performed with the program FigP (Biosoft, Cambridge, England).

Results

The c(t)-curves showed a high inter-patient variability. Typical curves for the three applications modes can be seen in Figures 1–6. Patients with short and long elimination phases (terminal half-life) are shown. The figures show the total as well as the "free" VP-16 levels in plasma and ultrafiltrate samples.

The terminal half-life, mean residence time (MRT), volume of distribution at steady state normalized to 1 kg BW, (Vss), plasma clearance normalized to 1 m^2 BSA (Clp) and area under the curve normalized to 30 mg/kg (AUC) values are given in Table 1. The pharmacokinetic parameters in case of 6 hour and 34 hour infusion were not significant different whereas the AUC, Vss and Clp were significantly different in case of the split mode application when compared either with the 6 hour infusion or the 34 hour infusion mode (Table 2).

VP-16 was detectable in 60% of all patients at the time of bone marrow transplantation. The blood levels of VP-16 at that time point varied between 80 to 820 ng/ml.

The overall time in hours for different VP-16 blood levels (0,05, > 0.1, > 1, > 10 and >100 µg/ml) are given in Table 3. The time (days) of leucocyte levels < 0.2, < 0.5 and < 1.0/nl in patients receiving ***allogeneic*** bone marrow related to the used VP-16 schedule is given in Table 4.

The time of detectable plasma levels was longest and significant different in case of the 34 hours infusion and in the 3 day split application mode when compared to the 6 hour infusion.

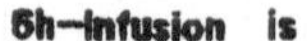

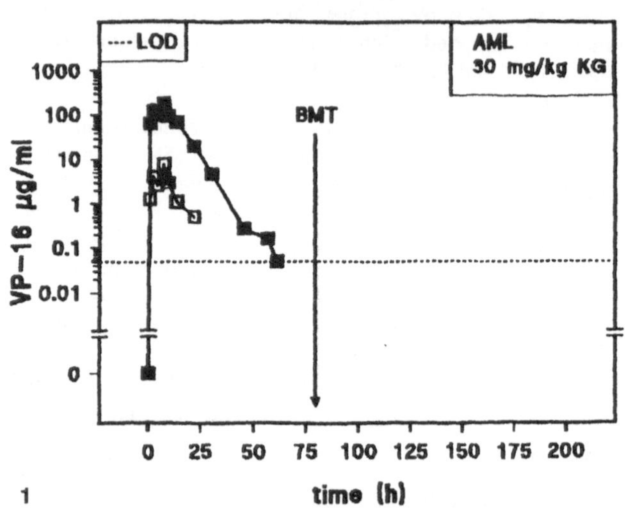

Figs. 1 and 2. c(t)-curves of VP-16 (6-hour infusion)

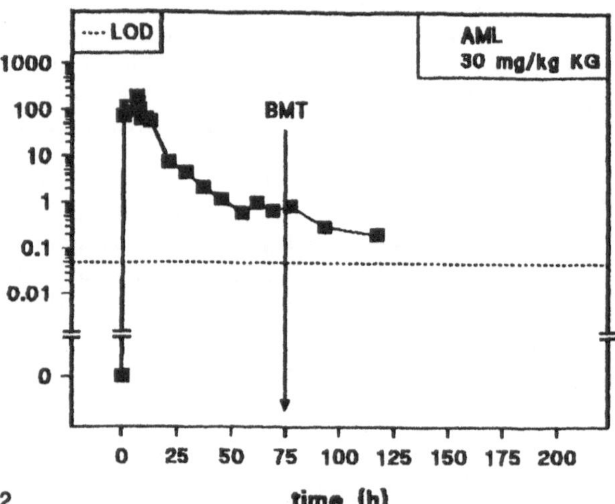

The longest aplasia and therefore greatest myelotoxicity was seen in case of the 3 discrete daily VP-16 pulses despite of the lowest systemic drug exposure and highest systemic clearance of this mode of application.

VP-16 plasma free samples (ultrafiltrate) showed that only a very minor part of about 1 to 3% of the total dose is "free" VP-16; most of the VP-16 is bound to protein (albumine). In case of the split mode the "free" fraction of VP-16 was twice the value obtained after a 34 hour infusion. At the time of BMT no "free" VP-16 was detectable in plasma samples.

Discussion

The results of these three pharmacokinetic studies [9–11] are interesting in several aspects. The volume of distribution as well as the systemic clearance of VP-16 is comparable to what was described in the literature (see in [7, 10]). A large variation of the pharmacokinetic parameters were found within each study and between studies. The elimination half-life which is longer than expected depends on the sensitivity of the used assay and different sampling periods. The assay used for the present study is sensitive

Figs. 3 and 4. c(t)-curves of VP-16 (34-hour infusion)

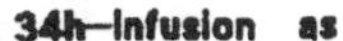

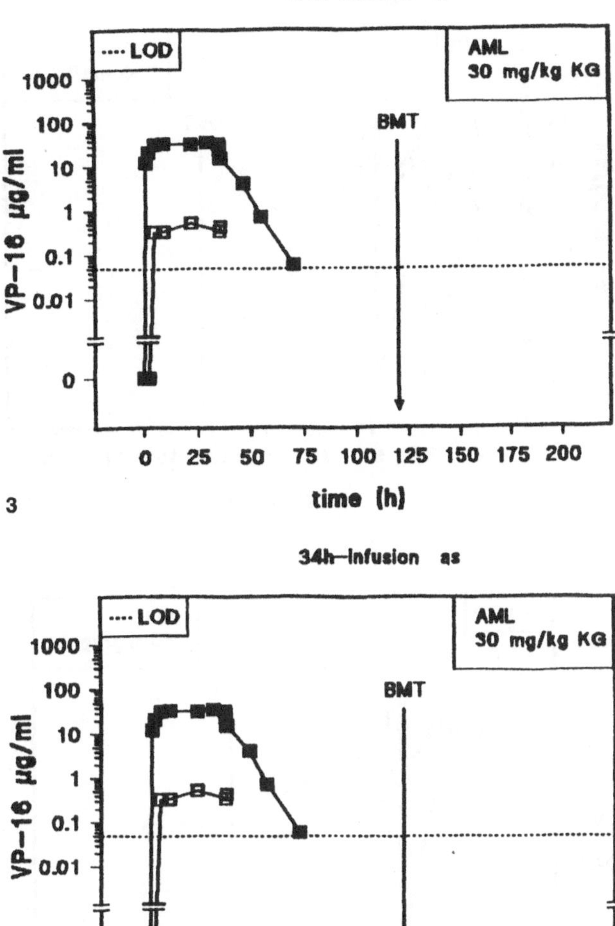

(much more than e.g. UV-detection) and the sampling period in this study was long enough to ensure precise determinations of the terminal half-life. In general the more sensitive assays use more complex models for pharmacokinetic analysis, consequently the half-life increases with the number of compartments used in the model. The majority of the pharmacokinetic studies of VP-16 have used a two-compartment model with a median half-life of 5.6 hours and, as anticipated, studies using three-compartment analysis have calculated longer terminal half-lives. The clinical relevance of using multicompartment analysis for calculating the terminal half-life of VP-16 has yet to be ascertained. The elimination phase represents only $7 \pm 5\%$ of the total drug exposure (AUC). If this small part of the total drug exposure is important for anti-cancer activity remains unknown.

The administration of high dose VP-16 within 6 hours is hampered by a large fluid volume because it is a common procedure to dilute VP-16 which is delivered in a complex solvent, highly concentrated (20 mg/ml) solution. This problem can be overcome by administration of the concentrated solution which is bioequivalent

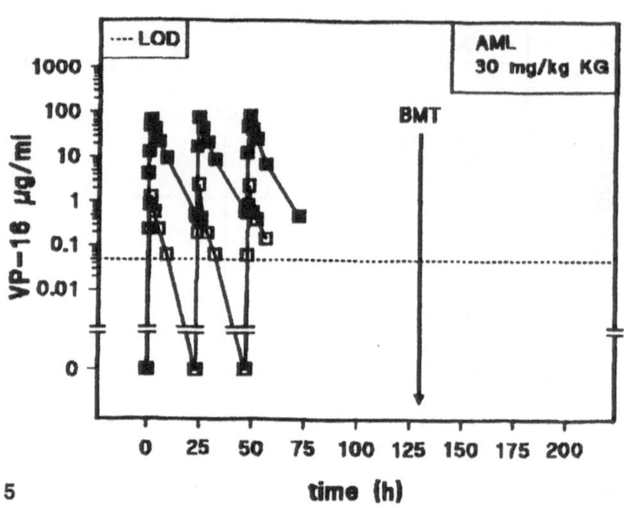

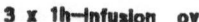

5

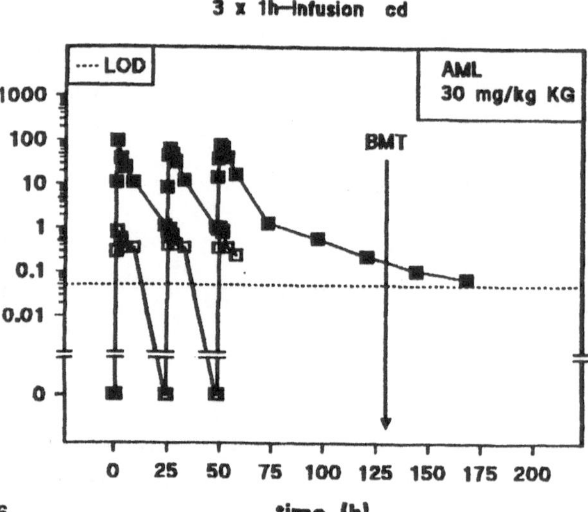

6

Figs. 5 and 6. c(t)-curves of VP-16 (1-hour, 3-day split)

Table 1. Pharmacokinetic results of three different schedule for high-dose VP-16 administration

	6h-infusion	34h-infusion	3 × 1h-infusion
	9	7	7
$t_{1/2\gamma}$ (h)	20.1 ± 12.8	20.8 ± 12.3	38.2 ± 24.3
MRT (h)	5.6 ± 1.5	5.2 ± 1.1	9.0 ± 2.8
V_{ss} (L/kg)	0.19 ± 0.08	0.14 ± 0.04	0.42 ± 0.22
Cl_p (ml/min/m*)	21.8 ± 7.6	19.1 ± 2.6	28.5 ± 8.0
AUC (µg/ml)h	1051 ± 344	1064 ± 199	706.0 ± 181

Table 2. Statistics of the pharmacokinetical comparisons

	6h vs 34h	6h vs 3 × 1h	34h vs 3 × 1h
$t_{1/2\gamma}$	not significant	$P<0.01$	not significant
MRT	not significant	not significant	$P<0.05$
V_{ss}	not significant	$P<0.05$	$P<0.05$
Cl_p	not significant	not significant	$P<0.05$
AUC	not significant	$P<0.05$	$P<0.05$

Table 3. Time of WBC below three cut-off levels. (Only allogeneic BMT)

WBC counts	6h-infusion	34h-infusion	3 × 1h-infusion
$<0.2\times10^9$/L	4 ± 4	8 ± 3	12 ± 4
$<0.5\times10^9$/L	8 ± 3	10 ± 3	14 ± 4
$<1.0\times10^9$/L	12 ± 4	14 ± 4	17 ± 4

Table 4. Time in hours for different VP-16 blood levels

Blood levels	6h-infusion	34h-infusion	3 × 1 h-infusion
>0.05 µg/ml	79 ± 21	114 ± 39	134 ± 28
>0.1 µg/ml	76 ± 24	101 ± 35	116 ± 34
>1.0 µg/ml	32 ± 8	45 ± 4	41 ± 20
>10.0 µg/ml	13 ± 3	35 ± 1	19 ± 7
>100.0 µg/ml	3 ± 2	0 ± 0	0 ± 0

in pharmacokinetic terms [9,12–13]. It is known from cell culture experiments as well as from clinical trials in the normal dose range that for the same cell kill in cancer cell lines, 100 times the dose of etoposide is required in a 1 hour exposure compared to a continuous incubation. This is consistent with the fact that VP-16 is a phase-specific drug. Results from cell culture experiments using original plasma samples of this pharmacokinetic study for CFU-C measurements indicate, that 0.38 µg/ml in plasma leads to an inhibition of 50% of the progenitor cells [14, 15]. In case of absence of albumine the IC^{50} is much lower as it was 0.01 µg/ml [16]. A significant correlation ($p<0.05$) between the CFU-C inhibition and the VP-16 concentration at the time of BMT as well as a significant correlation between the CFU-C inhibition at the time of BMT and the duration of time to an increase of WBC$>0.2\times10^9$/L was found. Patients with a long terminal half-life of VP-16 due to e.g. a reduced plasma clearance which leads to a significant VP-16 plasma level at the scheduled day of BMT have a higher risk for a prolonged aplasia time [15]. VP-16 drug monitoring (TDM) can help to reduce such risk and will be recommended.

The complete administration of the total drug amount within the shortest possible time is probably not the best schedule to reach the greatest efficacy in cancer cell kill. Cell cycle kinetics of tumor cells do not support such a procedure. Even more important than the cell cycle stage of tumor cells seems to be the proliferative state. Proliferative states may include a cycling or proliferative subpopulation, a non-cycling or quiescent subpopulation and a non-proliferating subpopulation destined to death. The greatest antitumor cell activity was observed in exponentially growing cells, non-proliferative cells were also killed as dose or drug exposure time of VP-16 was increased.

The measured myelotoxicity after 6 hour infusion of VP-16 is significantly less than after the split mode of administration. The 6 times longer infusion time (34 hour infusion) is in pharmacokinetic terms (AUC, Vss and Clp) identical with the 6 hour infusion. The only difference is the total time of detectable plasma levels, which is longer. Concentrations >10 μg/ml are twice longer if compared to the 6 hour infusion or to the split mode. Nevertheless, the myelotoxicity in patients treated with 34 hour infusion was not different if compared with the 6 hour infusion mode.

The 3 day administration mode offered three discrete, daily 1 hour pulses of VP-16 with a significant lower systemic exposure, a significant higher plasma clearance and a significant higher volume of distribution for etoposide. This schedule showed the greatest myelotoxicity with the longest aplasia time (at different leucocyte count thresholds). The pulsed administration mimics two different conditions: for a short respectively intermediate time high concentrations of a cytostatic agent as well as sustained low plasma levels. These features are optimal for a phase specific anti-cancer drug and to overcome resistance.

The reason for the higher Vss, the lower AUC and the greater Clp is not clear. The pharmacokinetic results were determined by use of the third VP-16 administration of the three day split mode to calculate the terminal phase correct. For the calculations 1/3 of the total dose was used which was 10–15 mg/kg. Nonlinear pharmacokinetics from about 15 mg/kg upwards would offer an explanation. Saturation effects for excretion, metabolization and tissue binding are factors which can influence the pharmacokinetics in these high dose ranges.

Up to now there is only one possible pharmacodynamic explanations for the greater efficacy in terms of different myelotoxicity: the presence of three separate daily exposures to VP-16. There was no greater duration of low plasma concentrations of drug>1.0 μg/ml in favour of one of the used schedules. The AUC which is the real drug exposure for the patient is obviously not the only determinant relevant for toxicity and for anticancer activity.

Still another point is the high and very variable amount of VP-16's binding to albumine [17]. The protein binding of etoposide is of such an order that it is likely to influence not only their pharmacokinetics in vivo, but also their cytotoxic effects. The "free" amount of VP-16 is very low (less than 5%). We have found in case of the split mode twice as much "free" VP-16 when compared to the 34 hour or 6 hour infusion mode. A significant higher amount of "free" VP-16 would offer another explanation for the differences in the myelotoxicity because "free" VP-16 is much more toxic than protein-bound VP-16. If the amount of "free" VP-16 is important for the anticancer activity, the higher "free" VP-16 fraction after the split mode would favour such a pulsed application mode. Within this context it is worthwhile to mention the inhibition of the formation of Ara-CTP, the intracellular phosphorylated Ara-C which is the prerequisite for its cytotoxic effects, by VP-16 in in-vitro studies [18]. This phenomenon can only be observed in the presence of "free" VP-16. In-vitro and invivo studies have shown that the high degree of protein (albumine) binding invivo (>96%) offsets the inhibitory effect on Ara-CTP formation [19]. The influence of VP-16 on ARA-C metabolism, shown in vitro, is a concentration-dependant event occurring when the cells are exposed to high levels of "free" drug. Therefore one can conclude that VP-16 administration to the patient has no adverse effect on Ara-C efficacy in case of a high albumine bound VP-16 fraction.

Another interaction with large influence on the pharmacokinetics of VP-16 is the co-administration of cyclosporin A. Resistance related to the multi drug resistance (MDR) gene and its gene product the drug efflux pump p-glycoprotein 170 (Pg-170) affects all natural anti-cancer drugs including VP-16. Several drugs (e.g. verapamil, tamoxifen, amphotericin B, cyclosporin A and others) can inhibit partly or complete this efflux pump in resistant cancer cells [20]. It was recently shown that cyclosporin A at steady state concentration of>2000 ng/ml increases VP-16 systemic exposure and hematological toxicity. The AUC of VP-16 was nearly doubled, the renal and nonrenal clearance was reduced which is consistent with inhibition of the multidrug transporter p-glycoprotein in normal tissue (in the liver and in the kidney) [21]. In case of implementation of resistance modifying agents (RMA's) into therapeutic concepts within high-dose regimen, careful pharmacokinetic and dynamic studies are necessary.

Conclusion

VP-16 has a long terminal half life, this can lead to significant VP-16 blood levels at the planned time of BMT. In case of detectable blood levels at the time of BMT, a longer aplasia phase is possible. The toxicity is schedule-dependant.

Three separate daily exposures to VP-16 are more toxic despite lower AUC if compared to 34-hour or 6-hour infusions. The administration of high-dose VP-16 should be done in a split mode to optimize the anticancer efficacy. In case of implementation of RMA's into conditioning regimen drug monitoring is highly recommended.

Acknowledgements. These studies were supported by Hamburger Krebsgesellschaft and Erich und Gertrud Roggenbruck Stiftung Hamburg. Many thanks to all members of the pharmacology laboratory and the bone marrow transplantation team of the department oncology and hematology.

Pure VP-16 and VM-26 necessary for the development of a VP-16 HPLC assay and for assay quality controls were kindly provided by Bristol Meyers Squibb.

References

1. Cockayne TO, Leech Book of Bald. Leechdon, Wartcunning and Starcraft of Early England. London, England, Holland Press 1961
2. Clark PI, Slevin ML, The clinical pharmacology of etoposide and teniposide. Clin Pharmacokinet 12: 223–253, 1987
3. Dombernowsky P, Nissen NJ, Schedule dependency of the antileukemic activity of the podophyllotoxin derivative VP 16–213 (NSC-141540) in L1210 leukemia. Acta Path Microbiol Scand Section (A) 81: 715–724, 1973
4. Roed H, Vindelov LL, Christensen IJ et al., The effect of the two epipodopyllotoxin derivatives etoposide (VP-16) and teniposide (VM-26) on cell lines established from patients with small cell carcinoma of the lung. Cancer Chemother Pharmacol 19: 16–20, 1987
5. Slevin ML, Clark PI, Joel SP et al., A randomized trial to evaluate the effect of schedule on the activity of etoposide in small cell lung cancer. J Clin Oncol 7: 1333–1340, 1989
6. Zander AR, Culbert S, Jagannath S, Spitzer G et al., High dose cyclophophamide, BCNU and VP-16 (CBV) as a condition regimen for allogenic bone marrow transplantation for patients with acute leukemia. Cancer 59: 1083–1086, 1987
7. Mross K, Bewermeier P, Hamm K et al., Pharmacokinetics of etoposide after high-dose chemotherapy conditioning regimen for bone marrow transplantation. In: Autologous bone marrow transplantation for Hodgkin's Disease, Non-Hodgkin's Lymphoma and Multiple Myeloma eds. Zander AR, Barlogie B, Springer, Berlin 54–67, 1993
8. Heinzel G, Woloszczak R, Thomann P, Pharmacokinetic and pharmacodynamic data analysis system for the PC, Fischer, Stuttgart, 1993
9. Mross K, Bewermeier P, Krüger M et al. Pharmacokinetics of undiluted or diluted high-dose etoposide with or without busulfan administered to patients with hematologic malignancies. J Clin Oncol 12: 1468–1474, 1994
10. Mross K Bewermeier P, Reifke J et al. Pharmacokinetics of high-dose VP-16: 6-hour infusion versus 34-hour infusion, Bone Marrow Transplantation 13: 423–430, 1994
11. Mross K., Reifke J, Bewermeier P et al., Pharmacokinetics of high-dose VP-16: 34-hour infusion versus 1-hour infusion split over 3 days (submitted 1994)
12. Ehninger G, Proksch B, Schmidt H et al., Unaltered pharmacokinetics after administration of high-dose etoposide without prior dilution. Cancer Chemother Pharmacol 28: 316–320, 1992
13. Creger RJ, Fox DRM, Lazarus HM, Infusion of high doses of undiluted etoposide through central venous catheters during preparation for bone marrow transplantation. Cancer Invest 8: 13–16, 1990
14. Baily-Wood R, Dallimore CM, Littlewood TJ et al., The effect of etoposide on human CFU-GM. Br J Cancer 52: 613–616, 1985
15. Postmus PE, De Vries EGE, De Vries-Hospers HG et al. Cyclophosphamide and VP-16 with autologous bone marrow transplantation. A dose escalation study. Eur J Cancer Clin Oncol 20: 777–782. 1984
16. Berger C, CFU-C Inhibition durch VP-16-haltige Plasmaproben: Biologische Aktivität von Etoposid (VP-16) in Plasmaproben nach hochdosierter Chemotherapie im Rahmen der Konditionierung vor der Knochenmarktransplantation, Dissertation, Universität Hamburg, Medizinische Fakultät 1993
17. Fleming RA, Evans WE, Arbruck SG et al. Factors affecting in vitro protein binding of etoposide in humans. J Pharmacetical Sciences 81: 259–264, 1992
18. Ehninger G, Proksch B, Wanner T et al., Intracellular cytosine arabinoside accumulation and cytosine arabinoside triphosphate formation in leukemic blast cells is inhibited by etoposide and teniposide. Leukemia 6: 582–587, 1992
19. Liliemark J, Knochenhauer E, Gruber A et al., On the interaction between cytosine arabinoside and etoposide in vivo and in vitro. Eur J Haematol 50: 22–25, 1993
20. Mross KB, Klinische und pharmakologische Untersuchungen zur Pharmakokinetik, Metabolisierung, Pharmakodynamik und Toxizität von Anthrazyklinen, Zuckschwerdtverlag, München. 1994
21. Lum BL, Kaubisch S, Yahanda AM et al., Alteration of etoposide pharmacokinetics and pharmacodynamics by cyclosporin in a phase I trial to modulate multidrug resistance. J Clin Oncol 10: 1635–1642, 1992

Acute Leukemias V
Experimental Approaches
and Management of Refractory Diseases
Hiddemann et al. (Eds.)

Targeted Drug Therapy in Childhood Acute Lymphoblastic Leukemia

Mary V. Relling, Ching-Hon Pui, and William E. Evans

Introduction

Pediatric acute lymphoblastic leukemia (ALL) is one of the most drug-responsive cancers, with approximately 70% of children being cured with chemotherapy alone (Pui and Crist, 1994). Focussing on the collective good responsiveness, however, may obscure the fact that there remain children who are not cured, and there are children who experience excessive toxicity from regimens that are well tolerated by the majority of children. Of the many factors that can affect how an individual responds to a particular ALL treatment regimen, one factor may be variability in the pharmacokinetics of antineoplastic agents. We describe herein our studies of whether overall clinical outcome is related to pharmacokinetic variability.

Background and Rationale

Several studies have suggested that disease-free survival of children with ALL is related to the pharmacokinetics of drugs that constitute a major component of treatment regimens. In our Study X for childhood ALL, a major component of therapy was 15 courses of high-dose methotrexate (1 g/m^2 over 24 hours), given in the first 72 weeks of continuation therapy. Relapse-free survival was significantly better in a group of 49 children whose median methotrexate Cp_{SS} exceeded 16 μM, compared to a group of 59 children whose median steady-state plasma concentration (Cp_{SS}) was <16 μM (Evans et al. 1986). Moreover, children with higher methotrexate Cp_{SS} had a significantly better continuous complete remission rate at 4 years (74%) than a historic control group (50%) who received similar therapy but *no* high-dose methotrexate (p=.004) (Evans et al. 1987; Abromowitch et al. 1988), suggesting that the addition of high-dose methotrexate is an important component of ALL regimens. The clinical antileukemic effect of high-dose methotrexate has also been suggested by Feickert et al. (1993), who reported improved event-free survival in children with T-cell ALL treated in a BFM regimen with 5 g/m^2 compared to 0.5 g/m^2. Notwithstanding these observations, methotrexate Cp_{ss} was not a prognostic indicator in patients with low-risk ALL (Camitta et al. 1989; Evans et al. 1990). Thus, the intensity of methotrexate treatment (e.g., systemic exposure) may be of greatest importance in the subgroup of patients at higher risk of treatment failure.

Teniposide (VM26) pharmacokinetics have also been shown to be of prognostic importance in a relatively small Phase I–II trial of escalating doses of teniposide (Rodman et al. 1987). In that study, 28 children, 13 of whom had relapsed ALL, were treated with teniposide at 300 to 750 mg/m^2 as a 72 hour continuous infusion. Both tumor response and toxicity were positively correlated with teniposide Cp_{SS}, while there was no significant relationship between dose and the same parameters. Most of the antitumor responses were found in the children with ALL, with the responses being more common in those

St. Jude Children's Research Hospital and Colleges of Pharmacy and Medicine, University of Tennessee, Memphis, USA

with teniposide Cp_{ss} > 12 mg/l. The substantial variability (4–6 fold) in clearance among patients resulted in wide overlap of systemic exposure at various dosage levels, rendering it difficult to recommended a Phase III dosage that would be optimal for all patients.

Another key component of continuation therapy for ALL is daily treatment with 6-mercaptopurine (6MP). In the United Kingdom's ALL (UKALL) trials VIII and X, oral 6-mercaptopurine and weekly methotrexate comprised the major components of therapy (Lennard et al. 1989). Red blood cell intracellular concentrations of 6-thioguanine nucleotides (active metabolites of 6-mercaptopurine) were evaluated as indicators of 6-mercaptopurine systemic exposure in 120 children. When children were divided into those whose 6-thioguanine nucleotide concentrations were greater than versus less than the median in the population, those children with higher 6-thioguanine nucleotides had a significant improvement in their long-term disease-free survival (Lennard et al. 1989). In a multivariate analysis, only red cell 6-thioguanine nucleotides, leukocyte count at diagnosis, and sex were significant predictors of relapse-free survival.

Thus, there is evidence that estimates of increased systemic exposure to anticancer drugs, given either chronically or in intermittent pulse fashion, are predictive of improved disease-free survival in children with ALL.

Prospective Trial at St. Jude Children's Research Hospital

Although retrospective studies suggested a pharmacodynamic relationship for antileukemic drugs, it is not known if it is feasible and effective to prospectively adjust doses of antineoplastics to achieve a target level of systemic exposure in children with ALL. Thus, we designed a Phase II trial (Study XII) of childhood ALL to adaptively control systemic exposure (i.e. AUC) for each intermittent pulse treatment of antineoplastics (Evans et al. 1991a). This randomized trial was designed to test the efficacy and toxicity of targeting systemic exposure versus conventional dosing methods. After a six-drug induction regimen (prednisone, vincristine, asparaginase, daunorubicin, teniposide and cytarabine), continuation therapy was given as weekly methotrexate (40 mg/m^2) and daily oral 6-mercaptopurine (75 mg/m^2/day) for 120 weeks, interrupted by five pulses of methotrexate (conventional dose = 1.5 g/m^2) alternated every 6 weeks with five pulses of teniposide (200 mg/m^2) plus cytarabine (AraC) (300 mg/m^2) for the first year of therapy. Importantly, the conventional dose of methotrexate was chosen so that the average methotrexate Cp_{SS} would exceed the 16 μM plasma concentration, which has been associated with favorable outcome in our previous study (Evans et al. 1986). Thus, the study was not biased toward under-treatment in the conventional arm. Likewise, the doses of teniposide and cytarabine were chosen so that a patient with average clearance of both agents would have an exposure expected to have an acceptable (but not a negligible) degree of toxicity. Moreover, the target AUC for teniposide was that associated with a higher probability of oncolytic response in our prior Phase I–II study (Rodman et al. 1987).

The major objective in the targeted arm was to avoid low systemic exposure (lowest 50th percentile, i.e. "below average") in children whose clearance of these agents was in the highest 50th percentile, and to avoid unusually high exposure (top 10th percentile of AUC) in those with very low clearance. The expected range of clearance (and thus AUC) estimates was based on several prior studies of methotrexate, teniposide, and cytarabine disposition in children (Sinkule et al. 1983, 1984; Evans et al. 1986; Rodman et al. 1987). Our goal was to avoid both sub-therapeutic and unusually high systemic exposure to the anticancer drugs comprising the pulse therapy. Although dosages of the weekly low-dose methotrexate and daily 6-mercaptopurine were not adjusted based on patient pharmacokinetics, red blood cell methotrexate polyglutamates and 6-thioguanine nucleotide metabolites were monitored at least 3 times per year in all children for their entire 120 weeks of continuation therapy. Interestingly, two of the 188 patients enrolled on Total XII (one received conventional and the other targeted therapy) were found to be phenotypically deficient in thiopurine methyltransferase, one of the key enzymes in the metabolism of 6-mercaptopurine (Evans et al. 1991b). Thus, both these children required a substantial reduction in 6-mercaptopurine dosages, allowing essentially normal delivery of their teniposide/cytarabine and methotrexate pulse therapy and weekly low-dose methotrexate injections.

Methotrexate was given as a 200 mg/m^2 intravenous (IV) loading dose over 1 hour and followed by 1300 mg/m^2 over the next 23 hours. Appropriate hydration, alkalinization, and leucovorin rescue were given. methotrexate was assayed in plasma samples obtained pre-dose and at 1, 6, and 23 hours from the start of each methotrexate infusion. In the 50% of children randomized to the targeted arm, methotrexate concentrations at 1 and 6 hours were used to estimate clearance and the predicted Cp_{SS}, and dosage adjustments were made by hour 8 of each 24 hour infusion. Pharmacokinetic parameters were estimated using a Bayesian algorithm and a two-compartment model (Evans et al. 1991a), using a modification of the ADAPT software (D'Argenio and Schumitzky, 1979) (USC, Los Angeles, USA). Parameter estimates were used to determine the infusion rate necessary to achieve a predicted AUC within the target range, which was 640 to 900 μM·hr. If the predicted AUC was within this range, no dosage adjustment was made, and the conventional dosing rate continued. Children with very low clearance estimates (about 10% of the population), such that their predicted AUC was > 900 μM·hr, had a reduction in infusion rate to achieve the target AUC of 800 μM·hr. However, the rate was not decreased to such an extent that the predicted Cp_{SS} would be < 20 μM. Children with clearance estimates higher than the population median, such that their predicted AUC was < 640 μM·hrs, had a rate increase (8 hours into the infusion) to achieve the target AUC of 800 μM·hr. In order to evaluate the achieved systemic exposure, pharmacokinetic parameters were estimated again using the 1, 6, and 23 hour methotrexate plasma concentrations and the Bayesian algorithm described above. This clearance estimate was then used to determine whether the patient would be predicted to achieve an AUC in the target range if they were given 1500 mg/m^2. If their clearance was estimated as either too high (> 86 ml/min/m^2) or too low (< 61 ml/min/m^2), then a dose for the subsequent course was chosen to achieve the target AUC of 800 μM·hr. The same process of measuring methotrexate plasma concentrations, estimating clearance, and adaptively controlling infusion rates was repeated with each of the 5 courses of high-dose methotrexate.

Teniposide and cytarabine were administered as concurrent 4 hour IV infusions on day 1 and day 3, every 12 weeks. In May of 1991, the protocol was amended to administer teniposide and cytarabine only on day 1 every 12 weeks, to decrease the frequency of fever and neutropenia following the teniposide/cytarabine pulses and to avoid the possible schedule-dependent risk of secondary acute myeloid leukemia following epipodophyllotoxin therapy (Pui et al. 1991). The conventional dose (and starting dose in the targeted patients) of teniposide was 200 mg/m^2, with 45% of the dose (90 mg/m^2) given over 1 hour, and the remainder given over the following 3 hours. The conventional dose of cytarabine was 300 mg/m^2, given as a 30 mg/m^2 loading dose IV push, with the remainder given as an IV infusion over the next 4 hours. Blood samples were obtained in all children with both Day 1 and Day 3 (when applicable) doses at 1 and 3 hours (both during the infusions), 8 hours, and approximately 20 hours from the start of the infusions, and assayed by separate HPLC assays for cytarabine and teniposide (Sinkule et al. 1983, 1984; Relling et al. 1992). Clearance was estimated as described above; a one-compartment model using the 1 and 3 hour concentrations was used for cytarabine and a two-compartment model with all 4 concentrations was used to obtain teniposide clearance estimates. For teniposide, the AUC target range was 400–500 μM·hr per dose, with the target AUC being 450 μM·hr. For cytarabine, the AUC target range is 25–57 μM·hr per dose, with the target AUC being 42 μM·hr. For children randomized to the targeted therapy, as for methotrexate, if the clearance estimates were such that the conventional dose would be predicted to produce an AUC within the target range, no dosage alteration was made for the subsequent dosages. If the clearance estimates were too high (> 49.3 l/hr/m^2 for cytarabine or > 12.7 ml/min/m^2 for teniposide) or too low (< 21.6 l/hr/m^2 for cytarabine or < 10.2 ml/min/m^2 for teniposide), the doses were appropriately adjusted with the next course. The process of measuring teniposide and cytarabine plasma concentrations and estimating clearance was repeated with every dose of every course, so that doses were continuously controlled adaptively in the targeted cases.

Some dosage adjustments were not based entirely on patient pharmacokinetics. For all children (conventional and targeted), if a child had two consecutive pulses that were followed by unacceptable toxicity, the dose was reduced by 25% from the toxic dose for all subsequent courses. Moreover, for teniposide and cytarabine (for which no rescue agent was available), the maximum dosage increase and decrease between any two dosages was 50% and 25%, respectively.

Preliminary Results

Because many patients remain on therapy, a full analysis of toxicities and long-term efficacy in the targeted versus the conventional arms is not yet available. However, the procedure of adaptively controlling systemic exposure to chemotherapy has proven to be feasible. We have now performed these dosage adjustments in over 425 courses of methotrexate and over 680 doses of teniposide/cytarabine. Adverse effects have been similar in the targeted and conventional arms, despite the fact that the average doses of methotrexate, teniposide, and cytarabine are about 1.4 times higher in the targeted arm for all 3 drugs. Although not yet proven, this equivalent tolerance between the two arms probably results from the avoidance of unnecessarily high AUC in the children on the targeted arm who have clearances in the lowest 10th percentile.

As anticipated, our preliminary analysis indicates that the target AUC was achieved in significantly more courses for the targeted arm than in the conventional arm for all three drugs: 87% versus 38% for methotrexate, 60% versus 42% for teniposide, and 62% versus 41% for cytarabine (all $p<.0001$ by chi square test). Thus, we were successful in achieving AUCs within the target range in the majority of patients on the targeted arm, and the distribution of AUCs achieved in the conventionally treated cases was as expected.

In summary, it is feasible to adaptively control patients' exposure to multiple anticancer drugs in a Phase III trial using limited sampling and a Bayesian algorithm to estimate clearances. Moreover, it is possible to avoid both very high and low systemic exposure in patients by this control strategy. Whether there are any long term-differences in overall toxicity or efficacy awaits longer follow-up.

Ackowledgements. We gratefully acknowledge the pharmacokinetic expertise of Drs. John Rodman, William Crom, Clinton Stewart, and our post-doctoral fellows; the technical assistance of the Pharmaceutical Department staff; the clinical care provided by the staff of SJCRH; and the participation of patients and their families in these studies.

Supported by NIH Leukemia Program Project Grant NCI PO1 CA-20180, NIH R29 CA51001, R37 CA36401, Cancer Center CORE grant CA21765, by a Center of Excellence grant from the State of Tennessee, and American Lebanese Syrian Associated Charities (ALSAC).

References

1. Abromowitch M, Ochs J, Pui C-H, Kalwinsky D, Rivera GK, Fairclough D, Look AT, Hustu O, Murphy SB, Evans WE, Dahl GV, Bowman WP. High-dose methotrexate improves clinical outcome in children with acute lymphoblastic Leukemia: St. Jude Total Therapy Study X. Med Pediatr Oncol 16: 297–303, 1988.
2. Camitta B, Leventhal B, Lauer S, et al. Intermediate-dose intravenous methotrexate and mercaptopurine therapy for non-T, non-B acute lymphocytic leukemia of childhood: a Pediatric Oncology Group study. J Clin Oncol 7: 1539–44, 1989.
3. D'Argenio DZ, A. Schumitzky. A program package for simulation and parameter estimation in pharmacokinetic systems. Computer Programs in Biomedicine. 9, 115–134 (1979).
4. Evans WE, Rodman JR, Relling MV, Crom WR, Rivera GK, Crist WM, Pui C-H. Individualized dosages of chemotherapy as a strategy to improve response for acute lymphocytic leukemia. Semin Hematology 1991a;28: (suppl 4) 15–21.
5. Evans WE, Crom WR, Abromowitch M, Dodge R, Look T, Bowman P, George SL, Clinical pharmacodynamics of high-dose methotrexate in acute lymphocytic leukemia: Identification of a concentration-effect relationship. N Engl J Med 314: 471–477, 1986.
6. Evans WE, Abromowitch M, Crom WR, Relling MV, Bowman WP, Pui C-H, Ochs J, Dodge R. Clinical pharmacodynamic studies of high-dose methotrexate in acute lymphocytic leukemia. NCI Monogr 5: 81–85, 1987.
7. Evans WE, Horner M, Chu YQ, Kalwinsky D, Roberts WM. Altered mercaptopurine metabolism, toxicity and dosage requirements in a thiopurine methyltransferase-deficient child with acute lymphocytic leukemia. J. Peds. 119: 985–989. 1991b.
8. Evans WE, Pui C-H, Schell MJ. MTX clearance more important for intermediate-risk ALL (Letter). J Clin Oncol 8: 1115–1116, 1990.
9. Feickert HJ, Bettoni C, Schrappe M, Reiter A, Ludwig W-D, Bode U, Ebell W, Riehm H. Event-free survival of children with T-cell acute lymphoblastic leukemia after introduction of high dose methotrexate in multicenter trial ALL-BFM 86. ASCO Proc 12: 317, 1993.

10. Lennard L, and Lilleyman JS. Variable mercaptopurine metabolism and treatment outcome in childhood lymphoblastic leukemia. J Clin Oncol 1989; 7: 1816–23.
11. Pui CH, Riberio R, Hancock ML, Rivera GK, Evans WE, Raimondi, S, David R. Head, Fred G. Behm, M. Hazem Mahmoud, John T Sandlund, William Crist: Acute myeloid leukemia in children treated with epipodophyllotoxins for acute lymphocytic leukemia. N. Engl. J. Med. 325: 1682–7, 1991.
12. Pui C-H, Crist WM. Biology and treatment of acute lymphoblastic leukemia. J Peds (in press) 1994.
13. Relling MV, Evans R, Desiderio D, Dass C, Nemec and J. Human cytochrome P450 metabolism of teniposide and etoposide. J Pharmacol Exp Ther 1992;261: 491–96.
14. Rodman JH, Abromowich M, Sinkule JA et al. Clinical Pharmacodynamics os Continuous Infusion Teniposide: Systemic Exposure as a Determinant of Response in a Phase I trial. J Clin Oncol. 7: 1007–1014, 1987.
15. Sinkule J, Evans WE. High performance liquid chromatography (HPLC) assay of cytosine arabinoside. J Chrom 274: 87–93, 1983.
16. Sinkule JA, Evans WE. High-performance liquid chromatographic analysis of the semi-synthetic epipodophyllotoxins, teniposide (VM26) and etoposide (VP16) using electrochemical detection. J Pharm Sci 73: 164–168, 1984.

Acute Leukemias V
Experimental Approaches
and Management of Refractory Diseases
Hiddemann et al. (Eds.)

Asparagine Levels in Children on E. Coli- and Erwinia-Asparaginase Therapy

J. Boos[1], G. Werber[2], E. Verspohl[2], E. Ahlke[1], U. Nowak-Göttl[1], and H. Jürgens[1]

Abstract. Asparaginase preparations from different biological sources are in therapeutical use. Questions remain regarding the comparability of pharmacodynamic effects. Therefore, blood concentrations of L-asparagine were monitored during therapy with Escherichia-coli asparaginase (Asparaginase Medac™, E.coli-asp) and Erwinia-caratovora asparaginase (Erwinase Porton, E-asp) on treatment according to the study ALL/NHL-BFM 90.

Erwinia-asparaginase was applied in case of allergic reaction to E.coli-asparaginase. The dose administered was 10000 U/m² on days 8,11,15 and 18 of protocol II. 6 children with E.coli-asp and 6 with E-asp were compared. Samples were taken immediately prior to application and the concentrations were monitored by HPLC.

With E.coli-asp asparagine levels were maintained above the detection limit (<0,1 μM) throughout therapy in only one child (0.08-0.2 μM), but there was no child with complete depletion in the E-asp group. The range was 0.18–92 μM on day 18 and 0.8–80 μM on day 22 in children receiving E-asp. The intensity and duration of asparagine depletion were significantly pronounced in children receiving E.coli-asp.

This finding may be due to the shorter biological half-life of E-asp and crossreacting antibodies might partly inactivate Erwinia-asp in children allergic to E.coli-asp. Therefore, substitution of different asparaginase preparations should take pharmacokinetic differences into account, and pharmacodynamic monitoring is warranted.

Introduction

L-asparaginase is a potent antileukemic enzyme used routinely in the treatment of acute leukemia in children. The enzyme catalyses the hydrolysis of L-asparagine into L-aspartic acid and ammonia [1].

Most tissues possess L-asparagine synthetase but leukemic lymphoblasts are thought to depend on exogenous asparagine related to a lack of L-asparagine-synthetase activity in sensitive cells [2]. Asparaginase therapy, therefore, aims at complete depletion of L-asparagine in plasma.

Asparaginase preparations from different biological sources are in therapeutical use. The original source for therapeutic use is the bacterium Escherichia coli but L-asparaginase obtained from Erwinia caratovora is commercially available as an alternative.

In the event of adverse reactions substitutions are widely used. Questions remain regarding the comparability of pharmacodynamic effects.

Patients

According to protocol ALL/NHL-BFM-90 therapy is initiated with E.coli-asparaginase (medac GmbH) and in case of allergic reaction substituted by Erwinia-asp (Erwinase Porton). All children underwent pharmacodynamic monitoring including serum asparagine (asn) levels. 6 children treated with E.coli-asp and 6 with

[1] Department of Pediatric Hematology/Oncology, University of Münster, 48149 Münster, Germany
[2] Institute of Pharmaceutical Chemistry, University of Münster, 48149 Münster, Germany

Erwinia-asp could be compared during consolidation therapy (protocol II). The dose administered was 10000 U/m² on days 8,11,15 and 18 of the protocol. Additional chemotherapy consisted of dexamethasone (daily), vincristine and adriamycin (once weekly).

Methods

Samples were taken immediately prior to the asparaginase application and if possible on additional days. Samples were centrifuged immediately, deproteinized with sulfosalicylic acid within 15 minutes and frozen < 80 °C. Asparagine was analyzed by HPLC following precolumn derivatization with o-phthaldialdehyde (OPA) according to Lenda and Svenneby [3]. The limit of detection is < 0,1 μM. Therefore, all samples with undetectable amounts are represented as values of 0.1 μM in Figure 1.

Results

In the group of children treated with Erwinia-asparaginase there was no child (0/6) with complete depletion (< 0,1 μM) of L-asparagine in the serum. The range was 0.18–92 μM on day 18 and 0.8–80 μM on day 22 in these children. In one child no change could be observed and the L-asparagine remained normal.

Under E.coli-asparaginase the L-asparagine levels remained measurable during therapy (0.08–0.2 μM) in only one child.

The intensity and duration of L-asparagine depletion were significantly pronounced in children receiving E.coli-asparaginase.

Discussion

We observed a marked difference in the depletion of L-asparagine between children treated with E.coli- and Erwinia-asparaginase.

While the depletion was complete with E.coli-asparaginase, there was a wide range of asparagine-levels in children treated with Erwinia-asparaginase. In one child L-asparagine levels remained normal.

Two aspects may contribute to this observation:

1. According to Asselin et al. the biological half-life of Erwinia-asparaginase is significantly shorter than that of E.coli-asparaginase [4]. In theory, substitution of a drug with a half-life of 1.3 days by one with a $t_{1/2}$ of 0.6 days requires changes in dose or interval of application.
2. The 6 children treated with Erwinia-asparaginase had shown allergic reactions to E.coli-asparaginase in the preceding induction phase of the protocol. None of them, however, had clinical signs of adverse reactions during the monitored consolidation therapy.

Crossreacting antibodies, however, might partly inactivate Erwinia-asparaginase in children allergic to E.coli-asparaginase.

In conclusion, substitution of different asparaginase preparations should take pharma-

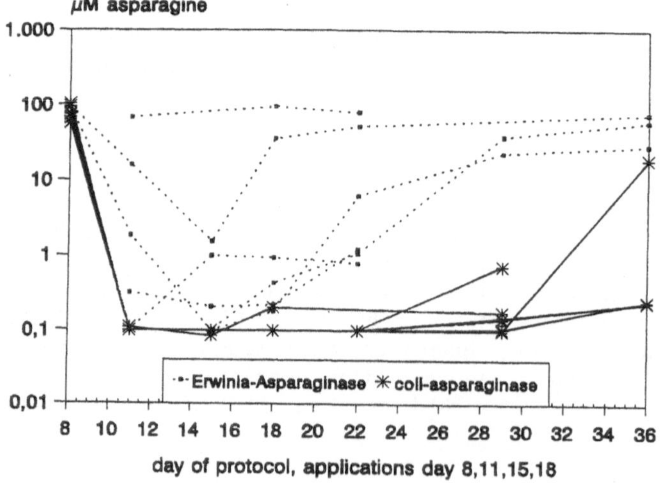

Fig. 1. L-Asparagine levels in patients with Erwinia-asparaginase or E.coli-asparaginase

cokinetic differences into account, and pharmacodynamic monitoring is warranted.

Acknowledgement. Supported by BMFT

References

1. Broome JD: L-Asparaginase: Discovery and development as a tumor-inhibiting agent. Cancer Treat Rep 65(Suppl4): 111–114; 1981
2. Charles LM, Bono VH: A review of the preclinical antitumor activity and toxicology of L-Asparaginase derived from E.coli. Cancer Treat Rep 65(Suppl 4):39–46; 1981
3. Lenda K, Svenneby G: . J Chromatogr 198: 516–519; 1980
4. Allelin BL, Whitin JC, Coppola DJ, Rupp IP, Sallan SE, Cohen HJ: Comparative pharmacokinetic studies of three Asparaginase preparations. J Clin Oncol 11: 1780–1786; 1993

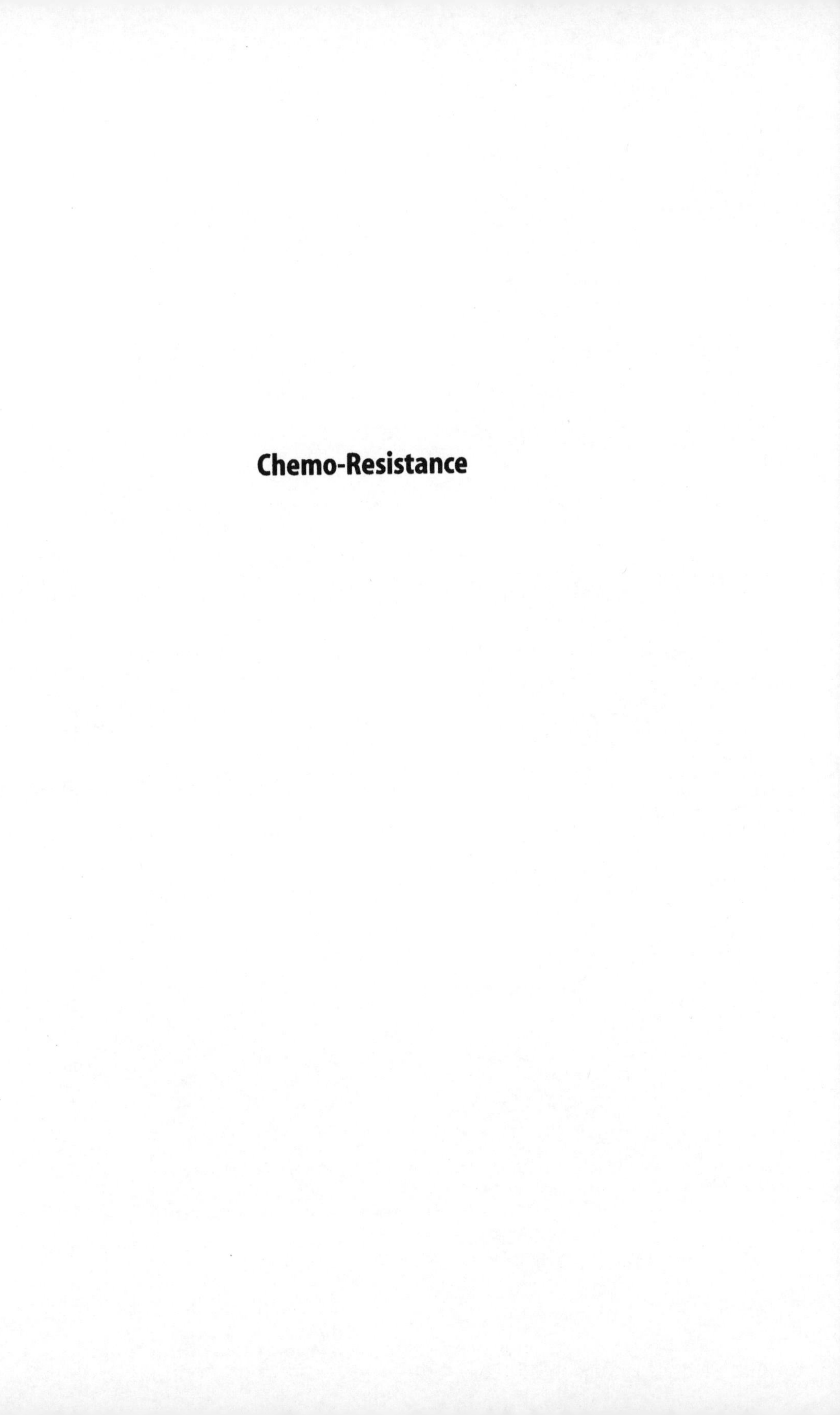

Chemo-Resistance

Acute Leukemias V
Experimental Approaches
and Management of Refractory Diseases
Hiddemann et al. (Eds.)

Pharmacologic Modulation of Multidrug Resistance in Acute Leukemia: Results and Challenges

Alan F. List, Betty Glinsmann-Gibson, and William S. Dalton

Introduction

The limited curative potential of conventional chemotherapy in patients with acute myeloid leukemia (AML) has directed attention to identification of cellular mechanisms contributing to treatment failure. Intrinsic and/or acquired resistance to antineoplastic remains a clinical challenge for patients with poor-risk AML and relapsed patients. Multidrug resistance (MDR) due to overexpression of the *mdr1* gene or its membrane product P-glycoprotein (P-gp), has been implicated as an important cellular mechanism of resistance that contributes to treatment failure in this disease [1]. Indeed, prospective studies in *de novo* AML have shown that overexpression of *mdr1* is associated with a lower complete remission rate and shorter remission duration in patients receiving conventional induction and post-remission therapy [2,3]. P-gp expression has been linked to a number of adverse prognostic variables including age, secondary leukemia, cytogenetic pattern, and a CD34 surface phenotype [3–6]. Evidence to date, indicates that *mdr1* expression is determined in part by the lineage and stage of cellular differentiation that mimics its physiologic regulation in blood cell development. Normal hematopoietic stem cells natively express high levels of *mdr1*, but a corresponding decrease in gene message is seen with myeloid maturation [7,8]. These observations suggest that expression of the MDR phenotype in AML, therefore, represents a conserved physiologic function.

Investigations of cellular pharmacodynamics of the anthracyclines have shown that blast concentrations of these agents may be a determinant of response to induction therapy [9]. Enhanced cellular extrusion of the anthracyclines is mediated in part by P-gp expression and contributes to the heterogeneity and drug retention observed in AML specimens [10, 11]. Indeed, cellular retention of daunorubicin is enhanced by exposure to P-gp antagonists such as verapamil or cyclosporin-A (Sandimmune) in blast subpopulation. These data, and observations that the decreased sensitivity to anthracyclines *in vitro* may be associated with the *mdr1* phenotype serve as the basis for testing agents capable of reversing *mdr1*-mediated drug resistance in clinical trials.

Clinical Trials

A number of noncytotoxic compounds serve as substrates for P-gp and competitively inhibit cellular extrusion of natural-product antineoplastics [12–14]. In non-Hodgkin's and multiple myeloma, verapamil has shown significant activity in restoring chemotherapy sensitivity, however, dose-related cardiovascular toxicity limits clinical application [15–17]. Cyclosporin-A is a potent inhibitor of P-gp *in vitro* at concentrations ranging from 500–2000ng/mL; concentrations that far exceed those targeted for its immunosuppressive properties [14,18]. On a molar basis, cyclosporine is a more potent

Section of Hematology/Oncology and Bone Marrow Transplant Program, Arizona Cancer Center and Departments of Medicine and Pharmacology/Toxicology, University of Arizona College of Medicine, Tucson, AZ

inhibitor of MDR both *in vitro* and in animal models compared to agents such as verapamil and quinidine. For this reason, cyclosporin-A was selected for testing in a Phase I/II trial performed at the Arizona Cancer Center in patients with poor-risk AML [19]. Patients received sequential treatment with high-dose cytarabine (3g/mg/m^2/day) daily for 5 days, followed by daunorubicin (45mg/m^2/day) administered concurrently with cyclosporin-A as a 72-hour continuous infusion. Cyclosporine dose escalations ranged from 1.5 to 20mg/kg/day. Leukemia specimens were analyzed for P-gp expression, and results confirmed by quantitative RNA polymerase chain reaction (PCR) assay for the *mdr1* gene message [20].

Forty-two patients enrolled in the trial were assessable for toxicity and response. P-gp expression was detected in over 70% of cases. Steady state blood concentrations of cyclosporin-A ranged from 500 to 3900ng/mL. Overall, 26 (62%) patients achieved a complete hematologic remission or restored chronic phase, and 3 patients achieved a partial remission for an overall response rate of 69%. Expression of P-gp did not adversely affect response to this treatment regimen. More importantly, gene message decreased at the time of disease progression in one patient achieving a partial remission, but was absent at relapse in specimens from 4 patients achieving complete hematologic remission, and remained undetectable at relapse in 2 patients who were MDR-negative prior to therapy (Fig. 1).

These results raise the possibility that this type of treatment may eliminate and/or minimize the emergence of *mdr1*-positive leukemia clones. Randomized trials are now in progress in the Southwest Oncology Group (SWOG) to determine the contribution of cyclosporine to this regimen in poor-risk AML.

Common toxicities of cyclosporine chemomodulation included nausea and vomiting (22%), hypomagnesemia (61%), burning dysesthesias (21%), and prolongation of myelosuppression. Transient hyperbilirubinemia developed in over 60% of treatment courses and was cyclosporine-dose dependent. Increased toxicity to organs that natively express P-gp, as might be expected with such a regimen, were uncommonly observed. Reversible azotemia developed during or immediately following cyclosporine administration in 2 patients receiving concurrent treatment with nephrotoxic antibiotics.

The etiology of cyclosporine-induced hyperbilirubinemia appears to result from a direct inhibitory effect on bilirubin transport. Cyclosporine is known to impair hepatic excretory function when administered on a chronic basis in patients receiving it for immunosuppression [21]. Immunodetection of P-gp is normally detected on the canalicular surface of hepatocytes [22]. However, investigations using isoform-specific antibodies indicate that the biliary form of P-gp is encoded for by the *mdr2* gene homologue, which does not confer multidrug resistance [23]. More recent studies sug-

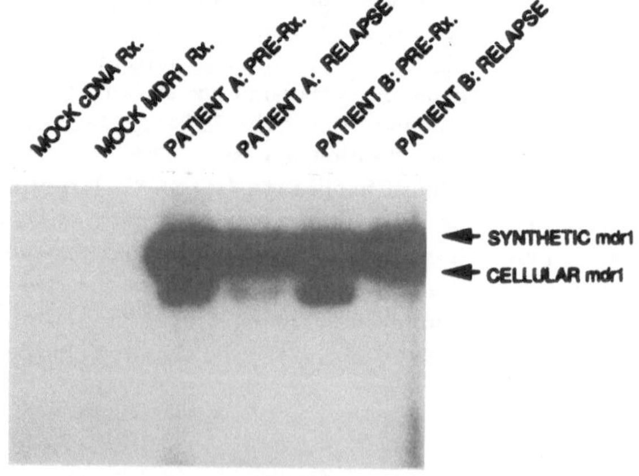

Fig. 1. Autoradiograph of RT-PCR amplification of AML patient specimens prior to treatment and at relapse. Upper band denotes synthetic mdr1 message as internal positive control; lower bands reflect cellular mdr1 gene message in patient specimens. Overexpression of mdr1 is seen prior treatment (PreRx) in both patients, but decreases or is absent in relapsed specimens

gest that the product represents only one of 5 or more biliary transport proteins that are sensitive to inhibition by cyclosporin-A. Other P-gp inhibitors may also share the cholestatic effects of cyclosporin-A. Transient hyperbilirubinemia was reported in a French trial using quinine as an MDR reversal agent when administered in conjunction with mitoxantrone [24].

It is not surprising then that hyperbilirubinemia was associated with higher plasma concentrations of daunorubicin in the Arizona trial due to presumed delay in hepatic drug clearance. Because of this, an improved response with MDR modulation might be ascribed to either increased systemic drug exposure or to MDR modulation. Likewise, results of randomized trials will also be influenced by the prevalence of *mdr1* gene overexpression in each treatment arm, the ability to achieve and sustain blood levels of chemomodulator that are effective in blocking P-gp, and/or the presence of non-MDR mechanisms of chemotherapy resistance. In the SWOG trial, cyclosporine blood levels and daunorubicin clearance will be assessed in each treatment arm, to permit valid comparison of response according to MDR phenotype and relative drug exposure.

New Agents and Strategies

The high concentrations of cyclosporine required to reverse MDR, its inherent immunosuppressive properties, and its nonspecific cholestatic effects encouraged the development of new compounds with greater P-gp specificity. Several compounds are currently in preclinical development [25,26]. One compound that has now entered clinical trials is PSC 833, an analogue of cyclosporin-D, selected because of its selective and potent inhibition of P-gp function. This compound lacks the immunosuppressive properties of cyclosporin-A but is a more potent inhibitor of P-gp function. On a molar basis, PSC 833 is approximately 5 to 10-fold more potent than the parent compound from which it is derived, cyclosporin-A [26–28]. The profound activity of this compound in reversing MDR at relatively low plasma concentrations as illustrated in Figure 2 makes it a much more attractive compound for clinical trials. In addition, preliminary results of Phase I trials in multiple myeloma have not demonstrated the cholestatic effects observed with cyclosporin-A. This agent is now being tested at the Arizona Cancer Center as a modulator of daunomycin resistance in patients with poor-risk AML.

An alternative to chemomodifiers is the selection of antineoplastics that are not P-gp substrates or are poorly pumped by P-gp. Idarubicin is a more potent cytotoxic than daunorubicin in both sensitive and MDR cell lines when compared at equal molar concentrations [29]. Preliminary investigations in our laboratory using steady state, physiologic concentrations have shown comparable activity in MDR cell lines [30]. Alkyl-substituted anthracycline analogues which exert their cytotoxic effects primarily by alkylation rather than DNA intercalation have preserved activity in MDR cell lines [31,32]. Similarly, liposome-encapsulated anthracyclines have superior activity in MDR cell lines justifying their consideration for clinical investigation in multidrug resistant leukemia.

Alternate Mechanisms of MDR

In addition to classical MDR mediated by P-gp, alternate mechanisms of MDR have been identified in selected drug-resistant cell lines. Altered catalytic activity in DNA cleavage by the nuclear enzyme Topoisomerase II is assumed to represent an important cellular mechanism of MDR in some cell lines [35, 36]. Assays to measure altered Topoisomerase II activity in clinical specimens have, to date, been problematic and its role in clinical drug resistance remains under investigation. The MRP gene, a new member of the ATP-binding cassette (ABC) transporter gene superfamily to which MDR belongs, was recently cloned from a doxorubicin-resistant human small cell lung cancer cell line by Cole and associates [37]. Overexpression of MRP is associated with a MDR phenotype to natural products and decreased nuclear drug accumulation. This drug resistance phenotype however is not sensitive to PGP inhibitors such as verapamil and cyclosporin-A. Its primary mechanism of resistance may relate to intracellular drug entrapment rather than a plasma membrane-based efflux pump. Using a reverse transcriptase PCR assay to measure MRP messenger RNA in 18 patients with high-risk AML, we could not detect overexpression in any patient specimen [38]. These specimens were selected because of their low prevalence of *mdr1* gene overexpression (22%) suggesting the presence of

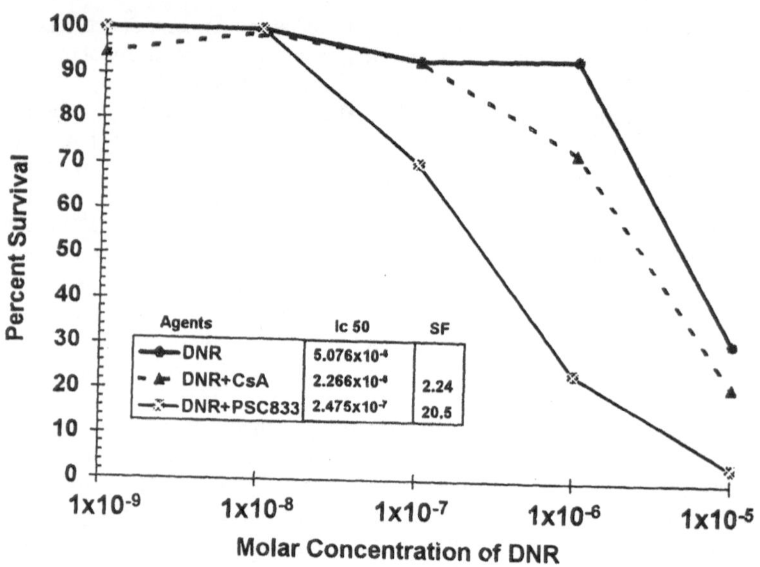

Fig. 2. Comparison of cyclosporin-A (CsA) and PSC 833 at equal molar concentrations (5005M) as modulators of daunorubicin (DNR) resistance in the K562/R cell line. IC50 denotes daunorubicin concentration producing 50% inhibition; SF denotes sensitization factor

an alternate mechanism of resistance. The role, if any, that MRP may play in leukemia requires further investigation.

The decrease or loss of *mdr1* gene overexpression in remitting patients receiving cyclosporinA, implicates the presence of alternate mechanisms of chemotherapy resistance. The monoclonal antibody LRP56 was selected against P-gp-negative tumor cell lines that display a classical MDR phenotype, associated with an energy-dependent reduction in cellular drug retention [39]. Like MRP, LRP56-positive cell lines are insensitive to chemosensitizers such as verapamil and cyclosporin-A and resistance may be mediated by intracellular entrapment in endomembrane structures. This mechanism of resistance was of particular interest in patients failing P-gp inhibitors because of the ability to select for this type of resistence in cell lines exposed concurrently to doxorubicin and verapamil (unpublished data). To evaluate the clinical relevance of this MDR phenotype, we evaluated the frequency of antibody staining and its prognostic significance in clinical specimens from patients with AML [38]. Immunostaining with LRP56 was analyzed immunocytochemically in 99 specimens from 82 patients. Diagnoses included *de novo* AML, secondary leukemia, AML in relapse, and blast phase CML (10 patients). Immunostaining with LRP56 was detected in 38% of patient specimens including 35% of cases with *de novo* AML, 48% of secondary AML, 38% of relapsed leukemias, and 1 of 10 patients with blast phase CML. Sixty-eight AML patients were evaluable for response to induction therapy. Among 41 patients who lacked LRP56 reactivity, 68% achieved a complete or partial remission compared to 36% of patients who were LRP56-positive ($p=0.003$). The significant difference in response to treatment resulted from a higher incidence of chemotherapy resistance in LRP56-positive patients (53% versus 15%). When analyzed according to LRP56 and P-gp phenotype, both markers had prognostic significance that appeared additive, with each marker identifying patients at greater risk for induction failure (Table 1). Progression-free survival was significantly longer in patients who lacked staining with LRP56 ($p=0.006$). Interestingly, prior treatment with mitoxantrone but not daunomycin or idarubicin was associated with positive staining for LRP56 in relapsed patients. Serial monitoring of 17 patients who received induction therapy with a cyclosporine-based regimen showed emergence of the LRP56 phenotype despite a decrease or loss of P-gp expression at the time of treatment failure ($p=0.026$). LRP56 overexpression was associated with a number of adverse prognostic features including P-gp, a

Table 1. Response to induction chemotherapy according to MDR phenotype

LRP56/P-gp phenotype	No.	Complete or partial remission	Resistant failure	Early death
LRP & P-gp-negative	27	20(74%)	3(11%)	4
LRP-negative/P-gp-positive	13	7(54)	4(31)	2
LRP-positive/P-gp-negative	11	5(45)	5(45)	1
LRP & P-gp-positive	18	5(28)	11(61)	2

CD7 surface phenotype, and age > 55 years, but not with CD34. This alternate MDR phenotype was an independent prognostic marker for progression-free survival when compared with P-gp ($p = 0.0015$). The clinical relevance of LRP56 will be further evaluated in SWOG as a prognostic marker for treatment failure in patients receiving cyclosporine chemomodulation. Nevertheless, it is clear from these preliminary data that LRP56 appears to be an important predictor of treatment outcome in AML that may be detected either *de novo*, or may be acquired after treatment with agents such as mitoxantrone or P-gp antagonists.

Summary

Multidrug resistance due to P-gp represents only one of possibly several cellular mechanisms contributing to anthracycline resistance in AML. Preliminary results of clinical trials using cyclosporine and other resistance-modifying agents are encouraging, but await results of randomized trials. Alternate MDR mechanisms such as that identified by LRP56 may be equally important in predicting treatment outcome in AML, and therefore may provide additional prognostic information applicable to decisions regarding high-dose consolidation. New antineoplastics with alternate mechanisms of action, or new resistance-modifying agents with broader specificity offer the greatest prospect for treatment advances.

References

1. List AF: Multidrug resistance and its clinical relevance in acute leukemia. Oncology 7: 23–32, 1993.
2. Pirker R, Wallner J, Geissler K, et al.: mdr1 gene expression and treatment outcome in acute myeloid leukemia. J Natl Cancer Inst 83: 708–712, 1991.
3. Campos L, Guyotat T, Archimbaud E, et al.: Clinical significance of multidrug resistance P-glycoprotein expression on acute nonlymphoblastic leukemia cells at diagnosis. Blood 79: 473–476, 1992.
4. Willman CL, Kopecky K, Weick J, et al. Riologic parameters that predict treatment response in *de novo* acute myeloid leukemia (AML): CD34, but not multidrug resistance (MDR) gene expression, is associated with a decreased complete remission (CR) rate and $CD34^+$ patients more frequently achieve CR with high dose cytosine arabinoside. Proc Am Soc Clin Oncol 1992; 11: 262a.
5. List AF, Spier CM, Cline A, et al. Expression of the multidrug resistance gene product (P-glycoprotein) in myelodysplasia is associated with a stem cell phenotype. Br J Haematol 1991; 78: 28–34.
6. Boekhorst PAW, de Leeuw K, Schoester M, et al. Predominance of functional multidrug resistance (MDR-1) phenotype in $CD34^+$ acute myeloid leukemia cells. Blood 1993; 82: 3157–3162.
7. Chaudhary PM, Roninson IB: Expression and activity of P-glycoprotein, a multidrug efflux pump, in human hematopoietic stem cells. Cell 66: 85–94, 1991.
8. Drach D, Zhao S, Drach J, Mahadevia R, Gattringer C, Huber H, Andreeff M: Subpopulations of normal peripheral blood and bone marrow cells express a functional multidrug resistant phenotype. Blood 80: 2729–2734, 1992.
9. Maruyama Y, Murohashi I, Nara N, Aoki N: Effects of verapamil on the cellular accumulation of daunorubicin in blast cells and on the chemosensitivity of leukemic blast progenitors in acute myeloid leukemia. Br J Haematol 72: 357–362, 1989.
10. Musto P, Melillo L, Lombardi G, Matera R, DiGiorgio G, Carotenuto M: High risk of early resistant relapse for leukemic patients with presence of multidrug resistance associated P-glycoprotein positive cells in complete remission. Br J Haematol 77: 50–53, 1981.
11. Kokenberg E, Sonneveld P, Delwel R, Sizoo W, Hagenbeek A, Lowenberg B: In vivo uptake of daunorubicin by acute myeloid leukemia (AML) cells measured by flow cytometry. Leukemia 2: 511–517, 1988.
12. Tsuruo T, Iida H, Tsukagishi S, Sakurai Y: Overcoming vincristine resistance in P388 leukemia in vivo and *in vitro* through enhanced cytotoxicity of vincristine and vinblastine by verapamil. Cancer Res 41: 1967–1972, 1991.
13. Tsuruo T, Iida H, Kitatani Y, Yokota K, Tsukagishi S, Sakurai Y: Effects of quinidine and related compounds on cytotoxicity and cellular accumulation

of vincristine and adriamycin in drug-resistant tumor cells. Cancer Res 44: 4303–4307, 1984.

14. Slater L, Sweet P, Stupecky M, Gupta S: Cyclosporin-A reverses vincristine and daunorubicin resistance in acute lymphatic leukemia *in vitro*. J Clin Invest 77: 1405–1408, 1986.
15. Dalton WS, Grogan TM, Durie BGM, Meltzer PS, Scheper RJ, Taylor CW, Miller TP, Salmon SE: Drug-resistance in multiple myeloma and non-Hodgkin's lymphoma: Detection of P-glycoprotein and potential circumvention by addition of verapamil to chemotherapy. J Clin Oncol 7(4): 415–424, 1989.
16. Miller TP, Grogan TM, Dalton WS, Spier CM, Scheper RJ, Salmon SE: P-glycoprotein expression in malignant lymphoma and reversal of clinical drug resistance with chemotherapy plus high dose verapamil. J Clin Oncol 9(1): 17–24, 1991.
17. Pennock GD, Dalton WS, Roeske WR, Appleton CP, Ryschon KL, Plezia P, Miller TP, Salmon SE: Systemic toxic effects associated with high dose verapamil infusion and chemotherapy administration. J Natl Cancer Inst 83(2): 105–110, 1991.
18. List AF, Glinsmann-Gibson B. Multidrug Resistance and its pharmacologic modulation in acute myeloid leukemia. In: Accomplishments in Cancer Research. Fortner JG and Rhoads JE (eds.). J. B. Lippincott Publishers, 1991, pp. 178–183. (Suppl 1) 1992.
19. List AF, Spier C, Greer, J, Wolff S, Hutter J, Dorr R, Salmon S, Futscher B, Baier M, and Dalton W. Phase I/II trial of cyclosporine as a chemotherapy-resistance modifier in acute leukemia. J Clin Oncol 11(9): 1652–60, 1993.
20. Futscher BW, Blake LL, Grogan TM, Gerlach TM, Dalton WS. Quantitative PCR analysis of mdr1 expression in multiple myeloma. Anal Biochem 213: 414–421, 1993.
21. Cadranel JF, Erlinger S, Desruenne M, et al.: Chronic administration of cyclosporin-A induces a decrease in hepatic excretory function in man. Dig Dis Sci 37: 1473–1476, 1992.
22. Thiebault F, Tsuruo T, Hamada H, et al.: Cellular localization of the multidrug-resistance gen product P-glycoprotein in normal human tissues. Proc Natl Acad Sci USA 84: 7735–7738, 1987.
23. Buschman E, Arceci RJ, Croop JM, et al.: mdr2 encodes P-glycoprotein expressed in the bile canalicular membrane as determined by isoform-specific antibodies. J Biol Chem 267: 18093–18099, 1992.
24. Solary E, Caillot D, Chauffert B, et al.: Feasibility of using quinine, a potential multidrug resistance-reversing agent, in combination with mitoxantrone and cytarabine for the treatment of acute leukemia. J Clin Oncol 10: 1730–1736, 1992.
25. Boesch D, Gavériaux C, Bénédicte J, Pourtier-Manzanedo A, Bollinger P, and Loor F: In vivo circumvention of P-glycoprotein-mediated multidrug resistance of tumor cells with SDZ PSC 833. Cancer Res 51: 4226–4233, 1991.
26. Hyafil F, Vergely C, Du Vignaud P, Grand-Perret T: In vitro and in vivo reversal of multidrug resistance by GF120918, an acridonecarboxamide derivative. Cancer Res 53: 4595–4602, 1993.
27. Keller RP, Altermatt HJ, Nooter K, Poschmann G, Laissue JA, Bollinger P, and Hiestand PC: SDZ PSC 833, a non-immunosuppressive cyclosporine: its potency in overcoming Pglycoprotein-mediated multidrug resistance of murine leukemia. Int J Cancer 50: 593–597, 1992.
28. Friche E, Jensen PB and Nissen NI: Comparison of cyclosporin A and SDZ PSC833 as multidrug-resistance modulators in a daunorubicin-resistant Ehrlich ascites tumor. Cancer Chemother Pharmacol 30: 235–237, 1992.
29. Berman E, McBride M: A comparative cellular pharmacology of daunorubicin and idarubicin in human multidrug-resistant leukemia cells. Blood 79: 3267–3273, 1992.
30. List AF, Grimm M, Glinsmann-Gibson B, Foley N, Dalton W: Relative cytotoxicity and P-glycoprotein binding avidity of idarubicin, daunorubicin and mitoxantrone in multidrug resistant (MDR) cell lines. Proc AACR 34: in press, 1993.
31. Coley HM, Twentyman PR, Workman P: 9-alkyl, morpholinyl anthracyclines in the circumvention of multidrug resistance. Euro J Cancer 26: 655–667, 1990.
32. Watanabe M, Komeshima N, Nito M, Isoe T, Otake N, Tsuruo T: Cellular pharmacology of mx2, a new morpholine anthracycline, in human pleiotropic drug-resistant cells. Cancer Res 51:157–161, 1991.
33. Mickisch GH, Rahman A, Pastan I, Gottesman MM: Increased effectiveness of liposome-encapsulated doxorubicin in multidrug-resistant-transgenic mice compared with three doxorubicin. J Natl Cancer Inst 84: 804–805, 1992.
34. Warren L, Jardillier J-C, Malarska A, Akeli M-G: Increased accumulation of drug in multidrug-resistant cells induced by liposomes. Cancer Res 52: 3241–3245, 1992.
35. Beck WT, Cirtain MC, Danks MK, et al.: Pharmacological, molecular and cytogenetic analysis of 'atypical' multidrug-resistant human leukemic cells. Cancer Res 47: 5455–5460, 1987.
36. Danks MK, Schmidt CA, Cirtain MC, Suttle DP, Beck WT: Altered catalytic activity of and DNA cleavage by DNA topoisomerase II from human leukemic cells selected for resistance to VM-26. Biochemistry 27: 8861–8879, 1988.
37. Cole SPC, Bhardwaj G, Gerlach JH, Mackie JE, Grant CE, Almquist KC, Stewart AJ, Kurz EU, Duncan AMV, Deeley RG: Overexpression of a transporter gene in a multidrug-resistant human lung cancer cell line. Science 258: 1650, 1992.
38. List AF, Spier CS, Abbaszadegan M, Grogan TM, Greer JP, Wolff SN, Scheper RJ, Dalton WS: Non-P-glycoprotein (Pgp) mediated multidrug resistance (MDR): identification of a novel drug resistance phenotype with prognostic relevance in acute myeloid leukemia (AML). Blood (Suppl 1) 82: 443a, 1993.
39. Scheper RJ, Broxterman HJ, Scheffer GL et al.: Overexpression of a M^r 110,000 vesicular protein in non-P-glycoprotein-mediated multidrug resistance. Cancer Res 53: 1475–1479, 1993.

Acute Leukemias V
Experimental Approaches
and Management of Refractory Diseases
Hiddemann et al. (Eds.)

Kinetic Resistance, Regrowth Resistance, and Multidrug Resistance in the Treatment of Acute Myelogenous Leukemia (AML)

Harvey D. Preisler and Azra Raza

Introduction

When kinetic resistance to treatment is considered, the focus is almost invariably on the relationship between the proliferative rate of the leukemia cells and "classical" drug resistance (the inability of cytotoxic therapy to kill leukemia cells) [1]. While there is a general relationship between the response to remission induction therapy of AML and cell proliferative rates (Table 1) [2], the concept that the higher the proliferative rate the greater the sensitivity of leukemia cells to cytotoxic agents has proven to be simplistic.

In the purest study of this proposition, patients with AML received a single course of high dose cytosine arabinoside, an S phase specific agent, and the effects of this agent on the number of leukemia cells in the bone marrow and on treatment outcome were carefully assessed. The study demonstrated that for the leukemia patient population considered as a whole, there was no relationship between the proliferative rate of the leukemia cells and treatment outcome [3]. On the other hand, a relationship between the reduction in marrow leukemia cells produced by therapy and proliferative rate was found, but only in those patients whose leukemia cells were sensitive to cytosine arabinoside [3].

This study demonstrated that the assumed relationship between classical drug sensitivity and proliferative rate exists, but is conditional upon the inherent metabolic sensitivity of the target cells to the cycle specific agent being administered. Previous studies which attempted to relate the proliferative characteristics of leukemia cells to treatment were flawed because they employed methods which could not accurately measure the percent S phase cells and because they assumed that the labeling index was equivalent to the cell cycle time. These methodological problems still confound many current studies which attempt to assess the effects of biological agents on the proliferative characteristics of leukemias and other neoplastic diseases [4]. The most important type of kinetic resistance, regrowth resistance, has been largely ignored [5].

With the sole exception of the radiotherapists [6,7], when oncologists consider why a cytotoxic therapy has been ineffective attention is almost invariably focused on the inability of the cytotoxic therapy to kill a sufficient number of malignant cells. As illustrated in Figure 1a, the

Table 1. Cell cycle time and prognosis in AML

	Tc (hrs)	
1. Newly Diagnosed		
a. Standard Prognosis	54 ± 4	$p = 0.09$
b. Poor Prognosis	64.2 ± 5.7	
2. Newly Diagnosed Poor Prognosis		
a. one risk factor	53.9 ± 7.3	$p = 0.03$
b. > one risk factor	83.5 ± 12.2	
3. 1st Relapse Disease		
a. good prognosis	35.2 ± 5.1	$p = 0.09$
b. poor prognosis	49.4 ± 4.5	

Rush Cancer Institute, Division of Hematology/Oncology and Rush-Presbyterian-St. Luke's Medical Center, Chicago, IL, USA

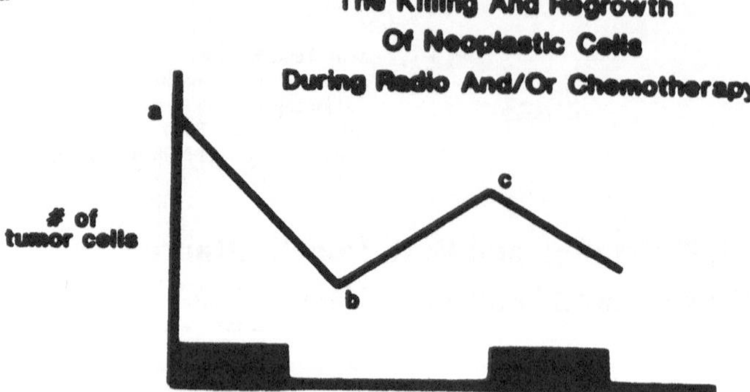

Fig. 1a,b. Theoretical effects of tumor regrowth between courses of cytotoxic therapy. NOTE: The reduction in tumor cell numbers is the same for each curve after each course of therapy. The only difference between the curves is the extent of tumor regrowth between each course of treatment.

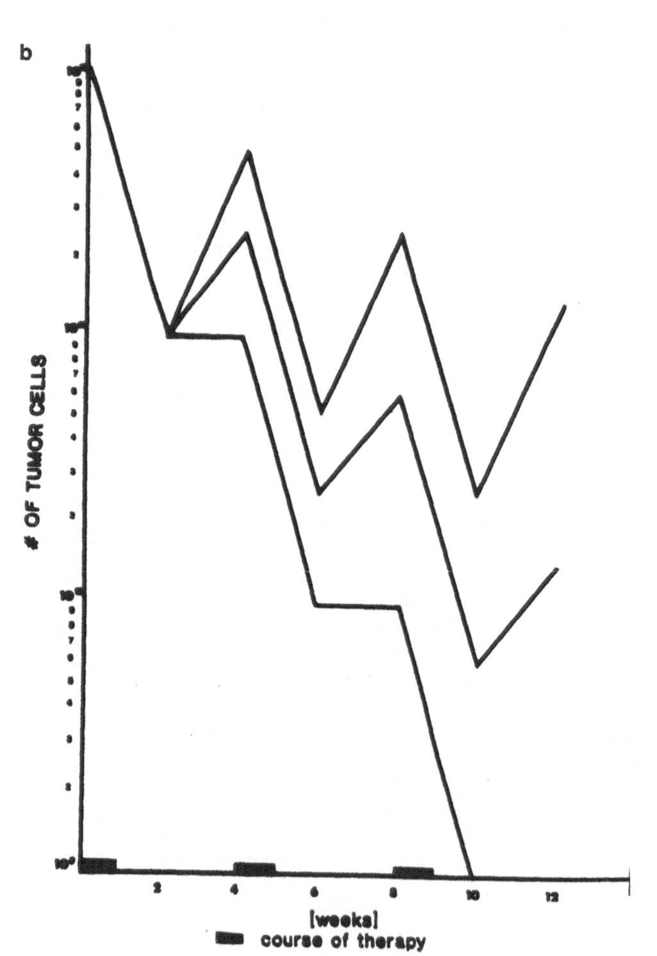

net effect of a course of therapy on a tumor is a function of both the number of malignant cells killed and the extent of malignant regrowth between courses of cytotoxic therapy (2, 5, 8–10). Figure 1b illustrates the theoretical effects of different rates of tumor regrowth between courses of therapy on the net effect of therapy. As can be seen, a sufficiently rapid regrowth rate can completely offset the effects of a course of cytotoxic therapy. Conversely, the inhibition of regrowth between courses of treatment could convert a noncurative therapy to a curative one.

Regrowth resistance, that is treatment resistance resulting from the regrowth of neoplastic cells between courses of therapy, is likely to be a significant contributor to treatment failure in a variety of neoplastic diseases (Table 2). These diseases share in common a high level of sensitivity to cytotoxic agents yet a low cure rate (except for testicular tumors). The reasons for the lack of attention paid to this cause of treatment failure has been speculated upon elsewhere [5].

The relative contribution of regrowth resistance to treatment failure in AML depends upon the category of AML being treated. The poor responsiveness of patients with poor prognosis newly diagnosed leukemia (leukemia subsequent to toxic exposure or to a myelodysplastic syndrome) is at least in part due to the rapid regrowth of the leukemia cells which begins as soon as the administration of the agents utilized in remission induction therapy is concluded. Regrowth resistance makes a significant contribution to remission induction failure in as many as one-half of the patients with this variety of leukemia [2,11]. Further, the rapid regrowth of leukemia cells once therapy ends undoubtedly also contributes to the short remission durations noted in these patients.

On the other hand, regrowth resistance is an infrequent cause of remission induction failure in newly diagnosed standard prognosis AML patients but plays an important role in determining remission duration in these patients [12]. Given that regrowth resistance is often a significant contributor to treatment failure in the leukemias, the reduction of or prevention of leukemia regrowth between courses of cytotoxic therapy would significantly increase the effectiveness of currently available therapies. Regrowth resistance is a general phenomenon having been also demonstrated in head and neck cancer where regrowth between individual doses of radiotherapy and during weekends in which radiotherapy is not administered have been demonstrated [13,14]. Similar phenomena undoubtedly occur in a variety of malignant diseases [10].

Cellular Determinants of Leukemia Regrowth Between Courses of Therapy

Cellular characteristics which may play a role in determining the rate of leukemia regrowth include the rate of cell birth, the rate at which leukemia cells leave the proliferating pool, the number of leukemia cells which survive therapy, the number of proliferating cells, and the proliferative rate (Table 3). Additionally the self-renewal capacity of the leukemia progenitor cells and their proliferative potential, that is the number of cells which a proliferating cell and its progeny produce during their reproductive life span, will help to define the regrowth rate.

Malignant cells can leave the proliferating pool via several different pathways. AML cells may differentiate, either spontaneously or under the influence of cytotoxic therapy [15], thereby reducing the number of proliferating cells. In the latter case, leukemias which are slowly proliferating are more likely to differentiate than rapidly proliferating leukemias [16]. Hence the long durations of remission of patients with

Table 2. Neoplastic diseases in which regrowth resistance is likely to affect treatment outcome

- Acute Myelogenous Leukemia
- Acute Lymphocytic leukemia
- Chronic Myelogenous Leukemia
- Intermediate and High Grade Lymphomas
- Small Cell Carcinoma of the Lung
- Ovarian Carcinoma
- Head and Neck Cancer
- Testicular Cancer
- Some Breast Cancers

Table 3. Determinants of regrowths rate

Cell production	Rate of express from the proliferative poor
1. proliferation pool size	1. cell differentiation
2. proliferative rate	2. apoptosis
3. sell renewal capacity	3. other types of cell death
4. proliferative potential	4. entry into Go (?)
5. growth factor independence	

slowly proliferating AML probably results from two phenomena: the slow proliferative rate of the cells and a constant removal of cells from the proliferative pool resulting from differentiation.

Apoptosis, Preleukemia, and the Development of AML

Recently the phenomenon of programmed cell death, of which apoptosis is one type, has received much attention. During this active process cells commit suicide [17]. It is of special interest that while both myelodysplastic disease and AML are characterized by rapidly proliferating cells, in the former the majority of cells are undergoing apoptosis while in the latter only rare cells are undergoing apoptosis [18]. These data strongly suggest that the evolution of myelodysplasia to AML involves two changes in cell behavior: a reduction in apoptosis and a loss or a reduction in the ability of myeloid progenitor cells to differentiate. It is possible that the initial lesion which causes the premalignant types of myelodysplastic diseases produces a high rate of apoptosis in the marrow. The high rate of apoptosis could then result in a compensatory increase in the proliferative rate of the myeloid cells resulting in the hypercellular marrows and ineffective hemopoiesis which characterize these syndromes [18]. Further the high proliferative rate and high death rate in myelodysplastic disease would predispose to the appearance of new genic abnormalities and evolution to acute leukemia. If this hypothesis is correct then the most appropriate therapy for myelodyplastic patients would be the suppression of apoptosis since this would abrogate the ineffective hemopoiesis and should reduce the proliferation rate of the myeloid elements to normal thereby reducing the likelihood of evolution to leukemia.

Apoptosis and the Treatment of AML

It is of interest that recent studies have demonstrated that at low and moderate dose levels many cytotoxic agents kill cells by inducing apoptosis [19,20]. It appears likely that cytotoxic agents cause apoptosis because the DNA damage which they produce triggers a normal mechanism by which organisms protect themselves against cells whose DNA has been damaged in the course of normal existence. In this setting the mechanism of apoptosis permits organisms to remove cells whose DNA damage is not reparable and therefore may lead to malignant transformation.

Additionally, the demonstration that cells can simultaneously be undergoing apoptosis while engaging in DNA synthesis [18] demonstrates that studies which only assess the proliferative characteristics of cells may provide misleading data regarding the growth characteristics of a cell population since even a highly proliferative cell population may produce few cells. As noted above, this is the case in myelodysplastic disease in which ineffective hemopoiesis is characterized by high proliferative rates and simultaneous high rates of apoptosis [18]. With respect to the treatment of the leukemias and other neoplastic diseases, the induction of apoptosis between courses of cytotoxic therapy would reduce neoplastic regrowth between courses of therapy.

Further, as discussed in detail below, the phenomena of leukemia cell differentiation and apoptosis link classical resistance and regrowth resistance since differentiation and apoptosis during and after treatment will result in a reduction of leukemia cell numbers during cytotoxic therapy and also in a reduction in regrowth rate between courses of therapy. To rationally develop potential therapeutic approaches, one should first consider the relationship between gene expression and treatment response in AML.

Genic Determinants of Response to Treatment

The expression level of several genes has been demonstrated to be associated with the response of AML to treatment (Table 4). High levels of expression of the multidrug resistance gene are

Table 4. Genes which influence treatment outcome

1. Multidrug resistance gene
2. c-myb
3. c-fms
4. bcl-2
5. c-myc
6. IL-1
7. p53

associated with reduction in both the likelihood of a patient entering remission and with short remissions [21]. The relationship of the expression of this gene to treatment outcome appears to be due to classical drug resistance resulting from the inability to maintain sufficiently high intracellular drug levels to permit the destruction of substantial numbers of leukemic cells.

a- myb. High levels of expression of the myb gene are associated with resistance to remission induction therapy manifested by low remission rates and by the relative resistance of leukemia cells to the cytotoxic effects of chemotherapy [22]. While the basis for resistance is unknown, several possible mechanisms would impact on the kinetic aspects of response. The constitutive expression of myb has been shown to prevent the induction of differentiation of myeloid leukemia cells in vitro. If the same were the case for AML cells in vivo, then the removal of leukemia cells from the proliferating pool by differentiation would be inoperative in leukemias with very high levels of expression of this gene.

As is the case for the myc gene, high levels of myb expression may be associated with relative or absolute growth factor independence and a high proliferative potential. These characteristics, with or without a reduced ability of the leukemia cells to differentiate, would contribute to kinetic resistance.

b- fms. Low levels of fms expression in standard risk AML cells are associated with a reduced likelihood of a successful outcome of remission induction therapy [23,24]. The percent of patients among poor prognosis AML whose cells express the fms gene is much less than in standard risk AML [2]. Hence the responses of patients within the group of standard risk AML patients and the differences in response between standard risk and poor prognosis AML patients parallel differences in the levels of fms expression. Studies monitoring the direct effects of remission induction therapy on the number of leukemia cells in the marrows of patients have demonstrated that low levels of fms expression are associated with classical resistance to cytotoxic therapy [24].

The phenomena responsible for these associations are unknown. Several possibilities suggest themselves. The first is related to the observation that high levels of fms expression are associated with an increased likelihood that leukemia cells will spontaneously differentiate in vitro [25]. It is possible that low levels of expression are associated with a reduced likelihood of spontaneous and drug induced differentiation in vivo, a phenomenon which would contribute to the relative kinetic resistance of leukemias which do not express fms or which express the gene at low levels.

A second possibility is suggested by the strong correlation between the level of fos expression and the level of fms expression [23]. Expression of the former gene is one of the early events associated with apoptosis. It is possible that the same is the case for expression of the fms gene and that high levels of fms expression is an indication that these leukemia cells are characterized by high levels of spontaneous apoptosis and/or that the leukemia cells are highly sensitive to the apoptotic triggering effects of chemotherapy.

A third possibility is the phenomenon of "fratricide" [24]. Studies in our laboratory have demonstrated that the marrow biopsies of many AML patients contain large numbers of monocytic/macrophage cells which contain nuclear debris [26]. These cells are present in sufficiently high numbers to suggest that they are of leukemic origin. The presence of nuclear debris within these cells indicates that the macrophages have phagocytosed dead or damaged cells. It is possible, therefore, that these differentiated leukemic macrophages are destroying damaged leukemia cells which otherwise might have been able to repair the damage produced by cytotoxic therapy. These observations suggest that high levels of fms expression, which is a marker for monocytic/macrophage differentiation, are associated with a good response to treatment because they indicate the presence leukemia cells which will differentiate during chemotherapy into monocyte/macrophages capable of committing fratricide. If this were the case then the efficacy of cytotoxic therapy would be increased since leukemia cells which were damaged but which were still viable would be killed by these cytotoxic cells of leukemic origin [24].

c- bcl-2. The expression of the bcl-2 gene is associated with protection against apoptosis. Given the evidence that apoptosis is a common mechanism through which cytotoxic agents kills target cells, it is not surprising that high levels of expression of this gene are associated with the resistance of AML to treatment [27].

d- myc. High levels of expression of the myc gene may contribute to treatment resistance through a variety of mechanisms. High levels are associated with reduced growth factor requirements and at times with growth factor independence, both of which could contribute to regrowth resistance [28,29]. High levels of expression are also associated with a reduced likelihood that leukemia cells will differentiate during remission induction therapy [24].

In a previous study we found that patients who entered remission and whose leukemia cells expressed myc at a high level had the greatest reduction in leukemic marrow cells during the first 6 days of remission induction therapy [23]. Recent studies have demonstrated that high levels of expression of the myc gene in the presence of inhibition of DNA synthesis are associated with apoptosis [30]. It is possible, therefore, that in patients with drug sensitive disease (as evidenced by the fact that the patient's leukemia entered complete remission)the high pretherapy levels of myc expression potentiated the effects of cytotoxic therapy by triggering apoptosis when DNA synthesis was inhibited during remission induction therapy.

e- IL1b. Evidence has been presented that high levels of expression in leukemia cells of the gene for IL1b are associated with short remissions [31]. This is not surprising since high levels of expression of this gene would be expected to be associated with the paracrine stimulation of leukemia cell regrowth. The lack of association of the level of expression of this gene and remission induction outcome [32] is surprising but simply may indicate that the effects of this gene on regrowth are not important relative to the other factors involved in determining remission induction outcome.

f- p53 gene. There have been no reports describing a relationship of the level of expression of the p53 gene and treatment outcome in AML. However while this gene is not often mutated in AML, it might be expected that the level of expression of the normal p53 gene would exert an influence on treatment outcome. High levels of expression in the presence of drug sensitive disease would be expected to potentiate the effects of cytotoxic therapy while low levels of expression or mutations of the gene would be expected to be associated with regrowth resistance (see below).

Multidrug Resistance and Regrowth Resistance

Multidrug resistance involving agents which have common mechanisms of cellular uptake or efflux or common mechanisms of producing DNA damage are readily understandable. Included in these categories are agents affected by the multidrug resistance efflux pump and by those agents which produce DNA damage by interacting with topoisomerase. On the other hand, initial observations that resistance to two cytotoxic agents with different mechanisms of uptake, efflux, and action, such as cytosine arabinoside and daunomycin [33], were difficult to understand beyond the obvious interpretation that there must be general mechanisms which confer resistance to different classes of action.

As described above, these latter associations of resistance exist in part because DNA damage, regardless of the causal insult, triggers a final common pathway of cell death, apoptosis. Phenomena which interfere with apoptosis will therefore contribute to resistance to many agents, regardless of the mechanism by which they produce DNA damage. Hence simultaneous resistance to cytosine arabinoside and daunorubicin are understandable since both act, at least in part, by triggering the apoptotic pathway.

As noted above, recent studies have demonstrated that the expression and/or alteration of several genes can affect both classical drug resistance and regrowth resistance. Overexpression of the bcl-2 gene can confer simultaneous resistance to a variety of cytotoxic agents by preventing apoptosis [20]. Additionally, in vitro studies have demonstrated that overexpression of this gene permits leukemia cells to resume proliferation as soon as exposure to cytotoxic agents ceases [27]. A similar effect in vivo would result in the rapid resumption of leukemia cell proliferation as soon as the administration of a course of cytotoxic therapy cases.

Mutation of the p53 gene would have a similar effect being associated with the prevention of apoptosis associated with cytotoxic therapy [19] as well as with the rapid proliferation of neoplastic cells between courses of cytotoxic therapy. Further, the delay in cell proliferation normally associated with DNA damage is dependent upon the presence of normal functioning p53 genes. This delay does not occur when a mutant p53 gene is present. Hence regrowth should resume sooner in leukemia cells bearing p53 mutations than in those containing normal p53 genes.

The involvement of the myc gene in both multidrug resistance and regrowth resistance would occur via a mechanism which is somewhat different from that described above for the bcl-2 gene and for mutated p53 genes. High levels of myc expression in the presence of inhibition of DNA synthesis can result in apoptosis [30]. On the other hand, high levels of expression of this gene in the presence of resistance to cytotoxic agents would associate regrowth resistance with classical resistance since myc expression would facilitate the former by reducing dependence upon growth factors or even conferring growth factor independence thereby increasing the proliferation potential of a tumor.

Finally, regrowth resistance per se is likely to facilitate the development of resistance to cytotoxic agents thereby providing another mechanism for the association of regrowth resistance and classical resistance to cytotoxic agents [10].

Strategies to Overcome Kinetic Resistance

a. Increasing the Proliferative Rate of AML Cells

Since one of the distinguishing general characteristics of treatment resistant categories of AML is a slow proliferative rate, it is possible that one might render these leukemias more amenable to treatment if one increased their proliferative rate. Attempts to increase proliferative rates have involved the administration of GM-CSF to leukemia patients prior to and during remission induction therapy. In the one study [34] and in an as yet unpublished study [35], remission rates were not increased. In the latter study clear cut evidence was obtained that the proliferative rates of the leukemia cells of patients were increased and yet treatment outcome was not improved [35].

There are several possible explanations for the failure of this strategy to improve treatment outcome. As noted above, the proliferative rate is relevant only if the leukemia cells are metabolically sensitive to the agents being administered. Without this precondition an increase in proliferative rate may in fact have an adverse effect since it will result in an increase in leukemia cell mass and in the regrowth of leukemia cells between courses of therapy and perhaps even between the administration of individual doses of chemotherapy agents. One problem with the use of cytokines to increase proliferative rates is that the categories of diseases which tend to have slow proliferative rates such as secondary AML and some relapsed AML, are those in which multidrug resistance is most common [21,36].

b. Recruitment of Cells into Cycle

Much has been made regarding the role which Go cells may play in causing resistance to treatment. The concept of Go leukemia cells traces its history to the original attempts 30–40 years ago to assess the proliferative rates of acute leukemia cells. In these studies the leukemia cells were either labeled in vivo or in vitro with 3HTdr and measurements were made on peripheral blood cells or on marrow aspirates. With labeling indices of 8–10% in the marrow aspirate and 0–2% in the peripheral blood it is easy to understand why it was assumed that many leukemia cells were not cycling.

Recently developed methods which permit the accurate assessment of the proliferative rates of leukemia cells in vivo in patients have presented a very different view of the kinetics of leukemia [37]. Unbeknownst to the early investigators leukemia is a highly proliferative disease with marrow leukemia cells having a labeling index of 25–30% and average cell cycle times of 55–60 hours. These data alone make the question of whether or not Go leukemia cells exist an open one. Unfortunately there are no markers available for identifying Go cells and the only recent data which have been used to suggest that Go leukemia cells exist in acute leukemia are based upon acridine orange staining and flow cytometry studies [38]. A recent study has, however, brought the interpretation of these reports into question [39]. At the present time the only data which suggest that Go cells may exist are the observations that leukemia cells in the peripheral blood are rarely in S phase, express high levels of the myc gene [22], and that they contain a subset of cells capable of producing leukemic colonies in vitro. Hence the possible role of Go cells in producing resistance to treatment remains to be defined.

c. Reducing Regrowth Resistance

Regrowth resistance could be reduced by slowing the proliferative rate of AML cells between courses of therapy and by reducing the activity of those genes whose expression appears to be associated with regrowth resistance. The administration of the combination of 13-cis retinoic acid and α-interferon has been shown to reduce the proliferative rate of both AML [40] and chronic myelogenous leukemia cells in vivo [41] and also to reduce the level of expression of the myc [42], bcl-2 [43], and IL1b genes [43] in the leukemia cells of some patients. Additionally, the administration of these two biological agents to patients results in an increase in apoptosis in leukemia cells in vivo in both acute [43] and chronic myelogenous leukemias [43]. Hence, with the rational administration of cytotoxic agents, it appears that it may be possible to reduce the regrowth rate of AML between courses of therapy and subsequent to the end of consolidation therapy. Studies of this proposition are in progress at the Rush Cancer Institute.

Summary

Whether or not current attempts to reduce regrowth resistance are successful, it is imperative that the important contribution which regrowth resistance makes to treatment failure in AML and in many other diseases be recognized. It is clear that the restraint of cell growth has great potential for increasing the efficacy of currently available cytotoxic agents and regimens. Unfortunately there has been little or no work in this area [5]. This situation is compounded by the fact that the evaluation of biological agents is currently based on the ability of these agents to induce remissions or to reduce the size of tumors. Clearly agents which restrain growth, while having great potential when administered between courses of therapy, will be deemed to be inactive when evaluated using these current criteria.

Appreciation of this type of kinetic resistance and the development of strategies to overcome regrowth resistance will result in a marked improvement of our ability to effectively treat patients with AML and other drug sensitive but usually incurable neoplastic diseases. To this end the system currently used to classify remission induction failures in the leukemias [44] has been modified so that the precise impact of regrowth resistance on treatment failure can be understood [9]. The use of this system will also help to evaluate therapeutic strategies designed to overcome regrowth resistance.

Finally, recent studies strongly suggest that multidrug resistance and regrowth resistance can result from abnormalities in bcl-2 expression and from mutations of the p53 gene. The association of these two types of resistance to treatment may account for those situations in which the resistance of leukemia to treatment appears to be absolute [3,11].

Acknowledgements. This work was supported by the National Cancer Institute Grants: CA60085, CA60086 and the Rice Foundation.

References

1. Preisler HD, Raza A, Wang Z, et al: Human Myeloid Leukemia Cells: Studies of Proto-oncogene Expression and Cell Differentiation In Vitro. In Waxman S, Rossi GB, Takaku F (eds): The Status of Differentiation Therapy of Cancer, Serona Symposia, Raven Press, 45: 79–93, 1988.
2. Preisler HD, Raza A, Gopal V, et al: Poor Prognosis Acute Myelogenous Leukemia. Leuk Lymp, 9: 273–283 1993.
3. Preisler, HD, Raza A, Larson R, et al: Some Reasons for the Lack of Progress in the Treatment of Acute Myelogenous Leukemia. Leuk Res, 15(9): 773–780, 1991.
4. Preisler HD and Raza A: Cell Cycle Studies in Acute Myelogenous Leukemia. Leukemia (Editorial) 6(8): 751–753, 1992.
5. Preisler HD and Gopal V: Regrowth Resistance in Cancer: Why Has it Been Largely Ignored? In press Cell Prolif, 1994.
6. Bentzen, SM and Thames, HD,: Clinical Evidence for Tumor Clonogen Regeneration: Interpretations of Data. Radiother Oncol, 22: 161–166, 1991
7. Fowler, JF,: Rapid Repopulation in Radiotherapy: A Debate on Mechanisms. Radiother Oncol, 22: 156–158, 1991.
8. Preisler HD, Raza A, Bacharani M, et al: Proliferative Advantage Rather Than Classical Drug Resistance as the Cause of Treatment Failure in Chronic Myelogenous Leukemia. Leuk Lymphoma, 11(1): 145–150, 1993.
9. Preisler HD and Gopal V: Regrowth Resistance in Leukemia and Lymphoma: The Need for a New System to Classify Treatment Failure and for New. Approaches to Treatment. In Press, Leuk Res, 1994.
10. Preisler HD, Raza A, Bonomi P, et al: Regrowth Resistance as a Major Contributor to Treatment Failure in Neoplastic Disease. In Press, Leukemia 1993.

11. Preisler HD, Larson RA, Raza A, et al: The Treatment of Patients with Newly Diagnosed Poor Prognosis Acute Myelogenous Leukemia: Response to Treatment and Treatment Failure. Br J Haematol, 79: 390–397, 1991.
12. Raza A, Preisler, HD, Day R, et al: Direct Relationship Between Remission Duration in Acute Myeloid Leukemia and Cell Cycle Kinetics. A Leukemia Intergroup Study. Blood, 76(11): 2191–2197, 1990.
13. Bentzen SM, Johansen LV, Overgaard, J. et al: Clinical Radiobiology of Squamous Cell Carcinoma of the Oropharynx. Int J Radiat Oncol Biol Phys, 20: 1197–1206, 1991.
14. Overgaard J, Hjelm-Hansen L, Vendelbo J, et al: Comparison of Conventional and Split-Course Radiotherapy as Primary Treatment in Carcinoma of the Larynx. Acta Oncol, 27: 147–152, 1988 Fasc 2.
15. Raza A, and Preisler HD: Evidence of In Vivo Differentiation in Myeloblasts Labeled with Bromodeoxyuridine. J Cancer, 1(1): 15–18, 1986.
16. Raza A, Preisler HD, Lampkin B, et al: Clinical and Prognostic Significance of in Vivo Differentiation in Acute Myeloid Leukemia. Am J Hematol, 42(2): 147–157, 1993.
17. Wyllie AH: Apoptosis and the Regulation of Cell Numbers in Normal and Neoplastic Tissues: An Overview. Cancer Met Rev, 11: 95–103, 1992.
18. Raza A, Mundle S, Iftikhar A, Gregory S, Marcus B, Adler S, Preisler HD: Extensive Apoptosis in Myelodysplastic Syndromes is the Probable Basis for Ineffective Hematopoiesis. Submitted to the 85th Annual Meeting of the American Association for Cancer Research, 1994.
19. Lowe SW, Ruley HE, Jacks T, et al: p53-Dependent Apoptosis Modulates the Cytotoxicity of Anticancer Agents. Cell, 74: 957–967, 1993.
20. Walton MI, Whysong PM, O'Connor D, et al: Constitutive Expression of Human Bcl-2 Modulates Nitrogen Mustard and Camptothecin Induced Apoptosis. Cancer Res, 53: 1853–1862, 1993.
21. Sato H, Gottesman MM, Preisler HD: Expression of the Multidrug Resistance Gene in Myeloid Leukemias. Leukemia Res, 1: 11–22, 1990.
22. Gopal V, Hulett B, Preisler HD et al: Myc and Myb Expression in Acute Myelogenous Leukemia. Leukemia Res, 10: 1003–1011, 1992.
23. Preisler HD, Raza A, Larson R, et al: Proto-Oncogene Expression and the Clinical Characteristics of Acute Nonlymphocytic Leukemia: A Leukemia Intergroup Pilot Study. Blood, 73: 255–262, 1989.
24. Preisler HD, Raza A, Larson R, et al: FMS Expression in Highly Predictive of Treatment Outcome in Standard Risk Newly Diagnosed Patients with Acute Myelocytic Leukemia. MYC Expression is Not. In press Leuk Lymphoma 1993.
25. Yin M, Gao XZ, Preisler HD, et al: Studies of the Proliferation and Differentiation of Immature Myeloid Cells in Vitro: 4. Preculture Characteristics and the Behavior of Myeloid Leukemia Cells in Vitro: Cell Biochem and Function, 9(1): 39–47, 1991.
26. Raza A, Lampkin BC, Preisler HD, et al: Infiltration of the Hematopoietic Microenvironment by Macrophages in Patients with Acute Promyelocytic Leukemia. In Press, Br J Hematol, 1992.
27. Miyashita T and Reed JC: Bcl-2 Oncoprotein Blocks Chemotherapy-Induced Apoptosis in a Human Leukemia Cell Line. Blood, 81: 151–157, 1993.
28. Gionti, E. et al: Avian Myelocytomatosis Virus Immortalizes Differentiated Quail Chondrocytes. Proc Natl Acad Sci, 82: 2756–2761, 1984.
29. Mougneau E, et al :Biological Activities of v-myc and Rearranged c-myc Oncogenes in Rat Fibroblast Cells in Culture. Proc Natl Acad Sci 81: 5758–5767, 1984.
30. Askew DS, Ashmun RA, Simmonds BC, et al: Constitutive c-myc Expression in an IL-3 Dependent Myeloid Cell Line Suppresses Cell Cycle Arrest and Accelerates Apoptosis. Oncogene, 6(10): 1915–1922, 1991.
31. Preisler HD, Raza A, Kukla C, et al: 1L1β Expression and Treatment Outcome in Acute Myelogenous Leukemia (AML). Blood, 78(3): 849–850, 1991.
32. Unpublished Observation.
33. Preisler HD, and Azarnia N: Assessment of the Drug Sensitivity of Acute Nonlymphocytic Leukemia Using the In Vitro Clonogenic Assay. Br J Haematol, 58(4): 633–640, 1984.
34. Estey E, Kurzrock R, Kantarjian H, et al: Treatment of Newly-diagnosed AML With GM-CSF Prior to and During Continuous-infusion High-dose ara-C + Daunorubicin: Comparison to Patients Treated without CM-CSF. Blood, 79: 2246–2255, 1992.
35. Mundle S, Sbalchiero J, Iftikhar A, Shetty V, Raza A: In Vivo Induction of Apoptosis in AML Cells by RA+IFNα Treatment. Submitted to the 18th Annual Meeting of the Cell Kinetics Society, 1994.
36. Sato H, Gottesman MM, Preisler HD, et al: Expression of the Mutidrug Resistance Gene in Myeloid Leukemias. Leuk Res, 14(1): 11–22, 1990.
37. Raza A, Maheshwari Y, Preisler HD: Differences in Cell Cycle Characteristics Amongst Patients with Acute Nonlymphocytic Leukemia. Blood, 69(6): 1647–1653, 1987.
38. Tofuri A, and Andreeff M,: Kinetic Rationale in Cytokine-induced Recruitment of Myeloblastic Leukemia Followed by Cycle-specific Chemotherapy in Vitro. Leukemia, 14: 826–834, 1990.
39. Preisler HD, Raza A, Gopal V, et al: The Study of Acute Leukemia cells by Means of Acridine Orange Staining and Flow Cytometry. In Press Leuk Lymphoma 1993.
40. Preisler HD, Raza A, Larson R: Alteration of the Proliferative Rate of Acute Myelogenous Leukemia Cells in Vivo in Patients. Blood, 80(10): 2600–2603, 1992.
41. Preisler HD, Kotelnikov V, Hegde U, et al: A Strategy Overcoming Regrowth Resistance in

Chronic Myelogenous Leukemia (SORRCML). Submitted to the Annual Meeting of the American Society of Hematology, September 1993.
42. Banavali S, Pancoast J, Preisler HD, et al: Serial Studies of C-MYC Expression in Bone Marrow Biopsies: Effects of Cytotoxic Agents, rhGM-CSF and Retinoic Acid-Interferon. In press Eur J of Cancer 1993.
43. Paper in preparation.
44. Preisler HD: Failure of Remission Induction in Acute Myelocytic Leukemia. Med Pediatr Oncol, 4: 275–276,1978.

Acute Leukemias V
Experimental Approaches
and Management of Refractory Diseases
Hiddemann et al. (Eds.)

Topoisomerases – from Basic Research to Clinical Implications

Frank Gieseler

Introduction

Topoisomerases (topos) are moved into the focus of haematologists and oncologists because they are interesting in several different aspects. These enzymes are life-important DNA-processing enzymes, their activity is necessary in every cellular action where alteration of the three-dimensional structure of the DNA is obligatory. Moreover, research on topos has a direct clinical aspect because topo I as well as topo II are target structures for several important cytostatics. In the following paper I will focus on the clinical part of this research area and will cover just the basic facts which are necessary to understand the clinical importance of these enzymes.

Biochemistry and mode of action. Controlling the three dimensional structure of the DNA is essential for every cell. This is true not only for cell division with the necessity for chromosome formation which does not work without topo activity (1) but also for gene transcription regulation since DNA-polymerases favour a certain degree of torsional stress in the DNA [2]. In these areas gene transcription is more likely to occur and, *vice versa* the synthesis of topoisomerases is influenced by the degree of DNA-relaxation [3].

Topos are a family of isoenzymes. As of now, we know of three different genes encoding for topos. The topo I-gene is located on chromosome 20, the one for topo II alpha is located on chromosome 17 and the one for topo II beta is located on chromosome 3 [4]. These genes encode for three different proteins that are additionally heavily posttranscriptionally modified. Ribosylation and phosphorylation, both with consequences for the enzymes' activity and their drug sensitivity have been described [5–9]. This might explain why we find several distinct topo-activities in intact cells.

The way of processing the DNA is obviously very similar for topo I and the topo II isoenzymes. We are able to differentiate at least six different steps which are important for the understanding of differences in the mode of action of inhibiting cytostatic drugs [10]:

- loose (non-covalent) binding of the enzyme to the DNA
- tight (covalent) binding
- DNA cleavage
- strand passage
- religation
- enzyme turn over.

This is of course a very theoretical model as it is extremely difficult to examine DNA-processing enzymes in vivo, that is inside the nucleus of a living cell. We must admit that we still do not know, how these enzymes work in intact human cells and several divergent models exist [11]. The principle difference between topo I and topo II is not their way of action *in vitro*, but probably their intranuclear localisation. In contrast to topo I, topo II is a major component of the nuclear matrix (NM) [12]. The DNA is organised in "loops" which are fixed to the NM at the "matrix attached regions" (MAR) [13]. At the footpoints of these loops topo II is localised, thus able to control the torsional stress of the attached DNA-loop [14]. This is true at least for

Medizinische Poliklinik, University Hospital, 97070 Würzburg, Germany

topo II alpha, its expression is tightly associated with proliferation and this isoenzyme seems to be the main target of the topo II inhibiting cytostatic drugs.

Our knowledge about topo II beta is even less. Obviously, this isoenzyme is more localised in the nucleolus of the cells [15]. Although we still do not know it's function, it seems to be more associated with cellular differentiation than with proliferation [16–18]. The fact that topo II alpha is found in all eukarionts whereas topo II beta is found only in vertebrates supports this suggestion [4]. Evidently, the cellular function of both isoenzymes can only be understood in the context of all DNA-binding proteins. In other words, purified topo does not necessarily act in the same way as it does in its physiological environment. This perception is important for the interpretation of *in vitro* experiments an the drawing of conclusions for therapy.

Clinical implications. Topo II inhibitors are well established therapeutics. They include substances from diverse chemical classes such as anthracyclines (adriamycin, daunomycin, idarubicin, epirubicin), the epipodophyllotoxines (etoposide, teniposide), the anthracenedions (mitoxantrone) and the acridines (amsacrine). Topo I inhibitors are derivatives from camptothecin (hypocamptamine-topotecan, CPT - 11) and are currently in clinical trials.

How do topo inhibitors work? The exact molecular events which finally result in apoptotic cell death are unknown. Obviously, the formation of a ternary complex between the DNA, the topo and the drug, called the "cleavable complex" (CC), is a prerequisite for all further steps. It has been shown that the CC can be repaired [19, 20], but without it's formation, genotoxicity of the drugs is not reasonable.

In Figure 1, some factors are named which are important for the formation of the CC. I think that the study of these factors is exceptionally important for the understanding of sensitivity or resistance of tumour cells to chemotherapy. A direct correlation between genotoxicity of the drugs and cytotoxicity has been shown and [21], moreover, cytotoxicity directly corresponds to the DNA binding of anthracyclines, being the first step in the formation of the CC [22, 23]. The cleavage potency of anthracyclines is a bell-shaped curve with its maximum at 1 μM for daunorubicin as well as for idarubicin [24]. At higher concentrations the intercalators inhibit DNA binding of topo II and consequently DNA cleavage. The interaction with podophyllotoxines which do not intercalate is different, these drugs are able to bind to topo II directly before the enzyme interacts with DNA.

Ole Westergaard from the university of Aarhus in Denmark has developed an experimental system to uncouple the DNA binding, cleavage and religation events of the topo II action (Fig. 2). The principle is, that a special DNA oligonucleotide with a topo II binding and cleavage site is used. After cleavage, a short fragment is liberated which can not be religated by the enzyme (Fig. 2, left panel). In agarose gel electrophoresis, the different states can be discriminated (Fig. 2, right panel). That is the DNA (lane A), the DNA bound topo (lane B) and the cleaved fragment (lane C). With this system, a number of Danish scientists and Robinson and Osheroff from Nashville, Tennessee examined different topo II inhibitors with respect to their mode of action [25, 26]. Interestingly enough, they found pronounced differences even within one chemical class, e.g. the anthracyclines (Fig. 3). Most anthracyclines such as daunorubicin, but also doxorubicin stabilise the cleavable complex before DNA-strand passage (CC1). In contrast, aclarubicin inhibits the binding of topo II. I have been mentioned before that there is a tight association between the concentration, the DNA intercalation and the cleavage potency of anthracyclines. The podophyllotoxines inhibit both, CC1 and CC2 and amsidyl stabilises CC2 resulting in inhibition of the religation step of the enzyme. Novobiocin is not used in therapy yet.

Consequences for therapy. These findings are not only of theoretical interests but have consequences for cellular sensitivity. Specific combinations, such as aclarubicin and daunorubicin, or aclarubicin and etoposide are not reasonable, in fact they inhibit one another which has been shown by Peter-Buhl Jensen from Copenhagen [27, 28]. Also, sensitivity to aclarubicin is not necessarily associated with sensitivity to other anthracyclines. In 1992 we published experiments describing a celline with altered topoisomerase II and multidrug resistance to daunorubicin, doxorubicin and idarubicin but still high sensitivity to aclarubicin [29]. Speaking of anthracyclines we should be aware

Fig. 1. The "cleavable complex" and factors important for its formation

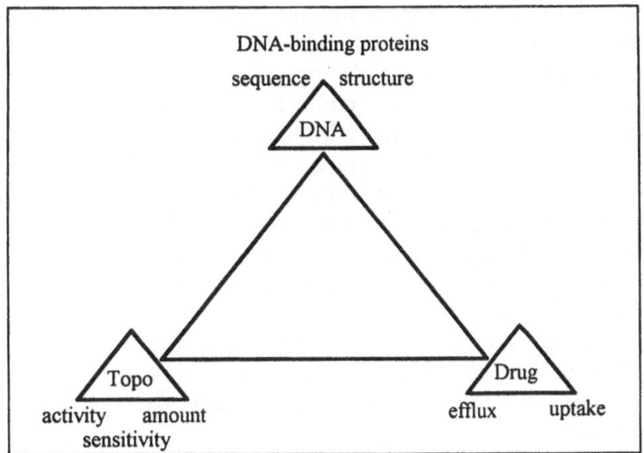

that these drugs do not only inhibit topo II but have additional intracellular effects such as direct membrane effects, they liberate free oxygen radicals, they intercalate into DNA and they inhibit the mitochondrial oxygen chain. Nevertheless, there are numerous indications that inhibition of topo II is the ultimate step for the induction of cell death.

These perceptions are important to design rational combination therapies especially when combining drugs with different intracellular targets. The mentioned interaction between nuclear matrix and topo II-function could be an example for the molecular background of combining taxol derivatives with topo II inhibitors. Also, it has been shown that prokaryotic topo I

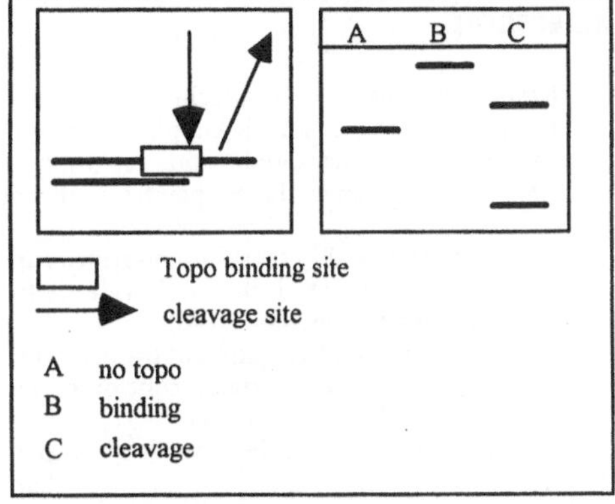

Fig. 2. Uncoupling the DNA binding, cleavage and religation events

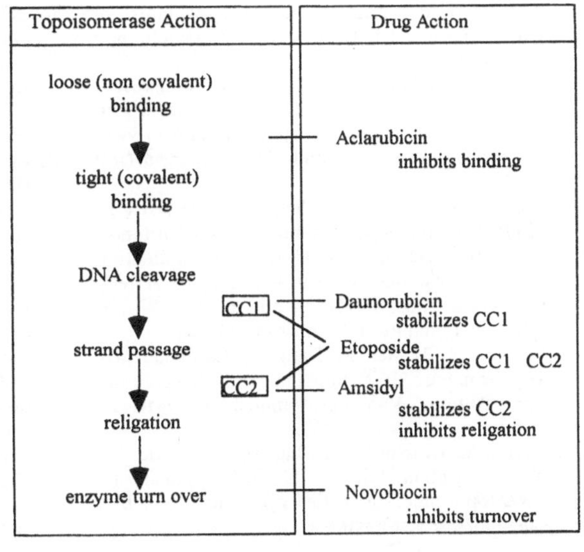

Fig. 3. Differences in the way of action of topo II inhibiting drugs. CC = cleavable complex

is able to substitute for a missing or defective topo II alpha. This might be interesting for chemotherapy now that we have potent topo I inhibitors which can be combined with topo II inhibitors. Another example is the combination of Ara C with topo II inhibitors. I does not seem to be reasonable to inhibit topo II before Ara CTP is incorporated into DNA but after this step, as the enzyme's function is necessary as well for the incorporation as for the following repair mechanisms. I hope these elucidations help to indicate the necessity to combine molecular-biological investigations with clinical studies, initiated by the doctor who treats the patients.

References

1. Uemura T, Ohkura H, Adachi Y, Morino K, Shiozaki K, Yanagida M. DNA topoisomerase II is required for condensation and separation of mitotic chromosomes in S. pombe. Cell 1987; 50: 917–925.
2. Tsao Y, Wu H, Liu LF. Transcription-driven supercoiling of DNA: direct biochemical evidence from in vitro studies. Cell 1989;56: 111–118.
3. Menzel R, Gellert M. Regulation of the genes for E. coli DNA gyrase: homeostatic control of DNA supercoiling. Cell 1983;34: 105–113.
4. Tan KB, Dorman TE, Falls KM, et al. Topoisomerase IIa and Topoisomerase IIβ Genes: Characterization and Mapping to Human Chromosomes 17 and 3, Respectively. Cancer Research 1992; 52: 231–234.
5. Takano H, Kohno K, Ono M, Uchida Y, Kuwano M. Increased Phosphorylation of DNA Topoisomerase II in Etoposide-resistant Mutants of Human Cancer KB Cells. Cancer Research 1991; 51: 3951–3957.
6. Samuels DS, Shimizu N. DNA topoisomerase I phosphorylation in murine fibroblasts treated with 12-O-tetradecanoylphorbol-13-acetate and in vitro by protein kinase. J Biol Chem 1992;267(16): 11156–62.
7. Schroder HC, Steffen R, Wenger R, Ugarkovic D, Muller WE. Age-dependent increase of DNA topoisomerase II activity in quail oviduct; modulation of the nuclear matrix-associated enzyme activity by protein phosphorylation and poly(ADP-ribosyl)ation. Mutat Res 1989;219(5–6): 283–94.
8. Gasser SM, Walter R, Dang Q, Cardenas ME. Topoisomerase II: its functions and phosphorylation. Antonie Van Leeuwenhoek 1992;62(1–2): 15–24.
9. Heck MM, Hittelman WN, Earnshaw WC. In vivo phosphorylation of the 170-kDa form of eukaryotic DNA topoisomerase II. Cell cycle analysis. J Biol Chem 1989;264(26): 15161–4.
10. Osheroff N. Eukaryotic topoisomerase II. J.Biol. Chem. 1986;261: 9944–9950.
11. Gieseler F, Boege F, Ruf B, Meyer P, Wilms K. Molecular pathways of topoisomerase II regulation and consequences for chemotherapy. In Hiddemann W. et al.: Leukemia IV, Springer Verlag 1993;in press.
12. Earnshaw WC, Halligen B, Cooke CA, Heck MM, Liu LF. Topoisomerase II is a structural component of mitoic chromosome scaffolds. J. Cell. Biol. 1985;100: 1706–1715.
13. Tsutsui K, Tsutsui K, Muller MT. The nuclear scaffold exhibites DNA-binding sites selective for supercoiled DNA. J. Biol. Chem. 1988;263: 7235–7241.
14. Laemmli UK, Gasser SM. A glimpse at chromosomal order. Trends in Genetics 1987;3.
15. Boege F, Kjeldsen E, Gieseler F, Alsner J, Biersack H. A drug-resistant variant of topoisomerase II alpha in human HL-60 cells exhibits alterations in catalytic pH optimum, DNA binding and subnuclear distribution. Eur. J. Biochem. 1993;218: 575–584.
16. Zwelling LA, Chan D, Hinds M, Mayes J, Silberman LE, Blick M. Effect of phorbol ester treatment on drug-induced, topoisomerase II-mediated DNA cleavage in human leukemia cells. Cancer Res 1988;48(23): 6625–33.
17. Gieseler F, Boege F, Clark M. Alteration of topoisomerase II action is a possible mechanism of HL-60 cell differentiation. Environ Health Persp 1990; 88: 183–185.
18. Gieseler F, Boege F, Biersack H, Spohn B, Clark M, Wilms K. Nuclear topisomerase II activity changes during HL-60 cell differentiation: alterations of drug sensitivity and pH-dependency. Leukemia and Lymphoma 1991; 5: 273–279.
19. Nishiyama M, Horichi N, Mazouzi Z, Bungo M, Saijo N, Tapiero H. Can cytotoxic activity of anthracyclines be related to DNA damage? Anticancer Drug Des 1990;5(1): 135–9.
20. Belvedere G, Suarato A, Geroni C, Giuliani FC, D'Incalci M. Comparison of intracellular drug retention, DNA damage and cytotoxicity of derivatives of doxorubicin and daunorubicin in a human colon adenocarcinoma cell line (LoVo). Biochem Pharmacol 1989;38(21): 3713–21.
21. Zunino F, Capranico G. DNA topoisomerase II as the primary target of antitumor anthracyclines. Anticancer Drug Des 1990;5(4): 307–17.
22. Gieseler F, Boege F, Biersack H, Mühlen I, Meyer P. Correlation between the DNA-binding affinity of anthracyclines and their cytotoxicity in vitro. Proc. Fourth Internatl. Congress on Anti-Cancer Chemotherapy. Paris, France 1993;: Abstr.169.
23. Gieseler F, Biersack H, Brieden T, Manderscheid J, Nüßler V. Cytotoxicity of anthracyclines: correlation with cellular uptake, intracellular distribution and DNA-binding. Ann. Haematol. 1994;supported.
24. Capranico G, Riva A, Tinalli S, Dasdia T, Zunino F. Markedly reduced levels of anthracycline-induced DNA strand breaks in resistant P388 leukemia cells and isolated nuclei. Cancer Res. 1987;47: 3752–3756.

25. Sorensen BS, Sinding J, Andersen AH, Alsner J, Jensen PB, Westergaard O. Mode of action of topoisomerase II-targeting agents at a specific DNA sequence. Uncoupling the DNA binding, cleavage and religation events. J Mol Biol 1992;228(3): 778–86.
26. Robinson MJ, Corbett AH, Osheroff N. Effects of topoisomerase II-targeted drugs on enzyme-mediated DNA cleavage and ATP hydrolysis: evidence for distinct drug interaction domains on topoisomerase II. Biochemistry 1993;32(14): 3638–43.
27. Jensen PB, Sorensen BS, Demant EJ, et al. Antagonistic effect of aclarubicin on the cytotoxicity of etoposide and 4′-(9-acridinylamino) methanesulfon-m-anisidide in human small cell lung cancer cell lines and on topoisomerase II-mediated DNA cleavage. Cancer Res 1990;50(11): 3311–6.
28. Jensen PB, Jensen PS, Demant EJ et al. Antagonistic effect of aclarubicin on daunorubicin-induced cytotoxicity in human small cell lung cancer cells: relationship to DNA integrity and topoisomerase II. Cancer Res 1991;51(19): 5093–9.
29. Erttmann R, Boetefür A, Erttmann KD, Gieseler F, Looft G. Conserved cytotoxic activity of aclacinomycin A in multifactorial multidrug resistance. Haematology and Blood Transfusion 1992;34: 49–55.

Acute Leukemias V
Experimental Approaches
and Management of Refractory Diseases
Hiddemann et al. (Eds.)

Mechanisms of Acquired ARA-C and DAC Resistance in Acute Myeloid Leukemia (AML): Development of a Model for the Study of Mutational Loss of Deoxycytidine Kinase (DCK) Activity

A. P. A. Stegmann, M. W. Honders, J. E. Landegent, and R. Willemze

Introduction

Complex and largely unknown mechanisms determine whether sufficient cyto-reduction occurs following chemotherapy for acute myeloid leukemia. The reasons for failure of induction treatment are related to patients' age. With the current supportive care measures, it is uncommon for patients <50 years of age to die from complications of the initial therapy; most of the 20% failure rate in this group is due to primary resistant leukemia. In contrast, in patients >60 years the cause of the failure rate (50%), can be equally divided between resistant leukemia and death occuring during marrow aplasia, due to the complications of pancytopenia. However, during subsequent relapses the majority of patients fails to respond due to drug resistance, and this is one of the major obstacles for long term disease free survival [1–3].

Deoxycytidine (dCyd) analogues, such as cytosine arabinoside (Ara-C) and 5-aza-2′-deoxycytidine (DAC), are currently used as the core drugs of most AML regimens [4, 5]. Resistance to these compounds has been explained by a variety of mechanisms. First, it may be that not all of the leukemic stem cells are proliferative and therefore are not likely to be eradicated by these S-phase specific drugs (cell kinetic resistance). Secondly, malignant cells may be present in certain anatomical sanctuaries, which protects them from the cytotoxicity of the chemotherapy (pharmacokinetic resistance). However, probably more important in explaining the development of resistance, are alterations in the basic metabolism of leukemic cells, that disturb the metabolic processing that both drugs need to undergo in order to acquire cytotoxicity (biochemical resistance). In general, the latter type of resistance may be the result of changes in genomic expression patterns, or disturbed regulation mechanisms leading to a decrease or increase of the activity of enzymes involved in drug metabolization [6, 7].

Metabolic Activation of Cytotoxic Potential

The metabolization of antiviral and anti-cancer purine and pyrimidine deoxynucleoside analogues is believed to be dependent on the activity of enzymes of the purine and pyrimidine salvage pathways [8–10]. A cascade of interacting enzymes normally controls the metabolization of the natural purines deoxyadenosine (dAdo) and deoxyguanosine (dGuo) and the pyrimidines, deoxycytidine (dCyd), thymidine (Thd) and deoxyuridine (dUrd). The initial phosphorylation of each of the purine and pyrimidine deoxynucleosides (dN) yields nucleotide monophosphates (dNMP) and is the rate limiting step in a biochemical sequale that eventually yields deoxynucleotide triphosphate residues (dNTP). dNTP's are essential for DNA synthesis in dividing cells. Hence synthesis and intracellular retention of Ara-C- and DAC-triphosphates, depends on the anabolic (phosphorylation) and catabolic (deaminating) activities of the pyrimidine pathway.

Dept. of Experimental Hematology, University Hospital Leiden, 2300 RC, Leiden, The Netherlands

Deoxycytidine is phosphorylated to deoxycytidine monophosphate (dCMP) by the rate limiting enzyme deoxycytidine kinase (DCK) [11]. dCMP is further phosphorylated by nucleoside mono- and diphosphate kinases to yield dCTP or deaminated into dUMP by dCMP-deaminase, which is the first step in the salvage pathway synthesis of dTTP-residues. dCTP acts as a feedback inhibitor of DCK (end product inhibition). Although the affinity of DCK for dC is highest, the enzyme also metabolizes the natural purine deoxynucleosides deoxyadenosine (dAdo) and deoxyguanosine (dGuo), as well as a variety of clinically relevant pyrimidine and purine nucleoside analogues, among them Ara-C and DAC [12].

A second enzyme however, the mitochondrial thymidine kinase-2 (TK2), is also capable of metabolizing dCyd, with an efficiency of 90% relative to its phosphorylating efficiency for Thd, whereas it is unable to use Ara-C as a substrate [13]. In general, the enzymes of the pyrimidine and of the purine salvage pathways display a broad substrate specificity and some substrates can be metabolized by more than one enzyme [13, 14]. Whether or not DAC is a substrate for TK2, is unknown, and DCK activity alone is believed to be essential for the potentiation of Ara-C and DAC mediated cytotoxicity.

Cytotoxic Mechanisms of Ara-C and DAC

The metabolic end-product of Ara-C, Ara-CTP, was found to be a weak inhibitor of DNA-polymerase alpha, that is required for its incorporation into newly synthesized DNA [15, 16]. When incorporated, Ara-CTP residues present at the 3′ end of a replicating strand of DNA, will serve as poor primer termini for further chain elongation, resulting in the termination of DNA synthesis [17]. The formation of (Ara-C)DNA correlates with the degree of cytotoxicity [18]. Recently, inhibition of DNA ligase by Ara-CTP was found to be partially responsible for Ara-C mediated toxicity [19, 20].

The DACTP residue on the other hand, has been shown to be actively incorporated into DNA [21]. Its cytotoxic effect occurs only after several cell cycles, and is believed to be due to its ability to cause hypomethylation of the replicating DNA through binding of the methyltransferase enzyme, a feature shared with other dCyd analogs containing chemical modifications of the 5-position of the cytosine ring [22, 23]. The methylation status of nuclear DNA has been shown to be an important regulator of gene expression, and perturbances of predetermined methylation patterns have been shown to induce unwarranted cellular differentiation processes [24].

DCK: Structural Properties and Kinetic Mechanism

Deoxycytidine kinase (DCK, EC 2.7.1.74) is a phosphotransferase enzyme of the pyrimidine salvage pathway. In its active form it is a dimer with a subunit molecular mass of 30.5 kDa [25]. It has been isolated from a variety of tissues and cell lines, such as calf thymus, human leukemic granulocytes, mouse spleen, monkey spleen, human tonsillar lymphocytes, and the cell lines MoltT4 (human lymphoblastic) and L1210 (mouse leukemic). In general thymus tissue preparations and T-lymphocytic lineages yield the highest amount of DCK [26–29].

Studies on the substrate binding affinity have revealed a relatively wide range of K_m-values for dC, AraC and DAC, much depending on the source and the degree of purification that was obtained. The reported K_m-values for dC vary from 0.3 μM to 14 μM. In one case, K_m-values as high as 300 μM–700 μM, were reported for measurements in crude cell-extracts of human malignant cell lines, such as HL60, OVCAR-5 and PANC-1 [30]. For Ara-C, K_m-values range from 8 μM to 175 μM. For DAC, only three reported K_m-values are known; 63 μM (calf thymus), 64 μM (mouse leukemic cell line L1210) and 29 μM (leukemic mouse spleen) [31, 32].

The kinetic properties of DCK, and the exact nature of its interaction with substrate(s) and phosphate-donor(s) is still a subject of debate. In several studies, particularly those in which crude enzyme preparations (e.g. whole cell extracts) were used, the enzyme has shown biphasic kinetics, with activity apparently being distributed between a high and a low range of substrate concentrations [33–35]. Keirdaszuk et al. measured the enzymes' intrinsic fluorescence pattern, that is quenched upon ligand binding and thus provides insight into the conformational behaviour of the protein. They found that the protein can adopt two distinct conformational statuses, with a high and a low affinity for the binding of dCyd, providing some experimental support for the observed non-linear kinetics [36]. However, in crude DCK preparations, the presence of other active nucleoside kinases (e.g. TK2) could explain the observed duality, due to the putative overlap in substrate specificity of the enzymes involved. Finally, the observed non-linear kinetics may be due to proteolytic cleavage that occurs during purification procedures. Studies with highly purified (up to 50,000-fold) DCK, do not show non-linear kinetics [26, 37, 25].

Results of steady-state initial rate kinetic analysis and inhibition studies using highly purified enzyme preparations, do agree on an ordered sequential pathway. Kim et al. claimed binding of ATP preceeding dC binding, as opposed to the latter, with dCTP acting as a multisubstrate analog, competitive towards ATP and non-competitive with dC [37]. Datta et al. proposed a sequential random Bi-Bi system, in which binding of dC is followed by binding of ATP and subsequent release of diphosphate and dCMP, with dCTP acting as a feedback inhibitor, competitive with dC and non-competetive with ATP [26]. A recent communication by Shewach et al. supports the findings of Datta et al, albeit with UTP instead of ATP as the preferred phosphate donor [38]. ATP is commonly used as a phosphate-donor in most assays to measure DCK-activity. It has been shown to be an efficient phosphate donor in various studies. However, the enzyme has been shown to also utilize UTP and GTP. Recently it was shown that the phosphorylation efficiency (V_{max} / K_m) for dC and AraC was greatest in the presence of UTP rather than ATP as the phosphate-donor [39, 40].

DCK as a Target for Resistance Research

Several of the enzymes and regulation systems in the pyrimidine salvage pathway have been targets for research into the mechanism of (acquired) Ara-C resistance. In Ara-C resistant leukemic cells of patients with a poor clinical response, dCyd-deaminase activity was found to be higher than in patients with a good response [50]. More recent reports however have not confirmed these findings and suggest a negligible role for dCyd deaminase in the development of Ara-C resistance [51]. An increased intracellular dCTP-pool size was found in Ara-C resistant cell lines and is believed to contribute to resistance through negative feedback inhibition of DCK as well as through competetive inhibition of DNA polymerases [52, 26]. However, the most consistent observation in Ara-C resistant leukemic cell lines, dating as far back as 1965, is the absence of measurable DCK activity [53, 35, 54]. DCK deficiency can be considered as a marker of Ara-C resistance in acute leukemia and DCK has become a prime target for research into the mechanism of Ara-C (and DAC-) resistance.

In 1978 Meyers & Kreis isolated the DCK-protein from an in vivo mouse neoplasm resistant to Ara-C (P815/AraC) and found its activity 90-fold decreased compared to the enzyme isolated from the same, but Ara-C sensitive neoplasm (P815). They argued that loss of function might be the result of a loss of structural features and demonstrated that the overall amino acid composition of the DCK protein isolated from the P815/AraC neoplasm differed from the protein of the sensitive cells [55, 35]. Based upon their observations they postulated a model of mutational inactivation of the DCK enzyme in Ara-C resistant cells.

It has not been untill recently, that genetic analysis of the DCK locus and of its transcriptional and translational control has been facilitated by the cloning of the human DCK-cDNA sequence and by the subsequent elucidation of the genomic structure of the human DCK gene [56, 57]. In addition, we were able to localize the DCK gene to chromosome 4 band q13.3-q21.1 by means of fluorescence in situ hybridization [58]. Owens et al. were the first to identify the molecular basis of DCK-deficiency in AraC-resistant T-lymphoblastic cell lines [59]. Two mutations could be characterized in cloned DCK complementary DNA's of the AraC-resistant cell line. One allele showed a 115 bp deletion corresponding to the fifth exon of the DCK gene, whereas the other allele carried a G to A transition at nucleotide 242, which is located in the concensus ATP-binding domain of the cDNA. Bacterial expression of both mutant DCK cDNA's showed an almost fully diminished catalytic activity of the mutant protein. To date, this has been the only published report describing mutational inactivation of DCK.

Development of a Model for the Study of Mutational Inactivation of DCK

Over the years, we have adapted and expanded an in vitro model of Ara-C resistant rat myeloid leukemia, consisting of numerous cell lines that are either resistant to AraC or DAC and that are either of clonal origin or cultured as heterogeneous cell populations. The model was derived from an in vivo model for acute myeloid leukemia in Brown Norway rats (BNML), that was originally developed at the Radiobiological Institute at TNO in Rijswijk (The Netherlands) [60, 61]. Within this model a cell line originating from the bone marrow of leukemic rats was propagated in vitro and named IPC-81 [62]. We now maintain this cell line as RCL/O (or BNML-Cl/O). Ara-C resistance was developed in vivo in the BNML model and an autonomously growing Ara-C resistant cell line was derived from it and named BNML-Cl/Ara-C [63]. We maintain this line as RCL/A [54].

In order to compare the phenotypic and the genotypic characteristics of Ara-C resistance, we cloned the RCL/A cell line in a limiting dilution assay (LDA) and obtained several homogeneous Ara-C resistant subclones: RA/1,2,4 and 7. Secondly, in vitro resistance to DAC was induced in the parent RCL/O cell line by exposing it to gradually increasing concentrations of the drug, over a 160-days period. We obtained a DAC-resistant cell line, RCL/D, and subsequently cloned it in a LDA, yielding the clonal lines RD/1 and RD/2. Cross-resistance was observed for both drugs in each of the resistant cell lines. We initially studied DCK inactivation in this model at the level of enzyme activity, and found that all Ara-C and DAC-resistant lines and clones were DCK deficient. Metabolization of either Ara-C or DAC was undetectable in the RCL/A, the RCL/D and the clonal sublines. We could still measure dC phosphorylation, but with calculated K_m-values increased 70- to 100-fold as compared to wild type RCL/O cells, showing a strongly decreased affinity of the enzyme for its natural substrate. Determination of kinetic constants revealed K_m-values of 9.4 μM (dC), 378.5 μM (Ara-C) and 31.2 μM (DAC) [54].

To be able to perform a genetic analysis of the DCK locus we developed a rat specific polymerase chain reaction (PCR) system. We synthesized oligonucleotide primers based on the human DCK-cDNA sequence as it was published by Chottiner et al. [56], and used them to perform PCR on rat cDNA on the assumption of conservation of the DCK sequence between man and rat. The PCR protocol permitted amplification of DCK-specific sequences from rat (and human) cDNA, that was reverse transcribed from poly(A)-mRNA isolated from all cell lines. We have recently obtained the full rat DCK-cDNA from a phage lambda rat lymphocyte cDNA library [64]. Sequence determination revealed a 89.7% homology at the nucleotide level, with only 21 out of the enzymes 260 amino acids different.

Currently we are undertaking detailed genetic analysis of this model. We are studying mRNA expression by PCR and Northern blotting, and will look for evidence of mutational events affecting the DCK locus by Southern blotting and by detection of Single Stranded Conformation Polymorphisms (SSCP). Our preliminary results, as presented in recent communications [65], support the possibility of mutational inactivation of DCK.

In order to be able to compare Ara-C and DAC resistance more precisely we will expand the model. We have cloned the RCL/O cell line and obtained the clones RO/1, 2 and 3. In each of these three genetically and phenotypically homogeneous clones we are currently inducing either Ara-C or DAC-resistance, following tightly scheduled induction schemes. Exposure will start at a level 100-fold below ID50 doses and will be increased at approximately 20 two week intervals up to otherwise lethal doses. We aim to identify mutational events affecting the DCK locus in each of the resulting resistant clones, and compare differences between individually generated clones as well as between Ara-C and DAC resistance.

Secondly, this model will facilitate understanding of the mechanism of resistance induction. If mutations can be induced by exposure to either AraC or DAC in cells of clonal origin, this will support the hypothesis that de novo mutations of the DCK gene can occur, as opposed to the idea of preferential outgrowth (from a heterogeneous population) of cells that already harbour such mutations (clonal selection). The latter might provide insight into the mechanism underlying primary drug-resistance in patients. During the course of induction of resistance, RNA and DNA samples can be collected before each dosis increase in order to determine whether or not mutations occur at a specific AraC- or DAC-dosis. We will also determine DCK activity at each interval, in order to determine at which drug-dosage DCK deficiency becomes apparent. From these experiments we hope to be able to determine the sequence of events that proceeds a resistant phenotype.

Finally, the model allows evaluation of cross resistance for more recently developed dCyd, dA and dGuo analogs that are used as anticancer or antiviral agents. 2′,2′-difluorodeoxycytidine (dFdC), used against several solid tumors, 2′,3′-dideoxycytidine (ddC), used as an anti HIV drug in AIDS treatment, and 2-chlorodeoxyadenosine (CdA), used for treatment of Hairy cell leukemia refractory to α-Interferon, are all substrates of DCK. The outcome of testing, within this model, for their potential to induce resistance could have prognostic significance for the choice of treatment and drug doses in each of these malignancies [66-68].

Through genetic analysis of the DCK locus during the course of resistance induction, within this well defined rat model for human AML, we hope to contribute to the identification of the events that eventually confer drug-resistance in AML.

References

1. Peters WG, Willemze, R & Colly LP. (1988) Results of induction and consolidation treatment with intermediate and high-dose cytosine arabinoside and m-Amsa of patients with poor risk acute myelogenous leukemia. Eur J Haematol 40: 198–204.
2. Schiller G, Gajewski J, Nimer S, Territo M, Ho W, Lee M & Champlin R. (1992) A randomized study of intermediate versus conventional-dose cytarabine cytarabine as intensive induction for acute myelogenous leukaemia. Br J Haematol 81 (2): 170–177.
3. Wiernik PH, Banks PL, Case DC jr., Arlin ZA, Periman PO, Todd MB, Ritch PS, Enck RE & Weitberg AB. (1992) Cytarabine plus idarubicin or daunorubicin as induction and consolidation therapy for previously untreated addult patients with acute myeloid leukemia. Blood 79 (2): 313–319.
4. Debusscher L, Marie JP, Dochin P, Blanc GM, Arrigo C, Zittoun R & Stryckmans P. (1989) Phase I-III trial of 5-Aza-2′-deoxycytidine in adult patients with acute leukemia. Proceedings: 5-Aza-2′-deoxycy-tidine, preclinical and clinical studies. Symposium, Amsterdam
5. Richel DJ, Colly LP, Kluin-Nelemans JC & Willemze R. (1990) The antileukaemic activity of 5-Aza-2′-deoxycytidine (Aza-dC) in patients with relapsed and resistant leukaemia. Br J Cancer 58: 144–148.
6. Hall A, Cattan AR & Proctor SJ. (1989) Mechanisms of drug resistance in acute leukemia. Leukemia Res 13 (5): 351–356.
7. Momparler RL, Onetto-Pothier N. (1989) In: D.Kessel, Ed. Drug resistance to cytosine arabinoside. Chapter 19; Resistance to antineoplastic drugs. CRC Press.
8. Reichard P. (1988) Interactions between deoxyribonucleotide and DNA synthesis. Annu Rev Biochem 57: 349–374.
9. Wasternack C. (1980) Degradation of pyrimidines and pyrimidine analogs: pathways and mutual influences. Pharmacol Ther 8 (3): 629–651.
10. Munch-Petersen A. (1983) Metabolism of nucleotides,nucleosides and nucleobases in microorganisms. London: Academic Press Inc. Ltd.
11. Momparler RL & Fischer GA. (1976) Mammalian deoxynucleoside kinases.I.Deoxycytidine kinase: Purification properties and kinetic studies with cytosine arabinoside. J Biol Chem 243: 4298–4304.
12. Kierdaszuk B, Bohman C, Ullman B & Eriksson S. (1992) Substrate specificity of human deoxycytidine kinase toward antiviral 2′,3′-dideoxynucleoside analogs. Biochem Pharmacol 43: 197–206.
13. Eriksson S, Kierdaszuk B, Munch-Petersen B, Oberg B & Johansson NG. (1991) Comparison of the substrate specificities of human thymidine kinase 1 and 2 and deoxycytidine kinase towards antiviral and cytostatic nucleoside analogs. Biochem Biophys Res Comm 176(2): 586–592.
14. Habteyesus A, Nordenskjold A, Bohman C & Eriksson S. (1991) Deoxynucleoside phosphorylating enzymes in monkey and human tissues show great similarities, while mouse deoxycytidine kinase has a different substrate specificity. Biochem Pharmacol 42(9): 1829–1836.
15. Tanaka M & Yoshida S. (1982) Altered sensitivity to 1-β-D-arabino-furanosylcytosine 5′-triphosphate of DNA polymerase from leukemic blasts of acute lymphoblastic leukemia. Cancer Res 42: 649–654.
16. Zittoun J, Marquet J, David J-C, Maniey D & Zittoun R. (1989) A study of the mechanisms of cytotoxicity of Ara-C on three human leukemic cell lines. Cancer Chemother Pharmacol 24 (4): 251–255.
17. Major PP, Egan EM, Herrick DJ & Kufe DW. (1982) Effect of Ara-C incorporation on deoxyribonucleic acid synthesis in cells. Biochem Pharmacol 31 (18): 2937–2940.
18. Major P, Egan E, Bearsley G, Minden MD & Kufe D. (1982) Lethality of human myeloblasts correlates with the incorporation of Ara-C into DNA. Proc Natl Acad Sci USA. 78: 3235–3239.
19. Gedik CM & Collins AR. (1991) The mode of action of 1-β-D-arabino-furanosylcytosine in inhibiting DNA repair; new evidence using a sensitive assay for repair DNA synthesis and ligation in permeable cells. Mutat Res 254 (3): 231–237.
20. Zittoun J, Marquet J & David J-C. (1991) Mechanism of inhibition of DNA ligase in Ara-C treated cells. Leukemia Res 15: 157–167.
21. Bouchard J & Momparler RL. (1983) Incorporation of 5-Aza-2′-deoxy-cytidine triphosphate into DNA. Interactions with mammalian DNA polymerase and DNA methylase. Mol Pharmacol 24: 109–114.
22. Jones PA & Taylor SM. (1980) Cellular differentiation, cytidine analogs and DNA methylation. Cell 20: 85–93.
23. Santi DV, Garret CE & Barr PJ. (1983) On the mechanism of inhibition of DNA-cytosine methyltransferase by cytidine analogs. Cell 83: 9–10.

24. Taylor SM. (1993) 5-Aza-2'-deoxycytidine: cell differentiation and DNA methylation. Leukemia 7 (suppl.): 3–8.
25. Datta NS, Shewach DS, Hurley MC, Mitchell BS & Fox IF. (1989) Human T-lymphoblast deoxycytidine kinase: purification and properties. Biochemistry 28: 114–123.
26. Datta NS, Shewach DS, Mitchell BS & Fox IH. (1989) Kinetic properties and inhibition of human T-lymphoblast deoxycytidine kinase. J Biol Chem 264(16): 9359–9364.
27. Bohman C & Eriksson S. (1988) Deoxycytidine kinase from human leukemic spleen: preparation and characterization of the homogenous enzyme. Biochemistry 27: 4258–4265.
28. Cheng Y-C, Domin B & Lee L-S. (1977) Human deoxycytidine kinase. Purification and characterization of the cytoplasmic and mitochondrial isozymes derived from blast cells of acute myelocytic leukemia patients. Biochim Biophys Acta 481: 481–492.
29. Kessel D. (1968) Properties of deoxycytidine kinase partially purified from L1210 cells. J Biol Chem 243: 4739.
30. Singhal RL, Yeh YA, Szekeres T & Weber G. (1992) Increased deoxycytidine kinase activity in cancer cells and inhibition by difluorodeoxycytidine. Oncology Res 4: 517–522.
31. Momparler RL & Derse D. (1979) Kinetics of phosphorylation of 5-Aza-2'-deoxycytidine by deoxycytidine kinase. Biochem Pharmacol 28: 1443–1444.
32. Vesely J & Cihak A. (1980) 5-Aza-2'-deoxycytidine: Preclinical studies in mice. Neoplasma 27: 112–119.
33. Ives DH & Durham JP. (1970) Deoxycytidine kinase. III Kinetics and allosteric regulation. J Biol Chem 245: 2285–2294.
34. Sarup JC & Fridland A. (1987) Identification of purine deoxynucleoside kinases from human leukemia cells: substrate activation by purine and pyrimidine deoxyribonucleosides. Biochemistry 26: 590–597.
35. Meyers MB & Kreis W. (1978) Comparison of the enzymatic activities of two deoxycytidine kinases purified from cells sensitive (P815) and resistant (P815/ara-C) to 1-β-D-Arabinofuranosylcytosine. Cancer Res 38: 1105–1112.
36. Kierdaszuk B, Rigler R & Eriksson S. (1993) Binding of substrates to human deoxycytidine kinase studied with ligand-dependant quenching of enzyme intrinsic fluorescence. Biochemistry 32: 699–707.
37. Kim M-Y & Ives DH. (1989) Human deoxycytidine kinase: kinetic mechanism and end product regulation. Biochemistry 28: 9043–9047.
38. Shewach DS, Reynolds KK, Hahn T. (1993) Apparent allosteric regulation of deoxycytidine kinase by UTP. Proc Am Assoc Canc Res 34: 10, abstract #55.
39. Shewach DS, Reynolds KK & Hertel L. (1992) Nucleotide specificity of human deoxycytidine kinase. Mol Pharmacol 42: 518–524.
40. White JC & Capizzi RL. (1991) A critical role for uridine nucleotides in the regulation of deoxycytidine kinase and the concentration dependance of 1-β-D-arabinofuranosylcytosine phosphorylation in human leukemia cells. Cancer Res 51: 2559–2565.
41. Steuart CD & Burke PJ. (1971) Cytidine deaminase and the development of resistance to cytosine arabinoside. Nature New Biol 233: 109–113.
42. Harris AL, Grahame-Smith DG, Potter CG & Bunch C. (1981) Cytosine arabinoside deamination in human leukemic myeloblasts and resistance to cytosine arabinoside therapy. Clin Sci 60: 191–196.
43. Momparler RL. (1968) Kinetic and template studies with cytosine arabinoside 5'-triphosphate and mamalian DNA polymerase. Mol Pharmacol 8: 362–367.
44. Chu Y & Fischer GA. (1965) Comparative studies of leukemic cells sensitive and resistant to cytosine arabinoside. Biochem Pharmacol 14: 333–341.
45. Stegmann, A.P.A., Honders, M.W., Kester, M.G.D., Landegent, J.E. and Willemze, R. Role of deoxycytidine kinase in an in vitro model for AraC- and DAC-resistance: substrate enzyme interactions with deoxycytidine, 1-β-D-arabinofuranosylcytosine and 5-aza-2'-deoxycytidine. (1993) Leukemia 7(7), 1005–1011.
46. Meyers MB & Kreis W. (1978) Structural comparison of deoxycytidine kinases purified from cells sensitive (P815) or resistant (P815/ara-C) to 1-β-D-arabinofuranosylcytosine. Cancer Res 38: 1099–1104.
47. Chottiner, E.G., Shewach, D.S., Datta, N.S., Ashcraft, E., Gribbin, D., Ginsburg, D., Fox, I.H. and Mitchell, B.S. (1991) Cloning and expression of human deoxycytidine kinase cDNA. PNAS 88: 1531–1535.
48. Song JJ, Walker S, Chen E, Johnson II EE, Spychala J, Gribbin T & Mitchell BS. (1993) Genomic structure and chromosomal localization of the human deoxycytidine kinase gene. PNAS 90: 431–434.
49. Stegmann APA, Honders MW, Bolk MWJ, Wessels J, Willemze R & Landegent J. (1993) Assignment of the human deoxycytidine kinase (DCK) gene to chromosome 4 band q13.3-q21.1. Genomics 17: 528–529.
50. Owens, J.K., Shewach, D.S., Ullman, B. and Mitchell, B.S. (1992). Resistance to 1-β-D Arabinofuranosylcytosine in human T-lymphoblasts mediated by mutations within the deoxycytidine kinase gene. *Cancer Res* 52: 2389–2393.
51. Martens ACM, Van Bekkum DW, Hagenbeek A. (1990) Review. The BN acute myelocytic leukemia (BNML) (A rat model for studying human acute myelocytic leukemia (AML)). Leukemia 4(4): 241–257.
52. Bekkum DW van & Hagenbeek A. (1977) Relevance of the BN leukaemia as a model for human acute myeloid leukemia. Blood Cells 3: 565–579.
53. Hagenbeek A, Martens ACM & Colly LP. (1987) In vivo development of cytosine arabinoside resistance in the BN acute myelocytic leukemia. Semin Oncol 14: 202–206.
54. Lacaze N, Gombaud-Saintonge G & Lanotte M. (1983) Conditions cotrolling long term proliferation of BN ratpromyelocytic leukemia in vitro:

primary growth stimulation by microenvironment and establishment of an autonomous BN "leukemic stem cell line". Leuk Res 7: 145–148.

55. Stegmann APA, Honders WM, Willemze R & Landegent J. Molecular cloning of rat deoxycytidine kinase (*dck*). Biochem Biophys Res Commun, submitted.
56. Stegmann APA, Honders WM, Willemze R & Landegent J. Mutations in the deoxycytidine kinase gene in acquired resistance to 1-β-D-arabinofuranosylcytosine and 5-aza-2′-deoxycytidine in acute myeloid leukemia. 22nd Annual Meeting of the International Society for Experimental Hematology (ISEH), Rotterdam, The Netherlands, August 1993. Oral presentation.
57. Heinemann V, Hertel LW, Grindey GB & Plunkett W. (1988) Comparison of the cellular pharmacokinetics and cytotoxicity of 2′,2′-difluorodeoxycytidine and 1-β-D-Arabinofuranosylcytosine. Cancer Res 48: 4024–4031.
58. Starnes MC & Cheng Y-C. (1987) Cellular metabolism of 2′,3′-dideoxycytidine, a compound active against human immunodeficiency virus in vitro. J Biol Chem 262(3): 988–991.
59. Beutler E. (1992) Cladribine (2-chlorodeoxyadenosine). Lancet 340: 952–956.

Acute Leukemias V
Experimental Approaches
and Management of Refractory Diseases
Hiddemann et al. (Eds.)

Expression of P-Glycoprotein in Children and Adults with Leukemia – Correlation with Clinical Outcome

Slawomir Kaczorowski [1], Maria Ochocka [2], Robert Aleksandrowicz [3], Maria Kaczorowska [4], Michal Matysiak [2], and Marek Karwacki

Abstract. The multidrug resistance (MDR) phenomenon has been shown to be associated with the expression of P-glycoprotein (P-gp), the product of mdr-1 gene. In the present study the expression of P-gp was investigated in 40 children, 21 adults' leukaemia and 10 healthy donors' samples. The presence of P-gp was evaluated by the immunohistochemical method (APAAP), with three different monoclonal antibodies (MAb's) directed against separate intra- (C219, JSB-1) and extra-cellular (MRK16) epitopes of P-gp. Human leukaemic cell line (K562) and Vincristine resistant (K562VCR) subline served as negative and positive controls for C219, JSB-1 and MRK16 staining, respectively. The expression of P-gp was found in 14 out of 40 (35%) children and in 8 out of 21 (38%) adults' leukemia cases. No expression of P-gp in 10 healthy donors' samples was observed. In children P-gp positive staining was detected in 3/8 Acute Myeloid Leukemia (AML), 8/26 Acute Lymphoblastic Leukemia (ALL), 1/1 Chronic Myeloid Leukemia (CML) and 2/5 Non Hodgkin's Lymphoma (NHL) cases. In adults P-gp positive staining was noticed in 7/17 AML, 1/4 ALL cases. In children and adults samples pattern of staining for P-gp was predominantly cytoplasmic, although a Golgi-associated dot like pattern of staining was also observed. Clinical follow up in children's and adults' leukemias reveals good response to induction chemotherapy both in P-gp positive and negative patients.

Introduction

The phenomenon of multidrug resistance (MDR) is one of the factors responsible for the lack of tumor sensitivity to cytotoxic drugs, potentially limiting the effectiveness of cancer chemotherapy. Treatment with one drug can cause cross resistance to a wide variety of structurally unrelated drugs with a different mode of action [1]. Drug resistance has been shown to be associated with the expression of P-glycoprotein (P-gp), the product of the mdr-1 gene [2]. In humans there are two closely related genes, the mdr-1 and mdr-3 [3]. Only the mdr-1 gene product has been linked to clinical and experimental multidrug resistance [4, 5]. The function of mdr-3 gene and its product remains unknown. Transfection experiments with mdr-1 gene provided the most direct evidence that P-glycoprotein overexpression is responsible for the MDR phenotype [2, 6]. Structural analysis of mdr-1 gene, encoding P-gp, reveals strong homology between P-gp and other transport proteins present in other organisms such as bacteria, yeast etc. [3, 7–9]. The P-gp is 1280 amino acids long, consists of two homologous parts of approximately equal length [7]. Structural analysis of

[1] Department of Immunology, Cancer Center and Institute of Oncology, Wawelska 15, 02-034 Warsaw, Poland
[2] Warsaw University Medical School, Department of Pediatric Hematology - Oncology, Dzialdowska 1, 01-184 Warsaw, Poland
[3] Department of Obstetrics and Gynaecology, Child and Mother Institute, Kasprzaka 17, Warsaw, Poland
[4] Department of Internal Medicine - Family Medicine, Postgraduate Medical Center, Czerniakowska 231, 00-416 Warsaw, Poland

P-gp demonstrates that each part of P-gp consists of hydrophobic and hydrophilic segments. Each half of P-gp includes a hydrophobic region with six predicted transmembrane segments as well as a hydrophilic region [3, 7]. It has been demonstrated that hydrophobic regions have binding sites for drugs as well as for ATP and express internal ATP-ase activity [10]. The P-gp functions as an energy dependent pump for the efflux of diverse anti cancer drugs i.e. Vincristine, Vinblastine, Adriamycin etc. from MDR cells. The overexpression of P-gp and expression of mdr-1 gene has been reported in drug resistant cell lines as well as in leukemias, lymphomas and solid tumors [4, 11–16]. The expression of P-gp was found in normal adult and foetal tissues with the highest level in the adrenal gland and organs with excretory function: liver, colon and kidney. In other organs and tissues the expression of P-gp is low, or P-gp is not detected [11, 15, 17, 18]. The protein shows polarised expression in a number of normal epithelial cells and in specialised capillary endothelium in brain, testis and some high endothelial venules in lymph nodes [15–17, 19, 20]. The physiologic role of P-gp and substrates for P-gp in normal cells are not known. P-gp plays probably an important role as one of the transport mechanisms within the tissues, or serves as one of the mechanisms protecting a normal or tumor cell from environmental toxins. The clinical importance of P-gp expression is being currently extensively studied. The aim of the present study was to investigate the expression of P-gp in leukemia cases using monoclonal antibodies (MAb's) directed against intra- (C219, JSB-1) and extra-cellular (MRK16) epitopes of P-gp. We would also like to compare the clinical outcome of patients with P-gp positive and negative staining.

Materials and Methods

Patients. Forty children at presentation and at different stages of disease; 8 (AML), 26 (ALL), 1 (CML) and 5 (NHL), (median age 8 9/12, range 1 8/12–14 5/12) and twenty one adults at the stage of presentation; 17 AML, 4 ALL (median age 45 6/12 range 18–77) were studied. Specimens obtained from ten healthy donors (6 children and 4 adults) were also studied. Adults' leukemia specimens for the study were retrieved from a blood bank. They were collected at the diagnosis stage. Children's material was obtained at different stages of disease; 31 cases at diagnosis, 3 at remission, 1 in first, 4 at second and 1 at third relapse. The diagnosis was made on the basis of bone marrow aspiration biopsy, by conventional clinical, morphologic, cytochemical and immunological criteria. The French-American-British (FAB) classification was used. A complete remission (CR) was determined as less than 5% of blasts counted in bone marrow smear [21]. All children investigated received treatment; in the case of AML and ALL it consisted of Berlin Frankfurt Münster (BFM) program BFM 83, BFM86 or BFM90 (Vincristine, Rubidomycin, Asparaginase, Cytarabin, Cyclophosphamide). NHL patients were treated with COAMP (Cyclophosphamide, Vincristine, Doxorubicin, Methotrexate, Prednisone). Adults with AML received treatment with either Rubidomycin – Vincristine – Cytarabin, or Mitoxantrone – Etoposid – Cytarabin or Thioguanin – Cytarabin – Daunorubicin. ALL patients received treatment with Daunorubicin – Cyclophosphamide – Vincristine – Prednisone – Asparaginase.

Methods

Antibodies. Three monoclonal antibodies, directed against separate epitopes of P-glycoprotein, were used; C219 (IgG2a) (Centocor, Diagnostics, USA) (13), JSB-1 (IgG1) (Sanbio/Monosan, Netherlands) [22] and MRK-16 (IgG2a) (kindly provided by Dr. T. Tsuruo, Cancer Chemotherapy Center, Japanese Foundation for Cancer Research, Tokyo, Japan) [23].

Preparation of blast cells. Peripheral blood mononuclear cells (PBMC) from patients were obtained by Ficoll/Hypaque (F/H) (Pharmacia, Sweden) gradient centrifugation. After F/H separation PBMC were washed three times in phosphate buffer saline (PBS). 1×10^6 cells were resuspended in PBS and cytospins were prepared (Shandon, UK). After drying at room temperature cytospins were fixed in acetone for 5 min., wrapped in Parafilm (American Can Company) and stored at (–) 70 °C until used.

Controls. Blasts from Vincristine (VCR) resistant human leukaemic cell line K562VCR, cultured in 150nM of VCR, and VCR sensitive K562 cell line were used as positive and negative controls, respectively. K562VCR cell line had been shown to have elevated levels of mdr-1 transcripts by solution hybridization (personal communication Dr. A. Gruber, Division of Medicine, Karolinska Hospital, Stockholm, Sweden). Ten PBMC separated from healthy donors, 6 children and 4 adults' specimens, were also studied.

Immunocytochemical staining. Before immunostaining cytospins were fixed once more in acetone for 5 min., rehydrated with Tris-buffered saline (TBS), preincubated with 1% Bovine Serum Albumin (BSA) and 1% normal human serum (NHS). Primary MAb's C219, JSB-1 and MRK16 were applied overnight at 4û C in a moist chamber. The Alkaline Phosphatase Anti Alkaline Phosphatase (APAAP) method was used [24]. Briefly after incubation with primary antibodies the slides were incubated with rabbit anti mouse immunoglobulins and APAAP complex both (Dakopatts, Glostrup, Denmark). The second and the third steps were repeated to enhance the reaction. Between consecutive steps slides were washed three times in TBS. A Vector SK5100 (Vector Lab., Burlingame, USA) red kit was used to develop the color product of enzymatic reaction. Nucleoli were counterstained with Mayer's Hematoxylin and were mounted with gelatine-glycerol mounting solution. The slides were evaluated at the light microscope. Appopriate positive and negative controls were also employed. Negative controls included omission of primary antibody as well as reconstitution of primary MAb's with irrelevant immunoglobulins of the same isotypes. We have considered, as a positive staining for P-gp, that case which was positive with at least two MAb's. Intensity of staining was evaluated as strong, moderate, weak and no staining on 200 cells counted at the light microscope in random choosen fields.

Results

Reactivity of MAb's on control slides. The Vincristine resistant K562VCR subline showed consistent reactivity with three antibodies. The intensity of staining varied from moderate to strong. Weak staining and occasionally no staining was also noticed. The cytoplasmic staining with C219 and JSB-1 MAb's and membrane staining with MRK-16 was observed. In Vincristine sensitive K562 cell line and ten PBMC samples obtained from healthy donors no reactivity with three antibodies was detected.

Reactivity with three MAb's on blast cells. Table 1 and 2 summarises clinical data and immunohistochemical staining for the P-gp. A positive staining for P-gp was detected in 14 out of 40 (35%) children's and in 8 out of 21 (38%) adults' cases. In children specimens staining for P-gp was detected in 10 out of 31 [32%) newly diagnosed cases and in 4 out of 9 [44%) cases during remission or relapse. One case, labelled in Table 1 "a"and "A", was P-gp positive at presentation and in relapse. In children's and adults' cases predominantly cytoplasmic and membrane staining was seen. A dot like - Golgi associated staining with JSB-1 and granular intracytoplasmic staining with C219 and JSB-1 antibodies was also observed. MRK-16 antibody displayed membrane staining. The intensity of staining with three antibodies varied within the cases examined and was labeled as weak (range 9%–79%) median 38,2 or moderate to strong (range 5%–47%) median 13,6. Commonly weaker

Table 1. Expression of P-gp in adult leukemias

Type/ No	FAB	P-gp(+)	Response	Stage	Bl. Group
AML 2	M1	–	CR	0	A
		+	CR	0	O
AML 5	M4	+	CR	0	O
		–	CR	0	O
		+	CR	0	A
		–	CR	0	O
		–	CR	0	A
AML 2	M5a	+	CR	0	O
		+	CR	0	nd
		–	CR	0	A
AML 3	M5b	–	CR	0	nd
		–	CR	0	O
		–	CR	0	nd
		–	CR	0	A
AML3	MDS	–	CR	0	O
		+	CR	0	nd
		+	CR	0	O
ALL 3	pre B	+	CR	0	A
		–	CR	0	A
		–	CR	0	B
All 1	T	–	CR	0	nd

AML–Acute Myeloid Leukemia, ALL–Acute Lymphoblastic Leukemia, MDS–Myelo Dysplastic Syndrome, CR–complete remision, (+)–positive staining for P-gp, (–)–negative staining for P-gp, Stage–stage of disease: 0–at presentation, B–B lymphocytes, T–T lymphocytes, nd–no data

staining with C219 MAb in comparison to staining of JSB-1 and MRK-16 MAb's was observed.

Correlation of P-gp staining with age, clinical outcome and ABO blood group. Forty children's specimens were investigated for the presence of P-gp Table 2. Thirty one cases of children, 10 P-gp(+) and 21 P-gp(–), were investigated at presentation. Complete remission was obtained in 7 P-gp(+) (22%) and 18 P-gp(–) (58%). In the three remaining P-gp(+) cases one CR was followed by death, in one death occurred without achieving of CR and one CR was followed by relapse and death. In 21 P-gp(–) cases at presentation CR was observed in 18 cases. In three remaining P-gp(–) cases one PR was followed by death, one case was a priori resistant to chemotherapy and was followed by death, and in one death occurred without achieving CR. Nine cases were examined at different stages of disease; 3 at remission, 2 at first relapse, 3 at second and 1 at third relapse. P-gp positive staining was detected in 4 out of 9 cases (two at remission, one at first relapse and two at second relapse). In 21 adults' samples examined at presentation Table 1.1 CR were observed in 8 P-gp(+) (38%) and 13 P-gp(–) (61%) cases. In the present study positive staining for P-gp was compared with ABO blood groups, FAB classification, and the age of the patients. No significant correlation between P-gp expression and these parameters was found.

Table 2. Expression of P-gp in childhood leukemias

Type/ No	FAB	P-gp (+)	Response	Stage	Bl. group
AML 1	M1/2	–	CR	II	A
AML 1	M3	–	PR#	o	A
AML 5	M4	–	RES#	o	A
		a+	CR	o	B
		A+	REL#	I	B
		+	CR	rem	A
		–	CR	o	B
AML1	M5	–	CR	o	A
ALL 5	L1	+	CR	o	A
		+	CR#	o	O
		–	CR/REL	III	B
		–	REL	II	A
		–	CR	o	O
ALL 7	L1/2	–	CR	o	A
		–	CR	o	A
		+	CR	o	nd
		+	CR	rem	A
		–	CR	o	O
		–	CR	o	A
		–	CR	o	A
ALL 11	L2	–	CR	o	AB
		–	CR	o	O
		–	CR	o	A
		–	CR	o	B
		+	CR	o	B
		+	CR	o	A
		+	CR	o	nd
		+	CR/REL#	o	B
		–	CR	o	A
		–	CR	o	A
		–	CR	o	A
ALL 2	L2/3	–	REL	II	O
		–	CR	rem	A
ALL 1	L3	–	CR	o	O
CML 1		+	CR	o	nd
NHL 5		–	CR	o	AB
		–	CR	o	nd
		+	#	o	A
		+	CR	I	A
		–	#	o	O

AML–Acute Myeloid Leukemia, ALL–Acute Lymphoblastic Leukemia, CML–Chronic Myelogenous Leukemia, NHL–Non Hodgkin's Lymphoma, CR–complete remission, PR–partial remission, REL–relapse, RES–resistant, (+)–positive staining for P-gp, (–)–negative staining for P-gp, Stage–stage of disease: o–at presentation, rem–at remission, I–at first relapse, II–at second relapse, III–at third relapse, a and A staining for P-gp at that same case n the interval of 13 months, #–death

Discussion

In recent years, significant advances have been made in our understanding of the biological behaviour of human tumor cells. Immunohistochemistry (IC), with specific monoclonal antibodies, plays a significant role in these studies. The sensitivity of IC methods is high enough to detect a small amount of the antigen(s), moreover it allows to determine the morphology of the cell [24]. P-glycoprotein is widely accepted, in vitro models, as a factor responsible for generating classical MDR phenotype [2, 5, 6]. The role of the P-gp in human tumors in vivo is currently being extensively studied [4, 12, 14–16, 25, 26]. This study reports expression of P-gp at high frequencies in 35% of children's and 38% of adults leukemias as detected with three monoclonal antibodies; C219, JSB-1 and MRK-16 [13, 17, 19, 22, 23, 27]. The specificity of these antibodies has not yet been fully characterised [19, 28]. The C219 MAb seems not only to detect the carboxy-terminal part of the protein, the product of mdr-1 gene, but also reacts with the mdr-3 gene product [11]. Thiebaut et al. report cross reactivity of C219 MAb with 200kDa (heavy chain) protein present in myosin molecules in the skeletal and heart muscle [19]. Cross blocking experiments reveal that the JSB-1 MAb react with epitope distinct from epitope recognised by C219 [28]. Weinstein et al. report predominant, Golgi associated staining with C219 and JSB-1 MAb's, with epithelial cells carrying antigens to blood group A. Further investigations revealed that some batches of MAb's C219 and JSB-1 contain technological contamination which cause unspecific bindings of MAb's to the particular A group structure present on the epithelium [29, 30]. The MRK-16 MAb reacts with the epitope localised on the external surface of the cell membrane [23, 27]. This part of the P-gp shows a weak sequence homology between mdr-1 and mdr-3 gene. This suggests that MRK-16 should not crossreact with the mdr-3 gene product. So far a few studies of multidrug resistance, related to expression of P-glycoprotein, in leukemias have been reported [31-35]. The expression of P-glycoprotein or amplification of mdr-1 gene have been studied in several hematologic malignancies and solid tumors with molecular biology and immunohistochemical techniques [4, 15, 16, 25, 26, 28, 34]. There were reports in which amplification of mdr-1 gene without the presence of P-gp was found [32]. In others the expression of P-gp was found without amplification of mdr-1 gene [31]. These reports point out that more complicated mechanisms are involved in mdr-1 gene regulation or imperfect methods for detection of mdr-1 mRNA or P-gp are used. An ideal assay should be able to discriminate between a product of mdr-1 and mdr-3 gene. Probably more specific new antibodies should be generated against P-gp molecule in the future. The clinical importance of immunostaining, showing only a few positive cells, is still unclear. Therefore in IC studies it is very important to establish a threshold level above which we will be able to enumerate our results as positive. On the other hand, clonal development of MDR cells between tumor cells raises the question whether 1 or 100 cells should be counted as a threshold level. Clonal growth may be an important factor in the further promotion of MDR phenotype from detected scattered P-gp positive cells. Goasguen et al. put the threshold level at 1% of P-gp positive cells in their studies [36]. We have reported variability in intensity of staining with three antibodies. Goasguen et al. report similar results. They also found a difference in intensity of staining with C219 and JSB-1 MAb's. The intensity of staining with JSB-1 was higher than with C219 MAb [36]. The first detection of MDR phenotype with C219 MAb was reported by Ma et al. in two longitudinally studied patients. They found an increasing proportion of P-gp (+) cells during chemotherapy [35]. In the present study P-gp was detected in high frequencies in children's (35%) and adults' (38%) leukemia cases. P-gp staining was compared to clinical response to chemotherapy. A significant increase of CR after chemotherapy in P-gp (−) patients in both studied groups in comparison to P-gp(+) cases was observed. Musto et al. report higher incidence of relapsed patients, while during the presentation or CR P-gp was detected in leukemic cells [34]. The present study reports variable expression of P-gp positive cells range from 9-79% labelled as weak and 5-47% as a moderate to strong staining. Musto et al. also report heterogenous expression of P-gp (+) cells range $<1\%$ to 100% in various hematologic malignancies [33, 34]. Zhou et al. too, found a high incidence of mdr-1 gene expression by IC 27% and by slot blot 43% in newly diagnosed and relapsed patients [37]. In the present study we have found a higher incidence of P-gp positive cases in relapsed patients than in the investigated cases at presentation. Similar results are reported by Zhou et al. Goasguen et al. [36, 37]. Kuwazuru et al. report higher refractoriness to chemotherapy in patients with P-gp(+) cases [38]. The presence of P-gp positive cells might identify a subset of patients with potential enormous risk of relapse. In the present study clinical follow up in children's and adults' leukemias reveals a good initial response to induction chemotherapy introduced to the newly diagnosed leukemias. Complete remission was higher in P-gp negative than in P-gp positive cases. In P-gp(+) relapsed cases of ALL and AML death occurred more frequently than in newly diagnosed cases.

Acknowledgements. This work was supported by KBN grant Nr 4 4198 91 02, MAb MRK-16 was generously provided by Dr. T. Tsuruo from Japanese Foundation for Cancer Research, Cancer Chemotherapy Center, Tokyo, Japan.

References

1. Riordan J.R., Ling V. (1985) Genetic and biochemical characterization of multidrug resistance. Pharmac. Ther., 28, 51–75
2. Deuchars K.L., Ling V. (1989) P-glycoprotein and multidrug resistance in cancer chemotherapy. Seminars in Oncology, 16, 156–165
3. Chen Ch., Chin J.E., Ueda K. et al. (1986) Internal duplication and homology with bacterial transport proteins in the mdr1 (P-Glycoprotein) gene from multidrug-rsistant human cells. Cell, 47, 381–389
4. Goldstein L.J., Galski H., Fojo A. et al. (1989) Expression of a multidrug resistance gene in human cancers. J. Natl. Cancer Inst., 81, 116–124
5. Van der Bliek A.M., Baas F., Van der Velde-Koerts T. et al. (1988) Genes amplified and overexpressed in human multidrug-resistant cell lines. Cancer Res., 48, 5927–5932
6. Shen D-W., Fojo A., Roninson I.B. et al. (1986) Multidrug resistance of DNA-mediated transformants is linked to transfer of the human mdr 1 gene. Mol. Cell. Biol., 6, 4039–4044
7. Gros P., Croop J., Housman D. (1986) Mammalian multidrug resistance gene: complete cDNA sequence indicates strong homology to bacterial transport proteins. Cell, 47, 371–380
8. McGrath J.P., Varshavsky A. (1989) The yeast STE6 gene encodes a homologue to the mammalian miltidrug resistance P-glycoprotein. Nature, 340, 400–404
9. Juranka P.F., Zastawny R.L., Ling V. (1989) P-glycoprotein: multidrug resistance and a superfamily of membrane associated proteins. FASEB J, 3, 2583–2592
10. Horio M., Gottesman M.M., Pastan I. (1988) ATP-dependent transport of vinblastine in vesicles from human multidrug-resistant cells. Proc. Natl. Acad. Sci. USA, 85, 3580–3584
11. Cordon-Cardo C., O'Brien J.P., Boccia J. et al. (1990) Expression of the multidrug resiatance gene product (P-glycoprotein) in human normal and tumor tissues. J. Histochem. Cytochem., 38, 1277–1287
12. Fojo A.T., Ueda K., Salmon D.J. et al. (1987) Expression of a multidrug-resistance gene in human tumors and tissues. Proc. Natl. Acad. Sci. USA, 84, 265–269
13. Kartner N., Evernden-Porelle D., Bradley G. et al. (1985) Detection of P-glycoprotein in multidrug resistant cell lines by monoclonal antibodies. Nature, 316, 820–823
14. Schlaifer D., Laurent G., Chittal S. et al. (1990) Immunohistochemical detection of multidrug resistance associated P-glycoprotein in tumour and stromal cells of human cancers. Br. J. Cancer, 62, 177–182
15. Pileri S.A., Sabattini E., Falini B. et al. (1991) Immunohistochemical detection of the multidrug transport protein P170 in human normal tissues and malignant lymphomas. Histopathology, 19, 131–140
16. Kaczorowski S., Porwit A., Christensson B. (1991) Expression of P-glycoprotein in Non-Hodgkin's lymphomas. Leukemia and Lymphoma, 5, 379–386
17. Thiebaut F., Tsuruo T., Hamada H. et al. (1987) Cellular localization of the multidrug-resistance gene product P-glycoprotein in normal human tissues. Proc. Natl. Acad. Sci. USA, 84, 7735–7738
18. Van Kalken C.K., Giaccone G., van der Valk P. et al. (1992) Multidrug resistance gene (P-glycoprotein) expression in the human fetus. Am. J. Pathol., 141, 1063–1072
19. Thiebaut F., Tsuruo T., Hamada H. et al. (1989) Immunohistochemical localization in normal tissues of different epitopes in the multidrug transport protein P170: evidence for localization in brain capillaries and crossreactivity of one antibody with a muscle protein. J. Histochem. Cytochem., 37, 159–164
20. Cordon-Cardo C., O'Brien J.P., Casals D. et al. (1989) Multidrug-resistance gene (P-glycoprotein) is expressed by endothelial cells at blood-brain barier sites. Proc. Natl. Acad. Sci. USA, 86, 695–698
21. Bennet JM, Catovsky D, Daniel MT et al. (1976) French American British (FAB) cooperative group proposals for the classification of acute leukemias. Br. J. Haematol., 33, 451–458
22. Scheper J.R., Bulte J.W.M., Brakee J.G.P. et al. (1988) Monoclonal antibody JSB-1 detects a highly conserved epitope on the P-glycoprotein associated with multi-drug-resistance. Int. J. Cancer, 42, 389–394
23. Hamada H., Tsuruo T. (1986) Functional role for the 170- to 180-kDa glycoprotein specific to drug-resistant tumor cells as revealed by monoclonal antibodies. Proc Natl Acad Sci USA, 83, 7785–7789
24. Cordell J.L., Falini B., Erber W.N. et al. (1984) Immunoenzymatic labeling of monoclonal antibodies using immune complexes of alkaline phosphatase and monoclonal anti-alkaline phosphatase (APAAP complexes). J. Histochem. Cytochem., 32, 219–229
25. Pirker R., Wallner J., Geissler K. et al. (1991) MDR 1 gene expression and treatment outcome in acute meloid leukemia. J. Natl. Cancer Inst., 83, 708–712
26. Sato H., Day H.P., Raza A. et al. (1990) MDR 1 transcript levels as an indication of resistant disease in acute myelogenous leukemia. Br. J. Haemat., 75, 340–345
27. Sugawara I., Kataoka I., Morishita Y. et al. (1988) Tissue distribution of P-glycoprotein encoded by a multidrug-resistant gene as revealed by monoclonal antibody MRK16. Cancer Res., 48, 1926–1929
28. Van der Valk P., van Kalken C.K., Katelaars H. et al. (1990) Distribution of multi-drug antibodies recognizing different epitopes of the P-glycoprotein molecule. Annals of Oncol., 1, 56–64
29. Weinstein R.S., Kuszak J.R., Jakate S.M. et al. (1990) ABO blood type predicts the cytolocalization of anti-P-Glycoprotein monoclonal antibody

reactivity in human colon and ureter. Hum Pathol., 21, 949–958
30. Finstad C.L., Yin B.W.T., Gordon C.M. et al. (1991) Some monoclonal antibody reagents (C219 and JSB-1) to P-glycoprotein contains antibodies to blood group A carbohydrate determinants: A problem of quality control for immunohistochemical analysis. J. Histochem. Cytochem., 39, 1603–1610
31. Ito Y., Tanimoto M., Kumazawa T. et al. (1989) Increased P-glycoprotein expression and multidrug resistant gene (mdr1) amplification are infrequently found in fresh acute leukemia cells. Cancer, 63, 1534–1538
32. Holmes J., Jacobs A., Carter G. et al. (1989) Multidrug resistance in haemopoietic cell lines, myelodysplastic syndromes and acute myeloblastic leukaemia. Br J Haematology, 72, 40–44
33. Musto p., Cascavilla N., Di Renzo N. et al. (1990) Clinical relevance of immunocytochemical detection of multidrug resistance associated P-glycoprotein in hematologic malignancies. Tumori, 76, 353–359
34. Musto P., Melillo L., Lombardi G. et al. (1991) High risk of early resistant relapse for leukaemic patients with presence of multidrug associated P-glycoprotein positive cells in complete remission. Br J Haematology, 77, 50–53
35. Ma D.D.F., Davey R.A., Harman D.H., et al. (1987) Detection of a multidrug resistant phenotype in acute non-lymphoblastic leukaemia. Lancet, 135–137
36. Goasguen J.E., Dossot J-M., Fardel O. et al. (1993) Expression of the multidrug resistance associated P-glycoprotein (P-170) in 59 cases of de novo acute lymphoblastic leukemia: prognostic implication. Blood, 81, 2394–2398
37. Zhou D-C., Marie J-P., Suberville A-M. et al. (1992) Relevance of mdr1 gene expression in acute myeloid leukemia and comparison of diagnostic methods. Leukemia, 6, 879–885
38. Kuwazuru Y., Yoshimura A., Hanada S. et al. (1990) Expression of the multidrug transporter P-glycoprotein in acute leukemia cells and correlation to clinical drug resistance. Cancer, 66, 868–873

Acute Leukemias V
Experimental Approaches
and Management of Refractory Diseases
Hiddemann et al. (Eds.)

Multidrug Resistance in Acute Myelogenous Leukemia: Relevance to Clinical and Laboratory Data

Andrey Zaritskey, Irina Stuf, Tatyana Bykova, Kirill Titov, Nadezhda Medvedeva, Natalya Anikina, and Boris Afanasiev

Introduction

MDR1 gene is responsible for resistance to a number of drugs conventionally used for the treatment of acute myelogenous leukemia in vitro and in vivo [1,2]. The clinical significance of this fact is still obscure. There are no consice clinical data, randomized trials and wide retrospective studies proving the necessity of adding drugs for overcoming MDR1 gene expression to conventional chemotherapy [2,3]. The possible role of other genes involved in cell cycle regulation and apoptosis (myc, p53, c-kit, TGF-beta)on the results of chemotherapy is also discussed [6]. Moreover it was shown that some of the above mentioned genes are mutually regulated [7].

That is why the aim of this study was the evaluation of MDR1, myc, TGF-beta genes in hemopoetic cells in AML patients in relation to prognosis, induction therapy and other clinical data.

Materials and Methods

28 patients with primary or pretreated AML were included in the current study (from 2 to 7 times). "7+3" and TAD-HAM regimens were used for treatment. A number of included patients were pretreated in other hospitals with less intensive regimens ("5+2", low doses Ara-C). Two patients successfully underwent autologous BMT. Gene expression was studied by the method of hybridization in situ [8] with some slight modifications.

Results and Discussion

Results of treatment of AML by "7+3" and TAD-HAM are presented in Figure 1 and 2. The more intensive regimen, TAD-HAM, seems to be more effective. At the onset of disease MDR1 gene expression was studied in 8 patients. Two of them expressed MDR1 in their hemopoetic cells. Both MDR1+ patients were treated by "7+3".

One of them entered a complete remission, the other failed. Six MDR1- patients were treated with "7+3" or TAD-HAM. CR was obtained in five of them. The study of MDR1 expression appeared to be nonsignificant in relation to obtaining CR ($p < 0.05$). So, MDR1+ phenotype is not frequent in primary patients and it seems to have no impact on the results of conventional chemotherapy.

Thereafter we have analyzed MDR1 gene expression in a population of patients earlier treated by regimens less intensive than "7+3" (Fig. 3). It appeared that this kind of therapy induces MDR1 expression. It stresses once more that intensive regimens should be used from the beginning. The possible role of the induction of MDR1 gene expression on further CR was studied. Patients treated by all types of regimens were included. In 12 patients with induced MDR1 9 failed to obtain CR. 8 patients with

BMT Centre for Advanced Medical Technologies, 1st Pavlov Medical Institute, Institute of Oncology, St. Petersburg, Russia

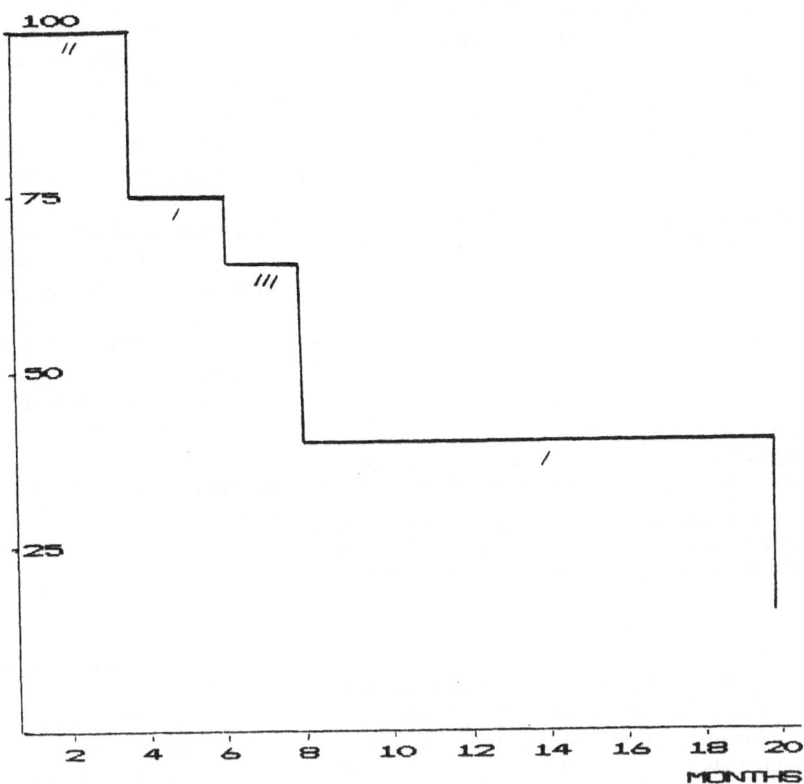

Fig. 1. AML remission duration "7+3" regimen

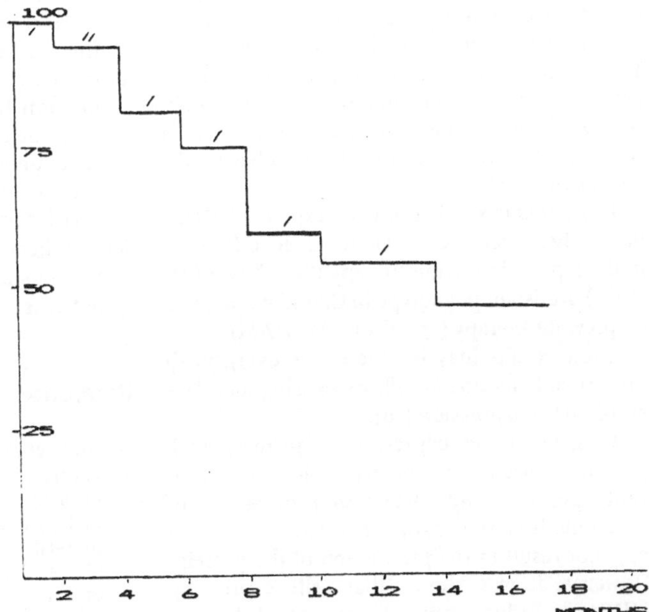

Fig. 2. AML remission duration TAD-HAM regimen

	MDR−1+	MDR−1−	TOTAL
NO PRETREATMENT	1	4	5
PRETREATMENT	9	2	11
TOTAL	10	6	16

Fig. 3. Expression of MDR1 in early stages of different regimens (before remission) in AML patients in relation to remission induction

	MDR−1+	MDR−1−	TOTAL
CR+	3	8	11
CR−	2	1	3
TOTAL	5	9	14

Fig. 4. Expression of MDR1 gene in early stages (before remission) in intensive regimens ("7+3" and TAD-HAM) in AML patients in relation to remission induction

absence of MDR1 induction entered CR (difference is statistically significant, $p < 0.01$).

When including patients only on intensive regiments ("7+3", TAD-HAM ($n = 14$)) the difference appeared to be not significant ($p < 0.05$, Fig. 4). So, it seems that the use of full dose intensive regimens reduces the value of MDR1 expression evaluation. In one patient with high MDR1 expression and resistant AML it was possible to overcome resistance by cyclosporin A. This did not result in any laboratory improvals. Three patients abrupted the expression of MDR1 gene after intensive chemotherapy used, only in two of them CR was obtained. Resistance in these patients were probably due to other mechanisms [9].

In 7 patients studied in CR 5 expressed MDR1 in their hemopoetic cells. There was no difference in the type of induction therapy ("7+3" or TAD-HAM). Resistant phenotype in CR did not depend on previous therapy ("7+3" or TAD-HAM).

These results may be due to the overgrowth of normal hemopoetic cells expressing high levels of MDR1 expression [10].

P53 gene was not expressed in 7 primary AML patients. Absence of its expression may prevent apoptosis and results in progression of leukemia. It is well known that RNA translation may not result in the production of the protein. However, it was shown that cells expressing MDR1 do produce appropriate protein [4].

Patients expressing MDR1 in CR did not differ in their response to the treatment in comparison to MDR1-patients. Some of them had undergone autoBMT, the rest were rotated according to the Buchner regimen.

P53 gene was not expressed in haemopoetic cells in AML patients before treatment. After initialization of chemotherapy the expression was found in 8/15 patients. This fact is coincident with the role of p53 in favouring programmed cell death in cells exposed to cytotoxic agents [6]. P53, TGF-beta genes expression appeared to be not significant in relation to CR. No relationship was found between the expression of above mentioned genes and MDR1 gene. This is coincident with the experimental data of no mutual regulation between MDR1 and p53 [11,12].

Conclusions

1. Primarily MDR1+ phenotype is rather rare in AML.
2. Not intensive chemotherapy can induce MDR1 gene expression.
3. Very intensive regimen (TAD-HAM] seems not be inductive for MDR1 gene expression.
4. Early induction of MDR1 expression on not intensive regiment is of predictive value for CR failure.
5. Discordant expression of MDR and p53 in AML claims no mutual regulation at least in this disorder.
6. Induction of MDR gene expression in postremission hemopoetic cells seems to be of no prognostic significance.
7. It appeared that 2/2 patients with high expression of myc resulted in early death on very intensive regimens (TAD-HAM).
8. TGF beta gene expression seems to be of no prognostic significance in primary AML patients.

References

1. Andreeff M., Zhao S., Drach D., Hegewish S. et al. Expression of multidrug resistance and p53 genes in hematological cell systems: implications for biology and gene therapy. Cancer Bull, 1993, v.45, p131–138.
2. Mc Lachlin Y.R., Englitis M.A.,Ueda K., Expression of a human complementary DNA for the multidrug resistance gene in murine hematopoetic

precursor cells with the use of retroviral gene transfer. J. Natl. Cancer Inst. 1990, v.82, p.1260.
3. Lum B.L., Kanbisch S., Yataha A.M. et al. Alter pharmacokinetics and pharmacodynamics by cyclosporine in a phase 1 trial to modulate multidrug resistance. Y. Clin. Oncol. 1992, v.10, p.1635.
4. Yahama A.M., Adler K.M., Fisher G.A. Phase I trial with etoposide with cyclosporin as modulator of multidrug resistance. Y. Clin. Oncol. 1992, v.10, p.1624.
5. Haber D.A., Multidrug resistance (MDR1) in leukemias: is it time to test. Blood 1992, v.79, p.259.
6. Sachs L., Lotem Y. Control of programmed cell death in normal and leukemic cells: new implications for therapy. Blood 1993, v.82, p.15.
7. Zhao Z, Drach D., Hu G., et al. Modulation of activity of the promoter of the human MDR1 gene by ras and p53. Science 1992, v.255, p.459.
8. Kunzl., Mielke R., Leohr G.W., Fauzer A.A. Detection of messenger RNAs within hybridization on small slide areas. Exp. Hematol. 1988, 16, 394–399.
9. Moscow J.A., Cowan K.H. Multidrug resistance. J. Natl. Cancer Inst. 1988, v.80, p.14–20.
10. Drach D., Zhao Z, Drach Y., Mahadevia R., Gatringer C., Huber H., Andreeff M. Subpopulations on normal peripheral blood and bone marrow cells express a functional multidrug resistant phenotype. Blood 1992, v.80, p.2729.
11. Andreeff M. Biological characterization and therapy monitoring of leukemia. In: Laerum O.D., Bierkues P., etc. Flow cytometry in hematology. London, England. Academia Press 1992, p.231.
12. Lotem Y., Such L. Regulation by bcl-2, myc and p53 of susceptibility to induction of apoptosis by heat shock and cancer chemotherapy compounds in differentiation component and defective myeloid leukemic cells. Cell Growth Differ 1993, v.4, p.41.

Acute Leukemias V
Experimental Approaches
and Management of Refractory Diseases
Hiddemann et al. (Eds.)

Mitoxantrone/Cytarabine with or without Quinine as a Potential MDR-Reversing Agent for the Treatment of Acute Leukemias

E. Solary[1], D. Caillot, F. Witz, P. Moreau, P. Genne, B. Desablens, J. Y. Cahn, A. Sadoun, B. Pignon, J. F. Abgrall, F. Maloisel, D. Guyotat, P. Casassus, N. Ifrah, P. Lamy, B. Audhuy, P. Colombat, and J. L. Harousseau

Abstract. We demonstrated previously that sera from quinine-treated patients reversed the MDR phenotype *in vitro*. Then, the combination of quinine with mitoxantrone (MTX) and cytarabine (Ara-C) was shown to be well-tolerated in patients with acute leukemias. To answer the question whether the response rate could be improved by quinine, we designed a phase III multicentric study. During the first year, the trial involved 112 adult patients (age 18–65y) with either relapsed or refractory acute myeloblastic or lymphoblastic leukemia or secondary leukemia or blastic transformation of myelodysplastic or myeloproliferative syndrome. All patients were treated with a combination of MTX (12 mg/m²/day – 4 days) and Ara-C (1 g/m²/12h – 5 days – 3 hrs iv infusion). After randomisation, 55 patients also received quinine (30 mg/kg/d – 5 days – beginning 24 hrs before MTX infusion). A 20% dose decrease was necessary in 14 patients due to vertigo or tinnitus and quinine was discontinued in 1 patient, due to excessive QT extension The remaining 57 patients received the chemotherapy alone. Toxic death was observed in 2 patients (one in each group) and ten patients (7 in quinine-treated group) died in aplasia before day 30. Response was assessable in 106 patients. As compared with the patients treated with MTX-Ara-C only, the patients treated with MTX-Ara-C plus quinine had a higher overall rate of response [29 / 52 (56%) versus 26 / 54 (48%)]. However, this difference is not significant. Quinine increased the duration of neutropenia (28,3 vs 23,9 days; $p<0.05$) and thrombopenia (35 vs 28,3; $p=0.02$). The incidence of nausea, vomiting and mucositis was also significantly higher in the quinine-treated group. This partial analysis confirmed the feasibility of using quinine in combination with MTX and Ara-C and suggested a trends for quinine to improve the response rate although these results have to be confirmed by the extended study.

Introduction

Failure of conventional regimens combining an anthracycline or an aminoanthraquinone with cytarabine or etoposide was related to primary or secondary resistance of leukemic cells to cytotoxic drugs [1]. Among the described mechanisms of resistance, the multidrug resistance (MDR) phenotype [2] has been identified in more than 50% of relapsed or refractory acute leukemias and related to lower response rate to conventional treatment [3–6]. The decreased intracellular accumulation of a variery of antineoplastic agents characteristic of this phenotype can be reversed *in vitro* by various noncytotoxic agents [7–12]. However, the *in vivo* use of most of these agents is precluded by serum protein binding or clinical toxicity [11,12].

We previously demonstrated that intravenous infusion of conventional doses of quinine allowed to reach sufficient concentration in serum to reverse the anthracycline resistance of rat colon cancer cells and MDR human leukemic cells [13,14]. Then, we defined the conditions for use of quinine as an MDR modifier [14]. We performed a phase I and II clinical trial to demon-

Clinical Hematology Unit, CHU Le Bocage, BP1542, 21034 Dijon, France, on behalf of the GOELAMS group

strate that quinine could be used safely in combination with mitoxantrone (MTX) and cytarabine (Ara-C) for the treatment of clinically resistant acute leukemias [15]. Here we report the partial analysis of a phase III multicentric study that was designed to answer the question whether the response rate could be improved by quinine. In this trial, patients with either relapsed or secondary or refractory acute leukemia were treated with a combination of MTX and Ara-C. After randomisation, half patients also received quinine as a potential MDR-reversing agent.

Patients and Methods

Patients. This study is an opened phase III trial with 15 participating medical centers, initiated in march 1992. Patients eligible for the study are those older than 14 and younger than 66 years of age with a bone-marrow diagnosis of acute non-lymphoblastic or lymphoblastic leukemia as defined by the French-American-British classification system. These patients either have relapsed from or are refractory to standard first line chemotherapy, which sometimes included bone-marrow transplantation. Patients with secondary leukemia or blastic transformation of myelodysplastic or myeloproliferative syndrome are also eligible.

Other eligibility criteria included adequate kidney and hepatic functions (creatinine clearance < 250 mol/L; serum bilirubin < 14 mg/L, transaminases < 4N), cardiac ejection fraction, and cumulative dose of anthracycline less than 400 mg/m^2 adriamycin-equivalent.

Regimen. The therapy regimen consisted of Ara-C 1 g/m^2 administered by 2-hour IV infusion twice a day on days 1 through 5 and mitoxantrone 12 mg/m^2 as a 30-minutes infusion on days 2 through 5. After randomisation, half patients received quinine formiate (Quinoforme; Vaillant-Defresne, Courbevoie, France) at a dosage of 30 mg/kg/d started 24 hours before the first dose of mitoxantrone and administered in continuous IV infusion until 24 hours after the end of the last mitoxantrone infusion. Toxicity was assessed according to the WHO grading system. Complete remission (CR) was defined by the disappearance of leukemic blasts from the bone-marrow and blood as well as possible extramedullary sites, including the cerebral fluid, and the normalization of peripheral granulocytes count to more than 1,500/μl. Partial response (PR) was defined by a percentage of bone-marrow blast cells lower than 25%, a percentage of peripheral-blood blast cells lower than 5%, and peripheral-blood granulocytes more than 1,000/μl. The duration of critical cytopenia was evaluated by the time for leukocyte (> 1000/μl), granulocyte (> 500/μl), and thrombocyte (> 100000/μl) recoveries from the onset of treatment.

Ex vivo assay. MDR-positive DXR/K12/PROb cells (2 × 10^5) were seeded in microtiter plates (24 wells/plate) and cultured for 24 hours as described [11]. Cells were incubated for 4 hours at 37 °C with 20 μM doxorubicin (97% non radioactive DXR; 3% [^{14}C]-DXR) diluted in 0.5 ml of serum-free Ham's F-10 medium or serum from patients. After incubation, cells were rinsed three times with ice-cold phosphate-buffered saline, trypsinized, and transferred into counting vials with 3 ml scintillant liquid (LKB, Stockholm, Sweden). The radioactivity was measured on a β scintillation counter (LKB 1214; Rackbeta, Stockholm, Sweden).

Statistical analysis. The characteristics of the patients before treatment and their response rates were compared by the Chi-squared test or the Fisher's exact test. Mann Whitney-test was used to compare quantitative parameters. A two-way analysis of variance was performed to compare hepatic enzymes and bilirubinemia changes induced by the treatments in quinine-treated and control groups.

Results

Patient's characteristics. From march 1992 to february 1993, 112 patients entered the trial (55 received quinine, 57 were treated without quinine). The clinical characteristics of the patients in the two treatment groups were similar (Table 1), excepted the duration of the first CR that was significantly longer in the control group (mean 26 months) compared to the quinine-treated group (mean 12 months; p=0.008). Two patients died before day 6 (one in each arm of the trial). Two patients did not receive the treatment in the quinine arm and the data from two patients from the control group were not obtained. Therefore, the analysis included 106

Table 1. Clinical characteristics of the patients according to treatment group

	Without Q (N=57)	With Q (N=55)
Mean age (yr)	47	43.7
Sex (male/female)	30/27	33/22
Relapsed AML	19	20
MDS (blastic transformation)	11	9
MPS (blastic transformation)	7	10
Refractory AML	10	4
Relapsed ALL	4	8
Secondary AL	2	3
Refractory ALL	2	1
Mean leukocyte count ($\times 10^9$/l)	31	23
Mean haemoglobin (g/l)	104	104
Mean platelet count ($\times 10^9$/l)	110	100
Karyotype (done/abnormal)	31/24	28/20
WHO performance status_2	50	46
Duration of first CR (months) (N=56)	26*	12

*p=0.08

patients (52 in the group given quinine, 54 in the control group).

Tolerance of quinine. Secondary effects due to quinine infusion were observed in 15 patients (27%) and included tinnitus, vertigo and tachycardia or bradycardia. In 14 patients, these effects disappeared or strongly decreased after a 20% quinine dose-decrease. In one patient, quinine infusion was stopped due to excessive QT increase.

MDR-reversing activity of sera. The ability of serum obtained at day 2 from quinine-treated patients to increase DXR accumulation in MDR-cells was compared to those of serum obtained before the beginning of quinine infusion (day 0). An MDR-reversing activity was observed in all quinine-treated patients, sera from quinine-treated patients inducing a two-fold increase of DXR uptake in MDR-positive cells. Sera from control patients were tested the same way and had no effect on DXR accumulation (Fig. 1).

Nonhematologic toxicity. Quinine infusion significantly increased the incidence and the duration of nauseas, vomiting and mucositiss (Fig. 2). By contrast, quinine had non influence upon renal and hepatic toxicity and did not induce significant increase of bilirubinemia. Although cardiac toxicity (WHO grade_2) was observed in 13 patients treated with quinine compared to 2 patients from the control group, the difference was not significant. Similarly, skin toxicity was slightly more frequent in quinine-treated patients. Quinine treatment had no influence upon the number of febrile episodes and the incidence of aspergillosis and candidosis.

Hematologic toxicity. Among responding patients, quinine significantly increased the duration of neutropenia ($p=0.05$) and thrombopenia ($p=0.02$). Two patients from the quinine-treated group never recovered a platelet count over 100x10^9/l. The increased duration of leucopenia and anemia was not statistically significant (Table 2).

Response to treatment. A response to therapy (CR+PR) was obtained in 55 of 106 (52%) assessable patients. The response rate was higher in quinine-treated group (29 of 52 patients – 56%) that in control group (26 of 54 patients – 48%). However, the difference between the two groups was not statistically significant.

Discussion

The combination of mitoxantrone and either intermediate-dose cytarabine or high-dose etoposide was shown to be an effective treatment of relapsed or refractory acute leukemias [16–18]. However, half patients did not respond and survival of responders did not excess a few months. Failure of these regimen was related to primary or acquired resistance of leukemic cells. Various mechanisms of resistance have been described, including MDR phenotype that could preclude mitoxantrone activity by reducing its accumulation in leukemic cells. The negative prognostic influence of MDR phenotype expression in response and survival for acute leukemias and the development of increased expression at the time of relapse after initial chemotherapy provide a rationale for the clinical study of MDR modulators. Among the modulators that have shown substantial ability to reverse drug resistance *in vivo* [10-12,19–21], we chose quinine because the concentration required to reverse MDR *in vitro* could be achieved clinically with doses previously used for the treatment of malaria [22] and its reversing activity was retained despite binding to plasma proteins [11,23].

Fig. 1. MDR-reversing activity of patients sera

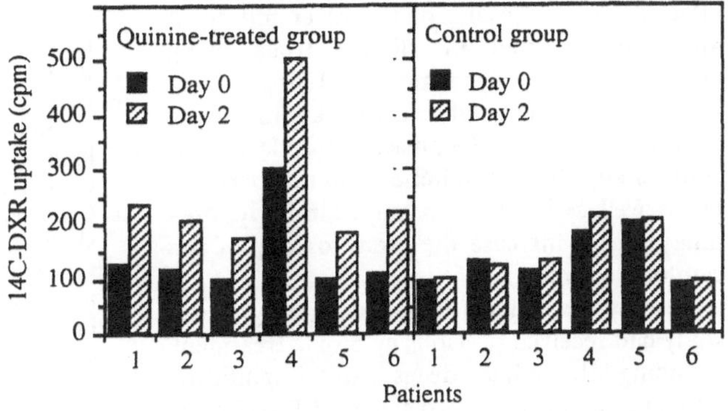

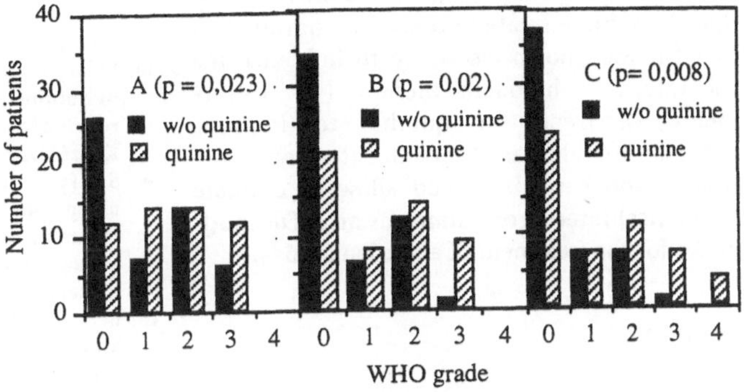

Fig. 2. Incidence of nauseas (A), vomiting (B) and mucositis (C) in control and quinine-treated groups

Table 2. Median duration of cytopenia (d: days)

	Without Q	With Q
Leukocytes $<10^9/l$	20.5 d	23.6 d
Granulocytes $<0.5\times10^9/l$	23.9 d*	28.3 d
Platelets $<100\times10^9/l$	28.3 d#	35.1 d
Hemoglobin <100 g/l	30.6 d	33.4 d

*p = 0.05 #p = 0.02

The present report describes the first partial analysis of a phase III randomized study that should include 300 patients on a 3-year period. Quinine-related toxicity included tinnitus and vertigo that disappeared after a 20% dose decrease [15,24]. Cardiac toxicity, that was observed in 13 patients from quinine-treated group compared to 2 patients from control group, could be explained by either a direct toxicity of quinine [24,25] or an interference of the reversing agent with the renal or hepatic elimination of mitoxantrone. Such a pharmacokinetic effect, that was demonstrated with other combination of reversing agents and MDR-related cytotoxic drugs [26–28], could also explain the significantly increased incidence of nauseas, vomiting and mucositis. The effect of quinine infusion on mitoxantrone pharmacokinetics as well as P-glycoprotein status of patients blast cells are currently in progress.

The alteration of mitoxantrone and cytarabine metabolism or excretion by normal tissues that express MDR phenotype could account also for the increased myelosuppression observed in quinine-treated patients. Other hypothesis include the reversion of P-glycoprotein function in the bone-marrow precursors or a direct effect of quinine on hematopoietic progenitors [29]. Increased duration of neutropenia and thrombopenia in quinine-treated patients was not associated with a significant increase of febrile episodes incidence.

In the previously reported phase I/II study of quinine-mitoxantrone-cytarabine combination, we described an increase of serum bilirubin in 6 of 15 patients. A modulation of P-glycoprotein transport of bilirubin in the lumenal surface of the canaliculi of the biliary tract was suggested since bilirubin was shown to be a substrate for the efflux pump [30]. Alternatively, such a toxic effect could be specific of the reversing agent and was reported in clinical trials using cyclosporine [12]. By comparing bilirubinemia in quinine-treated and control patients using analysis of variance, the present analysis did not confirm any effect of quinine upon this parameter as well as hepatic enzymes. Similarly, quinine did not increase the renal toxicity of the cytotoxic regimen.

Seventy-six patients included in the present study had received previous cytotoxic treatment including MDR-related drugs with no significant difference between the two groups. CR had been obtained in 56 of these patients. Duration of first CR was significantly longer in control group than in quinine-treated group. The duration of first CR was shown elsewhere to influence the CR rate to subsequent therapy [31]. Nevertheless, a trend for quinine to improve the response rate was observed. Extension of the trial to 300 patients should allow to evaluate the clinical interest of quinine as an MDR modulator for the treatment of acute leukemias.

References

1. Morrow CS, Cowan KH. Mechanisms and clinical significance of multidrug resistance. Oncology, 1988, 2: 55.
2. Moscow JA, Cowan KH. Multidrug resistance. J Ntl Cancer Inst 1988, 80: 14.
3. Pirker R, Wallner J, Geissler K et al. MDR1 gene expression and treatment outcome in acute myeloid leukemia. J Ntl Cancer Inst 1991, 83: 708.
4 Marie JP, Zittoun R, Sikic BI. Multidrug resistance (mdr1) gene expression in adult acute leukemias: correlations with treatment outcome and *in vitro* drug sensitivity. Blood 1991, 78: 586.
5. Campos L, Guyotat D, Archimbaud E et al. Clinical significance of multidrug resistance P-glycoprotein expression on acute nonlymphoblastic leukemia cells at diagnosis. Blood, 1992 79: 473.
6. Goasguen JE, Dossot JM, Fardel O et al. Expression of the multidrug resistance-asociated P-glycoprotein (P-170) in 59 cases of de novo acute lymphoblastic leukemia: prognostic implications. Blood 1993, 81: 2394.
7. Tsuruo T, Iida H, Tsukagoshi S, et al. Increased accumulation of Vincristine and Adriamycine in drug resistant P388 tumor cells following incubation with calcium antagonists and calmomodulin inhibitors. Cancer Res 1982; 42: 4730.
8. Chauffert B, Rey D, Coudert B et al. Amiodarone is more efficient than Verapamil in reversing resistance to anthracyclines in tumor cells. Br J Cancer 1987; 56: 119.
9. Nooter K, Oostrum R, Jonker R et al. Effect of cyclosporin A on daunorubicin accumulation in multidrug resistant P388 leukemia cells measured by real-time flow cytometry. Cancer Chemother Pharmacol 1989; 23: 296.
10. DeGregorio MW, Ford JM, Benz C et al. Toremifene: Pharmacologic and pharmacokinetic basis of reversing multidrug resistance. J Clin Oncol 1989; 9: 1359.
11. Genne P, Dimanche-Boitrel MT, Mauvernay RY et al. Cinchonine, a potent efflux inhibitor to circumvent anthracycline resistance *in vivo*. Cancer Res 1992; 52: 2797.
12. Lum BL, Fisher GA, Brophy NA et al. Clinical trials of modulation of multidrug resistance. Pharmacokinetic and pharmacodynamic considerations. Cancer 1993; 72: 3502.
13. Chauffert B, Corda C, Pelletier H, et al. Potential usefulness of quinine for the circumvention of the anthracycline resistance in clinical practice. Brit J Cancer 1990; 62: 395.
14. Solary E, Velay I, Chauffert B, et al. Sufficient levels of quinine in the serum circumvent the multidrug resistance of the human leukemic cell line K562/ADM. Cancer 1991, 68: 1714.
15. Solary E, Caillot D, Chauffert B et al. Feasibility of using quinine, a potential multidrug resistance-reversing agent, in combination with mitoxantrone and cytarabine for the treatment of acute leukemia. J Clin Oncol 1992, 10: 1730.
16. Bezwoda WR, Bernasconi C, Hutchinson RM et al. Mitoxantrone for refractory and relapsed acute leukemia. Cancer 1990; 66: 418.
17. Hiddemann W, Kreutzmann H, Sraif K et al High-dose cytosine arabinoside and mitoxantrone: a highly effective regimen in refractory acute myeloid leukemia Blood 1987; 69: 744.
18. O'Brien S, Kantarjian H, Estey E et al. Mitoxantrone and high-dose etoposide for patients with relapsed or refracory acute leukemia. Cancer 1991, 68: 691.
19. Sonneveld P, Nooter K. Reversal of drug resistance by cyclosporin-A in a patient with acute myelocytic leukaemia. Br J Haemat, 1990; 75: 208.
20. Bessho F, Kinumaki H, Kobayashi M et al. Treatment of children with refractory acute lymphocytic leukaemia with vincristine and diltiazem. Med Pediatr Oncol, 1985; 13: 199.
21. Benson AB, Trump DL, Koeller JM et al. Phase I study of vinblastine and verapamil given by concurrent IV infusion. Cancer Treat Rep, 1985; 69: 795.
22. Krogstad DJ, Herwaldt BL, Schlesinger PH Antimalarial agents: specific treatment regimens. Antimicrobial agents chemotherapy, 1988; 32: 957.
23. Silamut K, White NJ, Looareesuwan S. et al.. Binding of quinine to plasma proteins in falciparum malaria. J Trop Med Hygiene, 1985; 34: 681.
24. Boland ME, Brennand Roper SM et al. Complications of quinine poisoning. Lancet, 1985; i: 384
25. Holford NH, Coates PE, Guentert TW et al. The effect of quinidine and its metabolites on the electrocardiogram and systolic time intervals : concentration-effect relationship. Brit J Clin Pharmacol 1981; 11: 187.

26. Nooter K, Oostrum R, Deurloo J. Effects of verapamil on the pharmacokinetics of daunorubicin in the rat. Cancer Chemother Pharmacol. 1987, 20: 176.
27. Kerr DJ, Graham J, Cummings J et al. The effect of verapamil on the pharmacokinetics of adriamycin. Cancer Chemother Pharmacol.1986, 18: 239.
28. Yahanda AM, Adler KM, Fisher GA et al. A phase I trial of etoposide with cyclosporine as a modulator of multidrug resistance. J Clin Oncol 1992, 10: 1624.
29. Christen RD, McClay EF, Wilgus LL et al. In vivo modulation of doxorubicin by high dose progesterone. A phase I/pharmacokinetic study. Proc Am Soc Clin Oncol 1992; 11: 121.
30. Gosland M, Brophy N, Duran G et al. Bilirubin: a physiological substrate for the multidrug transporter. Proc Am Assoc Cancer Res 1991; 32: 426.
31. Harousseau JL, Reiffers J, Hurteloup P et al. Treatment of relapsed acute myeloid leukemia with idarubicin and intermediate-dose cytarabine. J Clin Oncol 1989, 7: 45.

Acute Leukemias V
Experimental Approaches
and Management of Refractory Diseases
Hiddemann et al. (Eds.)

In Vitro Modulation of Multidrug Resistance by BIBW22BS in Blasts of De Novo or Relapsed or Persistent AML

J. Schröder[1], M. Esteban[1], S. Kasimir-Bauer[1], U. Bamberger[2], A. Heckel[2], M. E. Scheulen[1], and S. Seeber[1]

Introduction

Drug resistance to chemotherapy is an important factor of treatment failure in acute myeloid leukemia (AML). One type of resistance, the multidrug resistance (MDR), can develop after exposure to certain natural chemotherapeutic agents such as vinca alkaloids, anthracyclines, actinomycin D, and epipodophyllotoxins (Biedler & Riehm 1970). MDR is associated with overexpression of a 170 kDa membrane glycoprotein (P170), which is encoded by the mdr1 gene located on the long arm of chromosome 7 (Bradley et al. 1988). Membrane transport studies have shown that calcium channel blocking agents such as verapamil (VER) inhibit drug efflux by direct binding to P170 causing increased intracellular drug accumulation (Willingham et al. 1986; Safa et al. 1987). Recent clinical studies have indicated that MDR is induced by treatment with anthracyclines and vinca alkaloids in several hematologic malignancies (te Boekhorst et al. 1993). Thus, the expression of mdr1 is detected in about 50% of patients with pretreated AML, in contrast to only 20% of patients with *de novo* AML (Marie et al. 1991). Patients with mdr1 gene expression had a significantly shorter overall survival compared with the mdr1-negative group (Pirker et al. 1991).

In the present study, we investigated the mode of action of the phenylpteridine derivative BIBW22BS (BIBW22), dexniguldipine (DEX), and VER as modifiers of MDR in blasts of *de novo* or relapsed or persistent AML *in vitro*, and also in a human MDR leukemia cell line. BIBW22 is a potent bifunctional modulator of drug resistance (Chen et al. 1993). The compound influences P170 mediated transport of cytostatic drugs and, in addition, nucleoside transport.

Patients and Methods

Patients. Thirty-five patients with AML, 15 *de novo* and 20 relapsed or persistent, were included in this study. Patients with prior hematologic disorders or known exposure to carcinogens were excluded.

Cell samples. Samples from bone marrow or blood were collected at diagnosis in heparinized tubes. Mononuclear cells were isolated from the samples by Ficoll-Hypaque density gradient centrifugation (density, 1.077 g/ml; Pharmacia, Uppsala, Schweden).

Cell lines. The CEM vinblastine-resistant cell line CEM-VBL was a generous gift from Dr. W. T. Beck, Memphis, Tennessee (Beck et al. 1979). CEM-VBL cells have been previously shown to express P170 on their surface membrane as determined by the monoclonal antibody HYB-241 (Meyers et al. 1989). The cell line was grown in RPMI 1640 (GIBCO; Karlsruhe, FRG) supplemented with 10% (v/v) heat-inactivated fetal calf serum (FCS; GIBCO) and 1% L-glutamine

[1]Innere Klinik und Poliklinik (Tumorforschung),Westdeutsches Tumorzentrum, Universitätsklinikum Essen, D-45122 Essen
[2]Dr. Karl Thomae GmbH, D-88397Biberach/Riß

(GIBCO) and incubated at 37 °C with 5% CO_2 and 95% humidified air.

Flow-cytometric determination of DNR, IDA and CD34 expression. Cells were washed in RPMI supplemented with 10% FCS. After washing, a suspension of 2×10^6 cells/ml was prepared. Fifty microliters of the cell suspension were incubated with 10 µl phycoerythrin-conjugated HPCA-2 (anti-CD34 PE; Becton Dickinson, San Jose, California) for 20 min at 4 °C. After washing, 5,000 events were counted using an ELITE flow-cytometer (Coulter Electronics, Hialeah, Florida). The PE fluorescence signal was logarithmically amplified. The blast populations were gated using scatter parameters. An irrelevant, isotype-matched MoAb was used as negative control. An expression of less than 10% was classified as negative. Data analysis was performed using ELITE software.

Cellular efflux studies. For efflux studies, cells at a concentration of 1×10^6/ml were incubated with either rhodamine 123 (R123), daunorubicin (DNR) or idarubicin (IDA) at a concentration of 5 µg/ml with or without BIBW22, DEX or VER. Drugs were diluted with RPMI containing 10% FCS before each experiment. After 15 min of incubation at 37 °C with 5% CO_2 and 95% humidified air, cells were washed and resuspended in ice-cold RPMI with 10% FCS alone or plus MDR-modifiers. Flow-cytometric analysis was performed at specified time points over a 30-minute period. The decrease of the fluorescence signal was measured after 15 min. Efflux was quantified as percent of the initial fluorescence intensity. All experiments were perfomed in triplicate. An efflux of more than 10% was classified as positive.

Chemicals. DNR and IDA were obtained from Farmitalia (Freiburg, FRG) and R123 from Sigma (München, FRG). BIBW22 was a gift from Dr. Karl Thomae GmbH (Biberach/Riss, FRG), DEX was a gift from Byk Gulden Pharmaceuticals (Konstanz, FRG), and VER was supplied by Knoll AG (Ludwigshafen, FRG).

Results

Effect of MDR-modifiers on R123 efflux in CEM-VBL cells. To determine an optimal MDR-modifier concentration for efflux studies BIBW22, DEX, and VER were analysed at concentrations ranging from 0.1 to 100 µM in the CEM-VBL cell line. Figure 1 shows R123 efflux in CEM-VBL cells exposed to R123 at a concentration of 5 µg/ml alone or in combination with MDR-modifiers. Effective efflux inhibitory concentrations for BIBW22, DEX, and VER could be demonstrated at 0.3 µM, 1 µM, and 10 µM, respectively.

Effect of MDR-modifiers on R123, DNR and IDA efflux in CEM-VBL cells. R123, DNR, and IDA efflux was determined in CEM-VBL cells exposed to either R123, DNR or IDA at concentrations of 5 µg/ml alone or in combination with 10 µM VER. As shown in Figure 2, CEM-VBL cells incubated

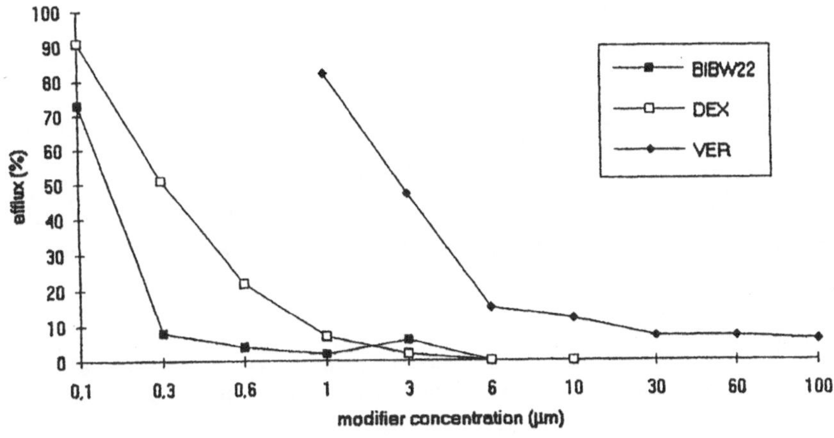

Fig. 1. R123 efflux in CEM-VBL cells after incubation with BIBW22, DEX, and VER as measured by flow-cytometric analysis

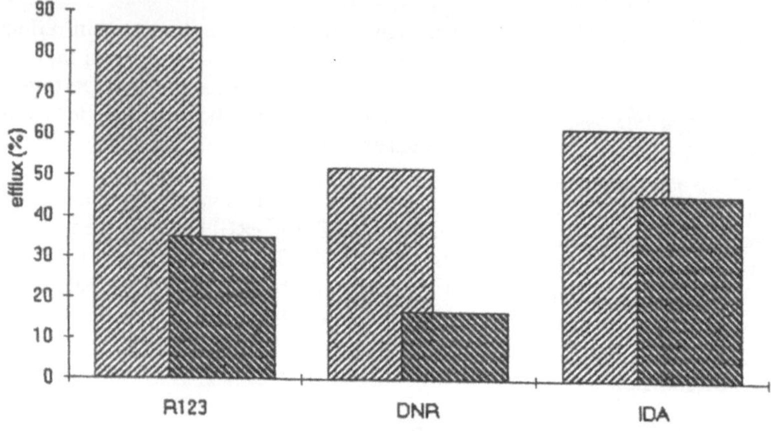

Fig. 2. R123, DNR, and IDA efflux in CEM-VBL cells after incubation with medium (light columns) or plus verapamil (dark columns) as measured by flow-cytometric analysis

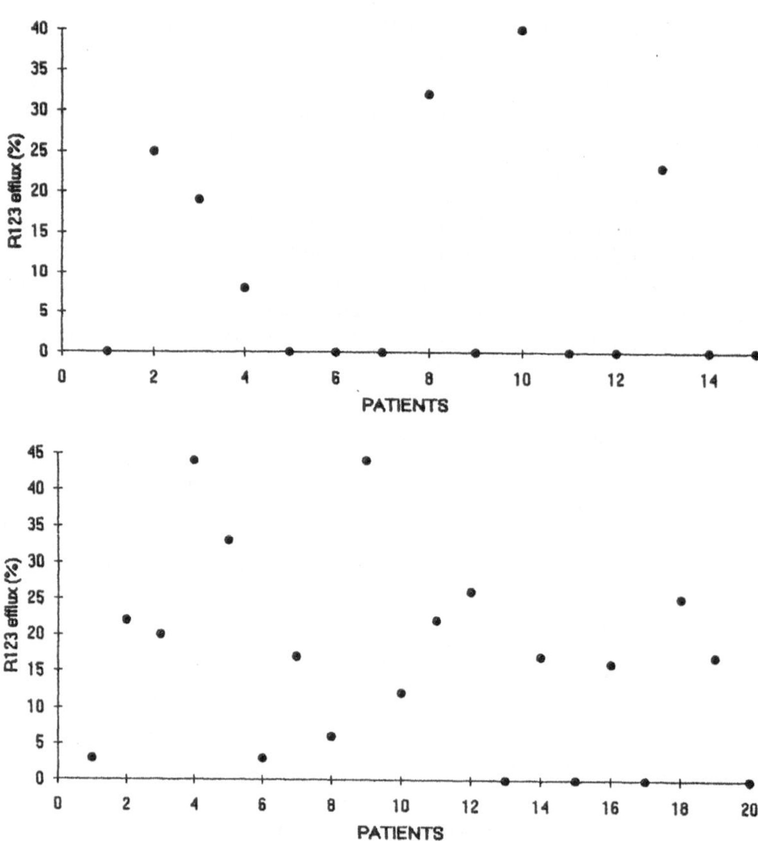

Fig. 3. R123 efflux in blast populations of *de novo* AML (top) or relapsed or persistent AML (bottom) as measured by flow-cytometric analysis

with R123, DNR or IDA for 15 min showed a rapid reduction in intracellular drug levels when incubated in fresh medium for 15 min. Approximately 14% of the initial R123, 48% of the DNR and 38% of the IDA concentration remained in these cells after 15 min. The addition of VER resulted in a 2.5-fold decrease in R123 efflux and in a 3.0-fold decrease in DNR efflux, respectively. In contrast, incubation of these cells with IDA and VER led only to a 1.3-fold decrease in IDA efflux.

Studies in AML blast cells. The results of R123, DNR, and IDA efflux studies in blast populations are illustrated in Figure 3. A total of 35 patients with AML, 15 *de novo* and 20 relapsed or persistent, was investigated. While only five out of 15 blast populations of *de novo* AML (33%) showed moderate efflux of R123 and DNR, 13 out of 20 blast populations of relapsed or persistent AML (65%) had a positive efflux within 15 min with maximum values of 45%. In these drug-resistant phenotype positive blast populations efflux of R123 (Fig. 4) and DNR (data not shown) could be significantly inhibited by 1 μM BIBW22, 1 μM DEX, and 10 μM VER, respectively. In contrast, for IDA we found an effusion of $45 \pm 9\%$ ($x \pm SD$) within 15 min, which could not be significantly inhibited by the modulators.

Correlation of CD34 expression and R123 efflux. Twenty-three consecutive patients with untreated or treated AML were evaluated. In 17 out of 23 blast populations the CD34 expression varied between 10 and 90% (mean, 57%). Eleven out of 17 CD34 positive blast populations (65%) showed a marked R123 efflux, while only two blast populations without CD34 expression (33%) were positive for R123 efflux (Fig. 5).

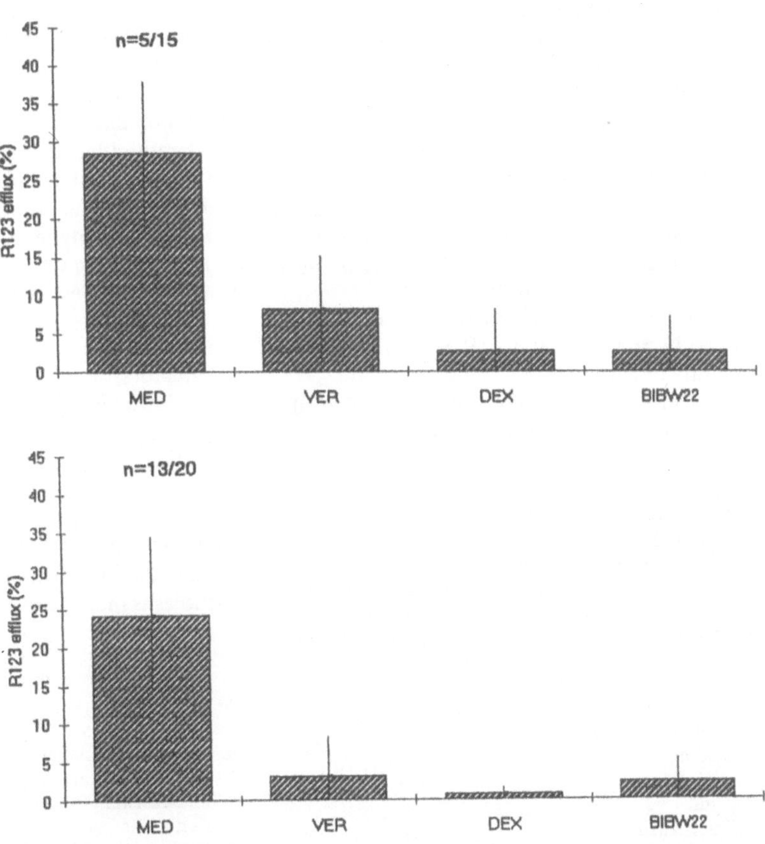

Fig. 4. R123 efflux in drug-resistant phenotype positive blast populations of *de novo* AML (top) or relapsed or persistent AML (bottom) after incubation with medium (MED) or plus modifier as measured by flow-cytometric analysis ($x \pm SD$)

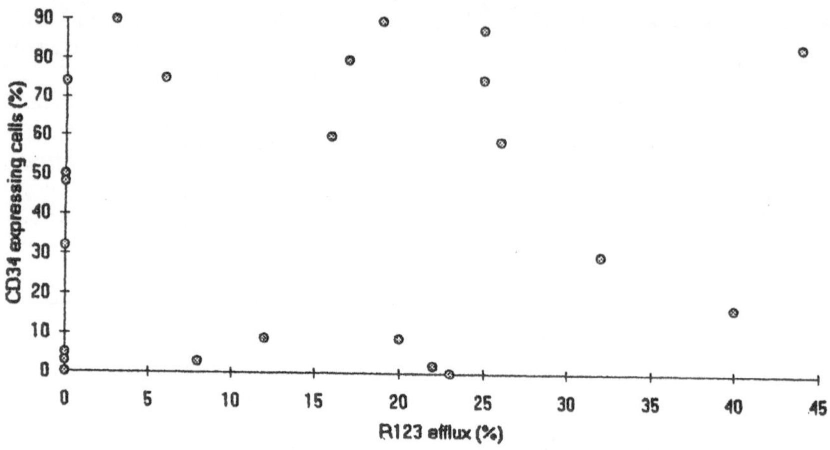

Fig. 5. Correlation between the proportion of R123 efflux and CD34 expression in AML blast populations

Discussion

Various compounds such as VER, DEX, tamoxifen, cyclosporin A and others have been demonstrated to modulate MDR by inhibiting the efflux of MDR-dependent drugs *in vitro* (Table 1).

Here we demonstrate that the phenylpteridine derivative BIBW22 (Chen et al. 1993) is an effective modifier of MDR in the human leukemia cell line CEM-VBL displaying the MDR phenotype, and also in blasts of *de novo*, relapsed or persistent AML *in vitro*.

The drug-resistant phenotype was determined by means of R123, DNR, and IDA efflux as a functional assay.

In CEM-VBL, the R123 and DNR efflux inhibiting potentional of BIBW22 was concentration dependent. There were no significant differences in the efflux inhibition for 0.3 μM BIBW22, 1 μM DEX, and 10 μM VER, respectively.

Table 1. Concentrations for MDR modulators (Kaye, 1990, modified)

Modulator	Optimal in in vitro concentration (μM)	Clinically achievabe plasma concentration (μM)
Verapamil	6–10	1–2
Dexverapamil	6–10	3
Dexniguldipine	0.5–1	0.3
Quinidine	4–6	3–10
Amiodarone	2	2–6
Bepridil	6	2–4
Trifluoperazine	2–12	0.3
Cyclosporin A	5	2–7
Cefoperazone	1	1
Tamoxifen	10	6

The efflux inhibition potential of VER, B935 and BIBW22 was also investigated in blast populations of 35 patients with AML. Only 33% of the blast populations from *de novo* AML showed moderate efflux of R123 and DNR. In contrast, 65% of the blast populations of relapsed or persistent AML functionally displayed the drug resistant phenotype. Efflux could be significantly inhibited by 1 μM BIBW22, 1 μM DEX, and 10 μM VER, respectively. For IDA we found an effusion of 45±9% in all blast populations which could not be significantly inhibited by the modulators.

We conclude that the application of BIBW22 might be a feasible approach to overcome MDR in patiens with AML, as it has a high efflux-inhibiting potential *in vitro*. However, the determination of the maximum tolerated dose, the clinically achievable plasma concentrations, and the therapeutic index of BIBW22 in clinical phase I-studies is mandatory for further assessment.

References

1. Beck WT, Mueller TJ, Tanzer LR (1979) Altered surface membrane glycoproteins in Vinca alkaloid-resistant human leukemic lymphoblasts. Cancer Res 39: 2070–2076
2. Biedler JL, Riehm H (1970) Cellular resistance to actinomycin D in Chinese hamster cells in vitro: Cross resistance, radioautographic and cytogenetic studies. Cancer Res 30: 1174–1184

3. Bradley G, Jurunka PF, Ling V (1988) Mechanism of multidrug resistance. Biochim Biophys Acta 948: 87–128
4. Chen HX, Bamberger U, Heckel A, Guo X, Cheng YC (1993) BIBW 22, a dipyridamole analogue, acts as a bifunctional modulator on tumor cells by influencing both P-glycoprotein and nucleoside transport. Cancer Res 53: 1974–1977
5. Kaye SB (1990) Reversal of multidrug resistance. Cancer Treat Rev 17 (Suppl A): 37–43
6. Marie J-P, Zittoun R, Sikic BI (1991) Multidrug resistance (mdr1) gene expression in adult acute leukemias: correlations with treatment outcome and in vitro drug sensitivity. Blood 78: 586–592
7. Meyers MB, Rittmann-Grauer L, O'Brien JP, Safa SR (1989) Characterization of monoclonal antibodies recognizing a Mr 180,000 P-glycoprotein: Differential expression of the Mr 180,000 and Mr 170,000 P-glycoprotein in multidrug-resistant human tumor cells. Cancer Res 49: 3209–3214
8. Pirker R, Wallner J, Geissler K, Linkesch W, Haas OA, Bettelheim P, Hopfner M, Scherrer R, Valent P, Havelec L, Ludwig H, Lechner K (1991) MDR1 gene expression and treatment outcome in acute myeloid leukemia. J Natl Cancer Inst 83: 708–712
9. Safa AR, Glover CJ, Sewell JL, Meyers MB, Biedler JL, Felsted RL (1987) Identification of the multidrug resistance-related membrane glycoprotein as an acceptor for calcium channel blockers. J Biol Chem 262: 7884–7888
10. te Boekhorst PAW, de Leeuw K, Schoester M, Wittebol S, Nooter K, Hagemeijer A, Löwenberg B, Sonneveld P (1993) Predominance of functional multidrug resistance (MDR-1) phenotype in CD34+ acute myeloid leukemia cells. Blood 82: 3157–3162
11. Willingham MC, Cornwell MM, Cardarelli CO, Gottesman MM, Pastan I (1986) Single cell analysis of daunomycin uptake and efflux in multidrug-resistant and -sensitive B cells: effects of verapamil and other drugs. Cancer Res 46: 5941–5946

Acute Leukemias V
Experimental Approaches
and Management of Refractory Diseases
Hiddemann et al. (Eds.)

In Vitro Drug Resistance Profiles in Childhood Acute Lymphoblastic Leukemia

R. Pieters[1], G. J. L. Kaspers[1], E. Klumper[1], E. R. van Wering[2], A. van der Does-van den Berg[2], and A. J. P. Veerman[1,2]

Abstract. In 1987, the short-term MTT assay was adapted in our laboratory to study in vitro cellular drug resistance in childhood acute lymphoblastic leukemia (ALL). In this paper, some clinically relevant data obtained with this method are summarized:

1. In a small retrospective study we showed that in vitro drug resistance was related to the long-term clinical outcome. In 1989 a nationwide, prospective study including 128 patients was started to confirm these data. Patients with cells relatively in vitro resistant to prednisolone had a significantly lower 2-year probability of disease-free survival (pDFS 0.67) than sensitive cases (pDFS 0.98). In vitro resistance to L-asparaginase and daunorubicin were also significantly related to outcome; for vincristine the relation was borderline significant. Combining the results for prednisolone, L-asparaginase and vincristine, the pDFS was 100% for the sensitive, 83% for the intermediately sensitive and 60% for the in vitro resistant patients ($p < .001$). In vitro drug resistance was an independent prognostic factor at multivariate analysis.

2. In vitro resistance of a group of 99 children with relapsed ALL was compared to that of 137 children with untreated ALL. Cells from children with relapsed ALL were significantly more in vitro resistant to corticosteroids, anthracyclines, antimetabolites and L-asparaginase but not to vinca-alkaloids, epipodophyllotoxins and ifosfamide. Resistance profiles and the degree of resistance highly differed between individual patients.

3. The prognostic significance of several cell biological features can mainly be explained by drug resistance. DNA hyperdiploid cases have a better prognosis than non-hyperdiploid cases. Hyperdiploid cALL cases were significantly more in vitro sensitive to the antimetabolites 6-TG, 6-MP and araC but not to other drugs. Immunophenotypic subgroups of ALL had their own specific drug resistance profiles that might explain the differences in prognosis related to phenotype.

Conclusions. Drug resistance measured with the MTT assay is an important predictor of clinical outcome in ALL and should be used for risk-group stratification in BFM-oriented treatment. Biological risk groups have their own specific in vitro drug resistance profiles that might be helpful in rational design of risk-group adapted therapies.

Introduction

About 70% of children with ALL is currently cured by chemotherapy. The remaining 30% is not cured despite intensive chemotherapeutic regimens. Many risk factors have been detected in the last two decades such as white blood cell count, age, sex, immunophenotype, DNA ploidy, structural chromosomal aberrations. Some of these have lost their prognostic relevance with more intensive treatment and differ between treatment protocols, implying that the

[1] Department of Pediatrics, Free University Hospital, 1007 MB Amsterdam
[2] Dutch Childhood Leukemia Study Group, The Hague, The Netherlands

prognostic value is treatment related. The underlying cause of the prognostic value of the factors mentioned above is not known. They must in some way reflect differences in the two factors that determine the clinical response to chemotherapy:

1. Pharmacokinetics that determines the amount of effective drug to which leukemic cells are exposed and the duration of exposure.
2. The intrinsic cellular sensitivity or resistance to these drugs.

We need more detailed knowledge about the clinical relevance of both factors to improve the chemotherapy for children with ALL instead of (or at least in addition to) simply increasing or reducing the intensity of chemotherapy protocols by trial and error.

Clonogenic assays have long been considered to be the gold standard for in vitro drug resistance testing. However, these assays are not applicable to samples of patients with ALL because ALL cells have a very low clonogenic capacity. Moreover, clonogenic assays are time consuming and laborious. Especially in the last decade, short-term assays have been developed that measure cell kill on the total cell population that is non-dividing. This is different from clonogenic assays that measure inhibition of proliferation on a small subset of cells that are selected by their characteristic of being easily induced to proliferation in vitro. There is growing evidence that the correlations between in vitro drug sensitivity and the clinical response to chemotherapy for short-term assays is at least as good as for clonogenic assays [1]. Moreover, it is more and more recognized that chemotherapy does not have its clinical effects only by acting on proliferating cells but also by directly killing non-dividing cells, e.g. by drug induced apoptosis or programmed cell death.

Our laboratory has adapted the socalled MTT assay for large scale in vitro drug resistance studies in childhood ALL [2]. In this assay, ALL cells are incubated in microculture plates containing six concentrations of a drug during 4 days. At present we test 20 different drugs. After 4 days the tetrazolium salt MTT is added which is exclusively reduced to a coloured formazan product by living cells. The cytotoxic effect is quantified by spectrophotometrically determining the formazan production. The LC_{50}, the drug concentration that kills 50% of the cells, is calculated and used as measure of drug resistance. In this way a drug resistance profile can be determined for each ALL patient. In this paper we will summarize some data obtained in our laboratory that will demonstrate the clinical relevance of this drug resistance profile.

Drug Resistance and Clinical Outcome

In 1991 we reported the relationship between in vitro drug resistance at initial diagnosis and long-term clinical outcome in 42 patients [3]. Cryopreserved cells of patients with a relatively high white blood cell count were used; the patients were treated according to several protocols of the early eighties. Because of this selection of patients, the overall clinical outcome was relatively low. Patients with cells that were in vitro relatively resistant to prednisolone had a significantly lower probability of 5 years continuous complete remission than patients with cells that were relatively sensitive to these drugs (Figure 1). The same was found for daunorubicin and thiopurines; For L-asparaginase and vincristine such a relation could not be detected. At stratification this prognostic relevance of in vitro resistance appeared to be independent from age, sex, white blood cell count, organomegaly and immunophenotype.

In 1989 we started a prospective nationwide study to confirm these findings. Material was received from 149 patients. The MTT assay was technically succesful in 80% of these cases. Major causes of technical failures were that too few ALL cells were available ($n=18$) or that they did not convert MTT ($n=12$). The patients were divided by the median LC_{50} value for a drug in two groups of equal size. Patients in vitro resistant to prednisolone had a lower 2-year probability of disease-free survival (pDFS 0.67) than sensitive patients (pDFS 0.98) ($p=.009$). Further subdivision in 3 groups of equal size also showed that the prognosis decreased with increasing in vitro resistance to prednisolone. In vitro resistance to dexamethasone, L-asparaginase, daunorubicin and mercaptopurine were also significantly related to outcome; for vincristine the relation was borderline significant. In vitro resistance to each of the other drugs (vindesine, doxorubicin, mitoxantrone, thioguanine, cytarabine and teniposide) was not significantly related to 2-year pDFS.

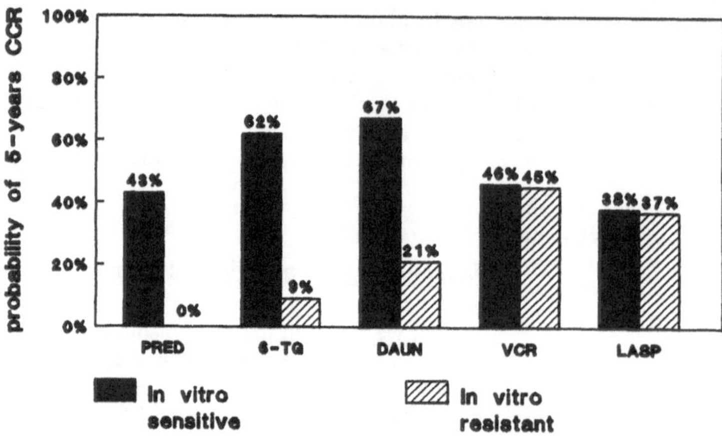

Fig. 1. Relation between in vitro drug resistance at initial diagnosis and probability of 5-years continuous complete remission (CCR) in childhood ALL. Data from a retrospective study; Adapted from Pieters et al. (Lancet 1991; 338: 399–403). Abbreviations: Prednisolone (Pred), 6-thioguanine (6-TG), daunorubicin (Daun), vincristine (VCR), L-asparaginase (LASP)

Combining the results for prednisolone, L-asparaginase and vincristine, the pDFS was 100% for the 38 in vitro sensitive, 83% for the 40 intermediately sensitive and 60% for the 23 resistant cases ($p<.001$). At multivariate analysis, the prognostic value of in vitro drug resistance was independent from age, sex, immunophenotype, DNA ploidy, white blood cell count, BFM risk factor and the clinical response to the first week monotherapy with prednisolone.

Drug Resistance in Relapsed ALL

We compared the in vitro drug resistance profiles of 99 children with relapsed ALL with that of 137 children with newly diagnosed, untreated ALL. The relative resistance of the relapsed samples was expressed by the resistance ratio which was defined as follows:

$$\text{Resistance Ratio} = \frac{\text{median } LC_{50} \text{ value of relapsed ALL}}{\text{median } LC_{50} \text{ value of untreated ALL}}$$

The results are summarized in Figure 2. In conclusion, the group of children with relapsed ALL was significantly more in vitro resistant to corticosteroids, anthracyclines, antimetabolites and L-asparaginase but not to vinca-alkaloids, epipodophyllotoxins and ifosfamide. However, these results are based on a group comparison. Resistance profiles and the degree of in vitro resistance turned out to vary widely between individual patients. This suggests that in some relapsed ALL cases still effective chemotherapy regimens might be composed while others are resistant to the whole spectrum of drugs. This has led to a clinical trial of tailored therapy in poor prognostic relapsed ALL in which part of the drugs is chosen by the individual in vitro drug resistance profile. This trial is a collaboration between the German BFM-ALL relapse section (Prof. G. Henze) and our laboratory.

DNA Ploidy and Drug Resistance

DNA hyperdiploidy is a favourable prognostic feature in childhood common ALL [4]. The explanation for this is not known although it is assumed that ploidy reflects differences in drug sensitivity. Recent support for this idea has come from in vitro drug sensitivity studies: Whitehead et al. [5] showed that hyperdiploid cases accumulated higher amounts of methotrexate polyglutamates, suggesting that hyperdiploid cases are more sensitive to this drug. They did not study other drugs. In a pilot study we compared the in vitro drug resistance profiles of 10 hyperdiploid cALL and 27 non-hyperdiploid cALL samples defined by a DNA-index of 1.16.

Hyperdiploid cases were significantly more in vitro sensitive to the antimetabolites 6-TG, 6-MP and araC but not to other drugs (Figure 3). The higher sensitivity of hyperdiploid cases for steroids and l-asparaginase did not reach

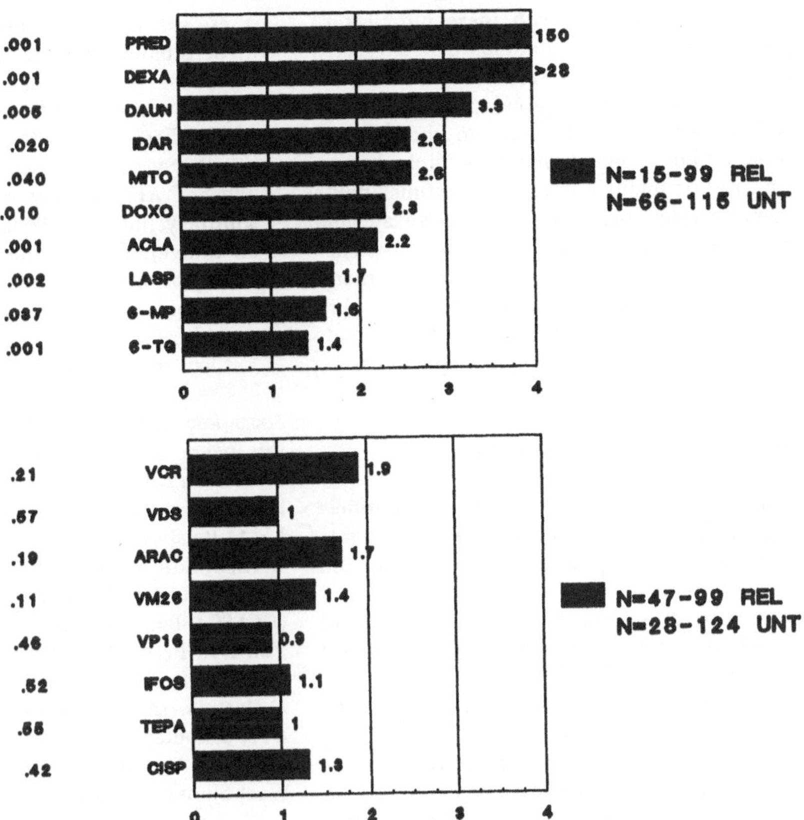

Fig. 2. In vitro drug resistance of a group of children with relapsed ALL compared to a group of children with newly diagnosed ALL. Given are the in vitro resistance ratio of drugs according to the definition in the text. Abbreviations: Prednisolone (Pred), dexamethasone (Dexa), daunorubicin (Daun), idarubicin (Idar), mitoxantrone (Mito), doxorubicin (doxo), aclarubicin (acla), L-asparaginase (LASP), 6-mercaptopurine (6-MP), 6-thioguanine (6-TG), vincristine (VCR), vindesine (VDS), cytosine arabinoside (AraC), 4-HOO-ifosfamide (Ifos), thiotepa (Tepa), Cisplatin (Cisp). P-values are shown on the left

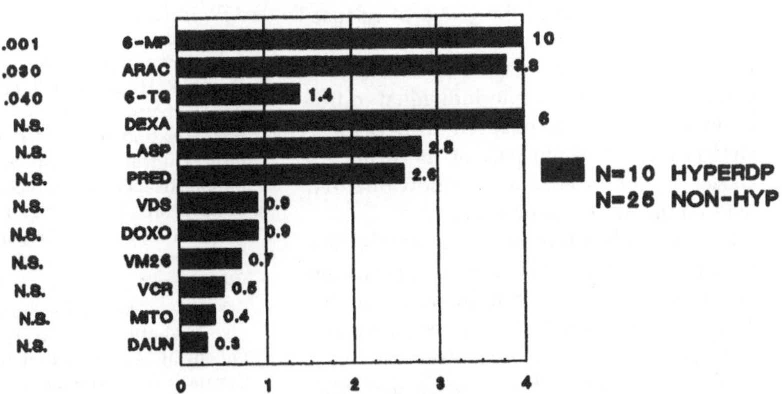

Fig. 3. Relation between in vitro drug resistance and DNA ploidy. For each drug the resistance ratio, i.e. the median LC50 value for the non-hyperdiploid common ALL group divided by the median LC50 value for the hyperdiploid common ALL group, is presented. For instance, non-hyperdiploid cases are median 2.6-fold more resistant to prednisolone than hyperdiploid cases. For abbreviations see Figure 2.

statistical significance with these numbers of patients. Also, these preliminary data suggested that hyperdiploid cases were not more sensitive to anthracyclines and epipodophyllotoxins but perhaps even more resistant to these drugs. Some authors suggest that hyperdiploid common ALL is highly curable with antimetabolite chemotherapy consisting of methotrexate and mercaptopurine [4,6]. Based on this experience and on the in vitro data shown above, it is therefore doubtful whether we should expose children with this type of ALL to very toxic agents such as anthracyclines and epipodophyllotoxins.

Conclusions and Perspectives

1. In vitro drug resistance testing is routinely possible in ALL with a technical success rate comparable to e.g. immunophenotyping and karyotyping.
2. In vitro drug resistance is an independent and important predictive factor of clinical outcome in childhood ALL.

   These two conclusions lead to the perspective that the in vitro drug resistance profile can be used for risk group stratification. A large group of patients at very low risk of relapse is currently treated with intensive chemotherapy with possible unnecessary side effects and even toxic deaths. The in vitro drug resistance assay is a suitable tool to identify these patients as low risk patients. On the other hand, patients with a poor prognosis in contemporary protocols, can also be recognized with the MTT assay.
3. The poor prognosis of the group of relapsed ALL patients is related to cellular resistance to several but not all classes of chemotherapeutic drugs. Large interindividual differences exist between relapsed ALL cases. A clinical trial in which part of the drugs are chosen by the in vitro assay (individualized, tailored therapy) is in progress.
4. The prognostic value of cell biological features such as DNA ploidy is at least partly due to cellular drug resistance. In earlier studies we have shown that each immunophenotypic and age group had its own drug resistance profile (Pieters 1993). This suggests that rational development of treatment protocols for specific biological subclasses or risk groups of ALL might be possible by using the knowledge of the in vitro drug resistance profiles of these subclasses. For instance, the profile of hyperdiploid common ALL supports the clinical observations that this form of ALL is highly curable with antimetabolite based chemotherapy and that it is very doubtful whether we should expose children with this type of ALL to very toxic agents such as anthracyclines and alkylating agents.
5. In individual cases, the in vitro drug resistance profile may contribute to palliative treatments with minimal side-effects in individual cases by omitting drugs that have no antileukemic activity in vitro.

Acknowledgements. Part of the results described in this paper were tested in connection with our studies on cellular drug resistance in childhood leukaemia in cooperation with the German ALL-BFM Relapse group (Prof. G. Henze), the German CoALL group (Prof. G.E. Janka-Schaub), and the Dutch Childhood Leukemia Study Group (DCLSG). Board members of the DCLSG are H Van Den Berg, MVA Bruin, JPM Bökkerink, PJ Van Dijken, K Hählen, WA Kamps, FAE Nabben, A Postma, JA Rammeloo, IM Risseeuw-Appel, AYN Schouten-Van Meeteren, GAM De Vaan, E Th Van't Veer-Korthof, AJP Veerman, M Van Weel-Sipman and RS Weening.

References

1. Veerman AJP, Pieters R. Drug sensitivity assays in leukemia and lymphoma. Br J Haematol 1990; 74: 381.
2. Pieters R, Loonen AH, Huismans DR, Broekema GJ, Dirven MWJ, Heyenbrok MW, Hählen K, Veerman AJP. In vitro drug sensitivity of cells from children with leukemia using the MTT assay with improved culture conditions. Blood 1990; 76: 2327.
3. Pieters R, Huismans DR, Loonen AH, Hählen K, van der Does-van den Berg A, van Wering ER, Veerman AJP. Relation of cellular drug resistance to long-term clinical outcome in childhood acute lymphoblastic leukemia. Lancet 1991; 338: 399.
4. Pui CH, Crist WM, Look AT. Biology and clinical significance of cytogenetic abnormalities in childhood acute lymphoblastic leukemia. Blood 1990; 76: 1449.
5. Whitehead VM, Vuhich M-J, Lauer SJ, Mahoney D, Carroll AJ, Shuster Esseltine DW, Payment C, Look AT, Akabutu J, Bowen T, Taylor LD, Camitta B, Pullen DJ. Accumulation of high levels of methotrexate polyglutamates in lymphoblasts from children with hyperdiploid (>50 chromosomes) B-lineage acute lymphoblastic leukemia: A Pediatric Oncology Group Study. Blood 1992; 80: 1316.
6. Pinkel D. Curing children of leukemia. Cancer 1987; 10: 1683.

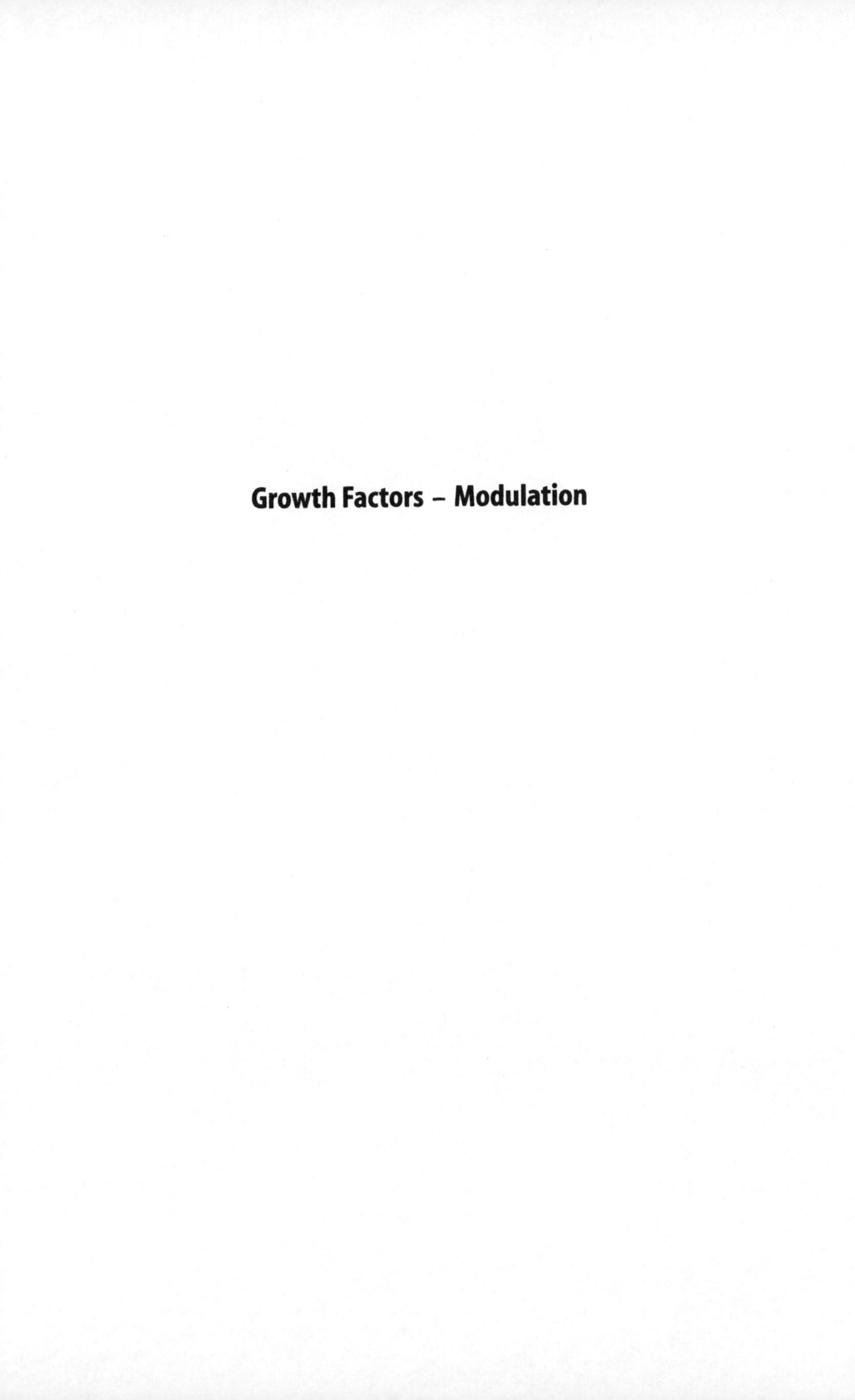

Growth Factors – Modulation

Acute Leukemias V
Experimental Approaches
and Management of Refractory Diseases
Hiddemann et al. (Eds.)

The Expression and Regulation of G-CSF and GM-CSF

E. Vellenga

Colony Stimulating Factors (CSF's) are important regulatory proteins that control the proliferation and differentiation of hematopoietic cells. At the moment, Granulocyte-CSF (G-CSF) and Granulocyte-Macrophage-CSF (GM-CSF) are applied to cancer patients for preventing pancytopenia after chemotherapy or for the isolation of peripheral blood stem cells [1]. Although the growth factors are exchangable in most cases with regard to the clinical applicability, distinct differences are noted in production and regulation under physiological circumstances. G-CSF is produced by different cell types like monocytes, endothelial cells and fibroblasts [2, 3]. In monocytes G-CSF mRNA expression is observed after 1–2 hrs of stimulation, followed by the secretion of the protein after 12–24 hrs. G-CSF mRNA can be upregulated by different cytokines like IL-1, IL-7, and by Lipopolysacccharide (LPS)[2–4]. The effect of LPS on monocytes is a direct effect mediated by binding to CD antigen [5]. However, a second peak in G-CSF expression can be observed after 15–18 hrs of stimulation which is due to the release of IL-1 in response to LPS stimulation and can subsequently be blocked by coculturing the cells with anti-IL-1 antiserum. However, LPS, IL-1 and IL-7 are not the only inducers of G-CSF protein by monocytes. Recently performed investigations have indicated that a naturally occurring bacterial cell wall breakdown product of peptidoglycan, N-acetylglucosaminyl-1,6 anhydro-N-acetylmuramyl-l-alanyl-D-isoglutamyl-m-diaminopimelyl-D-alanine G (Anh)Tetra is capable to induce cytokine mRNA [6] Monocytes stimulated by G(Anh)MTetra express cytokines such as G-CSF, IL-1, and IL-6. The response at mRNA level is comparable to LPS, and can be further enhanced by culturing the cells with LPS plus G(Anh)MTetra. These results indicate that besides LPS additional factors are released during bacteremia which modulate the cytokine release and subsequently the clinical course of septic patients. Additional studies with G(Anh)MTetra indicated that the expression of cytokines was in part due to stabilization of the cytokine mRNA at post-transcriptional level. However, an increase in the transcriptional rate of the cytokine genes was also demonstrated. This was associated with induction of different transcription factors such as activator protein-1 (AP-1) and nuclear factor-κB (NF-κB) whereas no change was observed in the expression of NF-IL

The expression of G-CSF in human monocytes can also be modulated by additional lymphokines. The T cell derived lymphokine Interferon-γ (IF-γ) has several effects on monocyte functions. For example IF-γ alone induces the expression of Macrophage-CSF (M-CSF) in human monocytes without inducing G-CSF transcripts [7]. However, monocytes primed with IF-γ for several hours and subsequently stimulated by LPS, demonstrate a marked increase in expression of G-CSF at mRNA and protein level compared to the effects of LPS alone [8]. These data underscore the role of IF-γ in cytokine secretion especially during bacteremia. This was already observed in experiments with mice by which treatment of

Department of Hematology, University Hospital Groningen, 9700 RB Groningen, The Netherlands

mice with anti-IF-γ significantly prolonged the survival [9].

The expression of G-CSF in monocytes is not only regulated by activators but also by repressor molecules. Especially the T cell derived lymphokine IL-4 suppresses the LPS and IL-1 induced expression of G-CSF [10, 11]. The inhibitive effect is most pronounced if the cells are pre-cultured for a short period in IL-4 containing medium and subsequently activated by LPS.

The suppressive effect of IL-4 can partially be ascribed to a reduced expression of transcription factors [12,13]. The transcription factor AP-1 which is encoded by the proto-oncogenes c-jun and c-fos, demonstrate a reduced expression compared to results of LPS alone. In addition a reduced expression of NF-κB has been demonstrated in the presence of IL-4. These data suggest that the control on transcription activity by IL-4, might be an important regulatory mechanism for controlling cytokine expression in human monocytes. An additional cytokine which suppresses the G-CSF expression is IL-10. IL-10 is secreted by different cell types such as T cells, monocytes, and mast cells [14]. In monocytes the expression of IL-10 mRNA is most prominent upregulated by Tumor Necrosis Factor (TNF)-α [15]. In addition it has been demonstrated that monocytes cultured in the presence of anti-IL-10, express significantly higher levels of IL-1, IL-6 and G-CSF mRNA in response to LPS stimulation indicating that IL-10 is an important autocrine repressor cytokine for human monocytes [16]. Although the effects of IL-10 and IL-4 are similar with regard to cytokine regulation, distinct differences are noticed in additional functions. For example CD expression on monocytes is down-regulated by IL-4 after 2–3 days of culture, whereas no change in CD expression is observed if the cells are exposed to IL-10. Furthermore it appeared that the suppressive effect of IL-4 and IL-10 on the monocytic lineage is not a general phenomenon in the hematopoietic system. This is illustrated by the fact that endothelial cells cultured with IL-4 or IL-10 express IL-6 mRNA [17]. In addition IL-4 enhances the G-CSF supported granulocytic colony formation from human bone marrow cells, tested in in vitro culture assay [18].

A second growth factor which is often applied to patients, is GM-CSF. GM-CSF is secreted by different cell types like monocytes, endothelial cells, fibroblasts, and T cells [1]. In contrast to G-CSF, GM-CSF mRNA is not induced by LPS stimulated monocytes. However, stimulating of the high affinity FcγRI on monocytes results in the production of significant amounts of GM-CSF protein [19]. T cells are also an important producer of GM-CSF. T cells stimulated with the lectin Concanavalin A, or triggering of the CD receptor complex, causes induction of GM-CSF transcripts [20]. Especially costimulation with the protein kinase C activator PMA or with anti-CD results in an strong enhancement in GM-CSF mRNA expression due to a strong increase in transcription rate of the GM-CSF gene and due to stabilization of the message at post-transcriptional level [21]. Additional cytokines that can modulate GM-CSF mRNA in activated T cells are IL-1, IL-2, IL-7 [22, 23]. The effect of IL-7 seemed to be a direct effect since blocking antibodies against several cytokines could not abrogate the response.

As described for G-CSF, the expression of cytokines is not only controlled by enhancers but also by repressor proteins. The involvement of the suppressive signaling pathway seemed to be cell type dependent. This is reflected by the fact the c-AMP dependent protein kinase A activation in monocytes enhances the expression of cytokine mRNA, whereas in T cells it is suppressive [24]. Recently performed studies in T cells have indicated that the c-AMP dependent signaling pathway strictly controls the GM-CSF mRNA expression as well in CD + as in CD + cells. The GM-CSF expression in activated T cells is downregulated if T cells are exposed to c-AMP analogues, or to prostaglandin E (PGE2) which elevates c-AMP by receptor mediated acitvation, or by isobutyl-methylxantin (IBMX) which inhibits phosphodiesterase activity [26]. However, different mechanisms seem to be involved in the suppressive effect of dibytyryl-cAMP (dbcAMP). In con A activated T cells db-cAMP significantly reduced the transcription rate of GM-CSF gene without affecting the half-life, while in con A plus PMA stimulated T cells, db-cAMP suppressed both the transcription rate and the half-life of the message indicating that the effector function of the PKA system depends on the stimuli presented to the T cell. This negative regulatory pathway might be an important negative feedback system since high concentrations of PGE are produced by monocytes and epithelial cells during an inflammatory response.

In summary these data indicate that the effects of hematopoietic growth factors are cell restricted which gives the opportunity to modulate several cellular processes in response to a limited number of cytokines.

References

1. Biesma B, Vellenga E, Willemse PHB, Vries de GE. Effects of hematopoietic growth factors on chemotherapy-induced myelosuppression. Critical Reviews in Oncology/Hematology 13: 107, 1992.
2. Vellenga E, Rambaldi A, Ernst TJ, Ostapovicz, Griffin JD. Independent regulation of M-CSF and G-CSF gene expression in human monocytes. Blood 71: 1529, 1988.
3. Schaafsma R, Falkenburg JHF, Duinkerken N, Van Damme J, Altrock BW, Willemze R, Fibbe WE. Interleukin-1 synergizes with granulocyte-macrophage colony-stimulating factor on granulocytic colony formation by intermediate production of granulocyte colony-stimulating factor. Blood 74: 2398, 1989.
4. Alderson M, Tough TW, Ziegler SF, Grabstein KH. Interleukin-7 induces cytokine secretion and tumoricidal activity by human peripheral blood monocytes. J.Exp.Med. 173: 923, 1991.
5. Hailman E, Lichenstein HS, Wurfel MM, Miller DS, Johnson DA, Kelley M, Busse LA, Zukowski MM, Wright SD Lipopolysaccharide (LPS)-binding protein accelerates the binding of LPS to CD14. J.Exp.Med. 179: 269, 1994.
6. Dokter WAH, Dijkstra AJ, Koopmans SB, Stulp BK, Kecks W, Halie MR, Vellenga E. G(Anh)MTETRA, a natural bacterial cell wall breakdown product, induces Interleukin-1 β and Interleukin-6 expression in human monocytes. Journal of Biological Chemistry. 269: 4201, 1994.
7. Rambaldi A, Young DC, Griffin J.D.Expression of M-CSF by human monocytes. Blood 69: 1409, 1987.
8. Wit de H, Dokter WHA, Esseling MT, Halie MR, Vellenga E. Interferon- γ enhances the LPS-induced G-CSF gene expression in human adherent monocytes, which is regulated at transcriptional and posttransscriptional levels. Experimental Hematology 21: 785, 1993.
9. Heremans H, Van Damme J, Dillen C, Dijkmans R, Billiau A. Interferon-γ, a mediator of lethal lipopolysaccharide-induced Shwartzman-like shock reactions in mice. J.ExpMed. 171: 1853, 1990.
10. Vellenga E, Vinne vd B, Wolf de JThM, Halie MR. Simultaneous expression and regulation of G-CSF and IL-6 mRNA in adherent human monocytes and fibroblasts. British Journal of Hematology 78: 14, 1991.
11. Vellenga E, Dokter W, Wolf de JThM, Vinne vd B, Esseling MT, Halie MR. Interleukin-4 prevents the induction of G-CSF mRNA in human adherent monocytes in response to endoxin and IL-1 stimulation. British Journal of Hematology 79: 22, 1991.
12. Dokter WHA, Esseling MT, Halie MR, Vellenga E. Interleukin-4 inhibits the lipopolysaccharide-induced expression of c-jun and c-fos messenger RNA and activator protein-1 binding activity in human monocytes. Blood 81: 337, 1993.
13. Donnelly RP, Crofford LJ, Freeman SL, Buras J.Remmers E, Wilder RL, Fenton MJ. Tissue-specific regulation of IL-6 production by IL-4. Journal of Immunology 151: 5603, 1993.
14. Rennick D, Berg D, Holland G. Interleukin 10: An overview. Progress in Growth Factor Research 4: 207, 1992.
15. Wanidworanun C, Strober W. Predominant role of tumor necrosis factor-α in human monocyte IL-10 synthesis. Journal of Immunology 151: 6853, 1993.
16. Waal de Malefyt RF, Abrams J, Bennet B, Figdor CG, Vries de JE. Interleukin 10 (IL-10) inhibits cytokine synthesis by human monocytes: An autoregulatory role of IL-10 produced by monocytes. J.Exp.Med. 174: 1209, 1991.
17. Sironi M., Muñoz C., Pollicino T., et al. Divergent effects of interleukin-10 on cytokine production by mononuclear phagocytes and endothelial cells. Eur.J.Immunol. 23: 2692, 1993.
18. Vellenga E, Wolf de JThM, Beentjes JAM, Esselink MT, Smit JW, Halie MR. Divergent effects of interleukin-4 (IL-4) on the granulocyte colony-stimulating factor and IL-3-supported myeloid colony formation from normal and leukemic bone marrow cells. Blood 75: 633, 1990.
19. Herrmann F, De Vos S, Brach M, Riedel D, Lindemann, Mertelsmann R. Secretion of granulocyte-macrophage colony-stimulating factor by human blood monocytes is stimulated by engagement of Fcγ receptors type I by solid-phase immunoglobulins requiring high-affinity Fc-Frγ receptor type I interactions. Eur.J.Immunol 22: 1681, 1992.
20. Chan JY, Slaman DJ, Golde DW, Gassan JC. Regulation of expression of human GM-CSF. Proc.Natl.Acad.Sci.USA. 83: 8669, 1986.
21. Dokter WHA, Sierdsema SJ, Esselink MT, Halie MR, Vellenga E. IL-7 enhances the expression of IL-3 and granulocyte-macrophage-CSF mRNA in activated human T cells by post-transcriptional mechanisms. Journal of Immunology 2584, 1993.
22. Sung SJ, Walter JA. Increased cyclic AMP levels enhance IL-1 α and IL-1 β mRNA expression and protein production in human myelomonocytic cell lines and monocytes. J.Clin. Invest. 88: 1915, 1993
23. Straaten van JFM, Dokter WHA, Stulp BK, Vellenga E. The regulation of Interleukin-5 and Interleukin-3 gene expression in human T cells. Cytokine (In press).
24. Borger P, Kauffman HF, Vijgen JLJ, Postma DS, Vellenga E. Activation of the c-AMP dependent signaling pathway inhibits the expression of IL-3 and granulocyte-macrophage-CSF in activated human T lymphocytes. (submitted)

Acute Leukemias V
Experimental Approaches
and Management of Refractory Diseases
Hiddemann et al. (Eds.)

In Situ Nick Translation as a Measure of Cell Death. Application to the Study of Growth Factors and Drug Sensitivity

Mark Minden, C. W. Wang, and E. A. McCulloch

Introduction

The role of growth factors in the expansion of a population of cells is two fold [1]. First, the growth factor provides a signal for the cell to enter and progress through the cell cycle. Second, the growth factor acts as a cell survival factor allowing the cell to maintain viability. In normal hematopoiesis and in the case of many leukemic cells withdrawal of growth factor results in the development of cell death through the process of apoptosis. Cells may also enter the process of programmed cell death as a result of treatment with ionizing radiation and chemotherapeutic agents of different classes [2,3].

Cells undergoing apoptosis may be recognized by their gross morphologic appearance, electron microscopy and by the development of DNA fragmentation as measured by DNA electrophoresis [2]. The above techniques are limited in sensitivity and are time consuming.

We have adapted in situ nick translation to identify cells undergoing apoptosis [4–7]. As DNA within a cell undergoing apoptosis is cleaved, sites of single stand breaks become targets for the entry of DNA polymerase I and for the synthesis of new DNA. We have taken advantage of this to incorporate biotinylated deoxynucleotides into newly synthesized DNA; this is then detected by fluorescent microscopy or flow cytometry. The technique is rapid, relatively inexpensive, and may be applied to many samples at once.

In the present manuscript we describe the assay and demonstrate its utility in measuring apoptosis in cells deprived of growth factor and cells treated with irradiation or the chemotherapeutic agent, cytosine arabinoside.

Materials and Methods

Cell lines and culture conditions. The murine IL-3 dependent cell line 32D was maintained in α-medium supplemented with 10% fetal calf serum (FCS)(growth medium) and murine IL-3 at a concentration of 10 U/ml [8]. For apoptosis experiments the cells were washed three times in growth medium without IL-3.

OCI/AML-2 is a human acute myeloblastic leukemia cell line developed at the Ontario Cancer Institute [9]. The cells are factor independent and are maintained in growth medium alone.

In situ nick translation. For each point $0.5^{-1} \times 10^6$ cells were washed and resuspended in phosphate buffered saline and then fixed and permeabilized in 1% paraformaldehyde for 5 minutes at room temperature and then 60% methanol at 4°C for 15 minutes. Cells could be left in 60% methanol for more than one week thus allowing batching of samples. To further permeabilize the cells they were treated in 0.1% Triton-X 100 in PBS for 15 minutes at room temperature. The nick translation reaction was carried out in a final volume of 50 µl containing 5 µM biotin dUTP (BioRad Laboratories, Richmond, CA), 5 µM biotin dATP (GIBCO-BRL, Burlington, Ont.) 5 µM dATP and dGTP and 1 µM dATP and

Department of Medicine and Medical Biophysics, 500 Sherbourne St., Toronto, Ont., Canada

dTTP (GIBCO-BRL, Burlington, Ont.), 50 mM Tris (pH7.5), 5 mM $MgCl_2$, 100 µg/ml bovine serum albumin (BSA) and 10 U of DNA polymerase I (GIBCO-BRL, Burlington, Ont.). The reaction was incubated at 37 °C for 1 hour. Cells were washed in PBS and then resuspended in 100 µl of PBS containing 6µl of Streptavidin-FITC (Amersham International, UK) and incubated in the dark at 4 °C for 1 hour. Cells were then washed in PBS and analyzed by flow cytometry or UV microscopy. The proportion of labelled cells was analyzed using a FACScan Flow Cytometer (Becton-Dickinson, Mountainview, CA). 1×10^4 cells were captured from each sample and analyzed using Consort 30 or Lysis II software.

Propidium iodide (PI) staining. The viability of cells and the integrity of the cell membrane was determined using PI staining. Cells were incubated in a solution of 50 µg/ml PI in PBS for 30 minutes and then used immediately for flow cytometry or washed and fixed prior to the nick assay [10].

DNA gel electrophoresis. To analyze DNA fragmentation 1×10^6 cells were lysed in 1% SDS and 50 mM EDTA pH 8.0 and incubated at 45 °C for 2 hours in the presence of 100 ug/ml of proteinase K. 100 U of RNAse was added for an additional 30 minutes. The DNA was then loaded onto a 1.8% agarose gel and electrophoresed. The DNA was visualized using ethidium bromide [2].

Results

To establish the method of in situ nick translation for detecting cells undergoing death due to DNA fragmentation we used the factor dependent cell line 32D. These cells grow well in the presence of IL-3, however they start to undergo cell death, as determined by light microscopy, within 18 hours of removal of IL-3. To determine whether the death of 32D cells involved DNA fragmentation we carried out DNA electrophoresis of uncut DNA. As can be seen in Figure 1 the

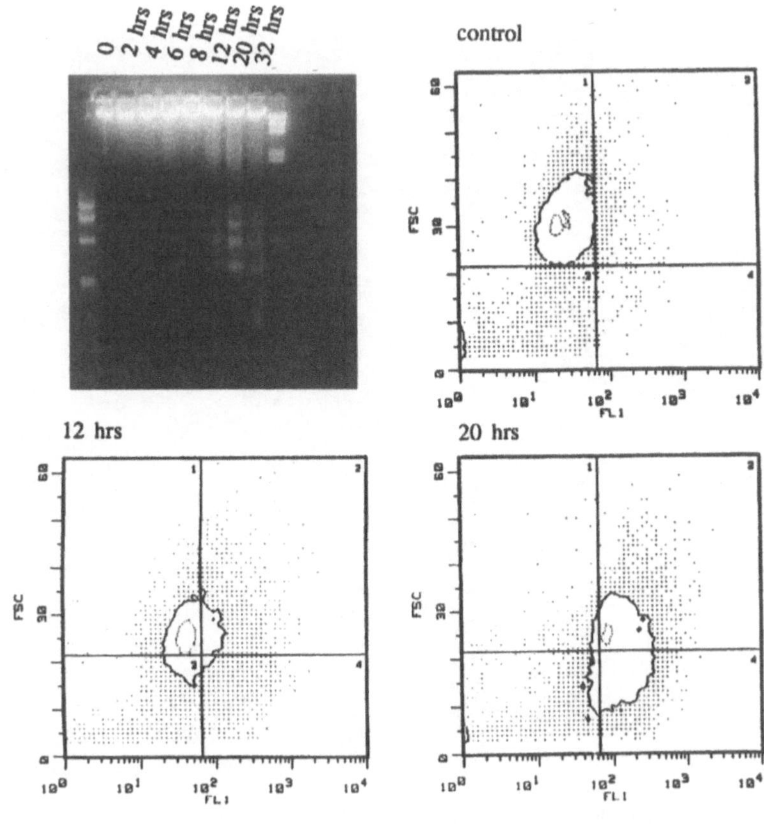

Fig. 1

DNA was intact up until 12 hours at which time a DNA ladder, typical of apoptotic cell death could be seen. The intensity of the ladder increased over time as more cells died (Fig. 1).

32D cells deprived of IL-3 for varying times up to 20 hours were fixed, labelled by in situ nick translation and analyzed either by flow cytometry or fluorescent microscopy. The results are presented as contour plots comparing fluorescent intensity (FL1) against forward scatter (FSC). As can be seen in figure 1 in the control panel cells maintained in IL-3 are not fluorescent; these are the cells in the left upper quadrant. Cells grown without IL-3 for 12 hours contain both unlabelled (left upper quadrant) and labelled cells (right upper quadrant). By 20 hours there are no unlabelled cells. In addition there is a decrease in the size of labelled cells (right lower quadrant); this is typical of cells undergoing apoptosis.

By fluorescent microscopy it was evident that the majority of the cells had labelled nuclei, while some cells did not contain appreciable amounts of label (Fig. 2). The finding of nuclear labelling is expected if the labelling is due to the production of new DNA. The labelling was shown to be dependant on the presence of polymerase I as when this enzyme was omitted there was no labelling of the cells (data not shown).

PI staining is commonly used as a simple measure of cell viability. To determine if cells labelled by the nick assay were also PI positive we carried out the following experiments. 32D cells deprived of IL-3 for 16 hours were stained with PI, fixed and then tested for the presence of DNA degradation. Using dual color fluorescence we found that cells labelled by in situ nick translation were PI negative while cells deprived of IL-3 for 24 hours were both nick translation and PI positive (data not shown).

The DNA fragmentation of 32D cells in the above experiments was due to the withdrawal of growth factor. To determine if other causes of apoptosis would have a similar effect we irradiated 32D cells to 600 cGy using a ^{60}Co source and then placed the cells in culture for 16 hours

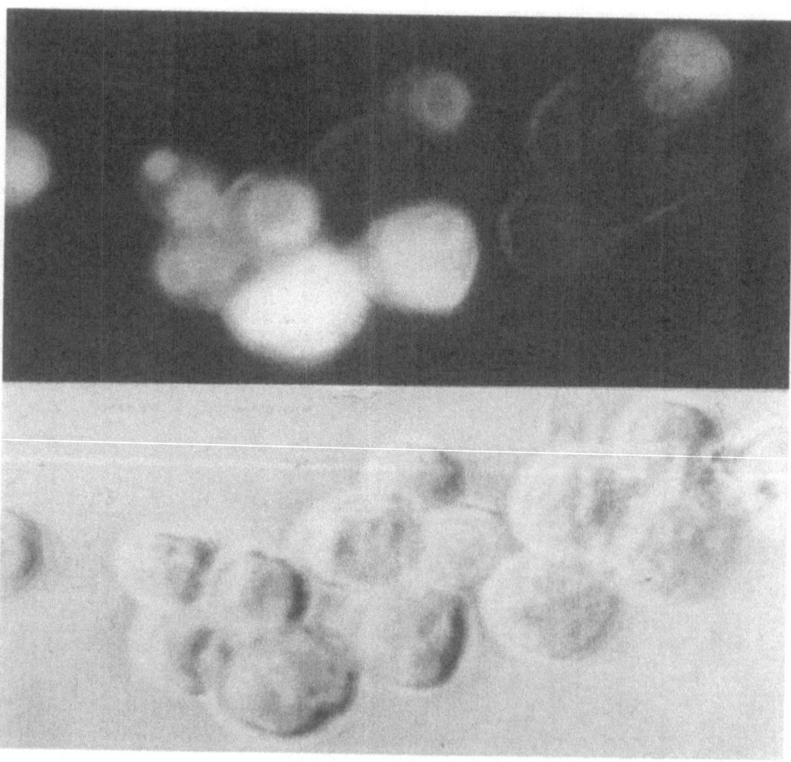

Fig. 2. Top panel phase contrast. Bottom panel fluorescent cells

with IL-3. The irradiated cells showed a similar pattern of labelling as cells deprived of IL-3 (data not shown).

A number of investigators have demonstrated that ara-C can induce DNA fragmentation [3,4]. As we planned to use the in situ nick translation assay as a rapid, inexpensive method for measuring the induction of apoptotic cell death we tested the effect of ara-C for its effect on nicking in a human leukemic cell line. OCI/AML-2 is a factor independent cell line that is highly sensitive to ara-C. Cells were treated for 24 hours in varying concentrations of ara-C and then tested for the degree of labelling. The results of this experiment are shown in figure 3. Control cells not exposed to ara-C had no appreciable labelling (Fig. 3A).

Cells exposed to a low dose of ara-C (2×10^{-6} M) for 24 hours were mainly unlabelled. However a small number of cells were labelled (Fig. 3B). Cells exposed to 1×10^{-5} M ara-C for 24 hours contained a large number of brightly labelled cells (Fig. 3C). It should also be noted that the size of the cells decreased, as determined by forward scatter.

Discussion

In this manuscript we describe a technique for detecting cells undergoing apoptosis. The method is simple, relatively inexpensive and rapid. In the experiments described here we

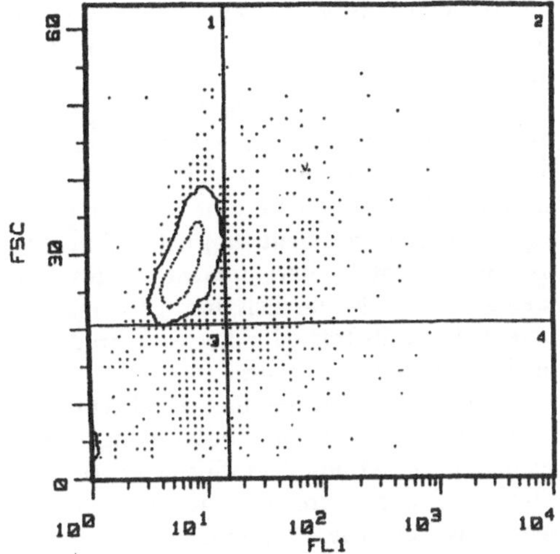

Fig. 3A

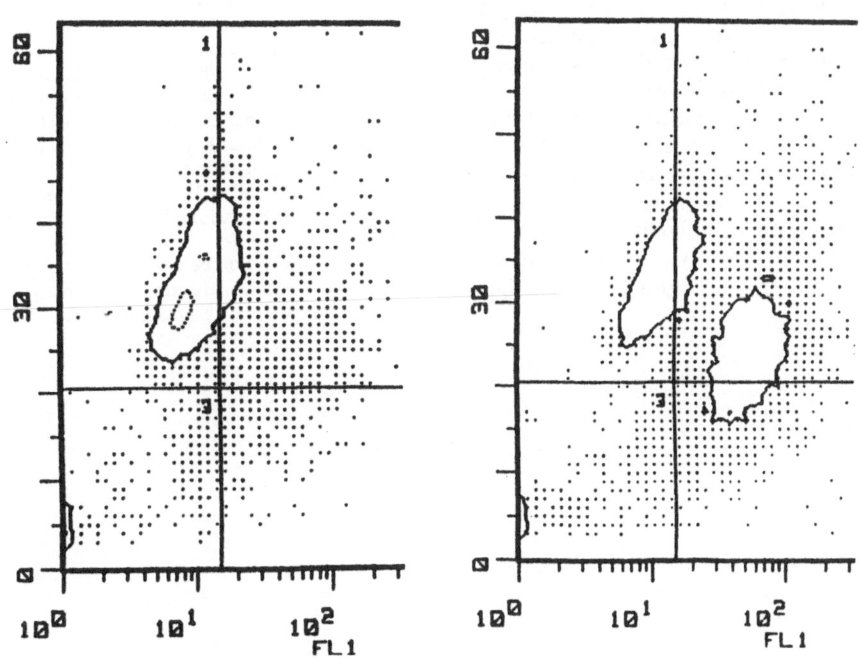

Fig. 3B, C

have shown that 32D cells deprived of growth factors undergo programmed cell death. The process begins approximately 10 hours after withdrawal of growth factor and proceeds over a period of 24 hours. When compared to the standard method of measuring apoptosis, DNA gel electrophoresis, both methods begin to detect DNA fragmentation beginning at about the same time. However, the gel method does not indicate that cells become apoptotic at different times. This is clearly evident in the flow cytometric analysis.

We also demonstrate that apoptosis induced by irradiation and chemotherapeutic agents can be detected with this method. Tests of cell death, such as colony assays are time consuming and expensive. In experiments not detailed here we have found that the development of DNA fragmentation closely parallels loss of clonogenic potential in cells treated either with irradiation or chemotherapeutic agents.

Previously we reported that the effect of ara-C on leukemic blast cells can be modulated by agents such as retinoic acid which increases sensitivity [11] and hydrocortisone which reduces sensitivity [9]. These experiments were done using clonogenic assays. In preliminary experiments we have found that the same protective and sensitizing effects observed with the clonogenic assays can be observed using the in situ nick translation assay. The total time for these experiments was 3 days as compared to 1–2 weeks with the clonogenic assay.

Another opportunity offered by the nick translation assay is that cells may be labelled with a monoclonal antibody prior to fixation. Then during the detection phase a second antibody with a different fluorescent tag can be added. In this way it is possible to identify specific subsets of cells undergoing apoptosis.

References

1. Williams GT, Smith CA, Spooncer E, Dexter MT: Haemopoietic colony stimulating factors promote cell survival by suppresing apoptosis. Nature 343: 76, 1990.
2. Williams GT: Programmed Cell Death – Apoptosis and Oncogenesis. Cell 65: 1097, 1991.
3. Lotem J, Sachs L: Hematopoietic cytokines inhibit apoptosis induced by transforming growth factor beta 1 and cancer chemotherapy compounds in myeloid leukemic cells. Blood 80: 1750, 1992.
4. Gorczyca W, Bigman K, Mittelman A, Ahmed t, Gong J, Melamud MR: Induction of DNA strand breaks associated with apoptosis during treatment of leukemia. Leukemia 7: 659, 1993.
5. Gorczyca W, Bruno S, Darzynkiewicz RJ, Gong J, Darzynkiewicz Z: DNA strand breaks occurring during apoptosis: their early in situ detection by the terminal deoxynucleotide transferase and nick translation assays and prevention by serine protease inhibitors. Int J Oncology 1: 639, 1992.
6. Wang C, McCulloch EA, Minden MD: Detection of DNA damage in myeloid hemopoietic cells during apoptosis using in situ nick translation. Blood 80: 148a (abst), 1992.
7. Masuck TM, Taylor AR, Lough J: Arabinosylcytosine induced accumulation of DNA nicks in myotube nuclei detected by in situ nick translation. J Cell Physiol 144: 12, 1990.
8. Greenberger JS, Sakakeeny MA, Humphries RK, Eaves CJ, Eckner RJ: Demonstration of permanent factor dependent multipotential (erythroid/neutrophil/basophil) hematopoietic progenitor cell lines. Proc Natl Acad Sci USA 80: 2931, 1983.
9. Yang GS, Wang C, Minkin S, Minden MD, McCulloch EA: Hydrocortisone in culture protects the blast cells in acute myeloblastic leukemia from the lethal effects of cytosine arabinoside. Journal of Cellular Physiology 148: 60, 1991.
10. Coligan JE, Kruisbeek AM, Margulies DH, Shevac EM, Strober W: Current protocols in immunology. New York, John Wiley and Sons, 1991.
11. Lishner M, Curtis JE, Minkin S, McCulloch EA: Interaction between retinoic acid and cytosine arabinoside affecting the blast cells of acute myeloblastic leukemia. Leukemia 3: 784, 1989.

Acute Leukemias V
Experimental Approaches
and Management of Refractory Diseases
Hiddemann et al. (Eds.)

Molecular Mechanisms of Ara-C Signalling: Synergy and Antagonism with Interleukin-3

Claus Belka, Claudia Sott, Friedhelm Herrmann, and Marion A. Brach

Introduction

Cytosine arabinosde (Ara-C) is the most widely used and most effective agent in the treatment of acute myelogenous leukemia [1]. Several lines of evidence have suggested that the efficacy of Ara-C may be enhanced by its combination with hematopoietic growth factors such as Interleukin (IL)-3 or Granulocyte-Macrophage Colony Stimulating Factor (GM-CSF) [2]. IL-3 has been shown by several laboratories to enhance Ara-C incoporation into DNA and Ara-C-mediated tumor cell kill by recruiting resting cells into the cell cycle but also by facilitating intracellular Ara-C metabolism into its active compound, Ara-CTP [3,4]. However, other reports have indicated that IL-3 may also confer resistance of acute myelogenous blasts to subsequent Ara-C [5]. It is thought that Ara-C exerts its cytotoxic effects after incorporation into DNA leading to inhibition of chain elongation [6,7]. In addition, more recent reports have indicated that Ara-C also induces features of apoptotic cell death including DNA fragmentation [8]. Ara-C modulates mRNA expression of several proto-oncogenes, such as c-jun, jun-B or c-myc [3,9,10]. Singaling events initiated by Ara-C, however, are still enigmatic. The present article explores signaling cascades initiated by Ara-C and point to their impact in mediating both synergistic and antagonistic effects of Ara-C and IL-3.

Modulation of the AP-1 Transcription Factor by Ara-C and IL-3

Upon exposure to Ara-C, human myeloid leukemia blasts display enhanced binding activity of the AP-1 transcription factor (Fig. 1). The capacity of Ara-C to increase binding activity is both time- and dose dependent. Enhanced binding activity of AP-1 is associated with functional activation in that insertion of the respective binding site 5' of a heterologous thymidine kinase promoter is sufficient to confer inducibility to the human growth hormone gene as a reporter gene by Ara-C. Activation of the AP-1 transcription factor furthermore leads to transcriptional activation of the c-jun gene resulting in enhanced formation of c-jun/AP-1 (not shown).

Binding activity of the AP-1 transcription factor is also enhanced upon exposure to IL-3 or GM-CSF (not shown), suggesting convergence of Ara-C- and IL-3 -initiated signaling events. In order to study the functional implication of enhanced AP-1 binding activity with respect to Ara-C-induced programmed cell death the antisense technique was employed. In the presence of an antisense-oligdeoxynucleotide to c-jun, the growth stimulatory interplay of TNF-α and IL-3 on early hematopoietic progenitor cells is abolished while in contrast an antisense c-jun oligodeoxynucleotide failed to interfere with the capacity of IL-3 to stimulate proliferation [12]. Likewise, an antisense to the c-jun component of the AP-1 transcription factor did not interfere

Department of Medical Oncology and Applied Molecular Biology, Universitätsklinikum Rudolf Virchow, Freie Universität Berlin and Max Delbrück Center for Molecular Medicine, Berlin, Germany

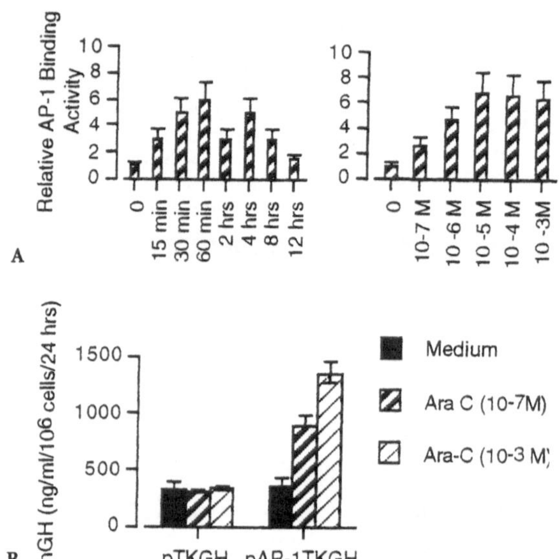

Fig. 1. Ara-C induces binding and spurs transcriptional activation activity of the AP-1 transcription factor. **A** KG-1 leukemia cells (10^6/ml) were exposed to Ara-C (10^{-5} M) for up to 12 hrs. Nuclear proteins were prepared and incubated with a synthetic oligonucleotide harboring the AP-1 recognition sequence as previously described [11]. Signal intensity of shifted bands was quantitated by laser densitometry and is expressed as fold-induction versus signals obtained with nuclear proteins extracted from cells exposed to medium only. **B** KG-1 cells were transiently transfected with a heterologous promoter construct containing (or not) the AP-1 recognition sequence 5' of the herpes thymidine kinase promoter linked to the human growth hormone gene as a reporter gene. Transfectants were split and either left in standard culture medium or exposed to Ara-C (10^{-5} M) for 24 hours. Human growth hormone activity was determined in cell culture supernatants by a commercially available enzyme immuno assay (EIA)

with the capacity of Ara-C to induce apoptotic cell death (Table 1).

KG-1 or MO7e cells were cultured in the presence of 10 μM of an antisense (AS) oligdeoxynucleotide targeting the translation inititating site of c-jun, the corresponding sense (S) oligodeoxynucleotide or an unrelated nonsense (NS) oligodeoxynucleotide with the same overall base-pair composition as the AS oligonucleotide as previously described [12] for 24 hours. Subsequently, cells were exposed to Ara-C (10^{-3} M) for additonal 12 hours and the percentage of apoptotic and viable cells was analyzed by FACS-analysis following propidium iodide staining.

Modulation of the NF-κB Transcription Factor by Ara-C and IL-3

Both hematopoietic growth factors such as IL-3 and Ara-C induce nuclear translocation of the NF-κB transcription factor leading to enhanced binding activity of NF-κB (Fig. 2). Introduction of the NF-κB recognition sequence 5' of a heterologous thymidine kinase promoter confers inducibility to the human growth hormone gene as a reporter gene (Fig. 2). Activation of the NF-κB transcription factor may contribute to the release of secondary cytokines such as IL-1, TNF, GM-CSF or IL-6 known to harbor functional active NF-κB binding sites in their promoters [13].

Table 1. Antisense to c-jun does not abolish the capacity of Ara-C to mediate apoptosis in myeloid leukemia cells

Exposure to:	AS-c-jun	S-c-jun	NS-c-jun
% viable cells :	23 ± 4	26 ± 7	22 ± 5

Signaling Pathways Involved in Ara-C-Mediated Transcription Factor Activation

NF-κB translocation has previously been linked to the intracellular formation of oxygen radicals, while in vitro data have also suggested that a Protein Kinase C (PKC)-mediated phosphorylation of the inhibitory IκB molecule may contribute to nuclear translocation of NF-κB [14]. Enhanced AP-1 binding has been shown in vitro to result from activation of the Mitogen Activated Protein kinase (15]. The following set of experiments aimed at further elucidating the signaling events leading to enhanced binding activity of AP-1 and NF-κB in response to Ara-C. Myeloid leukemia cells were either depleted of PKC through a 24 hrs incubation period with 12-O-tetradecanoylphorbol 13-acetate (TPA) present or were exposed to the oxygen scavenger N-acetyl-cystein (NAC) prior to exposure to Ara-C. The capacity of Ara-C to promote

Fig. 2. Ara-C induces binding and transcriptional activation activity of the NF-κB transcription factor. A KG-1 leukemia cells (10^6/ml) were exposed to Ara-C (10^{-5} M) for up to 12 hrs. Nucelar proteins were prepared and incubated with a synthetic oligonucleotide harboring the NF-κB recognition sequence as previously described [11]. Signal intensity of shiftet bands was quantitated by laser densitoemtry and is expressed as fold-induction versus control cells exposed to medium only. B KG-1 cells were transiently transfected with a heterologous promoter construct containing (or not) the NF-κB recognition sequence 5' of the herpes thymidine kinase promoter linked to the human growth hormone gene as a reporter gene. Transfectants were split and either left in standard culture medium only or exposed to Ara-C (10^{-5} M) for 24 hours. Human growth hormone activity in cell culture supernatants was determined by a commercially available EIA

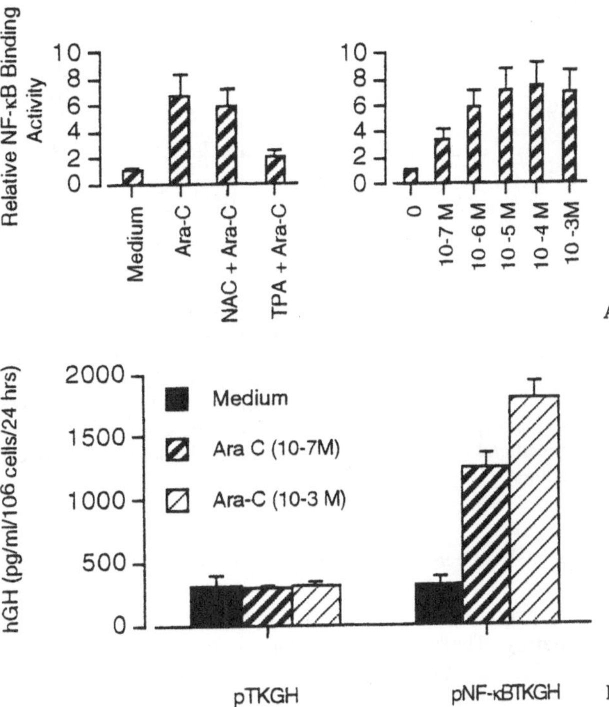

enhanced NF-κB binding activity was significantly reduced in the presence of NAC, while PKC depletion had no effect on Ara-C -induced NF-kB binding activity (Fig. 3). In contrast Ara-C-mediated AP-1 binding activity was only marginally affected by the presence of NAC, while depletion of intracellular PKC diminished Ara-C -induced AP-1 activation significantly (Fig. 3). These findings suggest that Ara-C may transmit signals into the nucleus by both PKC-dependent pathways as well as by engaging the intracellular formation of oxygen radicals.

KG-1 or MO7e leukemia cells were maintained in the presence or absence of TPA (1μM) for 24 hours or were pretreated with NAC (30 mM) for 30 minutes prior to exposure to Ara-C (10^{-6}M) for 30 minutes. Thereafter, nuclear extracts were prepared and binding activity of the AP-1 or the NF-κB transcription factor were analyzed by electrophoretic mobility shift asays as previously described [11]. Signal intensity of shifted bands was quantitated by laser densitometry and is expressed as fold enhancement versus medium-treated control cells.

Exposure of Myeloid Leukemia Cells to Ara-C Leads to Serine Phosphorylation of the Small Heat Shock Protein Hsp27

The exposure of human cells to stress signals such as heat or to cytotoxic cytokines has

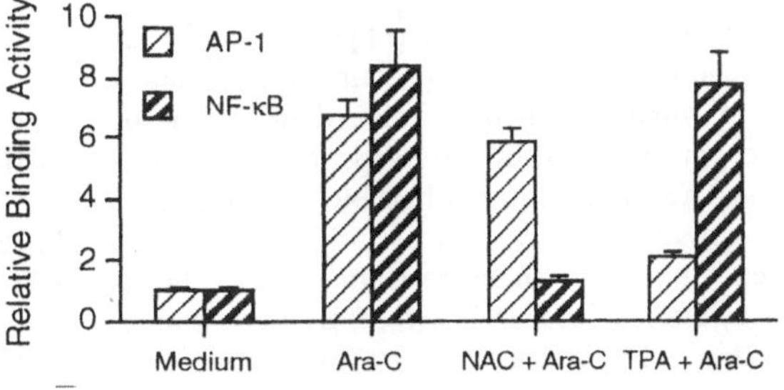

Fig. 3. Ara-C mediates binding activity of AP-1 and NF-κB through distinct intracellular pathways

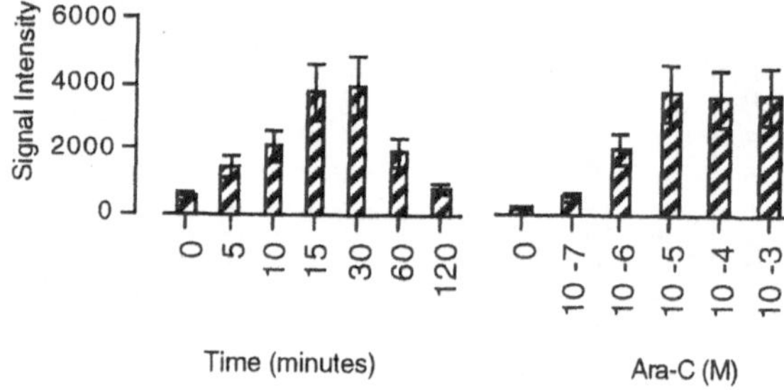

Fig. 4. Ara-C induces dose- and time-dependent phosphorylation of the small heat shock protein Hsp27.KG-1 or MO7e leukemia cells were serum- and factor-deprived for 16 hours prior to exposure to Ara-C in concentrations ranging from 10^{-7} M to 10^{-3} M for the time points indicated. Thereafter, cell lysates were prepared and fractionated by FPLC as previously described [19]. Fractions containing MAPKAP kinase 2 activity were employed for in vitro kinase assays using recombinant human Hsp27 as a substrate as described [19].Values are expressed as relative phosphorylation of Hsp27 which was analyzed by quantitation of photo-stimulated luminescence as described and values (signal intensity versus background) were expressed as means ± SD of three independent experiments

previously been demonstrated to result in enhanced phosphorylation of the small heat shock protein (Hsp)27 [16,17]. The major kinase mediating Hsp27 phosphorylation has been identified as the mitogen activated protein kinase activated protein (MAPKAP) kinase 2. [18] MAPKAP kinase 2 activation in myeloid leukemia cells results also from signaling cascades initiated by IL-3 or GM-CSF [19]. Moreover, exposure of myeloid leukemia cells to Ara-C also leads to dose and time-dependent phosphorylation of Hsp27 (Fig. 4). Hsp27 becomes phosphorylated in response to low-dose (10^{-7} M) of Ara-C. Dose escalation leads to enhanced phosphorylation of Hsp27 in concentrations of up to 10^{-5} M, while dose-dependency is lost when even higher concentrations are used. Hsp27 phosphorylation is observed within 5 to 10 minutes following exposure to Ara-C, peaks after 15 to 30 minutes and returns to starting levels thereafter.

Phosphorylation of Hsp27 Protects from Ara-C -Induced Apoptosis

Hsp27 acts as a molecular chaperone, and thus may be required to fold proteins appropriately or to modulate their cellular distribution or transportation. Although Hsps are well conserved during evolution, their biologic functions remain unclear. Overexpression of Hsp27 has been linked to chemoresistance [20]. Phosphorylation of Hsp27 has recently been shown to confer hyporesponsiveness of various cells towards TNF-α [21,22]. Myeloid leukemia cells respond to IL-3 with rapid and transient phosphorylation of Hsp27 [19]. When cells displaying phosphorylated Hsp27 are tackled by Ara-C they fail to respond to Ara-C with apoptotic cell death. Myeloid cells regain senstivity to Ara-C, when Ara-C is given at a time-point where phosphorylation of Hsp27 has returned to baseline levels (not shown). Detailed analysis will have to show whether this reflects a causal relationship or is merely a coincidence. The recent observation that constitutive activation of the mitogen activated protein kinase renders tumor cells resistant to X-radiation [23] is in support of the former hypothesis since activation of the MAP kinase may result in activation of MAPKAP kinase 2 and thereby stimulates Hsp27 phosphorylation [18]. Phosphorylation of Hsp27 in response to Ara-C occurs in cells which – by serum and factor-deprivation – are arrested in the Go/G1 phase of the cell cycle. In these cells Ara-C promotes Hsp27 phosphorylation without being incoporated into DNA These findings are consistent with the notion that Ara-C initiates signaling pathways at the membrane or cytosol and does not require incorporation into DNA.

Summary and Conclusion

In summary, we propose the following model of Ara-C/IL-3 interaction. Ara-C and IL-3 exert a series of overlaping signaling events in myeloid leukemia cells. Both compounds promote

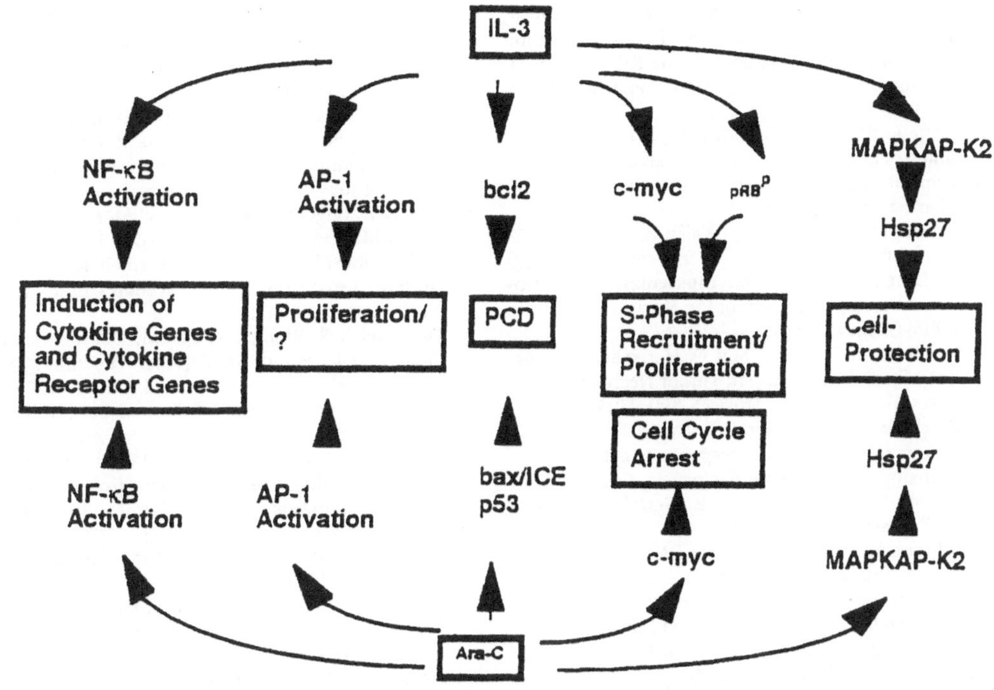

Fig. 5. Schematic representation of overlapping and distinct signalling pathways inititated by IL-3 or Ara-C in myeloid leukemia cells

enhanced binding activity of nuclear transcription factors such as AP-1 and NF-κB. Thereby, both modulate the expression of the c-jun gene and may also – by engaging NF-κB – contribute to the release of secondary cytokines such as GM-CSF, TNF-α, IL-1 or IL-6. Both pathways lead to phosphorylation of the small heat shock protein, which may protect myelogenous leukemia cells from Ara-C-induced apoptosis. In order to further elucidate signaling events that may counteract IL-3/Ara-C combination it will be necessary to investigate the modulation of those genes regulating the programmed cell death, such as the Interleukin-1β converting enzyme (ICE), the bax and bcl-2 gene as well as the p53 gene (Fig. 5).

References

1. Frei E, Bickers JN, Hewitt JS, Lane M, Leary WV, Tailley RW (1969) Dose-schedule and antitumor studies of arabinosyl cytosine. Canc Res 29: 1325–1332
2. Brach MA, Henschler R, Mertelsmann R, and Herrmann F. (1991) To overcome pharmacologic and cytokinetic resistance to cytarabine in the treatment of acute myelogenous leukemia by using recombinant interleukin-3. Semin Hematol 28: 39–47
3. Brach MA, Klein H, Platzer E, Mertelsmann R, Herrman F (1990) Effect of Interleukin-3 on cytosine-arabinoside-mediated cytotoxicity of leukemic myeloblasts. Exp Hematol 18: 748–753
4. Bhalla K, Holladay C, Arlin Z, Grant S, Ibrado AM, Jasiok M (1991) Treatment with Interleukin-3 plus Granulocyte-Macrophage Colony stimulating factors improve the selectivity of Ara-C in vitro against acute myeloid leukemia blasts. Blood 78: 2674–2679
5. Koistinen P, Wang C, Curtis JE, McCulloch EA (1991) Granulocyte-Macrophage Colony-Stimulating Factor and Interleukin-3 protect leukemia blast cells from Ara-C toxicity. Leukemia 5: 789–795
6. Major P, Egan EM, Beardsley G, Minden M, Kufe DW (1981) Lethality of human myeloblasts correlates with the incorporation of ara-C into DNA. Proc. Natl. Acad. Sci USA 78: 3233–3239
7. Ohno Y, Spriggs D, Matsukage A, Ohno T, Kufe D (1988) Effects of 1-ß-D-arabinosylcytosine incorporation on elongation of specific DNA sequences by DNA polymerase ß. Canc Res 48: 1494–1498
8. Gunji H, Kharbanda S, Kufe D (1991) Induction of internucleosomal DNA fragmentation in huzman myeloid leukemia cells by 1-ß-D-arabinofuranosylcytosine. Canc Res 51: 741–746

9. Henschler R, Brennscheidt U, Mertelsmann R, Herrmann F (1991) Induction of c-jun expression in the myeloid leukemia cell line KG-1 by 1-ß-D-arabinofuranosylcytosine. Mol Pharmacol 39: 171–176
10. Datta R, Kharbanda S, Kufe D (1990) Regulation of jun-b gene expression by 1-ß-D-arabinofuranosylcytosine in human myeloid leukemia cells. Mol Pharmacol 38: 435–439
11. Brach MA, Gruss HJ, Kaisho T, Asano Y, Mertelsmann R, Hirano T, Herrmann F (1993) Ionizing radiation induces Interleukin 6 transcription involving activation of the Nuclear Factor κ B. J. Biol Chem 268: 8466–8471
12. Brach M A., Gruss HJ, Sott C, Herrmann F (1993) The mitogenic response to Tumor Necrosis Factor-a requires c-jun/AP-1. Mol Cell Biol 13: 4824–4830
13. Brach M A., Herrmann F (1994).Transcription Factors in the mitogenic response to cytokines. In: Hematopoietic Growth Factors in Clinical Application (eds.: F. Herrmann, R. Mertelsmann) New York, Marcel Dekker, 63–83
14. Schreck R, Rieber P, Bäuerle PA (1991) Reactive oxygen intermediates as apparently widely used messengers in the activation of the NF-κB transcription factor and HIV-1. EMBO J 10:2247–2258
15. Pulverer BJ, Kyriakis JM, Avruch J, Nikolakaki E, Woodgett JR (1991) Phosphorylation of c-jun mediated by MAP kinases. Nature 353: 670–673
16. Landry J, Lambert H, Zhou M, Lavoie JN, Hickey E, Weber LA, Anderson CW (1992) Human HSP27 is phosphorylated at serines 78 and 82 by heat shock and mitogen-activated kinases that recognize the same amino acid motif as S6 kinase II. J Biol Chem 267: 794–803
17. Arrigo AP (1990) Tumor Necrosis Factor induces rapid phosphorylation of the mammalian heat shock protein hsp 28. Mol Cell Biol 10: 1276–1281
18. Stokoe D, Engel K, Campbell DG, Cohen P, Gaestel M (1992) Identification of MAPKAP kinase 2 as a major enzyme responsible for the phosphorylation of the mammalian small heat shock proteins. FEBS Lett. 313: 307–311
19. Ahlers A, Engel K, Sott C, Gaestel M, Herrmann F, Brach MA (1994) IL-3 and GM-CSF induce rapid serine phosphorylation of the small heat shock protein (hsp27) involving activation of the MAP-KAP kinase 2. Blood 83:1791–1798
20. Oesterreich S, Weng CN, Qiu M, Hilsenbeck SG, Osborne CK, Fuqua SAW (1993) The small heat shock protein hsp27 is correlated with growth and drug resistance in human breast cancer cell lines. Canc Res 53: 4443–4448
21. Jaattela M, Wissing D, Bauer PA, Li GC (1992) Major heat shock protein hsp70 protects tumor cells from tumor necrosis factor cytotoxicity. EMBO J. 11: 3507–3512
22. Konig M, Wallach D, Resch K, Holtmann H (1991) Induction of hyporesponsiveness to an early post-binding effect of tumor necrosis factor by tumor necrosis factor itself and interleukin-1. Eur. J. Immunol. 21: 1741–1745
23. Stevenson MA, Pollock SS, Coleman CN, Calderwood SK (1994) X-Irradiation, Phorbol Esters, and H_2O_2 stimulate mitogen activated protein kinase activity in NIH3T3 cells through the formation of reactive oxygen intermediates. Canc Res 54: 12–15

Acute Leukemias V
Experimental Approaches
and Management of Refractory Diseases
Hiddemann et al. (Eds.)

Hematopoietic Recovery and Priming – Therapeutic Effects of GM-CSF in the Treatment of AML

T. Büchner, W. Hiddemann, B. Wörmann, R. Rottmann, G. Maschmeyer, W.-D. Ludwig, M. Zühlsdorf, K. Buntkirchen, A. Sander, J. Aswald, I. Binder, S. Prisett, and M. C. Sauerland

Summary

After a first study showed that GM-CSF following chemotherapy effectively accelerated neutrophil recovery and reduced early mortality in high risk patients with AML, a second study was begun in which GM-CSF was applied preceeding chemotherapy and continuing until neutrophil recovery in the initial 5 chemotherapy courses for patients with newly diagnosed AML. The CR rate in patients of 16–75 (median 50) years is 79% in GM-CSF patients and 82% in controls. GM-CSF patients showed a trend to more frequent rapid blast clearance and fewer persistent leukemias and – in patients under age 60 – a significantly superior remission duration as of this update. It should be shown later by this study whether GM-CSF multiple course priming and longterm administration adds to the cure rate of patients with AML.

Introduction

When in 1987 human recombinant GM-CSF became available for clinical use the first attempt to apply it in AML was to possibly accelerate the recovery of neutrophils after chemotherapy in patients at high risk of mortality. The neutrophil recovery time could indeed be reduced by a median of 1 week when compared to control patients receiving chemotherapy alone which also resulted in a reduction in early deaths from 39% to 14% ($p=0.009$). In addition, this study documented a low risk of promoting the progression of leukemia by GM-CSF [1]. Similar results were obtained using G-CSF [2]. Using the same dosage and schedule of GM-CSF as in our study [1] in a placebo controlled trial in older age AML the ECOG found a significant reduction in neutropenia and infections and a prolongation of survival [3]. A non-significant trend in favour of GM-CSF was also seen in a trial by CALGB with some differences in the study design [4].

Besides this mainly supportive strategy other approaches with GM-CSF aim at an enhancement of the antileukemic effect of chemotherapy by a recruitment of chemoresistant resting leukemic cells into sensitive phases of the cell cycle. Even in vitro a kind of recruitment can be observed when AML blasts are stimulated by GM-CSF to multiply and produce colonies [5–8]. The GM-CSF induced increase in leukemic S-phase cells also increased the leukemic clonogenic cell kill by Ara-C [9].

Recruitment could then be demonstrated in vivo after a 24–48 hour infusion of GM-CSF prior to chemotherapy and appeared by a shift of leukemic blasts from G_0 to higher RNA and DNA content corresponding to the G_1 and S-phases and also by an increase in S-phase cells incorporating BrDU which was found in the majority of patients [10].

GM-CSF priming strategies as used in the above study may also benefit from an enhancement of antileukemic drug cytotoxicity. Thus, we could show that the incorporation of Ara-C into DNA in leukemic blasts in vitro was increased to 1.5–8.5 (median 2.0)fold by a 48 hour preincubation and simultaneous incubation together with

Department of Medicine, Hematology/Oncology, University of Münster, Germany

GM-CSF, an effect found in 23/28 cases. In 10/13 cases investigated GM-CSF increased the Ara-C mediated leukemic clonogenic cell reduction to 2.2–229 (median 3.2) fold [11].

In contrast, others discussed a protection of AML-cells against antileukemic agents by GM-CSF. Thus, AML blasts in vitro showed a substantial clonogenic cell kill after a 20 minutes pulse of Ara-C only if cultured in G-CSF and not in GM-CSF or IL-3. However, if the exposure to Ara-C was extended to 6 days there was a marked cell kill in all 3 growth factors even though the most expressed in G-CSF, and mixing together G-CSF and GM-CSF brought the result close to that of G-CSF [12]. These data suggest an enhancement of cytotoxicity by growth factors rather than a leukemic cell protection at least when Ara-C was present during an adequate period of time. In a clinical setting 56 patients with newly diagnosed AML received GM-CSF either 20 or 125 μg/m²/day during a period varying between 0 and 8 days prior to chemotherapy. This inhomogenous population showed the lowest CR-rate and shortest survival when compared to two historical control groups. The authors discussed a resistance of leukemic cells induced by GM-CSF [13].

Apoptosis or programmed cell death is a newly described effect of antileukemic chemotherapy. In a murine leukemic cell line nuclear condensation and fragmentation and DNA fragmentation as typical features of apoptosis were found induced by TGFβ and were prevented by GM-CSF. GM-CSF also inhibited apoptosis induced by Ara-C while the overall clonogenic cell reduction was not reduced. The authors discussed that apoptosis may be regulated independently from other mechanisms of cell kill [14]. In human AML cell lines apoptosis was even enhanced by a GM-CSF/IL-3 fusion protein. This effect also occured with an increase in clonogenic cell reduction [15].

Thus, in the therapeutic in vivo situation different effects of GM-CSF may interfere with each other. In addition, potential recruitment effects on early leukemic stem cells in vivo may not be detectable in vitro and may only be reflected by an improved longterm outcome of patients. We here present data from two therapeutic studies using GM-CSF with chemotherapy at two different time schedules.

Patients and Methods

The first study started in 1987 and was restricted to high risk AML including patients of 65+ years and patients with first relapse within 6 months or multiple relapse. GM-CSF 250 μg/m²/day started on day 4 after the end of induction chemotherapy and continued until neutrophil recovery. Patients with residual blasts after chemotherapy did not receive GM-CSF. The results including those of the patients not receiving GM-CSF were compared to a historical control group receiving the same chemotherapy in similar situations.

The second study started in 1990 and included only patients with newly diagnosed AML. GM-CSF 250 μg/m²/day started 24 hours before chemotherapy and then continued until neutrophil recovery. Patients were randomized to receive the same dose of GM-CSF either by continuous i. v. infusion or by one s.c. injection or devided into two s. c. injections. A fourth group received the same chemotherapy without GM-CSF. Chemotherapy was TAD [16] for the first induction course and the consolidation course, HAM [17,18] for the second induction course and AD-AT-AC for maintenance [16]. The second induction was given to patients at 60+ years only if the bone marrow still contained $>=5\%$ blasts, and to all patients under 60 years even in aplasia with no blasts.

Results

36 patients 27 to 84 (median 68) years of age entered the first study including 6 patients not receiving GM-CSF due to persistent bone marrow blasts. The historical controls comprised 56 patients. The CR-rate was 50% in the GM-CSF group and 32% in the controls ($p=0.09$) and the early death rate in the 2 groups was 14% and 39% ($p=0.009$) as published before [19]. A new update of remission duration shows 32% continuous remissions projected to 3 years in both the GM-CSF and the control group. As in the entire patient population remission duration is not different in either of the two subgroups of newly diagnosed AML at higher age and of relapsed AML.

Ninety five patients entered the second study, so far. Their median age is 50 (range 17–75) years. Since there is no difference in the results between the three different GM-CSF applications randomized all GM-CSF patients are compared with the controls as one single group. GM-CSF patients and controls are not different in neither age, WBC, Serum-LDH and FAB-subtype. Among hematologic effects the prechemotherapy administration of GM-CSF induced an increase in peripheral blood blasts to 1.2–14.0 (median 2.1)- fold the pretreatment levels. The recovery time of neutrophils to 500/cmm after the first induction course is reduced in the GM-CSF group when compared with the controls ($p = 0.007$), whereas the recovery time of platelets to 50 000/cmm is not different. After the second induction and the consolidation course recovery times of both cells show a trend to progressive prolongation in the control arm which is more expressed in the GM-CSF arm.

A reduction of the leukemic blasts to less than 5% in the day 16 bone marrow was found in 57% GM-CSF patients and in 42% controls. 79% and 82% of patients went into complete remission, whereas 4% and 15% exhibited persistent leukemia.

Remission duration shows 51% continuous remissions after 3 years in both arms. For patients under age 60 remission duration is shown in Figure 1. The 3 year remission rate is 70% in the GM-CSF and 50% in the control arm.

Discussion

As a first attempt in patients with AML and high risk of mortality GM-CSF following chemotherapy did prove effective in accelerating the recovery of neutrophils and in reducing patients mortality. Concerns regarding an activation of the disease were not confirmed in our first study since only 2/30 patients showed a leukemic regrowth under GM-CSF which was completely reversible in one case and appeared GM-CSF independent in the second case [19]. As from present update remission duration is not adversly effected by GM-CSF and shows identical 32% ongoing CR after 4 years in the two high risk populations with and without GM-CSF.

This study provided a basis for the new randomized study now performed in newly diagnosed AML extending GM-CSF to an administration simultaneous with and 24 hours preceeding each chemotherapy course in a total of 5 consecutive courses. An update presented here again gives no evidence that the disease progression is promoted by GM-CSF in this setting. In addition, a protection of the leukemic blasts against the antileukemic effects of drugs discussed by others [12–14] was not confirmed. In contrast, the trend to a more frequent rapid bone marrow blast clearance and less frequent persistent leukemia and in younger patients – they received more intensive chemotherapy – a significantly superior preliminary remission duration reflect an enhancement of the

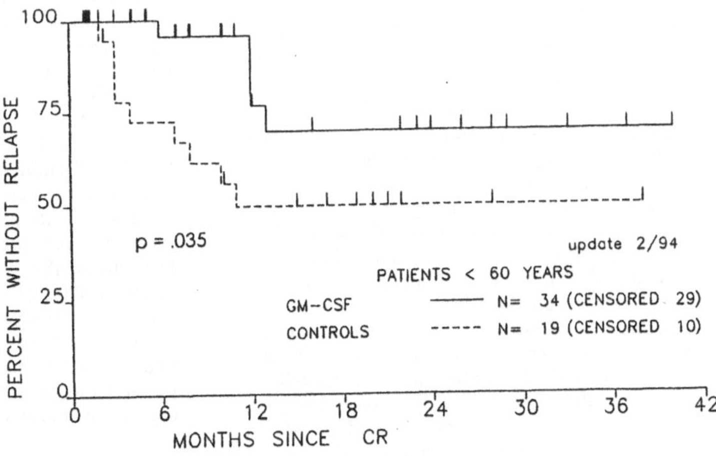

Fig. 1. Kaplan-Meier plots of remission duration. Censored are patients without relapse, also indicated by tic marks

antileukemic cytotoxicity by GM-CSF rather than a protective effect by GM-CSF. This can in part be explained by a modulation of the Ara-C metabolism resulting in an increased incorporation of Ara-C into DNA and the reduction of leukemic clonogenic cell growth [11]. A prolongation of remission duration - if holding up during the next years - also suggests a recruitment of resting early leukemic stem cells into chemosensitivity as an effect of the repeated "priming" by GM-CSF preceeding chemotherapy. That early progenitor or stem cells are involved in priming might also be concluded from the progressive impairment of both granulocytopoiesis and thrombocytopoiesis appearing more expressed in the GM-CSF patients than in the control group.

References

1. Büchner Th, Hiddemann W, Koenigsmann M et al. (1991) Recombinant granulocyte-macrophage colony-stimulating factor after chemotherapy in patients with acute myeloid leukemia at higher age or after relapse. Blood 78: 1190–1197
2. Ohno R, Tomonaga M, Kobayashi T et al. (1990) Effect of granulocyte colony-stimulating factor after intensive induction therapy in relapsed or refractory acute leukemia. N Engl J Med 323: 871–877
3. Rowe JM, Andersen J, Mazza JJ et al. (1993) Phase III randomized placebo-controlled study of granulocyte-macrophage colony stimulating factor (GM-CSF) in adult patients (55–70 years) with acute myelogenous leukemia (AML). A study of the Eastern Cooperative Oncology Group (ECOG). Blood 82 (1): 1299
4. Stone R, George S, Berg D et al. (1994) GM-CSF 'V' placebo during remission induction for patients > 60 years old with de novo acute myeloid leukemia: CALGB study #8923. Proc ASCO 13: 992
5. Griffin JD, Young D, Herrmann F et al. (1986) Effects of recombinant human GM-CSF on proliferation of clonogenic cells in acute myeloblastic Leukemia. Blood, 67: 1448–1453
6. Miyauchi J, Kelleher CA, Yang Y et al. (1987) The effect of three recombinant growth factors, IL-3, GM-CSF, and G-CSF, on the blast cells of acute myeloblastic leukemia maintained in short-term suspension culture. Blood 70: 657–663
7. Kelleher C, Miyauchi J, Wong G et al. (1987) Synergism between recombinant growth factors GM-CSF and G-CSF, acting on the blast cells of acute myeloblastic leukemia. Blood 69: 1489–1503
8. Vellenga E, Young DC, Wagner K et al. (1987) The effect of GM-CSF and G-CSF in promoting growth of clonogenic cells in acute myeloblastic leukemia. Blood 69: 1771–1776
9. Cannistra SA, Groshek P, Griffin JD (1989) Granulocyte-macrophage colony-stimulating factor enhances the cytotoxic effects of cytosine arabinoside in acute myeloblastic leukemia and in the myeloid blast crisis phase of chronic myeloid leukemia. Leukemia 3: 328–334
10. Bettelheim P, Valent P, Andreeff M et al. (1991) Recombinant human granulocyte-macrophage colony-stimulating factor in de novo acute myeloid leukemia, Blood 77: 700–711
11. Reuter CH, Auf der Landwehr U, Schleyer E et al. (1994) Modulation of intracellular metabolism of cytosine arabinoside in acute myeloid leukemia by granulocyte macrophage colony stimulating factor. Leukemia 8: 217–225.
12. Koistinen P, Wang C, Curtis JE et al. (1991) Granulocyte-macrophage colony-stimulating factor and interleukin-3 protect leukemic blast cells from ara-C toxicity. Leukemia 5: 789–795
13. Estey EH, Thall PF, Kantarjian H et al. (1992) Treatment of newly diagnosed acute myelogenous leukemia with granulocyte-macrophage colony-stimulating factor (GM-CSF) before and during continuous-infusion high-dose ara-C + daunorubicin: Comparison to patients treated without GM-CSF. Blood 79: 2246–2255
14. Lotem J, Sachs L (1992) Hematopoietic cytokines inhibit apoptosis induced by transforming growth factor β1 and cancer chemotherapy compounds in myeloid leukemic cells. Blood 80: 1750–1757
15. Bhalla K, Tang C, Ibrado AM et al. (1992) Granulocyte-macrophage colony-stimulating-factor/interleukin-3 fusion protein (pIXY 321) enhances high-dose ara-C-induced programmed cell death or apoptosis in human myeloid leukemia cells. Blood 80: 2883–2890
16. Büchner Th, Urbanitz D, Hiddemann W et al. (1985) Intensified induction and consolidation with or without maintenance chemotherapy for acute myeloid leukemia (AML): Two multicenter studies of the German AML Cooperative Group. J Clin Oncol 3: 1583–1589
17. Hiddemann W, Kreutzmann H, Straif K et al. (1987) High-dose cytosine-arabinoside and mitoxantrone: A highly effective regimen in refractory acute myeloid leukemia. Blood 69: 744–749
18. Büchner T, Hiddemann W, Löffler G et al. (1991) Improved cure rate by very early intensification combined with prolonged maintenance chemotherapy in patients with acute myeloid leukemia: Data from the AML Cooperative Group. Sem Hematol 28 (4): 76–79
19. Büchner T, Hiddemann W, Koenigsmann M et al. (1991) Recombinant human granulocyte-macro phage colony-stimulating factor after chemotherapy in patients with acute myeloid leukemia at higher age or after relapse. Blood 78: 1190–1197

Acute Leukemias V
Experimental Approaches
and Management of Refractory Diseases
Hiddemann et al. (Eds.)

Improved Antileukemic Activity of the Combination of Ara-C with GM-CSF and IL-3 Fusion Protein (PIXY321)

Kapil Bhalla, Ana Maria Ibrado, Gloria Bullock, Caroline Tang, Swapan Ray, Yue Huang, and Vidya Ponnathpur

Abstract. Co-treatment with GM-CSF/IL3 fusion protein pIXY321 significantly increased apoptosis and the loss of clonogenic survival of HL-60 cells due to a treatment with high dose Ara-C (100 μM) for 4 hours or prolonged treatment with lose dose Ara-C (10 nM) for 5 days. In contrast, pIXY321 inhibited high dose Ara-C-induced apoptosis in $CD34^+$ normal bone marrow cells. Combined treatment with staurosporine also enhanced Ara-C induced apoptosis in HL-60 cells. None of these modulations of Ara-C-induced apoptosis in the leukemic or normal cells was associated with appreciable alterations in intracellular p26BCL-2 levels.

Introduction

In human acute myeloid leukemia (AML) cells, high dose cytosine arabinoside (Ara-C) (>10 μM) has been demonstrated to overcome many of the known biochemical mechanisms of resistance observed for conventional doses of Ara-C [1]. Results of previous studies have also shown that by increasing the percentage of cycling AML cells in S phase, hemopoietic growth factors GM-CSF and/or IL-3 increase their sensitivity toward the S phase specific drug Ara-C, thereby potentially overcoming a cytokinetic mechanism of Ara-C resistance in AML cells [25]. In vitro cotreatment with GM-CSF plus IL-3 has been shown to significantly enhance the intracellular Ara-CTP/dCTP pool ratio and Ara-C DNA incorporation in AML but not normal human bone marrow mononuclear cells, and this was associated with an improved antileukemic selectivity of HIDAC against AML cells [6]. Treatment with HIDAC produces internucleosomal DNA fragmentation and the morphologic features of apoptosis in AML cells [7]. Recent reports have indicated that the enhancement of the antileukemic activity of HIDAC by GM-CSF and IL-3 may be partly due to their potentiation of HIDAC-induced internucleosomal DNA fragmentation and morphologic features of apoptosis in AML cells [6]. pIXY321 is a GM-CSF/IL-3 fusion protein which as a hemopoietic growth factor has greater receptor affinity and biologic activity than IL-3 and/or GM-CSF [8, 9]. Cotreatment with pIXY321 and HIDAC has been demonstrated to produce a greater loss of clonogenic survival of AML blasts than that of normal bone marrow progenitor cells [10]. In the present studies we have examined the effect of pIXY321 on Ara-C induced apoptosis in CD34+ normal human bone marrow mononuclear cells (NBMMC). Since modulations of the activities of intracellular protein kinases have been demonstrated to affect drug-induced apoptosis [11], we also examined the effects of staurosporine and phorbol myristate acetate (PMA), which affect protein kinases on HIDAC-induced apoptosis in AML cells. Results of these studies demonstrate that the cotreatment with staurosporine and PMA markedly enhance HIDAC-induced internucleosomal DNA fragmentation and apoptosis in AML cells. In contrast, co-treatment with pIXY321, which

Hematology/Oncology Division, Department of Medicine, Medical University of South Carolina, Charleston, SC 29425, USA

has been reported to increase HIDAC-induced apoptosis in AML cells [10], was found to significantly inhibit apoptosis due to HIDAC in CD34+ NBMMC.

Methods

AML cells. Human myeloid leukemia HL-60 cells were derived from the original cell line were maintained in suspension culture as described previously [12]. Logarithmically growing cells at a concentration of 3 to 5×10^5 cells/ml were utilized for all experiments.

Procurement of normal bone marrow progenitor cells. Bone marrow aspirate samples were obtained with informed consent from normal volunteers. Low density bone marrow cells are separated over Ficoll-Hypaque [13]. CD34 positive NBMMC are positively selected by indirect immune adherence utilizing immunomagnetic beads (Dynal Inc, Great Neck, NY), or anti-CD34 antibody coated columns (CELLPRO, Bothell, WA), as previously described [14,15].

Drugs. Ara-C hydrochloride staurosporine and PMA were purchased from Sigma Chemicals, St. Louis, MO. pIXY321 was kindly provided by Dr. Douglas E. Williams of Immunex Corp, Seattle, WA. The specific activity of pIXY321 is 1×10^6 units/μg of the protein [8]. pIXY321 concentration of 10 ng/ml was utilized for all experiments, since this was determined to have maximal biologic activity as a HGF in the colony culture assays of normal and leukemic bone marrow progenitor cells (data not shown).

Quantitative and qualitative analyses of taxol-induced internucleosomal DNA fragmentation. HL-60 or $CD34^+$ NBMMC were treated with the designated concentrations and schedule of pIXY321 and/or Ara-C, or alternatively with Ara-C and/or staurosporine or PMA. Subsequently, cells were trypsinized, pelleted and washed with PBS at 4 °C and disrupted by suspension for 20 minutes at 4 °C in 5 mM Tris-HCL buffer containing 0.5% (v/v) Triton-X-100 and 20 mM EDTA. The quantitative and qualitative assessment of internucleosomal DNA fragmentation was performed by a previously published method from our laboratory [10,16].

Internucleosomal DNA fragmentation in human bone marrow progenitor cells. To improve the sensitivity of detecting internucleosomal DNA fragmentation ladder associated with apoptosis in $CD34^+$ NBMPC, a slightly modified version of a previously described Southern blot method was used [10,17]. The DNA fragmentation was detected and estimated by a phosphoimager (Molecular Dynamics, Sunnyvale, CA).

Western blot analysis of p26BCL2 protein. The expression of p26BCL-2 oncoprotein in control or drug-treated HL-60 or $CD34^+$ NBMMC cells was determined by Western blot analyses by a previously described method, utilizing a monoclonal anti-BCL-2 antibody [18].

Colony culture of HL-60 and human bone marrow progenitor cells. Following incubations with Ara-C and/or PIXY321, HL60 cells were washed and their clonogenic survival was determined by a minor modification of a previously described method [16]. Colony growth of normal CFU-GEMM was also determined by a previously described method [13].

Assessment of the morphology of apoptosis and cell viability of leukemic cells. Briefly, following incubations with the designated concentrations and schedules of the drugs, cells were cytospun onto glass slides and stained with Wright stain. Cell morphology was determined by light microscopy. Five different fields were randomly selected for counting at least five hundred cells. Percentage of apoptotic cells was calculated for each experiment. Cells which displayed the characteristic morphologic features of apoptosis included those with cell volume shrinkage, chromatin condensation and the presence of membrane bound apoptotic bodies [10,16]. The assessment of the percentage of apoptotic cells was confirmed by an additional independent observer who was blinded to the results of the first observer. Alternatively, cells were stained with trypan blue to assess the percentage of dead cells unable to exclude the dye [16].

Statistical analysis. Significant differences between values obtained in a population of leukemic cells treated with different experimental conditions were determined by paired t test analyses.

Results

We examined the effects of pIXY321 on Ara-C-induced internucleosomal DNA fragmentation and the loss of clonogenic survival of HL-60 cells. Cells were exposed for 24 hours to pIXY321 (10 ng/ml) or 100 μM Ara-C alone for 4 hours, or 10 ng/ml pIXY321 for 20 hours followed by an additional exposure to pIXY321 plus Ara-C for 4 hours. Alternatively, cells were exposed to 10 ng/ml pIXY321 and/or 10 nM Ara-C for 5 days. Following these treatments, DNA was purified from the supernatant of lysed and pelleted cells, electrophoresed into agarose gels and stained with ethidium bromide. A more intensely stained internucleosomal DNA fragmentation ladder was observed in the lanes containing DNA from the cells treated with pIXY321 plus Ara-C versus Ara-C alone at high as well as the low concentrations of Ara-C (data not shown). Quantitative analysis of the fragmented DNA in the supernatant released from the pellets, expressed as the mean of % of the total starting DNA, is shown in Table 1. Exposure to 100 μM Ara-C for 4 hours or 10 nM for 5 days increased DNA fragmentation to 9.1 ± 1.0 and $10.4. \pm 5\%$, respectively. Treatments with pIXY321 alone for up to 5 days had no significant effect on the DNA fragmentation. Cotreatment with pIXY321 produced significant increases in the DNA fragmentation due to either of the treatment schedules of Ara-C. Table 1 also shows that although treatment with pIXY321 alone improved HL-60 colony growth, treatment with a combination of pIXY321 plus Ara-C (10 nM or 100 μM) versus Ara-C alone caused significantly greater loss of clonogenic survival of HL-60 cells.

Utilizing anti-BCL-2 monoclonal antibody, Western analyses did not demonstrate significant differences in the intracellular p26BCL-2 levels in HL-60 cells which had been exposed to the two schedules and concentrations of Ara-C and/or pIXY321 (data not shown).

Figure 1 shows that the $CD34^+$ NBMMC incubated in SFM for 24 hours demonstrated internucleosomal DNA fragmentation (lane 1), which further increased if 100 μM Ara-C was added for 4 hours to the SFM (lane 2). Addition of pIXY321 to the SFM for 24 hours markedly inhibited internucleosomal DNA fragmentation (lane 3). Importantly, in contrast to HL-60 cells, co-incubation of $CD34^+$ NBMMC with pIXY321 plus Ara-C significantly reduced the DNA fragmentation observed with Ara-C alone. Light microscopic assessment of the morphology of apopsis in $CD34^+$ NBMMC treated with identical concentrations and schedule of Ara-C and/or pIXY321 confirmed that pIXY321 cotreatment also significantly reduced the percentage of apoptotic $CD34^+$ NBMMC observed following their incubation in either SFM alone or Ara-C plus SFM (data not shown). These findings indicate that the combined treatment with pIXY321 improves the antileukemic selectivity of high doses of Ara-C at least partly by inhibiting its cytotoxic effects against $CD34^+$ NBMMC.

Table 1. Effect of pIXY321 on Ara-C

Condition	Fragmented DNA[a]	Colony Growth[b]
Control	0%	100
pIXY321 (10 ng/ml for 24 hours)	0.6	124.3 ± 3.1
pIXY321 (10 ng/ml for 5 days)	0.5	116.0 ± 7.0
Ara-C (10 nM) for 5 days)	10.4 ± 0.5	47.0 ± 2.1
Ara-C (100 μM for 4 hours)	9.1 ± 1.0	42.8 ± 2.4
pIXY321 (10 ng/ml) + Ara-C (10 nM) for 5 days	$15.3 \pm 0.6^*$	$27.0 \pm 2.3^*$
pIXY321 (10 ng/ml for 24 hours) + ara-C (100 μM for 4 hours)	$13.5 \pm 0.8^+$	$23.6 \pm 1.6^+$

[a] Mean percent of total DNA ± SEM (mean of 3 experiments)

[b] Mean percent of control colony growth ± SEM (mean of 3 experiments)

* Values significantly different ($p < 0.05$) from those in the cells treated with 10 nM Ara-C

\+ Values significantly different ($p < 0.05$) from those in the cells treates with 100 μM Ara-C

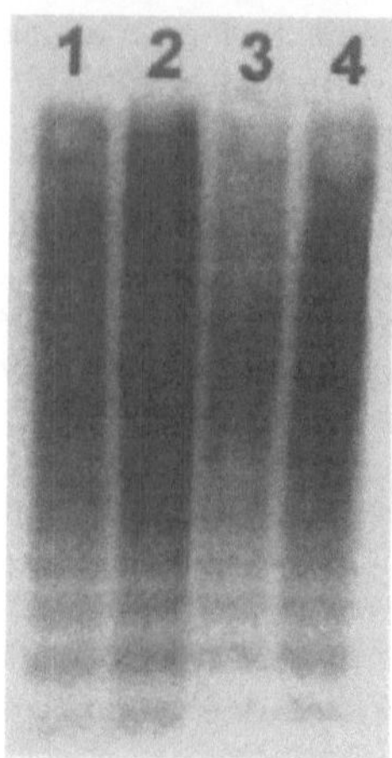

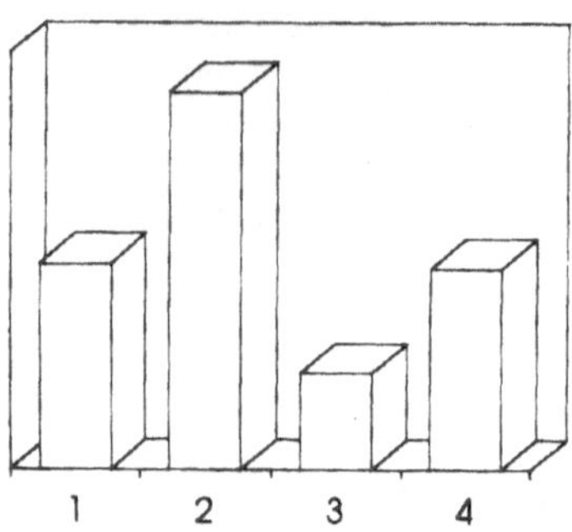

Fig. 1. Upper panel: Southern blotting and phosphoimage analysis of internucleosomal DNA fragmentation in CD34+ normal bone marrow mononuclear cells. Electrophoresed low molecular weight DNA in each lane was purified from the supernatant of lysed and pelleted 1×10^5 cells treated as follows: Lane 1, 24 hours in serum free medium (SFM); lane 2, 100 μM Ara-C added for 4 hours to SFM; lane 3, 10 ng/ml pIXY321 added for 24 hours to SFM and lane 4, pIXY321 for 20 hours followed by pIXY321 plus Ara-C added SFM for additional 4 hours. Lower panel: Quantitation by phosphoimager analysis of the image density in each lane, reflecting the amount of fragmented DNA in the cells treated with each of the conditions, as above

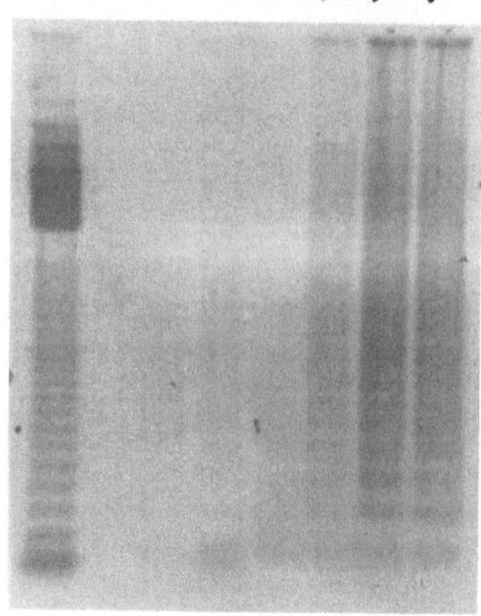

Fig. 2. HL-60 cells were treated with 5 or 50 ng/ml staurosporine and/or 10 μM Ara-C. The lanes contain ethidium bromide stained, electrophoresed fragmented DNA purified from the supernatant of cells treated as follows: untreated control cells, C; staurosporine alone, ST; 10.0 μM Ara-C alone, Ara-C; or co-treatment with Ara-C and ST. Lane M contains 123 base pair marker DNA ladder

Utilizing monoclonal anti-BCL-2 antibodies, Western analysis did not reveal significant differences in the intracellular p26BCL-2 levels in $CD34^+$ NBMMC treated with Ara-C alone versus pIXY321 plus Ara-C in the schedule and concentrations described above (data not shown).

We have also examined the effect of various modulators of protein kinase activity on high dose Ara-C-induced internucleosomal DNA fragmentation in HL60 cells. The microbial alkaloid staurosporine is a potent protein kinase C (PKC) inhibitor with IC_{50} value between 2 to 10 nM [19]. At higher concentrations, it is also known to inhibit the activity of other protein kinases [20]. Figure 2 demonstrates that the treatment with 5 or 50 ng/ml staurosporine for 4 hours did not produce internucleosomal DNA fragmentation in HL-60 cells, while exposure to 10 μM Ara-C for 4 hours produced the characteristic DNA fragmentation. Combined treatment with 5 or 50 ng/ml staurosporine and Ara-C significantly increased the intensity of DNA fragmentation ladder that was observed with Ara-C alone (Figure 2). Staurosporine plus Ara-C versus Ara-C alone was also associated with a twofold increase in the percentage of cells showing morphologic features of apoptosis. A similar enhancement of internucleosomal DNA fragmentation and apoptosis was also observed when HL-60 cells were treated with an identical schedule of Ara-C and 10 ng/ml PMA (data not shown). This increase in Ara-C-induced apoptosis by staurosporine and PMA was not associated with any significant alteration in the intracellular p26BCL-2 levels in HL-60 cells, as detected by Western analysis (data not shown).

Discussion

Programmed cell death or apoptosis is an active process of genedirected cellular selfdestruction [21]. The molecular signals or the gene-expressions which regulate this process may be subject to modulations by a variety of growth factors or mitogenic stimuli [11,21]. In human myeloid leukemia cells the exposure to clinically relevant, high concentrations of Ara-C results in internucleosomal DNA fragmentation and apoptosis [7]. Here, we report that cotreatment with pIXY321 significantly increased Ara-C-induced apoptosis of HL-60 cells, but inhibited HIDAC mediated apoptosis and loss of clonogenic survival of $CD34^+$ NBMMC. This differential in vitro effect of pIXY321 on HIDAC-mediated apoptosis in leukemic versus normal bone marrow progenitor cells may have several explanations, as described below.

Hemopoietic growth factors (HGFs) including IL-3 and GM-CSF are survival factors in that they suppress apoptosis induced by the withdrawal of HGFs in normal bone marrow progenitor cells [2,23]. This is supported by the evidence presented here that the addition of pIXY321 to SFM inhibits apoptosis observed when human $CD34^+$ NBMMC are cultured for 24 hours in SFM alone (Fig. 1). We have not observed a similar effect of pIXY321 on HL-60 cells or patient derived AML blasts (data not shown). This suggests that AML cells may have a blunted response with respect to the pIXY321-mediated intracellular protein phosphorylations which may regulate the activity of pIXY321 as a survival factor and inhibitor of apoptosis. In addition, GM-CSF plus IL-3 or pIXY321 has been demonstrated to enhance the intracellular metabolism of Ara-C in AML but not in NBMMC [6]. Since intracellular Ara-CTP/dCTP pool ratios and Ara-C DNA incorporation correlate with Ara-C-induced cytotoxicity and its ability to induce apoptosis [6, 24], taken together these observations may explain why cotreatment with pIXY321 may differentially increase Ara-C-induced apoptosis in AML cells. Following prolonged cotreatment with pIXY321 and low dose Ara-C versus treatment with Ara-C (10 nM) alone, the increased DNA fragmentation and apoptosis as well as the loss of clonogenic survival of HL-60 cells also has implications for the treatment of refractory anemia with excess of blasts (RAEB) or RAEB in transformation. In these clinical settings, pIXY321 plus low dose Ara-C may demonstrate an improved antileukemic selectivity.

A number of gene products have been implicated in regulating druginduced apoptosis in leukemic cells [25–27]. High intracellular levels of p26BCL-2 and the mutated p53 geneproduct have been shown to inhibit, while the overexpressions of c-myc, bcl-2 related bax gene or the wild-type p53 gene- product may promote apoptosis due to antileukemic drugs [27, 28]. Although the present studies utilizing Western analysis did not reveal significant differences in p26BCL-2 levels in HL-60 or $CD34^+$ NBMMC treated with pIXY321 plus Ara-C versus Ara-C alone, they did not rule out any differences in the expression of the other regulatory genes for apoptosis as possible mechanism(s) underlying the differential antileukemic activity of pIXY321 plus Ara-C. The possibility also exists that pIXY321 may differentially affect the function of p26BCL-2 in leukemic versus NBMMC.

Although several reports have indicated that the modulation of the activity of protein kinases can influence drug-induced apoptosis in a variety of cell lines [11, 19], the signalling pathway for the regulation of apoptosis have not clearly been defined [11]. Nonetheless, protein kinases, e.g. c-raf, MAP-kinase or PKC, are considered important links in the molecular signalling for the activation of the endonucleolytic DNA fragmentation and apoptosis [11, 21]. Recently, the activity of tyrosine kinases(s) have also been shown to regulate apoptosis and bcl-2 gene expression in growth factor dependent myeloid cell lines [29, 30]. Our results corroborate this by demonstrating that staurosporine, or a prolonged exposure to a phorbol ester, which down-regulate PKC-activity and by themselves do not induce internucleosomal DNA fragmentation, significantly enhance HIDAC-induced DNA fragmentation and apoptosis. The present and previous reports also underscore the potential linkage between protein kinases, cell cycle perturbations and the expression of genes which influence drug-induced apoptosis. It would be clearly important to examine such a linkage to define clinically applicable specific interventions which would differentially enhance druginduced apoptosis in cancer but not the normal host cells.

References

1. Bolwell, B. J., Cassileth, P. A., Gale, R. P. (1988) High dose cytarabine: A review. Leukemia, 2: 253–260.
2. Tafuri, A., Andreeff, M. (1990) Kinetic rationale for cytokine induced recruitment of myeloblastic leukemia followed by cycle specific chemotherapy in vitro. Leukemia, 4, 826–834.
3. Cannistra, S. A., Groshek, P., Griffin, J. D. (1989) Granulocyte macrophage colony stimulating factor enhances the cytotoxic effect of cytosine arabinoside in acute myeloblastic leukemia and in the myeloid blast crisis phase of chronic myeloid leukemia. Leukemia, 3, 328–334.
4. Brach, M., Klein, H., Platzer, E., Mertelsmann, R., Herrman, F. (1990) Effect of Interleukin-3 on cytosine arabinoside mediated cytotoxicity of leukemic myeloblasts. Exp Hematol, 18, 748–753.
5. Bernstein, S.H. (1993) Growth factors in the management of adult acute leukemia. Hem/Oncol Clin N Amer, 7, 255–74.
6. Bhalla, K., Holladay, C., Arlin, Z., Grant, S., Ibrado, A. M., Jasiok, M. (1991) Treatment with IL-3 plus GM-CSF improves the selectivity of Ara-C in vitro against AML blasts. Blood, 78, 2674–2679.
7. Gunji, H., Kharbanda, S., Kufe, D. (1991) Induction of internucleosomal DNA fragmentation in human myeloid leukemia cells by 1-B-D-arabinofuranosylcytosine. Cancer Res, 51, 741–743.
8. Curtis, B.M., Williams, D.E., Broxmeyer, H.E., Dunn, J., Farrah, T., Jeffery, E., Clevenger, W., DeRoos, P., Martin, U., Friend, D., Craig, V., Gayle, R., Price, V., Cosman, D., March, C., Park, L.S. (1991) Enhanced hematopoietic activity of a human granulocyte/macrophage colony-stimulating factor-interleukin 3 fusion protein. Proc Natl Acad Sci, 88, 5809–5813.
9. Williams, D.E., Park, L.S. (1991) Hematopoietic effects of a granulocyte-macrophage colony stimulating factor/interleukin3 fusion protein. Cancer, 67, 2705–2707.
10. Bhalla, K., Ibrado, A.M., Bullock, G., Tang, C.Q., Tourkina, E., Huang, Y. (1992) GM-CSF/IL-3 fusion protein (PIXY321) enhances high dose Ara-C induced programmed cell death or apoptosis in human myeloid leukemic cells. Blood, 80, 2883–2890.
11. Dive, C., Evans, C.A., Whetton, A.D. (1992) Induction of apoptosis - new targets for cancer chemotherapy. Semin Cancer Biol, 3, 417–427.
12. Gallegher, R., Collins, S., Triejillo, J., McCredie, K., Ahearn, M., Tsai, S., Metzgar, R., Aulakh, G., Ting, R., Ruscetti, F., Gallo, R. (1979) Characterization of the continuous differentiating myeloid cell line (HL-60) from a patient with acute promyelocytic leukemia. Blood, 54, 713–33.
13. Bhalla, K., Bullock, G., Lutzky, J., Holladay, C., Ibrado, A.M., Jasiok, M., Singh, S. (1992) Effect of combined treatment with interleukin-3 and interleukin-6 on 4-Hydroperoxycyclophosphamide mediated reduction in glutathione levels and cytotoxicity in normal and leukemic bone marrow progenitor cells. Leukemia, 6, 814–819.
14. Fackler, M.J., Civin, C.I., May, W.S. (1992) Upregulation of surface CD34 is associated with protein kinase C-mediated hyperphosphorylation of CD34. J Biol Chem, 25, 17540–17546
15. Petrini, M., Quaranta, M.T., Testa, U., Samoggia, P., Tritarelli, E., Care, A., Cianetti, L., Valtieri, M., Barletta, C., Peschele, C. (1992) Expression of selected human HOX-2 genes in B/T acute lymphoid leukemia and interleukin-2/interleukin-1 β-stimulated natural killer lymphocytes. Blood, 80, 185–193.
16. Bhalla, K., Ibrado, A.M., Tourkina, E., Tang, C.Q., Mahoney, M.E., Huang, Y. (1993) Taxol induces programmed cell death in human myeloid leukemia cells. Leukemia, 7, 563–568.
17. Facchinetti, A., Tessarollo, L., Mazzocchi, M., Kingston, D., Collavo, D., Biasi, G. (1991) An improved method for the detection of DNA fragmentation. J Immunol Methods, 136, 125–131.
18. Bhalla, K., Ray, S., Huang, Y., Tang, C., Self, S., Mahoney, M.E., Ponnathpur, V., Ibrado, A.M., Bullock, G., Willingham, M.C. (1994) Characterization of a human myeloid leukemia cell line highly resistant to taxol. Leukemia, 8, 465–475.
19. Grunicke, H.H., and Uberal, F. (1992) Protein kinase C modulation. Semin. Cancer Biology, 3, 351–360.
20. Gadbois, D.M., Hamaguchi, J.R., Swank, R.A., Bradbury, E.M. (1992) Staurosporine is a potent inhibitor of $p34^{cdc2}$ and $p34^{cdc2}$-like kinases. Biochem and Biophys Res Comm, 184, 80–85.
21. Waring, P., Kos, F.J., Mullbacher, A. (1991) Apoptosis or programmed cell death. Med Res Rev, 11, 219–236.
22. Williams, G.T., Smith, C.A., Spooncer, E., Dexter, T.M., Taylor, D.R. (1990) Hemopoietic colony stimulating factors promote cell survival by suppressing apoptosis. Nature, 343, 76–79.
23. Brandt, J.E., Bhalla, K., Hoffman, R. (1994) Effects of Interleukin-3 and c-kit ligand on the survival of various classes of human hematopoietic progenitor cells. Blood, 83, 1507–1514.
24. Bhalla, K., Tourkina, E., Huang, Y., Tang, C., Mahoney, M.E., Ibrado, A.M. (1993) Effect of hemopoietic growth factors G-CSF and pIXY321 on the activity of high dose Ara-C in human myeloid leukemia cells. Leukemia and Lymphoma, 10, 123–131.
25. Miyashita, T., and J.C. Reed. (1993) BCL-2 oncoprotein blocks chemotherapy-induced apoptosis in a human leukemia cell line. Blood, 81, 151–157.
26. Lowe, S.W., Ruley, H.E., Jacks, T., Housman, D.E. (1993) p53-Dependent apoptosis modulates the cytotoxicity of anticancer agents. Cell, 74, 957–967.
27. Lotem, J., Sachs, L. (1993) Regulation by bcl-2, c-myc, and p53 susceptibility to induction of apoptosis by heat shock and cancer chemotherapy compounds in differentiation-component and -defective myeloid leukemic cells. Cell Growth & Diff, 4, 41–47.

28. Oltvai, Z.N., Milliman, C.L., Korsmeyer, S.J. (1993) Bcl-2 heterodimerizes in vivo with a conserved homolog, Bax that accelerates programmed cell death. Cell, 74, 609–616.
29. Otani, H., Erdosd M., Leonard, W.J. (1993) Tyrosine kinases(s) regulate apoptosis and bcl-2 expression in a growth factordependent cell line. J Biolog Chem, 268, 22733–22736.
30. Laneuville, P., Timm, M., Hudson, A.T. (1994) bcr/abl expression in 32D cl3(G) cells inhibits apoptosis induced by protein tyrosine kinase inhibitors. Cancer Res, 54, 1360–1366.

Acute Leukemias V
Experimental Approaches
and Management of Refractory Diseases
Hiddemann et al. (Eds.)

A Double-blind Controlled Study of G-CSF Started Two Days Before Induction Chemotherapy in Refractory Acute Myeloid Leukemia

R. Ohno, T. Naoe, A. Kanamaru, M. Yoshida, A. Hiraoka, T. Kobayashi, T. Ueda, S. Minami, Y. Morishima, Y. Saito, S. Furusawa, K. Imai, Y. Takemoto, Y. Miura, H. Teshima, and N. Hamajima

Abstract. A prospective, double-blind controlled study was conducted to determine the efficacy of a recombinant granulocyte colony-stimulating factor (G-CSF, 200 μg/m²) starting daily from 2 days before an induction therapy until neutrophils recovered to above 1,500/μl or until 35 days after the therapy in 58 patients with relapsed or refractory acute myeloid leukemia (AML). Twenty-eight patients in the G-CSF group showed significantly faster recovery of neutrophils ($P < 0.001$) than 30 patients in the placebo group. The incidence of febrile episodes and of documented infections was almost the same in both groups. However, among 39 patients who did not show any infectious episodes during the 2 week-period after the start of chemotherapy, the incidence of documented infections after the third week tended to be lower in the G-CSF group, but not statistically significantly. There was no evidence that G-CSF stimulated the growth of AML cells in the bone marrow during the 2-day period prior to the chemotherapy, nor that G-CSF accelerated the regrowth of AML cells during the 5-week period after the therapy. Fifty percent of patients in the G-CSF group and 37% in the placebo group had complete remission (CR). Although the rate was higher in the G-CSF group, the difference was not statistically significant ($P = 0.306$). There was no difference between the two groups in event-free survival of all patients, and in disease-free survival of patients who had achieved CR.

Introduction

Granulocyte colony-stimulating factor (G-CSF) has been proved useful for the recovery of severe neutropenia after an intensive chemotherapy and BMT [1–3]. However, the clinical application of G-CSF in myeloid leukemia has been controversial, because it stimulates myeloid leukemia cells as well as normal granulocyte progenitors in vitro [4–6]. Although several investigators have reported that G-CSF does not stimulate AML cells in vivo if the drug is used in patients whose leukemia cells are highly reduced by chemotherapy [7,8], we sometimes experience patients whose AML cells increase during the G-CSF therapy, in case when patients have leukemia cells in the peripheral blood. On the other hand, if G-CSF really simulates leukemia cells, the stimulated leukemia cells may become more susceptible to cell-cycle dependent antitumor drugs, and better therapeutic results may be obtained.

In this preliminary double-blind controlled study in patients with relapsed or refractory AML, we asked two questions: 1) Does G-CSF given prior to the induction therapy stimulate leukemia cells *in vivo?* 2) Does G-CSF increase the complete remission rate by recruiting quiescent leukemia cells into chemotherapy-sensitive proliferating cells?

Patients and Methods

Patients were enrolled to this study from 23 institutions which belonged to the Leukemia Study Group of the Ministry of Health and Welfare (Kohseisho) between October 1990 and October 1992. Patients were eligible if they had AML which was refractory to 2 courses of the remission-induction therapy of Japan Adult

The Kohseisho Leukemia Study Group, the Department of Medicine, Hamamatsu University School of Medicine, Hamamatsu 431-31, Japan

Leukemia Study Group; the AML-89 study till December, 1991 and the AML-92 study from January 1992, relapsed from remission, relapsed and refractory to salvage therapy, or if they had AML arising from proven myelodysplastic syndromes (MDS). Patients were not eligible if their serum bilirubin was ≥ 2.0 mg/dl, blood urea nitrogen ≥ 35 mg/dl or serum creatinine ≥ 2.0 mg/dl, or if the ECOG performance status was 4. They were registered by telephone, and stratified according to the type of leukemia (AML or MDS), age (< 60 or ≥ 60 years) and the disease stage (relapsed or refractory). Informed consent was obtained from the patients or from the family members.

All patients received an induction therapy which consisted of mitoxantrone 7 mg/m² by 30 min i.v. infusion daily for 3 days, etoposide 100 mg/m² by 1 hr i.v. infusion daily for 5 days and behenoyl cytosine arabinoside (BHAC) 200 mg/m² by 2 hr i.v. infusion daily for 7 days. Beginning from 2 days before the start of induction therapy and continuing till 35 days after it, patients received either a recombinant human G-CSF (filgrastim, Kirin/Sankyo, Tokyo, 200 µg/m²) or placebo by 60-min i.v. infusion daily. The placebo contained the same amount of additives to the G-CSF preparation; polysorbate-80 and D-mannitol. The drug was discontinued earlier if peripheral neutrophil counts recovered to above 1,500/µl. After achieving CR, therapy with the same drugs was repeated until relapse.

This was a multicenter randomized, double-blind, placebo-controlled study in adult patients with relapsed or refractory AML to evaluate the effect of G-CSF on hematopoietic reconstitution after intensive remission induction therapy, on the growth of leukemia cells in bone marrow 2 days after the administration of G-CSF, on the regrowth of leukemia cells after the induction therapy, and on the incidence of infectious episodes during the 5-week period after the start of G-CSF therapy. Caution was taken to avoid unnecessary stimulation of neutrophil production by G-CSF. Bone marrow aspirations were done at day −2, day 0 (the day when chemotherapy was started), day 13, day 20, day 27 and day 35. Incidence of febrile episodes with temperature over 38 °C and of documented infections were recorded. When patients died before their blood counts recovered to the designated numbers, they were regarded as cases which showed no recovery during the study period. When patients did not achieve complete remission by one course of the induction therapy, they were regarded as failure cases in terms of remission induction. A complete remission was considered to be established when bone marrow contained less than 5% of blasts with normal level of peripheral neutrophils (> 1,500/µl) and platelet counts (> 100,000/µl). Statistical analysis was done by the chi-square test, the t-test, the Wilcoxon rank-sum test, the generalized Wilcoxon test or the log-rank test using the SAS computer program. The study was approved by the institutional review board at each institution.

Results

Sixty patients were registered to the study, but 2 patients did not receive the therapy due to the deterioration of their general condition. Thus, 58 patients were entered to the study. All of them completed the 7-day chemotherapy and were evaluated. Fifty patients had AML and 8 had AML arising from MDS (MDS-AML). Twenty-eight patients received G-CSF and 30 received placebo. Patient's characteristics were shown in Table 1. There was no statistical difference between two treatment groups in age, sex,

Table. 1. Patient's characteristics

	G-CSF	Placebo
entered	28	30
evaluable	28	30
M/F	14/14	15/15
Age (years old)		
median	43	47
range	18–63	16–66
Type		
AML	24	26
M0	0	1
M1	3	7
M2	14	11
M4	6	5
M5	1	1
M6	0	1
MDS	4	4
Stage		
primarily refractory	3	3
relapsed	19	18
relapsed & refractory	2	5
untreated	4	4
WBC (median/µl)	3,950	3,050
RBC (median/µl)	3,150	3,170
platelet (median/µl)	60	47
Blasts % in bone marrow (median)	64	47

type of AML, or stage of leukemia. One patient in the G-CSF group and two in the placebo group died of infection within 35 days after the start of induction therapy.

Recovery of neutrophil counts. The recovery of neutrophils over 500/μl and 1,000/μl (Fig. 1) was significantly faster in the G-CSF group than in the placebo group (P = 0.0001, respectively, by the log-rank test). The neutrophil count recovered to more than 500/μl in 25 patients in the G-CSF group within a median of 24 days, while it recovered in 18 patients in the placebo group within a median of 29 days. The neutrophil count recovered to more than 1,000/μl in 24 patients in the G-CSF group within a median of 25 days, while it recovered in 15 patients in the placebo group within a median of 32 days. There was no difference in the recovery of platelet counts to more than 100,000/μl between the two groups (P = 0.5186 by the log-rank test).

Incidence of infectious episodes and documented infection. Eight (29%) of 28 patients in the G-CSF group and one (3%) of 30 patients in the placebo group had already had febrile episodes at the start of G-CSF (P = 0.011 by the Fisher's exact test). Twenty-six (93%) patients in the G-CSF group and 27 (90%) in the placebo group had some febrile episodes during the 37-day study period. Mean total of febrile days (± standard deviation) was 11.3 ± 6.3 days in the G-CSF group, and 9.6 ± 6.4 in the placebo group. Documented infections were observed in 14 (50%) patients in the G-CSF group and 13 (43%) patients in the placebo group. There were 4 cases of septicemia, 3 pneumonia, 4 tonsillitis/ stomatitis, one liver abscess and one cellulitis in the G-CSF group, and 3 septicemia, 2 pneumonia, 6 tonsillitis/ stomatitis and 2 cellulitis in the placebo group. However, among 39 patients who did not show any infectious episodes during the 2 week-period after the start of chemotherapy, 2 (14%) of 15 patients in the G-CSF group and 7 (29%) of 24 patients in the placebo group presented infectious episodes (P = 0.460 by the Fisher's exact test), and one (7%) in the G-CSF group and 7 (29%) in the placebo group developed documented infections after the third week (P = 0.230). Among patients who did not have febrile episodes at the start of G-CSF, 18 (90%) of 20 patients in the G-CSF group and 26 (89%) 29 in the placebo group developed febrile episodes during the 37-day study period.

Growth of leukemia blasts in bone marrow two days after the start of G-CSF therapy. The growth of blasts was compared in the two groups by examining the bone marrow on the day when the G-CSF therapy was started (day −2) and on the day when the induction chemotherapy was started (day 0). Two-hundred-fifty cells on May-Giemsa-stained bone marrow aspirates were examined by blinded hematologists at each institution. In the G-CSF group, the mean and median percentages of blasts on day −2 were 54% and 63%, respectively, and those on day 0 were 54% and 62%, respectively. In the placebo group, the mean and median percentages of blasts on day −2 were 52% and 47%, respectively, and those on day 0

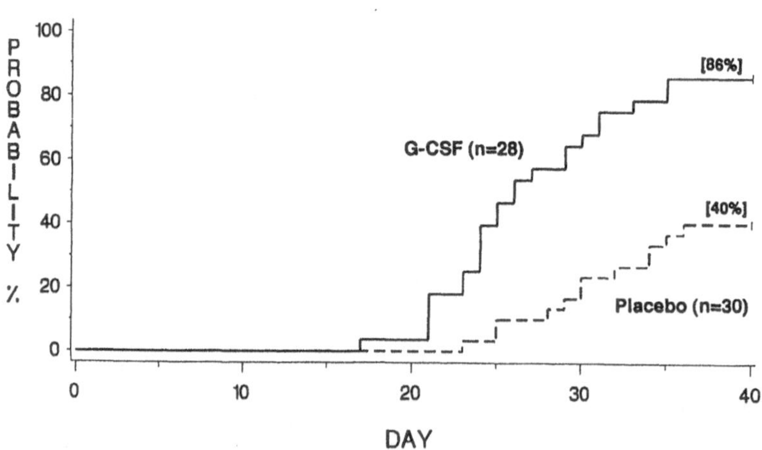

Fig. 1. The recovery of neutrophils over 1,000/μl

were 54% and 63%, respectively. There was some increase of blast percentages in the bone marrow on day 0 in both groups. However, the mean increase of the blast percentage from day 0 to day −2 was only 1.6% in the G-CSF group and 2.3% in the placebo group. The increase in individual patients showed no statistical significance by the paired t-test in both groups ($P=0.5603$ and $P=0.3870$, respectively).

Regrowth of leukemia blasts in bone marrow 3 to 5 weeks after the start of g-csf therapy. The regrowth of blasts was compared in the two groups by examining the bone marrow on day 21, day 28 and day 35 of the induction therapy. There was no difference between the two groups in the regrowth of blasts. The mean and median percentages of blasts on day 21 were 13% and 4% in the G-CSF group, and 15% and 5% in the placebo group, respectively. The mean and median percentages of blasts on day 28 were 15% and 3% in the G-CSF group, and 26% and 12% in the placebo group, respectively. The mean and median percentages of blasts on day 35 were 15% and 2% in the G-CSF group, and 20% and 2% in the placebo group, respectively. These values showed no statistical significance by the Wilcoxon rank-sum test. Three patients in the G-CSF group and 6 patients in the placebo group showed some increase of blasts during the study period.

Result of remission induction therapy. The result of remission induction therapy is shown in the left column of Table 2. Fifty percent of the patients in the G-CSF group had CR after one course of induction therapy, as compared to 37% of those in the placebo group. The rate of remission was higher in the G-CSF group, but the difference was not statistically significant, although the power is not strong due to small sample size ($\alpha=0.306$, $1\text{-}\beta=0.310$). Among patients with AML, 54% of 24 patients in the G-CSF group and 42% of 26 patients in the placebo group achieved CR. Among patients with MDS, one of 4 patients in the G-CSF group and none of 4 patients in the placebo group obtained CR. Among patients with MDS, two patients in each group had some chromosomal abnormality involving chromosome 7 or 8, but the patient who obtained CR had no such abnormality. One patient in the G-CSF group and 2 in the placebo group died of infections within 5 weeks after the induction therapy.

Event-free survival of all patients, and disease-free survival of complete remission cases. There was no difference between the two groups in EFS and DFS ($P=0.3642$ and $P=0.5449$, respectively, by the generalized Wilcoxon test) at the median follow-up of 24 months. Since no patient died before they relapsed, the continuing CR length was the same as DFS.

Toxicities of G-CSF. Only one patient in the G-CSF group complained of bone pain, and there was no other toxic effects reported in both groups.

Discussion

Acute leukemia is a cancer with highly proliferative potency, and it is not uncommon to see patients whose leukemia cells multiply daily in the peripheral blood, if antitumor drugs are not given. Therefore, in order to clarify whether G-CSF really stimulates leukemia cells in vivo, it was expected that only a randomized study would only answer this controversial question.

We previously conducted a prospective randomized study in relapsed or refractory acute

Table 2. Result of induction therapy in refractory acute myeloid leukemia. G-CSF started before or after induction therapy

		before chemotherapy			after chemotherapy		
	Type	No. of cases	No. of CR	(%)	No. of cases	No. of CR	(%)
G-CSF	AML	24	13	(54%)	30	17	(57%)
	MDS-AL	4	1	(25%)	2	0	(0%)
	Total	28	14	(50%)	32	17	(53%)
Control	AML	26	11	(42%)	31	12	(39%)
	MDS-AL	4	0	(0%)	–	–	
	Total	30	11	(37%)	31	12	(39%)

leukemia [7]. The study showed no difference between the two groups in the regrowth of leukemia cells within 40 days after the end of induction therapy, nor in the occurrence of relapse [7]. We also reported that there was no increase of leukemia relapse in newly diagnosed patients with AML who received G-CSF for life-threatening infection during remission induction or consolidation therapy in the AML-87 study of Japan Adult Leukemia Study Group [8]. Moreover, a meta-analysis of two double-blind controlled studies of G-CSF after allogeneic BMT [9,10] showed no difference of disease-free survival in patients with myeloid leukemia who received G-CSF or placebo [11].

However, there have been several reports that G-CSF stimulated growth of myeloid leukemia cells in vivo. Teshima et al. observed an increase of blasts with the parallel increase of neutrophils in a patient with CML in myeloid crisis during the G-CSF therapy [12]. Soutar also reported the development of secondary AML in a patient with Hodgkin's disease who had been receiving G-CSF for 6 weeks for an unexplained neutropenia [13]. We also experienced 2 patients with AML derived from MDS who had shown transient increases of peripheral leukemia blasts during the G-CSF therapy (unpublished data).

On the other hand, based on in vitro data which demonstrated that G-CSF or granulocyte-macrophage-colony stimulating factor (GM-CSF) recruited quiescent AML cells to become more sensitive to cell-cycle specific cytotoxic drugs and consequently promoted the drug-induced cell kill [14–18], several investigators have attempted to give GM-CSF before and during induction chemotherapy in order to increase remission rates. Bettelheim et al. reported 83% CR, higher than that of their historical control group, in 18 newly diagnosed patients with de novo AML by combination of standard induction chemotherapy and continuous infusion of GM-CSF from 48 to 24 hours before the chemotherapy until peripheral neutrophil recovered over 500/µl [19]. On the contrary, Estey et al. reported that administration of GM-CSF from 8 to 0 days before the start of induction chemotherapy resulted in a lower CR rate and a lower survival probability in newly diagnosed AML than those of their prognostically adjusted historical control patients receiving no GM-CSF [20]. Both of these studies are not randomized trials, and a well-controlled prospective study is needed to clarify whether CSFs produce any other therapeutic benefit besides the acceleration of neutrophil recovery.

The neutrophil recovery in the G-CSF group was significantly faster than that in the placebo group after the induction therapy. Nevertheless, overall incidence of febrile episodes or of documented infections was not different between two groups. This may come from the fact that 29% of the patients in the G-CSF group already had febrile episodes at the start of study compared to 5% in the placebo group. Furthermore, it is known that the neutrophil recovery after an intensive chemotherapy in acute leukemia usually takes place around 2 weeks after the start of G-CSF as being observed in the present study and in the previous study [7]. Therefore, the incidence of infectious episodes during the 2 week-period would not probably be different. When the patients who had not shown any infectious episodes during the 2 week-period after the start of chemotherapy were analyzed, the incidence of documented infections tended to be lower in the G-CSF group (7%) than in the placebo group (29%) due to the earlier recovery of neutrophils in the former group.

From this study, it has not been clarified whether the 2-day administration of G-CSF stimulated the growth of AML cells in vivo. At least there was no significant difference in the percentage of blasts in the bone marrow after the 2-day administration of drugs between two groups. There was neither any sign that G-CSF stimulated the regrowth of leukemia blasts in the bone marrow during the 28-day administration of G-CSF after the end of induction therapy.

Patients in the G-CSF group tended to have a higher CR rate (50%) than patients in the placebo group (37%). However, the current results showing a CR rate of 50% with G-CSF treatment given from 2 days prior to chemotherapy are very similar to the results obtained in our previous study in which G-CSF was given after bone marrow aplasia [7]. In the latter study, patients in the G-CSF group obtained a CR rate of 50% and those in the control group achieved a CR rate of 36% by an induction therapy with the same drug combination used in the present study, i.e., mitoxantrone, etoposide and behenoyl cytosine arabinoside [7] (Table 2). Therefore, it was not clear whether the tendency of a higher CR rate in the G-CSF group in the present study was due to the recruitment effect by G-CSF or due to the stimulatory effect of neutrophil production by G-CSF. In order to clarify this question, a randomized study will be necessary by giving G-CSF or placebo from day −2 till the last day of chemotherapy, and then giving G-CSF to both groups until neutrophil recovery.

There was no difference in disease-free survival (DFS) of patients in the G-CSF and the placebo groups who had obtained CR, which indicated that patients in the G-CSF group showed no earlier relapse due to the G-CSF administration. We already reported that newly diagnosed patients with AML who received G-CSF due to life-threatening infections showed no earlier relapse but rather tended to have better DFS than those who did not receive G-CSF [8].

From the present pilot, placebo-controlled study, no evidence was revealed to prove that the administration of G-CSF accelerated the regrowth of AML cells in vivo, and became harmful to patients. Furthermore, there was no convincing data that G-CSF at the standard dose for clinical use stimulated AML cells in vivo. For further clinical trials to recruit quiescent AML cells making more sensitive to cell-cycle specific cytotoxic drugs, GM-CSF instead of G-CSF might be more suitable, since there are ample evidences that GM-CSF stimulates AML colony-forming units more than G-CSF *in vitro*.

Even though there is no convincing *in vivo* data which demonstrate that G-CSF stimulates leukemia cells when this drug is used after intensive chemotherapy, when G-CSF is used for the accelerated recovery of neutrophils, caution must still be taken to avoid a possible stimulatory effect of AML cells *in vivo*, since G-CSF definitely stimulates AML cells *in vitro*. The dose of G-CSF to be utilized clinically should be a minimally required dose for an accelerated recovery of neutrophils, and the administration period should also be as short as possible. No more than 1,500/μl of neutrophils in the peripheral blood will be needed for the control of regular microbial infections [21]. From our experience, absence of AML blasts in the peripheral blood or less than 20% of AML blasts in hypoplastic bone marrow seems relevant for the starting time of the G-CSF therapy.

Moreover, until further randomized studies show whether G-CSF is really safely used in patients with AML, the clinical use of G-CSF should be limited to life-threatening infections or uncontrollable infections in severely neutropenic states in standard-risk AML. In case of high-risk AML, such as AML in elderly patients or relapsed and/or refractory AML, G-CSF can be used when patients have severe neutropenia, or even be given prophylactically, since early recovery from neutropenia or no development of neutropenia will permit dose-intensified chemotherapy in these patients, plausibly resulting in a better therapeutic outcome.

Acknowledgements. We thank all participating physicians from 23 institutions for their cooperation, and Tomoko Kawashima for the preparation of the manuscript. We are also indebted to Kirin Co. Ltd. and Sankyo Co. Ltd. for providing us the G-CSF and the placebo.

References

1. Groopman JE, Molina J-M, Scadden DT. Hematopoietic growth factors: Biology and clinical applications. New Engl J Med 321: 1449–1459, 1989.
2. Antman KS, Griffin JD, Elias A, Socinski MA et al. Effect of recombinant human granulocyte-macrophage colony-stimulating factor on chemotherapy-induced myelo-suppression. N Engl J Med 319: 593–598, 1988.
3. Sheridan WP, Morstyn G, Wolf M et al. Granulocyte colony-stimulating factor and neutrophil recovery after high-dose chemotherapy and autologous bone marrow transplantation. Lancet 2: 891–895, 1989.
4. Souza LM, Boone TC, Gabrilove JL et al. Recombinant human granulocyte colony-stimulating factor: Effects on normal and leukemic myeloid cells. Science 232: 61–65, 1986.
5. Griffin JD, Löwenberg B. Clonogenic cells in acute myeloblastic leukemia. Blood 68: 1185–1195, 1986.
6. Vellenga E, Young DC, Wagner K et al. The effect of GM-CSF and G-CSF in promoting growth of clonogenic cells in acute myeloblastic leukemia. Blood 69: 1771–1776, 1987.
7. Ohno R, Tomonaga M, Kobayashi T et al. Effect of granulocyte colony stimulating factor after intensive induction therapy in relapsed or refractory acute leukemia: A randomized controlled study. N Engl J Med 323: 871–877, 1990.
8. Ohno R, Hiraoka A, Tanimoto M et al. No increase of leukemia relapse in newly diagnosed patients with acute myeloid leukemia who received granulocyte colony-stimulating factor for life threatening infection during remission induction and consolidation therapy. Blood 81: 561–562, 1993.
9. Masaoka T, Moriyama Y, Kato S et al. A double-blind controlled study of KRN 8601 (rhG-CSF) in patients received allogeneic bone marrow transplantation. Kyo-no-Ishoku 3: 233–239, 1990.
10. Asano S, Masaoka T, Takaku F, Ogawa N. Placebo controlled double trial of recombinant human granulocyte colony-stimulating factor for bone marrow transplantation. Kyo-no-Ishoku 3: 317–321, 1990.

11. Ohno R, Masaoka T, Asano S, and Takaku F. G-CSF after intensive induction chemotherapy in refractory acute leukemia and bone marrow transplantation in myeloid leukemia. Haemat Blood Trans 34: 101–7, 1992.
12. Teshima H, Ishikawa J, Kitayama H et al. Clinical effects of recombinant human granulocyte colony-stimulating factor in leukemia patients: A phase I/II study. Exp Hematol 17: 853–858, 1989.
13. Soutar R. Acute myeloblastic leukaemia and recombinant granulocyte colony stimulating factor. Brit J Med 303: 123–124, 1991.
14. Cannistra S, Groshek P, Griffin J. Granulocyte-macrophage colony-stimulating factor enhances the cytotoxic effects of cytosine arabinoside in acute myeloblastic leukemia and in the myeloid blast crisis phase of chronic myeloid leukemia. Leukemia 3: 328, 1989.
15. Tafuni A, Andreeff M. Kinetic rationale for cytokine-induced recruitment of myeloblastic leukemia followed by cycle-specific chemotherapy in vitro. Leukemia 4: 826, 1990.
16. Santini V, Nooter K, Delwel R, Lowenberg B. Susceptibility of acute myeloid leukemia cells from clinically resistant and sensitive patients to daunomycin (DNR): Assessment in vitro after stimulation with colony stimulating factors. Leuk Res 14: 377, 1990.
17. Karp J, Burke P, Donehower R. Effects of rhGM-CSF on intracellular ara-C pharmacology in vitro in acute myelocytic leukemia: Comparability with drug-induced humoral stimulatory activity. Leukemia 4: 553, 1990.
18. Bhalla K, Birkhofer M, Arlin Z et al. Effect of recombinant GM-CSF on the metabolism of cytosine-arabinoside in normal and leukemic human bone marrow cells. Leukemia 2: 810, 1988.
19. Bettelheim P, Valent P, Andreeff M et al. Recombinant human granulocyte-macrophage colony-stimulating factor in combination with standard induction chemotherapy in de novo acute myeloid leukemia. Blood 77: 700–711, 1991.
20. Estey E, Thall PF, Kantarjian HM et al. Treatment of newly diagnosed acute myelogenous leukemia with and granulocyte-macrophage colony-stimulating factor (GM-CSF) before and during continuous-infusion high-dose ara-C + daunorubicin: comparison to patients treated without GM-CSF. Blood 79: 2246–2255, 1992.
21. Bodey GP. Infections in cancer patients. Cancer Treat Rev 2: 89–97,1975.

Acute Leukemias V
Experimental Approaches
and Management of Refractory Diseases
Hiddemann et al. (Eds.)

Effects of Growth Factors In Vitro on Acute Lymphoblastic Leukemia Cells

G. J. L. Kaspers[1], R. Pieters[1], C. H. Van Zantwijk[1], G. H. Broekema[1], K. Hählen[2], and A. J. P. Veerman[1]

Abstract. Growth factors may enhance the cytotoxicity of anticancer agents. Little is known about this effect of growth factors on acute lymphoblastic leukemia (ALL) cells. We studied the effects of interleukin-3 (IL-3), interleukin-7 (IL-7) and B-cell growth factor (BCGF) on cell survival and drug resistance in ALL samples, using the MTT assay.

Compared to drug-free culture without growth factors, the cell survival was significantly increased by IL-3, IL-7 and BCGF. Compared to growth factor-free drug incubations, the cytotoxicity of thioguanine was significantly enhanced by IL-3 and IL-7, and the cytotoxicity of cytarabine was significantly enhanced by IL-7. In contrast, the cytotoxicity of prednisolone was decreased by the growth factors in most ALL samples, and overall not significantly modulated.

We conclude that the MTT assay can be used to study the effects of growth factors on cell survival and drug resistance of ALL cells. This type of information may be useful for the design of clinical trials with growth factors in ALL.

Introduction

One of the applications of growth factors in hematopoietic malignancies is to increase the chemosensitivity of the malignant cells. This effect is assumed to be caused by the recruitment of non-proliferating cells into cycle. In vitro studies might identify growth factors which may be useful for this purpose. In addition, the results might even predict the clinically heterogeneic response to growth factors (Estrov et al., 1992).

The purposes of the present study were to investigate the effects of IL-3, IL-7, and BCGF on cell survival and on resistance to cytarabine, thioguanine, and prednisolone of ALL cells. For these purposes, the methyl-thiazol-tetrazolium (MTT) assay was used (Pieters et al., 1990).

Materials and Methods

Samples which had been cryopreserved in liquid nitrogen of 17 children with newly diagnosed ALL were successfully tested with the MTT assay at the research laboratory for pediatric hemato-onco-immunology of the Free University Hospital in Amsterdam. It concerned 15 precursor B-cell and 2 T-cell ALL samples. All samples contained ≥ 90% ALL cells after isolation and after 5 days of culture.

The ALL cells were cultured in flasks without or with growth factor (IL-3 30 IU/ml, IL-7 100 IU/ml, BCGF 10% v/v) in serum-free Iscove's modified Dulbecco's medium with supplements. After 24 hours, cells were plated in the wells of 96-well microculture plates and cultured for 4 more days in the continuous presence or absence of growth factor, without or with drug (each at 4 different concentrations).

The MTT assay was used to assess the degree of cell survival and to assess the cytotoxicity of

[1] Department of Pediatrics, Free University Hospital, 1081 HV Amsterdam,
[2] Sophia Children's Hospital, Subdivision Hemato-/Oncology, Rotterdam, The Netherlands

cytarabine, thioguanine and prednisolone as described previously (Kaspers et al., 1991). MTT is reduced to a coloured formazan by living but not by dead cells. The optical density (OD), which is linearily related to the number of living cells (Pieters et al., 1988), was measured spectrophotometrically. The LC50, the drug concentration lethal to 50% of the cells, was calculated from the dose-response curves and used as measure of resistance.

Stimulation indices were calculated by: (OD with growth factor)/ (OD without growth factor). A stimulation index of >1 indicates an increased cell survival.

Sensitization indices were calculated by: (LC50 without growth factor)/(LC50 with growth factor). A sensitization index of >1 indicates enhanced cytotoxicity.

Comparisons of cell survival and drug resistance with and without growth factor were done with the Wilcoxon's matched pair test.

Results

Effects of growth factors on cell survival. IL-3, IL-7, and BCGF induced a significantly increased ALL cell survival as assessed on day 5 by the MTT assay. An inhibitory effect of any growth factor on cell survival was very rarely seen in individual samples. Table 1 summarizes the results. BCGF had a greater effect on cell survival than IL-3 ($p=0.02$), while such a comparison between BCGF and IL-7 and between IL-3 and IL-7 was not significantly different.

Effects of growth factors on drug resistance. Incubation with any growth factor enhanced the cytotoxicity of cytarabine and thioguanine towards the ALL cells in most samples. For cytarabine this was significant for IL-7, and for thioguanine it was significant for IL-3 and IL-7. In contrast, the cytotoxicity of prednisolone was more often decreased, and overall not significantly modulated. An example of cytarabine cytotoxicity enhanced by IL-3, and an example of prednisolone cytotoxicity decreased by IL-7 are shown in Fig. 1 and Table 2 summarizes the overall results. IL-7 enhanced the cytotoxicity of thioguanine to a greater extent than IL-3 ($p=0.02$) and BCGF ($p=0.02$), and that of cytarabine to a greater extent than IL-3 ($p=0.03$).

Table 1. Effect of growth factors on ALL cell survival ($n=17$)

	IL-3	IL-7	BCGF
Stimulation Index			
median	1.4	1.4	2.1
range	0.7–3.8	1.0–7.3	1.4–6.6
P-value	0.002	0.001	0.001

Discussion

We studied the in vitro effects of IL-3, IL-7 and BCGF on cell survival and drug resistance of childhood ALL cells obtained at initial diagnosis. For these purposes, we used the colorimetric MTT assay, which is a rapid and objective assay suited to study proliferation (Mosmann, 1983) and drug resistance (Veerman & Pieters, 1990).

Cell survival was increased by each growth factor, especially by BCGF. Whether this is caused by a stimulatory effect on proliferation or by a decreased 'spontaneous' apoptosis remains to be elucidated. Stimulatory effects on proliferation of ALL cells have been reported by other authors for IL-3 (Uckun et al., 1989; Eder et al., 1990; Findley et al., 1990; O'Connor et al., 1991), IL-7 (Eder et al., 1990; Touw et al., 1990; O'Connor et al., 1991; Skjønsberg et al., 1991) and BCGF (Wörmann et al., 1987; Findley et al., 1990; Skjønsberg et al., 1991).

With respect to the modulation of drug resistance, we observed that the growth factors enhanced the cytotoxicity of cytarabine and thioguanine in most patient samples. A significant enhancement of the cytotoxicity of thioguanine was induced by IL-3 and IL-7, and that of cytarabine by IL-7. The reason for this enhanced cytotoxicity is not clear from this study. It is generally attributed to the recruitment of non-proliferating cells into cycle. However, other speculative effects of growth factors, e.g. on the expression on apoptosis-regulatory oncoproteins, may play a role. In this respect it is of interest that the cytotoxicity of prednisolone was more frequently decreased in case of co-incubation with growth factor. Similarly, a decreased cytotoxicity of cytarabine was occasionally observed. Similarly, it has been reported that IL-4 protected mouse thymocytes from dexamethasone-induced cell death by apoptosis (Migliorati et al., 1993). Koistinen et al. (1991) reported that IL-3 and granulocyte-macrophage

Fig. 1. Examples of the effect of growth factors on the cytotoxicity of drugs on ALL cells in individual samples. Top: enhanced cytoxicity of cytarabine by IL-3; bottom: decreased cytotoxicity of prednisolone by IL-7

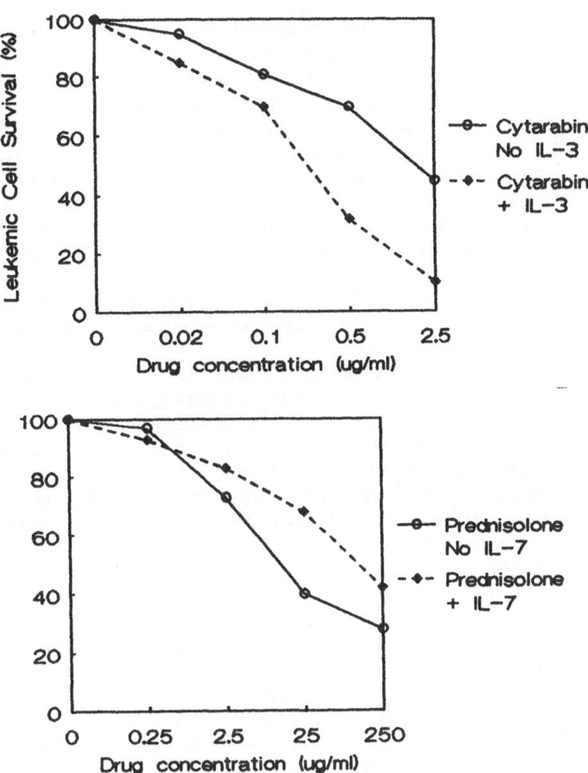

Table 2. Effect of growth factors on drug resistance of ALL cells (n = 17)

	IL-3	IL-7	BCGF
Cytarabine			
Sensitization Index			
median	1.0	1.1	1.0
range	0.3–7.4	0.4–31.3	0.5–7.4
P-value	0.93	0.04	0.58
Thioguanine			
Sensitization Index			
median	1.2	1.6	1.2
range	0.8–9.3	1.0–27.0	0.6–11.6
P-value	0.03	0.005	0.13
Prednisolone			
Sensitization Index			
median	1.0	1.0	0.8
range	0.3–8.1	0.01–50.0	0.1–10.9
P-value	1.0	0.17	0.14

colony-stimulating factor decreased cytarabine cytotoxicity in some patient acute myeloid leukemia samples, even when the cells were actively synthesizing DNA.

We conclude that the MTT assay can be used to study the effects of growth factors on cell survival and drug resistance of ALL cells. IL-3, IL-7 and BCGF increased ALL cell survival in nearly all samples tested. The cytotoxicity of thioguanine and cytarabine was enhanced by these growth factors in most ALL samples. However, a decreased cytotoxicity of cytarabine was seen in some samples, while a decreased cytotoxicity of prednisolone after exposure of the ALL cells to growth factors was seen in most cases. The results of this type of in vitro studies could be useful in the design of clinical trials in ALL in which growth factors are applied.

References

1. Eder M, Ottmann OG, Hansen-Hagge TE, Bartram CR, Gillis S, Hoelzer D, Ganser A. Effects of human IL-7 on blast cell proliferation in acute lymphoblastic leukemia. Leukemia 1990, 4: 533–540
2. Estrov Z, Estey EH, Andreeff M, Talpaz M, Kurzrock R, Reading CL, Deisseroth AB, Gutterman JU. Comparison of in vivo and in vitro effects of granulocyte-macrophage colony-stimu-

lating factor (GM-CSF) in patients with acute myeoid leukemia. Exp Hematol 1992, 20: 558–564
3. Findley Jr HW, Zhou M, Davis R, Abdul-Rahim Y, Hnath R, Ragab AH. Effects of low molecular weight B-cell growth factor on proliferation of leukemic cells from children with B-cell precursor-acute lymphoblastic leukemia. Blood 1990, 75: 951–957
4. Kaspers GJL, Pieters R, Van Zantwijk CH, De Laat PAJM, De Waal FC, Van Wering ER, Veerman AJP. In vitro drug sensitivity of normal peripheral blood lymphocytes and childhood leukaemic cells from bone marrow and peripheral blood. Br J Cancer 1991, 64: 469–474
5. Koistinen P, Wang C, Curtis JE, McCulloch EA. Granulocyte-macrophage colony-stimulatingfactor and interleukin-3 protect leukemic blast cells from ara-C toxicity. Leukemia 1991, 5: 789–795
6. Migliorati G, Nicoletti I, Pagliacci MC, D'Adamio L, Riccardi C. Interleukin-4 protects double-negative and CD4 single-positive thymocytes from dexamethasone-induced apoptosis. Blood 1993, 81: 1352–1358
7. Mosmann T. Rapid colorimetric assay for cellular growth and survival: Application to proliferation and cytotoxicity assays. J Immunol Methods 1983, 65: 55–63
8. O'Connor R, Cesano A, Lange B, Finan J, Nowell PC, Clark SC, Raimondi SC, Rovera G, Santoli D. Growth factor requirements of childhood acute T-lymphoblastic leukemia: Correlation between presence of chromosomal abnormalities and ability to grow permanently in vitro. Blood 1991, 77: 1534–1545
9. Pieters R, Huismans DR, Leyva A, Veerman AJP. Adaptation of the rapid automated tetrazolium dye based MTT assay for chemosensitivity testing in childhood leukemia. Cancer Lett 1988, 41: 323–332
10. Pieters R, Loonen AH, Huismans DR, Broekema GJ, Dirven MWJ, Heyenbrok MW, Hählen K, Veerman AJP. In vitro sensitivity of cells from children with leukemia using the MTT assay with improved culture conditions. Blood 1990, 76: 2327–2336
11. Skjønsberg C, Erikstein BK, Smeland EB, Lie SO, Funderud S, Beiske K, Blomhoff HK. Interleukin-7 differentiates a subgroup of acute lymphoblastic leukemias. Blood 1991, 77: 2445–2550
12. Touw I, Pouwels K, Van Agthoven T, Van Gurp R, Budel L, Hoogerbrugge H, Delwel R, Goodwin R, Namen A, Löwenberg B. Interleukin-7 is a growth factor of precursor B and T acute lymphoblastic leukemia. Blood 1990, 75: 2097–2101
13. Uckun FM, Gesner TG, Song CW, Myers DE, Mufosn A. Leukemic B-cell precursors express functional receptors for human interleukin-3. Blood 1989, 73: 533–542
14. Veerman AJP, Pieters R. Drug sensitivity assays in leukaemia and lymphoma. Br J Haematol 1990, 74: 381–384
15. Wörmann B, Mehta SR, Maizel AL, LeBien TW. Low molecular weight B cell growth factor induces proliferation of human B cell precursor acute lymphoblastic leukemias. Blood 1987, 70: 132–138

Acute Leukemias V
Experimental Approaches
and Management of Refractory Diseases
Hiddemann et al. (Eds.)

The Experience of Polish Children's Leukemia Lymphoma Study Group on G-CSF and GM-CSF Interventional Use in Neutropenia Associated with Chemotherapy of Childhood Acute Lymphoblastic Leukemia (ALL)

A. Chybicka[7], J. Boguslawska-Jaworska[7], J. Armata[1], W. Balwierz[1], K. Boruczkowski[3], J. Kowalczyk[2], M. Matysiak[4], M. Ochocka[5], U. Radwańska[3], and D. Sonta-Jakimczyk[3]

Abstract. The aim of this study was to determine a clinical efficacy and tolerance of G and GM-CSF in children with neutropenia and infectious complications, associated with chemotherapy of ALL. Total number of 38 courses of G (25) and GM-CSF (13) were applied in 29 children aged from 1–14 years, 17 boys and 12 girls. Twenty children with ALL served as historical control group. GM-CSF Leucomax Sandoz was given at dose 5 μg/kg, G-CSF Filgrastim Hoffman la Roche at dose 5–12 μg/kg daily sc. until the neutrocyte count reached at least 10×10^9/l for two consecutive days. Duration of therapy ranged from 2–16 days with median 6 days. The duration of granulocytopenia <500/mm^3 before cytokines therapy ranged from 3–16 days with median 5 days.

The mean and median numbers of total WBC, neutrophilis, monocytes and eosinophils increased after both G and GM-CSF therapy. The median time to neutropenic recovery was shorter in group of children treated with cytokines than in children from historical control group (4 vs. 14.5 days). Also shorter median time of febrile days in comparison with control group was observed (1 vs. 4 days). No significant differences between G and GM-CSF group were observed. All children tolerated cytokines treatment well. Our study have demonstrated a good efficacy of G and GM-CSF in reduction of the number of neutropenic and febrile days associated with chemotherapy of ALL.

Introduction

Modern intensive multi-drug chemotherapy and radiotherapy for children with ALL has significantly increased long-term event free survival EFS to 80% at 10 years [8, 26]. The myelotoxicity of these treatment, however, results in a substantial morbidity related primarily to infectious complications. Risk of infection is related to both the degree and length of neutropenia [6, 20, 28].

The increasing availability of molecularly cloned hematopoietic growth factors for clinical applications is one of the exciting recent developments in oncology [3, 18, 19]. A number of CSF and interleukins are being tested in patients with variety of conditions associated with bone marrow failure of different etiology including neutropenia associated with chemotherapy [2, 7, 11, 13, 15, 29].

Although the use of GM-CSF and G-CSF is becoming relatively widespread, the art and full potential of the utilization of these agents in children has not been completely defined yet [5, 10, 16, 26].

[1]Department of Children Hematology, Polish American Children's Hospital, M. Copernicus Institute of Pediatrics, Krakow, Poland
[2]Department of Children Hematology, Institute of Pediatrics, Faculty of Medicine, Lublin, Poland
[3]Department of Children Hematology and Oncology, Faculty of Medicine, Poznan, Poland
[4]Department of Children Hematology and Oncology, Faculty of Medicine, Warsaw, Poland
[5]Department of Children Hematology, Faculty of Medicine, Warsaw, Poland
[6]Department of Children Hematology and Oncology, Faculty of Medicine, Zabrze, Poland
[7]Department of Children Hematology and Oncology, Faculty of Medicine, Wroclaw, Poland

Aim of Study

The aim of this study was to determine a clinical efficacy and tolerance of G and GM-CSF in children with neutropenia and infectious complications, associated with chemotherapy of ALL.

Material and Methods

Patients. Total number of 29 children with ALL aged from 2–17 years, 17 boys and 12 girls were included to the study. Twenty children with ALL served as historical control group.

The ALL children were treated according to BFM 86 protocols for low risk group LRG and middle risk group MRG [25]. Children with ALL high risk group HRG were treated according to New York protocol. Children with ALL, relapse were treated according to BFM 85 relapse protocol.

Total number of 38 courses included G-CSF Filgrastim (Amgen Hoffman la Roche) (25 courses) and GM-CSF Leucomax (Sandoz) (13 courses). CSFs were applied during granulo cytopenic period after aggressive chemo and radiotherapy complicated with life threatening infection in children with ALL.

Clinical characteristics of children are presented in Tables 1 (Leucomax), 2 (Filgrastim) and 3 (control group).

Clinical and laboratory monitoring. The evaluations included regularly assessment of vital signs, physical examinations, and tests of hepatic and renal functions. Complete blood counts and differential counts were performed at least once daily during the whole period of the therapy.

Studydesign. GM-CSF-Leucomax Sandoz Schering Plough was given at dose 5 μg/kg/day, G-CSF Filgrastim Hoffman la Roche at dose 5–12 μg/kg daily sc. until the neutrocyte count reached at least 10×10^9/l for two consecutive days. Duration of therapy ranged from 2–16 days with median 6 days. The duration of granulocytopenia <500/mm3 before cytokines therapy ranged from 3–20 days with median 5 days. The time from the end of chemotherapy ranged from 2 to 14 with median 5.

Results

The results obtained in children with ALL treated with Filgrastim and Leucomax are separately presented in Table 4. The mean and median

ıble 1. clinical characteristics of children treated with GM-CSF (Leucomax) during neutropenia asociated with ALL ıemotherapy

No.	Initials	Age years	Sex	Diagnosis	cytokine dose/day	uration of therpy days	uration of febrile days	days to neutrocyte recovery
	A.P.	2	f	ALL-L G remission	75 g	7	2	6
	C.	2.5	m	ALL-M G remission	100 g	16	2	4
	P.	7	m	ALL-M G remission	100 g	5	0	4
	M.	7	f	ALL-M G remission	100g	4	0	–
	S.	5	f	ALL-M G remission	90 g	4	3	3
	C.	9	m	ALL-G remission	200 g	4	3	4
						5	3	3
	P.	12	m	ALL-G remission	150 g	13	0	1
						12	0	1
						10	0	1
						7	0	1
	S.	11	m	ALL relapse	120 g	8	7	7
	S.	8	m	ALL relapse	200 g	2	0	2
ıean		7.06				7.46	1.54	2.29
ıedian		7				7	0	2.5

no neutrocyte recover

Table 2. Clinical characteristics of children treated with G-CSF (Filgrastim) during neutropenia associated with ALL chemotherapy

P.N.	Initials	Age years	Sex	Diagnosis	Cytokine dose/day	Duration of therapy days	Duration of febrile days	Days to neutro-cyte recovery
1.	G.P.	3	f	ALL-LRG I remission	75 µg	2	1	2
2.	K.P.	8	m	ALL-LRG I remission	250 µg	12	4	12
3.	H.Sz.	5	f	ALL-MRG I remission	120 µg	6	2	5
4.	L.J.	6	f	ALL-MRG I remission	80 µg	5	3	4
5.	S.K.	5	f	ALL-MRG I remission	200 µg	16	10	15
6.	R.N.	6	m	ALL-MRG I remission	100 µg	10	0	10
7.	D.S.	4	m	ALL-MRG I remission	100 µg	11	6	10
8.	P.P.	7	m	ALL-MRG I remision	210 µg	7	0	5
9.	O.P.	3	f	ALL-MRG I remision	110 µg	2	0	2
10.	J.M.	3	f	ALL-MRG I remission	95 µg	4	0	4
					100 µg	3	0	3
11.	S.E.	10	f	ALL-MRG I remission	240 µg	6	0	6
12.	M.P.	4	m	ALL-HRG I remission	100 µg	6	1	5
						7	3	6
						2	0	2
						4	0	3
13.	W.D.	5	m	ALL-HRG I remission	160 µg	2	0	2
14.	W.M.	17	m	ALL-HRG I remission	200 µg	4	0	3
15.	K.K.	7	f	ALL relapse	180 µg	5	3	5
16.	K.Sz.	8	m	ALL relapse	200 µg	4	2	4
17.	Cz.D.	6	m	ALL relapse	210 µg	6	4	6
						4	0	4
18.	N.P.	7	f	ALL relapse	100 µg	5	1	5
19.	R.K.	8	m	ALL relapse	200 µg	7	1	7
20.	G.J.	13	m	ALL relapse	235 µg	4	0	4
mean		6.75				5.76	1.64	5.36
median		6				5	1	5

Table 3. Clinical characteristics of children with ALL in the control group

P.N.	Initials	Age years	Sex	Diagnosis	Duration of febrile days	Days to neutro-cyte recovery
1.	L.	6	m	ALL-LG remission	0	12
2.	S.	10	m	ALL-LG remission	3	9
3.	P.	9	m	ALL-MG remission	6	24
4.	..	2	m	ALL-MG remission	0	5
5.	M.G.	8	f	ALL-MG remission	3	7
6.	..	2	m	ALL-MG remission	0	5
7.	M.	7	f	ALL-MG remission	3	11
8.	G.	13	m	ALL-G remission	1	13
9.	G.	8	f	ALL-G remission	12	14
10.	..	11	m	ALL-G remission	7	14
11.	..	10	m	ALL-G remission	3	8
12.	A.G.	8	f	ALL-G remission	5	14
13.	P.	4	m	ALL-G remission	3	5
14.	P.	2	m	ALL relapse	3	8
15.	S.	16	m	ALL relapse	7	14
16.	S.	5	m	ALLrelapse	9	14
17.	A.L.	12	m	ALLrelapse	6	14
18.	T.S.	11	m	ALLrelapse	7	17
19.	S.P.	14	f	ALL relapse	19	21
20.	S.S.	14	m	ALL relapse	13	19
mean		8.6			5.5	12.4
median		8.5			4	13.5

Table 4. Results of G and GM-CSF therapy in children with ALL

Type of cytokine	Number of cycles	Values	Leukocyte count/mm³		Neutrophile count/mm³		Monocyte count/mm³		Eosinophile count/mm³		Platelet count/mm³	
			before therapy	day after	before therapy	day after	before therapy	day after	before therapy	day after	before therapy	day after
G-CSF	25	mean	575.0	4502.5	39.3	2681.1	12.3	334.6	29.0	226.3	42.6	84.4
Filgrastim		median	600.0	4100.0	0.0	2137.5	0.0	317.5	0.0	28.0	37.0	92.5
GM-CSF	13	mean	791.7	4604.2	131.7	2533.1	10.6	271.3	2.5	32.6	61.6	73.0
Leucomax		median	700.0	3950.0	30.0	1760.0	0.0	84.0	0.0	10.0	31.5	51.0

numbers of total WBCs, mature neutrophils, neutrophilic bands and eosinophils consistently increased during both G and GM-CSF administration. In both groups the greatest percentage increase in the neutrophil lineage was noticed between 2–15 days (Fig. 1 and 2). The median time to neutropenic recovery was shorter in group of children treated with GM-CSF than

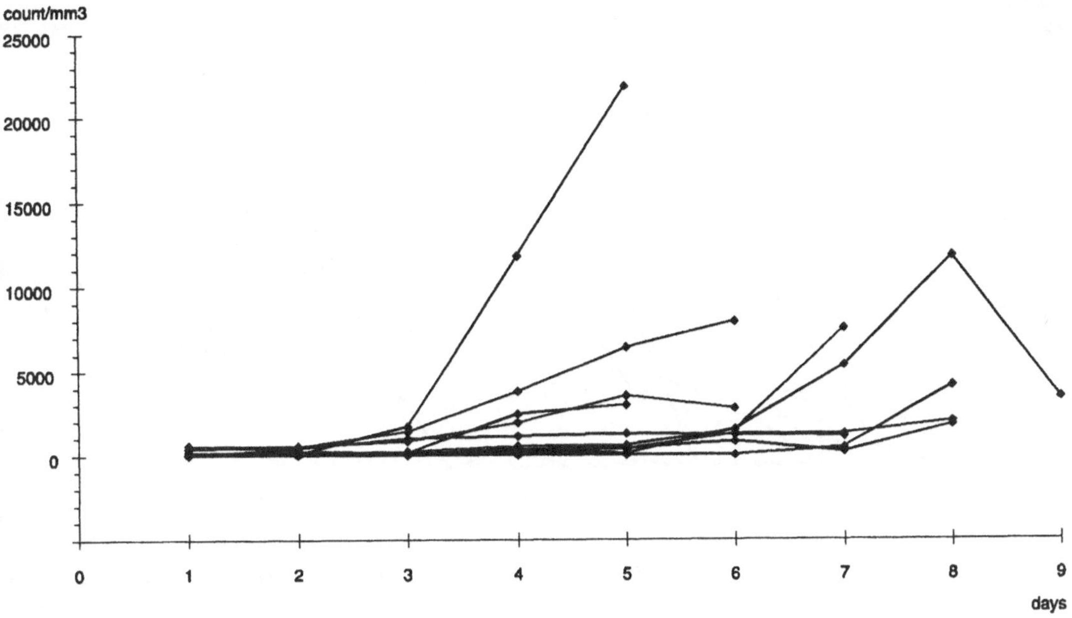

Fig. 1. Individual neutrophile count in children with ALL treated with GM-CSF (Leucomax)

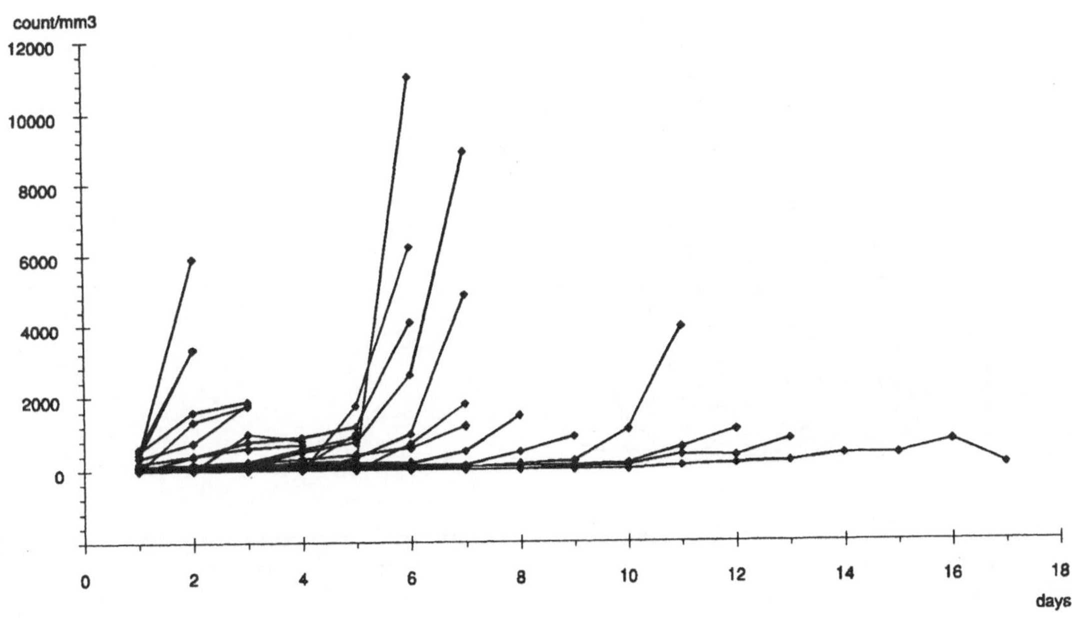

Fig. 2. Individual neutrophile count in children with ALL treated with G-CSF (Filgrastim)

with G-CSF and that in children from historical control group (2,5 days v 5 days v 13,5 days) (Table 1 and 2). Also consistent increase in the monocyte lineage was observed (Fig. 3 and 4).

In 9/11 children treated with G-CSF and in 4/7 treated with GM-CSF signs of infection disappeared even before granulocyte count increased. Also shorter median time of febrile days in com-

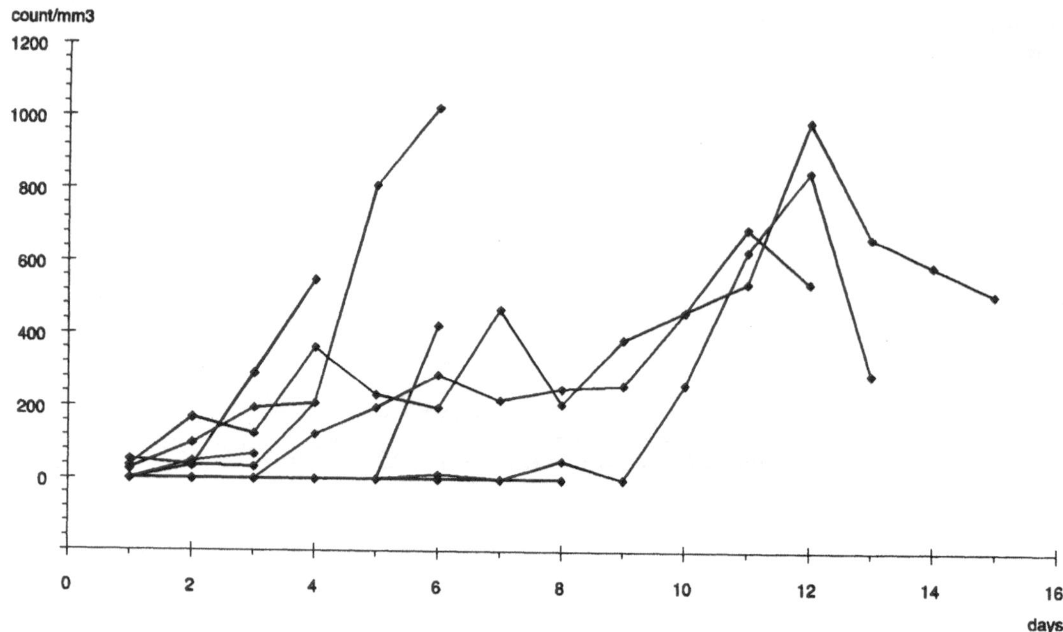

Fig. 3. Individual monocyte count in children with ALL treated with GM-CSF (Leucomax)

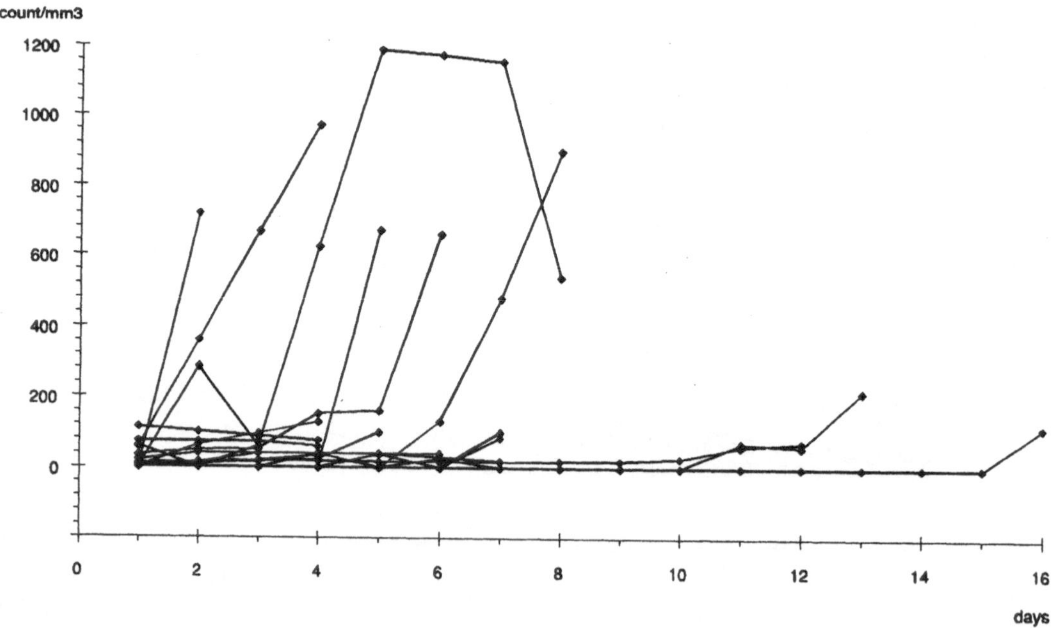

Fig. 4. Individual monocyte count in children with ALL treated with G-CSF (Filgrastim)

parison with control group was observed (GM-CSF-0 days vs. G-CSF-1 day vs. 4 days control group).

No serious side effects during cytokines therapy were noticed. In one patient local erythema in injection place was observed.

Discussion

The present study was designed to investigate a clinical efficacy and tolerance of GM-CSF and G-CSF in children with neutropenia associated with chemotherapy of ALL. Our results showed that both rh GM-CSF and G-CSF administered after chemotherapy in children with ALL produced increase of absolute neutrophils count and decreased severity and duration of infections.

This good results could be explained by stimulation with G and G-CSF of neutrophile proli feration and differentiation. In addition to its hematopoietic properties GM and G-CSF amplifies several important functions of mature leukocytes including the oxidative burst, adhesion, phagocytosis, degranulation and lipid mediator synthesis, in response to second signals of neutrophil [1, 4, 12, 23]. It is now established that neutrophile upon G and GM-CSF stimulation synthetize many important macromolecules including cytokines such as IL-1, IL-6, IL-8 [25].

Similar beneficial results of G and GM-CSF on neutrophile recovery in patients with granulocytopenia after chemotherapy were described by many authors [14, 16, 17, 21, 24, 27, 30].

In our study no serious side effects during cytokines therapy were noticed. In one patient local erythema in injection place was observed, however other studies showed serious side effects such as capillary leak syndrome [9].

The treatment with cytokines (GM-CSF and G-CSF) did not appear to compromise the ALL response rate. Ode and cow. have found using both DNA synthesis and clonogenic assays that G and GM-CSF did not stimulate the growth of leukemic BM cells from children with ALL [22] while stimulate AML cells [14]. Nevertheless larger number of patients and longer follow-up time are essential for drawing the proper conclusions in this aspect.

Conclusions

Our study have demonstrated a clear reduction of the number of febrile days, reduced incidence and shorter duration of bone marrow suppression, a decreased frequency of infectious complications.

Acknowledgement. The work was supported by grant no 4 0961 91 01.

References

1. Aglietta M., Felice L.D., Stacchini A., Petti M.C., Bianci A.C.M., Spiriti M.A., Sanavio F.C., Piacibello W., Apra F., Stern A.C, Gavosto F., Mandelli F. (1991) In vivo effect of granulocyte-macrophage colony stimulating factor on the kinetics of human acute myeloid leukemia cells. Leukemia, 5, 11: 979–984
2. Antman K.S., Griffin J.D., Elias A., Socinski M.A., Ryan L., Cannistra S.A., Oete D., Whitley M., Frei E., Schnipeper L.E., (1989) Effect of rh GM CSF on chemotherapy induced myelosuppresion. N Eng J Med, 319, 593–598
3. Asano S. Human granulocyte-colony stimulating factors: Its basic aspects and clinical applications. (1991) Amer. J Ped Hematol/Oncol. 13, 4 400–413
4. Azakami S., Eguchi M.,(1993) Ultrastructural and ultracytochemical alteration of rat neutrophils induced by G-CSF. Eur. J. Hematol. 51; 166–172
5. Borsi J.D., Ferencz T., Csaki C., Schuler D., (1992) Clinical pharmacological perspectives with use of hematopoietic growth factors in children with malignant diseases. The role of Clin. Pharmacol. in Ped. Oncol edd. Ricardi, Borsi, 68–77.
6. Bronchud M. (1992) Can haematopoietic growth factors be use to improve the success of cytotoxic chemotherapy? Anti-Cancer Drug, 4, 127–139
7. Büchner T., Hiddemann W., Koenigsmann M., Zühlsdorf M., Wörmann B., Boeckman A., Freire E.A., Inning G., Maschmeyer G., Ludwig W.D., Sauerland M.C., Heinecke A., Schultz G., (1991) Recombinant human granulocyte-macrophage colony stimulating factor after chemotherapy in patients with acute myeloid leukemia at higher age after relapse. Blood, 78, 1190–1197.
8. Demetri G.D., Morgan R., Mamaounas E. (1993) Progress in the delivery of high-dose chemothe rapy with haematopoietic support. Oncol. Review, 8, 2, 10–11
9. Emminger W., Emminger-Schmidmeier W., Peters Ch., Susani M., Hawliczek R., Hocker P., Gadner H., (1990) Capillary leak syndrome during low dose granulocyte macrophage colony-stimulating factor (rh GM-CSF) treatment of a patient in a continuous febrile state. Blood , 61, 219–221
10. Furman W.L., Crist W.M. (1991) Potential uses of recombinant human granulocyte-macrophage colony-stimulating factor in children. Am. J. Ped. Heamatol/Oncol. , 13, 4, 388–399
11. Gulati S.C., Bennet C.L. (1992) GM-CSF as adjunct therapy in relapsed Hodgkin's disease. J. Ann. Intern. Med. 1992, 16, 3, 177–182

12. Hamilton J.A. (1993) Colony stimulating factors, cytokines and monocyte-macrophages-some controversies. Immunol. Today, 14, 1, 18–23
13. Ho A., Del Valle F., Engelhard M. (1990), Mitoxantrone/high dose Ara C and rh GM-CSF in the treatment of refractory non-Hodgkin's lymphoma. Cancer 66, 423–430
14. Ishikawa I.,Yoshimura M., Matsunashi T., Tominaga N., Ashima N., Hiaroka A., Nakamura H., Shibata H., Masaoka T., Takaku U. (1991) Clinical effect of granulocyte colony-stimulating factor on neutrophils and leukemic cells in myelogenous leukemia. Jpn. J. Clin.Oncol., 21, 3, 169–175
15. Lanino E., Prasole R., Garaveta A., (1991) Treatment of poor risk neuroblastoma with intensive chemotherapy and rh GM-CSF. Ann. Hematol., 62, 6, 115
16. Linch D.C. (1993) Assessment of haematopoietic growth factors in clinical trials. Granulocyte reports, I, 2, 2–3
17. Mertelsmann R.,Kanz L. (1993) Hematopoietic growth factors in cancer chemotherapy. Handbook of chemotherapy ed. Cvitkoviæ, Droz, Armand, Khooury, 1–6
18. Metcalf D. The colony stimulating factors. (1990) Discovery, development and clinical applications. Cancer, 65, 2185–2194
19. Moore M.A.S. (1991). The future of cytokine combination therapy. Cancer, 67, 2718–2726
20. Morstyn G. (1992) Recommendations for the successful integration of recombinant G-CSF into current clinical practice in oncology. Clinician, 10, 2, 61–69
21. Neidhardt J.A. (1992) Hematopoietic colony stimulating factors. Uses in combination with standard chemotherapeutic regimens and support of dose intensification. Cancer, 70, 913–920.
22. Ode D.L., Zhou M., Findley H.W., Abdel-Mageed A., Ragab A.H. (1992) The effect of recombinant GM-CSF and G-CSF on the bone Marrow cells of children with acute lymphoblastic leukemia. Leukemia, 6, 1210–1211.
23. Ohsaka A., Saioni K., Sato N., Mori T, Ishimoto K, Inamatsu T., (1993) Granulocyte colony stimulating factor down regulates the surface expression of the human leukocyte adhesion molecule-1 on human neutrophils in vitro and in vivo. Brit. J. Hematol., 84, 574–580
24. Ottmann O.G., Ganser A., Freund M., Heil G., Hiddemann W., Heit W., Gracien E., Hoelzer D. (1993) Simultaneous administration of granulocyte colony stimulating factor (Filgrastim) and induction chemotherapy in acute lymphoblastic leukemia. Ann. Hematol., 67; 161–167.
25. Pouliot M., McDonald P., Khamzina L., Borgeat P., McColl R. (1994) GM-CSF enhances 5-Lipooxygenase levels in human polymorphonuclear leukocytes. J. Immunol. 152, 851 – 857
26. Riehm H., Gadner H., Henze G., Konhuber B., Lampert F., Niethammer D., Reiter A., Schellong G. (1990): Results and significance of six randomized trials in four consecutive ALL-BFM studies. In. Acute Leukemia's II Hem Blood Trans., Ed. Büchner T.,Schellong G., Hiddemann W., Ritter J. 33: 439–450.
27. Saarinen U.M., Hovi L., Riikonen P., Pihkala J., Juvonen E. (1992) Recombinant human granulocyte-macrophage colony stimulating factor in children with chemotherapy -induced neutropenia. Med. Ped. Oncol., 20, 489–496
28. Tesch H. (1993) HGF use in solid tumors and hematopoietic malignancies. Granulocyte reports I, 4, 8–10.
29. Trillet-Lenoir V., Green J., Manegold C., Pavel J., Gatzemeier B., Depierre A., Johnson P., Decoster G., Tomita D., Ewen C. (1993) Recombinant Granulocyte colony stimulating factor reduces the infectious complications of cytotoxic chemotherapy. Eur. J. Cancer, 29A, 3, 319–324
30. Wardrop C.A.J., Holland B. (1992) Hematopoietic growth factors. Current Opinion in Pediatrics, 4, 84–91

Acute Leukemias V
Experimental Approaches
and Management of Refractory Diseases
Hiddemann et al. (Eds.)

Induction Therapy with Idarubicin, Ara-C, and VP-16, Followed by G-CSF and Maintenance Immunotherapy with Interleukin-2 for High-Risk AML

A. Ganser[1], G. Heil[2], G. Seipelt[1], J. Th. Fischer[3], W. Langer[4], W. Brockhaus[5], K. Kolbe[6], T. H. Ittel[7], N. Brack[8], H. G. Fuhr[9], L. Bergmann[1], and D. Hoelzer[1]

Abstract. Aggressive chemotherapy followed by administration of G-CSF and maintenance therapy with interleukin-2 was evaluated in 16 patients with advanced myelodxysplastic syndrome, 47 patients with AML evolving from myelodysplastic syndromes, 3 patients with subacute myeloid leukemia and 5 patients with secondary AML. Median age was 59 years (range: 23 to 76 years). All patients achieving a complete remission (CR) after two induction courses went on to receive two consolidation courses, to be followed by randomization to either high-dose or low-dose IL-2 to evaluate the potential of IL-2 to eliminate residual leukemic cells and to prolong the duration of CR. Patients ≤ age 55 with an HLA identical sibling donor subsequently proceeded to allogeneic bone marrow transplantation. Sixty-eight of 71 patients are evaluluable on the chemotherapy arm. Thirty-one patients (46%) achieved a complete remission, 7 patients (10%) a partial remission, while 24 patients (35%) were treatment failures. Early death occurred in 6 pts (9%). Three patients with CR and 3 with PR underwent allogeneic bone marrow transplantation. Until now, 12 patients were randomized to receive four cycles of IL-2 treatment, either 9×10^6 or 0.9×10^6 IU/m^2/day IV, days 1–5 and 8–12. Eight patients relapsed, 6 prior to IL-2 maintenance therapy, and 2 after IL-2. Median relapse-free survival was 11 months. We conclude that aggressive chemotherapy with idarubicin/ara-C/VP-16 followed by G-GSF is both effective and well tolerated with a low rate of early death when compared to published trials without growth factor support, while the assessment of IL-2 treatment warrants additional patient accrual and longer follow-up.

Introduction

The use of multi-agent chemotherapy for patients with myelodysplastic syndromes (MDS) in transformation to acute myeloid leukemia (AML) or with AML that has evolved from MDS or has occurred after previous cytotoxic chemotherapy has generally been less effective than for patients with de novo AML (reviewed in [1,2]). Complete remission (CR) rates are lower and treatment-related deaths, especially from infections during prolonged neutropenia, are more frequent than in patients with primary AML. In addition, the duration of CR is shorter than 12 months in patients with these adverse subtypes of AML and thereby lower than in patients with de novo AML.

[1]Medizinische Klinik III, Klinikum der Universität Frankfurt
[2]Medizinische Klinik III, Klinikum der Universität Ulm
[3]II. Medizinische Klinik; Städtisches Klinikum Karlsruhe
[4]Abteilung für Hämatologie-Onkologie, Ev. Krankenhaus Essen-Werden
[5]2. Medizinische Klinik, Klinikum Nürnberg
[6]Abteilung für Hämatologie, III. Medizinische Klinik der Universität Mainz
[7]Medizinische Klinik II, Klinikum der RWTH Aachen
[8]Abteilung für Hämatologie-Onkologie, München-Harlaching
[9]Medizinische Klinik B, Klinikum Wiesbaden

Recent trials in elderly patients with high-risk AML have demonstrated that the rate of infection-related deaths during induction therapy can be reduced by using hematopoietic growth factors to accelerate of hematopoietic recovery [3,4]. In addition, treatment of AML patients with interleukin-2 (IL-2) has resulted in the induction of an anti-leukemic immune response and elimination of overt leukemic cells [5,6,7]. We have therefore initiated a phase III trial of aggressive chemotherapy followed by rescue with G-CSF in patients with high-risk AML. Patients achieving a complete remission are then randomly assigned to achieve either high-dose or low-dose IL-2 to further eliminate residual leukemic cells and thereby to prolong the duration of CR. The present report underscores the feasability of this therapeutic approach which had already been apparent at an early interim analysis [8].

Patients and Treatment Protocol

From January 1992 until December 1993, 71 patients with refractory anemia in transformation to acute leukemia (RAEB-T), subacute leukemia (stable clinical course for more than three months), AML evolving from MDS, or AML secondary to previous cytotoxic chemotherapy were entered into this study. The diagnosis was established by examination of blood and bone marrow aspirate and trephine biopsies.

The chemotherapy regimen for induction consisted of cytosine-arabinoside (ara-C) as a continuous IV infusion at a daily dose of 100 mg/m² for 7 days, idarubicin administered as IV bolus at 10 mg/m² days 1, 2, and 3, and VP-16 as 1-hour infusion at 100 mg/m² on days 3 to 7 (Table 1). Two early consolidation courses consisted of ara-C, 100 mg/m² CIVI, days 1–5, idarubicin, 10 mg/m² IV, days 1 and 2, and VP-16, 100 mg/m² IV, days 1–5. A late consolidation course included amsacrine, 60 mg/m², administered by IV bolus injection on days 1–5, and ara-C at a dose of 600 mg/m² as 2-hour infusion every 12 hours on days 1–5.

After each course of chemotherapy, patients received G-CSF until recovery of granulocyte counts. Starting 4–6 weeks after the late consolidation course, patients were randomized to four cycles of either high dose (9×10^6 IU/m²) or low-dose (0.9×10^6 IU/m²) recombinant interleukin-2 (rIL-2, provided by Hoffmann-LaRoche) as 1-hour infusion on days 1–5 and 7–13 [7]. Cycles were repeated at 6-week intervals. Eligible patients (below 55 years of age, HLA-identical donor) received an allogeneic bone marrow transplant after achieving CR or PR.

Table 1. Patient characteristics and treatment results

Number of patients	71 (68 evaluable)
Male/Female	34/37
Age (Years)	
median	59
range	23–76
Diagnoses	
AML after MDS	47
RAEB-T	16
secondary AML	3
subacute AML	5
Results of therapy	
CR	31(46%)
PR	7(10%)
Failure	24(35%)
Early death	6(9%)

Results

Until December 31, 1993, 71 patients have been entered into this study: 34 males and 37 females with a median age of 59 years (range, 23–76 years). The diagnoses and the treatment outcome are listed in Table 1. Thirty-one of the 68 evaluable patients (46%) achieved a complete remission. Seven patients obtained a partial remission after completion of the induction course, resulting in a total response rate of 56%. Twenty-four of the patients (35%) were non-responders, since their bone marrows were still cellular with more than 25% blasts. Early death occurred in only six patient (9%) during induction therapy. Six patients, three in CR and three in PR, underwent allogeneic bone marrow transplantation. In two patients, treatment with IL-2 had to be stopped because of recurrent cardiac arrhythmia, one patient in the high-dose and another one in the low-dose arm.

The median duration of relapse-free survival was 11 months with a median follow-up time in the patients achieving a CR of 11 months (range: 1–20 months). The median duration of continuous complete remission was not yet reached. Eight patients relapsed, six of them before and two after IL-2 maintenance therapy. One relapse each occurred after high-dose and low-dose IL-2.

Discussion

This study was prompted by reports that idarubicin is effective in patients with high-risk AML [9,10] and that the use of hematopoietic growth factors, e.g. G-CSF and GM-CSF, for acceleration of neutrophil recovery will reduce the rate of severe infections and early death [3,4]. The interim results in sixty-eight patients illustrate that the combination of idarubicin, ara-C, and VP-16 is highly effective for remission induction being in the upper range with regard to the rate of complete remission and the median duration of continuous complete remission or relapse free survival of what has been previously observed with other regimens [1,2].

In previous studies of aggressive chemotherapy in a comparable patient population, the rate of early death usually ranged between 20% and 40% [1,2]. Due to this high rate of death during induction therapy, many centers hesitate to treat these patients aggressively, but rather give low-dose chemotherapy or supportive care only. The low rate of early death in our patients which was not higher than in younger patients treated for de novo AML, might be due to the use of G-CSF after each chemotherapy cycle which by accelerating neutrophil recovery would prevent or ameliorate the course of infections, as previously shown by other authors [3,4]. Thus, the low rate of early death makes our protocol a suitable treatment regimen for the mainly elderly patients with high-risk AML.

Since the disease-free survival ranges between 0–20% in this patient population, all non-transplant-eligible CR patients were randomized to receive either high-dose or low-dose rIL-2 to elicit an immune response against minimal residual leukemic blast cells [5–7]. Although twelve patients have already been treated with either high-dose or low-dose IL-2, the results are still too preliminary and will require further follow-up before the value of this approach can be evaluated.

In conclusion, the early data of this treatment schedule suggest that improved treatment results can be obtained in patients with high-risk leukemia. This regimen will therefore allow the evaluation of immunotherapy with rIL-2 in a larger number of patients with high-risk AML who previously would have been excluded from myeloablative chemotherapy protocols.

References

1. Cheson BD. Chemotherapy and bone marrow transplantation for myelodysplastic syndromes. Semin Oncol 19: 85–94, 1992
2. Kantarjian HM, Estey E, Keating MJ. Treatment of therapy-related leukemia and myelodysplastic syndrome. Hematol/Oncol Clin North America 7: 81–107, 1993
3. Büchner T, Hiddemann W, Königsmann M, et al. Recombinant human granulocyte-macrophage colony-stimulating factor after chemotherapy in patients with acute myeloid leukemia at higher age or after relapse. Blood 78: 1190–1197, 1991
4. Ohno R, Tomonaga M, Kobayashi T, et al. Effect of granulocyte colony-stimulating factor after intensive induction therapy in relapsed or refractory acute leukemia. N Engl J Med 323: 871–877, 1990
5. Archimbaud E, Bailly M, Doré JF. Inducibility of lympholine activated killer (LAK) cells in patients with acute myelogenous leukaemia in complete remission and its clinical significance. Br J Haematol 77: 328–334, 1991
6. Foa R, Meloni G, Tosti S, et al. Treatment of acute myeloid leukemia patients with recombinant interleukin 2: a pilot study. Br J Haematol 77: 491–496, 1991
7. Bergmann L. Mitrou PS, Hoelzer D. Interleukin-2 in the treatment of acute myelocytic leukemias: in vitro data and presentation of a clinical concept. Haematol Blood Transfusion 34: 601–607, 1992
8. Ganser A, Heil G, Kolbe K, et al. Aggressive chemotherapy combined with G-CSF and maintenance therapy with interleukin-2 for patients with advanced myelodysplastic syndrome, subacute and secondary acute myeloid leukemia – initial results. Ann Hematol 66: 1234–126, 1993
9. Berman E, Heller G, Santorsa J, et al. Results of a randomized trial comparing idarubicin and cytosine arabinoside with daunorubicine and cytosine-arabinoside in adult patients with newly diagnosed acute myelogenous leukemia. Blood 77: 1666–1674, 1991
10. Carella AM, Berman E, Maraone MP, Ganzina F. Idarubicine in the treatment of acute leukemias. An overview of preclinical and clinical studies. Haematologica 75: 159–169, 1990

Acute Leukemias V
Experimental Approaches
and Management of Refractory Diseases
Hiddemann et al. (Eds.)

Incidence of Infections in Adult Patients (> 55 Years) with Acute Myeloid Leukemia Treated with Yeast-Derived GM-CSF (Sargramostim): Results of a Double-Blind Prospective Study by the Eastern Cooperative Oncology Group

J. M. Rowe[1], A. Rubin[2], J. J. Mazza[3], J. M. Bennett[1], E. Paietta[4], J. W. Anderson[5], R. Ghalie[2], and P. H. Wiernick[4]

Abstract. Between 9/90 and 11/92, the ECOG conducted a double-blind randomized trial of yeast-derived GM-CSF (Sargramostim) versus placebo in 124 patients age > 55–70 with *de novo* acute myeloid leukemia (AML). Induction therapy consisted of 1–2 courses of daunorubicin (60 mg/m²/day, days 1–3) and cytarabine (100 mg/m²/day, days 1–7). Consolidation therapy consisted of one course of high-dose cytarabine (1.5 g/m²/q12h × 12 doses). GM-CSF (250 µg/m²/day) or placebo was started on day 11 of the first course of induction therapy if the bone marrow on day 10 was hypoplastic and with < 5% leukemic cells. If marrow aplasia was not obtained, a second course of induction therapy was given and study drug begun 4 days later if the repeat bone marrow study showed < 5% leukemic cells. Of 117 eligible patients, study drug was given to 99 during induction therapy and to 47 during consolidation therapy. The same study drug given during induction therapy was also given after consolidation therapy. Following induction therapy, the median number of days to reach neutrophils > 500/mm³ and > 1,000/mm³ was shorter by an average of 4 and 7 days, respectively in the GM-CSF group (13 versus 17 days and 14 versus 21 days, $p \leq 0.004$). Patients given GM-CSF had significantly fewer grade 4, 5 infections (9.6% versus 36.2%, $p = 0.002$), fewer fatal infections during and within 30 days of completing study drug (5.8% versus 23.4%, $p = 0.019$), fewer fatal pneumonias (14.3% versus 53.8%, $p = 0.046$) among subjects who contracted a pneumonia, and fewer deaths associated with a fungal infection (1.9% versus 19.1%, $p = 0.006$). Fewer patients given GM-CSF died in the first 180 days of entry onto study (17.3% versus 42.6%, $p = 0.008$). There were no increase in the frequency of resistant or recurrent leukemia and in the incidence of adverse events ascribed to GM-CSF. In conclusion, GM-CSF is safe and effective in older patients undergoing induction therapy for AML and it significantly ameliorates infection rates and complications of infections. Its role in younger patients or in patients with recurrent disease needs to be investigated.

Introduction

Despite recent progress in antimicrobial therapy, infectious complications remain a major problem during the remission induction therapy of acute myeloid leukemia (AML). Severe infections, which occur in 40–80% of patients [1–3], represent a significant cause of morbidity, mortality, and resource utilization. Sepsis and pneumonia are the most common causes of early death following induction therapy, accounting for fatality rates of about 10–40% [4, 5]. The mortality from life-threatening infections is the highest among elderly patients [6–8] or in patients with recurrent or refractory leukemias

[1]University of Rochester Medical Center, Rochester, NY, USA
[2]Immunex Corporation, Seattle, WA, USA
[3]Marshfield Clinic, Marshfield, WI, USA
[4]Montefiore and Albert Einstein Cancer Center, Bronx, NY, USA
[5]Division of Biostatistics, Dana Farber Cancer Institute, Boston , MA, USA

[9, 10]. Because the longer the duration of neutropenia, the greater the risk of infections [11, 12], faster hematological recovery following induction therapy may decrease the risk of severe infections and improve the overall outcome of the therapy. Furthermore, amelioration of infectious complications may also decrease other causes of death due to toxicity, such as bleeding, multi-organ failure, and adult repiratory distress syndrome.

Sargramostim, a yeast-derived granulocyte-colony stimulating factor (GM-CSF), was shown to accelerate hematological recovery after bone marrow transplantation [13, 14] and dose-intensive chemotherapy for solid tumors [15, 16]. The effect of hematopoietic growth factors on hematological recovery following induction therapy for AML has only recently been evaluated. The main reason behind the delay in conducting clinical trials in AML was the concern of the potential for cytokine stimulation of acute leukemia. Nevertheless, small phase I-II studies, mostly conducted in high-risk AML patients, have suggested that cytokines administered after completion of chemotherapy do not adversely affect the response to induction therapy. To evaluate the safety and hematologic effect of GM-CSF in AML, the Eastern Cooperative Oncology Group (ECOG) was the first to conduct a placebo-controlled, double-blind study in adult patients over the age of 55 with *de novo* AML. The overall results of this study are presented elsewhere (Rowe et al, Blood, in press). This report focuses on the effect of GM-CSF on infectous complications and mortality from infections in this patient population.

Material and Methods

Patients. The study was conducted in 25 ECOG participating centers. Eligibility criteria for entry in the study included: 1) morphologic proof of AML (FAB type M0-M7); 2) age greater than 55 but not exceeding 70 years; 3) adequate renal, hepatic, and cardiac function; 4) no previous cytotoxic or radiation therapy; 5) no prior myelodysplasia; and 6) all patients were required to give informed consent prior to registration.

Chemotherapy regimens. Induction therapy consisted of daunorubicin given intravenously at 60 mg/m²/day, days 1 to 3 and cytarabine given intravenously at 25 mg/m² by push on day 1 followed by continuous infusion of 100 mg/m²/day, days 1 to 7. If the bone marrow on day 10 was not severely hypoplastic and revealed 5% or more residual leukemic cells, another identical course of induction chemotherapy was given. Patients achieving a complete remission after one or two courses of induction therapy were to receive a course of consolidation chemotherapy consisting of cytarabine, 1.5 g/m² by one-hour intravenous infusion every 12 hours for a total of 12 doses. Patients failing to achieve a complete remission after two courses of induction chemotherapy were removed from the study but were followed for survival.

Study drug. Patients were registered and randomized to the GM-CSF (Leukine®, Immunex Corporation, Seattle, WA) or placebo arm prior to the initiation of induction chemotherapy. The same study drug given after induction chemotherapy was also given after consolidation therapy. Study drug was started on day 11 of the first cycle of chemotherapy if the day 10 bone marrow was aplastic without residual leukemia. Otherwise, the study drug was withheld and started 3–4 days after completing the second course of induction chemotherapy if the bone marrow at that time was free of residual leukemia. For eligible patients, study drug was also started on day 11 of consolidation therapy. Study drug was given daily by 4-hour infusion until the absolute neutrophil count was >1,500/µL for three consecutive days or for a maximum of 42 days. Study drug was to be immediately discontinued in the presence of leukemic regrowth. The daily dose of GM-CSF was 250 µg/m² and the placebo product was delivered in an equal volume of identically-appearing solution.

Supportive care. A central venous catheter was placed for all patients. All patients with neutropenia received empiric broad spectrum antibiotics for fever >38 °C after appropriate cultures and radiographic studies were obtained. Selection of antibiotics was based on individual institutions policies, but usually consisted of an aminoglycoside and a cephalosporine or semisynthetic penicillin. Vancomycin was added to patients with methicillin-resistant Staphylococcus Epidermidis. Patients with documented fungal infections or with persistant unexplained fever received intravenous amphotericin B at a dose of 0.5–1.0 mg/kg/day. Patients with history of Herpex Simplex infection or who were sero-positive for Herpes Simplex were to be given Acyclovir prophylaxis (250 mg/m² IV TID) for 14 days.

Parameters evaluated. Complete remission was defined as a normocellular marrow containing less than 5% blasts and peripheral blood counts demonstrating no circulating blasts, neutrophils of greater than 1,500/µL, and platelets of greater than 100,000/µL. In order to obtain a uniform start-up time for evaluation of hematological recovery, this latter was measured from day 11 of the last cycle of induction therapy to the day of recovery. Treatment toxicity was graded by the NCI Common Toxicity Criteria. Using this scale, a grade 3 infection was characterized as a severe infection requiring intravenous antibiotics or antifungal therapy and a grade 4 infection was characterized as a life-threatening or disseminated multi-organ infection.

Statistical analysis. The sample size for the study was calculated to provide an 80% power to detect a 7–9 day reduction in the median duration of neutropenia. Univariate differences between dichotomous variables (infection rates, toxicity rates, deaths) were evaluated with Fisher's Exact Test. Survival curves were estimated by the method of Kaplan and Meier and comparisons between treatment made with the log-rank test. Survival was measured from day 1 of randomization and data were last updated in March 1995. Hematologic recovery times were compared with a standard stratified log-rank test where cases who died without recovery are censored. Analyses were computed using SAS, version 6.08 (SAS Institute, Gary , NC).

Results

Patient characteristics and drug assignment. Between September 1990 and November 1992, 124 patients were randomized into the study, 62 in each treatment arm. Seven patients were ineligible or non-evaluable after randomization for the following reasons: prior chemotherapy (one patient), no follow-up (two patients), and unconfirmed diagnosis (four patients). The median age of the study population was 64 years. The characteristics at presentation of the 117 evaluable patients were not significantly different between the two groups (Table 1). Of the 117 eligible patients, 18 did not receive study drug because of early death (14 patients), failure to achieve aplasia (3 patients), and treating physician's decision (1 patient). Thus 99 patients received study drug during induction. Thirteen of the 62 patients achieving a complete remission did not receive consolidation therapy, eight for medical reasons, four because of no follow-up, and one patient refusal. Two of the 49 patients receiving consolidation therapy were not given study drug (one death and one medical exclusion). Thus, 47 patients received study

Table 1. Characteristics of the 117 eligible patients

Characteristics	Level	GM-CSF n = 60	Placebo n = 57	Total (%)
Age	56–65	40	44	84(72)
	66–70	20	13	33(18)
ECOG Performance status	0–1	49	46	95(81)
	>1	11	11	22(19)
Bone marrow blasts	≤80%	42	41	83(71)
	>80%	18	16	34(29)
Circulating WBC	≤50,000/mm³	33	25	58(50)
	>50,000/mm³	27	32	59(50)
Circulating platelets	≤50,000/mm³	22	21	43(370
	>50,000/mm³	38	36	74(63)
FAB Classification	1–2	34	35	69(59)
	3	2	4	6(5)
	4–5	16	14	30(25)
	Other	8	4	12(10)

drug for both the induction phase and the consolidation phase of the therapy.

Response rates and treatment outcome. Overall, 62 patients (53%) achieved a complete remission, with a trend toward a higher response rate in the GM-CSF group (60% versus 46%). With a median follow-up of 18 months, the median survival for subjects given GM-CSF was 54 weeks compared to 38 weeks for subjects given placebo. Subjects given GM-CSF had a lower mortality rate in the first six months from entry onto study (9 of 52 given GM-CSF versus 20 of 47 given placebo, $p = 0.008$).

Hematologic recovery. GM-CSF resulted in faster hematologic recovery after induction therapy. A second course of induction therapy was required in 30% of patients and the hematologic recovery was longer in patients receiving two cycles of chemotherapy. Therefore, in all assessments of recovery of hematologic parameters, the data were stratified to take into account the number of cycles of induction therapy given. The median time for neutrophil recovery to $500/mm^3$ and $1{,}000/mm^3$ was reduced by an average of 4 and 7 days, respectively, in the GM-CSF group ($p \leq 0.004$ for both comparisons). The improved neutrophil recovery with GM-CSF remains atistically significant if patients given one or two courses of induction therapy are analyzed separately. There was no significant difference in recovery times to self-sustained platelets greater than $20{,}000/mm^3$ and to red blood cell transfusion independence. Following consolidation therapy, there was no significant differences in times to neutrophils, platelets, and red blood cell recovery.

Infection data (Table 2). Infections were assessed for the 99 subjects who received study drug from day 1 of chemotherapy through consolidation. The rate of grade 3–5 infections was similar in both treatment groups prior to the onset of study drug (31.6%). On the other hand, the incidence of grade 4–5 infections during induction therapy was significantly lower in the GM-CSF group, (9.6% versus 36.2%, $p = 0.002$). Overall, there were fewer grade 3–5 infections (51.9% versus 74.5%) and fatal infections (5.8% versus 17.0%) in the group given GM-CSF. Also, there were significantly fewer deaths from infection on study or within 30 days of completing study in the GM-CSF group (3/52 = 5.8% versus 11/47 = 23.4%, $p = 0.019$).

Systemic fungal infections and fatal fungal infections occured less frequently during induction therapy in patients given GM-CSF (Table 2). Eight patients given GM-CSF developed a grade 3–4 fungal infection, one of whom died of this infection. In contrast, 12 patients on placebo developed a grade 3–4 fungal infection, nine of whom died from their infection ($p = 0.02$). Also, there was an additional case of fatal disseminated apergillosis in the placebo group during consolidation therapy. The incidence of infectious pneumonias during induction therapy was similar in both groups. Fatal pneumonias, however, occurred less frequently in the GM-CSF group. Fourteen subjects given GM-CSF developed

Table 2. Rate of serious infections following induction therapy in subjects given study drug

	GM-CSF(n = 52)		Placebo (n = 47)		
	# patients	Incidence	# patients	Incidence	P*
Grade 3/4/5 infections	27/52	51.9 %	35/47	74.5 %	0.024
Grade 4/5 infections	5/52	9.6 %	17/47	36.2 %	0.002
Fatal infections while on study	3/52	5.8 %	8/47	17.0 %	0.110
Fatal infections during and within 30 days of completing study	3/52	5.8 %	11/47	23.4 %	0.019
Death from pneumonias in subjects with pneumonia	2/14	14.3 %	7/13	53.8 %	0.046
Death from fungal infections for all subjects given study drug	1/52	1.9 %	9/47	19.1 %	0.006
Fatal fungal infections in subjects with grade 3-4 fungal infection	1/8	12.5 %	9/12	75 %	0.02

*Fisher's Exact Test

pneumonia, two of whom died from this complication. By contrast, seven of the 13 subjects given placebo died from their pneumonia (p = 0.046).

Evaluation of study drug toxicity. Table 3 reports the frequency of adverse events (NCI grade 3–4) occurring during induction therapy in at least 5% of patients given study drug. During consolidation therapy, one patient given GM-CSF experienced dyspnea and bronchospasm requiring study drug discontinuation. There were statistically fewer hepatic, neurological, and hemorrhagic complications in the GM-CSF group. Otherwise, the incidence of clinical and laboratory adverse events were comparable in both groups. Similarly, the incidence of adverse events was similar in both treatment groups during consolidation therapy.

Discussion

In remission induction therapy of AML, it is necessary to ablate the leukemic cells in the bone marrow to permit regrowth of normal cells. During this period of aplasia lasting several weeks, deaths from infection, bleeding, and other complications usually exceeds 10–20%. The management of older patients with AML represents a particular challenge because of the higher risk for infection and other complications [8]. Since over half of the patients with AML are over the age of 60, progress in supportive care therapy is clearly needed.

Table 3. Number (%) of grade 3–4* adverse events during induction therapy

Event	GM-CSF (n = 52)	Placebo (n = 47)	p**
Pulmonary	8 (15)	13 (28)	
Hepatic	6 (12)	20 (43)	0.0006
Metabolic	6 (12)	9 (19)	
Neurologic	5 (10)	15 (32)	0.011
Cutaneous	5 (10)	8 (17)	
Cardiac	4 (8)	9 (19)	
Nausea	3 (6)	1 (2)	
Psychiatric	1 (2)	4 (9)	
Genito-urinary	1 (2)	4 (9)	
Hemorrhage	0	4 (9)	0.047
Stomatitis	1 (2)	3 (6)	
Diarrhea	0	3 (6)	

*NCI common toxicity scale
**Fisher's Exact Test (all others comparisons p >0.05)

This randomized study objectively demonstrated that yeast-derived GM-CSF improves the hematologic recovery and decreases the risk of life-threatening and fatal infections in older patients with AML undergoing standard induction therapy. Except for the age distribution, the characteristics of patients included in this study are similar to most AML reports [1–7]. In this study, GM-CSF accelerated neutrophil recovery over 500/μL and 1,000/μL following induction therapy by an average of four and seven days, respectively. Similar to bone marrow transplant data [14], GM-CSF did not abolish the period of aplasia but resulted in faster neutrophil recovery once normal hematopoiesis began. The lack of statistically significant effect on neutrophil recovery following consolidation therapy may be due to the small study sample size during this phase (n = 47 patients).

Patients receiving GM-CSF experienced fewer grade 3/4/5 severe, life-threatening, and fatal infections, fewer systemic fungal infections, and fewer fatal pneumonias than patients given placebo. Lower rate of life-threatening and fatal infections is probably due to faster neutrophil recovery, since the overall incidence of all infections was comparable in both group. Another possible explanation to this finding is increased anti-microbial activity of neutrophils and macrophages by GM-CSF, an effect previously reported in vitro [17, 18]. The reduction in fatal infections resulted in an overall improved survival at six months, although this benefit was not maintained with longer follow-up.

Yeast-derived GM-CSF was well tolerated and did not result in more side effects than placebo. On the other hand, more patients given placebo experienced hepatic, neurologic, and bleeding complications. Although there were a priori concerns that GM-CSF may protect leukemic cells from the antitumor effect of the cytoreductive therapy, this study clearly demonstrated that GM-CSF can be safely used following induction therapy, once aplasia had been documented. In fact, failure to eradicate leukemia was noted in equal number of patients in both groups and the number of relapses after achieving a complete remission was similar in both groups (data not presented).

This is the first randomized trial that clearly demonstrates the benefit of GM-CSF during induction therapy of older patients with AML. In 1991, Büchner et al [19] reported a phase 2 study of Sargramostim in 19 older patients with newly diagnosed AML and 11 patients in relapse. GM-CSF (250 μg/m²/day) was given four days after the end of the chemotherapy if the bone marrow was aplastic and with less than 5% blasts. Compared to matched historical controls, GM-CSF significantly accelerated neutrophil recovery, reduced the risk of early death, and improved complete remission rates. GM-CSF was well tolerated and did not increase the incidence of resistant leukemia.

Preliminary results of four large controlled trials of myeloid growth factors in AML patients have recently been reported [20-23]. Differences in the specific growth factor given (yeast-derived GM-CSF, E Coli-derived GM-CSF, G-CSF), dose and schedule, chemotherapeutic agents used, and study design prevent meaningful comparisons with our study. A significant difference among these trials is the timing of the onset of growth factor use, i.e., before, during, and after chemotherapy administration versus after aplasia has been documented.

In conclusion, yeast-derived GM-CSF is effective and well tolerated when used after achieving aplasia with standard induction therapy in older patients with do novo AML. Sargramostim significantly accelerates neutrophil recovery and decreases the incidence of severe and fatal infections. Its role in patients with recurrent AML or in patients under the age of 55 warrants further investigations.

References

1. Arlin Z, Case DC, Moore J, et al: Randomized multicenter trial of cytosine arabinoside with mitoxantrone or daunorubicin in previously untreated adult patients with acute nonlymphocytic leukemia (ANLL). Leukemia 4: 177-183, 1990
2. Preisler HD, Davis RB, Kirshner J, et al: Comparison of three remission induction regimens and two postinduction strategies for the treatment of acute nonlymsphocytic leukemia: A Cancer and Leukemia Group B Study. Blood 69: 1441-1149, 1987
3. Yates J, Glidewell O, Wiernick P, et al: Cytosine arabinoside with Daunorubicin or Adriamycin for therapy of acute myelocytic leukemia: A CALGB study. Blood 60: 454-462, 1982
4. Rai KR, Holland JF, Glidewell OJ, et al: Treatment of acute myelocytic leukemia: A study by Cancer and Leukemia Group B. Blood 58: 1203-1212, 1981
5. Estey EH, Keating MJ, McCredie KB, et al: Causes of initial remission failure in acute myelogenous leukemia. Blood 60: 309-315, 1982
6. Sebban C, Archimbaud E, Coiffier B, et al: Treatment of acute myeloid leukemia in elderly patients: A retrospective study. Cancer 61: 227-231, 1988
7. Rees JKH, Gray R: Comparison of 1+5 DAT and 3+10 DAT followed by COAP or MAE consolidation therapy in the treatment of acute myeloid leukemia: MRC ninth AML trial. Sem Oncol 14: 2(Supp 1): 32-36, 1987
8. Champlin RE, Gajewski JL, Golde DW: Treatment of acute myelogenous leukemia in the elderly. Sem Oncol 16: 51-56, 1989
9. Keating MJ, Kantarjian H, Smith TL, et al: Response to salvage therapy and survival after relapse in acute myelogenous leukemia. J Clin Oncol 7: 1071-1080, 1989
10. Davis CL, Rohatiner AZS, Lim J, et al: The management of recurrent acute myelogenous leukemia at a single center over a fifteen-year period. Br J Haematol 83: 404-411, 1993
11. Bodey GP: Infection in cancer patients. Am J Med 81(Suppl 1A): 11-26, 1986
12. Guiot HFL, Fibbe WE, van't Hout JW: Risk factors for fungal infection in patients with malignant hematologic disorders: Implications for empirical therapy and prophylaxis. Clin Infect Dis 18: 525-532, 1994
13. Nemunaitis J, Rabinowe S, Singer J, et al: Recombinant granulocyte-macrophage colony-stimulating factor after autologous bone marrow transplantation for lymphoid cancer. N Engl J Med 324: 1773-1778, 1991
14. Nemunaitis J, Singer JW, Buckner CD, et al: Use of recombinant human granulocyte-macrophage colony-stimulating factor in graft failure after bone marrow transplantation. Blood 76: 245-253, 1990
15. Vadhan-Raj S, Broxmeyer HE, Hittleman WN: Abrogating chemotherapy-induced myelosuppression by recombinant granulocyte-macrophage colony-stimulating factor in patients with sarcoma: Protection at the progenitor cell level. J Clin Oncol 10: 1266-1277, 1992
16. Neidhart JA, Mangalick A, Stidley CA, et al: Dosing regimen of granulocyte-macrophage colony-stimulating factor to support dose-intensive chemotherapy. J Clin Oncol 10: 1460-1469, 1992
17. Smith PD, Lamerson CL, Banks SM, et al: Granulocyte-macrophage colony-stimulating factor augments human monocyte fungicidal activity for Candida Albicans. J Infect Dis 161: 999-1005, 1990
18. Robi G, Markovich S, Athamna A, et al: Human recombinant granulocyte-macrophage colony-stimulating factor augments viability and cytotoxic activities of human monocyte-derived macrophages in long-term cultures. Lymphok Cytok Res 10: 257-263, 1991
19. B‚chner T, Hiddermann W, Koenigsmann M, et al: Recombinat human granulocyte-macrophage colony-stimulating factor after chemotherapy in patients with acute myeloid leukemia at higher age or after relapse. Blood 78: 1190-1997, 1991
20. Stone R, George S, Berg D, et al: GM-CSF v Placebo during remission induction for patients > 60 years

old with de novo acute myeloid leukemia: CALGB study # 8923. Proc ASCO, #992, 1994

21. Witz F, Harrousseau JL, Cahn JY, et al: GM-CSF during and after remission induction treatment for elderly patients with acute myeloid leukemia (AML). Blood 10 (Suppl 1): #908, 1994
22. Zittoun R, Mandelli F, de Witte T, et al: Recombinant human-granulocyte-macrophage colony-stimulating factor (GM-CSF) during induction treatment of acute myelogenous leukemia (AML). A randomized trial from EORTC-GIMEMA Leukemia Cooperative Groups. Blood 10 (Suppl 1): #909, 1994
23. Dombret H, Yver A, Chastang C, et al: Increased frequency of complete remission by Lenograstim recombinat human granulocyte colony-stimulating factor (rhG-CSF) administration after intensive induction chemotherapy in elderly patients with de novo acute myeloid leukemia (AML). Final results of a randomized multicenter double-blind controlled study. Blood 10 (Suppl 1): #910, 1994

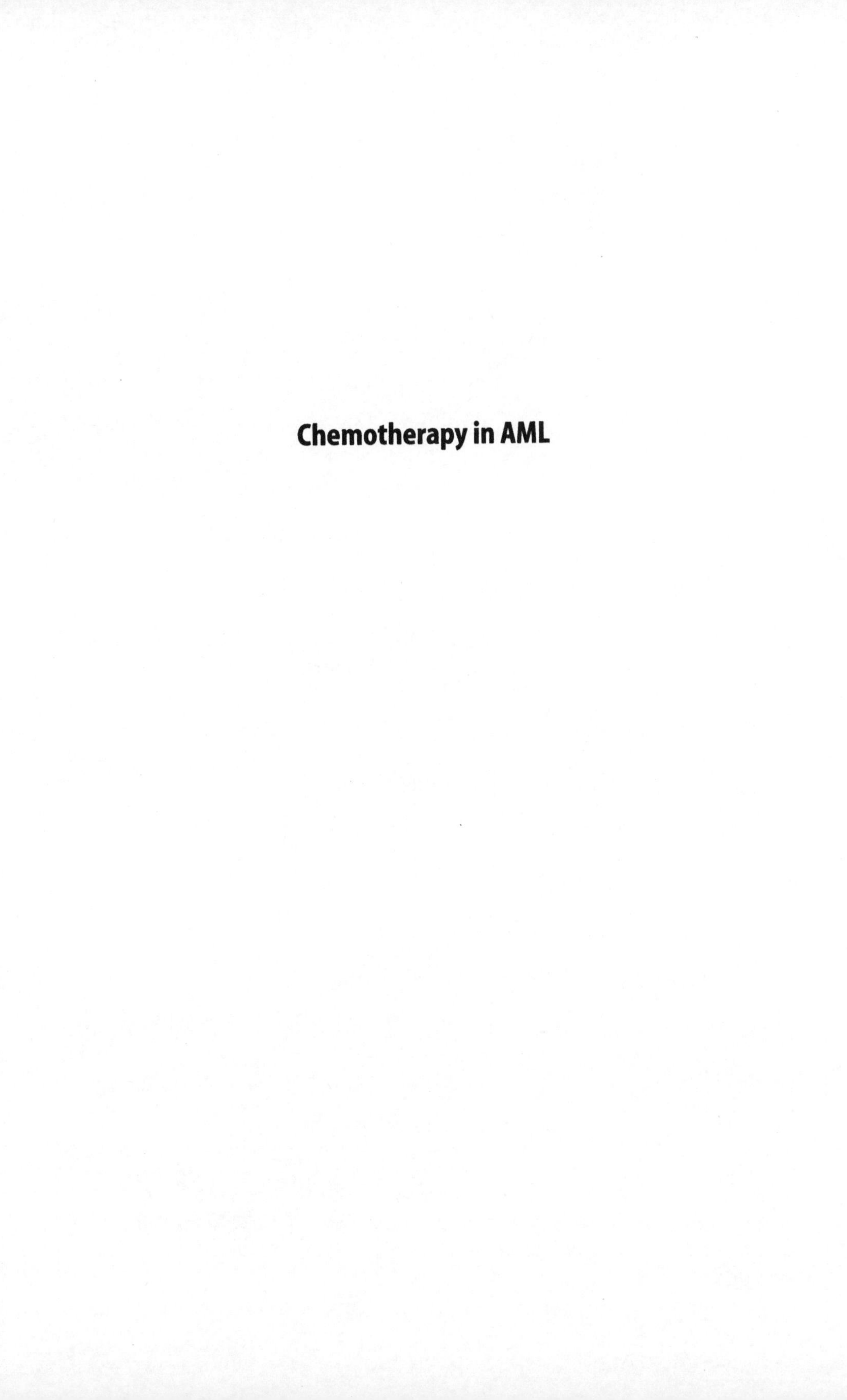

Chemotherapy in AML

Acute Leukemias V
Experimental Approaches
and Management of Refractory Diseases
Hiddemann et al. (Eds.)

New Approaches in the Treatment of AML and MDS

Michael J. Keating

Introduction

Despite recent advances in the genetics, biology, and diagnosis of acute myelogenous leukemias (AML) and myelodysplastic syndromes (MDS), clinical management of patients with both disorders still remains unsatisfactory. After start of treatment, the majority of patients temporarily achieve complete remission. However, between 10% and 20% of patients die during induction therapy, and 70% of patients who achieve complete remission eventually relapse. The incidence of long-term survivors in AML is about 20% for all patients and less than 5% after relapse (Champlin 1987).

A major intention of current clinical studies is to translate the progress in basic research, new drug development and pharmacology from bench to bedside. Clinical strategies including risk group adapted chemotherapy in AML, use of pharmacokinetically guided drug application schedules or application of hematopoietic growth factors in order to increase the cytotoxic efficacy of conventional antineoplastic drugs should be introduced into newly designed protocols for treatment of hematological neoplasias. New classes of compounds, like all-trans retinoic acid or purine analogs have enhanced the spectrum of single agent and combination chemotherapy approaches. High dose chemotherapy with peripheral blood progenitor cells has allowed for increased dose intensity in treatment of various disorders.

Treatment options for patients with acute myelogenous leukemia have considerably improved within the last three decades. In general, the therapeutic concept includes remission induction chemotherapy and a variety of post remission treatment strategies of consolidation, maintenance and intensification.

Induction of remission in AML is mainly achieved by administration of cytarabine and an anthracycline. In classical approaches, conventional doses of cytarabine (70 to 100 mg/m^2/d) were combined with daunorubicin. Modifications of the cytarabine dose led to concepts of intermediate dose (500 mg/m^2/d) or high dose (1000 mg/m^2/d) ara-C treatment. A number of new approaches have used novel agents such as amsacrine, mitoxantrone or newer anthracyclines with cytarabine in different doses and schedules.

The outcome of remission induction therapy at M.D. Anderson Cancer Center over a period from 1975 to 1993 is summarized in Table 1.

A total of 1244 patients were treated, 751 (60%) obtained a complete remission, while 324 patients (26%) died within the course of the first therapeutic regimen. A considerable portion (169 patients, 13%) of patients showed primary resistance to chemotherapy.

Analysis of treatment outcome for separate time periods did not reveal significant improvements with regard to induction chemotherapy within the last two decades. Overall, a stable CR rate of about 60% has been achieved since 1975.

These data include all patients diagnosed with acute myelogenous leukemia at M.D. Anderson Cancer Center between 1975 and 1993, irrespective of age, performance index or other exclusion criteria for chemotherapy. Higher

Department of Hematology, University of Texas M.D. Anderson Cancer Center, Houston, TX 77030, USA

Table 1. Outcome of remission induction therapy in AML

Patient group	Total n	CR n	CR %	Died n	Died %	Resistant n	Resistant %
Total	1244	751	60%	321	26%	169	13%
Patients according to month of treatment							
1/75–11/82	141	240	58%	116	28%	58	14%
12/82–11/88	415	253	61%	100	24%	62	15%
11/88–5/93	415	257	62%	112	27%	46	11%
Patients according to eligibility status 1, 2							
eligible	694	521	75%	104%	15%	69	10%
ineligible	550	226	41%	220	40%	104	19%

[1]eligibility for treatment studies as defined by the following criteria: patients of any age, without prior malignancies or myelodysplastic syndromes, without prior chemotherapy or radiotherapy, performance status (Zubrod) <3, serum bilirubin <2 mg/dl and serum creatinine <2 mg/dl

[2]difference in treatment outcome (eligible vs. ineligible patients) statistically significant ($p<0.0001$)

response rates after induction therapy with complete remission in 70% to 90% of patients have been reported for various experimental treatment protocols, however, definition of patient eligibility criteria (Table 1) frequently led to exclusion of high risk patients. If patients eligible for treatment studies of AML were analysed separately, superior response rates were demonstrated. Comparison of eligible and ineligible patients revealed significant differences ($p < 0.0001$) with regard to CR rate after induction therapy (75% vs. 42%) and long-term survival (20% vs. 7%).

These results emphasize the risk of patient selection for clinical studies and underline the bias due to definition of patient eligibility criteria.

Definition of Risk Groups for AML

The data as given above demonstrate only minor improvements with regard to remission rate and overall survival of patients with AML. However, further biological analysis of the malignant clones in acute myelogenous leukemias and myelodysplastic syndromes showed that the karyotype of malignant cells is strongly correlated with response and remission duration in previously untreated patients with AML (Keating 1987, Larson 1983).

Patients with low risk and higher probability of survival are characterized by specific cytogenetic categories like t(8;21), t(15;17), inv16 or diploidy. High risk situations are defined by trisomy 8, deletion of chromosome 5 or chromosome 7 as well as by antecedent hematological disorders (myelodysplastic or myeloproliferative syndromes).

The predictive value of AML risk groups was assessed in a historical control population of 807 patients treated between 1980 and 1990. In the low risk group, 583 patients were treated, 67% achieved complete remission after induction therapy, 21% died and 12% were primarily resistant. The high risk group consisted of 224 patients, 38% achieved complete remission, 38% died during the first course of chemotherapy and 24% were not responsive. Long-term survival was significantly different ($p < 0.0001$), observed in the low risk and high risk groups in 18% and 4% of the patients, respectively.

In conclusion, determination of cytogenetic abnormalities allows for definition of patient groups with "favorable" and "unfavorable" prognosis. The treatment protocols chosen within the last two decades seem to be of minor influence with regard to clinical outcome, and the lack of improvement in overall CR rate or survival illustrates the need for introduction of new agents into current or novel protocols.

In view of the data given above, at M.D. Anderson Cancer Center a concept for risk group adapted chemotherapy in AML and MDS was developed in 1990 (Table 2).

Idarubicin (4-demethoxy-daunorubicine) is a novel anthracycline which is characterized by

Table 2. Risk group adapted chemotherapy in AML and MDS (1990)

Low risk group: Idarubicin + high dose cytarabine
Idarubicin 12 $mg/m^2/day$, for 3 days, 30 minutes infusion once daily
Cytarabine 1.5 $g/m^2/day$, continuous infusion (3 days if age > 60 years)
High risk group: Fludarabine + intermediate dose cytarabine
Fludarabine 30 $mg/m^2/day$, for 5 days, once daily
Cytarabine 0.5 $g/m^2/h$, for 6 days, 2 to 6 hours daily

Treatment of AML with Idarubicin and Cytarabine

lipophilic behavior, high oral bioavailability and penetration of the CNS through the blood-brain barrier. As compared to daunorubicin, idarubicin demonstrated superior effects in various preclinical and clinical studies in AML and MDS. In randomized comparative trials, idarubicin showed a higher rate of complete remissions than daunorubicin, with more patients achieving CR after a single course of treatment (Berman 1991, Wiernik 1991). Idarubicinol, the main metabolite of idarubicin, has significant antileukemic activity, resulting in prolonged antileukemic efficacy of the drug after single application. Due to its high lipophility, idarubicin and idarubicinol show strong DNA-binding and intranuclear concentration (Plumbridge 1978, Capranico 1987). As compared to all other anthracyclines, idarubicin is less susceptible to P-glycoprotein-mediated drug transport (multidrug resistance) due to reduced cytoplasmic concentration of the drug (Berman 1992, Müller 1992, Gieseler 1994). Furthermore, idarubicin is well tolerated, resulting in a reduced need for intensive supportive care.

These data suggest idarubicin as the anthracycline of choice for combination regimens with cytarabine. At M.D. Anderson Cancer Center, a combination of idarubicin, 12 $mg/m^2/day \times 3$ (Table 2) was used as induction chemotherapy in low risk patients with AML. Results are detailed in Table 3.

Overall, 50 patients were treated with idarubicin and cytarabine. No eligibility criteria were applied, however, patients older than 59 years of age received ara-C for three days only. Thirty-eight patients (76%) achieved complete remission and 3 patients (6%) died after the first course of therapy. In seven patients a second course of treatment was applied, another 6 patients (12%) achieved CR. Three patients (6%) were completely resistant. These data demonstrate, that a combination of idarubicin and high dose cytarabine is effective to induce remission rapidly and with a high rate of CR in low risk patients with newly diagnosed AML. Analysis of different patient subgroups revealed that elder patients (> 60 years) tolerated

Table 3. Idarubicin + high dose cytarabine in AML

	Total	CR		Died		Resistant	
Patient group	n	n	%	n	%	n	%
Total	50	44	88%	3	6%	3	6%
Number of courses	1						
one course	43	38	88%	3	7%	2	5%
two courses	7	6	86%	–	0%	1	14%
Patients age							
<50 years	24	20	83%	3	13%	1	4%
50–59 years	7	7	100%	–	0%	–	0%
60–82 years	19	17	89%	–	0%	2	11%
Karyotype							
inv16	13	13	100%	–	0%	–	0%
diploid	20	17	85%	2	10%	1	5%
AHD[2]	17	14	82%	1	6%	2	12%

[1]43 patients underwent one course of induction therapy, in 7 patients a second course was applied. 38 patients achieved CR after the first course, 6 patients after the second course of treatment

[2]AHD antecedent hematological disorders (myeloproliferative or myelodysplastic)

treatment well. Prognosis in patients with antecedent hematological disorders (high risk group) was worse than in patients with karyotypic abnormalities indicating low risk, e.g. inv16.

Postremission schedules are still an important issue in treatment of leukemias and lymphomas. Until september 1991, at M.D. Anderson Cancer Center patients achieving complete remission upon induction treatment for AML with idarubicin and high-dose cytarabine (protocol "3+4": idarubicin 12 mg/m²/d × 3+cytarabine 1.5 g/m²/d × 4) were treated with the same protocol for two additional courses. Analysis of efficacy and tolerability of this regimen revealed high toxicity and made a change in postremission chemotherapy necessary. Since september 1991, treatment of all patients was continued by application of one course of low-dose cytarabine, 100 mg/m²/d for five days. If complete remission persisted, combined chemotherapy with idarubicin and high-dose ara-C was continued for two additional courses, however, dose levels of each individual course were reduced (treatment protocol "2+2": idarubicin 12 mg/m²/d × 2+cytarabine 1.5 g/m²/ d × 2). Overall, the median duration of remission in patients with AML after idarubicin and high dose cytarabine treatment was 18 months in patients 16 to 60 years of age. Elder patients showed a shorter median disease-free survival of 9 to 10 months.

Myelodysplastic Syndromes

Myelodysplastic syndromes (MDS) are clonal bone marrow disorders, characterized by ineffective hematopoiesis, peripheral blood cytopenias involving at least two hematopoietic cell lineages, and an increased risk of transformation to acute myeloid leukemia. In patients with these disorders, conventional chemotherapy usually yields results inferior to patients with de novo AML (List 1990). Prognosis is particularly poor in patients with more than 5% bone marrow blasts, whose median survival varies between 3 and 18 months (Aul 1992).

Therefore, classical treatment of myelodysplastic syndromes consisted mainly of red blood cell and platelet substitution, inadvertently resulting in iron overload and immunological rejection of donor platelets. However, recent data based on the availability of hematopoietic growth factors and the development of novel cytotoxic agents have stimulated new interest in potentially efficacious treatment modalities. In aggressively treated MDS patients, complete bone marrow remissions were achieved in up to 80% of cases (Michels 1989). Further studies on possible treatment strategies in myelodysplastic syndromes are necessary.

Treatment of MDS with Idarubicin and Cytarabine

A similar approach of combined chemotherapy with idarubicin and cytarabine (protocol "3+4": idarubicin 12 mg/m²/d × 3+cytarabine 1.5 g/m²/ d × 4) was chosen for patients with newly diagnosed myelodysplastic syndromes. Prognostic groups were defined according to the criteria as given above. A total of 15 patients were treated. In 13 low risk patients, application of idarubicin and high-dose cytarabine led to a complete remission rate of 92% (12/13 patients), one patient died during induction chemotherapy. Two patients fulfilled high risk criteria, both patients were primarily chemoresistant.

FLAG Protocol in MDS

In view of the high toxicity and disappointing efficacy of the combination of fludarabine and intermediate dose cytarabine (FLA protocol), especially in high risk situations, additional application of G-CSF was started in 89 patients with MDS (FLAG protocol). A complete remission rate of 64% (57 out of 89 patients) was achieved, 11 patients were primarily resistant to the FLAG regimen.

Treatment of AML with Fludarabine and Cytarabine

Fludarabine (9-β-D-arabinofuranosyl-2-fluoroadenine monophosphate) is a fluorinated analog of ara-adenine that is relatively resistant to adenosine deaminase (Lee 1960). Clinical application initially concentrated on treatment of low grade Non-Hodgkin's lymphoma and chronic lymphoproliferative disorders, e.g., chronic lymphocytic leukemia and hairy cell leukemia (Keating 1993). Previous in vitro studies demonstrated, that leukemia cells loade with arabinosyl-2-fluoroadenine 5'-triphosphate (F-ara-ATP) accumulated arabinosylcytosine 5'-triphosphate (ara-CTP) at a significantly higher range compared to control cells. These data strongly suggested, that a protocol designed to administer fludarabine prior to cytarabine infusion would augment ara-CTP accumulation by leukemic cells (Gandhi 1989, 1993). Consequently, various protocols were designed to evaluate the efficacy of fludarabine, alone and in combination with cytarabine and other agents in patients with acute myelogenous leukemia.

FLA Protocol in AML

Combined treatment with fludarabine, 30 mg/m²/day given once daily for 5 doses, and intermediate dose cytarabine, 0.5 g/m²/h for 2 to 6 hours daily for 6 doses (FLA protocol), was administered to 54 patients with acute myelogenous leukemia. Doses of fludarabine preceded those of ara-C by 4 hours. The CR rate was 52% (28/54 patients), however, 21 patients (39%) died during induction chemotherapy. Primary resistance was observed in 5 patients (9%). Median survival was short with 4 months in the high risk and 13 months in the low risk group, the difference being statistically significant. Long-term survival was achieved in only 14% (4/30) of patients in the high risk group (Figure 1).

FLAG Protocol in AML

A combination of fludarabine and ARAC with or without granulocyte colony-stimulating factor (G-CSF) was studied in 132 patients (FLAG protocol) (Table 4).

In subjects treated with fludarabine+ARAC alone, an overall complete remission rate of 52%

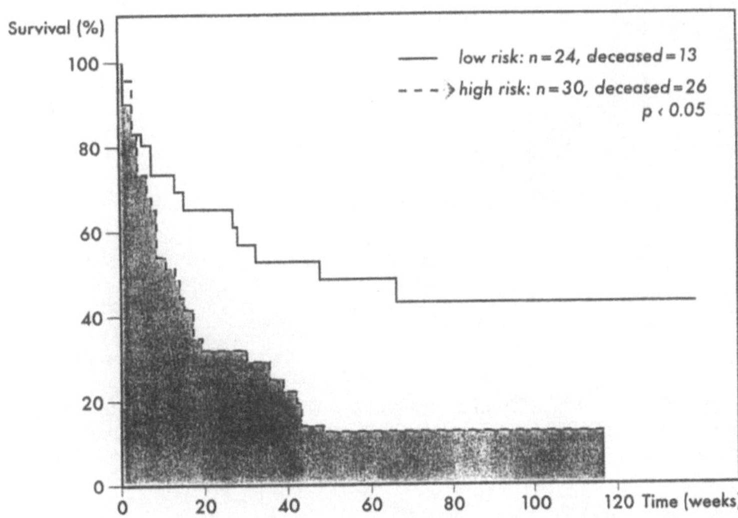

Fig. 1. Overall survival in AML high risk and low risk patients after treatment with fludarabine and intermediate dose cytarabine /(FLA regimen)

Table 4. Outcome of Fludarabine+ARAC ± G-CSF in treatment of AML

	Overall		Low risk group		High risk group	
Treatment group	CR/Total	%	CR/Total	%	CR/Total	%
Fludarabine+ARAC	28/54	52%	16/24	67%	12/30	40%
Fludarabine+ARAC+ G-CSF	50/78	64%	27/35	77%	23/43	54%

was achieved. The addition of G-CSF led to a significant increase in cytotoxicity: in patients treated with a combination of fludarabine and G-CSF a CR rate of 64% was achieved.

The increase in cytotoxic activity by addition of G-CSF was obvious in both low risk (CR rate 67% vs. 77%) and high risk patients (40 % vs. 54 %), respectively. No increase in toxicity was observed in the G-CSF combination regimen.

As compared to the FLA regimen, an increased median survival time and overall survival rate was achieved. After a median follow up of 1 year, a significant difference in survival was observed between high risk and low risk patients (Figure 2).

Treatment of AML with Fludarabine, Cytarabine and Idarubicin

Comparative evaluation of various protocols applied in treatment of patients with acute myelogenous leukemia between 1991 and 1993 is given in Table 5.

A lower complete remission rate and higher toxicity is obvious in patients treated according to the FLA and FLAG protocols. Furthermore, in both groups a considerable number of patients with primarily resistant leukemias is obvious. Most patients were high risk.

Toxicity analysis of fludarabine containing regimens shows a substantial rate of infectious

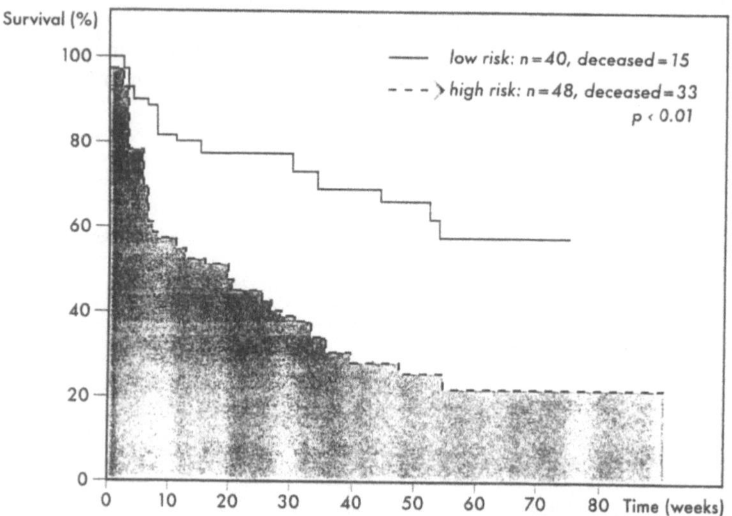

Fig. 2. Overall survival in AML high risk and low risk patients after treatment with fludarabine, intermediate dose cytarabine and G-CSF (FLAG regimen)

Table 5. Comparative evaluation of treatment results in AML by regimen, 1991–1993

Regimen	Total n	CR n	CR %	Died n	Died %	Resistant n	Resistant %
Idarubicin + hd cytarabine	62	53	86%	6	10%	3	5%
Fludarabine + id cytarabine (FLA)	54	28	52%	21	39%	5	9%
Fludarabine + id ara-C+G-CSF (FLAG)%	89	57	64%	21	24%	11	12%

hd high dose, id intermediate dose

complications. As the median count of T-helper cells is decreased to about 200/µl after fludarabine treatment, opportunistic infections due to cytomegalovirus, pneumocystis carinii or herpes zoster virus have been seen in few cases. However, the rate of life-threatening infectious complications in patients treated with fludarabine was not significantly increased. This may be due to the low doses of fludarabine used, as the drug was applied as a modulator of ara-CTP pharmacokinetics and not at doses required for cytotoxic efficacy.

Therefore, a new concept for risk group adapted chemotherapy was developed in 1993, based on additional treatment with hematopoietic growth factors in low risk and addition of an anthracycline to the FLAG protocol in high risk AML patients. The novel regimens are given in Table 6, detailing therapy with idarubicin, cytarabine and G-CSF in the low risk group and with FLAG + idarubicin in high risk patients.

Table 6. Risk group adapted chemotherapy in AML and MDS (1993)

Low risk group: Idarubicin+high dose cytarabine+G-CSF
Idarubicin 12 mg/m²/day, days 1–3, 30 minutes infusion once daily
Cytarabine 1.5 g/m²/day, days 1–4, continuous infusion (3 days if age > 60 years)
G-CSF 400 µg/m², days-1 to complete remission

High risk group: Fludarabine+intermediate dose cytarabine+idarubicin+G-CSF
Fludarabine 30 mg/m²/day, days 1–4, once daily
Cytarabine 2 g/m²/day, days 1–4, over 4 hours daily, 4 hours after fludarabine
Idarubicin 12 mg/m²/day, days 2–4, 30 minutes infusion once daily
G-CSF 400 µg/m², days-1 to complete remission

Between 1993 and 1994, 14 high risk patients have been treated with FLAG+idarubicin. A preliminary evaluation and comparison of the outcome of FLA, FLAG and FLAG+idarubicin in acute myelogenous leukemia is given in Table 7.

The high complete remission rate (79%) after treatment with FLAG+idarubicin should be noted. Moreover, so far no patient was primarily resistant to the regimen. Three patients (21%) died during induction chemotherapy. However, a higher number of patients should be included for final evaluation of cytotoxic efficacy and long-term results of this regimen.

Conclusions

As current standard protocols for therapy of acute myeloid leukemias and myelodysplastic syndromes have not resulted in significant improvements with regard to patient survival within the last two decades, new treatment strategies are necessary. Clinical studies involving hematopoietic growth factors, recent pharmacological concepts and new cytotoxic agents have been initiated at M.D. Anderson Cancer Center. It should be emphasized, that all patients with newly diagnosed AML were treated according to these protocols, irrespective of patient eligibility criteria. However, risk group adapted chemotherapy was performed according to cytogenetic characteristics and history of antecedent hematological disorders.

In low risk patients, combined chemotherapy with idarubicin and cytarabine was well tolerated and highly effective in remission induction and postremission therapy. The addition of idarubicin to treatment of AML has resulted in a significant difference in long-term survival. In high risk patients, modulation of cytarabine effects was achieved by pharmacokinetically

Table 7. Preliminary comparative evaluation of treatment results in high risk AML

Regimen	Total	CR		Died		Resistant	
	n	n	%	n	%	n	%
FLA	54	28	52%	21	39%	5	9%
FLAG	89	57	64%	21	24%	11	12%
FLAG+Idarubicin	14	11	79%	3	21%	–	0%

FLA fludarabine+intermediate dose cytarabine
FLAG fludarabine+intermediate dose cytarabine+G-CSF

guided application of fludarabine. Combined treatment with fludarabine, cytarabine and GCSF led to remission rates and overall survival similar to current standard protocols.

A new set of trials for risk group adapted chemotherapy has been opened in 1993. In the low risk group, G-CSF is applied together with idarubicin and cytarabine. High risk patients are treated with a combination of fludarabine, cytarabine, idarubicine and G-CSF. Preliminary evaluation of 14 patients treated according to this protocol revealed a high CR rate and a low number of primarily resistant AML cases at tolerable side effects.

References

1. Aul C, Gattermann N, Heyll A, Germing U, Derigs G, Schneider W. Primary myelodysplastic syndromes: Analysis of prognostic factors in 235 patients and proposals for an improved scoring system. Leukemia 1992;6: 52–59.
2. Berman E, Heller G, Santorsa JA, McKenzie S, Gee T et al. Results of a randomized trial comparing idarubicin and cytosine arabinoside with daunorubicin and cytosin arabinoside in adult patients with newly diagnosed acute myelogenous leukemia. Blood 1991;77: 1666–1674.
3. Berman E, McBride M. Comparative cellular pharmacology of daunorubicin and idarubicin in human multidrug-resistant leukemia cells. Blood 1992;79: 3267–3273.
4. Capranico G, Riva A, Tinelli S, Dasdia T, Zunino F. Markedly reduced levels of anthracycline-induced DNA strand breaks in resistant P388 leukemia cells and isolated nuclei. Cancer Res 1987;47: 3752–3756.
5. Champlin R, Gale RP. Acute myelogenous leukemia: Recent advances in therapy. Blood 1987;69: 1551–1562.
6. Gandhi V, Nowak B, Keating MJ, Plunkett W. Modulation of arabinosylcytosine metabolism by arabinosyl-2-fluoroadenine in lymphocytes from patients with chronic lymphocytic leukemia: implications for combination chemotherapy. Blood 1989;74: 2070–2075.
7. Gandhi V, Estey E, Keating MJ, Plunkett W. Fludarabine potentiates metabolism of cytarabine in patients with acute myelogenous leukemia during therapy. J Clin Oncol 1993;11: 116–124.
8. Gieseler F, Clark M, Wilms K. Cellular uptake of anthracyclines, intracellular distribution, DNA binding and topoisomerase II activity. Determinants for hematopoietic cell sensitivity in chemotherapy. Ann Hematol 1994;68(suppl.1): A24, abstract 95.
9. Keating MJ, Cork A, Broach Y et al. Toward a clinically relevant cytogenetic classification of acute myelogenous leukemia. Leuk Res 1987;11: 119–133.
10. Keating MJ, Kantarjian H, Smith TL, Estey E, Walters R, Andersson B, Beran M, McCredie KB, Freireich EJ. Response to salvage therapy and survival after relapse in acute myelogenous leukemia. J Clin Oncol 1989;7: 1071–1080.
11. Keating MJ, O'Brien S, Kantarjian H, Plunkett W, Estey E, Koller C, Beran M, Freireich EJ. Long-term follow-up of patients with chronic lymphocytic leukemia treated with fludarabine as single agent. Blood 1993;11: 2878–2884.
12. Larson RA, LeBeau MM, Vardiman JW et al. The predictive value of initial cytogenetic studies in 148 adults with acute nonlymphocytic leukemia: a 12 year study (1970–1982). Cancer Genet Cytogenet 1983;10: 219–236.
13. Lee WW, Benitz A, Goodman A, Baker BR. Potential anticancer agents LX: Synthesis of the β-anomer of 9-(d-arabinofuranosyl)adenine. J Am Chem Soc 1960;82: 2648.
14. List AF, Garewal HS, Sandberg AA. The myelodysplastic syndromes. Biology and implications for management. J Clin Oncol 1990;8: 1424–1441.
15. Müller MR, Lennartz K, Boogen C, Nowrousian MR, Rajewski MF, Seeber S. Cytotoxicity of adriamycin, idarubicin, and vincristine in acute myeloid leukemia: chemosensitization by verapamil in relation to P-glycoprotein expression. Ann Hematol 1992;65: 206–212.
16. Plumbridge TW, Brown JR. Studies on the mode of interaction of 4'-epi-adriamycin and 4-demethoxy-daunomycin with DNA. Biochem Pharmacol 1978, 27: 1881–1882.
17. Wiernik PH. New agents in the treatment of acute myeloid leukemia. Sem Hematol 1991;28(suppl.4): 95–98.

Acute Leukemias V
Experimental Approaches
and Management of Refractory Diseases
Hiddemann et al. (Eds.)

S-HAM Salvage Therapy of Relapsed and Refractory AML Followed by Interleukin 2 Postremission Therapy

W. Hiddemann[1], M. Unterhalt[1], M. Kemper[2], E. Schleyer[1], P. Schönrock-Nabulsi[3], L. Uharek[4], M. Fromm[5], D. Braumann[6], M. Planker[7], U. Kubicka[8], J. Karow[9], S. Lange[10], C. Tirier[11], B. Wörmann[1], C. Sauerland[12], A. Heinecke[12], and Th. Büchner[2] for the German AML Cooperative Group

Abstract. A preceding study of the German AML Cooperative Group with an age adjusted randomized comparison of high-dose versus intermediate-dose Cytosine Arabinoside (AraC) as part of the S-HAM protocol indicated a significantly higher antileukemic activity of AraC at a dose of 3.0 vs. 1.0 g/m^2 per single dose predominantly in patients with early relapse and second or subsequent recurrence of disease but also an increased rate of early deaths. Based on these results the current study aimed at taking advantage of the high antineoplastic activity of high dose AraC but to reduce the associated infectious complications by the posttherapeutic application of G-CSF. AraC dose was adjusted to disease status and age in that patients below 60 years of age with early relapse and second or subsequent recurrence received AraC at a dose of 3.0 g/m^2 while later first relapses and older patients were treated with AraC 1.0 g/m^2. Immediately after the end of S-HAM G-SCF was applied at a dose of 5 ug/kg until neutrophil recovery. Patients achieving a complete remission underwent randomization for postremission therapy with Interleukin 2 (IL2) 18×10^6 U/m^2/d over 5 days by cont. infusion or observation only. IL2 therapy was repeated at 4 week intervals. At the present time 53 patients have been entered into the study and 38 are evaluable for response and toxicity. 22 cases (58%) obtained a CR, 9 patients (24%) were NR and 7 cases (18%) died during the first six weeks (early deaths). Neutrophil recovery occured at a median of 28 days and was significantly shorter as compared to the preceding S-HAM therapy without G-CSF support. 8 patients have been randomized for IL2 postremission therapy. These results indicate a significant improvement of remission rate and a reduction of lethal complications by G-CSF administration as compared to the historic control. Further recruitment and a longer observation time are needed to substantiate these findings and to assess the impact of IL2 on remission duration.

Introduction

In spite of substantial improvements in the first line therapy of acute myeloid leukemia (AML) and increasing rates of long term remissions, the majority of cases still experience a recurrence of

[1]Department of Hematology and Oncology, University of Göttingen, Göttingen, Germany
[2]Department of Hematology and Oncology, University of Münster, Münster, Germany
[3]Department of Hematology and Oncology, St. Georg Hospital, Hamburg, Germany
[4]Department of Hematology and Oncology, University of Kiel, Germany
[5]Department of Hematology and Oncology, Technical University of München, München, Germany
[6]Department of Internal Medicine, Hospital Altona, Hamburg, Germany
[7]Department of Internal Medicine, Hospital Krefeld, Krefeld, Germany
[8]Central Hospital St. Jürgen, Bremen, Germany
[9]Department of Internal Medicine III; Hospital Düren, Düren, Germany
[10]Department of Hematology and Oncology, Hospital Hamm, Hamm, Germany
[11]Department of Internal Medicine, Hospital Essen-Werden, Essen-Werden, Germany
[12]Department of Biostatistics, University of Münster, Münster, Germany

their disease to which they ultimately succumb [1,2]. Hence, new and more effective antileukemic strategies are deeply warranted. These should not only aim at developing cytostatic regimens with a high antileukemic activity but must also improve the safety of such therapies currently associated with a considerable mortality mainly from infectious complications. This requirement is illustrated by the results of a preceeding study of the German AML Cooperative Group in relapsed and refractory AML randomly comparing Cytosine Arabinoside (AraC) at high or intermediate doses on the basis of the sequential high-dose Arac–Mitoxantrone protocol (S-HAM) [3, 4]. This trial indicated a higher antileukemic efficacy of high dose AraC especially in cases with refractory AML which did not translate into an increased remission rate due to a concomitant rise of treatment associated early deaths.

The main challenge of AML therapy, however, still remains the control and final eradication of residual leukemia in remission. Among different postremission strategies that have been explored prolonged monthly maintenance and intensive consolidation have proven beneficial [5,6,7]. The most effective treatment in remission remains allogeneic bone marrow transplantation (BMT) from a HLA identical sibling donor which can be applied, however, to a minority of cases, only. Increasing evidence strongly suggests that the antileukemic activity of allogeneic BMT is mediately in part through an activation of cellular defense mechanisms of the immune system in way of a "Graft versus Leukemia" reaction [8,9]. This effect is obviously not restricted to transplantation and may be augmented by cytokines such as Interleukin 2 (IL 2), in particular [10, 11, 12, 13].

The current protocol of the AMLCG aims at investigating both aspects of AML therapy by trying to reduce the S-HAM therapy associated mortality by the posttherapeutic application of Granulocyte-Colony Stimulating Factor (G-CSF) but also by investigating the feasibility and impact of IL 2 postremission therapy on remission duration and survival.

Patients, Treatment Protocol and Methods

Patients: The current study was designated to patients above 18 years of age with relapsed or refractory AML after first-line therapy according to the corresponding trials of the AMLCG. Diagnosis was based on the FAB classification and complementary cytochemical and immunological criteria.

Therapy: Therapy comprized the S-HAM regimen consisting of AraC on days 1, 2, 8 and 9 and Mitoxantrone on days 3, 4, 10, and 11, respectively [3]. The AraC dose was adjusted to disease status and age in that patients below 60 years of age with early first relapse and second or subsequent recurrences were classified as refractory AML and received AraC at a dose of 3.0 g/m^2 per single dose while first relapses occuring after a preceding complete remission of more than 6 months duration were considered as non-refractory AML and were treated with AraC 1.0 g/m^2 per dose. Patients above 60 years of age all received AraC at a dose of 1.0 g/m^2 per application irrespective of disease status.

Immediately after the end of the S-HAM course G-CSF was started in all patients at a dose of 5 ug/kg body weight until neutrophil recovery to more than 1500/mm^3.

All patients received glucocorticoid eye drops during AraC administration for the prophylaxis of photophobia and conjunctivitis. Antiemetic therapy consisted of ondansetron 8 mg twice daily on days 1–4 and 8–11.

Antileukemic response was judged according to CALGB criteria and side effects were evaluated following WHO definitions. The interval between the onset of therapy and the post treatment achievment of more than 20.000 thrombocytes/mm^3 and more than 500 granulocytes/mm^3 was defined as time to recovery (TR).

Patients achieving a complete remission were randomized for postremission therapy with IL 2 18×10^6 IU/m^2/d over 5 days by continuous infusion to be repeated every 4 weeks until relapse or untolerable toxicity or no further maintenance therapy.

Results

At present, 53 patients of ages 18 to 68 years have been entered into the study. According to the status of their disease 23 cases were classified as refractory AML while the remaining 30 patients had non-refractory leukemia (Table 1).

Thirty-eight patients are currently evaluable for response and toxicity. As indicated by Table 2 22 patients (58%) achieved a complete remission while 9 cases (24%) had persistant

Table 1

Patients characteristics n 53 age 16–68 years	
primary NR	5
early relapse < 6 months	18
relapse > 6 < 18 months	15
late relapse > 18 months	15

Table 2

Response rate		
randomized patients	53	
evaluable patients	38	
CR	22	(58%)
ED	7	(18%)
NR+PR	9	(24%)

leukemia or obtained a partial remission, only. Seven cases (18%) died during the first 42 days after the start of therapy and were considered as early deaths.

Non-hematologic toxicity consisted mainly of fever and infections, diarrhea, mucositis and liver enzyme elevation. Nausea and vomiting was also frequently observed but did rarely exceed WHO grades 2 and 3 (Table 3).

The median time of blood cell recovery to more than 20.000 thrombocytes/mm³ and 500 granulocytes/mm³ (TR) was 28 days with a range from 18 to 44 days, the median time to complete remission was 46 days (28–56 days). Table 4 depictes the respective values in comparison to the preceeding S-HAM trial in which no G-CSF was applied in the posttreatment period.

From the 22 patients achieving a complete remission 8 cases have been randomized to IL 2

Table 3

	Toxicity			
	WHO I/II		III/IV	
Nausea/vomiting	19	(50%)	4	(11%)
Mucositis	15	(39%)	6	(16%)
Hepatic	13	(34%)	3	(8%)
Diarrhea	16	(42%)	14	(37%)
Renal	4	(11%)	1	(3%)
Skin	3	(8%)	–	–
CNS	2	(5%)	1	(3%)
Infection	21	(55%)	17	(45%)

Table 4

	S-HAM	S-HAM+G-CSF
Recovery of blood cells	38(24–52)	28(18–44)
Time to complete remission	60(34–90)	46(28–56)

postremission therapy or observation, only. Because of the early stage of this trial no meaningful evaluation can be performed for this part of the study at the present time.

Discussion

Studies in relapsed and refractory acute leukemias are not only undertaken to salvage patients from first-line treatment failure but also to explore novel strategies including new drug combinations and cytokines such as hematopoietic growth factors and interleukins. These approaches were also followed by the German AMLCG and a series of phase II protocols were investigated including high-dose AraC based regimens and the combination of Etoposide with Aclacinomycin A or Idarubicin. These efforts lead to the incorporation of the high-dose AraC–Mitoxantrone regimen into first-line therapy and the development of double induction [2, 14]. In refractory AML, a timed-sequential modification of the two drug combination, the so called S-HAM regimen proved highly effective and was the basis for a prospective randomized comparison of high-dose versus intermediate-dose AraC [3, 4]. This study clearly indicated a dose response relation and a higher antileukemic effect of high-dose AraC which did not transplate into an improved remission rate because of an increased mortality mainly from severe infections during treatment induced aplasia. In addition, remission duration was short with a median of only 5 months and long term survival was observed in less than 10% of cases, only. Hence, the present trial was initiated with the goal to reduce the treatment related mortality but also to explore new ways of postremission control of residual leukemia through activation of cellular defense mechanisms by IL 2. This approach emerged from preceeding in vitro investigations demonstrating an antileukemic activity of autologous cytotoxic lymphocytes against leukemic blasts which could be augmented by IL 2 [15,16,17]. A subsequent clinical pilot study in 9 patients demonstrated the feasibility of high-dose IL 2 maintenance therapy in second or subsequent remissions and also suggested a potential prolongation of remission duration in single cases. This approach is investigated by the current trial in way of a prospective randomized comparison. Since only 8 patients have entered this trial so far no meaningful judgement about the feasibility and efficacy of this study part is possible at the present time.

A clear indication of a beneficial effect of G-CSF administration after initial cytoreductive S-HAM therapy, however, emerges from the analysis of the first 38 cases undergoing this treatment. The overall remission rate of 58% compares favorably with the preceeding experiences with the identical cytostatic combination achieving only 48% remissions without G-CSF support. This difference results from a shortening of the period of severe granulocytopenia from a median of 38 days to 28 days, respectively, which translates into a reduction of early deaths from 26% to 18%. These data thus confirm corresponding reports by other investigators [18] and also a preceeding study of the AMLCG exploring GM-CSF in high risk AML patients [19]. Hence, hematopoietic growth factors and G-CSF and GM-CSF in particular have convincingly shown to reduce intensive therapy associated mortality from infections and thus make AML therapy more safe and effective. On this basis new strategies can be further explored which will ultimately improve the long term perspectives in AML therapy.

References

1. Gale RP, Foon KA: Therapy of acute myelogenous leukemia. Semin Hematol 2224: 40–54, 1987
2. Büchner Th, Hiddemann W: Treatment strategies in acute myeloid leukemia – First line chemotherapy (AML), Blut 60: 61–67, 1990
3. Hiddemann W, Maschmeyer G, Pfreundschuh M et al: Treatment of refractory acute myeloid (AML) and lymphoblastic leukemia (ALL) with high-dose cytosine arabinoside (HD-AraC) and mitoxantrone: indication of increased efficacy by sequential administration. Proc Am Soc Clin Oncol 5: 189, 1988
4. Hiddemann W, Aul C, Maschmeyer G et al: High-dose versus intermediate dose cytosine arabinoside combined with mitoxantrone for the treatment of relapsed and refractory acute myeloid leukemia: Results of an age adjusted randomized comparison. Leukemia and Lymphoma 10: 133–137, 1993
5. Büchner Th, Urbanitz D, Hiddemann W et al: Intensified induction and consolidation with or without maintenance chemotherapy for acute myeloid leukemia (AML): Two multicenter studies of the German AML Cooperative Group. J Clin Oncol 3: 1583–1589, 1985
6. Büchner Th, Hiddemann W, Löffler H et al: Improved cure rate by very early intensification combined with prolonged maintenance chemotherapy in patients with acute myeloid leukemia (AML): Data from AMLCG. Semin Hematol, 28, Suppl. 4: 76–79, 1991
7. Stone RM, Mayer RJ: Treatment of the newly diagnosed adult with de novo acute myeloid leukemia. Hematol/Oncol Clin. North America: 47–64, 1993
8. Gale RP, Champlin R: How does bone marrow transplantation cure leukemia? Lancet 2: 28–30, 1987
9. Sullivan KM, Fefer A, Witherspoon R et al: Graft versus leukemia in man: Relationship of acute and chronic graft-versus-host disease to relapse of acute leukemia following allogeneic bone marrow transplantation. In: Truitt RL, Gale RP, Bortin MM eds. Cellular Immunotherapy of Cancer. New York, Alan R Liss: 391–399, 1987
10. Adler A., Chervenick PA, Whiteside TL et al: Interleukin 2 induction of lymphokine-activated killer (LAK) activity in the peripheral blood and bone marrow of acute leukemia patients. I. Feasability of LAK generation in adult patients with active disease and in remission. Blood 71: 709–716, 1988
11. Teichmann JV, Ludwig WD, Seibt-Jung H, Thiel E: Induction of lymphokine-activated killer cells against human leukemic cells vitro. Blut 59: 21–24, 1989
12. Lotzová E, Savary CA, Herberman RB: Induction of NK cell activity against fresh human leukemia in culture with interleukin 2. J Immunol 138: 2718–2727, 1987
13. Foa R, Fierro MT, Cesano A et al: Defective lymphokine-activated killer cell generation and activity in acute leukemia patients with active disease. Blood 78: 1041–1046, 1991
14. Büchner Th, Hiddemann W, Wörmann B et al: Chemotherapy intensity and long-term outcome in AML. In: Th. Büchner, W. Hiddemann, B. Wörmann, G. Schellong, J. Ritter (eds.): Acute Leukemias IV. Prognostic Factors and Treatment Strategies. Springer Verlag Heidelberg: 513–518, 1994
15. Pelzer P, Garritsen HSP, Wörmann B et al: Inhibition of colony formation of leukemic blasts in acute leukemia by interleukin 2 stimulated autologous lymphocyte subsets. Blut 61: 176, 1990
16. Garritsen HSP, Segers-Nolten GMJ, Radosevic K et al: Assessment of lymphokine-activated killer activity in myeloid leukemic blasts and the myeloid cell line K562 by flow cytometry. In: Hiddemann W et al. eds. Acute Leukemias.

Pharmakokinetics and Management of Relapsed and Refractory Disease. Berlin, Springer Verlag: 581–589, 1992
17. Garritsen HSP, Kaufhold E, Pelzer P et al: Prognostic relevance and specific cytotoxic lymphocyte subpopulations in patients with acute myeloid leukemia. Onkologie 14, suppl. 2: 50, 1991
18. Ohno R, Tomonaga M, Kobayashi T et al: Effect of granulocyte colony-stimulating factor after intensive induction therapy in relapsed or refractory acute leukemia. N Engl J Med 323: 871–877, 1990
19. Büchner Th, Hiddemann W, Koenigsmann M et al: Recombinant human granulocyte-macrophage colony-stimulating factor following chemotherapy in patients with acute myeloid leukemia at higher age or after relapse. Blood 78: 1190–1197, 1991

Acute Leukemias V
Experimental Approaches
and Management of Refractory Diseases
Hiddemann et al. (Eds.)

Mitoxantrone-Etoposide or HD-ARA-C/Mitoxantrone for Remission Induction in Children with First Relapse of AML

K. Stahnke[1], J. Ritter[2], J. Boos[2], and U. Creutzig[2]

Introduction

One third of children with AML, initially responding to chemotherapy encounter recurrence of their disease. An effective chemotherapeutic regimen with tolerable toxicity is needed for this group of heavily pretreated children. In the past AML-BFM protocols did not specify for a salvage therapy. Reinduction chemotherapy with High Dose Ara-C/Mitoxantrone (HAM) or Mitoxantrone/Etoposide (Mitox/VP) was proposed. We performed a retrospective analysis among patients with first relapse previously treated with the AML-BFM 87 protocol with respect to initial response rates, toxicity and long term survival comparing the different reinduction regimen.

Patients

Of 309 patients eligible for the study AML-BFM-87 232 (75%) achieved a complete remission. 134 patients were in continous complete remission within a median follow up of 37 months. Of 89 relapsed patients 28 patients were not treated further or were treated palliativelly while 61 children received a salvage therapy. Age at diagnosis of relapse was 1.1 to 18.3 years with a median of 7.1 years. 35 children (57.4%) were male, 26 (42.6%) were of female sex. Duration of first remission ranged from 2.6 months to 66.2 months with a median of 12.7 months.

Therapy

For remission induction in first relapse two different regimen were proposed:

A. Mitox/VP: VP-16 was given in a 5-day schedule (100 mg/m^2/12h) in order to have a longer duration of etopside plasma levels above 1µg/ml. Dosage of Mitoxantrone was 10 mg/m^2/day, applied on days 1 and 2.

B. HAM: Therapy consisted of High-Dose-Ara-C 3 g/m^2/12h, 3h-infusion on days 1–3 and Mitoxantrone 10 mg/m^2/day on days 3 and 4.

Several clinics applied various other chemotherapeutic regimen, including combinations of Daunorubicin/Ara-C/Thioguanin/VP-16, Aclacinomycin A/VP-16, High-Dose Ara-C/VP-16, High-Dose Ara-C/VP-16/Mitoxantrone, m-Amsa/Ara-C, Iphosphamide/VP-16 and High-Dose Ara-C/ Iphosphamide. These patients are summarized in *Group C. Other*.

Postremission therapy was heterogenous, most children were treated with a second or third course of polychemotherapy; 8 were allo- and 12 autografted in second CR.

Results

Response to salvage therapy. Complete remission was achieved in 34 of 61 pts. treated: Of 10 children with early relapse (< 6 month of 1. CR) only one responded to salvage therapy, while 18 of 32 pts.

[1]Universitäts-Kinderklinik Ulm, Abt. Kinderheilkunde II, D-89070 Ulm, Germany
[2]Universitäts-Kinderklinik Münster, D-48129 Münster, Germany

Table 1. Response to salvage therapy

	Duration of first remission			
	< 6 months	6–18 months	> 18 months	Total
A: Mitox/VP				
Pts. treated	1	7	5	13
2nd CR	0	4	5	9(69.0%)
B: HAM				
Pts. treated	3	12	9	24
2nd CR	0	8	7	15(62.5%)
C: Other Therapies				
Pts. treated	6	13	5	24
2nd CR	1	6	3	10 (41.6%)
all Patients	10	32	19	61
2nd CR	1	18	15	34(55.7%)

(56%) with an initial CR lasting 6–18 months and 15 of 19 children (79%) with late relaps (> 18 months) achieved a second remission.

Response rates were comparable for group A (Mitox/VP) and B (HAM) and tended to be lower in group C (various regimen).

Table 2. Toxicity observed during induction therapy

	Early death	Severe infection
Group A		
Mitox/VP 13 pts	1	1
Group B		
HAM 24 pts	0	4
Group C		
Other 24 pts	3	2
all Patients 61 pts	4	7

*Severe infection: sepsis, aspergillosis

Toxicity. The early death rate for the whole group (4/61) was within the range of other relapse regimen [1, 2, 3]. Three deaths in group C were caused by sepsis (2 pts.) and cerebral haemorrhage (1 pt.). With the proposed regimen Mitox/VP and HAM there was only one early death, this was due to measles pneumonia. 4 children had severe aspergillosis, 1 in group A and 4 in group B indicating long term bone marrow supression.

Survival. Of 61 patients treated 18 survived within a follow up ranging from 2.1 months to 48.6 months. Comparison of the induction protocols is problematic because different postremission regimen were applied. However, again there is a trend in favour of the proposed regimen HAM and Mitox/VP.

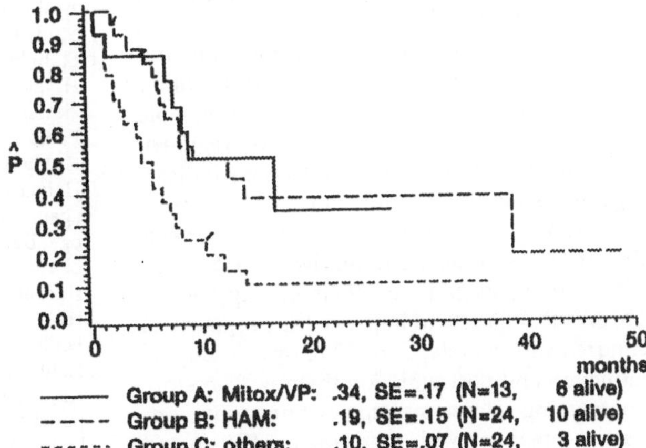

Fig. 1. Survival after salvage therapy

Table 3. Postremission therapy and survival

	no BMT	autologous BMT	allogeneic BMT	Total
A: Mitox/VP				
2nd CR achieved	2	4	3	9
alive	1	2	3	6
B: HAM				
2nd CR achieved	5	6	4	15
alive	5 (2 a.r.)	4 (1 a.r.)	1	10(3 a.r.)
C: Others				
2nd CR achieved	7	2	1	10
alive	2	0	1	3
All Patients				
2nd CR achieved	14	12	8	34
alive	7 (2 a.r.)	6 (1 a.r.)	5	18(3 a.r.)

(a.r.): after 2nd relapse

Postremission therapy and survival. Table 3 shows the survival rates broken down to treatment group and postremission therapy. 5 patients survived after allogeneic bone marrow tranplantation, while 10 patients are alive in CCR after autologous BMT or chemotherapy alone.

Discussion

We performed an analysis among all of the children relapsing after initial treatment with the BFM-87-protocol. Most of the patients (61/89) were treated with the intention to achieve a second remission. The choice of the induction protocol A: Mitox/VP, B: HAM or other regimen was done by the treating physican.

The analysis of initial response rates confirmed previous reports [4, 5, 6] indicating that long duration of first remission is a predictor for good response to salvage therapy. The proposed regimen were similar effective in inducing 2nd remission while results for the various other regimen were lower. Toxcity was acceptable with no toxic death in the proposed regimen, but with a high rate of fungal infections indicating longlasting myelosupression.

The analysis of postremission therapy reveals that there are long term survivors in 2nd CR with autologous BMT or chemotherapy alone. This result suggests to improve the prognosis of children with 1st relapse of AML by intensifying induction and postremission therapy. Therefore the ongoing relapse strategy of our group consists of a regimen with Mitoxantrone/VP-16 and HAM double induction therapy followed by autologous BMT using a Busulfan VP 16 preparative regimen.

References

1. Miller LP, Pyesmany AF, Wolff LJ, Rogers PCJ, Siegel SE, Wells RJ, Buckley JD, Hammond GD: Successful reinduction therapy with Amsacrine and Cyclocytidine in acute nonlymphoblastic leukemia in children. Cancer (1991) 67: 2235–2240
2. Mirro jr. J, Crom WR, Kalwinsky DK, Santane VM, Baker DK, Belt J: Targeted plasma drug concentration: a new therapeutic approach to relapsed nonlymphoblastic leukemia in children. Hematology and Blood Transfusion (1990) 32: 82–86
3. Movassaghi N, Higgins G, Pyesmany A, Baehner R, Chard R,Sather H, Hammond D Evaluation of Cyclocytidine in reinduction and maintenance therapy of children with acute nonlymphocytic leukemia previously treated with Cytosine Arabinoside: A Report from Children's Cancer Study Group. Med. Ped. Oncol. (1984) 12: 352–356
4. Stahnke K, Ritter J, Schellong G, Beck JD, Kabisch H, Lampert F, Creutzig U:Rezidivbehandlung bei akuter myeloischer Leukämie im Kindesalter. Klin. Pädiatr. (1992) 204: 253–257
5. Hiddemann W, Martin WR, Sauerland CM, Heinecke A, Büchner T: Definition of refractoriness against conventional chemotherapy in acute myelogenous Leukemia: A proposal based on the results of retreatment by Thioguanine, Cytosine Arabinoside, and Daunorubicin (TAD 9) in 150 patients with relapse after standardized first line therapy. Leukemia 4, (1990) 184–188
6. Kantarjian HM, Keatin MJ, Walters RS, McCredie KB, Freireich EJ: The characteristics and outcome of patients with late relapse acute myelogenous leukemia. JCO (1988) 6: 232–238

Acute Leukemias V
Experimental Approaches
and Management of Refractory Diseases
Hiddemann et al. (Eds.)

Sequential Mitoxantrone, Ara-C and VP-16 (s-MAV) Followed by Immuno-maintenance-Therapy with Interleukin-2 (IL-2) in the Treatment of Refractory and Relapsed Acute Myelogenous Leukemia

G. Hübner[1], J. Wendler[2], B. Otremba[3], I. Fackler-Schwalbe[4], and H. Link[1]

Introduction

With standard induction regimen combining anthracyclines and cytosine-arabinoside (Ara-C) complete remission (CR) rates of 60–80% can be achieved in previously untreated patients with acute myelogenous leukemia (AML). However, the majority of these patients eventually relapse. Repeated intensive induction therapy results in poorer CR-rates. Once remission is achieved, its duration is substantially shorter than the previous remission[1].

Recently, we have shown that MAV is an effective therapy for patients with refractory or relapsed AML, resulting in a complete remission rate of 58.3%. The disease-free interval, however, was only 4.5 months in median and lasted no longer than 12 months[2].

Aims of the Study

1. In vitro, etoposide was shown to inhibit the cellular ara-c uptake when given simultaneously[3]. In this trial we used a new sequential MAV regimen with non-parallel application of etoposide and ara-c to further improve the remission rate.
2. Recombinant IL-2 effectively enhances NK- and LAK-activity. AML-blasts are sensitive toward IL-2 activated effector cells in vitro[4]. In this trial, we applied IL-2 based immunotherapy as maintenance therapy in patients with high risk AML in remission to extend the remission duration.

Patients and Methods

Sixteen patients underwent s-MAV combination therapy. After induction of CR, 7 patients were treated with IL-2 immunomaintenance therapy.

Results

The results are shown in Tables 1–4 and Figs. 1–3.

Conclusions

Sequential MAV is an effective therapy regimen for patients with relapsed or refractory AML resulting in a complete remission rate of 62.5%.

Table 1. Patient characteristics

Median Age (range)	42.5(18–67)
Sex (m/f)	4/12
AML	
de novo/secondary	14/2
primary refractory	1/–
1st relapse	10/2
>2nd relapse	2/–
not known	1/–
Median duration of prior remission (range)	8(1–29)

[1]Dept. Hematology, Medical School Hannover, D-30623 Hannover, Germany
[2]Dept. Hematology, University Hospital, D-91054 Erlangen, Germany
[3]Dept. Hematology, Ev. Hospital, D-26122 Oldenburg, Germany
[4]Dept. Hematology, Central Hospital, D-86009 Augsburg, Germany

Table 2. Results: s-MAV

	MAVI n=16	MAVII n=7	total n=16
CR	11	5	10(62,5%)
PR	2		1(6,2%)
NR	3		3(18,8%)
Early death		2	2(12,5%)

- cause of death:
  - Septicemia 1 patient (CR after MAV I)
  - Pneumonia 1 patient (Pr after MAV I)
- One patient with PR entered CR after IL-2

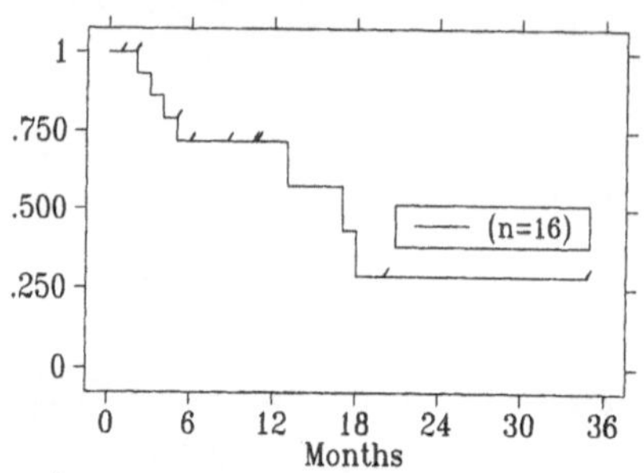

Fig. 1. Cumulative survival

Table 3. Results: IL-2

Pat.	AML	Status	Courses IL-2	Duration of remission	
				prior	post IL-2
F.G.	sec.	1st relapse	4+	8	6
J.U.	sec.	1st relapse	4	5	6
L.A.	de novo	2nd relapse	4	9	7
G.H.	de novo	1st relapse	3+	27	4
D.E.	de novo	3rd relapse	1	13	1
B.J.	de novo	2nd relapse	1	2	1*
W.R.	de novo	1st relapse	1/2ˣ		

+Dose reduced to one half after 1st course
*PR after MAV I, CR after IL-2
ˣthis pat. rejected treatment after 2 days of IL-2

Table 4. IL-2 treatment: toxicity (per patient)

	I°	II°	III°
Drug fever	–	5	2
Fluid retention	1	2	–
Blood pressure	3	–	–
Dyspnea	–	1	–
Skin rash	2	1	1
Local pain	1	3	–
Dry eye	–	1	–
Dry mouth	1	–	–
Nausea/vomiting	2	1	–
Diarrhea	1	–	–
Hematuria	1	–	–
CNS (weariness)	3	–	–
Hemoglobin	2	–	–
Thrombopenia	2	–	–
Alcaline phosphatase	–	1	–
Bronchitis	–	1	–

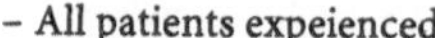

- All patients expeienced
  - temporary eosinophilia
  - local swelling at the injection site
- Toxicity was less in later courses

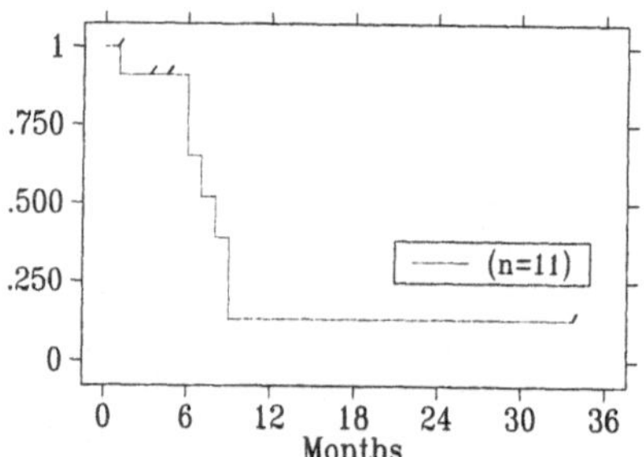

Fig. 2. Event-free survival

This CR-rate confirms the favourable result of our previous trial: 58,3% complete remissions in 36 patients after MAV reinduction therapy. Median duration of remission was 8 months. One patient is still disease-free with 34 months follow-up.

Immunomaintenance therapy with s.q. administration of IL-2 is a practical out-patient

Treatment Schedules

s-MAV:

Mitoxantrone	10 mg/m^2	d 1-5
Ara-C		
8.00:	100 mg/m^2	d 1-5
20.00:	100 mg/m^2	d 1-5
Etoposide	100 mg/m^2	d 1-5

Interleukin 2:

IL-2:	18 x 10^6 $U/m^2/d$	d 1-3
(s.q.,	9 x 10^6 $U/m^2/d$	d 4-5
1x/d)	P a u s e	
	9 x 10^6 $U/m^2/d$	d 8-12

IL-2 maintenance therapy is started after marrow regeneration (L>3000/µl)

Optionally, s-MAV II could be given in case of CR after s-MAV I

Treatment Plan

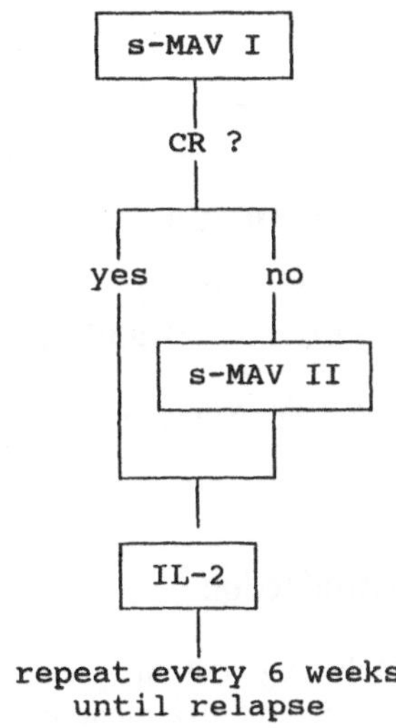

Fig. 3.

therapy. Toxicity is tolerable with no major adverse events. Duration of remission after treatment with IL-2 was generally short with two major exceptions: One patient who entered only PR after S-MAV went into CR after the first cycle of IL-2. Another patient experienced a longer duration of second than first CR; this patient eventually relapsed after 4 cycles of IL-2 treatment.

The treatment of further patients is necessary to evaluate the effect of IL-2 in immuno-maintenance therapy in AML.

References

1. Hiddemann W, Martin WR, Sauerland CM, et al: Definition of refractoriness against conventional chemotherapy in acute myeloid leukemia: a proposal based on the results of retreatment by thioguanine, cytosine arabinoside, and daunorubicin (TAD 9) in 150 patients with relapse after standardized first line therapy. Leukemia 4: 184–188, 1990.
2. Link H, Freund M, Diedrich H, et al: Mitoxantrone, cytosine arabinoside, and VP16 in 36 patients with relapsed and refractory acute myeloid leukemia. Acute Leukemias II Berlin, Springer, pp.322–325, 1990.
3. Ehninger G, Proksch B, Wanner T, et al: Intracellular cytosine arabinoside accumulation and cytosine arabinoside triphosphate formation in leukemic blast cells is inhibited by etoposide and teniposide. Leukemia 6: 582–587, 1992.
4. Oshimi K, Oshimi Y, Akutsu M, et al: Cytotoxicity of interleukin 2-activated lymphocytes for leukemia and lymphoma cells. Blood 68: 938–948, 1986.

Acute Leukemias V
Experimental Approaches
and Management of Refractory Diseases
Hiddemann et al. (Eds.)

Mitoxantrone, Etoposide and Cyclosporine A Therapy for Relapsed and Refractory Acute Myelogenous Leukemia, A Pediatric Oncology Group Phase II Trial

G. V. Dahl[1], N. Brophy[2], H. Grier[3], H. Weinstein[3], B. Sikic[2], and R. Arceci[3]

Introduction

Multidrug resistance remains a major obstacle to effective treatment of patients with Acute Myelogenous Leukemia (AML). A growing body of evidence indicates that over-expression of the MDR1 gene, which encodes the multidrug transporter P-glycoprotein(P-gp), contributes to the resistance of human cancers to many anti-cancer drugs [1,2]. One strategy currently being explored to overcome this resistance is the co-administration of non-cytotoxic drugs that bind to and inhibit the function of P-gp, thereby rendering the cells sensitive to concurrently administered chemotherapy. The Pediatric Oncology Group Phase II clinical trial reported here was designed to test the safety and efficacy of this strategy. Among the agents that are currently approved for clinical trials, Cyclosporine A (CSA) is the most potent inhibitor of P-gp. CSA has been shown to reverse chemotherapeutic resistance due to expression of the MDR1 P-gp both in vitro and in animal models. Phase I trials have demonstrated that blood levels of CSA similar to those required to modulate MDR in vitro can be achieved with acceptable toxicity. Alterations in the pharmacokinetics of MDR related drugs have been reported so that chemotherapy doses need to be chosen carefully to prevent undue toxicity [5].

Mitoxantrone and etoposide are chemotherapy drugs with proven effectiveness in AML They are also known to be substrates for P-gp and are actively transported from cells that over-express MDR1. Mitoxantrone and etoposide combinations have been used to successfully treat relapsed and refractory AML by several investigators. A 5 day induction course of 10 mg/m^2/day mitoxantrone and 100 mg/m^2/day etoposide resulted in CR for 42% of the relapsed adult patients[6]. A prolonged aplastic phase followed this therapy and a high incidence of infections was reported. Such effects of myelotoxicity may be a special hazard of this combination although in general it was highly active and well-tolerated by the patients with refractory and poor-risk AML.

Our hypothesis is that high expression of MDR1 in some leukemias results in clinical resistance to certain drugs, e.g. etoposide, mitoxantrone, doxorubicin and vincristine. CSA administration during chemotherapy with such agents may reverse this resistance by inhibiting the P-gp efflux pump[7]. Reports indicating expression of MDR1 in relapsed AML and evidence for in vitro reversal of clinical resistance by CSA provide an additional rationale for this approach[8]. A pilot protocol designed to modulate MDR1 with CSA performed at our institutions demonstrated that continuous infusions of CSA plus mitoxantrone and etoposide could induce remissions with acceptable toxicity.

The objectives of this study are to 1) determine the remission induction rate and toxicity to mitoxantrone, etoposide and Cyclosporine A (MEC), 2) achieve a steady state Cyclosporine A

[1]Pediatric Hematology/Oncology Division, Stanford University, Stanford, CA 94305
[2]Medical Oncology, Stanford University, Stanford, CA 94305
[3]Pediatric Oncology, Dana-Farber Cancer Institute, Boston, MA 02115

(CSA) level of >2400 ng/ml, 3) determine MDR1 mRNA and protein expression in leukemic blasts and 4) determine the ability of CSA to increase intracellular drug in vitro.

Methods and Materials

Patients. As of June 1993, 38 eligible patients with refractory or relapsed AML were treated with the MEC regimen at POG institutions after informed consent was obtained. All patients had failed prior therapy one or more times prior to MEC therapy. The median patient age was 5 years with a range of 1 to 21 years. Male to female ratio was 21:17 and the FAB types included Mo [2], M1–M2 [17], M3 [2], M4–M5 [12], M7 [3], RAEB [1] and treatment related second malignancy AML [1]. All patients were heavily pretreated with the following failure types: on therapy relapse 20 (53%), induction failures 7 (18%) and off therapy relapse 11 (29%). For those who had achieved a first remission the median duration of initial CR was 5 months.

MDR assays. MDR1 P-gp surface expression was determined by flow cytometry using the anti-MDR1 P-gp mouse monoclonal antibody, 4E3. The testing of the in vitro ability of CSA at 2.5uM to increase intracellular accumulation of 3H-daunorubicin was determined on samples from the study patients. Expression of MDR1 mRNA and the recently cloned Multidrug Resistance Associated Protein (MRP) mRNA were determined by PCR.

Study Design. CSA 10 mg/kg bolus was given over 2 hours as a loading dose and followed by 30 mg/kg/day continuous infusion for 98 hours (total 100 hours). The CSA dose was adjusted at hours 14, 26, 38 ,50 and 74 to maintain a steady state serum CSA level above 2.5 uM (3000 ng/ml to 5,000 ng/ml). If the serum CSA level was below 3,000 ng/ml, the infusion dose was increased by 25%; if the serum CSA level was >5,000 ng/ml the infusion was stopped until the next level was known. Mitoxantron 6 mg/m^2 and etoposide 60 mg/m^2 were given IV daily for 5 days . The first doses were given just after the 2 hour loading dose. A bone marrow aspirate and biopsy were taken at diagnosis and leukemia cells analyzed for MDR1 expression and function. Repeat marrow aspirate and biopsy were performed on day 14 from the start of therapy. If cellularity was greater than 20% and/or leukemia cells were identified in the aspirate, a second full course was given and appropriate CSA dose levels were chosen from the initial course. A repeat course of MEC was given as consolidation therapy for those who achieved remission. Patients in CR or PR received bone marrow transplants once they recovered from consolidation.

Results

Since this study is open and accruing patients the response rate is masked. Preliminary results indicate that complete remissions are occurring in these heavily pretreated patients and induction failures. Remissions have been attained in MDR positive and negative patients but the early proportion of patients identified as MDR positive is too small to perform a meaningful analysis. All patients achieved serum levels of CSA determined to be effective in modulating MDR1 in vitro. There was great interpatient variability but the median CSA level during the 100 hour infusion was 3,187 ng/ml (2.7uM). All patients manifested increases in serum bilirubin which returned to baseline within 1–3 days of completing the CSA infusion. For the patients who achieved remission the count recovery was as follows: Neutrophils >500 in 26 days [23–33], Platelets >100,000 in 34 days [23–34], Complete remission in 33 days [28–43].

Studies used to detect multidrug resistance were, as indicated earlier, the analysis of leukemia cell RNA and immunodetection and functional assays. The results of the MDR1, MRP and CSA reversal are detailed in Table 1. Seven of 25 samples were MDR positive and 18 were MDR negative. The detection of MDR by monoclonal antibody and flow cytometry indicated a similar proportion of positive samples with 6 of 25 patient samples positive for the 4E3 mouse monoclonal antibody. PCR determination for

Table 1. MDR1, MRP & CsA reversal study results

	Positive	Negative
MDR (PCR)	7/25(28%)	18/25(72%)
MDR (4E3)	6/25(24%)	19/25(76%)
MPR (PCR)	14/25(56%)	11/25(44%)
CsA reversal	11/25(44%)	14/25(56%)

MRP indicated that 14 of 25 leukemia cell samples demonstrated increased expression. Reversal of ^{3}H-daunorubicin efflux was identified in vitro in 11 of 25 patients.

The significant toxicities of this regimen were limited to myelosupression, mucositis and cardiotoxity. Grade IV mucositis requiring intravenous hyperalimentation developed in 22% of the patients, an additional 24% reported Grade I–III mucositis. Clinical heart failure was reported in 4 of 38 patients who had received daunorubicin prior to MEC treatment at cumulative dose levels of 405, 405, 210 and 405 mg/m^2 respectively. Three of the four children received two cycles of MEC before developing heart failure and one of the three developed heart failure only after recovering from a bone marrow transplant.

Discussion

Drug resistance, which may arise by somatic mutations during tumor growth or be present de novo, is an important cause of failure of cancer chemotherapy. Since our understanding of the mechanisms of drug resistance is based on laboratory models, the relationship of the models to the clinical setting has been difficult to prove. Few clinical trials have been designed to answer specific questions related to drug resistance. Since combination chemotherapy is often used, the contribution of one drug is difficult to assess. An increasing body of evidence implicates MDR1 expression as a determinant of both intrinsic and acquired drug resistance in human cancers.

Several non-cytotoxic drugs, such as verapamil, phenothiazines and CSA have been shown to modulate MDR in part by competitive inhibition of P-gp function. Verapamil and phenothiazines modulate MDR at drug concentrations which produce unacceptable clinical toxicities in vivo. CSA concentrations which reverse MDR in vitro are 1 to 2 uM, levels that were easily achievable in the patients reported here.

The patients admitted to this protocol were heavily pretreated with extensive use of prior anthracyclines and ara C. Most patients received etoposide prior to MEC and many received prior mitoxantrone. Marrow hypoplasia was induced in all patients treated and usually after only one course of MEC. The addition of CSA to the two drug five day mitoxantrone, etoposide regimen most certainly contributed to this response. Pharmacokinetic studies have shown increased AUC when CSA is given concomitantly with etoposide. The pharmacokinetics of mitoxantrone is likely affected similarly although studies have not been reported. The combined effect of increased AUC and P-gp modulation may be the significant contribution of the MEC therapy.

Serum levels of CSA >3,000 ng/ml and greater were achieved over a 5-day period. Hepatic toxicity was only manifested by hyperbilirubinemia and was reversible. Only two patients suffered renal abnormalities that were also reversible and likely related to tumor lysis and fluid deficit. Serious cardiotoxity was identified in 4 of 38 patients treated. The cardiotoxicity is likely related to the heavy use of anthracyclines prior to MEC although the role for mitoxantrone and the possible increased AUC of this agent needs to be taken into consideration. Presently we are studying the pharmacokinetics of mitoxantrone and etoposide in patients entering this protocol in an attempt to understand any contribution mitoxantrone may make to the cardiotoxicity seen in these patients. Whether or not CSA inhibition of P-gp leads to increased cardiotoxicity because of increased intracellular mitoxantrone levels or decreased clearance of mitoxantrone from inhibition of bilirubin excretion is at present unknown.

Initial results show that MDR can be detected in at least one quarter of patients and MRP in over one half. Studies to correlate the significance of MDR1 and MRP expression and in vitro drug uptake reversal by CSA and clinical response are underway.

These early results of a phase II study show that serum levels of CSA capable of reversing MDR are achievable in children with acceptable toxicity. Mucositis and heart failure were found to be major treatment related toxicity's in this heavily pretreated population. The response rate of this study is presently masked as the study remains open for accrual. Preliminary results show complete remissions in heavily pretreated patients and induction failures with AML. Remissions have been achieved in MDR positive and negative patients.

References

1. Fojo AT, Veda K., Slamon DJ., Poplack DG, Gottesmann MM and Pastan I: Expression of a multidrug-resistance gene in human tumors and tissues. Proc Natl. Acad. Sci. USA, 84: 265–269, 1987

2. Pastan I and Gottesman MM. Multi-drug resistance in human cancer. N. Engl. J. Med, 316: 1388–93, 1987
3. Slater LM, Sweet P, Stupecky M, and Gupta S: Cyclosporine A reverses vincristine and daunorubicin resistance in acute lymphatic leukemia in vitro. J. Clin. Investig. 77: 1405–1408, 1986
4. Marie JP, Zittoun R, and Sikic BI: Multidrug resistance (mdr1) gene expression in adult acute leukemias: correlations with treatment outcome and in vitro drug sensitivity. Blood 78: 586–592, 1991
5. Lum BL, Kaubisch S, Yahanda AM, Adler KM, Jew L, Ehsan MNAlterations of etoposide pharmacokinetics and pharmacodynamics by cyclosporine in a phase I trial to modulate multidrug resistance. J. Clin Oncol: 1635–42, 1992
6. Ho A, Lipp T, Ehninger G, et al: Combination mitoxantrone and etoposide in refractory AML- an active well-tolerated regimen J. Clin. Oncol.6: 213–217, 19887
7. Oseika R, Seeber S, Pannenbacker R, Soll D, Glatte P, and Schmidt CG: Enhancement of etoposide-induced cytotoxicity by cyclosporine A. Cancer Chemother Pharmacol. 18: 198–202, 1986
8. Marie J-P, Bastie JN, Coloma F, Just-Landi S Filleul S, Catalina J, et al. A phase I-II trial of cyclosporine with etoposide and mitoxantrone in advanced acute leukemia. Proc Am Soc Clin Oncol 11: 275, 1992

Acute Leukemias V
Experimental Approaches
and Management of Refractory Diseases
Hiddemann et al. (Eds.)

Sequential Chemotherapy with Mitoxantrone, Etoposide and Cytarabine for Previously Treated Acute Myeloid Leukemia: EMA 86 Regimen

Eric Archimbaud[1], Xavier Thomas[1], Véronique Leblond[2], Mauricette Michallet[3], Pierre Fenaux[4], François Dreyfus[5], Xavier Troussard[6], Catherine Cordonnier[7], J. Jaubert[8], P. Travade[9], Jacques Troncy[1], David Assouline[1], Denis Fière[1]

Abstract. EMA 86 regimen, associating mitoxantrone, 12 mg/m²/day on days 1–3, etoposide, 200 mg/m²/day as a continuous infusion on days 8–10 and cytarabine, 500 mg/m²/day as a continuous infusion on days 1–3 and 8–10, was administered to 133 patients. 70 patients had refractory AML and 63 had late first relapse. 60% achieved complete remission (CR), including 44% of refractory patients and 76% late first relapse patients ($p=0.0002$). 11% died from therapy-related toxicity. Median survival is 7 months, with 11% survival at 5 years. Median disease-free survival (DFS) is 8 months, with 20% DFS at 5 years.

Introduction

The principle of timed sequential chemotherapy (TSC), used in the therapy of acute myeloid leukemia (AML), is to recruit leukemic cells in the cell cycle using a first sequence of chemotherapy, then to administer a second sequence, using cycle active drugs, at the time of peak cell recruitment in order to increase efficacy [1]. Initially described TSC regimen, which included daunorubin and cytarabine in the first sequence and cytarabine alone in the second sequence, have shown efficacy when used both as first line therapy [2], and in previously treated patients [3]. EMA 86 regimen includes mitoxantrone instead of daunorubicin in the first sequence and associates etoposide to cytarabine in the second sequence. After encouraging initial results in 72 patients [4], we report here on 133 patients treated with this regimen.

Patients and Methods

Patients. Patients had AML non responsive to previous chemotherapy or in first or subsequent relapse. Only patients with a performance status of 2 or less and no grade >2 organ failure according to the World Health Organization (WHO) grading system could enter the study. Refractoriness was defined, according to Hiddeman et al [5], as (a) nonresponse, (b) early first relapse, occurring after a first CR of less than 6-month duration or while the patient is still on therapy, and (c) second and subsequent relapses.

Treatment regimen. Induction included a first sequence of chemotherapy combining mitoxantrone, 12mg/m²/day, administered IV as a

[1]Service d'Hématologie, Hôpital Edouard Herriot, 69437 Lyon, France
[2]Groupe Hospitalier Pitié-Salpêtrière, Paris
[3]Hôpital André Michallon, Grenoble
[4]Hôpital Claude Huriez, Lille
[5]Hôpital Cochin, Paris
[6]C.H.U., Caen
[7]Hôpital Henri Mondor, Créteil
[8]Hôpital Nord, Saint-Etienne
[9]Hôtel-Dieu, Clermont-Ferrand

short infusion over 3 days, and cytarabine, 500mg/m²/day IV as a continuous infusion over the same period. The second sequence, administered after a 4-day free interval, consisted in etoposide, 200 mg/m²/day IV as a continuous infusion over 3 days (days 8 to 10) and cytarabine, as in the first sequence. Post-induction therapy varied according to individual policies at each of the centers participating to this collaborative study. Most patients received a second course of chemotherapy identical to induction. Alternatively, patients received monthly maintenance courses with reduced dosages of drugs used during induction regimen, autologous bone marrow transplantation (BMT), or allogeneic BMT.

Results

Patient population. One hundred thirty-three patients entered the study, 16 of them with secondary AML or AML following a previous myelodysplastic syndrome. Seventy patients (53%) were classified as refractory and 63 had late first relapse. Median age of the patients was 46 years (range 15 to 70 years), 22 patients were aged over 60 years. Twelve patients had non M1-M6 AML.

Results of induction. Overall 79 patients (60%) achieved CR, 2 of them after 2 courses of chemotherapy, including 44% of refractory patients and 76% of late first relapses ($p = 0.0002$). Ten (46%) of 22 patients aged over 60 years and 12 (75%) of 16 patients with secondary AML or AML following a previous MDS achieved CR. Median duration of granulocyte count below 0.5×10^9/l was 31 days (range 11 to 64 days) and of platelet count below 20×10^9/l 29 days (range 12 to 85 days). WHO grade >2 extra-hematologic toxicity of induction included infection (54% of patients), oral mucositis (23%), vomiting (9%), hyperbilirubinemia (8%), bleeding (6%), cutaneous rash (5%), diarrhea (3%), complex metabolic disorders (2%) and cerebellar syndrome (1%). Fifteen patients (11%) died from toxicity.

Results of postinduction. Among the 79 complete remitters, 17 received no additional therapy, 27 received a second course of intensive chemotherapy using the same regimen as for induction, 10 received maintenance chemotherapy, 13 patients younger than 50 years received allogeneic BMT from a family-related donor, and 12 patients aged up to 64 years received autologous BMT.

At a median follow-up of 50 months, when patients receiving BMT are censored at the time of transplant, overall survival of the whole group of patients is 11% at 5 years, with a median survival of 7 months. Disease-free survival of the patients who achieved CR is 20% at 5 years, with a median DFS of 8 months. Five year overall survival is 3% in refractory patients and 20% in late first relapse patients ($p = 0.0002$). Five year DFS is 12% and 25% respectively ($p = 0.02$). One patient relapsed before scheduled intensive consolidation and 4 before autologous BMT. DFS at 5 years for patients younger than 60 years in whom intended post-induction therapy was intensive chemotherapy, autologous BMT or allogeneic transplantation are 24%, 15% and 46% respectively ($p = NS$).

Discussion

These results confirm that observed in the initial cohort of 72 patients treated according to EMA86 regimen [4], showing high initial antileukemic efficacy of this regimen including in selected patients aged more than 60 years. Furthermore, EMA 86 regimen induces 20% long term DFS, a rate higher than that observed in older series of relapsed patients [6,7]. The role of cell recruitment in the efficacy of daunorubicin and cytarabine-based TSC has been established [8]. If recruitment is to play a role in the efficacy of this particular regimen, CR rate might be increased, particularly in refractory patients, by the use of CSFs between the 2 sequences in order to potentially increase recruitment [9]. A pilot study has shown no increased toxicity when administering GM-CSF between the 2 sequences of EMA regimen [10]. This association is therefore being evaluated in a randomized trial (EMA 91 trial).

References

1. Vaughan WP, Karp JE, Burke PJ: Long chemotherapy-free remissions after single-cycle timed sequential chemotherapy for acute myelocytic leukemia. Cancer 45: 859–865, 1980

2. Vaughan WP, Karp JE, Burke PJ: Two-cycle timed-sequential chemotherapy for adult acute nonlymphocytic leukemia. Blood 64: 975–980, 1984
3. Fiere D, Campos L, Vu Van H, Guyotat D, et al: Intensive timed chemotherapy protocol for 37 resistant or relapsing acute myeloid leukemias. Cancer Treat Rep 70: 285–286, 1986
4. Archimbaud E, Leblond V, Michallet M, et al: Intensive sequential chemotherapy with mitoxantrone and continuous infusion etoposide and cytarabine for resistant or relapsing acute myelogenous leukemia. Blood 77: 1894–1900, 1991
5. Hiddemann W, Martin WR, Sauerland CM, Heinecke A, Büchner Th: Definition of refractoriness against conventional chemotherapy in acute myeloid leukemia: a proposal based on the results of retreatment by thioguanine, cytosine arabinoside, and daunorubicin (TAD 9) in 150 patients with relapse after standardized first line therapy. Leukemia 4: 184–188, 1990
6. Keating MJ, Kantarjian H, Smith TL, et al: Response to salvage therapy and survival after relapse in myelogenous leukemia. J Clin Oncol, 7: 1071–1080, 1989
7. Davis CL, Rohatiner AZS, Lim J, et al: The management of recurrent acute myelogenous leukemia at a single center over a fifteen-year period. Br J Haematol 83: 404–411, 1993
8. Karp JE, Donehower RC, Enterline JP, Dole GB, Fox MG, Burke PJ: In vivo cell growth and pharmacologic determinants of clinical response in acute myelogenous leukemia. Blood 73: 24–30, 1989
9. Tafuri A, Andreeff M: Kinetic rationale for cytokine-induced recruitment of myeloblastic leukemia followed by cycle-specific chemotherapy in vitro. Leukemia 4: 826–834, 1990
10. Archimbaud E, Fenaux P, Reiffers J, Cordonnier C, Leblond V, Travade Ph,Troussard X, Tilly H, Auzanneau G, Marie JP, Berger E. Granulocyte-macrophage colony-stimulating factor in association to timed-sequential chemotherapy with mitoxantrone, etoposide and cytarabine for refractory acute myelogenous leukemia. Leukemia 7: 372–373, 1993.

Acute Leukemias V
Experimental Approaches
and Management of Refractory Diseases
Hiddemann et al. (Eds.)

Treatment of Childhood Acute Nonlymphoblastic Leukemia – Final Results of the Austrian-Hungarian Study AML-IGCL-84

F. M. Fink[1], G. Mann[2], P. Masát[3], E. R. Panzer-Grümayer[2], P. Kajtar, G. Kardos, Ch. Urban, D. Schuler[4], and H. Gadner[2] for the IGCI[5] Pediatric Study Group

Introduction

In the treatment of childhood acute nonlymphoblastic leukemia remission rates of 70 to 80 percent can be achieved by a variety of intensive induction chemotherapy regimens [1–5]. Anthracycline antibiotics are among the most effective agents for the treatment of ANLL. Therefore these drugs or related compounds are used in high doses.

Aclarubicin (ACR) – a newer generation anthracycline – has been introduced to clinical use more than ten years ago. Phase I and II studies had shown a significant anileukemic activity of the drug, particularly against acute nonlymphoblastic leukemia [6–8].

In 1984 a cooperative multicentric study (AML-IGCI-84) was initiated which applied ACR in combination with cytosine arabinoside and etoposide in children with acute nonlymphoblastic leukemia.

Patients, Treatment and Methods

Children with newly diagnosed untreated ANLL were eligible for the study. They were treated at several pediatric clinics in Austria and Hungary. Leukemias were classified according to the cytologic and cytochemical criteria of the FAB group [9, 10]. In addition, in most cases, immunologic classification of cell surface markers, determination of terminal deoxynucleotidyl transferase (TdT), and cytogenetic analysis were performed.

From January 1984 until November 1989 95 children with ANLL – 46 boys, 49 girls, median age 7;06 years (1 day - 17;01 years) – were treated. FAB subtypes included M_1 (n=29), M_2 (n=13), M_3 (n=1), M_4 (n=26), M_5 (n=20), M_6 (n=2) and M_7 (n=4). The median initial white blood count was 18.6 G/l (1.4–1350.0), 3 patients showed initial CNS-involvement.

Study design: The back-bone of the protocol was identical with the german therapy study AML-BFM-83 (Fig. 1) [5]. In contrast to the BFM-83 protocol, however, all patients received induction 1 (Ara-C, ACR, VP-16; Fig. 2).

Children in complete remission after I1 (<5% blasts in the bone marrow aspirate) proceeded to the intensive BFM-83-consolidation (a modified childhood BFM-ALL-protocol: prednisone 40mg/m² daily p.o. days 1–28, 6-thioguanine (6-TG) 60mg/m² daily p.o. days 1–56, vincristine 1.5 mg/m² i.v. and doxorubicin 25 mg/m² i.v. days 1, 8, 15, 22, cytosine arabinoside (Ara-C) 75 mg/m² i.v. on 4 consecutive days starting on days 3, 10, 17, 24, 31, 38, 45, 52, respectively, cyclophosphamide 500 mg/m² i.v. on days 29 and 57, age-dependent inthrathecal Ara-C on days 31, 38, 45 and 52: <1 year 20 mg, 1 – 2 years 26 mg, 2–3 years 34 mg, >3 years 40 mg). The consolidation protocol included cranial irradiation with age-dependent dose (<1 year 12 Gy, 1–2 years 15 Gy, >2 years 18 Gy) [6].

[1]Dept. of Pediatrics, University of Innsbruck, Innsbruck, Austria
[2]St.Anna Children's Hospital, Vienna, Austria
[3]Teaching Hospital Szombathely, Szombathely, Hungary
[4]Semmelweis University Medical School Budapest, Budapest, Hungary
[5]Internationale Gesellschaft für Chemo- und Immunotherapie

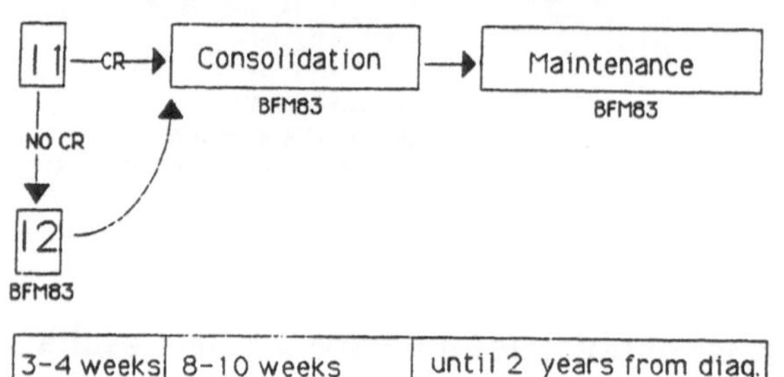

Fig. 1. Study design: I1, induction 1; I2, induction 2; CR, complete remission; NO CR, no CR achieved

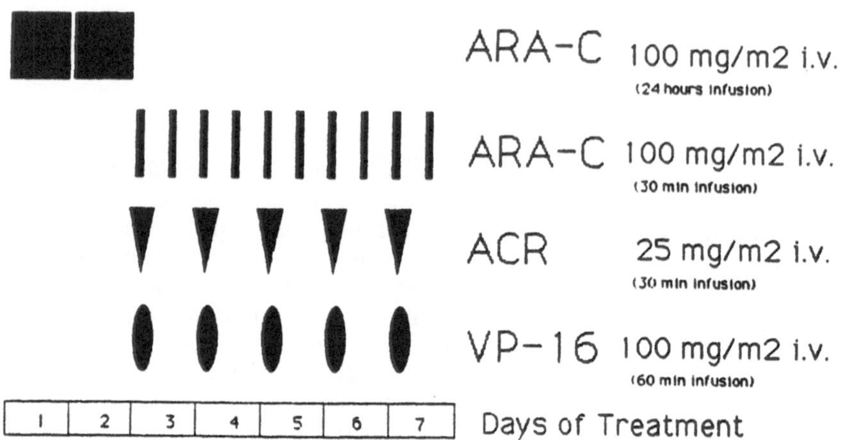

Fig. 2. Induction I1: ACR, aclarubicin; ARA-C, cytosine arabinoside; VP-16, etoposide

Children not in complete remission after I1 received an induction I2 (BFM-83: Ara-C 100 mg/m^2 24-hour infusion days 1 and 2, 100 mg/m^2 i.v. twice daily days 3–8, daunorubicin 60 mg/m^2 i.v. days 3–5, VP-16 150 mg/m^2 days 6–8) before consolidation [6].

Maintenance was started 2 weeks after the end of the consolidation therapy with daily 6-TG (40 mg/m^2 p.o.), Ara-C (40 mg/m^2 s.c.) for 4 days every 4 weeks, and doxorubicine (25 mg/m^2 i.v every 8 weeks 4 times only (during the first year). Maintenance was stopped 2 years after diagnosis.

I2, consolidation and maintenance were original protocols of the study AML-BFM-83 [6].

Patients with high initial white blood cell counts (WBC) (>50.000/μL) and/or extensive organomegaly received a cytoreductive pretreatment with 6-TG and Ara-C.

Results

64 patients (67%) achieved complete remission (CR), 47 (49%) by I1, 16 patients (17%) by I2, 1 patient by the consolidation course. Induction failure was caused by early death in most cases: 5 patients died within one week from diagnosis, 16 pts. during bone marrow aplasia following I1, and 10 pts. died later without having ever achieved remission.

7 pts. proceeded to bone marrow transplantation (BMT) in first CR (allogeneic n = 2, syngeneic n = 1, autologous n = 4), they were censored for survival analyses at the date of grafting. By the date of evaluation (December 1993) 27 relapses had occurred, 5 patients died in CR. 30 patients remain in first CR. Probability of event free survival is .30 (SE .05, Fig. 3), of event free interval .44 (SE .07) at 9 years after diagnosis or CR, respectively (Life table analysis, median follow up in CR 6;05 years).

Infants less than 12 months of age at diagnosis represented a remarkably high proportion of the study population (n = 12, 13%) and had a dismal prognosis, only one patient autografted in first CR survived. Initial leukocyte count, FAB-subtype and gender had no significant impact on the outcome.

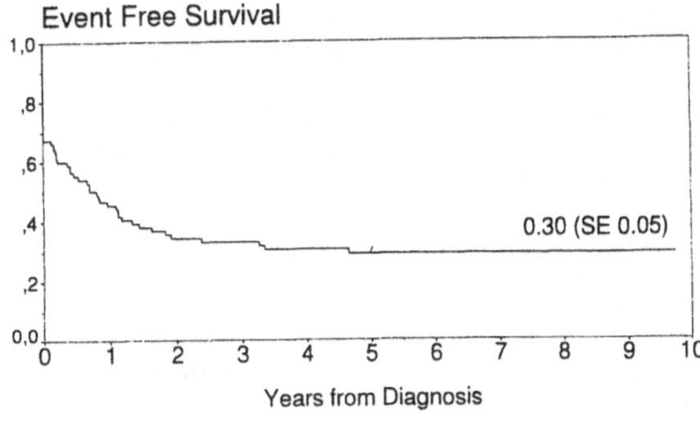

Fig. 3. Survival analysis (life-table method) of study AML-IGCI-84 (n = 95)

Discussion

The induction chemotherapy including ACR as first line anthracycline was effective. Three quarters of all remissions were already achieved by the ACR-containing induction regimen. In addition, a considerable percentage of children remained in long-term remission. These results compare well with those published for other protocols for childhood ANLL [1–6].

In adults, the value of ACR for the treatment of acute myelogenous leukemia has already been demonstrated in refractory disease as well as in front line therapy. Rowe et al. showed a high remission rate induced by a combination of high dose ACR and etoposide in patients with refractory acute myelogenous leukemia [11]. In a randomized trial of Hanson et al. the ACR-containing induction course yielded a significantly higher remission rate than the one with daunorubicin [12].

However, compared with the original BFM-83 protocol the results of our study were still inferior [6]. This might partially be explained by the high proportion of infant leukemia. Secondly, a high rate of early deaths due to uncontrolled infections before remission as well as a nearly 8 % rate of deaths in complete remission turned out to be the main problems to be solved in future protocols.

Acknowledgement. We would like to thank colleagues in Austria and Hungary who entered patients in our cooperative study for their kind cooperation. We acknowledge the support by Prof. D. Lutz during the planning and initiation of the study.

References

1. Creutzig U, Ritter J, Riehm H, Langermann HJ, Henze G, Kabisch H, Niethammer D, Jürgens H, Stollmann B, Lasson U, Kaufmann U, Löffler H, Schellong G (1985) Improved treatment results in childhood acute myelogenous leukemia. Blood 65: 298
2. Weinstein HJ, Mayer RJ, Rosenthal DS, Coral FS, Camitta BM, Gelber RD (1983) Chemotherapy for acute myelogenous leukemia in children and adults: VAPA update. Blood 62: 315–319
3. Buckley JD, Chard RL, Baehner RL, Nesbit ME, Lampkin BC, Woods WG, Hammond GD (1989) Improvement in outcome for children with acute nonlymphocytic leukemia. A report from the Children's Cancer Study Group. Cancer 63: 1457–1465
4. Amadori S, Ceci A, Comelli A, Madon E, Masera G, Nespoli L, Paolucci G, Zanesco L, Covelli A, Mandelli F (1987) Treatment of acute myelogenous leukemia in children: results of the Italian cooperative study AEIOP/LAM 8204. J Clin Oncol 5: 1356–1363
5. Creutzig U, Ritter J, Schellong G (1990) Identification of two risk groups in childhood acute myelogenous leukemia after therapy intensification in study AML-BFM-83 as compared with study AML-BFM-78. Blood 75: 1932–1940
6. Warrell RP, Arlin ZA, Zempin SJ, Young CW (1982) Phase I–II evaluation of a new anthracycline antibiotic, aclacinomycin A, in adults with refractory leukemia. Cancer Treat Rep 66: 1619–1623
7. Yamada K, Nakamura T, Tsurno T, et a. (1980) A phase II study of aclacinomycin A in acute leukemia in adults. Cancer Treat Rev 7: 177–182
8. Pedersen-Bjergaard J, Brincker H, Ellegard J, Drivsholm A, Freund L, Jensen KB, Jensen MK, Missen NI (1984) Aclarubicin in the treatment of acute nonlymphocytic leukemia refractory to treatment with daunorubicin and cytarabine.: a phase II trial. Cancer Treat Rep 68: 1233–1238
9. Bennett JM, Catovsky D, Daniel MT, Flandrin G, Galton DAG, Gralnick HR, Sultan C (1976)

Proposals for the classification of the acute leukemias. French-American-British (FAB) cooperative groups. Br J Haematol 33: 451–458

10. Bennett JM, Catovsky D, Daniel MT, Flandrin G, Galton DAG, Gralnick HR, Sultan C (1985) Criteria for the diagnosis of acute leukemia of megakaryocytic lineage (M7). A report of the French-American-British cooperative group. Ann Intern Med 103: 460
11. Rowe JM, ChangAY, Bennett JM (1988)Aclacinomycin A and etoposide (VP-16-213): an effective regimen in previously treated patients with refractory acute myelogenous leukemia. Blood 71: 992–996
12. Hansen OP, Pedersen-Bjergaard J, Ellegaard J, Brincker H, Boesen AM, Christensen BE, Drivsholm A, Hippe E, Jans H, Jensen KB, et al. (1991) Aclarubicin plus cytosine arabinoside versus daunorubicin plus cytosine arabinoside in previously untreated patients with acute myeloid leukemia: a Danish national phase III trial. The Danish Society of Hematology Study Group on AML, Denmark. Leukemia 5: 510–516

Acute Leukemias V
Experimental Approaches
and Management of Refractory Diseases
Hiddemann et al. (Eds.)

TAD Double Induction, HDAra C Consolidation, Rotation Maintenance in ANLL: the Results and Prophylaxis of Hepatitis and Fungal Infection

S. Pushkareva[2], N. Gorbounova[1], E. Oboukhova[2], A. Davtian[1], M. Kontchalovski[1], G. Selidovkin[1], and A. Baranov[1]

Introduction

In the last 10 years the results of the treatment of ANLL became much better because of the intensification of chemotherapy programs even without the use of new medicines [1]. In our clinic we also constantly try to optimise the treatment, so, last years it is in many parts similar to 1985 study of AMLCG [2] - TAD double induction and consolidation on the base of high-dose cytosine arabinoside (HDAra C).

There are our experience of treatment adult ANLL and results of prophylaxis with amphotericin B (ampho-B) inhalation and parenteral recombinant human α-interferon (rHuIFN-α) of systemic mycoses and viral hepatitis.

Materials and Methods

Patients. Between January 1990 and December 1993 79 newly diagnosed ANLL patients (pts) were admitted. 56 of them were under the age of 60 (14–59, med. - 39 y.o.). Male - 27, female - 29. The FAB variants of leukaemia: were M_1- 4, M_2- 20, M_3-2, M_4-23, M_5- 6, M_6- 1.

Besides 7 patients were treated with the same program in 1988-89 years and had age 14–51 (med. 36 y.o., M_2- 3, M_3- 1, M_4- 3).

Treatment. In 1990 we used double TAD-7 for remission induction: cytarabine (Ara C) 100 mg/m² (4 h-infusion, b.i.d.), d 1–7; 6-mercaptopurin (6MP) 75 mg/m²,, b.i.d., p.o., d 1–7; daunorubicin (DNR) 60 mg/m², d 5–7. In 1991–92 VP-16 100 mg/m² was added to TAD-7 in 8, 9 days of treatment. From July 1992 remission induction included two TAD-9: Ara C 100 mg/m² (24 h-infusion in 1, 2 days and 1 h-infusion every 12h in d 3–8), 6-thioguanin 100 mg/m² or 6MP 75 mg/m², b.i.d., p.o., d 3–9; DNR 60 mg/m², d 3–5. Period between induction courses was not regulated strictly but it was tried to be not more than 30 days.

For consolidation high-dose Ara C (1 g/m², ¹h-infusion, every 12h, d 1–4) and DNR 45 mg/m², d 5–7, were used. One consolidation cycle was done in 2 months after induction of CR upto July 1992, then two such cycles has been desided to de done in six month CR period.

Long-term maintenance treatment was used only in patients with poor prognosis (hyperleukocytosis, hepatosplenomegalia, skin infiltration) and in patients which treatment program was not fulfilled in planned period of time. Maintenance included Ara C 50 mg/m², t.i.d., s.c., d 1–5, every 6 weeks. Second medicine was alternated - DNR 30 mg/m², d 1; or cyclophosphamide 750 mg/m², d 1; or 6MP 75 mg/m², t.i.d., d 1–5.

Hepatitis and its prophylaxis. The diagnosis of acute viral hepatitis (AVH) was made when AST and/or ALT were over 10 times of upper normal value (10N). The rise of AST and/or ALT level till 10N was called as "hyperaminotranspheremia of unknown origin" (HaUO).

For hepatitis prophylaxis patients received the rHuIFN-α (1–2 × 10⁶ iU, e.o.d., i.m.) from the

[1]Clinical Department of Institute of Biophysics
[2]Clinical Hospital No 6, Marshal Novikov St., 23, 123098 Moscow, Russia

first day of 1st induction cycle and it was continued all time untill inpatient staying for induction and consolidation courses.

Systemic fungal infection and prophylaxis of aspergillosis. The diagnosis of systemic (invasive) fungal infection was undoubted if fungi were discovered in blood or in species of material from lesion's place (bacteriological, bacterioscopical, histological investigations). Fungal pneumonia was suspected in cases with typical X-ray film: spherical lesions and cavities with so-called "fungus ball" (aspergillosis) [3]. The effect of ampho-B treatment conformed the diagnosis.

The aspergillosis prophylaxis was made with ampho-B inhalations through the whole periods of patient's hospitalisations (ultrasonic inhaler, 5 mg of ampho-B in 10 ml of distilled water, b.i.d.) [4].

Results

Remission induction. Remission rate in 56 patients under 60 is 65%, in all cases after first TAD. Intensification of induction therapy increased the remission rate and decreased the number of resistant cases, but there were no differences in mortality (Table 1).

The time between TAD courses is a characteristic of induction's intensity (Table. 2). Only in 20% of patients it was possible to begin the second induction course in month after the first one. So, intensity of induction treatment was much less if compared with planned. Up to the moment of consolidation 36 patients (65%) were alive.

Remission consolidation. Consolidation with HDAra C+DNR performed in 23 from 36 patients, of the other ones: 3 received BMT, 2 had early relapse, 5 refused the treatment and 3 are on consolidation just now. Seven more patients in 1988–89 completed such program of induction and consolidated. They are joined (23+7) for analysis. Most (22 from 30) patients received first consolidation in 6 month from remission (Table 3). In other 4 cases it performed some later because they had severe hepatitis. Three patients died during first consolidation (hepatorenal failure, intracerebral hemorrhage, sudden cardiac death).

Second consolidation course was performed only in 10 from 27 patients which were alive after the previous one. In first 10 cases (before 1992) second consolidation was not planed, 3 patients are on the treatment now, but 1 patients had the relapse after first consolidation, in 2 cases treatment delayed because of chronic active hepatitis. One patient died during second consolidation (*Pseudomonas* sepsis).

Table 1. Results of induction treatment

	Induction course			
	TAD-7	TAD+VP-16	TAD-9	Total
No. of patients	23	19	14	56
Complete remission	13(56%)	13(68%)	12(86%)	38(68%)
Death in 1 induct.	5(22%)	3(16%)	2(14%)	10(18%)
Death in 2 induct.	0	0	2[a](14%)	2(4%)
Resistant cases	5(22%)	3(16%)	0	8(14%)

[a]patients died in first remission

Table 2. Interval between TAD cycles

	Time between cycles, days			
	⩾21–30	⩾31–40	⩾41–50	>50
Patients. of 1988–89, n=7	0	2	4	1
Patients. of 1990–93, n=38	9	10	1	18
Total, n=45	9(20%)	12(27%)	5(11%)	19(42%)

Table 3. Time between remission and HDAra C+DNR consolidations

	Interval remission to consolidation, months						
	⩾2–4	>4–6	>6–8	>8–10	>10–12	>12	Total
First consolidation[a]	16	6	2	2	2	2	30
Second consolidation[a]	–	1	3	4	1	1	10

[a]number of patients

Maintenance chemotherapy. Maintenance chemotherapy is conducted in 13 from 26 patients, who finished the program of TAD double induction and one or two courses of HDAra C+DNR consolidations. Most of the patients come over the treatment satisfactorily, only 3 patients are needing to prolong intervals between cycles because of long aplasia.

Probability of disease free survival. There is a curve of DFS of 26 ANLL patients, who were alive after double TAD-induction and one or two courses of consolidations by HDAra C+DNR (see Fig. 1): median is 22 months, the plateau started after 30 months, on the level of 39%.

Hepatitis and prophylaxis with rHuIFN-α. The rate of hepatitis and the results of its prophylaxis were studed in two groups: first group included 40 patients of 1990–93 years, which were alive more then 4 months and only half of them completed program of chemotherapy and second group of 30 patients, who have performed both induction and cosolidation treatments (Table 4).

Different kinds of liver damages appeared in 87% of patients, AVH was in 52–57% of patients. Hepatitis began in a period from 1 to 12 month, the half of all cases had the beginning this complication in 4–6 mo, and about 30% of patients-in 2–3 months after induction. rHuIFN-α-prophylaxis decreased hepatitis rate, but not reduced the portion of patients, who needed chemo-therapy reduction because of liver damages. Only 6 of all patients had normal amynotranspheras level through the whole period of treatment, 5 of them received rHuIFN-α prophylaxis.

Fungal infection and its prophylaxis. Systemic or severe invasive mycoses were diagnosed in 21 (26%) from 79 adult ANLL patients, treated in 1990–93 (Table 5). There were candidosises in 13 patients (4-septicaemia, 8-pneumonia, 1-oesophageal ulceration with massive bleeding). In all patients complications disappeared with amphotericin B treatment and after granulocyte level normalisation. Treatment of candidosis was the reason to delay next course of chemotherapy in 3 patients. Aspergillosis pneumonia occurred in 8 patients, in 4 cases it was the main cause of the death.

Aspergillosis appeared in our department only from 1992. Frequency of this complication and efficiency of its prophylaxis were analysed in 44 patients, treated in this period. In group with ampho-B prophylaxis aspergillosis was diagnosed in 2 from 18 patients (11%), the complications occurred in first induction course and in one case it was the cause of the death. In group without prophylaxis 6 from 26 (23%) patients had this complication (3 patients – in first induction of the first remission and 3

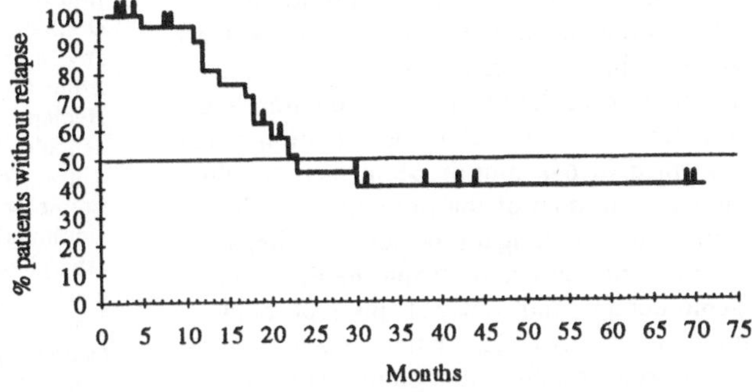

Fig. 1. Probability of DFS in group of 26 ANLL patients, who were alive after TAD double induction and 1 or 2 courses of HDAra C+DNR consolidations

Table 4. Acute viral hepatitis (AVH), hyperaminotranspheremia of unknown origin (HaUO) and rHuIFN-α prophylaxis in two groups of ANLL patients

	Induction-Consolidation			
	Pts. on prophylaxis		Pts. after prophylaxis	
	yes	no	yes	no
No.of patients.:	17	23	10	20
- AVH	7(40[a])	14(70)	3(30)[b]	14(70)
- HaUO	12(70)	19(85)	7(70)	19(85)
- No.of pts. needed chemotherapy reduction:	6(35)	7(30)	3(30)	8(40)
- because of AVH	5	6	2	6
- because of HaUO	1	1	1	2

[a]per cent of the patients;
[b]$p < 0.05$ [5]

Table 5. Patients with systemic mycoses in 1990–1993

	1990	1991	1992	1993
No patients:	4	2	7	8
- with Candidosis	4	2	4	3
- with Aspergillosis	0	0	3	5

patients – in induction of the second remission). 3 patients died because of aspergillosis, others were cured and proceeded chemotherapy. There were no relapses of aspergillosis, but it was necessary to delay the beginning of the next course.

Discussion

From current data we know that the rate of remission and its duration depend on the intensity of the treatment in cycles of induction and consolidation. But intensity of the treatment is determined not only by the doses of medicines, but by intervals between courses of chemotherapy. For example, 1985 trail of AMLCG lay out 21-days period between two induction courses TAD-9 and 6–8 weeks till next consolidation.

The results of similar treatment of ANLL are presented in this article. Only in 25% of patients the program of double TAD-9 induction and 2 courses of HDAra C+DNR consolidation can be performed in 6–8 month. Main factors, which influence the time of the program were in our circumstances – fungal infections and hepatitis. The first ones occurred during the first cycle of chemotherapy and delayed interval between induction courses. The latter appeared most often during second induction or just after it, so 6–8 week intervals between next courses were unreal.

Viruses of hepatitis B and C were the cause of hepatitis in our patients. We suppose also that the same viruses are the cause for the most part of HaUO, but could not prove it. The time of starting of hepatocellular damages from the beginning of chemotherapy and massive haemotransfusion (1.5–3 months for HaUO, and 3–6 month for hepatitis) is the reason for this suspicion.

Prophylaxis of aspergillosis with ampho-B inhalations and of hepatitis with rHuIFN-α, which were used in our clinic last years, decreased the rate of aspergillosis and the rate and severity of hepatitises. It is necessary to improve these prophylaxis treatments to get the better results from intensive chemotherapy of ANLL.

References

1. Büchner T – Acute leukemia. Current opinion in Hematology, 1993, 172–182.
2. Büchner T, Hiddemann W., Löffler G. et al. – Improved cure rate by very early intensification combined with prolonged maintenance chemotherapy in patients with acute myeloid leukemia: Data from the AML cooperativ group; Seminars in Hematology, 1991, 28, Suppl 4 (July), 76–79.
3. Salfelder K. – Atlas of fungal pathology, p. 38–43, Kluver Acad. Publ., 1990, 200 p.
4. Connealy E., Cafferkey M., Daly P. et al. – Nebulized amphotericin B as prophylaxis aganst invasive aspergillosis in granulocytopenic patients.Bone marrow transplantation, 1990, 5, 403–406.
5. Fimrey D., Latscha R., Bennet B., Hsu P. – Tables for testing significane in a 2×2 contingency Table. Cambridge, Univ Press, 1963.

Chemotherapy in ALL

Acute Leukemias V
Experimental Approaches
and Management of Refractory Diseases
Hiddemann et al. (Eds.)

Salvage Therapy of Childhood ALL: Prognosis of Marrow Relapse After Intensive Front-line Therapy

G. Henze, R. Hartmann, and R. Fengler on behalf of the BFM Relapse Study Group

Introduction

Bone marrow (BM) is the most frequent relapse site in childhood acute lymphoblastic leukemia (ALL). In the experience of the ALL-REZ BFM relapse trials the marrow was involved in 80% of relapse patients. The following report summarizes the results of four consecutive trials for treatment of relapsed ALL and addresses the question whether bone marrow transplantation (BMT) is required in any case of systemic recurrence.

Patients and Methods

Between 1983 and 1993, 540 children and adolescents up to the age of 18 years having experienced their first marrow relapse were enrolled in four consecutive multicentric relapse trials of the BFM Study Group. Median age was 8.2 years (range 1.5–18), 315 patients (58.3%) were boys and 94% had been initially treated according to intensive front-line therapy as used in the German BFM and COALL trials. Isolated BM relapse (leukemia only detectable in the marrow, >25% BM blasts) was diagnosed in 380 patients (70.4%). 160 patients had combined relapses (cytologically or histologically proven extramedullary leukemia with at least 5% BM blasts). The most frequent concomitantly involved site was the central nervous system (CNS), followed by the testicles and other regions such as skin, mediastinum, pleura, ovaries or the prostatic gland.

Late relapse (beyond six months after the end of front-line therapy) was present in 315 patients. In 63 children the relapse had occurred during the first 18 months of first complete remission (CR), in the following referred to as very early relapse, and in 162 patients the time of relapse was in between (early relapse). As previously shown, children with very early systemic relapse or any relapse of T-cell ALL have a dismal prognosis [7]. Therefore, these patients were termed Poor Prognosis Group (PPG). Detailed patient characteristics are shown in Table 1.

Treatment consisted of alternating short-term multidrug chemotherapy courses, four R1 and R2 courses each in studies ALL-REZ 83, 85 and 87[4]. In study ALL-REZ 90 which is still open for patient entry course R3 (main constituents: VP16 and high-dose ARA-C) was introduced such that three of each R1, R2 and R3 courses are administered up to a total of nine. In the first three trials, children with early or very early marrow relapse received an initial induction protocol[6]. Different in the study design were the methotrexate (MTX) doses used within the R-courses. However, up to now no differences in outcome depending on MTX dosage could be shown[8, 11].

After completion of R-courses maintenance therapy consisting of daily oral thioganine and biweekly intravenous MTX at conventional doses was given for 2 years. Radiation therapy to extramedullary involved sites was performed at the end of R-courses. Because of a high rate of second relapses in the CNS following first isolated marrow relapse in study ALL-REZ 85 radia-

Dept. of Pediatric Hematology/Oncology, Rudolf-Virchow Medical Center, Berlin, Germany

Table 1. Patient characteristics

Bone marrow relapse		No. of pts	%
Total	age 8.2 yrs	540	100
boys	8.2 yrs	315	58.3
girls	8.3 yrs	225	41.7
study ALL-REZ	BFM 83	58	10.7
	BFM 85	112	20.7
	BFM 87	156	28.9
	BFM 90	214	39.6
isolated	BM	380	70.4
combined	BM+CNS	92	17.0
	BM+testicular	45	8.3
	BM+other	17	3.1
	BM+2 sites	6	1.1
late relapse		315	58.3
early relapse ≥ 18 months 1st RD		162	30.0
early relapse < 18 months 1st RD		63	11.7
poor prognosis group		73	13.5
allogeneic bone marrow transplant		77	14.3

tion therapy to the CNS was strongly recommended during the course of study ALL-REZ 87 and became a firm constituent of study ALL-REZ 90[3, 6].

Patients having a matched sibling donor were to be transplanted soon after 2nd CR had been achieved but not earlier than after 2 courses of chemotherapy. If no place for BMT was available at that time chemotherapy had to be continued according to the protocol until BMT could be performed. Autologous BMT was optional as was the decision for matched unrelated BMT.

Life-table curves were constructed according to the Kaplan-Meier procedure and results compared by the logrank test. Estimates for the probability of event-free survival (p-EFS) include all adverse events, i.e., nonresponse, induction death, death in 2nd CR, and relapse at any site. Results obtained with chemotherapy were estimated by censoring transplanted patients at the time of BMT. Estimates for the probability of disease-free survival (p-DFS) include all adverse events from achievement of CR.

Results

A total of 478 out of 540 patients (89%) achieved a second CR. Remission rate was highest in children with late relapse and clearly worse in patients with shorter first remission duration. The main reason for failure to achieve 2nd CR was nonresponse (NR) to treatment (Table 2).

Likewise, as well as final outcome as the duration of 2nd CR are strongly dependent on time. As shown in Fig. 1 prognosis is better with longer time off front-line therapy. Furthermore there are additional pretreatment parameters significantly influencing the prognosis such as T-cell phenotype, involvement of extramedullary sites concomitant to BM relapse and the number of circulating blood leukemic cells in children with late marrow relapse. The most important treatment variable was found to be radiation therapy to the CNS in patients with late isolated BM relapse. Respective figures are given in Table 3.

Out of 77 patients who were referred to allogeneic BMT 36 were transplanted for early BM relapse. The median time to BMT was 150 days. At that time 93 children with early marrow relapse were still in 2nd CR lacking a matched donor and therefore remaining on

Table 2. Remission rates in trials ALL-REZ BFM 83–90

	no 2nd CR			2nd CR	
Type of relapse	n	ED	NR	n	%
Late BM	315	11	8	296	94
Early BM	162	7	16	139	86
Very early BM	63	5	15	43	68
Total	540	23	39	478	89

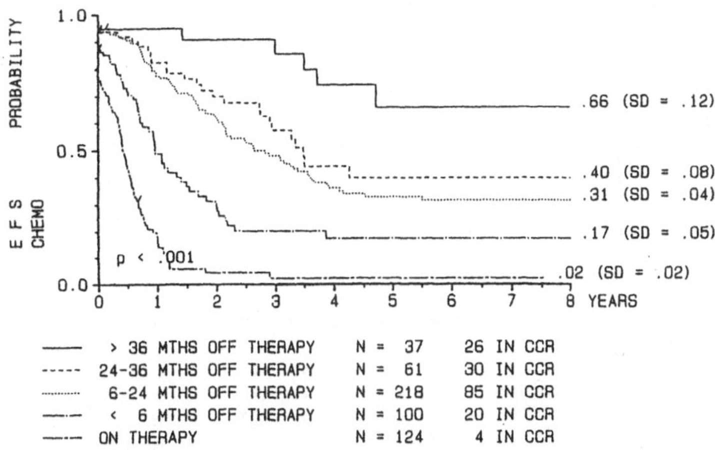

Fig. 1. Probability of event-free survival dependent on length of first remission. Patients who received BMT are censored. Curves have been cut at 8 years. Tick mark represent last follow-up

Table 3. Pretreatment and therapeutic prognostic parameters: Kaplan-Meier estimates for chemotherapy (transplanted patients censored)

Parameter	n	p-EFS ± SD
T-cell phenotype	30	0.04 ± 0.04***
Non-T-cell phenotype	481	0.28 ± 0.03
Isolated BM early	152	0.01 ± 0.01***
Combined BM early	73	0.24 ± 0.06
Isolated BM late	130	0.29 ± 0.05*
Combined BM late	54	0.51 ± 0.07
Late BM, blasts > 10 G/L	54	0.19 ± 0.08
Late BM, blasts < 10 G/L	259	0.41 ± 0.04
Late isolated BM, no CNS Rx[§]	74	0.21 ± 0.06**
Late isolated BM with CNS Rx[§]	87	0.47 ± 0.07

[§]DFS from end of R-courses (earliest time for CNs irradiation)
*p<0.05, **p<0.01, ***p<0.001

chemotherapy. The Kaplan-Meier estimates show a highly statistically significant difference in outcome between both groups (Fig. 2). In contrast, allogeneic BMT is not superior to chemotherapy in children with late BM relapse who had received radiation therapy to the CNS for either isolated or combined marrow relapse. For 16 children who had been more than 3 years off front-line therapy the prognosis is even .82 ± .11 with chemotherapy (Fig. 3). The curve for all patients transplanted for late relapse ends at a plateau of .55 ± .08, and there are four late second events which are not to be seen in children transplanted for early relapse.

Fig. 4 shows EFS curves for all 540 patients. The lower curve reflects results obtained with chemotherapy (BMT patients censored), and in the upper curve all transplanted patients are counted as transplants. It can be seen that BMT

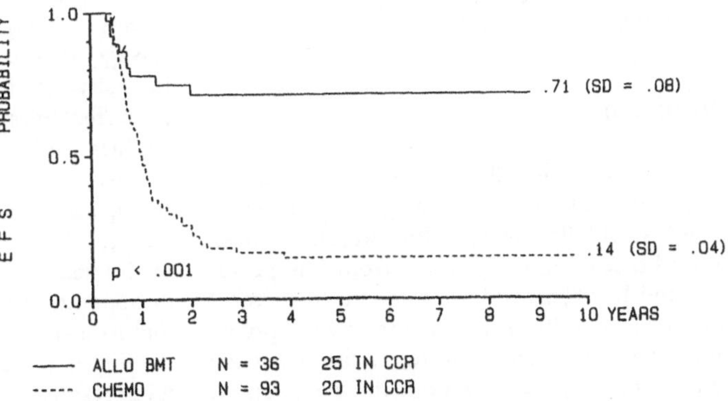

Fig. 2. Comparison of the probability of event-free survival between chemotherapy and allogeneic BMT for patients with early BM relapse. Tick mark respresents last follow-up

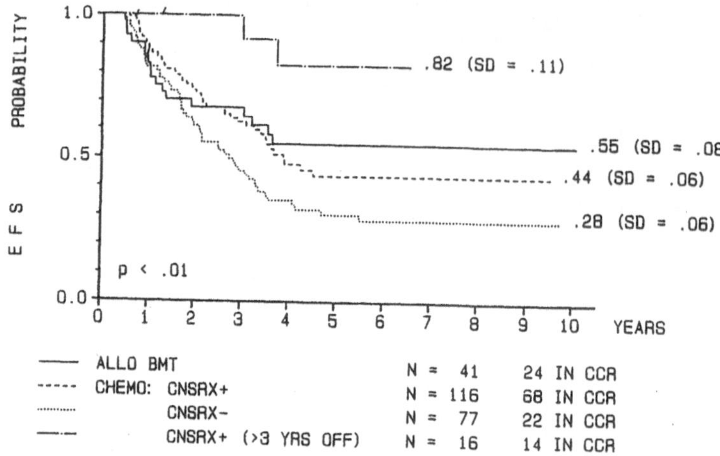

Fig. 3. Comparison of the probability of event-free survial between chemotherapy and allogeneic BMT for patients with late BM relapse. Chemotherapy treated patients are splitted according to whether or not they had received CNS irradiation and to time off front-line therapy. Tick mark respresents last follow up

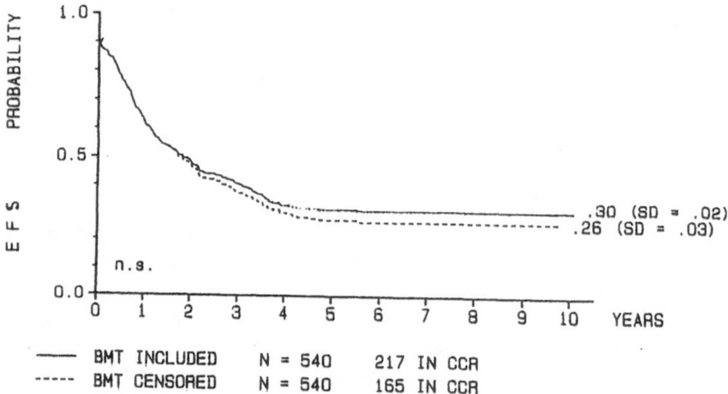

Fig. 4. Probability of event-free survival for all BM relapse patients. The lower curve reflects results obtained with chemotherapy (allogeneic BMT patients censored). The upper curve includes BMT patients and represents the overall treatment result. Tick mark represents last follow-up

yields only a 4% gain to the prognosis of the total group.

Discussion

To our knowledge this report represents the largest quite uniformly treated group of children with first ALL BM relapse who had initially been treated according to intensive front-line protocols and have been followed for up to 10 years after relapse. With front-line therapy as applied in these patients long-term remission is already in the range of 70%. About one third of relapsed children is apparently curable at the second attempt. The question whether or not results of salvage therapy are really influenced by the intensity of front-line treatment cannot be answered properly because there is no trial to confirm this assumption. But theoretically intensive first-line therapy is likely to exert a strong selection pressure leading to highly resistant residual leukemic cells, and clinical trials on intensively pretreated patients have shown disappointing results[5, 10]. At least, it appears that front-line therapy may not be irrelevant for the discussion and comparison of salvage treatment results.

Several strong pretherapeutic and therapeutic prognostic factors could be determined which have to be considered, in particular as to the question whether or not patients should be referred to matched sibling donor BMT or even matched unrelated BMT.

In this large series of patients it is possible to demonstrate that prognosis is more or less steadily improving with longer duration of first remission preceding relapse. Nearly all patients of the ALL-REZ trials had received front-line treatment for 2 years, some of them only 18 months. This has to be considered when comparing results of different trials for relapse. Definitions for late and early relapse may be seemingly the same, i.e., later than six months after the end of front-line therapy or earlier. However, since the duration of front-line therapy varies in different study groups duration of first remission may differ considerably despite the "same" definition[2, 9]. Nevertheless, time remains the strongest independent prognostic variable in case of relapse. Obviously 2nd CR rates are much lower in early relapse indicating drug resistance of the leukemic cell population. This has also been described by other authors [1], whereas also overall remission rates of 87% have been reported in early marrow relapse patients[2]. However, since in all trials 2nd remission durations are short for these children, achieving 2nd CR may be only a poor parameter to assess the quality of therapy.

In patients with late first relapses remission rates are higher but they tend to experience again late 2nd relapses. Surprisingly, this is not only observed in chemotherapeutically treated patients but also following allogeneic BMT. The finding that with either treatment modality the period at risk is different between early and late relapses probably reflects different proliferation kinetics of the leukemic cell population.

The second independent adverse prognostic factor is T-cell phenotype. Recurrence of T-ALL indicates a very poor outcome. Remission rate was only 70% in our patients and the median time to subsequent relapse was as short as 3 months. Overall data of the ALL-REZ trials – not only from protocol patients – point in the direction that also allogeneic BMT has disappointing results in T-ALL. Only 1 out of 14 patients remained in CR following BMT (data not shown). It appears, therefore, that recurrent T-ALL is highly resistant to any treatment modality.

The observation that combined BM relapse carries a significantly better prognosis than isolated BM relapse was recently published[4]. It could be shown that this is not dependent on the degree of BM infiltration as one would argue. A more likely explanation is that occult extramedullary leukemia exists in a number of patients presenting with apparent isolated BM relapse and has not been treated accordingly, whereas additional leukemic manifestations are known and locally treated in children with overt extramedullary and BM relapse. This assumption would be in context with the finding that the prognosis was markedly improved by effective preventive radiation therapy to the CNS in children with late isolated marrow relapse[3]. However, since prognosis was not improved for children with early isolated BM relapse by this measure there must be additional factors, presumably different drug resistance profiles, to satisfactorily explain the observed phenomena.

Allogeneic BMT may be of high value for individual patients. The greatest benefit in our series could be shown for children with early BM relapse whereas no difference exists in late relapse. Because numbers of transplanted patients are still small one can only speculate about these findings. Differences in proliferation kinetics as mentioned above might be a reason that in early relapses leukemic cells are more susceptible to high-dose chemo-/radio-conditioning therapy than in late relapse, where dormant cells might survive even ablative therapy. There is no reason to believe that the BMT-linked immunotherapy, i.e., the GvL effect would be different in late or early relapses. According to our data matched sibling donor BMT is definitely indicated in early relapse. In late relapse, however, there is no proof for improvement of prognosis. By no means matched unrelated BMT would be justified in a child with late BM relapse since the mortality related to this procedure is presently still in the range of about 40%.

The positive impact of BMT on the prognosis of the total population of relapse patients is only marginal. Only 14% of children were finally transplanted despite a statistical chance of about 25% to find a matched sibling donor. Major reasons for the low transplantation rate are that either a stable 2nd remission was not achieved or the duration of 2nd CR was too short for timely referral of patients to BMT. Thus, BMT remains only a relative treatment option and transplantation results are based on a selected group of patients.

In summary, curative retreatment is possible for about one third of children with ALL marrow relapse. Independent prognostic factors are duration of first remission and T-cell immunophenotype. Prognosis in marrow relapse is superior if extramedullary sites are concomitantly involved. Effective preventive therapy to the CNS is essential for successful retreatment. Allogeneic BMT, though highly effective in individual patients, contributes only marginal to the prognosis of the total relapse population and should be carefully considered based on the individually underlying conditions.

Acknowledgements. This work was supported by grants from the Deutsche Krebshilfe.

We are indebted to the principal investigators, physicians and nurses at the 101 participating BFM institutions in and outside Germany who cared for the patients and contributed to the submission of data.

References

1. Behrendt H, VanLeeuwen EF, Schuwirth C, et al. (1990): Bone marrow relapse occurring as first relapse in children with acute lymphoblastic leukemia. Med Pediatr Oncol, 18, 190–196
2. Buchanan GR, Rivera GK, Boyett JM, et al. (1988): Reinduction therapy in 297 children with acute lymphoblastic leukemia in first bone marrow relapse: a Pediatric Oncology Group study. Blood, 72, 1286–1292
3. Bührer C, Hartmann R, Fengler R, et al. (1994): Importance of effective central nervous system therapy in isolated bone marrow relapse of childhood acute lymphoblastic leukemia. Blood, 83, 3468–3472
4. Bührer C, Hartmann R, Fengler R, et al. (1993): Superior prognosis in combined compared to isolated bone marrow relapses in salvage therapy of childhood acute lymphoblastic leukemia. Med Pediatr Oncol, 21, 470–476
5. Culbert SJ, Shuster JJ, Land VJ, et al. (1991): Remission induction and and ontinuation therapy in children with their first relapse of acute lymphoid leukemia. A Pediatric Oncology Group study. Cancer, 67, 37–42
6. Fengler R, Hartmann R, Bode U, et al. (1990): Risk of CNS relapse after systemic relapse of childhood acute lymphoblastic leukemia. Haematol Blood Transfus, 33, 511–515
7. Henze G, Fengler R, Hartmann R, et al. (1991): Six-year experience with a comprehensive approach to the treatment of recurrent childhood acute lymphoblastic leukemia (ALL-REZ BFM 85). A relapse study of the BFM Group. Blood, 78, 1166–1172
8. Henze G, Fengler R, Hartmann R, et al. (1994): High dose versus intermediate dose MTX for relapsed childhood ALL: interim results of the randomized multicentric trial ALL-REZ BFM 90 (abstr). Med Pediatr Oncol, 23, 190
9. Sadowitz PD, Smith SD, Shuster J, et al. (1993): Treatment of late bone marrow relapse in children with acute lymphoblastic leukemia: a Pediatric Oncology Group study. Blood, 81, 602–609
10. VonDerWeid N, Wagner B, Angst R, et al. (1994): Treatment of relapsing acute lymphoblastic leukemia in childhood. III. Experiences with 54 first bone marrow, nine isolated testicular, and eight isolated central nervous system relapses observed 1985–1989. Med Pediatr Oncol, 22, 361–369
11. Wolfrom C, Hartmann R, Fengler R, et al. (1993): Randomized comparison of 36-hour intermediate-dose versus 4-hour high-dose methotrexate infusions for remission induction in relapsed childhood acute lymphoblastic leukemia. J Clin Oncol, 11, 827–833

Acute Leukemias V
Experimental Approaches
and Management of Refractory Diseases
Hiddemann et al. (Eds.)

Salvage Therapy of Adult ALL

M. Freund[1], G. Heil[2], K. Pompe[2], R. Arnold[2], C. Bartram[3], Th. Büchner[4], H. Diedrich[1], C. Fonatsch[5], A. Ganser[6], W. Hiddemann[4], P. Koch[4], K. Kolbe[7], H. Link[1], H. Löffler[8], W. D. Ludwig[9], G. Maschmeyer[9], N. Schmitz[8], M. Schwonzen[10], E. Thiel[11], and D. Hoelzer[6] on behalf of the German Relapsing Acute Lymphocytic Leukemia Study Group (GRALLSG)

Abstract. In a first study (1986 to 1992) the German Relapsing ALL Study Group (GRALLSG) has treated 67 adult patients with a first relapse of ALL. A first phase of induction consisted of vindesine, daunorubicin, asparaginase, and prednisone, a second phase of high-dose cytosine-arabinoside (Hd ara-C) and VP16. Results: 45 CR, 2 PR, 13 failures, 7 early death. 25 patients received a BMT. 10 had an allogeneic BMT in CR, 5 after another relapse or with refractory disease. Of 10 with autologous BMT 8 have been in 2nd CR. Only 4 of all 67 patients are surviving without relapse: One after unrelated BMT (36+mo), two after autologous BMT in 2nd CR (46+,64+mo), and one after chemotherapy (61+mo). One patient has been lost in relapse. The median survival is 7.2 months and the overall survival 4% after 5 years. The duration of the first CR was an important risk factor for response to induction. Patients are accordingly stratified in a new protocol. Patients with a preceding 1st CR<18 months receive Hd ara-C/idarubicin. The others are treated with the phase I of the previous protocol and a consolidation of Hd MTX, ifosfamide, prednisolone, ara-C and VP16. Furtheron a phase I/II trial is performed in patients with refractory disease or multiple relapses to evaluate the activity of 2-CDA.

Introduction

The primary treatment of acute lymphocytic leukemia (ALL) has been considerably improved. Therefore allogeneic BMT has been postponed to 2nd remission by the German Multicenter ALL Study Group for patients with T-ALL and low risk patients. However the prognosis of relapsing acute lymphocytic leukemia is still very poor. Salvage therapy for these patients is clinically important and challenging.

The German Relapsing Acute Lymphocytic Leukemia Study Group has tested several approaches to this problem on which we hereby report.

[1]Abteilung Hämatologie und Onkologie, Medizinische Hochschule Hannover, D-30625 Hannover
[2]Medizinische Klinik und Poliklinik, Universität Ulm, D-89081 Ulm
[3]Sektion Molekularbiologie, Abteilung Kinderklinik II, Universität Ulm, D-89075 Ulm
[4]Medizinische Universitätsklinik und Poliklinik, Abteilung A, D-48149 Münster
[5]Institut für Humangenetik, Arbeitsgruppe Tumorzytogenetik, Medizinische Universität Lübeck, D-23538 Lübeck
[6]Zentrum Innere Medizin, Abteilung Hämatologie, Johann-Wolfgang-Goethe-Universität, D-60590 Frankfurt am Main
[7]Abteilung für Hämatologie, Johannes-Gutenberg-Universität, D-55131 Mainz
[8]II. Medizinische Universitäts- und Poliklinik, D-24116 Kiel
[9]Universitätsklinikum Rudolf Virchow der Freien Universität, Standort MDC – Robert Rössle Klinik, Hämatologie/Onkologie, Abteilung Molekularbiologie, D-13125 Berlin
[10]Medizinische Universitätsklinik, D-50931 Köln
[11]Universitätsklinikum Steglitz, Innere Medizin mit Schwerpunkt, Hämatologie und Onkologie, D-12203 Berlin

Long-Term Results of Study 01/87

Patients and methods. In a first study sixty-seven patients have been treated for first relapse of acute lymphocytic leukemia. All patients have been pretreated with the BMFT-regimen [8–10].

The patients have been recruited in 18 centers. There were 47 men and 20 women. The patients' median age was 29.7 years (range 16.0 to 62.2 years) and the mean duration of the preceding remission was 21 months (range 1 to 80 months). Forty patients had a B-precursor ALL, 5 of them identified as being Ph'+. Twenty-two patients had a T-precursor ALL, 4 o-ALL and in one patient the immunophenotype has not been identified.

Induction phase I consisted of prednisone (60 mg/m² PO on days 1–21), vindesine (DVA 3 mg/m² IV on days 1, 8, 15), daunorubicin (DNR 45 mg/m² IV on days 1, 8, 15), and erwinia-asparaginase (10,000 U/m² IV on days 7, 8, 14, 15). For CNS-prophylaxis methotrexate was given i.t. (MTX 15 mg on days 1, 8). In patients with no detectable remaining bone marrow infiltration on day 21 hematopoietic recovery was allowed before start of the second induction phase. Patients with remaining blast infiltration were started with phase II of induction after recovery from organ-toxicity and after stabilization of the clinical status. Induction phase II consisted of high-dose cytosine-arabinoside (Hd ara-C 3 g/m² as a 3 h infusion 2 times daily on days 1–4), and etoposide (VP16 100 mg/m² IV on days 1–5). In patients over 50 years intermediate-dose (Id) ara-C was given (1 g/m² 2 times daily on days 1–4). In some patients a consolidation was given as previously reported [2].

Results. Forty-five (67%) of 67 patients achieved a complete remission: 35 patients after phase I, and 10 after phase II of induction. Two patients had a partial remission, and 13 patients did not respond. Seven patients died during treatment (10.4%). Details on the treatment results in subgroups are given below.

Toxicity data on the regimen have been previously published [2]. In this progress report we will concentrate on the long-term prognosis of the patients.

The median duration of disease-free survival (DFS) was 3.6 months with only 13% of the patients remaining disease-free at 5 years (Figure 1). The median overall survival (OAS) was 7.2 months ending at 4% at 5 years (Figure 2).

Table 1. Treatment results in study 01/87 for several subgroups

Subgroup	n	CR	PR	NR	ED
B-Precursor	40	73%	3%	20%	5%
T-Precursor	22	55%	5%	18%	23%
Preceding CR < 18 mo	36	56%	6%	25%	14%
Preceding CR > 18 mo	31	81%*	–	13%	6%
Ph'+	5	40%	20%	40%	–

*Difference statistically significant (Chi-square test)

Twenty-five patients have been submitted to bone marrow transplantation (BMT). Allogeneic BMT in 2nd CR: 10, autologous BMT in CR: 8, allogeneic later or with refractory disease: 5, autologous BMT later: 2 patients. The influence of BMT on the survival of the whole patients' group is shown in Figure 3. When patients with BMT are not censored the median survival is unchanged and the longterm prognosis drops to 0 due to a late death of a patient after allogeneic BMT. However with longer observation time there may be a favourable trend for BMT.

Currently only four of the 67 patients are alive: 2 after autologous BMT, one after HLA-matched unrelated BMT and one after chemotherapy alone. A single patient has been lost when returning to Turkey with refractory disease. In all other patients follow-up is complete and updated on February 1st, 1994.

Study 02/92

In 1992 a second study was started. It had the rationale to shorten the induction period and to bring as much patients as possible forward to intensive consolidation with autologous or allogeneic bone marrow transplantation.

Patients and methods. Patients with a 1st preceding CR below 18 months receive an induction therapy with three days of 2 × 3 g/m² Hd ara-C and 12 mg/m² idarubicin IV followed by filgrastim 5 µg/kg SC daily. In patients over 50 years the doses are reduced to 2 × 1 g/m² (Id araC) and to 8 mg/m² idarubicin.

Currently 23 patients have been enroled (16 men and 7 women). The patients' mean age is

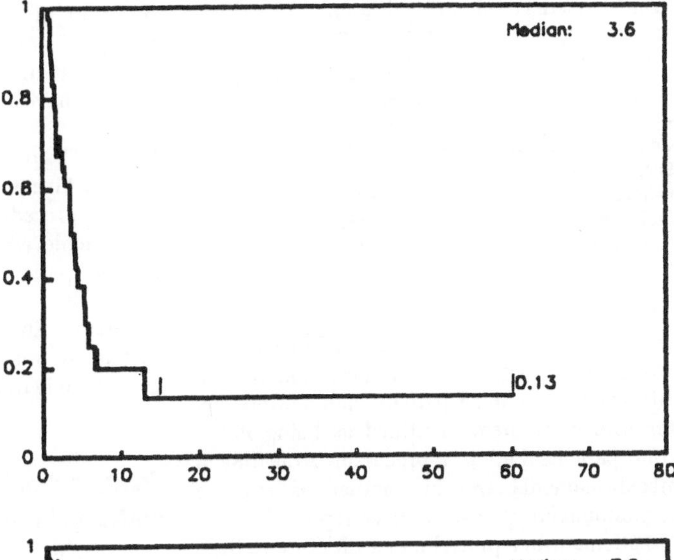

Fig. 1. Disease-free survival of 67 patients treated for 1st relapse of ALL (study 01/87). Patients with BMT are censored at the time of the procedure

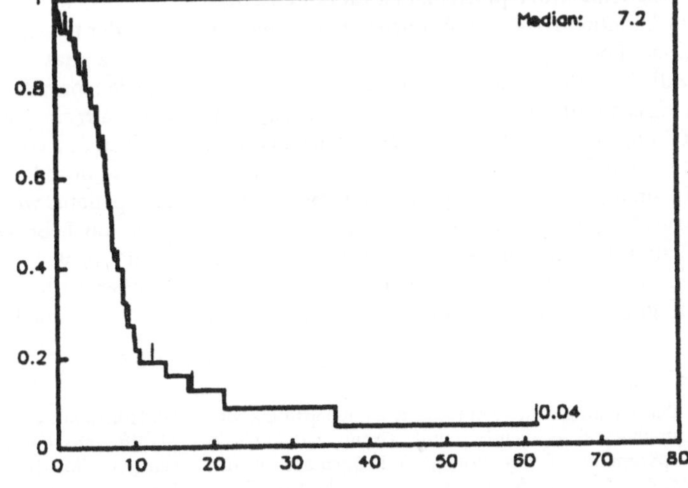

Fig. 2. Overall survival in study 01/87 (patients with BMT censored)

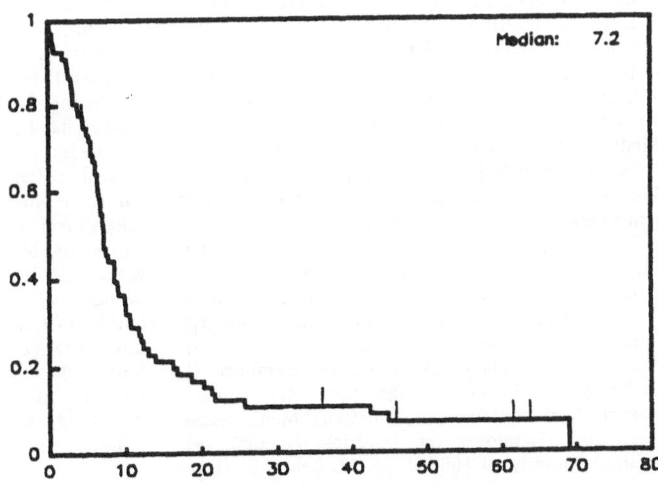

Fig. 3. Overall survival in study 01/87 including the results of all performed BMT (patients with BMT are not censored). Four patients are alive and disease-free

Table 2. Interim results for study 02/92

	Preceding CR			
	< 18 mo		> 18 mo	
Complete remission	10	43%	5	71%
Partial remission	–		–	–
Failure	11	48%	–	–
Early Death	1	4%	1	14%
Not evaluable	1	4%	1	14%

37.5 years (range 21 to 59 years). The mean duration of the preceding remission was 8 months in this group. Seventeen patients had a B-precursor ALL, 7 of them identified as being Ph[1]+. Four patients had a T-precursor ALL, one a mixed leukemia and in another patient the immunophenotype has not been reported.

Patients with a preceding 1st CR of more than 18 months receive the unchanged induction phase I of the protocol 01/87 and a consolidation with Hd MTX (5 g 24 h infusion day 1 with a reduced folinic acid rescue), ifosfamide (1.5 g/m² IV days 1–4), prednisolone (60 mg/m² PO days 1–4), ara-C (500 mg/m² escalated to 1,000 mg/m² IV on days 3–4) and etoposide (100 mg/m² escalated to 250 mg/m² IV on days 3–4).

In this arm of the study 7 patients have been enroled (3 men and 4 women) with a mean age of 30.5 years (range 17 to 49 years). The mean duration of the preceding remission was 28 months. Three patients had a B-precursor ALL, none of them identified as being Ph[1]+. Each 2 patients have a T-precursor and a 0-ALL.

Results. The treatment results are summarized in Table 2. Five of the seven Ph[1]+ ALL in the group with a preceding remission below 18 months have achieved a complete remission (1 PR, another patient too early to evaluate). The follow-up is too short for a valid information on remission duration or survival. By now, the results are not significantly different to the preceding study 01/87.

Treatment of Refractory ALL with 2-Chlorodeoxyadenosine

In order to evaluate the activity of new cytotoxic drugs a phase I-II study has been started with 2-chlorodeoxyadenosine (2-CDA) for patients with refractory ALL or multiple relapses. 2-CDA is given as a continuous 24 h IV infusion for five days at dose levels of 11, 13 and 15 mg/m² daily. Five patients will be treated on each dose-step.

As on February 1st, 1994 four patients have been enroled, 3 with refractory disease and another with 2nd early relapse. Two patients have responded with a reduction of the periph-

* Participating Centers in the German Relapsing Acute Lymphocytic Leukemia Study Group (GRALLSG): Departments of Hematology and Oncology at the RWTH Aachen (S. Handt, H.G. Sieberth); Freie Universität Berlin, Klinikum Steglitz (W. Knauf, J. Maurer, E. Thiel); Krankenhaus St. Jürgen Strafle, Bremen (U. Kubica, H. Rasche); Universität Düsseldorf (A. Heyll, W. Schneider); St. Johannes-Hospital, Duisburg (C. Schadeck-Gressel, M. Westerhausen); Universität Erlangen (M. Gramatzki, J.R. Kalden); Medizinische Klinik und Poliklinik, Gesamthochschule Universität Essen (C. Kasper, G. Brittinger); Westdeutsches Tumorzentrum, Gesamthochschule Universität Essen (M.R. Nowrousian, S. Seeber); Evangelisches Krankenhaus Essen-Werden (C. Tirier, W. Heit); Universität Frankfurt (B. Völkers, H. Martin, A. Ganser, D. Hoelzer); Universität Freiburg (L. Kanz, R. Mertelsmann); Universitätsklinikum Hamburg-Eppendorf (S. Peter, J. Dierlamm, D.K. Hossfeld); Allgemeines Krankenhaus St. Georg, Hamburg (J. Dethling, R. Kuse); Evangelisches Krankenhaus Hamm (A. Grote-Metke, L. Balleisen); Medizinische Hochschule Hannover (H. Diedrich, H. Link, M. Freund); Universität Heidelberg (M. Bentz, R. Haas, W. Hunstein); Universität Homburg/Saar (R. Schmits, M. Pfreundschuh); Städtisches Krankenhaus Kaiserslautern (M. Hartmann); II. Medizinische Klinik, Klinikum Karlsruhe (S. Wilhelm, Th. Fischer); Städtische Kliniken Kassel (B. Eggeling, W.D. Hirschmann); Universität Kiel (W. Gassmann, N. Schmitz, H. Löffler); Universität Köln (M. Schwonzen, V. Diehl); Städtische Krankenanstalten Krefeld (M. Weitmann, M. Prumbaum, K. Becker); Medizinische Universität Lübeck, Arbeitsgruppe Tumorzytogenetik (H. Rieder, C. Fonatsch); Universität Mainz (K. Kolbe, C. Huber); Onkologisches Zentrum der Fakultät für Klinische Medizin, Mannheim (W. Queifler); Technische Universität München (A. Hanauske, J. Rastetter); Universität Münster (P. Koch, Th. Büchner, J. van de Loo); 5. Medizinische Klinik, Klinikum Nürnberg (H. Wandt, W.M. Gallmeier); Diakonissen-Krankenhaus Stuttgart (R. Mück, M. Siegel, E. Heidemann); Robert-Bosch-Krankenhaus Stuttgart (B. Löffler, K. Schumacher); Universität Ulm (G. Heil, R. Arnold, K. Pompe, C.R. Bartram, H. Heimpel); Universität Würzburg, Medizinische Poliklinik (P. Meyer, K. Wilms).

eral blast counts. No neurotoxicity has been observed. Further patients are currently recruited.

Discussion

Despite all progress in the primary treatment of ALL the prognosis of patients with relapsing disease is very poor.

Eleven studies on modern combination chemotherapy with more than 20 adult patients with relapsing or refractory ALL have been published [1,3–7,11–15]. CR-rates from 26 to 75% have been reported. Comparable results have been achieved in the studies of the German Relapsing Acute Lymphocytic Leukemia Study Group*. In patients with a preceding remission below 18 months the remission rate reported by Giona [4] has been exactly reproduced.

Sufficient data on the remission duration and the long-term survival are rarely given in studies on relapsing ALL. With the data of our first study being now mature it is obvious that only few patients will achieve long-term survival despite intensive induction therapy and despite the intent to offer high-dose chemotherapy with allogeneic or autologous bone marrow transplantation to as many patients as possible. A comparable long-term follow-up is given only in the publication of the GIMEMA/AIEOP [5]. Although children are included, the longterm survival has been similar as in our study ranging from 7% to 18% at 3 to 4 years according to subgroups.

We conclude that we have the obligation to systematically investigate novel treatment concepts for relapsing acute lymphocytic leukemia including new cytotoxic drugs, immunotherapy and high-dose chemotherapy. Relapsing acute lymphocytic leukemia is a disease extremely resistant to chemotherapy and easy to detect with molecular biologic approaches. It can serve as a model to study new strategies for the cancer problem.

References

1. Arlin ZA, Feldman E, Kempin S, Ahmed T, Mittelman A, Savona S, Ascensao J, Baskind P, Sullivan P, Fuhr HG, Mertelsmann R (1988) Amsacrine with high-dose cytarabine is highly effective therapy for refractory and relapsed acute lymphoblastic leukemia in adults. Blood 72: 433–435
2. Freund M, Diedrich H, Ganser A, Gramatzki M, Heil G, Heyll A, Henke M, Hiddemann W, Haas R, Kuse R, Koch P, Link H, Maschmeyer G, Planker M, Queißer W, Schadeck-Gressel C, Schmitz N, von Verschuer U, Wilhelm S, Thiel E, Hoelzer D (1992) Treatment of relapsed or refractory adult acute lymphocytic leukemia. Cancer 69: 709–716
3. Garay G, Milone J, Dibar E, Pavlovsky S, Kvicala R, Sackmann Muriel F, Montres Varela D, Eppinger-Helft M (1983) Vindesine, prednisone, and daunomycin in acute lymphoblastic leukemia in relapse. Cancer Chemother Pharmacol 10: 224–226
4. Giona F, Testi AM, Amadori S, Meloni G, Carotenuto M, Resegotti L, Colella R, Leoni P, Carella AM, Grotto P, Miniero R, Mandelli F (1990) Idarubicin and high-dose cytarabine in the treatment of refractory and relapsed acute lymphoblastic leukemia. Ann Oncol 1: 51–55
5. Giona F, Testi AM, Annino L, Amadori S, Arcese W, Camera A, Cordero di Montezemolo L, Ladogana S, Liso V, Meloni C, Moleti M:, Rondelli R, Zanesco L, Pession A, Mandelli F (1994) Treatment of primary refractory and relapsed acute lymphoblastic leukaemia in children and adults: the GIMEMA/AIOP experience. Br J Haematol 86: 55–61
6. Harousseau JL (1991) Intermediate dose cytarabine in the treatment of relapsed and refractory acute myeloid leukemia (AML). Ann Hematol 62: A32 (Abstract)
7. Hiddemann W, Buchner T, Heil G, Schumacher K, Diedrich H, Maschmeyer G, Ho AD, Planker M, Gerith Stolzenburg S, Donhuijsen Ant R, et al. (1990) Treatment of refractory acute lymphoblastic leukemia in adults with high dose cytosine arabinoside and mitoxantrone (HAM). Leukemia 4: 637–640
8. Hoelzer D, Thiel E, Loeffler H, Bodenstein H, Plaumann L, Buechner T, Urbanitz D, Koch P, Heimpel H, Engelhardt R, Müller U, Wendt F-C, Sodomann H, Rühl H, Herrmann F, Kaboth W, Dietzfelbinger H, Pralle H, Lunscken Ch, Hellriegel K-P, Spors S, Nowrousian RM, Fischer J, Fülle H, Mitrou PS, Pfreundschuh M, Görg Ch, Emmerich B, Queisser W, Meyer P, Labedzki L, Essers U, König H, Mainzer K, Herrmann R, Messerer D, Zwingers T (1984) Intensified therapy in acute lymphoblastic and acute undifferentiated leukemia in adults. Blood 64: 38–47
9. Hoelzer D, Thiel E, Löffler H, Büchner T, Ganser A, Heil G, Koch P, Freund M, Diedrich H, Rühl H, Maschmeyer G, Lipp T, Nowrousian MR, Burkert M, Gerecke D, Pralle H, Müller U, Lunscken C, Fülle H, Ho AD, Küchler R, Busch FW, Schneider W, Görg C, Emmerich B, Braumann D, Vaupel HA, von Paleske A, Bartels H, Neiss A, Messerer D (1988) Prognostic factors in a multicenter study for treatment of acute lymphoblastic leukemia in adults. Blood 71: 123–131
10. Hoelzer D, Thiel E, Löffler H, Büchner T, Ganser A, Heil G, Kurrle E, Heimpel H, Koch P, Lipp T,

Kaboth W, Kuse R, Küchler R, Sodomann H, Maschmeyer G, Freund M, Diedrich H, von Paleske A, Weh J, Kolb H, Müller U, Bross K, Fuhr G, Gassmann W, Gerecke D, Kress M, Fusch FW, Nowrousian RM, Schneider W, Aul C, Rühl H, Bartels H, Harms F, Weiss A, Löffler B, Glöckner W, Fülle H, Pralle H, Ho AD, Bonfert B, Emmerich B, Braumann D, Brenner-Serke M, Planker M, Straif K, Meyer P, Greil R, Petsch S, Görk C, Grüneisen A, Vaupel HA, Bodenstein H, Overkamp F, Schlimock G, Augener W, Öhl S, Nowicki L, Raeth U, Zurborn KH, Neiss A, Messerer D (1987) Teniposide (VM-26) and cytosine arabinoside as consolidation therapy in adult high-risk patients with acute lymphoblastic leukemia. Semin Oncol 14: 92–97

11. Kantarjian HM, Estey EH, O'Brien S, Anaissie E, Beran M, Rios MB, Keating MJ, Gutterman J (1992) Intensive chemotherapy with mitoxantrone and high-dose cytosine arabinoside followed by granulocyte-macrophage colony-stimulating factor in the treatment of patients with acute lymphocytic leukemia. Blood 79: 876–881
12. Kantarjian HM, Walters RS, Keating MJ, Barlogie B, McCredie KB, Freireich EJ (1989) Experience with vincristine, doxorubicin, and dexamethasone (VAD) chemotherapy in adults with refractory acute lymphocytic leukemia. Cancer 64: 16–22
13. Ryan DH, Kopecky KJ, Head D, Gumbart CN, Grever MR, Karnes C, Weick JK, Coltman Jr. CA (1987) Phase II evaluation of teniposide and ifosfamide in refractory adult acute lymphocytic leukemia: A southwest oncology group study. Cancer Treat Rep 71: 713–716
14. Terebolo HR, Anderson K, Wiernik PH, Cuttner J, Cooper RM, Faso L, Berenberg JL (1986) Therapy of refractory adult acute lymphoblastic leukemia with vincristine and prednisolone plus tandem methotrexate and L-asparaginase. Results of a Cancer and Leukemia Group B Study. Am J Clin Oncol 9: 411–415
15. Yap BS, McCredie KB, Keating MJ, Bodey GP, Freireich EJ (1981) Asparaginase and methotrexate combination chemotherapy in relapsed acute lymphoblastic leukemia in adults. Cancer Treat Rep (Suppl 1) 65: 83–87

Acute Leukemias V
Experimental Approaches
and Management of Refractory Diseases
Hiddemann et al. (Eds.)

Protocol RACOP in the Treatment of Resistant and Relapsed ALL

R. A. Kutcher, V. G. Isaev, V. G. Savchenko, E. N. Parovitchnikova, L. S. Lubimova, and L. P. Mendeleeva

Introduction

A considerable success was achieved in adult ALL treatment, as the long-term disease-free survival for CR patients is reported to be 19–72% according to the risk factors [1,2,3]. But still relapses occur in many patients and account for most treatment failures. Another category of poor prognosis patients are those withrefractory disease (10–15%). The majority of treatment schedules for relapsed and resistant ALL now include high dose ARA-C (HD ARA-C) in combination with different cytostatic drugs and provide 38–64% of second CR [4,5,6,7] Taking in consideration the sufficient toxic (especially non-hematologic) effects of HD ARA-C regimens we introduced a new protocol RACOP and evaluated its efficacy in the high risk groups of patients.

Patients and Methods

Between August 1987 and August 1993, 34 patients with advanced ALL (16 men, 18 women; median age 26 years; range 16 to 60 years) were enrolled in the study. 17 patients with refractory disease were hardly pretreated: median duration of previous treatment was 7 months (range 2 to 12 months) and it consisted of vincristine, daunorubicin, prednisone for 4 weeks followed by cytarabine, 6-mercaptopurine, cyclophosphamide for 4 weeks, or short repeated courses with the same drugs in different combinations (COAP, VAMP). It should be noted that in many of these cases the doses of cytostatic drugs were not adequate as the majority of patients were treated in the regional hospitals before being admitted to the department of hematological oncology and BMT of National Research Center for Hematology. So refractorness was sometimes determined according to the duration of previous uneffective treatment (more than 2 months). CNS prophylaxis was carried out with intrathecal methotrexate, cytarabine and prednisone. 17 patients had a relapsed ALL: median duration of the first CR was 8 months; range 2 to 30 months. Only one patient had a prolonged 1 CR – 30 months, all the others – less than 12 months. And one patient was in his second relapse (1 CR–22 months, 2 CR – 20 months).

Remission induction consisted of one or two courses RACOP: rubomycine (daunorubicin) 45 mg/m^2 i.v. 1–3 days, ara–c 100 mg/m^2 i.v. bid 1–7 days, cyclophosphamide 400 mg/m^2 i.v.1–7 days, oncovin 2 mg i.v.1,7 days, prednisone 60 mg p.o. 1–7 days. The following postremission therapy was conducted according to the same protocol, but 1/3 dose reduction of cyclophosphamide and ara-c was needed in some patients during maintenance. The intervals between reinduction courses were 4–5 weeks.

Evaluations with physical examination, standard laboratory tests and bone marrow aspirates were done before each course of treatment. Toxicities were evaluated according to World Health Organization (WHO) criteria and response according to the criteria of the Cancer and Leukemia Group B (CALGB). Survival was analyzed according to Kaplan and Meyer.

National Research Center for Hematology, Moscow, Russia

Patients undergoing BMT were censored for overall and disease-free survival.

Results

Thirty four patients have been treated, sixteen patients were in first relapse, one patient was in second relapse, seventeen had no complete remission after primary induction treatment.

All patients received RACOP as induction treatment. Detailed information on the extent of treatment administered and the reasons for termination are given in Table 1.

Toxicity during and after applied treatment was evaluated in all patients. Except nausea and vomiting (WHO Grade 1–2 in 15 pts, Grade 3 in 2) there were no direct toxic effects of the regimen. The main side effects were due to myelotoxicity with subsequent infections and hemorrhages that became the cause of death in 8 patients. The median duration of granulocytopenia WHO Grade 4 was 18 days, Grade 3–4 – 21 days. Thrombocytopenia WHO Grade 4 was encounted in all patients. Results of induction treatment according to the stage of ALL are reflected in Table 2.

Survival for all patients who entered the study (overall survival) and for those in whom CR was obtained (disease-free survival) is represented on Figure 1. and Figure 2. Patients with autologous BMT in CR are censored at time of BMT. The median duration of CR for resistant ALL was 8 months and for relapsed ALL – 6 months. One patient with refractory disease is alive and well for 86 months and one patient with her first relapse, subsequent 2 CR and autologous BMT is alive and well for 78 months.

Discussion

Primary therapy for acute lymphoblastic leukemia is now well established, and high remission rates and long-term survival are seen in large proportion of adults. At the time of relapse, patients frequently can achieve second remission with the same drugs that had induced remission initially [7,8] But long-term results are poor so high-dose ARA-C was introduced in the protocols for advanced ALL. Rates of CR were reported from 38% to 72% [4,5,6,7]. Nevertheless prolonged survival and duration of 2 CR remains poor – 2–7 months. It was proved that the duration of first remission (more or less than 12 months) had a significant impact on 2 CR length [4,6,7]. In this aspect the group of patients reported here represent mostly unfavorable category of patients with advanced ALL. It's a pity but we don't possess an information on immunophenotyping of leukemic cells. But it appeared that there were no striking differences in 2 CR rate and survival in respect with immunophenotype of ALL [6] . Another point is non-hematological toxicity of high-dose ARA-C that limits the wide use of this approach. It is noticed that diarrhea WHO grade 1–3 occurs in 57%–63% of patients, mucositis WHO Grade 1–4 – in 97%, hepatic toxicity WHO Grade 1–3 – in 67%, cutaneuos reactions WHO grade 1–3 – in

Table 1. Status of treatment and reasons for discontinuation of therapy

Treatment	Treatment plan completed	Reasons for discontinuation			
		Death	Refractory	BMT	Relapse
RACOP-induction	34	8	10	–	–
Postremission	16	–	–	2	12

BMT: bone marrow transplantation

Table 2. Results of induction in relapsed and resistant ALL

Acute Lymphocytic Leukemia	Complete Remission		Death		Refractory	
	No	Percent	No	Percent	No	Percent
Relapsed (n = 17)	7	41	4	23,5	6	35,5
Resistant (n = 17)	9	53	4	23,5	4	23,5
Total (n = 34)	16	47	8	23,5	10	28,5

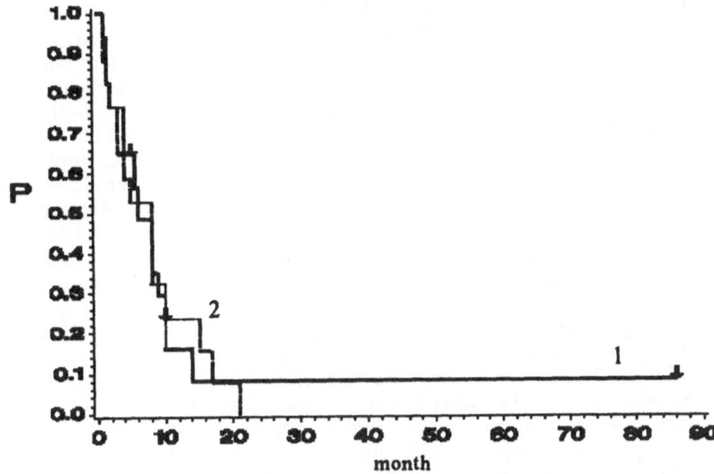

Fig. 1. Overall survival after RACOK treatment for 17 resistant (1) and 17 relapsed (2) ALL patients

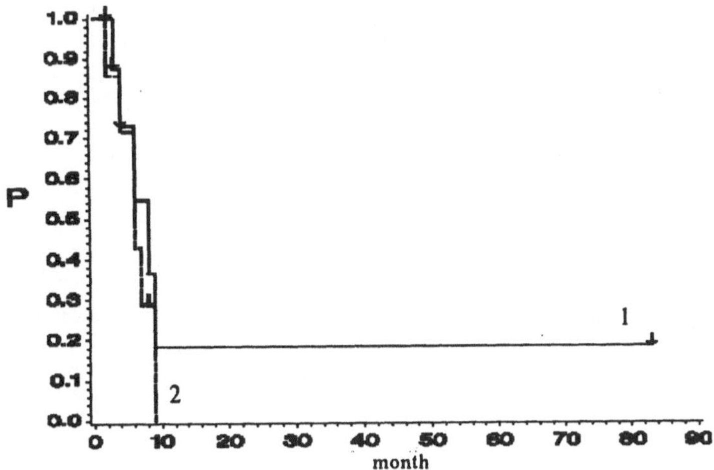

Fig. 2. Disease-free survival after RACOP treatment for 9 resistant (1) and 7 relapsed (2) ALL patients

51%, eyes involvement WHO Grade 1–2 – in 5%-22%, cerebellar WHO Grade 1–3 – in 8% [4,6]. Therefore mainly myelosuppressive effect of RACOP was considered to be an advantage of this schedule. Surely prolonged cytopenia and profound immunosuppression particularly due to high dose cyclophosphamide contributes to a high rate of infectious complications, but antileukemic effect of this course was found to be satisfactory. The median duration of 2 CR or CR in resistant ALL is among the best ever reported. From our point of view these results can be explained by maintenance treatment after CR achievement and perhaps by different state of refractorness in our patients. Of course further studies are needed especially in the groups of homogeneously pretreated patients.

References

1. Hoelzer D., Thiel E., Ludwig W.D., Loffler H., Buchner T., Freud M., Heil G., Hiddemann W., Maschmeyer G., Volkers B. Results of the German Multicenter Trials for Adult ALL. Haematological 1991; 76 (suppl 4): 106

2. Larson R.A., Burns C.P., Dodge R.K., George S.L., Bloomfield C.D., Davey F.R., Hooberman A.L.; Sobol R.E., Schiffer C.A. A 5-Drug Induction Regimen with Intensive Consolidation for Adult Acute Lymphoblastic Leukemia (ALL): Cancer and Leukemia Group B. Proc.Am.Soc.Clin.Oncol. 1992; 11: A864
3. Hoelzer D., Arnold R., Aydemir U., Buchner T., Freud M., W.Glassmann. N.Gokbuget, Hiddemann W., Koch P., Loffler H., Ludwig W.D., Maschmeyer G., Thiel E., Volkers B. Results of Intensified Consolidation Therapy in Four Consecutive German Multicenter Studies for Adult ALL. Blood 1993; 82(suppl 1): 193 a (N 758)
4. Arlin Z.A., Feldman E., Kempin S., Ahmed T., Mittelman A., Savona S., Ascensao J., Baskind P., Sullivan Ph., Fuhr H.G., Mertelsmann R. Amsacrine with High-dose Cytarabine is Highly Effective Therapy for Refractory and Relapsed Acute Lymphoblastic Leukemia in Adults. Blood 1988; 72 (2) pp 433–435
5. Kantarjian H.M., Estey E.H., O'Brien S., Anaissie E., Beran M., Rios M.B., Keating M.J., Gutterman J. Intensive Chemotherapy with Mitoxantrone and High-dose Cytosine Arabinoside Followed by Granulocyte-Macrophage Colony-Stimulating Factor in the Treatment of Patients with Acute Lymphocytic Leukemia. Blood 1992; 79(4) pp 876–881
6. Freund M., Diedrich H., Ganser A., Gramatzky M., Heil G., Heyll A., Henke M., Hiddemann W., Haas R., Kuse R. et al Treatment of Relapsed or Refractory Adult Acute Lymphocytic Leukemia. Cancer 1992; 69 (3) pp 709–716
7. Giona F., Annino L., Ferrari A., Crescenzi S., Aloe Spiriti M.A., Arcese W., Meloni G., Pigna M., Testi A.M., Mandelli F. Adult Acute Lymphoblastic Leukemia (ALL) Refractory or in Relapse: Results of Treatment over 17-yr Period. Haematological 1992; 76 (suppl 4): 67
8. Elias L., Shaw M.T., Raab S.O. Reinduction Therapy for Adult Acute Leukemia with Adriamycin, Vincristine, an Prednisone: a Southwest Oncology Group Study. Cancer Treat.Rep. 1979; 63 pp 1413–1415

Acute Leukemias V
Experimental Approaches
and Management of Refractory Diseases
Hiddemann et al. (Eds.)

Treatment of Philadelphia Chromosome Positive ALL with Interferon Alpha

J. L. Harousseau[1], F. Guilhot, P. Casassus, and D. Fière

Abstract. Philadelphia positive (Ph) Acute Lymphoblastic Leukemia (ALL) constitutes 20 to 25% of adult ALL. The management of Ph + ALL is difficult and even if complete remissions (CR) can be achieved with conventional chemotherapy, they are usually short and the long-term disease free survival is less than 10%. Following the initial report by Ohyashiki et al. (Leukemia 1991, 5: 611,) showing encouraging results in 3 patients, we have tried to maintain CR induced by conventional chemotherapy with a Interferon. Eight patients (5 male, 3 female) aged 38–66 years (med 57) who had achieved CR with various induction regimen received a Interferon (α IFN) after consolidation chemotherapy. Six patients were in first CR of de novo Ph positive ALL, one patient was in second CR after a relapse post allogenic bone marrow transplantation, one was in CR after lymphoid blast cusis of chronic myeloid leukemia (CML). The dose of α IFN varied from 3 M IU/m² 3 times weekly (4 patients) to 5 M IU/m² daily. Of the 8 patients 6 relapsed 1 to 11 months (median 3) after initiation of α IFN therapy. In 2 cases hematological relapse was preceded by cytogenetic relapse (4 and 3 months before). Two patients remain in continous CR at 8 and 14 months. These preliminary results do not appear to confirm the initial positive results. However, more patients are needed to assess the exact place of α IFN in Ph + ALL.

Introduction

Philadelphia Chromosome positive ALL remains one of the most difficult issues in the therapy of ALL [1]. The incidence of Ph positive ALL increases from less than 5% in children to more than 40% in patients over the age of 50 [2, 4]. The overall incidence of Ph positive cases in adult ALL is estimated around 25%. The prognosis of Ph positive ALL remains very poor. The complete remission (CR) rate appears to be somewhat lower than in other adult ALL (50–80%) but mostly the duration of remission is shorter. With conventional chemotherapy, the Leukemia free survival (LFS) does not exceed 20% at 2 years and is 0% at 5 years [1, 5].

Recently Roberts et al. have reported 4 long term remissions out of 11 children with Ph positive ALL treated with aggresive induction/consolidation followed by rotational treatment with non cross resistant drugs [6]. However the role of intensive chemotherapy remains to be determined, specially in adult patients.

Autologous bone marrow transplantation is another approach but preliminary experience is in favour of a high relapse rate despite intensive preparative regimen [7, 9]. Allogenic bone marrow transplantation is the only possibility for obtaining long term remissions [10, 11]. Data from the International Bone Marrow Transplant Registry show a 2 year actuarial probability of LFS of 38% for patients in first CR [11].

Alpha Interferon (α IFN) is an effective treatment of CML [12]. It frequently induces hematological remissions and sometimes complete cytogenetic responses. This observation led several authors to use α IFN in Ph1 positive ALL after relapse [13, 14] or in first CR [15]. We report here our experience on 8 adult patients with ALL in CR treated with α IFN as maintenance therapy.

[1] Department of Hematology, Hôtel Dieu, CHU Nantes, 44035 Nantes, France

Clinical Observations

We have collected the records of 8 adult patients with Ph positive ALL in CR treated with α IFN as maintenance therapy.

One 38 year old man was treated with a combination of Hydroxyurea and α IFN for CML. Nine months after the diagnosis of CML he was in blast crisis of ALL type. After failure of a Vincristine-Prednisone regimen he achieved CR with a combination of Mitoxantrone-Intermediate dose ARAC-C. He was treated immediately with rα2b IFN (5MU/m²/Day) but relapsed 2 months later.

One 30 year old man was treated for de novo pre B Ph positive ALL. He achieved CR with a combination of Idarubicin and Intermediate Dose ARA-C. He then underwent an allogenic bone marrow transplantation but relapsed 5 months later. A second CR was obtained by Vincristine and Prednisone. He received maintenance treatment with rα2b IFN (5MU/m²/Day) but relapsed within six weeks.

Six patients were treated in first CR of de novo Ph positive ALL. Their clinical data are in Table 1.

Four of the 6 patients relapsed at 4 weeks, 13 weeks, 16 weeks and 47 weeks. Two patients remain in hematological remission (32 weeks, 14 months) but one is in cytogenetic relapse.

Discussion

Partial or complete loss of α and β IFN genes located on chromosome 9 has been demonstrated in malignant cells from patients with ALL [16, 17]. Moreover even in patients with apparently normal IFN genes, other abnormalities of the interferon system (IFN production, α IFN receptors, IFN induced enhancement of 2′5′ A synthetase) have been described [18]. Finally, evidence of direct in vitro cytotoxicity against ALL blasts has been reported recently [19]. These observations may represent a rationale for the use of α IFN a least in some subgroups of ALL. Ph1 positive ALL could be one of these subgroups since α IFN induces hematological responses and partial or even complete cytogenetic responses in Ph1 positive CML [12]. However it should be noticed that α IFN is usually not effective in CML in blast crisis.

Table 1. Ph⁺ ALL IN FIRST CR

	Age	WBC	Induction	Consolidation	aIFN	Remission Duration
1	52	2.4	D, V, Asp, P Asp, I, Ara	P, Ara, Mi, E ABMT	3M/D	4W
2	56	35.4	Mi, V, P I, Ara	P, Ara, Mi, VP Ad, Asp, Ara	V. P. 3 MU/m²/D	16W
3	43	3.4	D, V, P	Ad, P, V BEAC	3 MU/m² 3T week MTX	47W*
4	63	33.6	D, V, C, P	D, Ara, Asp	3MU/m² 3T week 6MT+MTX	13W
5	66	22	D, V, C, P	D, Ara, Asp	3MU/m² 3T week 6MP+MTX	32W+**
6	58	5	D, V, C, P	D, Ara, Asp	3MU/m² 3T week 6MT+MTX	14M+

*Cytogenetic relapse after 25 W; **Cytogenetic relapse

Abbreviations:

WBC: White Blood Cells
D: Daunorubicine
V: Vincristine
Asp: Asparaginase
P: Prednisone
C: Cyclophosphamide
AIFN: a Interferon
Arc: ARA-C
Mi: Mitoxantrone
Ad: Adriamycine
MTX: Methotrexate
GMP: G Mercaptopurine
E Etoposide
B: BCNU
W: Week
M: Month

Several investigators have used α IFN in the treatment of Ph positive ALL. Ochs et al. have given α IFN to 31 children with ALL in first on chemotherapy marrow relapse as the sole treatment (30MU/m²/day intravenously) before standard chemotherapy. They have obtained only 2 partial remissions. Out of the 23 patients achieving CR with subsequent chemotherapy, 22 received α IFN maintenance at a dose of 30 MU/m²/day for 3 consecutive days every 3 weeks in combination with multiagent chemotherapy. Five patients remained in continuous CR for 26 to 35 months. The administration of α IFN did not compromise the intensity of chemotherapy but the interest of this combination is questionable in this study.

Haas et al. have treated 2 patients with recombinant α2c IFN. One in second marrow remission relapsed rapidly under α IFN therapy (2×10^6 U/D). In the other case, chronic phase CML evolved six months after the end of ALL therapy. Daily treatment with 2 MU α IFN was initiated after failure of Hydroxyurea and hematological remission was achieved. When the daily dose was increased to 4 MU a nearly complete cytogenetic remission was obtained and had been maintained for 22 months at the time of publication.

Ohyashiki et al reported the results of α IFN as maintenance therapy in 3 out of 7 patients with Ph positive ALL. Two of them were in hematological CR but their marrow caryotype was Ph positive.

Reduction of the percentage of Ph positive marrow metaphases was obtained by α IFN therapy and they remained in remission for 8 months and 13 months. The third one was treated with α IFN immediatly after achieving CR but the follow up was only 3 months at the time of publication. In a more recent paper, the same authors stated that the 3 patients were still alive but did not give information on their hematological and cytogenetic remission status [20].

Our results appear to be rather disappointing since 6 out of 8 patients relapsed (5 within 4 months of α IFN maintenance therapy). Of the 6 patients in first CR only two remain in hematological CR for 8 and 14 months and one of them is in cytogenetic relapse. These 2 patients actually received a combination of a α IFN and classical maintenance treatment with mercaptopurine and methotrexate.

The apparent discrepancy between our experience and Ohyaskiki's paper [15] cannot probably be explained by the dose of α IFN. We have used doses ranging from 3 MU/m² 3 times a week to 5M/m²/Day. The doses used in favourable cases range from 2 MU/D to 4 MU/D [14, 15]. Another explanation is proposed by Ohyashiki [20]. At the molecular level Ph positive ALL consists of two subsets [2, 5]. In the first subtype, the molecular defect is identical to that seen in CML in which the breakpoints on chromosome 22 are within the major breakpoint cluster region (M-BCR). In this subtype the fusion gene is translated into a 210 KD chimeric protein. In the second subtype the chromosome 22 breakpoint is upstream of the M-BCR region in a region called minor breakpoint cluster region. In this subtype, a 190 KD protein is produced. The vast majority of pediatric Ph positive ALL and 50–70% of adult cases are of the P190 type.

Ohyashiki stated that the biological behaviour of Ph positive ALL could pastly depend on the type of molecular defect and that α IFN therapy could be useful in cases with the molecular defect seen in CML. The 3 cases he reported as well as the case described by Haas had the M-BCR rearrangement.

This hypothesis should be confirmed by larger series. Currently the results are not sufficient to propose α IFN maintenance for all adult patients with Ph positive ALL.

References

1. Hoelzer D. Therapy of acute lymphoblastic leukemia in adults. Leukemia, 1992, 6, Supp 2: 132–135.
2. Secker-Walker LM, Craig JM, Hawkins JM, Hoffbrand AV. Philadelphia positive acute lymphoblastic leukemia in adults: age distribution, BCR breakpoint and prognostic significance. Leukemia, 1991, 5: 196–199.
3. Berger R, Chen SJ, Chen Z. Philadelphia positive acute leukemia cytogenetic and molecular aspects. Cancer Genet Cytogenet, 1990, 44: 143–152.
4. Ribeiro RC, Abramovitch M, Raimondi SC, et al. Clinical and biologic hallmarks of the Philadelphia Chromosome in childhood acute lymphoblastic leukemia. Blood 1987, 70: 948–953.
5. Grigg AP. Approaches to the treatment of Philadelphia positive acute lymphoblastic leukemia. Bone Marrow Transplant, 1993, 12: 431–435.
6. Roberts WM, Rivera GK, Raimondi SC. Intensive chemotherapy for Philadelphia chromosome positive acute lymphoblastic leukaemia. Lancet 1994, i: 331–332.

7. Brennan C, Weisdorf D, Kersey J et al. Bone marrow transplantation for Philadelphia positive acute lymphoblastic leukemia. ASCO Proc, 1991, 10: 222 (abstract N °766).
8. Sebban C, Lepage E, Vernant JP et al. Allogenic bone marrow transplantation is the best post-remission therapy for high risk adult acute lymphoblastic leukemia: a study from the French Group of adult ALL. ASCO Proc. 1992, 11: 159 (abstract N °847).
9. Miyamura K, Tanimoto M, Morishina Y et al. Detection of Philadelphia Chromosome positive acute lymphoblastic leukemia by polymerase chain reaction: possible eradication of minimal residual disease by marrow transplantation. Blood, 1992, 79: 1366–1370.
10. Forman SJ, O'Donnell MR, Nademanee AP et al. Bone marrow transplantation for patients with Philadelphia Chromosome positive leukemia. Blood, 1987, 70: 587–588.
11. Barrett AJ, Horowitz MM, Ash RC et al. Bone marrow transplantation for Philadelphia Chromosome positive acute lymphoblastic leukemia. Blood, 1992, 79: 3067–3070.
12. Talpaz M, Kantarjian H, Kurzrock R et al. Interferon-alpha produces sustained cytogenetic response in chronic myeloid leukemia. Ann Intern Med, 1991, 114: 532–538.
13. Ochs J, Brecher HL, Mahoney D et al. Recombinant interferon alpha given before and in combination with standard chemotherapy in children with acute lymphoblastic leukemia in first marrow relapse: a Pediatric Oncology Group pilot study. J. Clin. Oncol,, 1991, 5: 777–782.
14. Haas OA, Mor W, Gadner H, Bartram CR. Treatment of Ph Positive Acute Lymphoblastic Leukemia with α Interferon. Leukemia, 1988, 2: 555.
15. Ohyashiki K, Ohyashiki JH, Tanchi T et al. Treatment of Philadelphia Chromosome Positive Acute Lymphoblastic Leukemia: A pilot study with raises important questions. Leukemia, 1991, 5: 611–614.
16. Einhorn S, Grandér D, Björk o, Söderhäll S. Loss of α and β interferon genes in malignant cells from children with acute lymphocytic leukemia. J. Interferon Res, 1989, 9: 105.
17. Diaz MU, Rubin CM, Harden A et al. Deletion of interferon genes in acute lymphoblastic leukemia. New Engl. J. Med, 1990, 322: 77–82.
18. Grandér D, Heyman M, Bröndum-Nielsen K et al. Interferon system in primary acute lymphoblastic leukemia cells with or without deletions of Ph1 α-β Interferon genes. Blood, 1992, 79: 2076–2083.
19. Manabe A, Campan AD. Cytotoxic activity of interferon α on normal and leukemic immature human B lineage cells. Blood, 1992, 80 (suppl 1): 35a (abstract 130).
20. Ohyashiki K, Ohyashiki JH, Toyama K. Therapy for Philadelphia Chromosome Positive Acute Lymphoblastic Leukemia: Possible list of Interferon on the basis of some navel concepts. Leukemia and Lymphoma, 1993, 9: 43–48.

Acute Leukemias V
Experimental Approaches
and Management of Refractory Diseases
Hiddemann et al. (Eds.)

Six Years' Experience with Treatment of Recurrent Childhood Lymphoblastic Leukemia. Report of the Polish Children's Leukemia/Lymphoma Study Group

J. Boguslawska-Jaworska[7], A. Chybicka[7], J. Armata[1], W. Balwierz[1], H. Bubala[4], B. Filiks-Litwin[2], J. Kowalczyk[2], D. Lukowska[4], M. Ochocka[5], U. Radwanska[3], R. Rokicka-Milewska[4], D. Sonta-Jakimczyk[6], W. Stronjny[4], and E. Zelenay[4]

Abstract. Between June 1987 and April 1993, 147 children aged from 2–18 years (47 girls and 100 boys) with first relapse of acute lymphoblastic leukemia were included to the study. The children were treated according to the BFM 85 ALL relapse protocol. There were 91 cases with early and 56 cases with late relapse (BM-72, local-50, combined-22, others-3). The probability of EFS were calculated according to Kaplan-Meier method. The overall second complete remission (CR) rate in early relapse was 79.12% and in late relapse 85.71%. The probability of overall event free survival (EFS) after 6 years was 25.52%. The EFS achieved in children with late relapses was four times higher when compared with early relapses 46.55% vs. 11.47% ($p = 0.05$).

The results obtained with BFM 85 chemotherapy in children with first late relapse are acceptable. For children with early relapses, other chemotherapy methods together with BMT in second remission should be introduced.

Introduction

Many factors within the past ten years have contributed to a marked improvement in the prognosis of childhood acute lymphoblastic leukemia (ALL): an increasing number of effective chemotherapeutic agents, combination chemotherapy, modified dose schedules, intensive treatment during remission, CNS prophylaxis and vigorous supportive care. Over 80% children now become long term survivors [4, 11]. Relapse has to be considered as the most important obstacle in the way of curing all children with ALL [3, 10, 16, 17].

154 of 1600 children treated for ALL in seven centres of The Polish Children's Leukemia Lymphoma Study Group between 1981–1993 according to the BFM protocols, relapsed during therapy or after its discontinuation.

Material and Methods

Patients and definition. Between June 1987 and April 1993, 147 children aged from 2–18 years (47 girls and 100 boys) with first relapse of acute lymphoblastic leukemia were included to the study. Initial characteristics of the children at first presentation of the disease and at relapse are presented in Table 1.

T cell ALL at 25% and B cell ALL at 21% of children were recognized.

At their first presentation children were treated according to the BFM 83 or 86 protocols [15], at relapse according to the BFM 85 relapse protocol [12].

[1]Department of Children Hematology, Polish American Children's Hospital, M. Copernicus Institute of Pediatrics, Krakow, Poland
[2]Department of Children Hematology, Institute of Pediatrics, Faculty of Medicine, Lublin, Poland
[3]Department of Children Hematology and Oncology, Faculty of Medicine, Poznań, Poland
[4]Department of Children Hematology and Oncology, Faculty of Medicine, Warsaw, Poland
[5]Department of Children Hematology, Faculty of Medicine, Warsaw, Poland
[6]Department of Children Hematology and Oncology, Faculty of Medicine, Zabrze, Poland
[7]Department of Children Hematology and Oncology, Faculty of Medicine, Wroclaw, Poland

Table 1. Initial characteristics of 147 children (100 boys, 68.03%; 47 girls, 31.97%) with first ALL relapse

		at first diagnosis	at relapse
age	<2 years	10(6.80%)	2(1.36%)
	2–10 years	115(78.23%)	102(69.39%)
	>10 years	22(14.97%)	43(29.25%)
clinical classification	LRG	41/131(31.30%)	
	MRG	56/131(42.75%)	
	HRG	34/131(25.95%)	
FAB classification	L1	40/84(47.62%)	21/80(26.25%)
	L2	42/84(50.00%)	56/80(70.00%)
	L3	2/84(2.38%)	3/80(3.75%)
immunological classification	B	6/54 (11.11%)	6/28(21.43%)
	pre B	11/54(20.37%)	12/28(42.86%)
	T	16/54(29.63%)	7/28(25.00%)
	Common	21/54(38.89%)	3/28(10.71%)

Early relapses were those, which occurred at the patients still on therapy or up 6 months after stopping front line treatment. The reminder were termed as late relapses.

Isolated bone marrow relapse was diagnosed in the presence of 25% bone marrow blasts with the absence of any other clinically proven leukemic extramedullary infiltration's.

Isolated extramedullary marrow relapses were those with clinically overt manifestations of leukemia or histologically/cytologically proven leukemic infiltration's at any site except bone marrow.

Marrow involvement was diagnosed in children with proven leukemia at extramedullary sites and at least 5% blasts in bone marrow.

Type and time of first ALL relapse in childhood are presented in Table 2. The predominance of early relapses was observed in our material. There were 91 cases with early and 56 cases with late relapse. Most of early relapses were isolated BM (51.65%), followed by isolated CNS (17.58%) and testes (16.48%). The total proportion of early mixed relapses was 10,99%.

In the group of late relapses predominated also isolated BM (44.64%) involvement followed

Table 2. Type and time of first ALL relapse treated according to BFM-85 protocol

type of relapse	early relapses n=91(61.90%)		late relapses n=56(38.10%)		total n=147(100%)	
isolated:						
BM	47	51.66%	25	44.64%	72	48.98%
CNS	16	17.58%	6	10.7%	22	14.96%
testes	15	16.48%	13	23.21%	28	19.05%
others*	3	3.30%	0		3	2.04%
total	81	89.01%	44	78.57%	125	85.03%
mixed:						
BM+CNS	5	5.49%	4	7.14%	9	6.12%
BM+testes	4	4.40%	8	14.29%	12	8.16%
BM+CNS+testes	1	1.10%	0		1	0.67%
total:	10	10.99%	12	21.43%	22	14.97%

*ovaries, tumor reg. sacralis, kidney

by isolated testes (23.21%) relapse, combined BM+testes (14.29%) and BM+CNS, and then isolated CNS.

Statistical analysis. The probability of EFS were calculated according to the Kaplan-Meier method [13].

Treatment. Patients were stratified into three treatment groups A, B and C (Fig. 1).

Regimen A was given to children with early combined BM relapse, regimen B to patients with late isolated or combined BM relapse, and regimen C to children with isolated extramedullary relapses, irrespective of the time of occurrence. In all patients treatment was started with a 5-day phase of prednisone (2 mg/kg/d). This was done to reduce the initial mass of leukemic cells and to stabilize the patients general condition.

Main elements of treatment for induction and consolidation were alternating courses of intensive polychemotherapy (R1 and R2) and in children with early BM relapse a separate induction protocol F (Table 3). All children with BM relapse were treated with eight R-blocks, whereas only six such courses were administered to children with isolated extramedullary relapse.

All the end of the intensive phase the systemic chemotherapy was supplemented by cranial irradiation in children with CNS relapse, as well as by testicular irradiation in boys with testicular relapse. Cranial irradiation was administered at dose 24 Gy to non preirradiated patients. Standardized dose reductions were made according to age of patients and doses previously applied.

In boys with unilateral testicular relapse the involved testis was surgically removed and biopsy was taken from clinically non involved testis. If the biopsied testis proved histologically to be free of leukemia, radiotherapy was administered to the remaining testis at dose of 18 Gy. In patients with bilateral testicular relapse either both testicles were to be removed or irradiated at a dose of 24 Gy.

After the end of the intensive phase of treatment the children received maintenance therapy with daily 6-tioguanine (50 mg/m^2) and biweekly iv Mtx (50 mg/m^2).

The duration of maintenance therapy was 2 years for children with BM relapse and 1 year for patients with isolated extramedullary relapse. Triple intrathecal therapy in 6-weeks intervals up to the end of the first year of treatment were administered to children with CNS relapse.

Response Criteria

In children with BM relapse remission was diagnosed, if there were less than 5% blast cells in an otherwise normocellular marrow. CNS remission was defined by the absence of leukemic cells in CSF.

In boys with isolated testicular relapses remission was achieved by orchiectomy, or in non-orchiectomised patients if the size of the involved testis (es) had returned to normal.

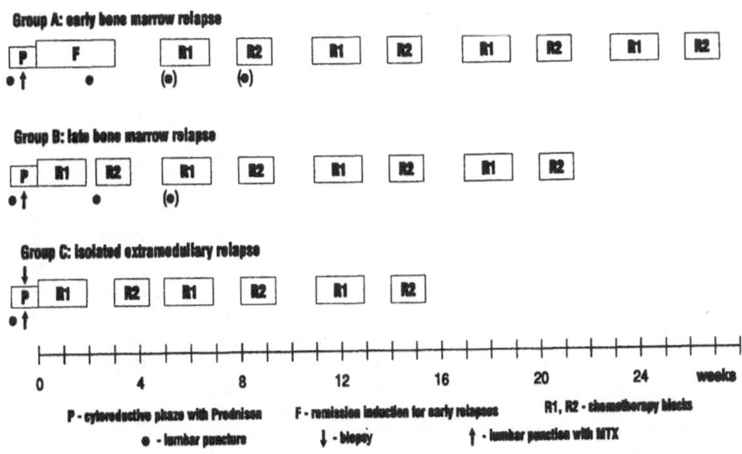

Fig. 1. Design of study relapse ALL BFM-85

Table 3. Treatment courses

	drugs	dosis	administered on day
induction F	Prednisone	100 mg/m²	1–7, 15–21
	Vincristine	1.5 mg/m²	1,8, 15,22
	Methotrexate	ID lub (or) HD	1
	HD-cytarabine	3 g/m²co 12h	15,16
	L-asparaginase	10,000 U/m²	2,3,17,18
block R1	Prednisone	100 mg/m²	1–5
	Mercaptopurine	100 mg/m²	1-5
	Vincristine	1.5 mg/m²	1
	Methotrexate i.v.	1 g/m²	1
	Methotrexate i.t.	12 mg*	1
	Cytarabine	300 mg/m²	5
	Teniposide	165 mg/m²	5
	L-asparaginase	10,000 U/m²	6–8
block R2	Dexamethasone	20 mg/m²	1–5
	Thioguanine	100 mg/m²	1–5
	Vindesine	3.0 mg/m²	1
	Methotrexate i.v.	1 g/m²	1
	Methotrexate i.t	12 mg*	1
	Ifosfamide	40 mg/m²	1–5
	Daunorubicin	50 mg/m²	5

*Methotrexat: dose 10/8/6 mg in children 3/2/1 years.

Complete remission (CR) had to be achieved after application of two treatment elements, i.e. in patients with early BM relapse after protocol F and block R1 or in other patients after Block R1 and R2. Patients in non remission at that time were termed non responders, even if CR was achieved later.

Results

A summary of the treatment response is shown in Table 4.

Table 4. Summary of results to treatment of first ALL relapse treated BFM-85 protocol

Type of relapse	N	CR		no CR		II relapse		death		still in CR	
		n	[%]	n	[%]	n	[%]	n	[%]	n	[%]
early:	91	72	79.12	19	20.88	38	41.76	64	70.33	27	19.67
BM	47	33	70.21	14	29.79	19	40.42	39	82.98	8	17.02
extram.	34	32	94.12	2	5.88	15	44.12	18	52.94	16	47.06
CNS	16	16	100.0	0		6	37.50	8	50.00	8	50.00
testes	15	15	100.0	0		8	53.33	7	46.67	8	63.33
other	3	1	33.33	2	66.67	1	33.33	3	100.0	0	
mixed	10	7	70.00	3	30.00	4	40.00	7	70.00	3	30.00
late:	56	48	85.71	8	14.29	17	30.36	21	37.50	34	62.50
BM	25	22	88.00	3	22.00	7	28.00	10	40.00	15	60.00
extram.	19	16	84.21	3	15.79	6	31.58	5	26.32	13	73.68
CNS	6	5	83.33	1	16.67	1	16.67	1	16.67	5	83.33
testes	13	11	84.61	2	15.39	5	38.46	4	30.77	9	69.23
other	0	0		0		0		0		0	
mixed	12	10	83.33	2	16.67	4	33.33	6	50.00	6	50.00

duration of II RC: 1–60 months, median 12 months; early relapses: 1–55 months, median 11 months; late relapses: 1–60 months, median 20 months

Overall Results

The overall second complete remission (CR) rate was 120 of 147 patients (81.63%).

The overall second complete remission (CR) rate in early relapse was 79,12% and in late relapse 85,71%. There are 27 children with early and 34 with late relapse still in II CCR.

Early death analysis in children with first ALL relapse is presented in Table 5.

Late death analysis in children with first ALL relapse is listed in Table 6.

The probability of overall event-free survival (EFS) after 6 years was 25,52% (Fig. 2).

The EFS achieved in children with late relapses was four times higher when compared with early relapses 46,55% v 11,47% (p=0,05) (Fig. 3).

The EFS achieved in children with isolated late BM relapses was four times higher when

Table 5. Early death (first 4 weeks) analysis in children with first ALL relapse (n=15/147)

	early relapse		late relapse	
	n	[%]	n	[%]
progression of disease	2	13.3	0	
aplasia+infection	4 1 E. coli. seps. 1 St. aureus seps. 1 Pseudom. seps. 1 Meningitis	26.7	3 1 Pneumona 1 sepsis	20.0
therapy toxicity diathesis heamorrhagica	1	6.7	1 toksycznoœæ po MTX+HD toxicity after MTX+HD	6.7
infection	1 CNS+seps. Proteus	6.7	1 sepsis Pseudom. aerug.	6.7
pure diathesis haemorrhagica	1	6.7	0	
therapy toxicity after PL	1	6.7	0	
TOTAL	10	66.67	5	33.33

Table 6. Last death analysis in children with first ALL relapse (n=70/147)

	early relapse		late relapse	
	n	[%]	n	[%]
progression of the disease	48	68.57	14	20.00
I relapse	12	17.14	0	
II relapse	36	51.43	14	20.00
death in CR	6	8.57	2	2.86
infection	3 1 seps. st. aureus 1 seps. ent.+E.c. 1 seps. sept.	4.29	2	2.86
therapy toxicity	2 1 after MTX 1 after PL	2.86	0	
coma hepatious	1	1.43	0	
TOTAL	54	77.14	16	22.86

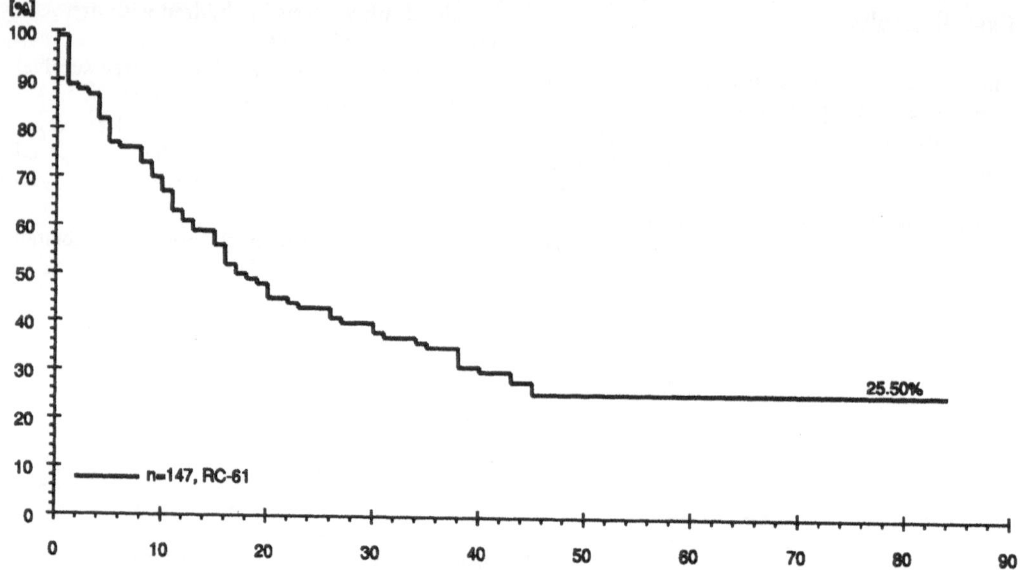

Fig. 2. Event-free survival of children with first relapse of ALL treated according to BFM-85 protocol

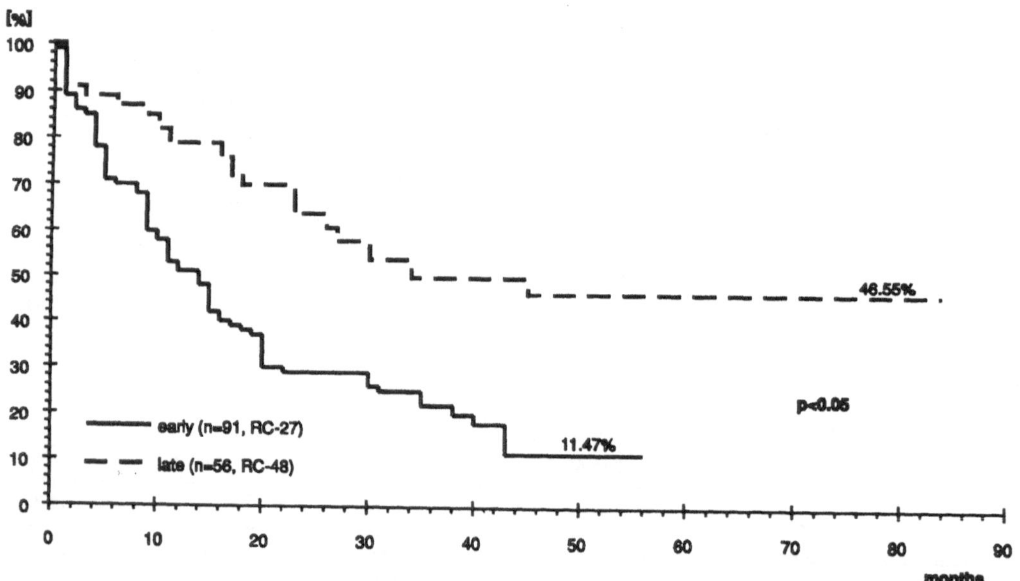

Fig. 3. Event-free survival of children with first early and late relapse of ALL treated according to BFM-85 protocol

compared with isolated early BM relapses 46,55% v 11,47% (p = 0,05) (Fig. 4).

The EFS achieved in children with very early relapse was 8.84% (Fig. 5).

The EFS achieved in children with late extramedullary relapses was two times higher when compared with extramedullary early relapses 58.13% v 20.15% (p = 0,1) (Fig. 6).

The EFS achieved in children with isolated late testes relapses was two times higher when compared with isolated early testes relapses 51.85% v 32.31% (p = 0,1) (Fig. 7).

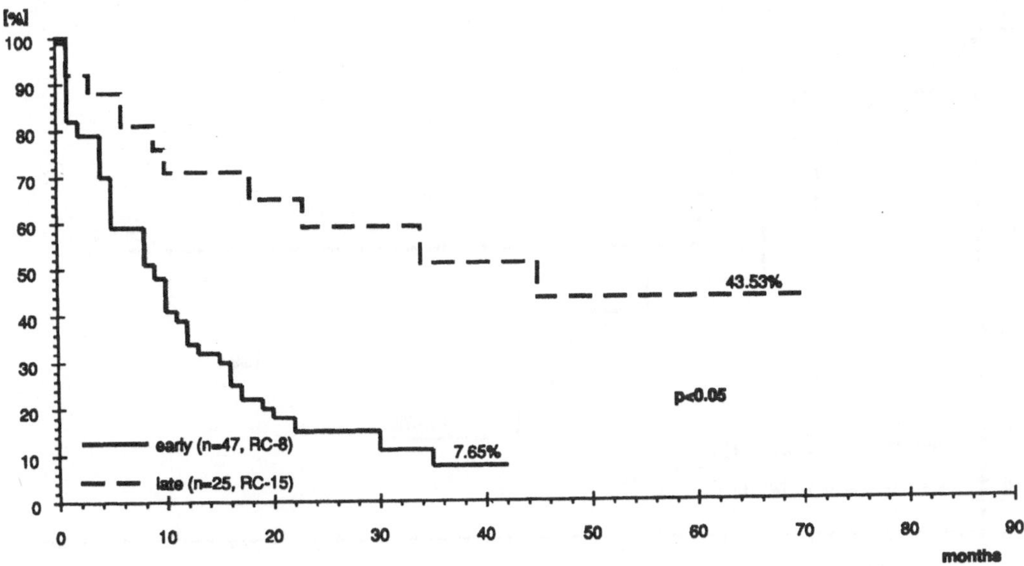

Fig. 4. Event-free survival of children with first BM relapse of ALL treated according to BFM-85 protocol

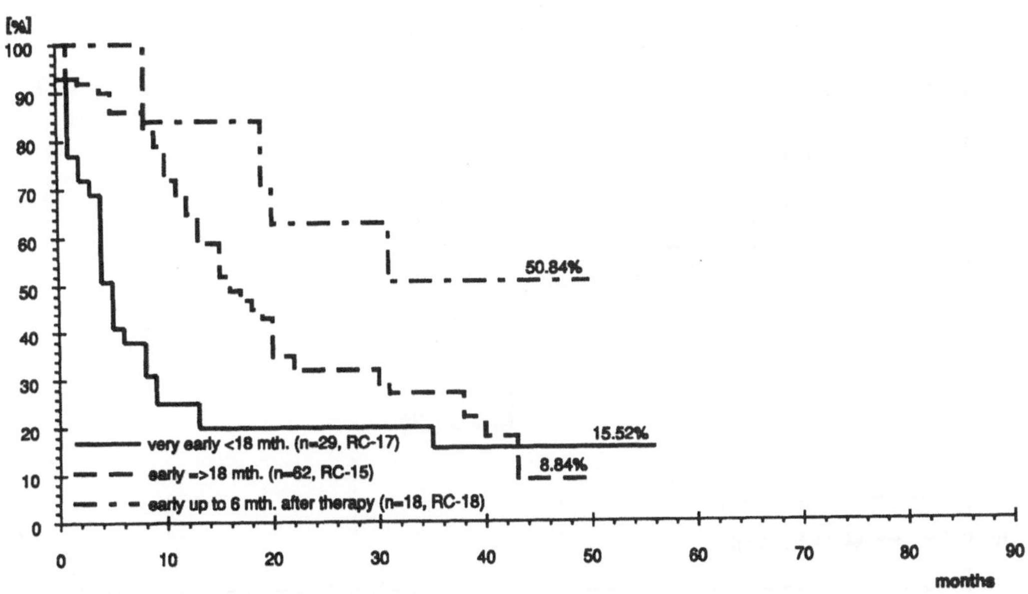

Fig. 5. Event-free survival of children with first early relapse of ALL treated according to BFM-85 protocol

The EFS achieved in children with isolated late CNS relapses was two times higher when compared with isolated early CNS relapses 83.33% v 41.65% (p = 0,1) (Fig. 8).

The EFS achieved in children with mixed late relapses was one and half times higher when compared with mixed early relapses 40.00% v 25.00% (p = 0,1) (Fig. 9).

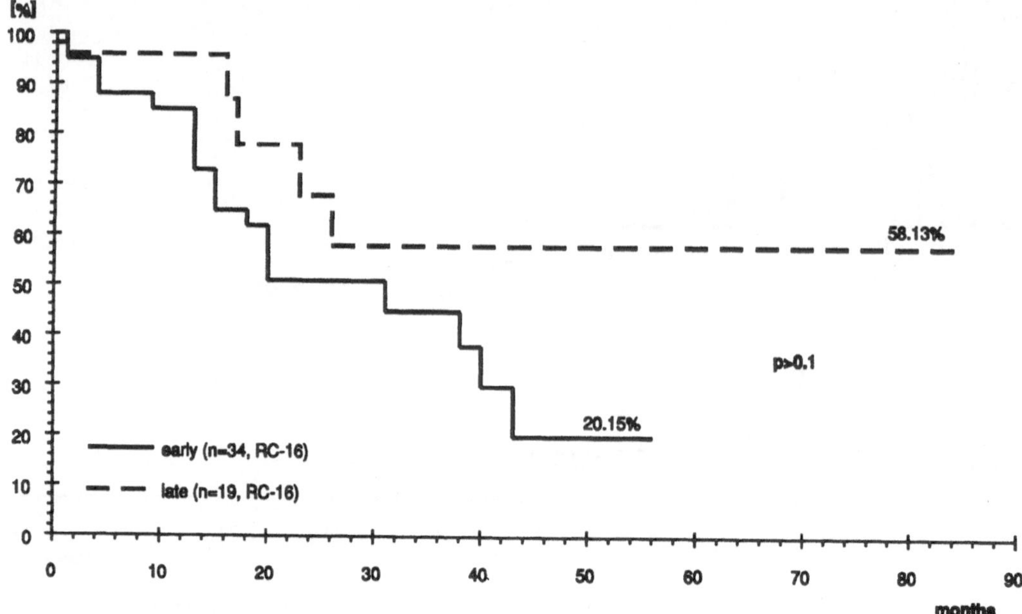

Fig. 6. Event-free survival of children with first extramedullary relapse of ALL treated according to BFM-85 protocol

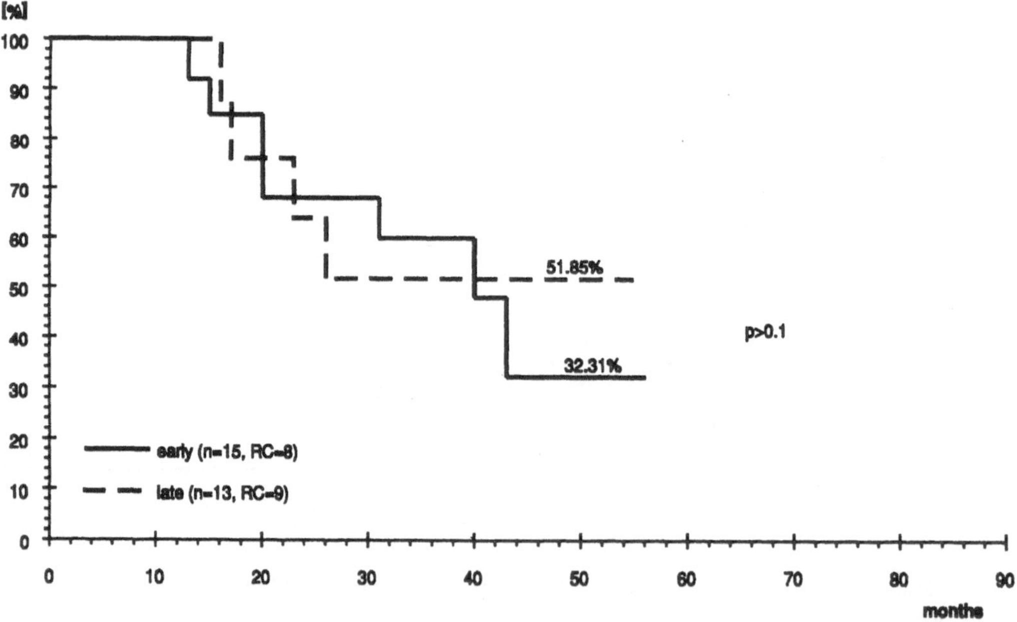

Fig. 7. Event-free survival of children with first testes relapse of ALL treated according to BFM-85 protocol

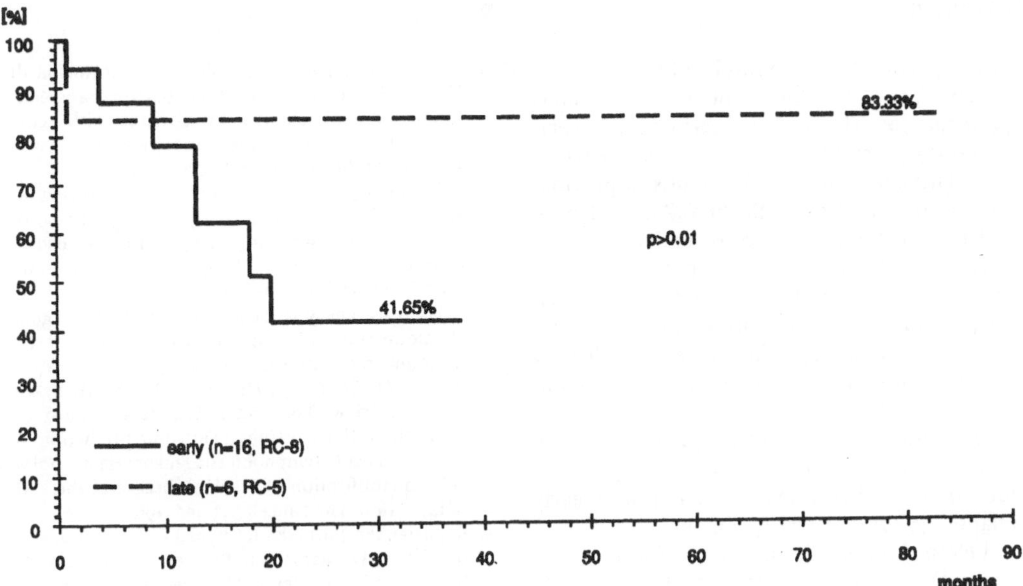

Fig. 8. Event-free survival of children with first CNS relapse of ALL treated according to BFM-85 protocol

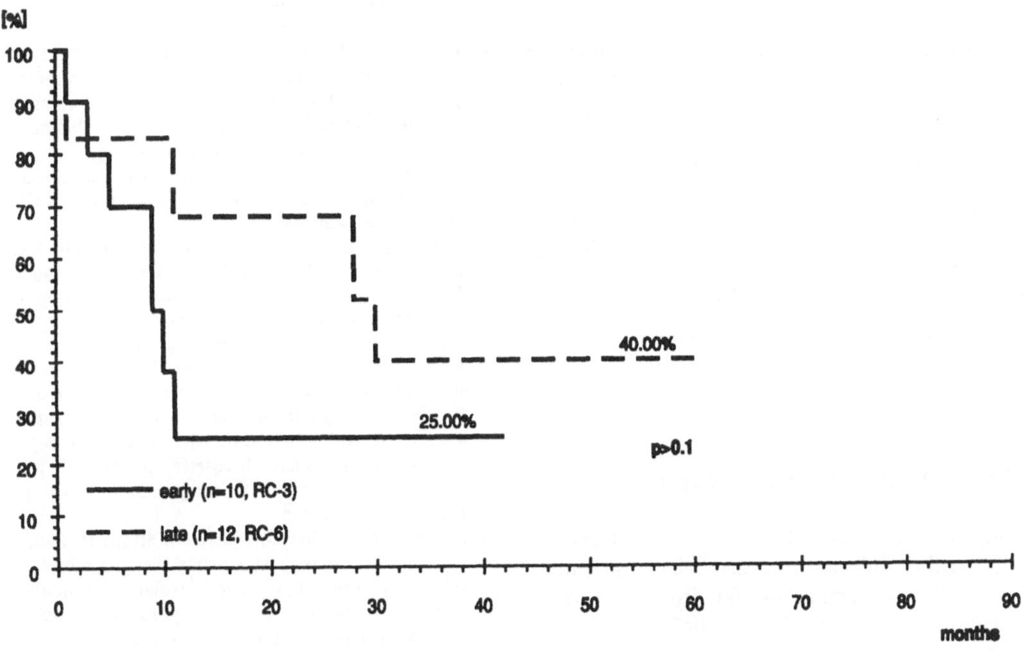

Fig. 9. Event-free survival of children with first mixed relapse of ALL treated according to BFM-85 protocol

Discussion

This report presents the results of the multicenter study and the efficacy of the BFM relapse protocol 1985. The trial was performed in years 1987–1993 in children with first recurrence of ALL. This study confirm the results of previous studies on children with first ALL relapses, which have shown that these patients do not make up a homogenous group [9, 18, 19]. It became clear that children, who developed their relapse during initial maintenance treatment and up to six months after the end of therapy (early relapse) have a worse prognosis compared with children, who relapse more than 6 months after cessation of therapy (late relapse). EFS achieved in children with late relapses was four times higher when compared with early relapses 46,55% v 11,47% ($p = 0,05$).

EFS in children with isolated BM relapse was 7,65%. Others have reported equally bad results in similar subgroup [2, 6, 17]. Until recently, the outcome in these children was unifoly dismal, with most patients succumbing to progressive and refractory disease within 12 months from the time of relapse [8, 14, 16].

It was shown in our previous study that the BFM protocol produced improvement of EFS in children with first relapse in comparison with chemotherapy previously used by the Polish Children's Leukemia Lymphoma Study Group [5].

The best therapy for children with late relapses, who achieved second remission is still controversial. Some findings suggest that bone marrow transplantation (BMT) is better than chemotherapy, whereas other do not [1, 7, 10, 13].

Conclusions

The results obtained with BFM 85 chemotherapy in children with first late relapse are acceptable. One must conclude that the treatment results obtained in children with early relapse, although gradually improving are far from satisfying. New treatment strategies together with BMT in second remission must be designed for this group of children.

References

1. Alarcon PA,Trigg ME, Giller ME, Rumelhardt Holida M, Wen B (1990): Bone marrow transplantation improves survival for children with acute lymphoblastic leukemia in relapse. Am.J. Ped.Hematol/Oncol, 12, 468–471
2. Behrendt H, Leeuven E Schurwirth C, Verkes R, Hermans J, Does van der Berg, Wering ER (1990): Bone marrow relapse occurring as first relapse in children with acute lymphoblastic leukemia Med.Oed.Oncol.,18,190–196
3. Belasco JB, Luery N, Scher Ch (1990): Multiagent chemotherapy in relapsed acute lymphoblastic leukemia in children. Cancer 66,2492–2497
4. Brisco MJ, Condon J, Hughes E, Neoh SH, Sykes PJ, Seshadri R, Toogood I, Waters K, Tauro G, Ekert H, Morley AA (1994): Outcome prediction in childhood acute lymphoblastic leukaemia by molecular quantification of residual disease at the end of induction. The Lancet, 343, 196–199
5. Boguslawska-Jaworska J, Chybicka A, Kazanowska B, Pietras W, Armata J, Balwierz W, Bubala H, Jackowska T, Koehler T, Michalewska D, Ochocka M, Radwanska U, Rokicka-Milewska R, Rytlewska M, Skomra S, Œladkowska G, Zelenay E (1990): The results of ALL relapses treatment according to BFM protocol in experience of the polish children's leukemia/lymphoma study group. Prac. Nauk. A.M., Suppl. 88–95
6. Buchanan GP, Riviera GK Boyett J,M Chauvent AR, Crist WM, Vietti TJ (1988): Reinduction therapy in 297 children with acute lymphoblastic leukemia in first bone marrow relapse: A Pediatric Oncology Group Study Blood,72,1286–1292
7. Butturini A (1987) Which treatment for childhood acute lymphoblastic leukemia in second remission? Lancet, 429–432
8. Culbert J, Schuster J, Land VJ, Wharam D, Thomas Rm, Nitschke R, Pinkel D, Vietti T (1991): Remission induction and continuation therapy in children with their first relapse of acute lymphoblastic leukemia. Cancer, 67, 37–42
9. Falleta JM, Schuster JJ, Crist WM, Pullen J, Bortowitz MJ, Wharam M, Patterson R, Foreman E, Vietti TJ (1992): Different patterns of relapse associated with three intensive treatment regiments for pediatric E-rosette positive T-cell leukemia: a Pediatric Oncology Study Group. Leukemia, 6, 541–546
10. Finkelstein J, Miller D, Feusner J, Stram D, Baum E, Shina D, Johnson D, Gyepes M, Hammond D (1994): Treatment of overt isolated testicular relapse in children on therapy for acute lymphoblastic leukemia. Cancer ,73, 219–223
11. Gale RP,Simone JV, Hoelzer D, Frei E (1991): Curing leukemia. Leukemia, 5, 632–635

12. Henze G (1991): 6-year experience with comprehensive approach to the treatment of recurrent childhood acute lymphoblastic leukemia (ALL-REZ. BFM 85). A relapse study of BFM Group. Blood 78, 1166–1292
13. Kaplan EL, Meier P (1958): Non parametric estimation from incomplete observations.J.Am.Stat. 53, 457–466
14. Pui Ch, Bowman P, Ochs J, Dodge RK, Riviera G (1988): Cyclic combination chemotherapy for acute lymphoblastic leukemia recurring after elective cessation of therapy. Med. Ped. Oncol. 16,21–26
15. Riehm H (1986): Treatment protocol ALL BFM-83. Klin. Pediatr., 199, 151–160
16. Riviera GK, Santana V, Mahmoud H, Buchanan G, Crist WM (1989): Acute lymphoblastic leukemia of childhood: the problem of relapses. BMT, 4, 80–85
17. Sauerbrey A,Zintl F, Malke H, Reimann M, Maaser M, Domula M, Dorffel W, Eggers G, Exadaktylos P Kotte W (1993): Results and experiences with a modified BFM protocol for treatment of recurrence in children with acute lymphoblastic leukemia in East German areas. Klin. Padiatr.,205, 281–287. Cancer,73, 219–223
18. Steinhertz P, (1989): Reinduction therapy for advanced or refractory acute lymphoblastic leukemia of childhood Cancer 63,1472–1476
19. Uderzo C, Zurlo MG, Adamoli L, Zanesco L, Calculi A, Comelli A, Montemezemolo L. Di Tulio M, Guazelli C, Donfrancesco A, Werner B (1990): Treatment of isolated testicular relapse in childhood acute lymphoblastic leukemia: An Italian Multicenter Study. J Clin Oncol, 8, 672–677

Acute Leukemias V
Experimental Approaches
and Management of Refractory Diseases
Hiddemann et al. (Eds.)

Interim Results of a Phase II Study with Idarubicin in Relapsed Childhood Acute Lymphoblastic Leukemia

A. Neuendank[1], R. Hartmann[1], R. Fengler[1], R. Erttmann[2], R. Dopfer[3], F. Zintl[4], E. Koscielniak[5], and G. Henze[1]

Introduction

Anthracyclines are effective drugs used for induction therapy of acute lymphoblastic leukemia (ALL). Since one of their major drawbacks is the well-known cardiac toxicity [11,14,17], other substances with similar antileukemic potency have been investigated to reduce this severe side effect. Additionally, cardiotoxicity can be reduced by prolonging the period of administration [10]. The new anthracycline analogue 4-demethoxydaunorubicin (idarubicin, IDR) may have some potential advantages compared to the "classic" compounds. Cardiotoxicity is possibly lower, and the main metabolite 13-hydroxyidarubicin (idarubicinol, IDRol) to which IDR is rapidly metabolized has the same cytotoxicity as IDR; however, the half-life is prolonged to 45–63 hours [1,8,13] and, furthermore, IDRol is capable of crossing the blood brain barrier, this having some protective effect against CNS leukemia [12]. IDR has proven its efficacy in the treatment of acute myelogenous leukemia, which has mostly been combined with cytarabine (Ara-C)[2,4,9,16]. But only few reports exist on the application of IDR in children with acute lymphoblastic leukemia [3, 5]. Testi et al. reported complete remission (CR) in 77% of intensively pre-treated children with ALL (n=31) by the combination of Ara-C and IDR [15]. To evaluate the toxicity and effectiveness of IDR monotherapy in ALL we designed a prospective, non-randomized multicenter study including 50 children with poor prognostic recurrences. This report describes interim results of the first 30 sequentially accrued patients.

Patients and Treatment

Idarubicin was given to 30 children with isolated or combined bone marrow (BM) relapse as monotherapy at a single dose of 24 mg/m^2 as 48 hour continuous infusion. These children were excluded from the regular ALL-REZ BFM protocol, because of standard exclusion criteria:

- refractory initial ALL
- very early BM relapse (previous remission duration < 18 months)
- relapse of T-cell phenotype
- second or multiple BM relapse

Characteristics of the patients are shown in Table 1. Previously, all children had received aggressive front-line therapy including anthracyclines. After the IDR pre-induction phase, treatment was continued with at least 3 courses of short-term intensive polychemotherapy to finally achieve CR, which is the prerequisite to perform either allogeneic or autologous bone marrow transplantation.

Methods

We performed a prospective study to evaluate the efficacy and toxicity of IDR in a therapeutic window as monotherapy. All patients were clinically monitored for signs of toxicity according

Dept. of Pediatric Hematology and Oncology, University Medical Centers of Berlin (UKRV),[1] Hamburg,[2] Tübingen,[3] Jena,[4] Olga Hospital Stuttgart,[5] Germany

Table 1. Patient characteristics

	First relapse	Multiple relapses	Total
patients (m:f)	18 (14:4)	12 (7:5)	30 (21:9)
median age	6 yrs (2–16)	10 yrs (1–13)	8 yrs (1–16)
previous CR duration	13 mos (4–32)	8 mos (2–32)	11 mos (2–32)
very early relapse	14 (78%)	11 (92%)	25 (83%)
T-cell phenotype	9 (50%)	–	9 (30%)
isolated BM relapse	14 (78%)	10 (83%)	24 (80%)
anthracycline pretreatment:			
< 200 mg/m²	1 (6%)	2 (7%)	3 (10%)
200–290 mg/m²	17 (94%)	4 (33%)	21 (70%)
300–390 mg/m²	–	6 (50%)	6 (20%)

to WHO criteria and were subjected to continuous clinical examination. The cardiac diagnostics consisted of E.C.G., M-mode echocardiography and chest X-ray. To assess the response to the drug, bone marrow aspirates were done before and 2 weeks after IDR infusion.

Response criteria:

1. Non Response (NR): stable/progressive disease
2. Minor Response: significant blast reduction (BM or peripheral blood)
3. Partial Remission (PR): blast redution < 25% in the BM
4. Complete Remission (CR): blast reduction < 5% in the BM and recovering hematopoesis

Table 2. Toxicity during or after IDR infusion

	WHO-grade					No. of patients
	0	1	2	3	4	
WBC	–	1	3	9	17	30
platelets	–	–	4	16	9	29
hemoglobin	–	1	13	13	3	30
infection	10	3	12	5	–	30
cardiac	27	2	–	1	–	30
neurologic	27	2	1	–	–	30
liver	16	8	4	1	–	29
kidney	28	2	–	–	–	30
nausea	16	5	7	2	–	30
stomatitis	14	9	6	1	–	30

Results

Serious toxic side effects, besides the desired blood-cell reduction were not observed (Table 2). No patient succumbed to therapy-related early death. In 26 of 30 patients, the leukocyte count fell below 1,000/μL with a nadir at day 10 (range day 5 to 17) accompanied by infection in 17 cases (57% of all patients). In the majority of patients, no organism could be proved in blood cultures. Non-hematology WHO-Grade 2 –3 toxicity (nausea, stomatitis and liver dysfunction) was seen in < 30% of patients.

Cardiac dysfunction was noticed in three patients. One child developed transient tachycardia during IDR infusion. In another case, pericardial effusion and diastolic dysfunction requiring glycoside therapy were observed 16 days after IDR administration, coinciding with aspergillus septicemia. The third patient exhibited signs of relative cardiac insufficiency pretherapeutically and showed unchanged cardiac function parameters and chest X-rays subsequent to the IDR infusion. Echocardiographic shortening fraction was determined in 25 children. All values were in the normal range (>30%) prior to and after IDR.

Complete or partial remission were seen in 1 and 10 patients, respectively, documented by day 15 bone marrow aspirates. One of the 10 partial responders whith aplastic marrow at day 15 attained a 2nd CR after one additional week without any further treatment. Neither responses to IDR were observed in 15 children licensed by significant reduction of leukemic blast cells, and only 4 patients had no objective response (Fig. 1).

The subsequent multidrug induction courses (scheduled at day 15 after IDR infusion) were delayed in 12 children (40%), because of prolonged aplasia (8 patients), infection (1 patient)

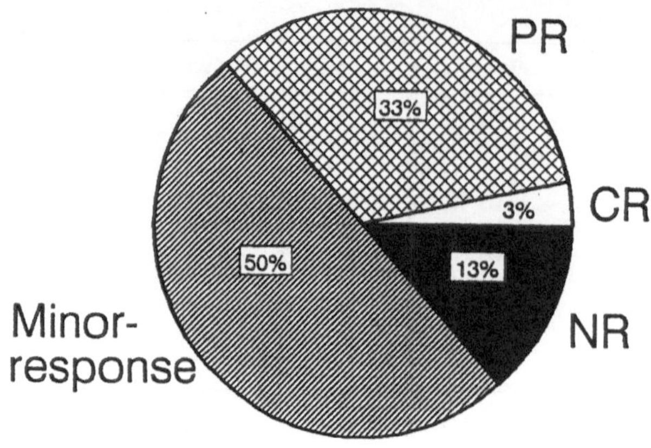

Fig. 1. Response to IDR monotherapy as documented by bone marrow puncture at day 15. CR, complete remission [1/30]; PR, partial remission [10/30]; Minor-response, significant blast cell reduction [15/30]; NR, non-response [4/30].

or combination of both (3 patients). In median, treatment could be continued after 21 days (range 11 to 41 days).

Discussion

Successful retreatment of children with relapsed ALL is obviously possible with chemotherapy, except for the subgroup of patients with very early or multiple relapses and for T-cell disease [7]. For these children, BMT in remission is indicated if possible. However, frequently remission may not be adviced in this subset of patients, suggesting that they suffer from highly refractory disease. The objective of this study was to evaluate the response to IDR given as monotherapy, an anthracycline which has not been used during previous therapy in these children. 11 of 30 patients showed a substantial response after IDR treatment as monotherapy, indicating that IDR is still an effective drug with antileukemic activity.

Only few data are available on the effective drug concentration of this new anthracycline in ALL, when used as single drug. Clinical phase I studies showed that the maximum tolerated drug concentration of IV IDR as monosubstance ranged between 30–40 mg/m^2 [6]. With dose escalation, haematologic toxicity was dose-limiting. IDR dose below 20 mg/m^2 in total showed no CR in patients with ALL [18]. Since all of our patients had previously been treated with daunorubicin or doxorubicin with a median cumulative dose of 270 mg/m^2 we have chosen 24 mg/m^2 of IDR as a propably safe dose in respect to cardiotoxicity while still having antileukemic potency in ALL. No additional severe drug related cardiotoxicity was seen in this study suggesting a favourable therapeutic index for IV IDR at the scheduled dose.

At this early stage, results are still preliminary. However, there is evidence for IDR being active in poor prognosis ALL relapse with tolerable cardiac and non-cardiac side effects.

Appendix

Participating centers and main investigators: Aarau (P. Imbach, MD), Berlin (G. Henze, MD), Berlin (W. Dörffel, MD), Berlin (G. Gaedicke, MD), Bremen (H. J. Spaar), Chemnitz (K. Hofmann, MD), Essen (B. Stollmann-Gibbels, MD), Erlangen (J. D. Beck, MD), Freiburg (C. Niemeyer, MD), Giessen (F. Lampert, MD), Göttingen (M. Lakomek, MD), Hannover (A. Reiter, MD), Heidelberg (B. Selle, MD), Homburg/Saar (N. Graf, MD), Jena (F. Zintl, MD), Koblenz (M. Rister, MD), Leipzig (M. Domula, MD), Linz (K. Schmitt, MD), Mainz (P.Gutjahr, MD), Rostock (M. Hagen, MD), Sankt Gallen (A. Feldges, MD), Stuttgart (E. Koscielniak, MD), Schwerin (B. Neubert, MD), Tübingen (D. Niethammer, MD).

References

1. Ames MM, Spreafico F: Selected pharmacologic characteristics of idarubicin and idarubicinol. Leukemia 6 Suppl 1: 70–75 (1992)
2. Berman E: New drugs in acute myelogenous leukemia: a review. J Clin Pharmacol 32: 296–309 (1992)
3. Carella AM; Berman E; Maraone MP; Ganzina F: Idarubicin in the treatment of acute leukemias. An

overview of preclinical and clinical studies. Haematologica (Pavia) 75: 1–11 (1990)

4. Carella AM; Carlier P; Pungolino E; Resegotti L; Liso V; Stasi R; Montillo M; Iacopino P; Mirto S; Pagano L et al: Idarubicin in combination with intermediate-dose cytarabine and VP-16 in the treatment of refractory or rapidly relapsed patients with acute myeloid leukemia. Leukemia 7: 196–199 (1993)
5. Erttmann R; Bode U; Erb N; Forcadell De Dios P; Gutjahr P; Haas R; Kuhn N; Siewert H; Landbeck G: Antineoplastische Wirksamkeit und Toxizität von Idarubicin (4-Demethoxydaunorubicin) bei rezidivierten akuten Leukämien des Kindesalters. Klin Padiatr 200: 200–204 (1988)
6. Feig SA; Krailo MD; Harris RE; Baum E; Holcenberg JS; Kaizer H; Steinherz L; Pendergrass TW; Saunders EF, Warkentin PL; Bleyer WA; Hammond GD: Determination of the maximum tolerated dose of idarubicin when used in a combination chemotherapy program of reinduction of childhood ALL at first marrow relapse and a preliminary assessment of toxicity compared to daunorubicin. Med Pediatr Oncol 20: 124–129 (1992)
7. Henze G; Fengler R; Hartmann R; Kornhuber B; Janka-Schaub G; Niethammer D; Riehm H: Six-year experience with a comprehensive approach to the treatment of recurrent childhood acute lymphoblastic leukemia (ALL-REZ BFM 85). A relapse study of the BFM Group. Blood 78: 1166–1172 (1991)
8. Kuffel MJ; Reid JM; Ames MM: Anthracyclines and their C-13 alcohol metabolites: growth inhibition and DNA damage following incubation with human tumor cells in culture. Cancer Chemother Pharmacol. 30: 51–57 (1992)
9. Kusnierz-Glaz CR; Normann D; Weinberg R; Fuchs R; Flasshove M; Hiddemann W; van de Loo J; Buchner T: Subcutaneous low dose arabinosylcytosine and oral idarubicin in high risk adult acute myelogenous leukemia. Hematol Oncol 11: 73–80 (1993)
10. Legha SS; Benjamim RS; Mackay B; Ewer M; Walace S; Valdivieso M; Rasmussen SL; Blumenschein GR; Freireich EJ: Reduction of doxorubicin cardiotoxicity by prolonged continuous intravenous infusion. Ann Intern Med 96: 133–139 (1982)
11. Lipshultz SE; Colan SD; Gelber RD; Perez-Atayde AR; Sallan SE; Sanders SP: Late cardiac effects of doxorubicin therapy for acute lymphoblastic leukemia in childhood. N Engl J Med 324: 808–815 (1991)
12. Reid JM; Pendergrass TW; Krailo MD; Hammond GD; Ames MM: Plasma pharmacokinetics and cerebrospinal fluid concentrations of idarubicin and idarubicinol in pediatric leukemia patients: a Childrens Cancer Study Group report. Cancer Res 50: 6525–6528 (1990)
13. Robert J: Clinical pharmacokinetics of idarubicin. Clin Pharmacokinet 24: 275–28 (1993)
14. Sperber AD; Cantor AA; Biran H; Keynan A: Selective right ventricular dysfunction following doxorubicin therapy. Isr J Med Sci 23: 896–899 (1987)
15. Testi AM; Moleti ML; Giona F; Iori AP; Meloni G; Miniero R; Pigna M; Amadori S; Mandelli F: Treatment of primary refractory or relapsed acute lymphoblastic leukemia (ALL) in children. Ann Oncol 3: 765–767 (1992)
16. Vogler WR; Velez-Garcia E; Weiner RS; Flaum MA; Bartolucci AA; Omura GA; Gerber MC; Banks PL: A phase III trial comparing idarubicin and daunorubicin in combination with cytarabine in acute myelogenous leukemia. J Clin Oncol 10: 1103–1111 (1992)
17. VonHoff DD; Rozencweig M; Layard M; Slavik M; Muggia FM: Daunomycin-induced cardiotoxicity in children and adults. A review of 110 cases. Am J Med 62: 200–208 (1977)
18. Zanette L; Zuchetti M; Freshi A; Eranti D; Tirelli U; D`Incalci M: Pharmacokinetics of 4-demethoxydaunorubicin in cancer patients. Cancer Chemother Pharmacol 25: 445–448 (1990)

Acute Leukemias V
Experimental Approaches
and Management of Refractory Diseases
Hiddemann et al. (Eds.)

Leukemia-Lymphoma in Children with Primary Nodal Peripheral and Mediastinal Involvement

M. Matysiak and M. Ochocka

Introduction

Non-Hodgkin Lymphoma (NHL), which is the third most common malignant disease in children, after leukemia and CNS tumors, is distinguished by many primary sites, different histologic subtypes and clinical stages.

The clinical findings at diagnosis are determined by the primary tumor site.

In an SJCRH review of 338 patients [1] the most frequent sites of involvement were the abdomen (31,4%), the mediastinum (26%) and the head and neck region, including Waldeyer's ring and /or cervical lymph nodes (29%). Peripherial lymph nodes outside the neck were the primary tumor site in only 6,5% of cases.

Nodal lymphomas constitute a group of lymphomas with primary sites either in peripherial nodes or the mediastinum.There are primary nodal lymphomas of the abdomen, but they should be considered as a part of the intraabdominal group of NHL (at the time they are diagnosed, the extranodal extension is such that determining a primary site is difficult, if not impossible) [2].

The bone marrow is frequently involved at diagnosis in children with NHL.

In 1976 , when the philosophy of treatment for leukemia-lymphoma had not yet evolved completely, Wollner et al. [2,3] proposed staging system for NHL, where the bone marrow involvement (Stage IV), can be subclassified as follows: Stage IV A – when the bone marrow or bone marrow sites contain clumps of extrinsic cells but less than 25% and Stage IV B – when the bone marrow or different bone marrow sites contain 25% or more blasts (leukemia-lymphoma syndrome).

While laboratory and clinical studies have demonstrated the close relationship between childhood NHL and acute lymphoblastic leukemia (ALL) , the criteria utilized to distinguish between these two categories of disease have been arbitrary and not uniformly accepted.

The distinction between NHL and ALL is currently based on the degree of infiltration of the bone marrow.

Children who have more than 25% infiltration of their marrow with blasts are considered to have ALL, while those with a bulky primary tumor and between 5 and 25% blast cells in the marrow are considered to have Stage IV NHL.

In our series of 100 pediatric patients with NHL studied from 1977–1992, 34 patients had nodal lymphomas. Five of these (5%) had peripherial nodal lymphomas and 29 (29%) had mediastinal nodal disease. Bone marrow involvement were observed in 20 patients (58,8%) with nodal lymphomas.

Five children had Stage IV A disease and 15 patients had Stage IV B using the Wollner's subclassification. This 15 children with leukemia-lymphoma syndrom will be presented in this paper.

Material and Methods

15 children with leukemia-lymphoma syndrom were treated from 1977 to 1992. There were 2

Department of Pediatric Hematology Warsaw University Medical School Warsaw, Poland

female patients and 13 male patients, aged from 3 to 16 years. The median age for the group was 9 years.

Five children lived in the country and 10 lived in the town.

In all patients except 2 children, diagnosis was obtained by a lymph node biopsy. In two boys, because of mass causing midairway obstruction, shortness of breath and evidence of superior vena cava obstruction, the diagnosis of NHL, was obtained by cytologic examination of pleural fluid.

All slides were reviewed using the Kiel classification.There were 10 children with NB-NHL and 3 patients with B-NHL among this group. In two cases, because of technical difficulties, the lymphoma could not be classified.

The clinical staging was done according to the criteria of Wollner [2,3].

Eight children were treated with the modified LSA2L2 protocol [3,4,5], six patients with BFM protocol [6,7] and one child with COAMP protocol [4,8].

Result

Symptoms at diagnosis were nonspecific (Table 1). The duration of symptoms before diagnosis ranged from 14 to 90 days, with a median of 36 days.

12 children (80%) had enlarged lymph nodes only above the diaphragm.

Mediastinal adenopathy was found in 13 children (86,6%).

In 3 children (20%) the disease was disseminated above and below the diaphragm.

Hepatosplenomegaly was presented in 13 patients (86,6%). One child had renal involvement.

Table 1. Symptoms at diagnosis

Symptom	No.of patients	% of total
Weakness	13	86,6
Loss of appetite	10	66,6
Fever	9	60,0
Weight loss	8	53,3
Large nodes	8	53,3
Cough	7	46,7
Difficult breathing	7	46,7
Pain	2	13,3
Nausea	1	6,6

Hematologic data at diagnosis are shown in Table 2.

13 children (86,6%) among 15 patients with leukemia-lymphoma syndrom achieved complete remission (CR). There were 2 children with B-NHL (from 3 children with B-NHL) and 9 patients with NB-NHL (from 10 patients with NB-NHL).

Two children did not respond to the therapy and died without I CR.

Six children relapsed . Three of them relapsed in first 6 months of treatment. Three relapses occured later (after 12 month of treatment).

All this children died during relapse due to initial tumor failure and infections (bacterial and fungial sepsis).

There were 6 children treated with LSA2L2, and 2 treated with BFM protocol among all died patients.

Seven children are still alive (2 from LSA2L2 group, 4 from BFM patients and 1 treated with COAMP).

We observed anemia, leukopenia and thrombocytopenia during therapy,which were dangerous for children and remained from 7 till 25 days.

Fever developed from cytosine arabinoside, and fever from unknown origin, bacterial pneumonia and sepsis were also observed.

No late toxic effects has been observed .

The event-free survival rate (EFS) for all 15 patients with leukemia-lymphoma syndrom is 44,4%.

Figure 1 shows the event-free survival rate of patients with leukemia-lymphoma syndrom and with primary nodal peripherial and mediastinal involvement.

Table 2. Hematologic data at diagnosis

Hemoglobin level (g/dl)	
Median	11,35
Low	6,6
High	15,6
Leukocyte count ($10^3/mm^3$)	
Median	35,64
Low	2,4
High	112,0
Platelet count ($10^3/mm^3$)	
Median	151,4
Low	19,0
High	275,0

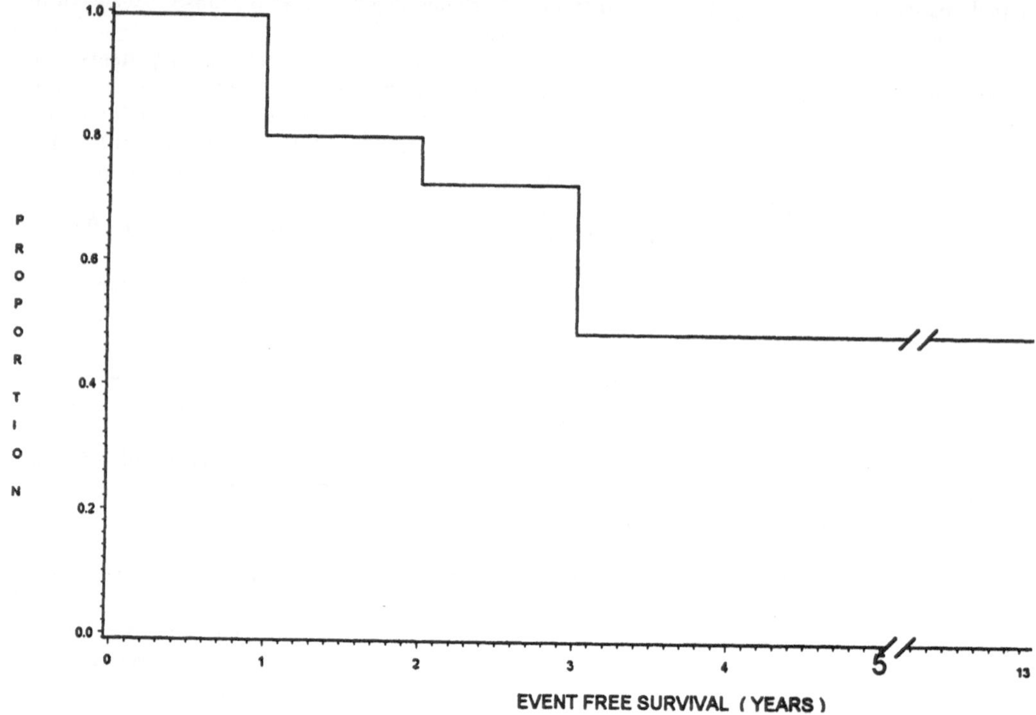

Fig. 1. Event free survival rate of patients with leukemia-lymphoma syndrom and with primary nodal peripheral and mediastinal involvement

Discussion

In discussing the reported results first of all we would like to point that our group has been too small to allow us to make a general conclusions. We have only confirmed in our patients, tendency observed by other authors on a big group of patients.

Primary nodal lymphoma usually is diagnosed when advanced, because the symptoms are usually unspecified. Sometimes the antibiotic therapy can cause a clinical response and therefore delay diagnosis and effective treatment. Duration of symptoms before diagnosis is usually long (Wollner – median 30 days [2], in our group median 36 days) what have a great influence on worse prognosis. Although Wollner and others [2] achieved EFS = 75% our results and results achived by the Polish Children's Leukemia / Lymphoma Study Group [4,5,9] had not been so successful, and were very similar to those reported by Murphy in 1989 [1].

Some authors suggest that dose intensity of chemotherapy influenced survival by promoting rapid and more complete cell kill, helping prevent the emergence of resistant cells [1].

We fully share this point of view.

The arbitrary distinction between leukemia and lymphoma,based on whether there is more or less than 25% involvement of the marrow, has not generally been found to be of prognostic significance[10].

On the other side Sullivan on behalf of POG [11] reported that patients with greater than 25% blast cells in the marrow and associated lymphomatous masses did appear to have a worse prognosis. For many patients, marrow involvement may simply represent further clinical evolution of lymphoma.

In our experience,the children with stage IV A peripherial nodal lymphoma, had the same bad prognosis, as the patients in stage IV B (unpublished data). Among 5 children with stage IV A peripherial nodal lymphoma, we observed 5 complete remissions followed by 4 lethal relapses.

In our opinion the distinction between stage IV A and IV B is out of prognostic significance, because of bad prognosis in both of them.

The distinction between NHL and ALL is at best ill-defined, and there is little evidence that within a single histologic or immunologic subgroup, patients with leukemia and lymphoma require dissimilar therapies [12]. The experience of BFM group reflect this view.

Conclusions

1. Bone marrow involvement either as clumps of extrinsic cells, but less then 25% of blasts or as leukemia-lymphoma syndrom (25% or more blasts) seems to have the same negative prognostic significance.
2. The duration of symptoms before diagnosis was extended (median 96 days) often because of antibiotic therapy.
3. T-cell lymphomas are the most common peripherial NHL.
4. Hepatosplenomegaly usually goes together with peripheral nodal lymphoma.

References

1. Murphy SB. et al.; Non-Hodgkin's lymphomas of childhood; an analysis of the histology, staging, and response to treatment of 338 cases at a single institution. J. Clin. Oncol. 1989, 7; 186
2. Wollner N, Exelby P. Lindsley KL, et al; Primary peripherial nodal lymphoma in children. Cancer, 1993, 71, 11, 3670.
3. Wollner N, Burchenal JH, Lieberman PH, et al: Non-Hodgkin's lymphoma in children; a comparative study of two modalities of therapy. Cancer, 1976, 37; 123
4. Boguslawska-Jaworska J, Rodziewicz B, Kazanowska B et al; Progress in treatment of advanced Non-Hodgkin's lymphoma in children-report on behalf of the Polish Children's Leukemia/Lymphoma Study Group.; Haematology and Blood Transfusion, 1987, vol.31; 39
5. Boguslawska-Jaworska J, Koefficielniak E, Sroczyñska M, et al: Evaluation of the LSA2L2 protocol for treatment of childhood Non-Hodgkin's lymphoma. Amer. J. Pediat. Hematol/Oncol., 1984, 6, 4: 363 [235]
6. Müller-Weihrich S, Beck J, Henze G, Jobke A. et al.: BFM-Studie 1981/83 zur Behandlung hochmaligner Non-Hodgkin-Lymphome bei Kindern: Ergebnisse einer nach histologisch-immunologischem Typ und Ausbreitungsstadium stratefizierten Therapie. Klin. Pädiat., 1984, 196: 135
7. Müller-Weihrich S, Henze G ,Odenwald W i wsp: BFM trials for childhood non-Hodgkin's lymphomas, in Cavalli F, Bonadonna G, Rosenswieg M: Malignant lymphomas and Hodgkin's disease: Experimental and therapeutic advances, Boston, Martinus Nijhoff, 1985: 633
8. Anderson JR, Jenkin R, Wilson JF, et al.: Long-term follow-up of patients treated with COMP or LSA2L2 therapy for childhood non-Hodgkin's lymphoma: A report of CCG-551 from the Childrens Cancer Group. J. Clin. Oncol. 1993, 11, 6; 1024
9. Boguslawska-Jaworska J, Kazanowska B, Rodziewicz-Magott B. et al.; Treatment results of Non-Hodgkin's lymphoma in the experience of the Polish Children's Leukemia/Lymphoma Study Group. Post. Med. Klin. Doœw. 1992, 1, supl.; 59
10. Bernard A, Boumsell L, Patte C. et al.: Leukemia versus lymphoma in children; a worthless question? Med. Pediatr. Oncol., 1986, 14; 148
11. Sullivan MP, Boyett J, Pullen J: Pediatric Oncology Group experience with modified LSA2L2 therapy in 107 children with Non-Hodgkin's lymphoma (Burkitt's lymphoma excluded). Cancer, 1985, 55; 323

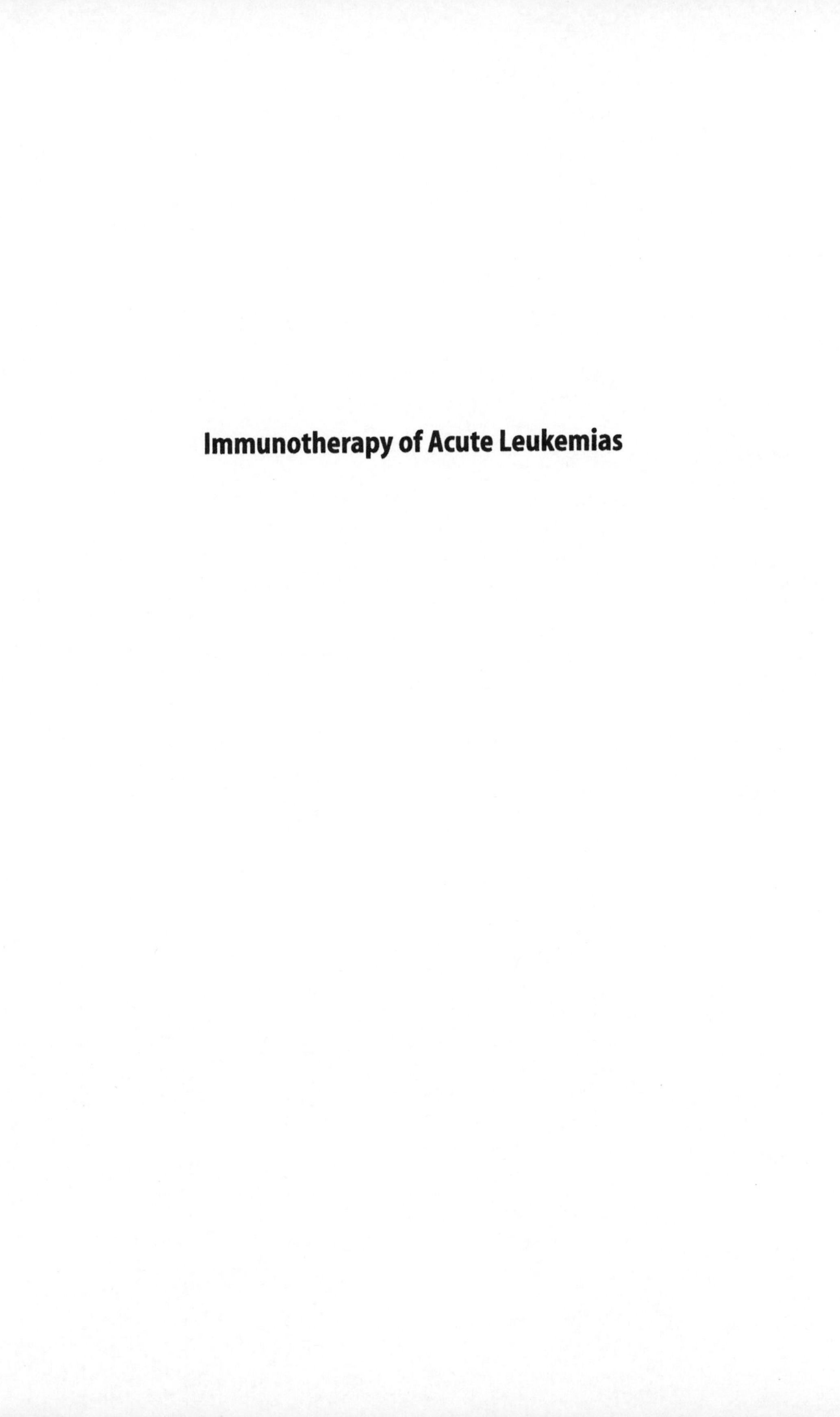

Immunotherapy of Acute Leukemias

Acute Leukemias V
Experimental Approaches
and Management of Refractory Diseases
Hiddemann et al. (Eds.)

Induction of Immunity Against Leukemia

S. de Vos[1], D. B. Kohn[2], W. H. McBride[3], and H. P. Koeffler[1]

Abstract. Great strides have been made in the chemotherapeutic treatment of acute lymphocytic leukemia (ALL) and moderate success has been made in treatment of acute myelogenous leukemia (AML). At this time, progress using chemotherapy has plateaued. Novel approaches to these diseases are required. Recent experiments have shown that several poorly immunogenic solid tumors can be recognized by MHC-class I restricted $CD8^+$ cytotoxic T lymphocytes (CTL) if the tumors are engineered by genetransfer to produce one of several cytokines, including IL-2, IL-4, IL-6, IL-7, GM-CSF, TNF-α, IFN-α and -γ, or B7/BB1. The local secretion of lymphokines, critical for CTL activation, appears to bypass a deficient helper T-cell arm of the immune system. In addition, secretion of cytokines by the tumor cells stimulates the host immune system to identify and kill the untransduced parental cells upon subsequent reimplantation; and even of potential more importance, a rejection of established cancer can occur by inducing a systemic anticancer immune response by vaccination with cytokine transduced tumor cells. We studied two different murine myeloid leukemia models using WEHI3 and C1498 cell lines, transduced with a retroviral vector coding for human IL-7 (JZEN hIL/tk neo), resulting in cytokine production up to 13 ng/10^6 cells/24 hrs. NIH-3T3-fibroblasts, transduced with a vector coding for human IL-2 (G1Na CV hIL-2), producing up to 21 ng/10^6 cells/24 hrs, mixed with parental WEHI3 leukemia were used for vaccination-studies as well. Vaccination with IL-7 producing WEHI3 clones (weekly s.c. injections of 106 cells over a period of one month) resulted in a 43% survival of mice, subsequently challenged with a lethal dose of parental leukemic cells (5]104 i.v.). Vaccination with a mixture of IL-2 producing NIH-3T3-fibroblasts and parental WEHI3 cells resulted in a systemic protection of 60% of lethally challenged mice. The same experiments performed with the C1498-model showed a strong inherent immunogenicity of irradiated parental cells, as 4 out of 5 mice survived in this group. Surprisingly, all mice died in the group vaccinated with an IL-7 producing subclone. This illustrates that the process of selecting a high-cytokine producing subclone can result in clones that no longer represent the antigenic spectrum of the parental cells.

Taken together, we show that induction of a specific anti-leukemia immune response may be effective treatment for AML, especially when the tumor burden is low.

Introduction

The central hypothesis underlying specific anticancer immunotherapy is that tumor cells express antigenic determinants, not expressed on their counterpart normal adult cells. Those antigenic determinants must be immunogenic in the host for an effective attack by the immune system [1–2].

[1] Division of Hematology/Oncology, Cedars-Sinai Medical Center, UCLA, Los Angeles, CA
[2] Children's Hospital, Los Angeles, CA
[3] Department of Radiation Oncology, UCLA, Los Angeles, CA

Cancer results from a series of mutational events within a cell that can result in the production of genetically altered proteins [3]. Peptides from these mutated proteins may bind to major histocompatibility complex (MHC) class I molecules and in this context may serve as targets for specific cytotoxic T cells (CTL) [45]. Tumor-associated antigens that provoke tumor rejection in the host have been demonstrated in experimental, chemically or viraly induced tumors. But in most experimental, spontaneous tumor systems (resembling the situation found in patients), tumor-associated antigens usually can not be detected. This resulted in speculations that either the host immune system fails to recognize neoplastic cells, or that neoplastic growth can thrive in the presence of an inefficient host immune response.

Recent experiments have shown that several poorly immunogenic solid tumors can be recognized by MHC-class restricted $CD8^+$ CTL, if the tumors are engineered to secrete one of several cytokines, including IL-2 [5–9], IL-4 [10–12], IL-6 [13], IL-7[14–15], GMCSF [16], TNF-α [17–18] and-γ [19–20], or B7/BB1 [21]. The mechanisms involved are bypassing a deficient helper T-cell arm of the immune system by local secretion of lymphokines, critical for CTL-activation, upregulation of MHC-molecules, second signal induction for CTL-activation, and enhancement of antigen-presentation by host antigen presenting cells (APC). In addition, secretion of cytokines by the tumor cells stimulated the host immune system to identify and kill the untransduced parental cells upon reimplantation; and even more, a rejection of established cancer can occur by inducing a systemic anticancer immune response by vaccination with cytokine-transduced tumor cells [12].

Anecdotal evidence that the immune system may help to eradicate leukemia is provided by occasional reports of improved survival following postinduction immunization with unspecific immunostimulators [22–24], although convincing evidence is still lacking. The graft versus leukemia (GvL) phenomenon after allogeneic BMT is the most striking evidence of a role of the immune system in controlling leukemia [25–26]. Alloreactive T-cells are not the only mediators of the GvL-effect; GvHD and GvL may, therefore, be separable [27]. Several studies have shown that lymphokine activated killer cells (LAK) from patients with acute leukemia lyse autologous blast cells [28–32]. Murine models have shown IL-2 to be effective in preventing relapse after BMT in a B-cell leukemia (BCL1)[33]; combined IL-1/IL-2 therapy inhibited metastatic tumor growth of Friend erythroleukemia cells (FLC)[34]; continuous coadministration of M-CSF and IL-2 protected mice against a lethal dose of T-cell leukemic cells (EL4)[35]; IFN- gene transfer into Friend erythroleukemia cells (FLC) abrogated tumorigenicity and injections of those IFN-α producing cells were effective in inhibiting tumor growth in mice with established metastatic tumors [36].

Among the various cytokines tested, IL-2 and IL-7 elicited antitumor effects primarily through T-cell involvement. IL-7 was originally described as a bone marrow stromal cell-derived growth-factor of pre–B-cells [37]. It was subsequently found also to function as a growth factor for thymocytes [38–39] and mature $CD4^+$ and $CD8^+$ T-cells [40–41] and to stimulate resting T-cells to proliferate both directly and through an IL-2 dependent pathway [40–45]. This latter activity can be attributed to IL-7 induced expression of IL-2 receptors. IL-7 has also been shown to help in the generation of CTL [38,46–48] and lymphokine activated killer (LAK) cells [47,49–50]. IL-2 is a growth-factor for CTL [51], helper T-cells [52], natural killer (NK)cells [53] and LAKcells [54], thereby stimulating specific as nonspecific immune response mechanisms. In addition it induces the secretion of secondary cytokines by IL-2-responsive cells.

Most of the described murine models used virally or chemically induced leukemias, which are therefore already immunogenic when simply irradiated [16]. We have developed a model system to study this tumor-vaccination approach using non-immunogenic, spontaneous murine WEHI3 leukemia cells.

Material and Methods

Mice. Pathogen-free female BALB/c and C57 B1/6 mice, 10–14 weeks old, were obtained from Harlan-Sprague Dawley (Indianapolis, IN).

Leukemia lines. WEHI3: a rapidly fatal acute myelomonocytic leukemia, spontaneously developed and of Balb/c origin, cells are non-immunogenic and express class I MHC molecules [55]. C1498: acute myeloblastic leukemia of C57B1/6 origin [56]. Both lines were obtained from ATCC and were maintained in IMDM/10% fetal calf serum (FCS). Cells were washed 3 times in PBS before injected into mice.

Retroviral vectors. Vectors used for transduction were the LN-based G1Nab CVhIL-2 (titer range 1 to 5×10^4 cfu/ml) vector in which the neoR selectable marker was driven by the Moloney murine leukemia virus long terminal repeat (LTR), and the human IL-2 cDNA driven by the cytomegalovirus (CV) early enhancer/promoter. The vector was provided as frozen supernatant from Genetic Therapy, Inc. (Gaithersburg, MD). The JZEN hIL-7/tk neo (titer range 1 to 10×10^6 cfu/ml) was constructed with the neoR gene driven by the thymidine kinase promoter, and the hIL-7 cDNA under the transcriptional control of the myeloproliferative sarcoma virus LTR (Graeme J. Dougherty, Terry Fox Lab., Vancouver, Canada)[23]. This construct was packaged in the GP + env AM 12 amphotrophic cell line and subcloned to produce high-titer stocks [57] (Fig. 1).

Gene transfer. About $1–2 \times 10^6$ exponentially growing leukemic target cells were grown in 10 ml supernatant of high titer retroviral-packaging cell lines in the presence of 4–8 µg/ml polybrene for 2–18 hrs. Following selection in cultures containing the neomycin-analog G418 (0.5–1.0 mg/ml bioactive G418) for 1–2 weeks, the surviving successfully transduced cells were subcloned by methylcellulose soft-gel-culture. Individual colonies were plucked and expanded in liquid culture. Using ELISA-assays (hIL-2- and hIL-7-Quantikine, R+D Systems) to measure the protein expression, high/low-cytokine producing clones were identified, expanded and viably frozen.

Vaccination and leukemia challenge. Either cytokine-producing leukemic cells or a mixture of cytokine-producing NIH-3T3-fibroblasts with unaltered parental leukemic cells were used for immunization. After irradiation (WEHI3: 1,000 rad; C1498: 3,000 rad; NIH-3T3-fibroblasts: 10,000 rad) to inhibit in vivo growth while preserving cytokine-production, the vaccine-preparation was injected s.c. every 7 days for up to 4 weeks. One week later, mice were challenged s.c. or i.v. with non-transduced, parental leukemic cells. Mice were followed up for local tumor-growth, development of leukemia and survival.

Results

Murine leukemia models. Survival of mice injected with increasing doses of syngeneic leukemia cells (WEHI3, C1498) is shown in Table 1.

Leukemia vaccines. The WEHI3 and C1498 leukemia lines were transduced with either the JZEN hIL-7/tk neo or only the neoR-encoding control retroviral vectors. Table 2 shows the cytokine production of 10^6 cells/24hrs from stably transduced subclones. In addition, a subclone of NIH-3T3-fibroblasts, transduced with the G1Na CVhIL-2 retroviral vector is shown.

Characterization of these subclones showed no difference in either morphologies or in vitro growth-rates in comparison to the parental cells. The hIL-7 production was stable over months. Following irradiation, the cytokine-production continued for up to a week at a level of 2/3 of the non-irradiated cells. These clones were used for further in vivo experiments.

In vivo growth of hIL-7 transduced leukemia clones compared to the parental cell line. As

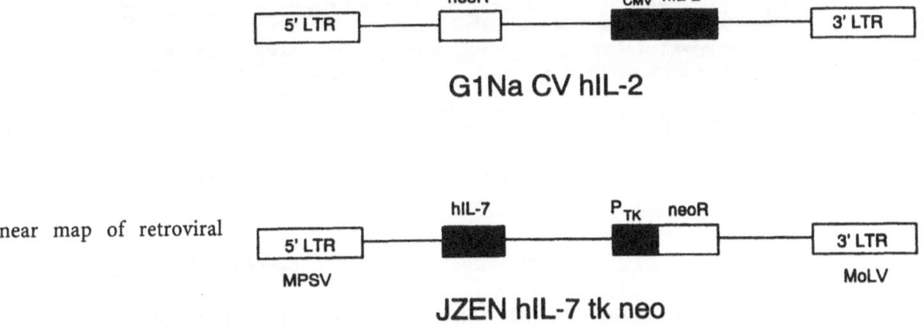

Fig. 1. Linear map of retroviral vectors

Table 1. Leukemogenicity of WEHI3- and C1498-cell lines in syngeneic hosts

number of i.v. injected Cells/mouse	survival after leukemia cell injection (days)	
	C57BI6–C1498	Balb/c–WEHI3
10^7	14	11
10^6	20	16
10^5	22	20
10^4	27(50% survival)	27(50% survival)
10^3	100% survival	100% survival
10^2	100% survival	100% survival

The data represent the medium survival in days of 4 mice per dose. Shown are the Balb/c derived WEHI3 leukemia and the C1498 derived C1498 leukemia

Table 2. Subclones genetically engineered to produce hIL-2 or hIL-7

transduced cell line	retroviral vector	subclone⁺	cytokine-production of 10^6 cells//24 hrs
C1498	JZEN hIL-7	#7	9870 pg
		#15	13730 pg
WEHI3	JZEN hIL-7	#23	2680 pg
		#2	8250 pg
		polyclonal	7860 pg
NIH-3T3	G1Na CV IL-2	#5	21,000 pg

shown in Figure 2 for the WEHI3- and in Figure 3 for the C1498-models, no statistically significant differences could be observed in the survival times of mice injected with unirradiated hIL-7 transduced subclones in comparison to unaltered parental cells.

No growth difference could be observed, when the same cell preparations were injected s.c. (1×10^6)(data not shown).

Vaccination studies. Mice were vaccinated with 4 s.c. injections ($1-5 \times 10^6$ cells; one injection

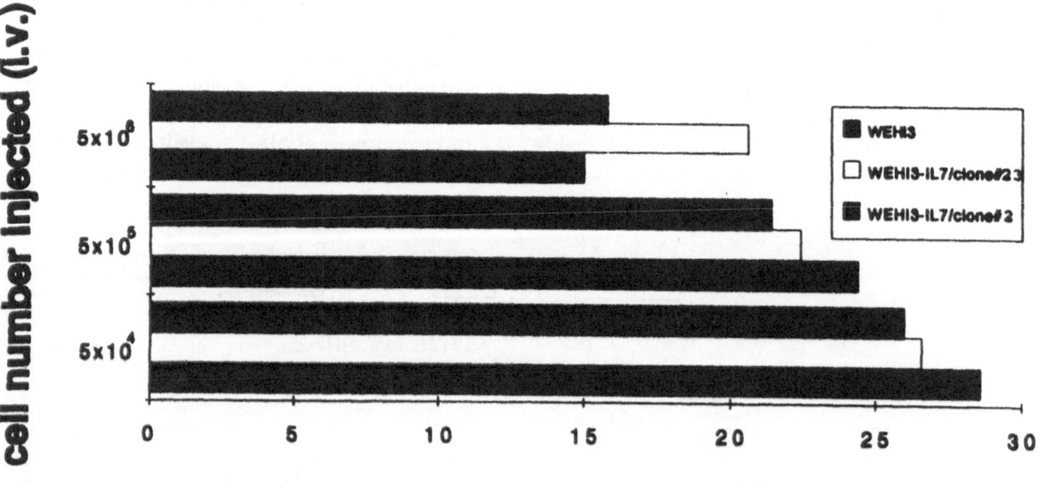

Fig. 2. Survival of Balb/c mice i.v.-injected with WEHI3-leukemia or IL-7 producing subclones

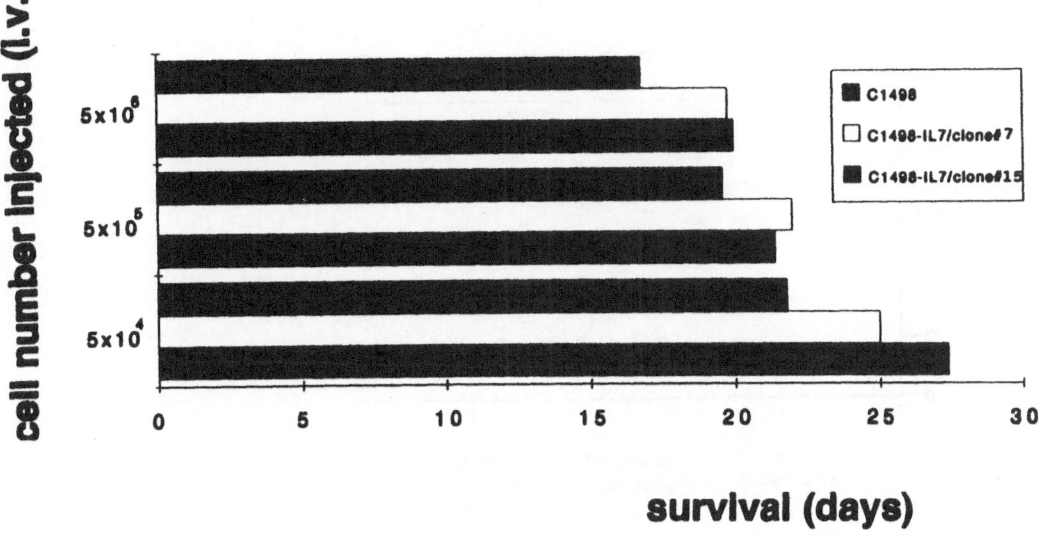

Fig. 3. Survival of C57Bl/6 mice i.v.-injected with C1498-leukemia or IL-7 producing subclones

weekly) of a panel of different vaccine-preparations. Subsequently, the mice were challenged with s.c.-injections ($2.5 \times 10^5 - 10^6$, in a volume of 100 μl) or i.v.-injections (5×10^4, in a volume of 300 μl) of the parental cell line.

Figure 4 confirms that WEHI3 is a non-immunogenic cell line. Balb/c mice vaccinated with high-IL-7-producing WEHI3 cells (clone #23 and the polyclonal preparation) showed systemic protection and rejected an i.v. challenge

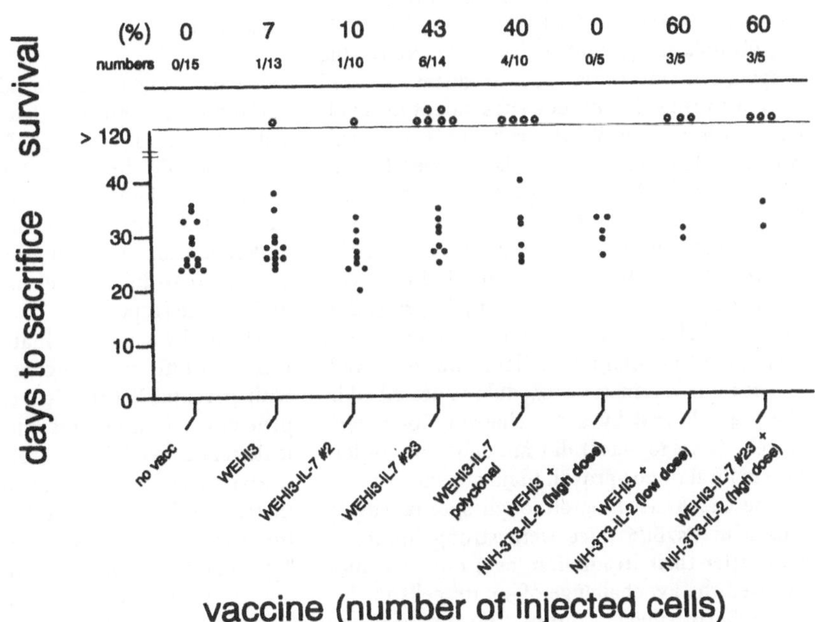

Fig. 4. Survival of vaccinated and i.v.-challenged Balb/c mice.10^6 leukemic cells and 5×10^5 (low dose) or 5×10^6 (high dose) IL-2 producing fibroblasts were used in the vaccine-preparation

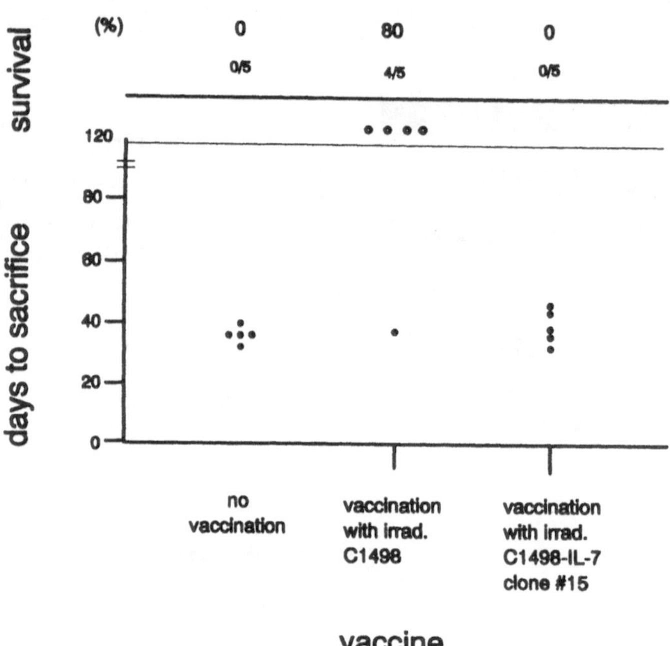

Fig. 5. Survival of vaccinated and i.v.-challenged C57Bl/6 mice

with 5×10^4 parental WEHI3 cells (43% and 40% survival, respectively). Vaccination with a low-IL-7-producing WEHI3 clone (clone #2) showed no protection.

When vaccinated with a mixture of 10^6 parental WEHI3 cells and IL-2 producing NIH-3T3-fibroblasts (5×10^5 or 5×10^6), only the preparation with 5×10^5 IL-2-producers showed systemic protection upon a subsequent i.v. challenge with parental WEHI3 cells (60% survival); with a 10-fold higher local IL-2 "dose" (5×10^6 IL-2-producing cells) this protective effect was lost again.

When mixing (5×10^6) IL-2-producing NIH-3T3 cells (no protection when used alone) with 10^6 IL-7-producing WEHI3 cells (43% protection when used alone) for vaccination, an increase in survival to 60% after i.v. challenge was observed.

The same vaccination-schedule as described in Figure 4 followed by a s.c. challenge of parental cells ($2.5 \times 10^5 - 10^6$) did not show any difference in local tumor-growth (data not shown).

The C1498 cell line, although spontaneously arosen in C57Bl/6 mice were strong immunogenic after their irradiation, as 4 out of 5 mice survived the i.v. challenge of 5×10^4 cells in this group. Surprisingly, 4 out of 5 mice died in the group vaccinated with the hIL-7 producing subclone (Fig. 5). This illustrates that the process of selecting a high cytokine producing subclone can result in a clone that no longer represents the antigenic spectrum of the parental cells.

Discussion

We have shown that transduction of the non-immunogenic murine leukemia line WEHI3 with the gene for human IL-7 elicits a systemic anti-leukemic immune response and causes rejection of leukemia in vaccinated syngeneic hosts. This effect was dose-dependent; only leukemic cells expressing high levels of IL-7, as compared to lower-level producers, stimulated an immune response.

Using the same vaccination approach with a mixture of hIL-2 producing NIH-3T3-fibroblasts with parental WEHI3 leukemic cells, we saw a protective immune-response against WEHI3 leukemia as well. The observation that the protective vaccination-effect vanishes with a 10-fold increase of local IL-2 production at the vaccination site, is in accord with previous reports of an "optimal dose" of local IL-2 production with no protective effect below or above this "window"[58].

Although it was possible to vaccinate successfully with irradiated IL-7 producing leukemia cells, no differences in development of leukemia and survival-times could be detected when these IL-7-producers were i.v. injected and compared to the unaltered parental leukemia. As has been seen in other leukemia models [59], the leukemia most likely develops too rapidly to give any emerging immune response time to prevent leukemia outgrowth.

We observed protective effects of our vaccination-protocol in i.v. - but not in s.c. - challenged mice. The reason is most likely, that 2.5×10^5 cells s.c. are too large of a tumor-load to detect an immune response in our model.

The C1498/C57Bl/6 leukemia model has not proven to be suitable for our vaccination studies because of strong inherent immunogenicity of irradiated cells. In addition, this model illustrates the hazard of loosing the antigenic heterogenicity when subcloning steps are included in the preparation of the vaccine. Prior studies have noted that it was not uncommon for a single spontaneous tumor to elicit heterogeneity in regard to antigen-expression or sensitivity to immune effector mechanisms [60-61]. Use of "polyclonal" vaccine-preparations and a combination of induction of different effector mechanisms may eventually overcome these difficulties. We are now examining various immunological parameters of our model, as well as studying B7/BB1- and mGM-CSF-vaccines as well as different vaccine combinations.

References

1. Marx J. Cancer vaccines show promise at last news. Science 244: 813-815, (1989)
2. Mathe G. Active immunotherapy. Adv.Cancer Res 14: 136, (1971)
3. Townsend ARM, Rothbard J, Gotch FM, Bahadur G, Wraith D, McMichael AD. The epitopes of influenza nucleoprotein recognized by cytotoxic T lymphocytes can be defined with short synthetic peptides. Cell 44: 959-968, (1986)
4. Fearon ER, Vogelstein BV. A genetic model for colorectal tumorigenesis. Cell 61: 759-767, (1990)
5. Lurquin, Van Pel A, Mariame B, De Plaen E, Szikora JP, Janssens C, Reddehase MJ, Lejeune J, Boon T. Cell 58: 293-303, (1989)
6. Fearon ER, Pardoll DM, Itaya T, Golumbek P, Levitsky JW, Simons H, Karasuyama H, Vogelstein B, and Frost P. Interleukin2 production by tumor cell bypasses T helper function in the generation on an antitumor response. Cell 60: 397-403, (1990)
7. Gansbacher B, Zier K, Daniels B, Cronin K, and Gilboa E. Interleukin 2 gene transfere into tumor cells abrogates tumorigenicity and induces protective immunity. J. Exp. Med. 172: 1217-1224, (1990)
8. Russel SJ, Flemming, Eccles SA, Johnson C, Collins MKL. Transfere and expression of the human IL-2 gene in a transplantable rat sarcoma. Cellular Immunity and Immunotherapy of Cancer, pp275-278, WileyLiss, Inc., (1990)
9. Bubenik J, Simova J, and Jandlova T. Immunotherapy of cancer using local administration of lymphoid cells transformed by cDNA and constitutively producing IL-2. Immunol Lett. 23: 287-292, (1990)
10. Tepper RI, Pattengale PK, and Leder P. Murine interleukin-4 displays potent antitumor activity in vivo. Cell 57: 503-512, (1989)
11. Li W, Diamantstein T, and Blankenstein TH. Lack of tumorigenicity of interleukine 4 autocrine growing cells seems related to the antitumor function of IL-4. Mol. Immunol. 27: 1331-1337, (1990)
12. Golumbek PT, Lazenby AJ, Levitzky HI, Jaffee LM, Karasuyama H, Baker M, Pardoll DM. Treatment of established renal cancer by tumor cells engineered to secrete interleukin4. Science 25: 713-716, (1991)
13. McBride WH, Thacker JD, Comora SH, and Dougherty GJ. Inhibitory effect of locally produced IL-6 on tumor growth in vivo. Abstr., International conference on gene therapy of cancer, San Diego, (1992)
14. McBride WH, Thacker JD, Comora S, Economou JS, Kelley D, Hogge D, Dubinett SM, and Dougherty GJ. Genetic Modification of a murine fibrosarcoma to produce Interleukin 7 stimulates host cell infiltration and tumor immunity. Canc. Res. 52: 3913-937, (1992)
15. Hock H, Dorsch M, Diamantstein T, Blankenstein T. Interleukin 7 induces $CD4^+$ T cell-dependent tumor rejection. J. Exp. Med. 174: 1291, (1991)
16. Dranoff G, Jaffee E, Lazenby A, Golumbek P, Levitsky H, Brose K, Jackson V, Hamada H, Pardoll D, Mulligan R.C. Vaccination with irradiated tumor cells engineered to secrete murine granulocyte-macrophage colony-stimulating factor stimulates potent, specific, and long-lasting antitumor immunity. Proc Natl Acad Sci USA 90: 3539, (1993)
17. Blankenstein T, Qin Z, Uberla K, Muller W, Rosen H, Volk HD, and Diamantstein T. Tumor suppression after tumor cell-targeted tumor necrosis factor alpha gene transfere. J. Exp. Med. 173: 1047-1052, (1991)
18. Asher AL, Mule JJ, Kasid A, Restifo NP, Salo JC, Reichert CM, Jaffe G, Fendy B, Kriegler M, and Rosenberg SA. Evidence for a paracrine immune effect of tumor necrosis factor against tumors. J. Immunol. 146: 3227-3234, (1991)
19. Gansbacher B, Bannererij R, Daniels B, Zier K, Cronin K, and Gilboa E. Retroviral vector-mediated interferon-gamma gene-transfere into tumor cells generates potent and long lasting antitumor immunity. J. Exp. Cancer Res. Med. 50: 7820-7825, (1990)
20. Watanabe Y, Kuribayashi K, Miyatake S, Nishihara K, Nakayama E, Taniyama T, and Sakata T.

Exogenous expression of mouse IFN gamma cDNA in mouse neuroblastoma 1300 cells results in reduced tumorigenicity by augmented anti-tumor immunity. Proc. Natl. Acad. Sci. USA, 86: 9456–9460, (1989)
21. Townsend SE, Allison JP: Tumor rejection after direct constimulation of CD8$^+$ T cells by B7-transfected melanoma cells. Science 259: 368–370, (1993)
22. Wittaker JA. Annotation: Immunotherpay in the treament of acute leukemia. Br. J Haematol 45: 859–65, (1980)
23. Reizenstein P. Adjuvant immunotherapy with BCG of acute myeloid leukemia: a 15-year followup. Br J Haematol 75: 288–99, (1990)
24. la Cour Petersen E, Hokland P, Ellegaard J. Adjuvant stimulation with Corynbacterium parvum during maintenance chemotherapy of acute leukemia. Cancer Immunol Immunother 16: 88–92, (1983)
25. Morstyn G, Campbell L, Souza LM, Alton NK, Keech J, Green M, Sheridan W, Metcalf D, Fox R: Effect of granulocyte colony stimulating factor on neutropenia induced by cytotoxic chenotherpay. Lancet 1: 667, (1988)
26. Trillet-Lenoir V, Green J, Manegold C, Von Pawel J, Gatzemeier U, Lebeau B, Depierre A, Johnson P, Decoster G, Tomita D, Ewen C: Recombinant granulocyte colony stimulating factor reduces the infectious complications of cytotoxic chemotherpay. Eur J Cancer 29A: 319, (1993)
27. Brenner MK, and Heslop HE: Immunotherpay of leukemia. Leukemia 6: 76–79, (1992)
28. Lotzova E, Savary Ca, Herberman RB. Induction of NK cell activity against fresh human leukemia in culture with interleukin 2. J Immunol. 138: 2718–2727, (1987)
29. Dawson MM, Johnston D, Taylor GM, Moore M. Lymphokin eactivated killing of fresh human leukaemias. Leuk Res. 10: 683–688, (1986)
30. Oshimi K, Oshimi Y, Akutsu M, Takei Y, Saito H, Okada M, Mozoguchi H: Cytotoxicity of interleukin-2-activated lymphocytes for leukemia, and lymphoma cells. Blood. 68: 938–948, (1986)
31. Adler A, Chervenick PA, Witeside TL, Lotzova E, Herberman RB. Interleukin 2 induction of lymphokine-activated killer (LAK) activity in the peripheral blood and bone marrow of acute leukemia patients: II. Feasibility of LAK gneration in children with active disease and in remission. Blood 74: 1690–1697, (1989)
32. Archimbaud E, Bailly M, Dore JF. Inducibility of lymphokine activated killer (LAK) cells in patients with acute myelogenous leukaemia in complete remission and its clinical relevance. Br J Haematol 77: 328–334, (1991)
33. Ackerstein A, Kedar E, and Slavin S: Use of recombinant human interleukin-2 in conjunction with syngeneic bone marrow transplantation in mice as a model for control of minimal residual disease in malignant hematologic disorders. Blood 78: 1212–1215, (1991)
34. Ciolli V, Gabriele L, Sestili P, Varano F, et al.: Combined interleukin 1/interleukin 2 therapy of mice injected with highly metastatic friend leukemia cells: host antitumor mechanisms and marked effects on established metastases. J. Ex. Med. 173: 313–322, (1991)
35. Vallera DA, Taylor PA, Aukerman SL, and Blazar BR: Antitumor protection from the murine T-cell leukemia/lymphoma EL4 by the continuous subcutaneous coadministration of recombinant macrophage-colony stimulating factor and interleukin-2. Cancer Res. 53: 4273–4280, (1993)
36. Ferrantini M, Proietti E, Santodonato L, Gabriele L, et al.: α-Interferon gene transfer into metastatic friend luekemia cells abrogated tumorigenicity in immunocommpetent mice: antitumor therapy by means of interferon-producing Cells. Cancer Res. 53: 1107–1112, (1993)
37. Namen AE, Schierer AE, March CJ, Overell RW, Park LS, Urdal DL and Mochizuki DY: B cell precursor growth-promoting activity. Purification and characterization of a growth factor active on lymphocyte precursors. J. Exp. Med., 167: 988–1002, (1988)
38. Widmer MB, Morrissey PJ, Namen AE, Voice RF, and Watson JD: Interleukin 7 simulates growth of fetal thymic precursors of cytolytic cells; induction of effector function by interleuin 2 and inhibition by interluekin 4. Int. Immunol., 2: 1055–1061, (1990)
39. Okazaki H, Ito M, Sudo T, Hattori M, Kano S, Katsura Y and Minato N: IL-7 promotes thymocyte proliferation and maintains immunocompetent thymocytes bearing αβ or γδ T cell receptors in vitro: synergism with IL-2. J. Immunol., 143: 2917–2922, (1989)
40. Welch PA, Namen AE, Goodwin RG, Armitage R and Cooper MD: Human IL-7: a novel T cell growth factor. J. Immunol., 143: 3562–3567, (1989)
41. Grabstein KH, Namen AE, Shanebeck K, Voice RF, Reed SG and Widner MB: Regulation of T cell proliferation by IL-7. J. Immunol., 144: 3015–3020, (1990)
42. Armitage RJ, Namen AE, Shanebeck K, Voice RF, Reed SG and Widmer MB. Regulation of T cell proliferation by IL-7. J. Immunol., 144: 938–941, (1989)
43. Chazen GD, Pereira GMB, LeGros G, Gillis S, and Shevach EM. Interleukin 7 is a T cell growth factor. Proc. Natl. Acad. Sci. USA, 86: 5923–5927, (1989)
44. Morrissey PJ, Goodwin RG, Nordan RP, Anderson D, Grabstein KH, Cosman D, Sims J, Lupton S, Acres B and Reed SG: Recombinant interleukin 7, pre-B cell factor, has costimulatory activity on purified mature cells. J. Exp. Med., 169: 707–716, (1989)
45. Widmer MB, Morrissey PJ, Goodwin RG, Grabstein KH, Park LS, Watson JD, Kincade PW, Conlon PJ and Namen AE: Lymphopoiesis and IL-7. Int. J. Cell Cloning 1: 168–170, (1990)
46. Hickman CJ, Crim JA, Mostowski HS and Siegel JP: Regulation of human cytotoxic T lymphocyte development by IL-7. J. Immunol., 145: 2415–2420, (1990)
47. Alderson MR, Sassenfeld HM and Widmer MB. Interleukin 7 enhances cytotoxic T lymphocyte

generation and induces lymphokine-activated killer cells from human peripheral blood. J. Exp. Med., 172: 577–587, (1990)
48. Bertagnolli M, and Herrmann S. IL-7 supports the generation of cytotoxic T lymphocytes from thymocytes. J. Immunol., 145: 1706–1712, (1990)
49. Lynch Dh and Miller RE. Induction of murine lymphokine-activated killer cells by recombinant IL-7. J. Immunol. 145: 1983–1990, (1990)
50. Stotter H, Custer MC, Bolton ES, Guedez L, and Lotze MT: IL-7 induces human lymphokine-activated killer cell activity and is regulated by IL-4. J. Immunol., 146: 150–155, (1991)
51. Erard F, Corthesy P, Nabholz M, Lowenthal JW, Zaech P, Plaetinck G, and MacDonald HR: Interleukin 2 is both necessary and sufficent for the growth and differentiation of lectin-stimulated cytolytic T lymphocyte precursors. J. Immunol. 134: 1644, (1985)
52. Mosmann TR, and Coffman RL: Two types of mouse helper T-cell clone. Immunol. Today. 8: 223, (1987)
53. Trinchieri G: Biology of natural killer cells. Adv. Immunol. 47: 187, (1989)
54. Rosenberg SA, and Lotze MT: Cancer immunotherapy using interleukin-2 and interleukin 2 activated lymphocytes. Annu. Rev. Immunol. 4: 681, (1986)
55. Ralph P, Nakoinz I. Direct toxic effects of immunopotentiators on monocytic, myelomonocytic, and histiocytic or macrophage tumor cells in culture. Canc. Res. 37: 546–550, (1977)
56. Ichikawa Y. Differentiation of a cell line of myeloid leukemia. J. Cell. Pysiol. 74: 223–234, (1969)
57. Markowitz D, Goff S, Bank A: Construction and use of a safe and efficient amphotropic packaging cell line. Virology 167: 400, (1988)
58. Miller AR, McBride WH, Moen RC, Schuck BC, Glasby SE, Economou JS.Interleukin-2 producing fibroblast cell line abrogates tumorigenicity in a murine tumor model: colon. An approach to genetically engineered vaccines. Surgical Forum 49: 512, (1993)
59. Hagenbeck A, de Grot CJ, Martens ACM: Cytokine gene mediated immunotherapy of leukemia. Studies in the Brown Norway Rat acute myelomonocytic leukemia employing the Interleukin-2 gene. Blood 82(supp.): 1000, (1993)
60. Miller FR: Intratumor immunologic heterogeneity. Cancer Metast Rev 1: 319, (1982)
61. Miller FR, Heppner GH: Antigenic heterogeneity and metastasis. In Immune Responses to Metastasis (Heberman R, Wiltrout R, Govelik E, eds.) Boca Raton, FL: CRC Press, pp 23–33, (1987)

Acute Leukemias V
Experimental Approaches
and Management of Refractory Diseases
Hiddemann et al. (Eds.)

IL2 in Acute Leukemia

D. Blaise, A. M. Stoppa, M. Attal, J. Reiffers, J. Fleury, M. Michallet, E. Archimbaud, R. Bouabdallah, J. A. Gastaut, and D. Maraninchi

Introduction

Immunotherapy is a logical approach for the strategy of a currative treatment for acute leukemia since allogeneic bone marrow transplantation had demonstrated the benefit of graft versus host disease (GVHD) to reduce the relapse rate [1,2]. In vivo administration of rIL2 is able to induce complete response in acute myeloid leukemia and in non Hodgkin lymphoma however usually with a short duration of response. Minimal residual disease obtained after autologous bone marrow transplantation (ABMT) seems the best situation to test the capacity of IL2 to mimic graft versus leukemia effect (GVL). We present here a summary of the activity of rIL2 administration in relapsed and refractory leukemia, and the preliminary data on follow up of patients receiving IL2 after ABMT in first complete remission (CR1).

Activity of IL2 in Refractory or Relapsed Acute Leukemia

Patients and methods. Table 1 shows the characteristics of the population, underlying the fact that 67% of the patients had been heavily pretreated with autologous or allogeneic BMT, and that 43% of the patient were in second relapse. rIL2 (Roussel Uclaf 49637) has a specific activity of 10×10^6 biological response modifier units per milligram of protein and was administrated as a 15 min bolus. Treatment consisted of three cycles of 5 days starting D1, D15 and D29 and rIL2 was given at the dose of 8 millions of international units (MIU)/m²/bolus three times per day (15 bolus) during cycle 1 and twice daily (10 bolus) for cycle 2 and 3. Toxicity management has been detailed previously [3,4].

Patients were scheduled to receive at least two cycles in the absence of serious toxicity, the third cycle was given only in stable or responsive disease.

Results. 34% of the patients received three cycle and 70% received at least two cycles. When cycles were began, the dose administrated was 80, 78, 70% of the scheduled dose for cycle 1, 2, 3 respectively.

Table 1. Characteristics of the patients

	AML	ALL
n	30	19
Age	39 (4–65)	28 (12–48)
<15 y	2	3
16–59 y	23	16
>60 y	3	0
no BMT	18	8
Allo	5	0
Auto	7	11
primary Refractory	4	0
Relapse first/second	16/10	11/8
Fab	M0 = 3 M1 = 4 M2 = 4 M4 = 6 M5 = 9 M6 = 1	L1 = 6 L2 = 13 T = 4 CD10 and/or CD 19 = 14

Institut Paoli Calmettes, 13273 Marseille Cedex 9, France

Incomplete administration of IL2 was related to classical reversible adverse effects of IL2 previously described (mainly capillary leak syndrom). Two patients died of interstitial pneumopathy (documented with CMV in one case). Thrombopenia occured in all patients and required platelet transfusions.

Phenotype lymphocyte analysis and cytotoxicity against K562 and Daudi cell lines was performed on day 0 and 8 on some patients as previously described. This analysis showed a 2 fold increase of CD3+ lymphocytes, a 2.5 fold increase of CD56+ CD3− lymphocytes, a 1.4 increase of LAK activity and a 2.5 increase of NK activity.

Bone marrow aspiration were performed at D1, D15 and D35. Table 2 shows the results of the antileukemic activity of IL2.

Complete and partial response were observed in 15% of AML. Eleven additional patients showed also clearance of blast cells (Preisler relative resistance type II = transient clearance; relative resistance type III = pancytopenia without blasts cells). This lead to an overall 41% and 21% evidence of activity in acute myeloblastic and lymphoblastic leukemia repectively. Complete and partial response were observed usually rapidly after the first cycle, never last more than three months and correlation with immune activation could not be established [3,4].

IL2 Administration after Auto BMT for Acute Leukemia in First Remission

Patients and methods. Our institution had conducted various trial of unique (6–12 days) administration or sequential administration (5 cycles) of escalating doses of IL2 after ABMT [5,6]. Table 3 show the characteristics of a selected population of patients with: 1) AL in CR1; 2) after CyTBI conditioning regimen for unpurged ABMT; 3) enrolled in various phase I and III trial of sequential IL2; 5) with a minimal follow up since ABMT of 12 months.

Table 2. Anti leukemic activity of IL2

	AML	ALL
n	30	19
Inadequate trial	3	0
Evaluable	27	19
Absolute resistance	16	15
CR	3	0
PR	1	0
Relative resistance type II/III	7	4
Overall response	11/27 (41%)	4/19 (21%)

Table 3. Characteristics of the patients

	AML	ALL
n	15	26
Age	41 (17–55)	28 (16–59)
FAB M1–M3/M4-M5/MoM7/L1/L2	5/7/3	12/14
WBC at diagnosis ($\times 10^9$/l)	26 (1–157)	30 (2–230)
t(9,22) or t(4,11)	0/8	6/15
Diag-ABMT (months)	4.3 (3–8)	5.2 (3–10)
ABMT-IL2 (months)	2.4 (1.4–4)	2.2 (1–3)
Scheduled level of IL2		
Level 12:	11	19
16/20/24	2/1/1	2/1/4

Therapy before ABMT consisted homogenously of a BFM like regimen (induction, consolidation, interval therapy) for ALL patients and standard induction and consolidation with intermediate dose of ARAC (500 mg/m^2 × 8 doses) for AML patients.

Roussel Uclaf rIL2 was administered after complete hematologic reconstitution. Treatment consisted in five cycles beginning D1, D15, D29, D43, D57. Cycle 1 consisted in five days therapy and the other four cycles of 2 days of therapy. IL2 was given in continuous 24 hours infusion at doses ranging from 12, 16, 20 to 24 MIU/m^2 per day.

Results. Figure 1 and 2 describe feasability of the scheduled treatment wich was slightly better for ALL (total dose 132 MUI/patient) than for AML (115 MIU/patient). However overall, the daily dose per patient was constantly inferior to lowest level of dose initially prescribed (10 MIU/day/m^2 for ALL, 8.8 MIU/day/m^2 for AML).

Toxicities leading to discontinuation of IL2 have been described (on the totality of the population of the phase I trial) and occured in 6%, 11%, 16% and 36% of the patients for the 12, 16, 20, 24 MIU dose level respectively [6].

Beside the constitutional syndrom and the hemodynamical toxicities, unusual neurotoxicity (seisure, coma, 12%) have been observed for

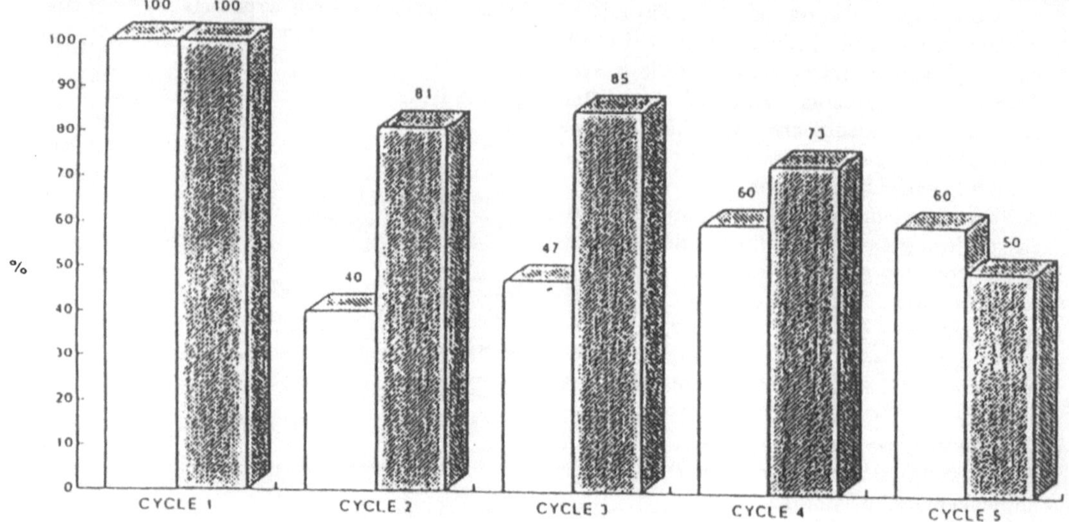

Fig. 1. Patients starting a cycle (ratio). □ LAM, ■ LAL

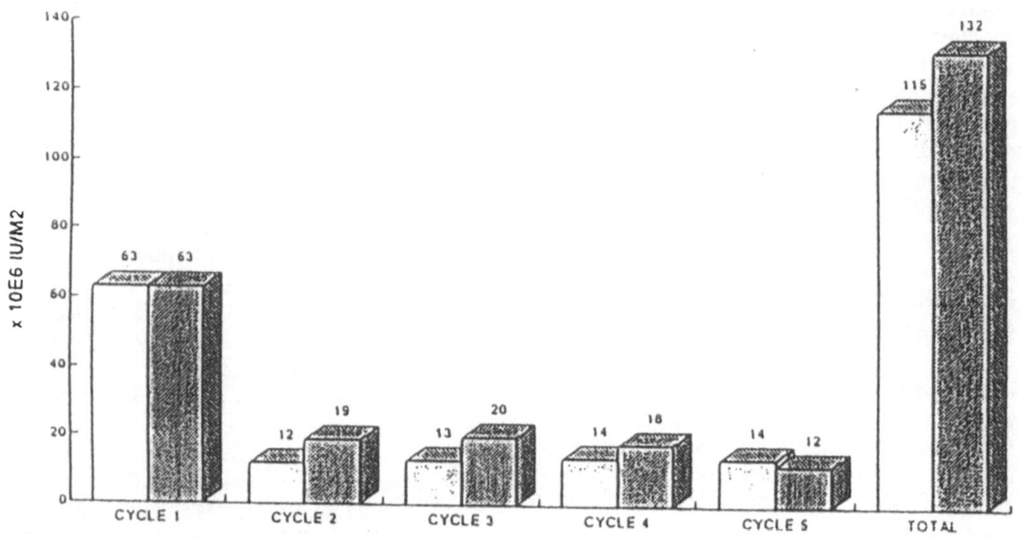

Fig. 2. Dose of rIL2 infused to patients (average)

the highest level of dose and for patients receiving IL2 earlier than 2 months after TBI. Secondly, unusual rate of gram negative (9%) septicemia in non neutropenic patient have been observed.

Immune activity had been sequentially studied and showed rapid and sustained stimulation of NK and LAK activity with 3 and 2 fold increase of the K562 and Daudi cell line cytolysis respectively.

Table 4 describes the early follow up of the patients and shows a higher relapse rate for ALL than for AML. With a median follow up of two years, probability for relapse and survival are 27% and 87% for AML and 55% and 63% for ALL.

Table 4. Outcome of ABMT patients after IL2

	AML	ALL
n	15	26
Follow up (months)	22 (13–54)	29 (14–56)
Relapse: n	7	14
Time of relapse (months from ABMT)	4-0-13 5-15-27 33	4-4-4-4 66-88-9 10-12-14-16
Remission duration med/months	23/20	20/14
Alive: n	12	14
Alive in CCR: n	8	12
KM probability of relapse at 2 y	27%	52%
KM probability of survival	87%	63%

Discussion

We have presented here up dated data on activity of IL2 in acute leukemia conducted in France since 1990.

The results of the phase II study in refractory or relapsed acute leukemia confirm that high dose rIL2 :

- is able to induce stimulation of lymphokine activated killer and natural killer cell activity,
- is able to induce complete remission in AML (15%). Mechanism of response to IL2 is not elucidated and may involved, apart the immune activation, upregulation of cell surface adhesion molecule ICAM1 and LFA3 on leukemia cells and facilitation of their clearance [7].

Since the first results [3, 4, 8], other observations of complete response in AML and myelodysplasia has been reported with low dose rIL2 [7–10]. On the other hand only minimal response has been observed in acute lymphoid leukemia despite increased immunological effectors. We also report a summary of feasability of rIL2 after ABMT. Immediate administration after TBI conditioning regimen has been reported as toxic in a pediatric population [11] and current strategy lead to administer continuous infusion after full hematologic reconstitution for a two to 3 months exposure [12, 13].

We report that 10 to 12 MIU/m²/day is usually regularly tolerated for AML or ALL after ABMT in CR1 in sequential administration of 13 days over a two months period. This schedule provide a high degree of LAK and NK activity.

On a population of adult patients in CR1 with a median follow up of two years, probabilities for relapse and survival are 27% and 87% for AML and 52 and 63% for ALL respectively.

There results challenge with historical control and do not show at the present time – at least for ALL patients – evidence of improvement. This observation is in agreement with the results of the phase II trial which show lower activity of IL2 in ALL than AML.

A European randomized study in CR1 adult AL has been closed in september 93 including 190 patients and results should be waited.

In vivo IL2 administration is the first step of active immunotherapy in acute leukemia. Major non specific immune activation has been clearly obtained. Specific antileukemia activity should certainly be also the goal of future clinical research.

References

1. Maraninchi D, Gluckman E, Blaise D et al. Impact of T cell depletion on outcome of allogeneic BMT for standard risk leukemia. Lancet, 1987, 2: 175–177.
2. Brenner MK, Heslop H. Immunotherapy of leukemia. Leukemia, 1992, vol 6, Suppl 1: 76–79.
3. Maraninchi D, Blaise D, Viens P, Brandely M, Olive D, Lopez M et al. High dose recombinant interleukin-2 and acute myeloid leukemias in relapse. Blood, 1991, 78, 9: 2181–2187.
4. Blaise D, Stoppa AM, Olive D, Brandely M, Gastaut JA, Sainty D et al. Treatment of relapsed acute leukemias with systemic recombinant interleukin-2 (RU 49637). Cytokines in hemopoiesis, oncology and AIDS. Ed Freund/Link/Schmidt/Welte. Springer Verlag, Berlin Heidelberg, 1992: 761–768.
5. Blaise D, Viens P, Olive D, Stoppa AM, Gabert J, Pourreau CN et al. Recombinant interleukin-2 (rIL-2) after autologous bone marrow transplantation (BMT) : a pilot study in 19 patients. Eur. Cytokine Net. 1991, Vol 2, n° 2: 121–129.
6. Blaise D, Olive D, Brandely M, Stoppa AM, Gabus R, Tiberghien P. Use of recombinant interleukin-2 (RU 49637) after autologous bone marrow transplantation in patients with hematological disease : phase I-II study. Cytokines in Hemopoiesis oncology and AIDS. Ed Freund/ Link/ Schmidt/ Welte, Springer Verlag, Berlin Heidelberg, 1992: 769–774.
7. Olive D, Lopez M, Blaise D, Viens P, Stoppa AM, Brandely M et al. Cell surface expression of ICAM-1 (CD34) and LFA-3 (CD58), two adhesion molecules, is up-regulated on bone marrow leukemic blasts after in vivo administration of high dose recombinant interleukin-2. Journal of Immunotherapy, 1991, 10: 412–417.
8. Foa R, Meloni G, Tosti S, Novarino A, Fenu S, Gavosto F, Mandelli F. Treatment of acute myeloid

leukaemia patients with recombinant interleukin-2 : a pilot study. British Journal of Haematology, 1991, 77: 491–496.

9. Toze CL, Barnett MJ, Klingemann HG. Response of therapy related myelodysplasia to low dose interleukin-2. Leukemia, 1993, 7, 3: 463–465.
10. Stoppa AM, Olive D, Mannoni P, Barouki K, Osterwalder B, Blaise D, Maraninchi D. Low dose IL2 induces prolonged complete remission in a refractory acute myeloid leukemia. Leukemia and lymphoma, Vol 13, Suppl 1: p115 (a).
11. Weisdorf DJ, Anderson PM, Blazar BR, Uckun FM, Kersey JH, Ramsay NKC. Interleukin-2 immediately after autologous bone marrow transplantation for acute lymphoblastic leukemia. A phase I study. Transplantation, 1993, vol 55, n° 1: 61–66.
12. Bosly A, Guillaume T, Brice P, Humblet Y, Staquet P, Doyen C. Effects of escalating doses of recombinant human interleukin-2 in correcting functional T-cells defects following autologous bone marrow transplantation for lymphomas and solid tumors. Exp Haematol, 1992, 20: 962–968.
13. Soiffer RJ, Murray C, Cochran K, Cameron C, Wang E, Schow P et al. Clinical and immunologic effects of prolonged infusion of low dose recombinant interleukin-2 after autologous and T-cell depleted allogeneic bone marrow transplantation. Blood, 1992, 79, 2: 517–526.

Acute Leukemias V
Experimental Approaches
and Management of Refractory Diseases
Hiddemann et al. (Eds.)

Is There a Role for Interleukin-2 Gene Transfer in the Management of Acute Leukemia?

Robert Foa[1,2], Alessandro Cignetti[1], Anna Gillio Tos[1], Anna Carbone[1], Paola Francia do Celle[1], and Anna Guarini[1]

Abstract. The limitations encountered with the administration of high dose exogenous interleukin-2 (IL-2) have triggered the search for alternative immunotherapeutic approaches or delivery modalities. Studies carried out in experimental tumor models suggest that the tumorgenic potential can be reversed following transduction of different cytokine genes into the DNA of the neoplastic cells. Transfer of the IL-2 gene has also been associated with the generation of anti-tumor specificity and anti-tumor memory. These findings have led to the activation of the first clinical vaccination protocols with human tumor cells engineered to release IL-2 in patients suffering from different tumors. Here, we shall report on the feasability of inserting the IL-2 gene into human acute leukemia cells and the possibility of using this approach for the management of patients with acute leukemia.

Introduction

Immunotherapy with exogenous interleukin-2 (IL-2), with or without the concomittant administration of ex-vivo generated lymphokine activated killer (LAK) cells, has enabled objective clinical responses in a proportion of patients with renal cell carcinoma and metastatic melanoma which can be estimated in the range of approximately 5 to 20 % [1–3]. Although these figures are relatively low, it should be noted that these responses have been long-lived.

Extensive pre-clinical studies, followed by the first clinical applications, have led to the belief that IL-2 based immunotherapy can be considered as a therapeutic option also for the management of a proportion of acute leukemia patients (for review see 4). This is based initially on experiments performed in vitro and in vivo in immunosuppressed nude mice [5–8], and, thereafter, on the first pilot studies carried out in acute leukemia patients [9–14]. These latter have allowed over the years to draw a number of conclusions. First, it has been shown that high doses of IL-2 can be administered to acute leukemia patients. In our experience, side effects have been acceptably managed using a continuous i.v. infusion and a daily dose-escalating protocol. In general, the clinical responses have been scarce in patients with a large leukemic mass, while complete remissions have been documented in acute myeloid leukemias (AML) with a limited proportion of residual bone marrow blasts. We have recently updated our results in 14 AML patients with less than 30 % residual bone marrow blasts and treated with high dose IL-2 [14]. Eight of the patients achieved a complete remission (CR) with IL-2 alone and in 5 this persists between 15 and 69 months later. In all 5 patients the IL-2-induced remission has been the longest in the natural history of the disease. These encouraging results need now to obtain further confirmation through randomized studies in 1st or 2nd remission AML. In Italy we are currently conducting a multicenter study in AML patients in 2nd CR (remission induced with the same re-induction protocol) who are

[1] Dipartimento di Scienze Biomediche e Oncologia Umana, Sezione Clinica
[2] Centro NR Immunogenetica e Oncologia Sperimentale, University of Turin, Turin, Italy

randomized to receive or not two cycles of high dose IL-2 and, thereafter, a monthly "maintenance" protocol with lower doses of IL-2.

Another obvious condition of potential immunotherapeutic intervention is in the setting of autologous bone marrow transplantation in the hope of boosting the immune system of the host to control or eradicate the disease at a time of minimal tumor burden. The results so far accumulated indicate that IL-2 may be administered to autografted patients of both adult and childhood age [15–19], though no clearcut evidence of a beneficial clinical response has so far been provided. There is still no uniform consensus on the optimal timing and doses of IL-2 given post-transplantation.

Both in solid tumors and in acute leukemia patients the administration of high doses of IL-2 is coupled with notable phenotypic and functional changes within the immune system of the recipient [20–23]. The most relevant changes are the increased natural killer (NK) and LAK functions, as well as the generation of endogenous LAK effectors. Studies carried out in acute leukemia patients have shown that these changes occur also in bone marrow lymphocytes [23]. A cascade of different cytokines is also induced in vivo in the treated patients ([24], and own data). These include interferon (IFN)-γ, tumor necrosis factor (TNF)-α, Il-3, IL-5, GM-CSF and are likely to play a primary role in some of the side effects and clinico-hematological changes which occur in patients treated with IL-2. Unfortunately, these immunological modifications appear to take place in practically all leukemic patients treated with IL-2 and no correlation has so far been observed with the clinical response to IL-2 [23], although the degree of immune response appears greater in patients with more limited disease [14]. The functional changes that occur in autografted patients are more evident than in non-grafted ones [17], demonstrating the presence in the former of an expanded NK and LAK cell compartment.

Despite some quite unequivocal objective and prolonged remissions in different tumors, a wider use of high dose IL-2 in the management of neoplastic patients has been hampered by at least three relevant considerations: 1) the more or less severe toxicity that affects all patients; 2) the heterogenous and so far unpredictable response to IL-2, and 3) the lacking demonstration that the administration of exogenous IL-2 is capable of activating cytotoxic T-lymphocytes (CTL) directed specifically against the tumor of the treated patient. These considerations have prompted the search for possible alternative administration modalities, including the use of lower doses of IL-2 over a longer time period, the subcutaneous adminstration route and the combined utilization of IL-2 with cytotoxic drugs and other biologic response modifiers or with the hormone melatonin [25].

Over the last few years it has been shown that cytokine genes can be productively inserted into the DNA of animal and human tumor cells. This has opened innovative theoretical and practi cal prospects in the treatment of patients with cancer.

Cytokine Gene Transfer into Tumor Cells

It has been convincingly shown that the genes for practically all cytokines and growth factors can be successfully introduced into the genome of experimental tumor cells (for reviews see [26–28]). Through different mechanisms the release of the related protein leads in most cases to a reduced abrogated tumor growth capacity. In addition to exploring the modifications induced in the tumorgenic potential of the engineered cells. cytokine gene transfer technologies have introduced new ways of assessing the immunogenicity of the neoplastic cells. Indeed, particularly with the IL-2 gene two of the primary goals of any immunotherapeutic protocol have been fulfilled, since in different experimental models it could be shown that the constitutive release of low doses of IL-2 was combined with anti-tumor immunologic memory [29–31].

As a follow-up of the studies carried out in animal tumors, efforts have aimed at assessing whether human neoplastic cells could also be transduced with cytokine genes. The results so far obtained indicate that human tumor cell lines of various origin can be successfully engineered to release different cytokines (for review see [26]). In view of the results obtained in a proportion of cancer patients with the administraton of exogenous IL-2, the majority of studies have aimed at investigating the IL-2 gene. It has, thus, been shown that following retroviral vector mediated gene tranfer human melanoma and renal cell carcinoma cell lines may be induced to release variable amounts of IL-2 [32–35]. When studied in nude mice, the IL-2 gene transduced neoplastic cell lines no longer grew in vivo. Recent evidence suggests that in some human melanoma lines the IL-2 released by the engineered cells may induce, in co-culture experminets with autologous lymphocytes, the generation of CTL directed specifically against the autologous tumor cells [36].

Based on the results obtained in experimental tumor models and, more recently, with human cancer cells it appears that at least two major limitations associated with the administration of high doses of exogenous IL-2, i.e. toxicity and generation of a specific anti-tumor response, may be potentially circumvented following transduction of the IL-2 gene into the neoplastic cells. Thus, vaccination protocols aimed at immunizing patients with different tumors, largely melanoma and renal cell carcinoma, with IL-2 gene transduced allogeneic cell lines have been designed and activated both in the US and in Europe. These are phase I pilot studies aimed at investigating the feasibility of such an approach. Immunological monitoring of the treated patients will also allow to verify whether through this therapeutic strategy a specific anti-tumor response can be generated. Should this be the case, cytokine gene therapy will gain further impetus and protocols aimed at treating neoplastic patients with less advanced disease will be justified.

IL-2 Gene Transfer of Human Acute Leukemia Cells

The clinical results and limitations recorded with the exogenous administration of high doses of IL-2 and the knowledge that the IL-2 gene can be inserted into DNA of different human tumor cell lines prompted our group to investigate whether the same gene tranfer approach could be extended to acute leukemia cells. The results so far observed [37] which are summarized in Table 1, indicate that using retroviral vectors the IL-2 gene can be successfully inserted into the DNA of acute leukemia cell lines. This holds true for lines of both myeloid and lymphoid origin. Evidence of DNA integration of the IL-2 gene is shown in Figure 1.

Though the overall levels of IL-2 released by the leukemic cell lines appear to be lower compared to those from cell lines derived from solid tumor patients (Table 2), the engineered cells can be subcloned by limiting dilution in order to obtain clones which produce variable amounts of IL-2. Horizontal studies have shown that the transduced cells continue to release consistent amounts of IL-2 for at least four months. An important issue that needed to be verified was the possibility that the integration of the IL-2 gene and subsequent protein release could modify the properties of the parental cells. Extensive studies have shown that the phenotypic features of the transduced cells do not change; furthermore, the alpha and beta chains of the IL-2 receptor are not upmodulated, nor could changes in the mRNA expression of different cytokine and growth factor genes analysed by RT-PCR be documented. Finally, the proliferative status of the parent and engineered cells remained unmodified. In order to establish whether the IL-2 producing leukemic cells changed their tumorgenic potential experiments were set in immunosuppressed nude mice, which represent the best model to study "in vivo" human acute leukemia cells. The results obtained demonstrate that while the parent leukemic cells induce the formation of a leukemic mass in nude mice, the IL-2 gene transduced clones show a reduced or abrogated tumorgenicity which parallels the levels of IL-2 released by the leukemic

Table 1. Results obtained following retroviral vector transfer of the IL-2 gene into human acute leukemia cells

a) Acute leukemia cell lines of both myeloid and lymphoid origin may be transduced with the IL-2 gene
b) This leads to the constitutive release of variable amounts of IL-2
c) The transduction of the IL-2 gene does not modify the phenotypic or proliferative properties of the engineered cells
d) The tumorigenic potential of IL-2 gene transduced cells is reduced or abrogated

Table 2. Levels of IL-2 released by human tumor cell lines transduced with the IL-2 gene

Cell lines studied (No.)	IL-2 released (U/10^6 cells/48h)
Melanoma (6)	1–139*
Renal cell carcinoma (7)	4–72*
Neuroblastoma (1)	220*
Lung adenocarcinoma (1)	200*
Acute leukemia (5)	1–20*°

*Range of IL-2 secretion from the different lines
°Subclones: 0.3–90 U of IL-2

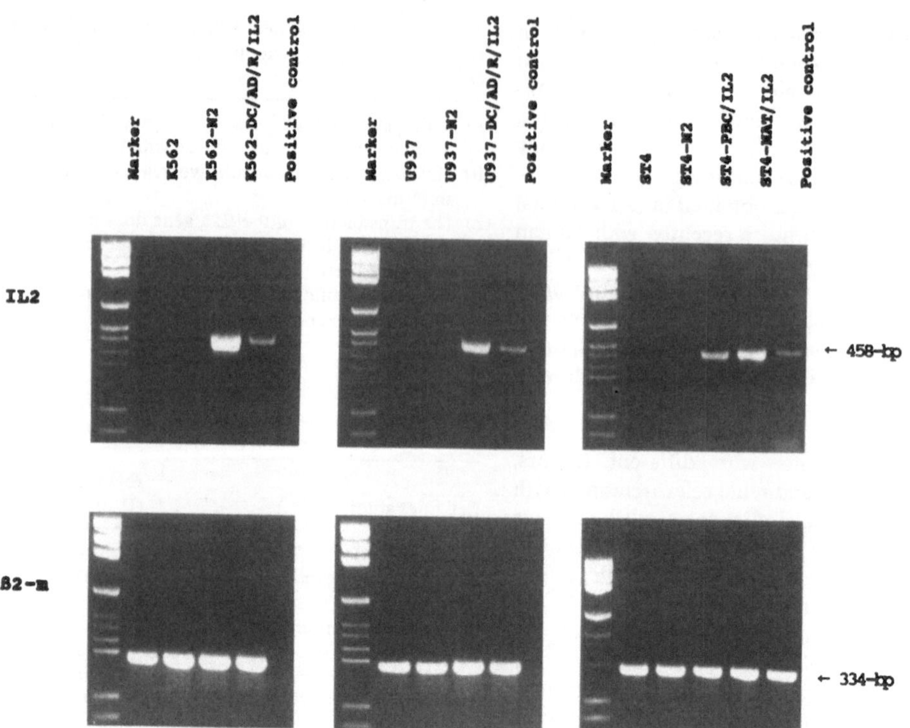

Fig. 1. IL-2 gene expression in parental and transduced leukemic cell lines analyzed by RT-PCR. N2 = control vector

clones. Since the nude mice employed are deficient in T and NK cells histological sections were performed and it was shown than the IL-2 gene transduced tumor cells were capable of recruiting monocyte macrophages.

Future Perspectives

The preliminary results so far obtained in melanoma and renal cell carcinoma patients vaccinated with allogeneic tumor cells transduced with the IL-2 gene indicate that this approach is feasible in terms of individual tolerability. Systemic side effects have not been observed and the only recorded changes have been local erythematous rashes. On clinical grounds some evidence of disease stabilization has been suggested. Phenotypic and functional studies of the immunologic compartment of the treated patients are being carried out in order to assess the effectiveness of the low quantities of IL-2 released in vivo by the engineered tumor cells. While this new therapeutic approach can thus be considered safe for the patients and easily carried out on an out-patient basis, in view of the clinical status of the patients so far enrolled, i.e. with advanced and resistant disease, it is less likely that significant clinical and biological information will be obtained. Several data, in fact, indicate that should immunotherapy have a role in the management of patients with cancer this is likely to occur in the setting of limited or minimal disease. This has been convincingly shown on clinical grounds in acute leukemia [11,14]. Furthermore, in vitro data indicate that the IL-2 stimulated cytotoxic compartment of the host directed against the autologous leukemic blasts is most often depressed in patients with advanced disease, while frequently restored in patients in remission of their disease [38].

Based on several considerations, acute leukemia patients, particularly of myeloid origin, represent potentially ideal candidates of a vaccination scheme with IL-2 gene transduced tumor cells. These include the evidence that: 1) long-lasting complete remissions have been obtained in AML with limited bone marrow disease with high dose exogenous IL-2; 2) IL-2 may generate, in complete remission patients, LAK directed activity against autologous tumor cells; 3) the kinetics and overall prognosis of adult AML allow to consider the enrolment of patients in remission (this is less realistic for patients with solid tumors). The pre-clinical results so far obtained indicate that acute leukemia cell lines may be successfully transduced to release constitutively relatively low amounts of IL-2, which, in turn, are capable of hampering the tumorigenic potential of the leukemic blasts without changing the phenotypic and functional properties of the engineered cells. Experiments are currently underway to assess whether through this approach the generation of specific anti-leukemic CTL may be documented. Should this be the case, on the one hand the possibility of designing pilot studies of cytokine gene therapy for the management of acute leukemia patients will gain further strength, and, on the other hand a technical tool aimed at a better definition of the immunogenicity of human leukemic cells may be made available.

Acknowledgements. This work was supported by "Associazone Italiana per la Ricerca sul Cancro" (AIRC), Special Program on "Gene Therapy", Milan, by Consiglio Nazionale dell Ricerche (CNR), Program on "Applicazioni Cliniche della Ricerca Oncologia", Rome, Italy. A. Carbone, A Cignetti, P. Francia di Celle are in receipt of fellowships from "AIRC", Istituto Superiore di Sanita' and Ministro dell'Universita'e della Ricerca Scientifica, respectively. A. Gillio is a PhD in Oncology at the University of Turin.

References

1. Rosenberg SA, Lotze MT, Muul LM et al (1987): A progress report on the treatment of 157 patients with advanced cancer using lymphokine-activated killer cells and interleukin-2 or high-dose interleukin-2 alone. New England Journal of Medicine 316: 889–897
2. West WH, Tauer KW, Yannelli JR et al (1987): Constant-infusion recombinant intelreukin-2 in adoptive immunotherapy of advanced cancer. New England Journal of Medicine 316: 898–905
3. Rosenberg SA, Lotze MT, Anyg JC et al. (1989): Experience with the use of high-dose interleukin-2 in the treatment of 652 cancer patients. Annals Surgery 210: 474–484
4. Foa R (1994):Does Interleukin-2 have a role in the management of acute leukemia? Journal of Clinical Oncology 11: 1817–1825
5. Oshimi K, Oshimi Y, Akutsu M et al (1986): Cytotoxicity of interleukin 2 activated lymphocytes for leukemia and lymphoma cells. Blood 68: 938–948
6. Lotzova E, Savary CA, Herberman RB (1987): Inhibition of clonogenic growth of fresh leukemia cells by unstimulated and IL-2 stimulated NK cells of normal donors. Leukemia Research 11: 1059–1066
7. Fierro MT, Xin-Sheng L, Lusso P et al. (1988): In vitro and in vivo susceptibility of human leukemic cells to lymphokine activated killer activity. Leukemia 2: 50–54
8. Foa R, Caretto P, Fierro MT et al. (1990): Interleukin 2 does not promote the in vitro and in vivo proliferation and growth of human acute leukaemia cells of myeloid and lymphoid origin. British Journal of Haematology 75: 34–40
9. Foa R, Caretto P, Tosti S et al. (1990): Induction and persistence of complete remission in a resistant acute myeloid leukemia patient following treatment with recombinant interleukin 2. Leukemia and Lymphoma 1: 113–177
10. Meloni G, Foa R, Tosti S et al. (1990): IL-2 in the treatment of chronic myeloid leukemia after lymphoid blast crisis: a pilot study. Haematologica 75: 502–505
11. Foa R, Meloni G, Tosti S et al (1991a): Treatment of acute myeloid leukaemia patients with recombinant interleukin 2: a pilot study. British Journal of Haematology 77: 491–496
12. Maraninchi D, Blaise D; Viens P et al. (1991): High-dose recombinant interleukin-2 and acute myeloid leukemias in relapse. Blood 78: 2182–2187
13. Lim SH, Newland AC, Kelsey S et al (1992): Continuous intravenous infusion of high-dose recombinant interleukin-2 for acute myeloid leukaemia – a phase II study. Cancer Immunology and Immunotherapy 34: 337–342
14. Meloni G, Foa R, Vignetti M et al (1994): Interleukin 2 may induce prolonged remissions in advanced acute myelogenous leukaemia. Blood, in press
15. Blaise D, Olive D; Stoppa AM et al. (1990) Hematologic and immunologic effects of the systemic administration of recombinant interleukin-2 after autologous bone marrow transplantation for hematologic malignancies. Blood 76: 1092–1097
16. Higuchi CM, Thompson JA, Petersen FB, Bruckner CD, Fefer A (1991): Toxicity and immunomodulatory effects of interleukin-2 after autlogous bone marrow transplantation for hematologic malignancies. Blood 77: 2561–2568
17. Meloni G, Foa R, Tosti S et al (1992): Autologous bone marrow transplantation followed by interleukin-2 in children with advanced leukemia: a pilot study. Leukemia 6: 780–785
18. Soiffer RJ, Murray C, Cochran K et al (1982): Clinical and immunologic effects of prolonged infusion of low-dose recombinant interleukin-2 after autologous and T-cell depleted allogeneic bone marrow transplanation. Blood 79: 517–526
19. Benyunes MC, Massumoto C, Higuchi CM et al. (1993): Interleukin-2 with or without lymphokine-

activated killer cells as consolidative immunotherapy after autologous bone marrow transplantation for acute myelogenous leukemia. Bone Marrow Transplantation 12: 159–163
20. Sondel PM, Kohler PC, Hank JA et al. (1988): Clinical and immunological effect of recombinant interleukin 2 given by repetitive cycles to patients with cancer. Cancer Research 48:: 2561–2567
21. Favrot MC, Combaret V, Negrier S et al. (1990): Functional and immunophenotypic modifications induced by interleukin-2 did not predict response to therapy in patients with renal cell carcinoma. Journal of Biological Response Modifiers 9: 167–177
22. Gottlieb DJ, Prentice HG, Heslop HE et al. (1989): Effects of recombinant interleukin-2 administration on cytotoxic function following high-dose chemo-radiotherapy for hematological malignancy. Blood 74: 2335–2342
23. Foa R, Guarini A; Gillio Tos A et al. (1991b): Peripheral blood and bone marrow immunophenotypic and functional modifications induced in acute leukemia patients treated with Interleukin 2: Evidence of in vivo lymphokine activated killer cell generation. Cancer Research 51: 964–968
24. Heslop HE, Gottlieb DJ, Bianchi ACM et al. (1989): In vivo induction of gamma interferon and tumor necrosis factor by interleukin-2 infusion following intensive chemotherapy or autologous marrow transplantation. Blood 74: 1374–1380
25. Lissoni B, Barni S, Tancini G et al. (1994): A randomised study with subcutaneous low-dose interleukin-2 alone versus interleukin-2 plus the pineal neurohormone melatonin in advanced solid neoplasms other than renal cancer and melanoma. British Journal of Cancer 69: 196–199
26. Foa R, Guarini A, Cignetti A et al. (1994): Cytokine gene therapy: a new strategy for the management of cancer patients. Natural Immunity 13: 65–75
27. Colombo MP, Forni G (1994): Cytokine gene transfer inhibition and tentative tumor therapy: where are we now? Immunology Today 15: 48–51
28. Forni G, Parmiani G, Guarini A, Foa R (1994): Gene transfer in tumor therapy. Annals of Oncology, in press
29. Fearon ER, Pardoll DM, Itaya T et al. (1990): Interleukin-2 production by tumor cells bypasses T helper function on the generation of an antitumor response. Cell 60: 3997–403
30. Gansbacher B, Zier K, Daniels B et al. (1990): Interleukin-2 gene tranfer into tumor cells abrogates tumorigenicity and induces protective immunity. Journal of Experimental Medicine 172: 1217–1224
31. Ley V, Langlade-Demoyen P, Kourilsky P, Larsson-Sciard L (1991): Interleukin 2-dependent activation of tumor-specific cytotoxic T lymphocytes in vivo. European Journal of Immunology 21: 851–854
32. Gansbacher B, Zier K, Cronin K et al. (1992): Retroviral gene tranfer induced constitutive expression of interleukin-2 or interferon-γ in irradiated human melanoma cells. Blood 80: 2817–2825
33. Gastl G, Finstad CL, Guyrini A et al. (1992): Retroviral vector-mediated lymphokine gene transfer into human cancer cells. Cancer Research 52: 6229–6236
34. Foa R, Guarini A, Gansbacher B (1992): IL2 treatment for cancer: from biology to gene therapy. British Journal of Cancer 66: 992–998
35. Belldegrun A, Tso C-L, Sakata T et al. (1993): Human renal carcinoma line tranfected with interleukin-2 and/or interferon α gene(s): implications for live cancer vaccines. Journal of the National Cancer Institute 85: 207–216
36. Guarini A; Gansbacher B, Cronin B et al. (1994): Specific T lymphocyte reactivity to IL-2 gene transduced human melanoma cells. In: Forni G, Foa R, Santoni A, Frati L (eds): Cytokine Induced Tumor Immunogenicity, London, UK: Academic Press, 403–413
37. Cignetti A, Guarini A; Carbone A et al. (1994): Tranduction of the IL2 gene into human acute leukemia cells: induction of tumor rejection without modifying cell proliferation and IL2 receptor expression. Journal of the National Cancer Insitute 86: 785–791
38. Foa R, Fierro MT, Cesano A et al. (1991c): Defensive lymphokine-activated killer cell generation and activity in acute leukemia patients with active disease. Blood 78: 1041–1046

Acute Leukemias V

Experimental Approaches
and Management of Refractory Diseases
Hiddemann et al. (Eds.)

Use of Roquinimex in the Myeloid Leukemias

J. M. Rowe[1], B. I. Nilsson[2], and B. Simonsson[3]

Introduction

The increasing use of allogeneic bone marrow transplantation has led to unequivocal evidence for the efficacy of immunotherapy in the treatment of acute leukemia. It is now known that syngeneic transplantation, T lymphocyte depletion and the absence of graft-versus-host disease all increase the risk of relapse following allogeneic transplantation for the myeloid leukemias, both acute and chronic. Leukemia-specific immune responses appear to play a major role in the therapy of the myeloid leukemias. In recent years attempts have been made to better characterize and effectively utilize these antileukemic immune responses. A beneficial effect is more likely to be seen when the tumor burden is low and such efforts have therefore concentrated on clinical states of minimal residual disease. This review will discuss the role of the novel immunomodulator roquinimex following autologous bone marrow transplantation for myeloid leukemias, and will focus on recent experience and ongoing clinical trials in acute myelogenous leukemia and chronic myelogenous leukemia.

Immunotherapy for Myeloid Leukemias

Historically, the concept of immunotherapy for myeloid leukemia had been investigated in several clinical trials [1–3], but critical evaluations could not establish a clear role for such therapy [4,5]. Nevertheless, *bona fide* anecdotal reports of spontaneous remission in AML continued to appear in the literature [6–9], all of these occurring in the setting of infection, consistent with the observation that antibody responses to *pseudomonas* may be correlated with improved probability of chemotherapy-induced complete remission [10].

With the advent of allogeneic bone marrow transplantation as curative therapy for AML, the role of immunotherapy in the myeloid leukemias became unequivocally established [11–19]. The data supporting the role of a graft-versus-leukemia [GVL] effect emanated from an increased rate of leukemia relapse following syngeneic transplants or after T cell depletion for allogeneic transplantation and the apparently beneficial effect of graft-versus-host disease [GVHD] in maintaining a long-term disease-free survival. Other clinical data supporting a GVL effect have come from reports of patients with recurrent disease who enter remission after a flare-up of GVHD or after induction of GVHD with infusion of peripheral blood buffy coat cells, or following withdrawal of immune suppressive therapy [20–26]. Due to the close association of GVHD and GVL it was initially thought that any beneficial effect of GVL could only be demonstrated in the allogeneic bone marrow transplant setting. It was presumed that GVHD and GVL are mediated by the identical subset of cells. However, only about 20–30% of patients have a histocompatible sibling and,

[1] Hematology Unit, University of Rochester Medical Center, Rochester, NY, USA
[2] Pharmacia Oncology, Helsingborg, Sweden and Columbus, OH, USA
[3] Division of Hematology, University Hospital, Uppsala, Sweden

although the use of matched unrelated donors is increasing [27–29], the toxicity associated with these procedures is often prohibitive. Attempts have therefore been made to identify the effector cell, or cells, associated with GVL and develop methods to induce their proliferation or reactivity in circumstances devoid of classic GVHD such as autologous bone marrow transplantation. The theoretical advantages are enormous in that the hitherto main cause of treatment failure after autologous bone marrow transplantation - high relapse rate - may be significantly lowered. Additionally, the toxicity from autologous transplantation, both morbidity and mortality, is far less than from any form of allogeneic bone marrow transplantation. Furthermore, this would considerably widen the availability of this form of therapy, as all patients can be their own donors and the upper age limit can often be extended to approximately 65 years.

Advances in the clinical use of immunotherapy have evolved around a clearer understanding of immunocompetent cells, and the various immunomodulatory substances collectively known as immunomodulating agents. The most important cells and agents involved in this complex set of reactions and under active preclinical and clinical investigation are listed in Table 1.

Immunocompetent Effector Cells Associated with Eradication of Minimal Residual Disease

Natural killer (NK) and lymphokine activated killer (LAK) cells. NK cells are known to have an inhibitory effect on normal hematopoiesis [30–31] as well as leukemic hematopoiesis [32] and established leukemia cell lines [33]. The ability of NK cells to lyse K562, a cell line derived from a patient with CML, suggests that enhancing NK cell number or activity might be clinically useful. Both NK and LAK cells are capable of lysing allogeneic and autologous leukemia cells. Following allogenic, and to a lesser extent, autologous bone marrow transplantation, there is a marked increase in the number of endogenously generated activated NK cells [34–35]. These NK cells are often capable of lysing cryopreserved, recipient CML cells *in vitro* as well as inhibiting leukemic progenitor colony growth without affecting colony-forming unit granulocyte-macrophage (CFU-GM) [36–37].

Table 1. The most important immunotherapeutic mediators in the myeloid leukemias

Immunocompetent cells	Immunomodulating agents
T-lymphocytes	IL-2
NK cells	Roquinimex
Macrophages	Interferons
	Cyclosporine A

Data are available which suggest that the best prospect for enhancement of NK cell activity are in complete clinical remission or minimal residual disease [38]. Furthermore, studies on NK cell function in patients with acute myelogenous leukemia (AML) after autologous bone marrow transplantation demonstrate an inverse relationship between NK cell activity and the risk of leukemia relapse. Thus, low NK cell activity after autologous bone marrow transplantation is likely to predict for a higher rate of relapse, and vice versa [39].

T lymphocytes. It has been shown that antigenic tumors can be completely eradicated by the transfer of T cells specifically immune to the tumor-associated antigens [40–42]. The role of T lymphocytes and minimal residual disease in leukemias has now been established based on the previously cited data demonstrating that allogeneic transplantation with T lymphocyte depletion from the donor marrow leads to significantly decreased incidence and severity of GVHD as well as reduced GVL, leading to a higher leukemic relapse rate. The initial interpretation of these data were that T-lymphocytes, in some way, mediate both GVHD and GVL and the two are interdependent. However a large survey from the international bone marrow transplant registry (IBMTR) [43] reported that the *relative risk* for relapse for patients receiving T-lymphocyte-depleted marrow transplants was greater than that observed for patients undergoing syngeneic transplants and both were significantly greater than the risk of relapse in patients undergoing allogeneic transplantation without T cell depletion in whom GVHD did not develop. This suggests a T-lymphocyte-mediated antileukemic effect that may be *independent* of GVHD or, at least, clinically apparent GVHD [44]. It is highly likely that GVHD and GVL are not mediated by identical cells, but rather overlapping subsets of cells. Supporting these clinical observations are experimental data showing antileukemic activity for both CD4+ and CD8+ alloreactive cytotoxic lymphocytes [45–46], although the CD4 cytotoxic lymphocytes (CTL) appear to play a greater role than the CD8 CTL [47]. Clinical data that may support the preferential GVL effect of CD4+ cells have been suggested from results of marrow purging with anti-CD8 monoclonal antibodies [48]. In this report, although the residual CD4 T-cell were capable of causing GVHD, the incidence of GVHD was lower than expected with pharmacologic prophylaxis, and the relapse rate was much lower than expected.

Macrophages. NK and LAK cells, macrophages can also be cytotoxic for tumor cells independent of the major histocompatibility complex (MHC). Published reports [49–51] describe the multiple potential effects of macrophages. They can be phagocytic, mediate antibody-dependent cellular toxicity, or, like NK cells, macrophages may be preferentially cytotoxic for tumor cells upon direct contact even in the absence of antibody. Numerous cytotoxic mediators have been implicated including cytolytic proteases, tumor necrosis-factor alpha (TNF-α) and related factors, interferon alpha (IFN-α), interleukin-2 (IL-2), reactive oxygen intermediates, arginase, thymidine and lysosomal enzymes [52].

Roquinimex as an Immunomodulating Agent

While several immunomodulating agents have been described, this report will focus on the preclinical data and clinical studies using roquinimex.

Preclinical data with roquinimex. Roquinimex (Linomide) is a quinoline derivative (Fig. 1) that is orally active.

Fig. 1. The structure of roquinimex

This novel immunomodulator enhances T-cell, NK cell and monocyte/macrophage activity [53–57]. The broad immunomodulatory properties of roquinimex have been associated with therapeutic effects in both primary tumors and metastases as well as parasitic and viral infections in several rodent models [56,58–60].

In a pilot study of patients with myeloid leukemia following autologous bone marrow transplantation, eleven patients were treated with roquinimex. The compound was administered intermittently, being given for three weeks then held for the other three weeks. In this way the patients acted as their own controls enabling an accurate assessment of the activity of roquinimex [61,62]. Figures 2 and 3 show that the classic NK immunophenotypes, CD16+ and CD56+/CD3−, were found to increase significantly during treatment cycles.

These quantitative observations were accompanied by functional studies which also indicated enhanced cytotoxic activity of patient cells against the NK-sensitive K562 cell line (Fig. 4).

Similar effects could be repeatedly observed with subsequent administrations of roquinimex (Fig. 5).

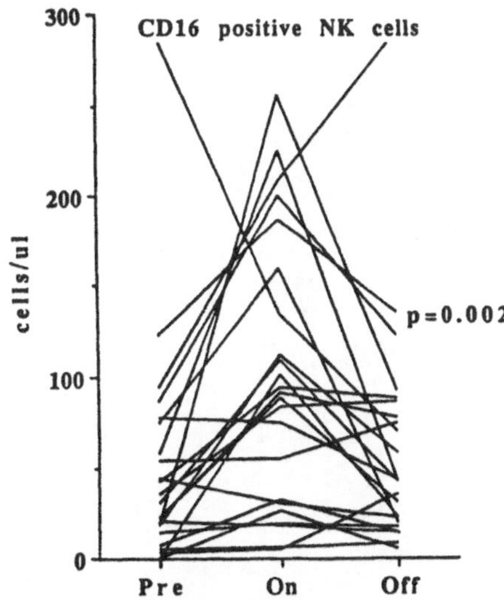

Fig. 2. Absolute numbers (cells/μL) of CD16+ NK-like cells in peripheral blood before, during and after roquinimex therapy. Pre-treatment values were obtained during the week preceeding the start of roquinimex therapy and on-treatment are from the week following the last dose in each treatment cycle. Off-treatment values were obtained 2–3 weeks after cessation of roquinimex. Reproduced with permission [62]

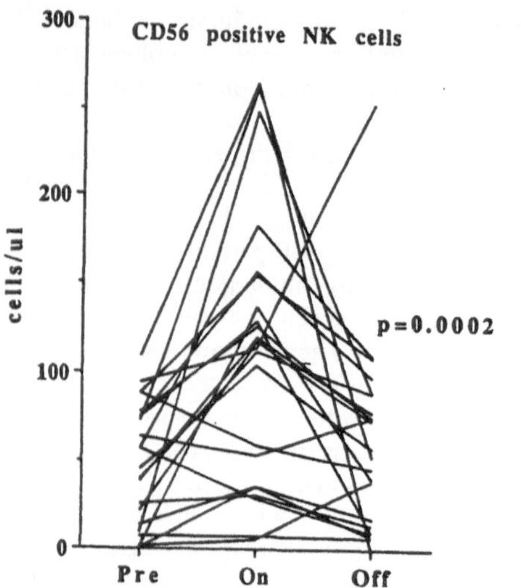

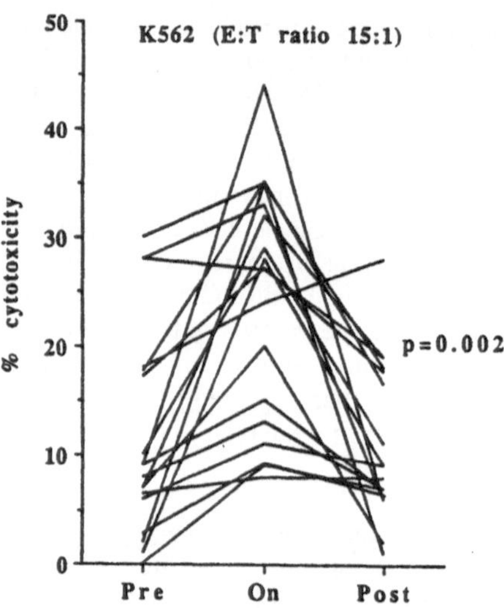

Fig. 3. Absolute numbers (cells/μL) of CD56+/CD3− NK-like cells in peripheral blood before, during and after roquinimex therapy. Other details as in legend to Figure 2. Reproduced with permission [62]

Fig. 4. Changes in the cytotoxic activity of patient cells during roquinimex therapy. Cytotoxic activity was measured in the standard chromium release assay against the NK-sensitive K562 cell line. Reproduced with permission [62]

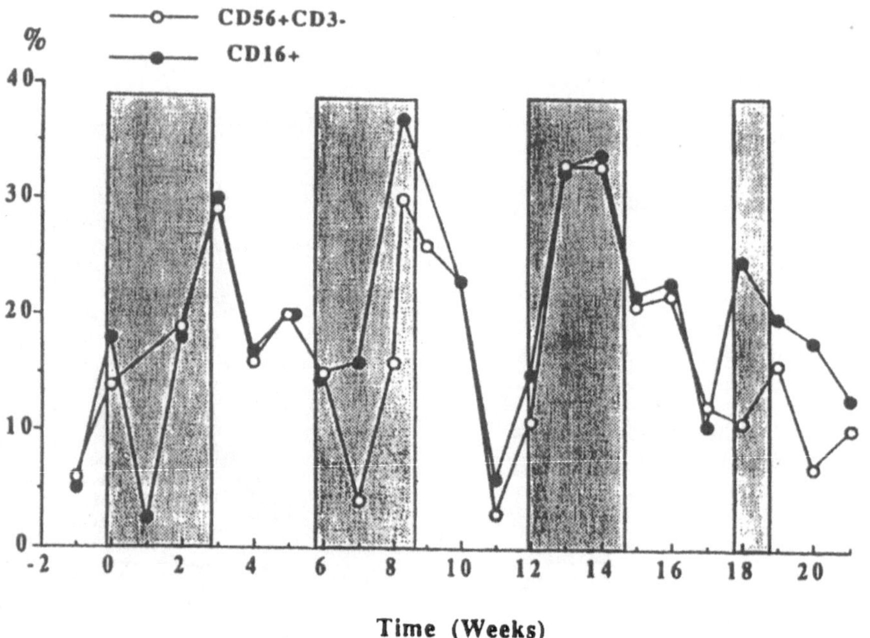

Fig. 5. Prospective monitoring of the percentage of CD16+ and CD56+/CD3− cells in peripheral blood in one patient. Treatment periods are indicated by shaded areas. Reproduced with permission [61]

The cyclic effect on the CD14+ monocytic cells was also observed (data not shown).

In these pilot studies, no harmful effects on engraftment were observed and the side effects in general were mild to moderate. These consist mainly of musculoskeletal aches, nausea, vomiting, edema, skin rash and diarrhea – all of which were usually easily managed with symptomatic treatment.

In addition to the enhancement of NK cell, T-cell and monocytic activity, roquinimex also enhances the delayed hypersensitivity reaction, the ability of lymphocytes to respond to B and T-cell mitogens and has adjuvant effects on antibody production (Table 2) [53–56].

Table 2. Immunological effects of roquinimex

1. Increase of NK cell precursors.
2. Augmentation of NK cell activity.
3. Increased delayed type hypersensitivity (DTH) reaction.
4. Increased proliferative response to T cell mitogens.
5. Cyclosporine antagonism.
6. Increased in vitro production of TNFa, IL-1 and IFNγ.
7. Increased IL-6 serum levels.

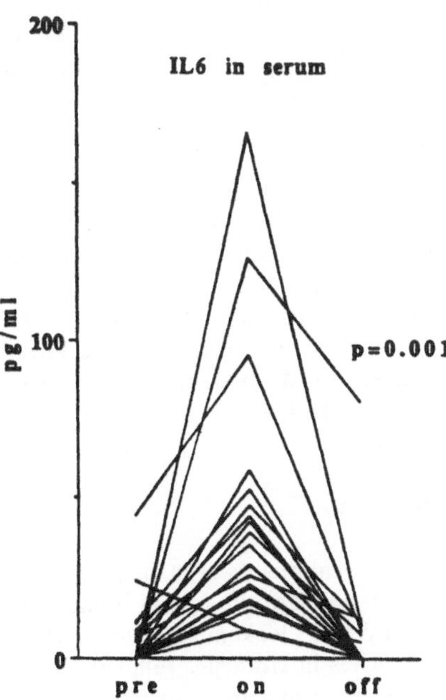

Fig. 6. Levels of IL-6 in peripheral blood before, during and after roquinimex therapy. Reproduced with permission [62]

Furthermore, it has recently been reported that IL-6 levels are also increased in the serum during treatment with roquinimex (Fig. 6) [62].

The mechanism of action of roquinimex is not well understood, and it is thought to represent a cascade-like effect since several different steps in macrophage and lymphocyte function are stimulated by roquinimex [53,56,59,63]. Roquinimex is well absorbed after oral administration with a plasma half-life in man of approximately 30-60 hours. The bioavailability of roquinimex after oral administration exceeds 90%. These features make it very practical to administer and conduct clinical trials.

The pharmacokinetics of roquinimex are not dose-dependent. In human phase I studies, NK cell number and function increased at dose levels of 0.2 and 0.3 mg/kg. Administration of higher doses do not lead to further enhancement of NK number and activity.

Clinical Trials with Roquinimex

Acute myelogenous leukemia. The availability of roquinimex to enhance immunocompetent cells such as T-cell, NK cells and macrophages – coupled with its relatively low toxicity profile and ease of administration, has led to several well designed major clinical trials evaluating the role of roquinimex and minimal residual disease [64]. In order to evaluate the activity of roquinimex in the treatment of minimal residual disease in patients with AML, two major international prospective phase III placebo-controlled double-blind studies are now underway studying the activity of roquinimex when administered post autologous bone marrow transplantation for patients in first or subsequent clinical remission. In a multi-center trial in the USA/Canada/Australia (Fig. 7) roquinimex is administered as soon as engraftment of 100 neutrophils/μL has occurred.

The starting dose of roquinimex is 0.05 mg/kg given orally twice a week and this is rapidly escalated, over two weeks, to 0.2 mg/kg which is the dose given for 12 months. An international study in Europe is very similar in design with the exception that roquinimex administration is started on day 14 irrespective of the level of engraftment and this is continued for a two year period. The European study has now accrued over 250 patients and the USA/Canada/Australia study has accrued over 150

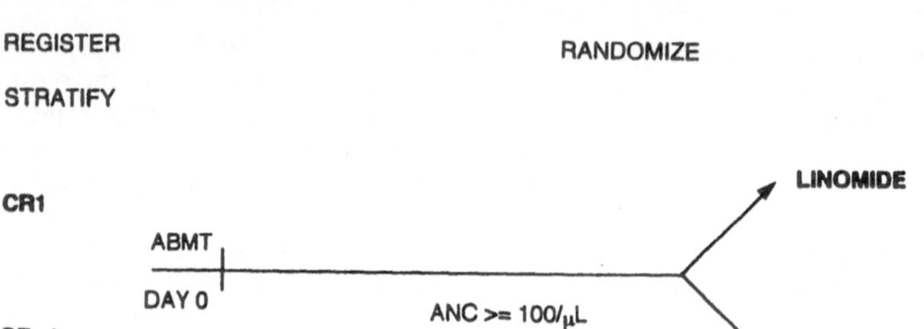

Fig. 7. Design of a current multi-institutional phase III study using roquinimex post-ABMT for AML patients in complete remission. US-Canadian-Australian international study (T91OL01)

patients. Because both studies are blinded, no interim efficacy data are available on the relapse rate or the time to relapse. However, the overall hematopoietic recovery pattern is typical of that seen post-ABMT without roquinimex. Correlative immunological studies are being performed in these phase III double-blind clinical studies and the results of these studies are anxiously awaited and should provide important information on the role of immunotherapy with roquinimex in acute myelogenous leukemia.

Chronic myelogenous leukemia. The activity of roquinimex in the myeloid leukemias may not be limited to AML. There is evidence that of all hematopoietic neoplasms, chronic myelogenous leukemia (CML) may be particularly susceptible to immune regulation [44]. The increased relapse rate post allogeneic transplantation in T-cell depleted donor marrow is greatest in CML patients [43,65]. Additionally, as previously described, patients relapsing after allogeneic BMT for CML have recently been shown to respond to infusions of donor T-lymphocytes with complete reversal of all cytogenetic abnormalities [21,26]. In a recent summary of the published literature regarding the therapeutic use of buffy coat infusions for patients who relapse after allogeneic BMT [25], it was reported that in a total of 46 patients, the overall clinical response was 83% with a cytogenetic remission reported in 20 of 25 evaluable patients (80%). 80% of patients were also reported to have suffered from grade 1–4 acute graft-versus-host disease. These data suggest that CML may be a particular candidate for immunomodulation following autologous bone marrow transplantation. A pilot study has been initiated in 1992 at the University of Rochester, Rochester, NY, USA, with a study design that was quite similar to the phase III study in AML (Fig. 7). Open-label roquinimex was used and all patients were conditioned with busulfan 1 mg/kg po q6h for four days followed by cyclophosphamide 60 mg/kg/day for two days. Unmanipulated bone marrow was used as the source of stem cells. Following engraftment (absolute neutrophil count >100/μL), patients are treated with roquinimex for two years. The pilot study is still at its infancy, but 12 patients have entered this study and some significant clinical as well as cytogenetic responses have been observed [66]. These initial results are intriguing and further accrual and follow-up is needed before any definitive conclusions can be made. Whether or not a true graft-versus-leukemia effect can be induced in CML patients receiving roquinimex remains to be seen.

Summary

Rapid developments over the past decade in our understanding of the role of immunotherapy in the myeloid leukemias have led to novel approaches in strategies following chemotherapy and bone marrow transplantation. The lack of an immunotherapeutic effect has been considered one of the main reasons for the high rate of leukemia relapse following autologous bone marrow transplantation. This review summarizes the rationale for studying the use of immunotherapy following autologous bone marrow transplantation through efforts to stimulate the immune responses after identifying the most important immunocompetent cells and immunomodulating agents. This is a novel area that has generated much enthusiasm and it is likely that its use will be further enhanced following the results of ongoing major clinical trials. Roquinimex appears to be one promising such agent because of its wide spectrum of immunomodulatory activity, low toxicity profile, and ease of administration.

References

1. Gutterman JU, Hersh RM, Rodriguez V, McCredie KB, Mavligit G, Reed R, Burgess MA, Smith T, Gehan E, Bodey GP, Sr. Freireich EJ (1974) Chemoimmunotherapy of adult acute leukaemia. Lancet, 2, 1405–9
2. Whiteside MG, Cauchi MN, Paton C, Stone J (1976) Chemoimmunotherapy for maintenance in acute myeloblastic leukemia. Cancer, 38, 1581–6
3. Whittaker JA (1980) Immunotherapy in the treatment of acute leukaemia. British Journal of Haematology, 45, 187–93
4. Galton DAG, Kay HE, Reizenstein P, Penchansky M, Vogler WR, Whittaker JA (1977) Infection and second-remission rates in patients having immunotherapy for acute myeloid leukemia. Lancet, 2, 973
5. Bennett JM, Begg CB (1981) Eastern Cooperative Oncology Group study of the cytochemistry of adult acute myeloid leukemia by correlation of subtypes with response and survival. Cancer Research, 41, 4833–7
6. Ifrah N, James JM, Viguie JPM, Marie JP, Zittoun R (1985) Spontaneous remission in adult acute leukemia. Cancer, 56, 1187–90
7. Enck RE (1985) Spontaneous complete remission in acute promyelocytic leukemia. New York State Journal of Medicine, 88, 662–3
8. Takaue Y, Culbert SJ, van Eys J, Dalton WT Jr, Cork A, Trujillo JM (1986) Spontaneous cure of end-stage nonlymphocytic leukemia complicated with chloroma (granulocytic sarcoma) Cancer, 58, 1101–5
9. Jehn UW, Mempel MA (1986) Spontaneous remission of acute myeloid leukemia. Blut, 52, 165–8
10. Passe S, Mike V, Mertelsmann R, Gee TS, Clarkson BD (1982) Acute nonlymphoblastic leukemia: prognostic factors in adults with long-term follow-up. Cancer, 50, 1462–71
11. Weiden PL, Sullivan KM, Flournoy N, Storb R, Thomas ED (1981) Antileukemic effect of chronic graft-versus-host disease: contribution to improved survival after allogeneic marrow transplantation. New England Journal of Medicine, 304, 1529–33
12. Sullivan KM, Fefer A, Witherspoon R (1987) Graft-versus-leukemia in man: Relationship with acute and chronic graft-versus-host disease to relapse of acute leukemia following allogeneic bone marrow transplantation in Cellular Immunotherapy of Cancer edited by RL Truitt, RP Gale and MM Bortin, pp. 391–399, New York: Alan R. Liss, Inc
13. Horowitz MM, Gale RP, Sondel PM, Goldman JM, Kersey J, Kolb HJ, Rimm AA, Ringden O, Rozman C, Speck B (1990) Graft-versus-leukemia reactions after bone marrow transplantation. Blood, 75, 555–62
14. Weisdorf DJ, Nesbit ME, Ramsay NKC, Woods WG, Goldman AI, Kim TH, Hurd DD, McGlave PB, Kersey JH (1987) Allogeneic bone marrow transplantation for acute lymphoblastic leukemia in remission: prolonged survival associated with acute graft-versus-host disease. Journal of Clinical Oncology, 5, 1348–55
15. Butturini A, Bortin MM, Gale RP (1987) Graft-versus-leukemia following bone marrow transplantation. Bone Marrow Transplantation, 2, 233–42
16. Fefer A, Sullivan KM, Weiden P, Buckner CD, Schoch G, Storb R, Thomas ED (1987) Graft versus leukemia effect in man: the relapse rate of acute leukemia is lower after allogeneic than after syngeneic marrow transplantation. Progress in Clinical & Biological Research, 244, 401–8
17. Sullivan KM, Storb R, Buckner CD, Fefer A, Fisher L, Weiden PL, Witherspoon RP, Appelbaum FR, Banaji M, Hansen J et al. (1989) Graft-versus-host disease as adoptive immunotherapy in patients with advanced hematologic neoplasms. New England Journal of Medicine, 320, 828–34
18. Goldman JM, Gale RP, Horowitz MM, Biggs JC, Champlin RE, Gluckman E, Hoffmann RG, Jacobsen SJ, Marmont AM, McGlave PB (1988) Bone marrow transplantation for chronic myelogenous leukemia in chronic phase. Increased risk for relapse associated with T-cell depletion. Annals of Internal Medicine, 108, 806–14
19. Butturini A, Gale RP (1987) The role of T-cells in preventing relapse in chronic myelogenous leukemia. Bone Marrow Transplantation, 2, 351–4
20. Odon LF, August CS, Githens JH, Humbert JR (1981) "Graft-versus-leukemia" reaction following bone marrow transplantation for acute lymphoblastic leukemia in Graft-versus-leukemia in man and animal models edited by O'Kunewick JT, Meredith RF, pp. 25–31, Boca Raton FL: CRC
21. Kolb HJ, Mittermuller J, Klemm C, Heller E, Ledderose G, Brehm G, Heim M, Wilmann SW (1990) Donor leukocyte transfusions for treatment of recurrent chronic myelogenous leukemia in marrow transplantations. Blood, 76, 2462–2465
22. Drobyski WR, Keever CA, Roth KS, Koethe S, Hanson G, McFadden P, Gottschall JL, Ash RC, vanTuinen T, Horowitz MM, Flomenberg N (1993) Salvage immunotherapy using donor leukocyte infusions as treatment for relapsed chronic myelogenous leukemia after allogeneic bone marrow

transplantation: Efficacy and Toxicity of a defined T-cell dose. Blood, 82, 2310–2318
23. Szer J, Grigg AP, Phillips GL, Sheridan WP (1993) Donor leucocyte infusions after chemotherapy for patients relapsing with acute leukemia following allogeneic bone marrow transplant. Bone Marrow Transplantation, 11, 109–111
24. Bar BM, Schattenberg A, Mensink EJ, Geurts van Kessel A, Smetsers TF, Knops EH, Linders EH, DeWite T (1993) Donor leukocyte infusions for chronic myeloid leukemia relapsed after allogeneic bone marrow transplantation. Journal of Clinical Oncology, 11 (3), 513–519
25. Antin JH. (1993) Graft-versus-leukemia: No longer an epiphenomenon. Blood, 82, 2273–2278
26. Cullis JO, Jiang YZ, Schwarer AP, Hughes TP, Barrett AJ, Goldman JM (1992) Donor leukocyte infusions for chronic myeloid leukemia in relapse after allogeneic bone marrow transplantation. Blood, 79, 1379–1381
27. Ash RC, Casper JT, Chitambar CR, Hansen R, Bunin N, Truitt RL (1990) Successful allogeneic transplantation of T-cell-depleted bone marrow from closely HLA-matched unrelated donors. New England Journal of Medicine, 322, 485–494
28. Beatty PG, Hansen JA, Longton GM, Thomas ED, Sanders JE, Martin PJ (1991) Marrow transplantation from HLA-matched unrelated donors for treatment of hematologic malignancies. Transplantation, 51, 443–447
29. Kernan NA, Bartsch G, Ash RC, Beatty PG, Champlin R, Pilipovich A (1993) Analysis of 462 transplantations from unrelated donors facilitated by the National Marrow Donor Program. New England Journal of Medicine, 328, 593–602
30. Vinci G, Vernant JP, Nakazawa M, Zohair M, Katz A, Henri A, Rochant H, Breton-Gorius J, Vainchenker W (1988) In vitro inhibition of normal human hematopoiesis by marrow CD3+, CD8+, HLA-DR+, HNK1+ lymphocytes. Blood, 72, 1616–21
31. Vinci G, Vernant JP, Cordonnier C, Henri A, Breton-Gorius J, Rochant H, Vainchenker W (1987) In vitro inhibition of hematopoiesis by HNK1, DR-positive T cells and monocytes after allogeneic bone marrow transplantation. Experimental Hematology, 15, 54–64
32. Lotze MT, Grimm EA, Mazumder A, Strausser JL, Rosenberg SA (1981) Lysis of fresh and cultured autologous tumor by human lymphocytes cultured in T-cell growth factor. Cancer Research, 41, 4420–5
33. Lotzova E, Savary CA, Herberman RB (1987) Induction of NK cell activity against fresh human leukemia in culture with the interleukin 2. Journal of Immunology, 138, 2718–27
34. Reittie JE, Gottlieb D, Heslop HE, Leger O, Drexler HG, Hazelhurst G, Hoffbrand AV, Prentice HG, Brenner MK (1989) Endogenously generated activated killer cells circulate after autologous and allogeneic marrow transplantation but not after chemotherapy. Blood, 73, 1351–8
35. Hauch M, Azzola MV, Small T, Bordignon C, Barnett L, Cunningham I, Castro-Malaspinia H, O'Reilly RJ, Keever CA (1990) Anti-leukemia potential of interleukin-2 activator natural killer cells after bone marrow transplantation of chronic myelogenous leukemia. Blood, 75, 2250–2254
36. Jiang YZ, Cullis JO, Kanfer EJ, Goldman JM, Barrett AJ (1993) T-cell and NK cell mediated graft-versus-leukemia reactivity following donor buffy coat transfusion to treat relapse after marrow transplantation for chronic myeloid leukemia. Bone Marrow Transplantation, 11, 133–136
37. MacKinnon S, Hows JM, Goldman JM (1990) Induction of *in vitro* graft-versus-leukemia activity following bone marrow transplantation for chronic myeloid leukemia. Blood 76, 2037–2040
38. Simonsson B, Nilsson BI, Rowe JM (1992) Treatment of minimal residual disease in acute leukemia – focus on immunotherapeutic options. Leukemia, 6 (Suppl 4), 124–34
39. Pizzolo G, Trentin L, Vinante F, Agostini C, Zambello R, Masciarelli M, Feruglio C, Dazzi F, Todeschini G, Chilosi M, et al (1988) Natural killer cell function and lymphoid subpopulations in acute non-lymphoblastic leukaemia in complete remission. British Journal of Cancer, 58, 368–72
40. Fefer A, Cheever M, Greenberg P (1982) Lymphocyte transfer as potential cancer immunotherapy, in Immunological Approaches to Cancer Therapeutics edited by Mihiche, pp. 299–332. New York: John Wiley and Sons
41. Fefer A, Cheever M, Greenberg P (1982) Overview of prospects and problems of lymphocyte transfer for cancer therapy, in Progress in Cancer Research and Therapy: The Potential Role of T-cells in Cancer Therapy, Vol 22 edited by Fefer A, Goldstein AL, pp. 126, New York: Raven Press
42. Rosenberg S, Packard B, Aebersold P (1988) Use of tumor-infiltrating lymphocytes and interleukin-2 in the immunotherapy of patients with metastatic melanoma: A preliminary report. New England Journal of Medicine, 319, 1676–1680
43. Horowitz MM, Gale RP, Sondel PM, Goldman JM, Kersey J, Kolb HJ, Rimm AA, Ringden O, Rozman C, Speck B (1990) Graft-versus-leukemia reactions after bone marrow transplantation. Blood, 75, 555–62
44. Barrett A, Jiang YZ (1992) Immune responses to chronic myeloid leukaemia. Bone Marrow Transplantation, 9, 305–11
45. Sosman JA, Oettel KR, Smith SD, Hank JA, Fisch P, Sondel PM (1990) Specific recognition of human leukemic cells by allogeneic T-cells: II. Evidence for HLA-D restricted determinants on leukemic cells that are crossreactive with determinants present on unrelated nonleukemic cells. Blood, 75, 2005–16
46. Falkenberg JHF, Goselink HM, Van der Harst D, Faber L, Fibbe WE, Willemze R, Brand A, Goulmy E (1990) Specific lysis of clonogenic leukemic cells (CLC) by cytotoxic T lymphocytes (CTL) against minor histocompatibility (MH) antigens: An *in vitro* model for graft vs leukemia (GVL). Experimental Hematology, 18, 682(abstract)
47. Jiang YZ, Kanfer E, Macdonald D, Cullis JO, Goldman JM, Barrett AJ (1991) Graft-versus-

leukaemia effect following allogeneic bone marrow transplantation: emergence of cytotoxic T lymphocytes reacting to host leukaemia cells. Bone Marrow Transplantation, 8, 253–8
48. Champlin R, Ho W, Gajewski J, Feig S, Burnison M, Holley G, Greenberg P, Lee K, Schmid I, Giorgi J, Yam P, Petz L, Winston D, Warner N, Reichert T (1990) Selective depletion of CD8+ T lymphocytes for prevention of graft-versus-host disease after allogeneic bone marrow transplantation. Blood, 76, 418–422
49. Melzer MS, Nacy CA (1989) Delayed type hypersensitivity in the induction of activated, cytotoxic macrophages, in Fundamental Immunology edited by P. Wee, pp. 735–764. New York: Raven Press
50. Fidler IJ, Schroit AJ (1988) Recognition and destruction of neoplastic cells by activated macrophages: discrimination of altered self. Biochimica et Biophysica Acta, 948, 151–73
51. Drysdale BE, Agarwal S, Shin HS (1988) Macrophage-mediated tumoricidal activity: mechanisms of activation and cytotoxicity. Progress In Allergy, 40, 111–61
52. Wunderlich JR, Hodes RJ (1991) Principles of tumor immunity: Biology of cellular immune responses in Biologic Therapy of Cancer edited by V.T. DeVita, S. Hellman, and S.A. Rosenberg, pp. 3–21. Philadelphia: J.B. Lippincott Co
53. Kalland T (1990) Regulation of natural killer progenitors. Studies with a novel immunomodulator with distinct effects at the precursor level. Journal of Immunology, 144, 4472–6
54. Larsson EL, Joki A, Stalhandske T (1987) Mechanism of action of the immunomodulator LS 2616 on T cell responses. International Journal of Immunopharmacology, 9, 425–31
55. Stalhandske T, Kalland T (1986) Effects of the novel immunomodulator LS 2616 on the delayed-type hypersensitivity reaction to Bordetella pertussis in the rat. Immunopharmacology, 11, 87–92
56. Kalland T (1986) Effects of the immunomodulator LS 2616 on growth and metastasis of the murine B16-F10 melanoma. Cancer Research, 46, 3018–22
57. Kalland T, Alm G, Stalhandske T (1985) Augmentation of mouse natural killer cell activity by LS 2616, a new immunomodulator. Journal of Immunology, 134, 3956–61
58. Kalland T, Maksimova A, Stalhandske T (1985) Prophylaxis and treatment of experimental tumors with the immunomodulator LS 2616. International Journal of Immunopharmacology, 7, 390
59. Stalhandske T, Jansson AH, Karlstrom R, Maksimova A, Wigow U, Kalland T (1985) Restoration of suppressed immune response with a new modulator quinoline-3-carboxamide (LS 2616) during experimental trypansoma infection. International Journal of Immunopharmacology, 7, 391
60. Ilback NG, Fohlman J, Slorach S, Friman G (1989) Effects of the immunomodulator LS 2616 on lymphocyte subpopulations in murine Coxsackievirus B3 myocarditis. Journal of Immunology, 142, 3225–8
61. Bengtsson M, Simonsson B, Carlsson K, Nilsson B, Smedmyr B, Termander B, Oberg G, Totterman T (1992) Stimulation of NK cell, T cell, and monocyte functions by the novel immunomodulator Linomide after autologous bone marrow transplantation. A pilot study in patients with acute myeloid leukemia. Transplantation, 53, 882–8
62. Nilsson BI, Simonsson B, Bengtsson M, Tötterman TH, Johansson C, Rowe JM (1993). Immunotherapy of AML after ABMT – Scientific rationale and early experiences with Linomide in Sixth International Symposium on Autologous Bone Marrow Transplantation, eds. Dicke KA, Keating A. Cancer Treatment Research Education Fund, Arlington TX, pp. 38–44, 1993
63. Tarkowski A, Gunnarsson K, Stalhandske T (1986) Effects of LS-2616 administration upon the autoimmune disease of (NZB × NZW) F1 hybrid mice. Immunology, 59, 689–94
64. Rowe JM, Nilsson BI, Simonsson B (1993) Treatment of minimal residual disease in myeloid leukemia – the immunotherapeutic options with emphasis on Linomide. Leukemia & Lymphoma, 11, 321–329
65. Apperley JF, Jones L, Hale G, Waldmann H, Hows J, Rombos Y, Tsatalas C, Marcus RE, Goolden AW, Gordon-Smith EC, et al (1986) Bone marrow transplantation for patients with chronic myeloid leukaemia: T-cell depletion with Campath-1 reduces the incidence of graft-versus-host disease but may increase the risk of leukaemic relapse. Bone Marrow Transplantation, 1, 53–66
66. Rowe J, Ryan D, DiPersio J, Gaspari A, Nilsson B, Larsson L, Liesveld J, Kouides P, Simonsson B (1993) Autografting in chronic myelogenous leukemia followed by immunotherapy. Stem Cells, 11 (Suppl 3), 34–42

Acute Leukemias V
Experimental Approaches
and Management of Refractory Diseases
Hiddemann et al. (Eds.)

The Inhibition of Lymphokine Activated Killer Cell Activation Mediated by AML Culture Supernatants Might Be Due to Transforming Growth Factor Beta1

D. K. Schui, J. Brieger, E. Weidmann, P. S. Mitrou, D. Hoelzer, and L. Bergmann

Introduction

The cytotoxic activity of peripheral mononuclear cells (PMNC) from patients with acute myelogenous leukemia (AML) is usually reduced at time of diagnosis [1, 2]. Production and release of immunosuppressive cytokines by leukemic blast cells might be a cause for impaired cytotoxic activity and immunosurveillance of leukemic cells. Indeed, soluble but yet undefined factors secreted by AML blasts have been described to be reponsible for inhibited cytotoxic activity in AML patients [3, 4]. Transforming growth factor beta (TGF-β) has been reported to be a strong inhibitor of cytotoxic activity of lymphokine activated killer (LAK) cells [5–9]. In ovarian carcinoma, increased TGF-β secretion was shown to suppress various immune functions [10]. It may be suggested that TGF-β may be an important factor in AML, too, causing immunosuppression.

Therefore, the present study was designed to examine the possible effects of AML culture supernatants on LAK cell activity and to investigate the expression of mRNA and release of TGF-β_1 protein by leukemic blast cells.

Material and Methods

PCR. Total RNA was extracted from leukemic blast cells and reverse transcribed. The obtained cDNA was used for amplification with TGF-β_1 spezific oligonucleotides. The amplification was initiated at 94 °C for 5 min. prior addition of polymerase, followed by 35 cycles of amplification. Each cycle was started by denaturating the DNA for 30 sec. at 94°C, followed by the annealing reaction for 30 sec. at 62°C and an extending reaction for 30 sec. at 72°C. After the last cycle a final extension reaction for 7 min. at 72°C was applied. The amplification products were separated by electrophoresis on an 1% agarose gel.

Northern blot analysis. 10 mg samples of total RNA were separated by electrophoresis and blotted on nylon membrane for hybridization. TGF-β_1 spezific mRNA was detected using 32P labeled TGF-β_1 cDNA.

Culture supernatants. Leukemic blast cells were isolated from bone marrow or peripheral blood from patients with untreated AML using Ficoll separation. The cells were cultured in AIM-V Medium. After 24h of culture at 37°C and 5% CO_2 supernatants were harvested and frozen at −20 °C until further use.

TGF-β Bioassay. TGF-β protein concentration was measured by growth inhibition of mink lung epithelial cells CCL 64. After trypsination, cells were cultured for 24 hours. Supernatants and TGF-β_1 standards were cocultured for further 24 hours. Subsequently ^{3}H-thymidine was added, cultured for 8–16 hours and counted on a beta counter.

Generation of LAK effector cells. After Ficoll separation of peripheral blood from normal donors mononuclear cells were cocultured at a concen-

Medical Clinic III, Hematology/Oncology, J. W. Goethe University, Frankfurt/M., Germany

tration of 2×10^6 cells/mL with 25U/mL recombinant interleukin 2 (rIL-2; EuroCetus, Frankfurt, FRG) and culture supernatants (5Vol%, 10Vol% or 25Vol%) in RPMI 1640 medium containing 10% FCS. AML culture supernatants were heated for 5 min. at 80 °C to activate latent TGF-β prior to addition to LAK cultures [11]. PMNCs were cultured for three days at 37 °C in 5% CO_2.

51Cr release assay. A 51Cr release assay was performed as described elsewhere [12]. NK resistant Daudi cells were used as targets. After radiolabeling with 100 mL sodium chromate (51Cr 100 Ci/mL) per 2×10^6 cells at 37 °C. After 2h target cells were washed three times and resuspended in RPMI 1640 medium at a concentration of 0.2×10^6 cells/mL. Effector cells from LAK cultures were added to target cells in effector to target ratios of 20:1, 10:1, 5:1 and 1:1. The assays were performed in duplicates. After 3h incubation at 37 °C 100L aliquots of supernatants were harvested and counted on a gamma counter.

Results

Expression of TGF-β_1 mRNA. Total RNA of leukemic blast cells of 13 patients with untreated AML was extracted and examined for TGF-β_1 mRNA expression using RT-PCR and Northern blotting. All investigated cases of AML blasts expressed detectable levels of TGF-β_1 mRNA. To ascertain that leukemic blasts are the source of TGF-β_1 mRNA, FACS sorted blast cells (purity >95%) were additionally analysed for TGF-β_1 mRNA expression. The data confirmed those of unseparated blast cells. Additionally, four leukemic cell lines (HL-60, K562, HEL92.1.7 and KG1) were analysed for TGF-β_1 mRNA by RT-PCR. In all four cell lines TGF-β_1 mRNA was demonstrable (Table 1).

Release of TGF-β protein. Leukemic blast cells from 10 patients with untreated AML were cultured in serum free AIM-V Medium at a concentration of 2×10^6 cells/mL. After 24 hours incubation at 37 °C supernatants were harvested and explored for TGF-β protein and effects on LAK activity. The TGF-β concentration of culture supernatants was measured by growth inhibition of mink lung epithelial cells CCL64. In all tested AML culture supernatants TGF-β protein could be detected in concentrations from 0.6 to 6.8 ng/ml (Table 2).

Table 1. Expression of TGF-β_1 mRNA and release of TGF-β protein by leukemic cell lines

Cell line	TGF-β_1 PCR	TGF-β concentration (ng/ml)
K562	+	n.d.
HL-60	+	7.5
KG1	+	5.6
HEL92.1.7	+	12.0

n.d. = not done

Table 2. TGF-β concentration of AML culture supernatants and their inhibitory effects on LAK activity

Culture supernatants of AML patients	TGF-β concentration (ng/mL)	LAK activity (20LU/10^7)	LAK activity after addition of Anti-TGF-β_1
Controls (mean)	–	307	n.d.
AH	3.0	150[a]	n.d.
WK	0.9	100	n.d.
ML	2.6	150	n.d.
ES	3.3	170	n.d.
AM	6.8	48	n.d.
RE	1.8	70	n.d.
RW	2.2	110	n.d.
WS	5.2	115	n.d.
HR	n.d.	50	350
HM	0.6	150	300
CH	2.9	125	275

[a]Culture supernatants were added to PMNCs in three different concentrations (5 Vol%, 10 Vol% and 25 Vol%). Shown are only lytic units of the concentration in which inhibition occurred

Supernatants of three leukemic cell lines (HL-60, KG1 and HEL92.1.7) and FACS sorted blast cells (purity > 95%) from four patients were examined for TGF-β protein, too, to confirm leukemic cells as the source of TGF-β. Culture supernatants from FACS sorted cells contain TGF-β in concentrations between 1.3 to 6.0 ng/mL and all three examined leukemic cell lines produced and secreted high levels of TGF-β (5.6 to 12 ng/mL) (Table 1).

Inhibition of LAK activity by AML culture supernatants. To investigate the effects of AML culture supernatants on LAK activity, PMNCs from healthy donors were cocultured with different concentrations of culture supernatants in the presence of 25U/mL IL-2. After three days of incubation at 37 °C the LAK activity of cultured cells were measured using an 51Cr release assay against Daudi targets. Culture supernatants of AML patients reduced LAK activity down to 37% (mean of 11 patients, range from 16% to 55%) of control (100%) (Table 2). PMNCs cocultured with 25U/ml rIL-2 were used as controls.

The concentration of TGF-β in AML culture supernatants was measured by growth inhibition of CCL 64 cells. LAK activity was determined by 51Cr release assay against Daudi target cells. Effector cells were obtained from healthy donors PMNCs cocultured with AML culture supernatants and 25U/mL IL-2 for 3 days. PMNCs cocultured with 25U/mL rIL-2 were used as controls. In additional experiments TGF-β_1 neutralizing antibodies were added.

Reversibility of impaired LAK activity by addition of neutralizing TGF-β_1 antibodies. In additional experiments, PMNCs from healthy persons were cocultured with 25U/mL rIL-2, AML culture supernatants with or without addition of neutralizing TGF-β_1 antibodies. In this allogeneic system, the LAK activity could also be inhibited by AML culture supernatants in a dose dependent manner. If neutralizing antibodies to TGF-β_1 were added, the impaired LAK cell activity could totally be restored indicating TGF-β to be the most relevant inhibiting factor in AML culture supernatants.

Discussion

In acute leukemias unknown soluble factors have been described to reduce cytotoxic activity [3, 13, 14]. Since TGF-β_1 is known to be a strong inhibitor of cytotoxic activity, this study was performed to investigate the expression and protein release of TGF-β_1 by leukemic blast cells and to explore the effects of AML culture supernatants on generation of LAK cells [5, 6]. In all examined patients TGF-β_1 mRNA was detectable. To exclude that TGF-β_1 was produced and secreted by other cells than leukemic blast cells, four leukemic cell lines and FACS sorted blast cells (purity > 95%) from five patients were tested and in all of them TGF-β_1 mRNA was demonstrable. Besides transcription of TGF-β_1 mRNA, production and release of TGF-β protein could be detected in all examined culture supernatants from AML patients, leukemic cell lines and FACS sorted blast cells.

PMNCs from healthy donors cocultured with AML culture supernatants in the presence of IL-2 show strongly inhibition of LAK activity in comparison to control cultures incubated with IL-2 only. The inhibition of LAK activity by AML culture supernatants could be restored by addition of antibodies directed against TGF-β_1. These data taken together strongly suggest that TGF-β_1 expressed and released by leukemic blast cells might be involved in the mechanism of immunosuppression observed in acute leukemias. Investigations of a possible regulation of TGF-β release in AML blasts by cytokines as described for IL-2 and IFN-α in LAK cells may be interesting especially in regard to immunotherapeutic approaches in AML [15, 16]. The data of our study may be a further step in the understanding of cytokine network involved in immunosuppression by acute myeloid leukemias.

Acknowledgement. Supported by Deutsche Krebshilfe grant W22/92.

References

1. Foa R., Fierro M.T, Cesano A., Guarini A., Bonferroni M., Raspadori D., Miniero R., Lauria F., Gavosto F., Defective lymphokine activated killer cell generation and activity in acute leukemia patients with active disease (1991) Blood, 78: 1041–1046.
2. Archimbaud E., Bailly M., Doré J.F., Inducibility of lymphokine activated killer (LAK) cells in patients with acute myelogenous leukemia in complete remission and its clinical relevance (1991) Brit. J. Haematol 77: 328–334.

3. Chiao J.W., Heil M., Arlin Z., Lutton J.D., Choi Y.S., Leung K., Suppression of lymphocyte activation and functions by a leukemia cell derived inhibitor (1986) Proc. Natl. Acad. Science, 83: 3432–3436.
4. Archimbaud E., Thomas X., Campos L., Fiere D., Doré J.F. Susceptibility of acute myelogenous blasts to lysis by lymphokine-activated killer (LAK) cells and its clinical relevance (1992) Leuk. Res., 16: 673–680.
5. Kasid A., Bell G.I., Director E.P. Effects of transforming growth factor-β on human lymphokine-activated killer cell precursors (1988) J. Immun, 141: 690–698.
6. Jin B., Scott J.L., Vadas M.A., Burns G.F. TGFβ down-regulates TLiSA1 expression and inhibits the differentiation of precursors lymphocytes into CTL and LAK cells (1989) Immunol., 66: 570–576.
7. Smyth M.J., Strobl S.L., Young H.A., Ortaldo J.R., Ochoa A.C. Regulation of lymphokine-activated killer activity and pore-forming protein gene expression in human peripheral blood CD8+ T lymphocytes (1991) J. Immunol., 146: 3289–3297.
8. Mulé J.J., Schwarz S.L., Roberts A.B., Sporn M.B., Rosenberg S.A. Transforming growth factor-beta inhibits the in vitro generation of lymphokine-activated killer cells and cytotoxic T cells (1988) Cancer Immunol. Immunother., 26: 95–100.
9. Brooks B., Chapman K., Lawry J., Meager A., Rees R.C. Suppression of lymphokine-activated killer (LAK) cell induction mediated by interleukin-4 and transforming growth factor-β_1: effect of addition of exogenous tumour necrosis factor-alpha and interferon-gamma, and measurement of their endogenous production (1990) Clin. Exp. Immunol., 82: 583–589.
10. Hirte H., Clark D.A., Generation of lymphokine-activated killer cells in human ovarian carcinoma ascitic fluid: identification of transforming growth factor-β as a suppressive factor (1991) Cancer Immunol. Immunother., 32: 296–302.
11. Brown P.D., Wakefield L.M., Levinson A.D., Sporn M.B., Physicochemical activation of recombinant latent transforming growth factor-beta's 1, 2 and 3 (1990) Growth Factors, 3: 35–43.
12. Bergmann L., Fenchel K., Enzinger H.-M., Weidmann E., Jahn B., Jonas D., Mitrou P.S. Daily alternating application of high dose interferon-alpha2b and interleukin-2 bolus infusion in metastatic renal cell carcinoma (1993) Cancer, 72: 1733–1742.
13. Lim S.H., Worman C.P., Jewell A., Goldstone A.H. Production of tumor-derived suppressor factor in patients with acute myeloid leukemia. (1991) Leuk. Res., 15: 263–268.
14. Adler A., Albo V., Blatt J., Whiteside T.L., Herberman R.B. Interleukin-2 induction of lympokine-activated killer activity in the peripheral blood and bone marrow of acute leukemia patients: II. Feasibility of LAK generation in children with active disease and in remission (1989) Blood, 74: 1690–1697.
15. Jahn B., Brieger J., Fenchel K., Bergmann L., Mitrou P.S.: In vivo regulation of transforming growth factor-β_1 mRNA in combined cytokine therapy: Interleukin-2 impairs interferon-a stimulated increase in transforming growth factor steady state mRNA levels. Cancer Immunol. Immunother., in press.
16. Bergmann L., Heil G., Kolbe K., Lengfelder E., Brücher J., Lohmeyer J., Mitrou P.S., Hoelzer D.: Interleukin-2 as consolidation treatment in 2nd remission of AML. Blood 82 Suppl. (1993), 130a.

Acute Leukemias V
Experimental Approaches
and Management of Refractory Diseases
Hiddemann et al. (Eds.)

Natural Killer Cell Alloreactivity Against Acute Leukemia Blasts: The Level of Activity Depends on the Individual Target-Effector Pair

B. Glass[1], L. Uharek[1], H. Ullerich[2], T. Gaska[2], H. Löffler[1], W. M. Müller-Ruchholtz[2], and W. Gassmann[1]

Abstract: Natural killer (NK) cells appear to be involved in graft-versus-leukemia activity after allogeneic bone marrow transplantation. Since recent findings suggest that NK cells can exert specific activity against allogeneic leukocytes, we tested 10 subjects for differences in their NK and lymphokine-activated killer (LAK) cell activity against 4 allogeneic leukemia cell targets and the cell line K562. Our results support the hypothesis that NK cells can react against allogeneic leukemia cells specifically. Only three of the donors demonstrated either generally high or low NK cell activity and none of the leukemias turned out to be principally resistant or sensitive towards NK cell-mediated lysis. Thus, most of the variance must be explained by specific NK cell/target cell interactions resulting in a complex pattern of high or low NK cell-mediated cytotoxicity. There was no clear correlation between lytic activity against a certain leukemia target and lysis of K562 or between lytic activity and the percentage of CD16- or CD56-positive cells. Future studies with larger data samples might allow the definition of distinct groups according to the pattern of alloreactivity observed. Our findings are of relevance for the application of allogeneic NK cells in the context of cellular immunotherapy for hematological malignancies.

Introduction

Treatment of leukemia with allogeneic bone marrow transplantation (BMT) results in a substantial proportion of long-term survivors [1]. Besides intensified chemoradiotherapy, a contribution to the reduced relapse risk after BMT may be made by the transfer and activation of antileukemic effector cells [2,3,4]. Particular interest has emerged on the role of cytokines and activated natural killer cells that do not induce graft-versus-host disease but might be relevant for the elimination of residual leukemic blasts after BMT [5,6].

Although it is known for many years that NK cells exhibit cytolytic activity against different types of autologous and allogeneic leukemia targets, the precise mechanism of natural killing is still unclear [7,8,9]. In contrast to T cells, NK cells characteristically lyse allogeneic and autologous target cells without prior sensitisation, without MHC-restriction and seemingly without a highly refined antigen recognition system. Recent findings, however, demonstrated that the ability of NK cells to lyse allogeneic leukocytes is intraindividually a clonally distributed function and that NK cell clones can be separated into different groups according to their capacity to lyse only certain allogeneic targets [10,11,12]. Interindividual differences in the susceptibility or resistance of leukemia cells to lysis by allogeneic natural killer cells from different donors might also be expected. To test this hypothesis, we investigated the natural and lymphokine activated killer cell activity of 10 subjects against peripheral blasts of 4 patients with acute leukemias.

II. Medizinische Klinik[1] und Institut für Immunologie[2], Christian-Albrechts-Universität Kiel, Germany

Methods

Leukemia cell targets. The human erythroleukemic cell line K562 was maintained in continuous culture in RPMI 1640 supplemented with 10% fetal calf serum (FCS) and 2 mmol/l L-glutamine. Leukocytes of 4 patients with newly diagnosed acute leukemia were isolated from heparinized venous blood by centrifugation on standard Ficoll gradients. Specific characteristics of the leukemias are shown in Table 1. Approximately 85–95% of the cells from the gradient interphase were blasts. The cells were washed and resuspended in RPMI 1640 plus 10% FCS to a concentration of 1×10^7 cells/ml. Using 10% dimethylsulfoxide (DMSO), aliquots of 2×10^7 cells were stored in liquid nitrogen. Prior to their use in cytotoxicity assays, cells were thawed rapidly in a 37 °C water bath and were cultured for 24 hrs. Viability, determined by trypan blue dye exclusion, was at least 80%.

Isolation of effector cells. PBMC were isolated from blood donor buffycoats by centrifugation on Ficoll gradients. Cells collected from the gradient interphase were washed twice in RPMI 1640 Medium and were frozen in 10% DMSO. They were stored up to 150 days in liquid nitrogen. Viability and functional effectiveness was not essentially altered by the freezing procedure, since fresh and frozen effector cells of 3 individuals showed essentially the same reactivity against K562 target cells. The immunophenotypical characterisation of the effector cells is shown in Table 2.

Chromium release assay. Target cell sensitivity to NK-mediated cytolysis was determined in a standard 4-hr ^{51}Cr release assay. After 1 day of culture in RPMI 1640 supplemented with 10% fetal calf serum, frozen human leukemia target cells were washed and labeled with 100–150 uCi of ^{51}Cr sodium chromate for 1–2 hrs at 37 °C.

Table 1. Immunophenotype of the leukemia target cells

	Leukemia cells			
Antigen	L1 (AML M2)	L2 (AML M1)	L3 (AML M2)	L4 (ALL, Ph+)
CD 2	0	1	2	8
CD 3	0	0	2	6
CD 10	2	2	1	54
CD 11a	92	26	34	nd
CD 13	72	80	68	60
CD 14	74	10	2	nd
CD 18	94	24	36	nd
CD 19	0	15	4	78
CD 33	30	40	4	10
CD 34	0	63	3	22
CD 54	35	69	25	nd
HLA Kl.1	74	86	84	nd
HLA DR	9	6	8	5

Table 2. Immunophenotype of the lymphocyte effector cell samples

	% positive cells (for each subject investigated)									
Antigen	S1	S2	S3	S4	S5	S6	S7	S8	S9	S10
CD2	82	85	82	82	86	55	77	82	84	86
CD3	71	72	70	73	81	79	76	77	71	70
CD4	40	51	49	41	42	51	53	40	36	49
CD8	33	38	24	46	42	37	19	33	27	36
CD16	15	15	16	8	6	8	9	15	15	16
CD56	22	24	30	23	11	22	18	23	22	17
CD16/56	11	6	12	5	5	6	9	11	4	10
CD3/56	6	4	1	4	1	4	1	6	3	2

Washed target cells (1×10^4 cells/well) were added to wells of U-bottomed 96-well plates and incubated with effector cells at effector: target (E:T) ratios ranging from 50:1 to 6:1. Maximal release and spontaneous release were determined by incubating the cells with 5% Triton-X or medium alone, respectively. All determinations were made in quadruplicate. Radioactivity was determined in a gamma-counter and percentage of specific lysis according to the formula: %specific lysis = (experimental cpm – spontaneous cpm)/(maximum release cpm – spontaneous cpm). Spontaneous release was usually in the range of 5 to 15%. Tests with a spontaneous release exceeding 20% were excluded from the analysis. To detect artefacts due to differences in effector cell viability, all tests were performed against noncultured human leukemia cells and K562 simultaneously. The standard deviation of activity against K562 is depicted in Figure 1 and 2. In 24 effector/target combinations tests with noncultured human

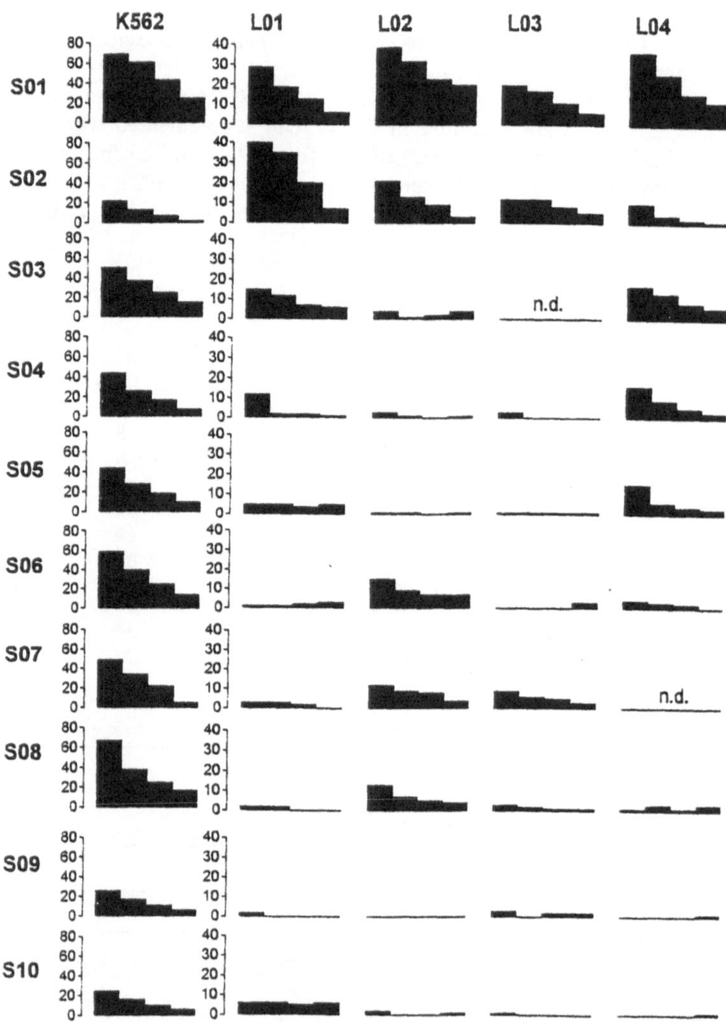

Fig. 1. NK-cell-mediated lysis of the standard taget cell line K562 and four samples of fresh acute leukemia blasts (L01–L04) by allogeneic, HLA different effector cells (S01–S10). These are results obtained with a standard 4 h Cr-release assay. Notice the different scales for the specific lysis of the experiments with the K562 cell line (0–80%) and the fresh leukemia blasts (0–40%). The four columns of each graph represent the specific lysis (%) obtained with an effector-target ratio of 100:1, 50:1, 25:1 and 12:1, respectively

leukemia cells were performed twice. The retest reliability calculated from these data was r = 0.94 (+/- 0.07).

Generation of LAK cells. Using 50 ml flasks (Greiner, Frickenhausen, Germany), 1×10^6 cells/ml were incubated as suspension cultures in RPMI 1640 at 37°C in humidified atmosphere of 5% CO_2. Purified human rIl- was added to a concentration of 200 U/ml. After 3 days of culture, nonadherent cells were decanted and centrifuged.

Flow cytometry analysis. 10 cells were stained with the appropriate mAb followed by flouresceinated goat-anti mouse Ig. Control aliquots were stained with the flourescent reagent alone. All samples were then analyzed on a flow cytometer (FACS Scan, Beckton Dickinson). Gates were used to exclude nonviable cells.

Results

Phenotypic characterisation of leukemia blasts and effector cells and correlation with lytic activity. Characteristics of the four leukemias are shown in Table 1, the phenotypic characterisation of the effector cells is shown in Table 2.

The number of CD56+ cells in the effector populations varied between 11 and 30% (mean 21.2

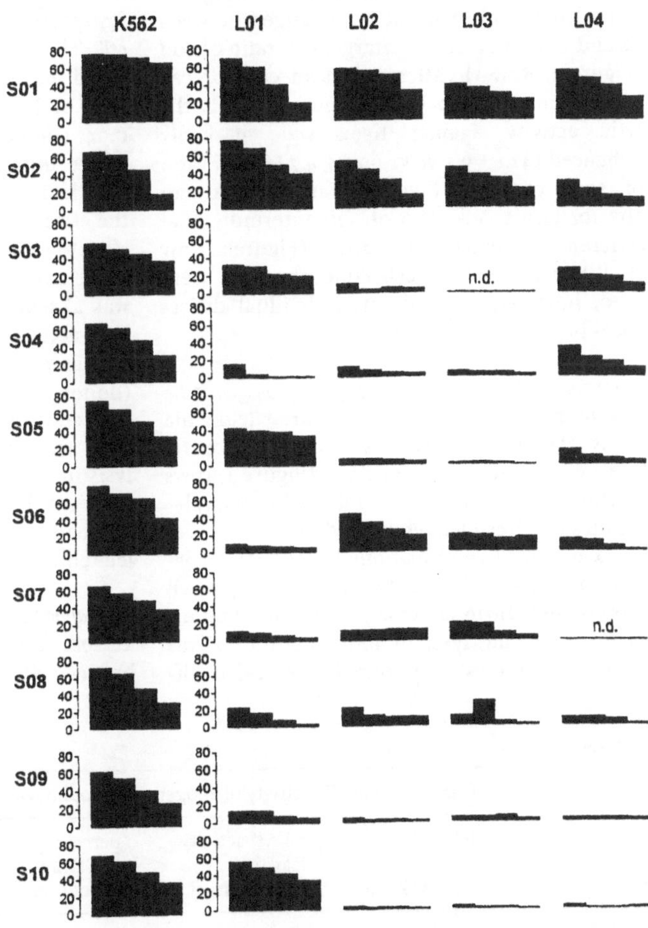

Fig. 2. LAK-cell-mediated lysis of the standard taget cell line K562 and four samples of fresh acute leukemia blasts (L01–L04) by allogeneic, HLA different effector cells (S01–S10). The effector cells were incubated with 200 IU/ml IL-2 for 3 days. Here, all scales for the specific lysis are identical and run from 0 to 80%. The four columns of each graph represent the specific lysis (%) obtained with an effector target ratio of 100:1, 50:1, 25:1 and 12:1, respectively

±3.6%). No statistically significant correlation between the number of cells positive for CD56, CD16, CD8, or any other surface marker and level of lytic activity against one of the leukemia targets was observed, though the percentage of CD16+ and CD56+ effector cells showed a trend towards positive correlation with the lytic activity against all 3 acute myelogenous leukemias (Table 3).

Susceptibility of K562 to lysis by allogeneic NK and LAK cells. Unmanipulated peripheral blood mononuclear cells were isolated on Ficoll gradients from buffy coats of ten healthy donors. The cells were used as effector cells in a conventional 4 hr ^{51}Cr release assay against K562 target cells. The interindividual variability in natural killing was remarkably high. Specific lysis ranged between 22 and 68% at an effector/target cell ratio of 50:1 (Figure 1, Row 1). After 3 days of effector cell incubation with 200 U/ml of human rIL-2, the lytic activity against K562 was markedly enhanced (42.1±9.5 % vs 69.7±4.7 %, E:T ratio of 50:1, compare Figure 1 and 2). At an effector/target cell ratio of 50:1 interindividual differences were less pronounced (Figure 2, Row 1). When lower LAK cell concentrations were used, however, marked interindividual differences became apparent again.

Susceptibility of leukemia blasts to lysis by allogeneic NK cells. In general, lysis of noncultured leukemia blasts (Figure 1, rows 2–5) was significantly lower compared to that of K562 (Figure 1, rows 1). However, in a limited number of cases, relevant lysis of fresh leukemia blasts was observed. In six out of 38 combinations tested (16%) specific lysis exceeded 20% at an effector/target cell ratio of 50:1. In 16 effector/target combinations (42%) a specific lysis of more than 10% was seen. Most interestingly, our data revealed different patterns of NK cell reactivity against different allogeneic leukemia blasts. Whereas two subjects (S09 and S10) exerted virtually no NK cell activity against the four targets tested, NK cells of donors S01 and S02 were shown to be effective against all targets. The other donors, however, demonstrated a complex pattern of reactivity. Subjects S03, S04, and S05 showed NK cell activity against leukemia L04 and (to some degree) against leukemia L01 but were unable to lyse leukemia L02 and L03. Subjects S06, S07, S08 exerted NK cell activity mainly against leukemia L02. All other targets were completely resistant, with the exception of leukemia L03 where effector cells of donor S07 showed some cytotoxicity.

Susceptibility of leukemia blasts to lysis by allogeneic LAK cells. The pattern of LAK activity against noncultured leukemia blasts was highly correlated to that of NK cell-mediated activity (r=0.81 to 0.94, compare Figs. 1 and 2). In those 16 cases where untreated effector cells induced significant leukemia cell lysis (10%, E:T ratio of 50:1), the effect was enhanced by IL-2 incubation (21.3 ±7.2% vs 40.1±10.1%). Of the 22 effector/target combinations in which NK cell mediated lysis was absent, ten demonstrated slightly elevated lytic activity in the range of 10 to 20%. Only in two cases of primarily resistant combinations (donor S10/leukemia L01 and donor S05/leukemia L01) the lytic activity was dramatically enhanced by IL-2 treatment: the specific lysis increased from 6% to 42% and 7% to 56%, respectively. Interestingly, the effect of IL-2 incubation was generally most pronounced with leukemia L01 as target.

Correlation between susceptibility of K562 and noncultured leukemia blasts. We observed no correlation between NK cell activity against the classical tar-

Table 3.

	Correlation of NK activity of allogeneic lymophocyte samples against leukemia blasts with:				
Target	NK cell activity against K562	LAK activity against same target	percentage of CD16+ effector cells	percentage of CD56+ effector cells	percentage of CD8+ effector cells
L1 (AML)	−0.57	0.81	0.33	0.35	0.12
L2 (AML)	−0.10	0.90	0.32	0.40	−0.21
L3 (AML)	−0.48	0.84	0.48	0.42	−0.21
L4 (Ph+ALL)	−0.22	0.94	−0.13	−0.02	0.23
K562		0.55	−0.38	0.03	0.18

get K562 and natural cytotoxicity against the four leukemias tested (Table 3). There were cases in which relatively high activity against K562 was associated with low activity against noncultured targets (subject S06 and S08). On the other hand, low NK cell activity against K562 did not exclude high activity against noncultured blasts (subject S02). However, in three cases (subjects S01, S09 and S10) remarkably high or low activity levels against K562 corresponded with the activity observed against allogeneic leukemia blasts.

Discussion

Several studies have demonstrated marked differences in the lysis of human leukemia cells by allogeneic NK and LAK cells [13,14,15,16,17]. This phenomenon is of particular interest in the context of allogeneic BMT, since resistance to natural killing appears to be associated with an increased risk of leukemic relapse [15]. Theoreticallly, differences in NK cell-mediated lysis of allogeneic leukemia cells can depend on three factors: (1) on the numerical and functional characteristics of the donor's NK cell pool, (2) on the susceptibility of leukemia cells towards natural killing and, (3) on the peculiar interaction between specific NK cell populations and a certain leukemia target.

The present study was mainly designed to investigate the third aspect, i.e. the hypothesis that specific NK cell/target cell interactions are involved. Until recently it appeared that the antileukemic activity of NK cells is largely nonspecific with the degree of cytolysis primarily reflecting the donor's "NK cell activity level" (usually defined by lysis of K562) and the target cell susceptibility to NK-mediated lysis. There is now accumulating evidence, however, that NK cells express surface receptors for different specificities and are capable of specific cytolytic activity against foreign cells [10,11]. Using peripheral blood-derived CD3-CD16+ NK cells that were stimulated in a mixed leukocyte culture, Ciccione et al. [11] showed that the ability of NK cells to lyse allogeneic PHA-induced blasts is a clonally distributed function. Their data further suggest that NK cell clones can be seperated into different groups according to their ability to lyse only certain allogeneic targets [12]. Moreover, the analysis of informative families indicated that the "sensitivity to lysis" of target cells maps to the MHC class I region [17]. It can be speculated that the ability of human CD3-CD56+ NK cells to recognize alloantigens may represent the human counterpart of murine hybrid resistance [11], a phenomenon that might be responsible for GvH-independent GvL-activity observed in murine systems [18].

The data presented here support the hypothesis that NK cells can recognize allogeneic leukemia cells specifically. Using peripheral blood lymphocytes of 10 healthy individuals as effector cells and the peripheral blasts of 4 patients with acute leukemias as targets, we observed a complex pattern of high and low NK cell-mediated cytotoxicity. Only three of the donors demonstrated either generally high (donor S01) or generally low (donors S09 and S10) NK cell activity and none of the leukemias turned out to be principally NK resistant or NK sensitive. Thus, most of the variance depend on specific NK cell/target cell interactions. It was behind the scope of the present study to categorize distinct patterns of reactivity definitively. Future studies with larger data samples, however, might allow the definition of diverse groups according to the pattern of alloreactivity observed.

Although the present study is based on relatively few effector/target combinations, it clarifies and confirms two important points that have been widely ignored in many investigations. On the one hand, NK cell activity against one target (e.g. K562) allows no conclusion regarding the level of NK activity against other targets. On the other hand, resistance towards NK cell-mediated lysis, determined with effector cells from one individuum, does not exclude high susceptibility to lysis by NK cells from another subject. These differences are less impressive for LAK cell mediated lysis as reported by others [16].

At least four principal questions arise from the data presented here. First, is the lysis of allogeneic leukemia target cells related to the phenomenon of NK-mediated specific lysis of "normal" (PHA-stimulated) allogeneic leukocytes? Ciccione et al. [17] demonstrated that NK clones with no activity against PHA-stimulated lymphocytes effectively lysed ovarian carcinoma cells. Although their data thus suggest that NK cell-mediated recognition of normal allogeneic cells can be distinguished from lysis of allogeneic tumor cells, it is not yet clear whether this holds also true for neoplasms of the hematopoietic system. Second, is the relationship between donor and leukemia MHC-class I alloantigens of relevance, as suggested by recent findings? Unfortunately, we have yet only incomplete data on the HLA-pattern of the subjects and leukemias tested. Third, the role of sensitization remains to be defined. Whereas all results indicating specific recognition of alloantigens by NK cell lines or clones were based on cells that had been previously sensitized, we tested allogeneic lymphocytes in a classical assay without prior sensitization. Thus, it is possible that two completely distinct mechanisms are responsible for the phenomena described by Ciccione et al. and for our results, i.e. MHC-restricted specific recognition of alloantigens after prior sensitization vs. MHC-unrestricted cytolytic activity directed against tumor targets. Fourth, specific recognition of alloantigens, as reported by Ciccione et al., referred to the clonal level. The individual reactivity pattern, however, represents the sum of activity of all NK cell populations reacting against the target cells. It is yet not clear to what extend the reported differences on the clonal level correspond to overall NK cell activity against a certain target.

Nevertheless, with regard to clinical BMT the present data implicate that if NK-reactivity of a marrow donor should be tested, leukemia or lymphoma cells of the patient should be used whenever possible. Predictive conclusions from the NK-activity against K562 appear to be of very limited value as demonstrated in a recent clinical trial [5]. More importantly, the findings of Ciccione et al. [11] and our results suggest that the in vivo antileukemic activity of allogeneic effector cells might be enhanced by preferring donors with optimal NK-cell activity against the patients leukemia cells. Since there is usually no possibility to choose between different marrow donors, the finding of specific alloreactivity might be more relevant for the application of allogeneic NK or LAK cells in the context of cellular immunotherapy after chemotherapy for hematological malignancies.

References

1. Transplant or chemotherapy in acute myelogenous leukaemia. International Bone Marrow Transplant Registry. Lancet 1:1119, 1989
2. Weiden PL, Flournoy N, Thomas ED, Prentice R, Fefer A, Buckner CD, Storb R: Antileukemic effect of graft-versus-host disease in human recipients of allogeneic-marrow grafts. N Engl J Med 300:1068, 1979
3. Horowitz MM, Gale RP, Sondel PM, Goldman JM, Kersey J, Kolb HJ, Rimm AA, Ringden O, Rozman C, Speck B, et al : Graft-versus-leukemia reactions after bone marrow transplantation. Blood 75:555, 1990
4. Gale RP, Butturini A: How do transplants cure chronic myelogenous leukemia? Bone Marrow Transplant 9:83, 1992
5. Hauch M, Gazzola MV, Small T, Bordignon C, Barnett L, Cunningham I, Castro Malaspinia H, O'Reilly RJ, Keever CA: Anti-leukemia potential of interleukin-2 activated natural killer cells after bone marrow transplantation for chronic myelogenous leukemia. Blood 75:2250, 1990
6. Keever CA, Welte K, Small T, Levick J, Sullivan M, Hauch M, Evans RL, O'Reilly RJ: Interleukin 2-activated killer cells in patients following transplants of soybean lectin-separated and E rosette-depleted bone marrow. Blood 70:1893, 1987
7. Lotzova E: Role of interleukin-2 activated MHC-nonrestricted lymphocytes in antileukemia activity and therapy. Leuk Lymphoma 7:15, 1992
8. Robertson MJ, Ritz J: Biology and clinical relevance of human natural killer cells. Blood 76:2421, 1990
9. Richards SJ, Scott CS: Human NK cells in health and disease: clinical, functional, phenotypic and DNA genotypic characteristics. Leuk Lymphoma 7:377, 1992
10. Suzuki N, Bianchi E, Bass H, Suzuki T, Bender J, Pardi R, Brenner CA, Larrick JW, Engleman EG: Natural killer lines and clones with apparent antigen specificity. J Exp Med 172:457, 1990
11. Moretta L, Ciccone E, Moretta A, Hoglund P, Ohlen C, Karre K: Allorecognition by NK cells: nonself or no self? Immunol Today 13:300, 1992
12. Moretta A, Bottino C, Pende D, Tripodi G, Tambussi G, Viale O, Orengo A, Barbaresi M, Merli A, Ciccone E, et-al : Identification of four subsets of human CD3−CD16+natural killer (NK) cells by the expression of clonally distributed functional surface molecules: correlation between subset assignment of NK clones and ability to mediate specific alloantigen recognition. J Exp Med 172:1589, 1990
13. Oshimi K, Oshimi Y, Motoji T, Kobayashi S, Mizoguchi H: Lysis of leukemia and lymphoma cells by autologous and allogeneic interferon-activated blood mononuclear cells. Blood 61:790, 1983
14. Archimbaud E, Bailly M, Dore JF: Inducibility of lymphokine activated killer (LAK) cells in patients with acute myelogenous leukaemia in complete remission and its clinical relevance. Br J Haematol 77:328, 1991
15. Adler A, Chervenick PA, Whiteside TL, Lotzova E, Herberman RB: Interleukin 2 induction of lymphokine-activated killer (LAK) activity in the peripheral blood and bone marrow of acute leukemia patients. I. Feasibility of LAK generation

in adult patients with active disease and in remission. Blood 71:709, 1988

16. Teichmann JV, Ludwig WD, Thiel E: Susceptibility of human leukemia to allogeneic and autologous lymphokine-activated killer cell activity: analysis of 252 samples. Nat Immun 11:117, 1992

17. Ciccone E, Pende D, Viale O, Tambussi G, Ferrini S, Biassoni R, Longo A, Guardiola J, Moretta A, Moretta L: Specific recognition of human CD3-CD16+ natural killer cells requires the expression of an autosomic recessive gene on target cells. J Exp Med 172:47, 1990

Acute Leukemias V
Experimental Approaches
and Management of Refractory Diseases
Hiddemann et al. (Eds.)

Cellular Immunotherapy of Acute Leukemias After High Dose Chemotherapy with Cytarabin (ARA-C) and Cyclophosphamide (CY) in a Murine Model

Lutz Uharek[1], Bertram Glass[1], Tobias Gaska[2], Matthias Zeis[2], Helmut Löffler[1], Wolfgang Müller-Ruchholtz[2], and Winfried Gassmann[1]

Abstract. Allogeneic lymphocytes are able to eradicate resistant leukemia cells after bone marrow transplantation. We developed a murine model to investigate their effectiveness for the prevention of leukemia relapse after high dose chemotherapy. Method: 1 × 105 A20 leukemia cells (H-2^d, B cell neoplasm) were injected into Balb/c (H-2^d) mice. Five days later, animals were treated with ARA-C (2 × 150 mg/kg i.p. daily; day 1–3) which provides high antileukemic activity against A20. To ensure sufficient immunosuppression, increasing doses of CY (60 to 125 mg/kg i.p.) were additionally given at day 4+5. At day 8 and 11, 2 × 107 either allogeneic MHC-mismatched (C57Bl/6, H-2^b) or allogeneic, MHC-matched (DBA, H-2^d) spleen cells were injected intravenously. Leukocyte counts were determined every three days. Leukemia relapse was defined as death with spleen weight > 0.15g and visible tumor nodules. Results: Without further therapy, relapse free survival was 0% with a median survival time (MST) of 21 days. Treatment with ARA-C and 2 × 60, 2 × 100, or 2 × 125 mg/kg CY cured 29%, 38% and 75% of the animals (MST = 45, 56, >200 days), respectively. After additional injection of MHC-mismatched allogeneic spleen cells, similar leukemia free survival (LFS) rates were observed: 38%, 45%, and 86% (MST = 52, 47, >200 days). Analysis of leukocyte counts revealed that 2 × 125 mg/kg CY were necessary to induce severe lymphocytopenia (<500/nl) in the majority of animals. Thus, at least in the groups treated with lower doses of CY, our negative findings could be explained by insufficient immunosuppression of the recipient (resulting in rapid rejection of allogeneic effector cells). When cells with a lower immunogenetic barrier to the recipient were used (DBA) after immunosuppression with 2 × 60 mg CY, a significant reduction of the relapse rate from 71% to 56% was observed. Conclusions: Our preclinical model allows the investigation of cellular immunotherapy after chemotherapy. Future studies will focus on the development of preparative regimens with better immunosuppressive potential. The separation and stimulation of allogeneic NK cells with antileukemia activity will enable us to transfer large effector cell numbers without GvHR.

Introduction

The antileukemic effect of allogeneic lymphocytes in the context of bone marrow transplantation is a well known phenomenon [3]. This graft-versus-leukemia effect has been attributed to the cytotoxic effects of T-lymphocytes or NK cells [4,7]. Although the graft-versus-leukemia effect is often combined with graft-versus-host disease [14], there is evidence from clinical observations as well as from animal experiments that GVHR is no prerequisite for GVL activity [8,6]. Recently, an extension in the use of allogeneic lymphocytes for immunotherapy of leukemias has been demonstrated by the use of donor buffy coat cells for relapsed leukemias after allogeneic BMT [11]. Here we describe an experimental model which allows the investiga-

II. Medizinische Klinik[1] und Institut für Immunologie[2], Christian-Albrechts-Universität Kiel, Germany

tion of a further extension of immunotherapy: The use of allogeneic lymphocytes after high dose chemotherapy but without transplantation of hematopoetic stem cells.

Methods

Animals: Balb/c (H-2^d), DBA (H-2^d) and C57Bl/6 (H-2^b) mice were bred and kept at the animal facilities of our institute. All animals were housed in conventional cages, seven to 10 animals to a cage, and were given non-sterilized food and water ad libidum.

Tumor cells: A20 is a B-cell lymphoma of Balb/c origin that occurred spontaneously in a 15 month old mouse [10]. The cells were maintained in culture in RPMI 1640+5% FCS at 37 °C and 5% CO_2. We performed an in-vivo passage of these cells by i.v. injection into Balb/c animals. After the mice had developed hepatosplenomegaly, they were killed in terminal stage of their disease and the spleens were removed. Spleen cell suspensions containing nearly 100% of this in-vivo passaged leukemia/lymphoma cells were stored in liquid nitrogen and used for further experiments.

Tumor diagnostics: The animals were examined daily and necropsied after death. Death due to leukemic relapse was defined as death with macroscopic proof of tumor and liver weight more than 1.5 g and spleen weight more than 0.15 g. Histologic examination of liver and spleen was performed for some animals in each group. Animals with hepatosplenomegaly were found to have infiltrations of leukemic cells in any case. Healthy mice of the same age were found to have a liver weight of 1.3 g ±0,2 g and a spleen weight of 0.1 g±0.02 g.

Chemotherapy: Cytarabin (Alexan, Fa. Mack) and Cyclophosphamide (Endoxan, Asta Medica) were purchased in convential aliquots for clinical use. Alexan was used undiluted and Endoxan was diluted in aqua dest. as recommended by the manufacturer. Before injection of the cytostatic agent, the body weight of the animals was determined and the dose adjusted. Both drugs were injected i.p. in general ether anesthesia.

Allogeneic lymphocytes: The donor mice for the allogeneic lymphocytes were C57BL/6 or DBA mice, respectively. The animals were killed under anesthesia and the spleens were removed under germ-free conditions. A single-cell suspension was prepared and the mononuclear cells were isolated by density gradient centrifugation.

Blood cell counts: Peripheral blood was collected by puncture of the tail veins. The total white cell count was done in a Thoma chamber. Pappenheim stains of blood smears were performed and the percentage of lymphocytes and granulocytes was determined.

Experimental system: Female Balb/c mice, 8–12 weeks of age, were i.v. injected with 1×10^5 cells of the B-lymphocytic leukemia A20 5 days prior to the start of the chemotherapy. The day when chemotherapy started was termed day 0. Cytarabin was given i.p. in a fixed dose of 150 mg/kg body weight twice daily on day 0–2. The animals received a total Cytarabin dose of 900 mg/kg body weight. Cyclophosphamide was given i.p. once daily on day 4 and 5. The doses were 2×60 mg/kg, 2×100 mg/kg and 2×125 mg/kg, respectively. At days 8 and 12, 2×10^7 allogeneic mononuclear spleen cells were injected i.v. in some groups. In the groups receiving 2×60 mg/kg, 2×100 mg/kg and 2×125 mg/kg Cyclophosphamide, spleen cells from allogeneic, MHC-mismatched C57Bl/6 donors were used. One experimental group received allogeneic MHC-matched spleen cells from DBA donors after immunosuppression with Cytarabin and 2×60 mg/kg cyclophosphamide. At days 0, 3, 7, 10, and 13 leukocyte counts were performed. The animals were observed until day 200 post leukemia injection.

Statistics: The survival data and the data for "freedom from leukemia" were calculated according to the method of Kaplan and Meier. The groups were compared using the Wilcoxon test. The calculations were done on a PC with the NCSS statistical software.

Results

Antileukemic effectiveness of high dose chemotherapy: After injection of 1×10^5 A20 cells, all animals receiving no further treatment died after a median survival time of 26 days (Fig. 1). The application of 6×150 mg/kg cytarabin and

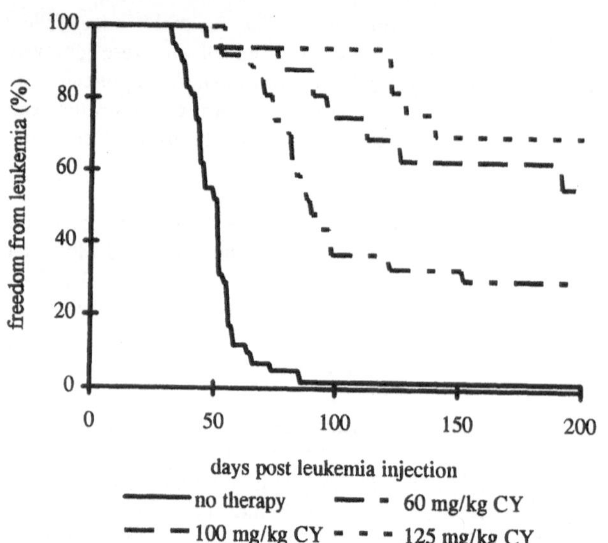

Fig. 1. Freedom from relapse after injection of 1 × 105 A20 leukemia cells into Balb/c mice 5 days prior to beginning of the chemotherapy. The animals received a fixed dose of 6 × 150 mg/kg ARA-C and 2 × 60 mg/kgCy (n = 12), 2 × 100 mg/kg (n = 16) or 2 × 125 mg/kg Cy (n = 9), respectively

2 × 60 mg/kg cyclophosphamide prolonged the median survival to 53 days and reduced the relapse rate to 71% ($p < 0.01$). Escalatating doses of cyclophosphamide in addition to the fixed dose of cytararabin further improved the survival. A dose of 2 × 100 mg/kg cyclophosphamide was followed by a relapse rate of 42% ($p < 0.05$). The highest dose of 6 × 150 mg/kg cytarabin plus 2 × 125 mg/kg cyclophosphamide resulted in a relapse rate of 25%.

Bone marrow depression: A dose response to cyclophosphamide on the leukocyte counts could be observed (Fig. 2). Mice receiving a dose of 2 × 60 mg of cyclophosphamide showed only a slight and short-term depression of the leukocyte counts. The nadir was reached 7 days after the start of chemotherapy. The leukocyte count dropped from 8000/μl to 4200/μl in median. The dose of 2 × 125 mg cyclophosphamide resulted in a more pronounced decrease of the leukocyte count. The median leukocyte count was 800/μl. Some animals could not be evaluated since they were in a very bad condition at the time of the critical blood sample and no material could be obtained. For that reason, the median of the leukocyte count probably underestimates the bone marrow depression of this group.

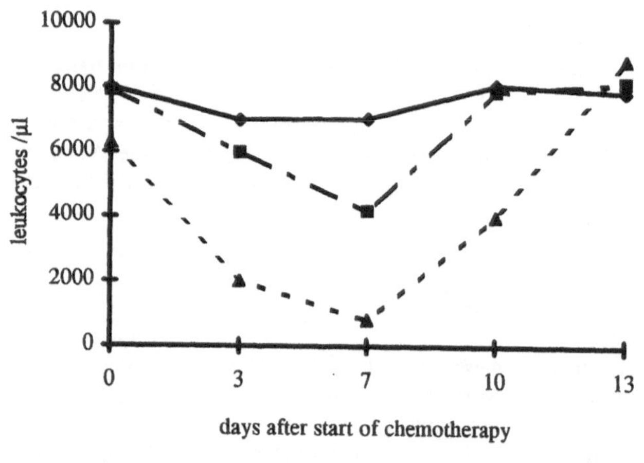

Fig. 2. Median leukocyte counts of Balb/c mice after administration of 6 × 150 mg/kg ARA-C and 2 × 60 mg/kg (n = 16) or 2 × 125 mg/kg (n = 9) Cy, respectively

Fig. 3. Survival of Balb/c mice injected with A20 leukemia cells. One group received no treatment (n = 20), the second group received 6 × 150 mg/kg ARA-C and 2 × 60 mg cyclophosphamide and the third group received MHC-matched (n = 12) allogeneic spleen lymphocytes on day 8 and day 12 after start of the same chemotherapy

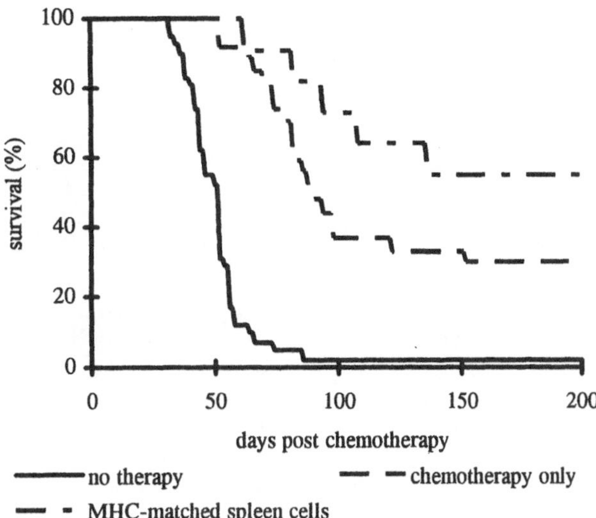

Antileukemic activity of allogeneic, MHC-matched leukocytes: The addition of MHC-matched allogeneic spleen cells after a chemotherapy with ARA-C and 2 × 60 mg/kg reduced the relapse rate from 71% to 42% compared to animals receiving chemotherapy only ($p < 0.05$). In these two groups, no lethal toxicity of the treatment protocol was observed. Animals which received fully allogeneic MHC-mismatched spleen cells died after a median survival time of 54 days. This group did even worse than the group receiving chemotherapy alone (Fig. 3). In a control group, receiving chemotherapy and fully allogeneic spleen cells but no leukemia, some animals showed weight loss and died after 18–50 days (data not shown).

MHC-mismatched spleen cells did not exert antileukemic activity after chemotherapy: We treated animals with higher immunosuppressive doses of cyclophosphamide (2 × 100 mg/kg and 2 × 125 mg/kg, respectively) in addition to ARA-C and injected allogeneic MHC-mismatched spleen cells of C57 donors. There was no advantage for these animals with respect to the relapse rate (Fig. 4). In both groups, we observed a major toxicity due to the application of the allogeneic spleen cells. Compared to animals receiving chemotherapy alone, the mortality increased from 8% to 42% for mice receiving 2 × 100 mg/kg and from 12% to 53% for animals receiving 2 × 125 mg cyclophosphamide. This effect was not observed for animals receiving the lowest dose of 2 × 60 mg cyclophosphamide (Fig. 5).

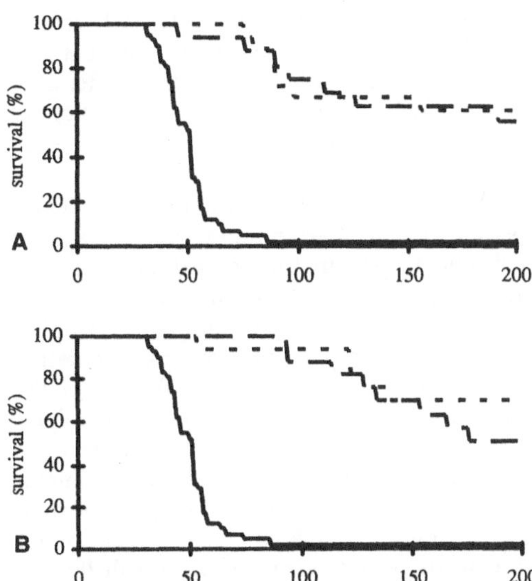

Fig. 4. Survival of Balb/c mice injected with A20 leukemia cells. The animals received either 100 mg/kg (**a**) or 150 mg/kg (**b**) cyclophosphamid in addition to ARA-C starting 5 days post leukemia injection. Some mice were injected with allogeneic, MHC-mismatched spleen cells at day 8 and 12 after start of the chemotherapy

Discussion

The antileukemic effect of allogeneic bone marrow cells after BMT is a well recognized phenomenon and intensive research is under way to define the effector cell population [5,12], the

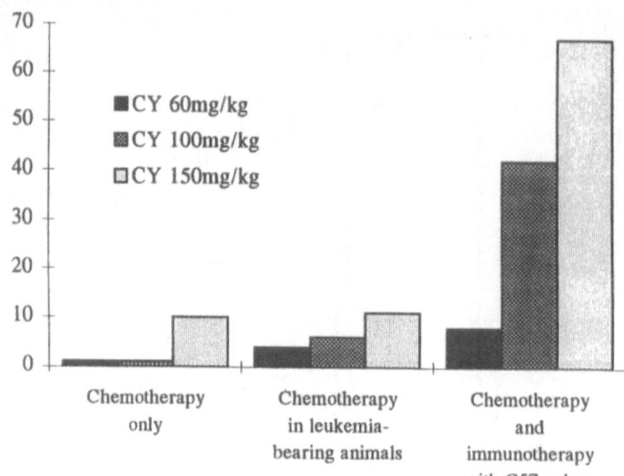

Fig. 5. Mortality not related to leukemia in Balb/c mice after chemotherapy with ARA-C, 150 mg/kg twice daily from day 1–3 and the indicated dose of cyclophosphamide on day 4–5. One group received chemotherapy only, the second group was injected on day −5 with A20 leukemia cells and treated with chemotherapy and the third group received leukemia cells, chemotherapy and MHC-mismatched cells of C57 origin

specificity of the effectors [1] and the relationship of this antileukemic effect to graft-versus-host disease [9]. By using donor buffy coat cells for the treatment of leukemic relapse after allogeneic BMT, a first successful application of these immunological phenomenons has been made.

We developed a murine model for the investigation of cellular immunotherapy against leukemia targets in the context of high dose chemotherapy. Our attempt was made to exploit the cytotoxic potential of allogeneic lymphocytes outside the bone marrow transplantation situation. By avoiding long-term chimerism, the use of fully allogeneic, MHC-mismatched lymphocytes should be possible. Intermediate immunosuppression and depression of hematopoiesis would allow allogeneic cells to exert their effects within a few hours or days. Thereafter autologous hematopoetic recovery will lead to rejection of allogeneic cells and will prevent GVHD.

A model for testing this approach has to meet several requirements. First, a leukemia and chemotherapy model has to be developed that simulates relapse rates comparable to those after chemotherapy of human leukemias and lymphomas. In our model, the murine B-lymphocytic leukemia A20 was used and dose dependent relapse rates of 70% to 30% were generated.

Secondly, chemotherapy induced immunosuppression and depression of the hematopoetic system should last at least for some days and allow the allogeneic cells to do their work. In our model, chemotherapy with ARA-C and cyclophosphamide induced a depression of the white cell count below 1/nl. A significant reduction of the white cells lasted for 4–7 days and a dosage effect of the chemotherapy was seen.

Thirdly, to determine the risk of GVHD makes it neccessary to have at least one allogeneic model in which GVHD effects are observable. In our model, injection of allogeneic, MHC-mismatched C57 lymphocytes after chemotherapy resulted in higher mortality rates as chemotherapy only. This difference was more pronounced in the groups with the highest immunosuppression. The clinical impressing of the animals (weight loss, hair loss) suggests GVHD as cause of death. GVHD occured in these animals very quickly after injection of the lymphocytes, resembling transfusion related GVHD in the human situation [13]. In future studies we will try to use lymphocyte subset depletion to reduce GVHD without impairment of the immuntherapeutic effect.

A model for immunotherapy should be able to demonstrate an immuntherapeutic effect at least in one basic donor-recipient combination. In our model, injection of allogeneic, MHC-matched lymphocytes significantly reduced the relapse rate after chemotherapy with ARA-C and cyclophosphamide. This effect, causing a 25% reduction of the relapse rate, is comparable to an enhancement of the cyclophosphamide dosage from 2 × 60 mg/kg to 2 × 100 mg/kg body weight. After injection of fully allogeneic, MHC-mismatched lymphocytes we were not able to detect such an antileukemic effect. This fact seems to be in contradiction to clinical results of allogeneic BMT with unrelated, MHC-matched or partially mismatched BM [2]. On the other hand, there is a stronger host-versus-graft reaction in the mismatched situation. Since in our model, the immunosuppression was lower than in the BMT situation MHC-mismatched cells might have been rejected after very short time.

Further investigations will focus on more intense immunosupression to prevent rapid lymphocyte rejection. Furthermore T-cell depletion of MHC-mismatched lymphocytes will be applied to avoid GVHD. We hope to create a preclinical model for immunotherapy of hematopoetic malignancies without the restrictions in donor selection which have to be taken into account in bone marrow transplantation.

References

1. Aizawa S, Sado T (1991) Graft-versus-leukemia effect in MHC-compatible and -incompatible allogeneic bone marrow transplantation of radiation-induced, leukemia-bearing mice. Transplantation 52: 885–889
2. Beatty PG (1992) Results of allogeneic bone marrow transplantation with unrelated or mismatched donors. Semin Oncol 19: 13–19
3. Butturini A, Bortin MM, Gale RP (1987) Graft-versus-leukemia following bone marrow transplantation. Bone Marrow Transplantation 2: 233
4. Butturini A, Gale RP (1987) The role of T-cells in preventing relapse in chronic myelogenous leukemia. Bone Marrow Transplantation 2: 351–354
5. Falkenburg JH, Goselink HM, van-der-Harst D, van-Luxemburg-Heijs SA, Kooy-Winkelaar YM, Faber LM, de-Kroon J, Brand A, Fibbe WE, Willemze R, et al (1991) Growth inhibition of clonogenic leukemic precursor cells by minor histocompatibility antigen-specific cytotoxic T lymphocytes. J Exp Med 174: 27–33
6. Glass B, Uharek L, Gassmann W, Focks B, Bolouri H, Löffler H, Müller-Ruchholtz W (1992) Graft-versus-leukemia activity after bone marrow transplantation does not require graft-versus-host disease. Ann Hematol 64: 255–259
7. Hauch M, Gazzola MV, Small T, Bordignon C, Barnett L, Cunningham I, Castro Malaspinia H, O'Reilly RJ, Keever CA (1990) Anti-leukemia potential of interleukin-2 activated natural killer cells after bone marrow transplantation for chronic myelogenous leukemia. Blood 75: 2250–2262
8. Horowitz MM, Gale RP, Sondel PM, Goldman JM, Kersey J, Kolb HJ, Rimm AA, Ringden O, Rozman C, Speck B, et al (1990) Graft-versus-leukemia reactions after bone marrow transplantation. Blood 75: 555–562
9. Johnson BD, Truitt RL (1992) A decrease in graft-vs.-host disease without loss of graft-vs.-leukemia reactivity after MHC-matched bone marrow transplantation by selective depletion of donor NK cells in vivo. Transplantation 54: 104–112
10. Kim KJ, Kannellopoulus-Langevin C, Mervin RM, Sachs DH, Asofsky R (1979) Establishment and characterization of Balb/c lymphoma lines with B cell properties. J Immunol 122: 549–554
11. Kolb HJ, Mittermuller J, Clemm C, Holler E, Ledderose G, Brehm G, Heim M, Wilmanns W (1990) Donor leukocyte transfusions for treatment of recurrent chronic myelogenous leukemia in marrow transplant patients. Blood 76: 2462–2465
12. Okunewick JP, Kociban DL, Machen LL, Buffo MJ (1991) The role of CD4 and CD8 T cells in the graft-versus-leukemia response in Rauscher murine leukemia. Bone Marrow Transplant 8: 445–452
13. Spitzer TR, Cahill R, Cottler Fox M, Treat J, Sacher R, Deeg HJ (1990) Transfusion-induced graft-versus-host disease in patients with malignant lymphoma. A case report and review of the literature. Cancer 66: 2346–2349
14. Sullivan KM, Weiden PL, Storb R, Witherspoon RP, Fefer A, Fisher L, Buckner CD, Anasetti C, Appelbaum FR, Badger C, Beatty P, Bensinger W, Berenson R, Bigelow C, Cheever MA, Clift R, Deeg HJ, Doney K, Greenberg P, Hansen JA, Hill R, Loughran T, Martin P, Neiman P (1989) Influence of acute and chronic graft-versus-host disease on relapse and survival after bone marrow transplantation from HLA-identical siblings as treatment of acute and chronic leukemia. Blood 73: 1720–1728

Acute Leukemias V
Experimental Approaches
and Management of Refractory Diseases
Hiddemann et al. (Eds.)

Interleukin-2 Bolus Infusion as Consolidation Therapy in 2nd Remission of Acute Myelocytic Leukemia

Lothar Bergmann[1], Gerhard Heil[2], Karin Kolbe[3], Eva Lengfelder[4], Ellen Puzicha[1], Hans Martin[1], Jürgen Lohmeyer[5], Paris S. Mitrou[1], and Dieter Hoelzer[1]

Introduction

In acute myelocytic leukemia (AML) the disease-free survival (DFS) is still unsatisfactory despite some advantages by intensification of chemotherapeutic strategies and/or bone marrow transplantation (BMT)[1]. Alternative immunotherapeutic approaches have been supported by BMT data indicating a correlation between graft versus host (GvH) reaction and DFS [2, 3]. The GvH reaction is supposed to be associated with a graft versus leukemia (GVL) reaction, which may be responsible for the elimination of minimal residual leukemic blast populations by activation of cytotoxic cells and secretion of cyctokines as TNF-α and IFN-γ [4–6].

Therefore, therapeutic approaches imaging a GvL-like reaction in AML patients to prolong DFS or even to cure the patients are desirable. In this regard interleukin-2 (IL-2) has been described to activate previously unrecognized populations of cytotoxic cells to trigger lytic activity against myelocytic blasts [7–9]. So far, clinical trials with IL-2 have demonstrated that complete remissions (CR) can be achieved in patients with AML in partial remission (PR) with limited tumor burden (<20% blasts in BM) [10]. Various clinical trials with IL-2 in AML with or without autologous BMT have been dealing with the feasibility of this approach [10–12]. However, a clear benefit for DFS has not yet been confirmed.

Here the results of a multicenter clinical phase II trial for AML patients in 2nd remission with recombinant IL-2 (rIL-2) as consolidation therapy with or without autologous BMT are reported.

Patients and Methods

Patients. All patients included into this study received an identical induction (2 cycles) and early consolidation (1 cycle) chemotherapy with intermediate high-dose cytosin-arabinoside (iHDAraC) and etoposide (VP-16). In detail, AraC was administered at a dosage of 2 × 600 mg/m^2 on day 1–4 as 2h infusion and VP-16 at a dosage of 100 mg/m^2 on day 1–7 as 1h infusion. In all patients, who achieved 2nd CR, IL-2 consolidation therapy was scheduled to be started within 4–6 weeks after peripheral reconstitution following the last chemotherapy cycle or autologous BMT (ABMT). rIL-2 (EuroCetus, Frankfurt, FRG) was administered in a dosage of 9 MIU/m^2 as 1h bolus infusion on day 1–5, 8–12. This schedule was repeated every six weeks up to a maximum of four cycles. Complete remission was defined according to the Eastern Cooperative Group criteria. To ascertain CR during consolidation therapy, complete blood counts were monitored weekly and bone marrow aspiration was repeated before rIl-2 therapy, after 2 cycles and after 4 cycles of rIL-2 and every 3 months in follow-up.

[1] Medical Clinic III, J.W. Goethe University, Frankfurt, FRG
[2] Div. of Hematology, University Hospital, Ulm, FRG
[3] Div.of Hematol., J. Gutenberg University, Mainz, FRG
[4] Div. of Hematol., University Hospital, Mannheim, FRG
[5] Division of Hematology, University Hospital, Gießen and the South German Hemoblastosis Group (SHG)

Totally, 36/59 (61%) patients with first relapse of de novo AML achieved CR by induction chemotherapy. The median age was 52 [23–68] years. Patients achieving 2nd remission were treated with rIL-2 late consolidation therapy. Meanwhile 20 patients including four patients, who received ABMT, entered late consolidation with rIL-2. Four patients are too early for evaluation, six patients relapsed before starting IL-2 therapy, two received allogeneic BMT and four patients refused IL-2 treatment.

Statistical analysis. Student's t test was used to calculate significant differences between lymphocyte subsets of various patient groups and Kaplan-Meier test for probability of survival.

Results

All patients entered into this study received a uniform induction therapy consisting of iHD AraC/VP-16 with or without following ABMT. Twenty patients with 2nd remission of de novo AML (including 4 autografted patients) received rIL-2 late consolidation therapy. Sixteen patients received three and more cycles rIL-2. Four patients received less than three cycles due to early relapses. In 15/69 (22%) cycles rIL-2, the planned dose had to be reduced due to subjective or objective toxicities.

The median duration of DFS in the IL-2 treated group was 11 (4–46+) months and the probability for 12 and 24 months DFS was 52% and 21%, respectively. Up to now 4/20 (20%) patients, who received rIL-2 late consolidation therapy, the 2nd remission duration reached or exceeded that in 1st remission (Table 1). One patient with M4 AML is in ongoing 2nd CR for more than 46 months. 7 patients are in still ongoing 2nd remission (5+–46+).

The side effects were moderate (Table 2). No grade IV toxicity was observed. In one patient recovering from autologous BMT, grade III desquamative erythrodermia was noted, associated with a concomittant allergic reaction against cotrimoxazol. One autografted patient with granulocytes >500/µl developed

Table 1. 1st and 2nd remission duration (RD) of patients with rIL-2 late consolidation therapy in 2nd remission of AML

Patient	FAB	age/sex (years)	1st RD (months)	2nd RD (months)	present status/ survival (months)	
1	M4	58, m	17	46+	CR	48+
2*	M5	33, f	33	35+	CR	36+
3	M4	66, f	16	18	dead in relapse	28
4*	M4	44, f	9	22	dead in relapse	29
5*	M4	28, f	39	20+	CR	22+
6	M1	58, f	18	16+	CR	18+
7	M4	67, f	13	10+	CR	12+
8	M2	56, f	16	11+	CR	14+
9	M1	54, f	11	5+	CR	6+
10*	M2	23, f	59	13	dead in relapse	20
11	M5	55, f	15	5	dead in relapse	10
12	M1	57, f	17	9	dead in relapse	21
13	M1	62, f	16	11	dead in relapse	17
14	M4	37, m	15	12	dead in relapse	18
15	M4	60, m	14	13	dead in relapse	20
16	M2	45, m	12	5	dead in relapse	9
17	M2	55, f	11	5	dead in relapse	9
18	M2	53, f	11	4	dead in relapse	5
19	M4	56, m	8	6	alive in relapse	8
20	Mx	27, f	21	6	alive in relapse	16+

*patients with autologous BMT in 2nd remission
RD = remission duration
CR = complete remission
overall survival = survival from time of starting chemotherapy
Patients 1–4 have a longer 2nd than 1st remission duration, patients 5–9 have a still ongoing CR but have not yet reached 1st RD

Table 2. Side effects during 69 cycles bolus infusion IL-2 in AML patients

	Side effects (WHO %)				
	0	I	II	III	IV
fever	23	10	64	3	0
chills	75	25	0	0	0
nausea	54	16	13	1	0
arthralgia	70	16	13	1	0
skin	75	14	9	1	0
hypotension	84	9	7	0	0
diarrhoeas	84	12	4	0	0
infection	90	1	1	8	0
cardiotoxicity	83	17	0	0	0
fluidretention	84	13	3	0	0
neurotoxicity	97	3	0	0	0
creatinine	91	9	0	0	0
sGOT/sGPT	51	36	12	1	0
AP	71	22	7	2	0
thrombopenia	83	13	4	0	0
granulocytopenia	94	3	3	0	0
eosinophilia	86	1	10	3	0

septicaemia (staphylococcus aureus) via central venous catheter during two cycles of IL-2 therapy requiring cessation of rIL-2 infusion. Altogether it seemed that subjective and objective side effects of IL-2 were much more pronounced in patients after autologous BMT than in patients without (data not shown). In the latter group rIL-2 was partially administered in an outside patient setting.

Discussion

The rationale for therapeutic approaches with IL-2 in patients with AML is based on several experimental and clinical data demonstrating the susceptibility of leukemic blasts to lymphokine-activated killer (LAK) cells and on the presence of cytotoxic precursor cells in bone marrow and peripheral blood of the patients [7, 8, 13, 14]. In vivo, administration of IL-2 has been shown to be feasible in AML patients with or without ABMT using various schedules [11, 12, 15]. Foa et al [10] demonstrated an antileukemic effect of IL-2 therapy by inducing CRs in AML patients with partial remission and less than 20% blasts in the BM but not in patients with higher tumor burden. The latter may find support by various observations describing an inhibitory effect of leukemic AML blast by soluble factors on immune reactions, resulting in reduced cytokine synthesis of lymphocytes and impaired cytotoxic activity at acute phase of disease leukemic blasts on cytotoxic cells [16–19].

In contrast to most other studies with IL-2 maintenance therapy, the patients in this study received a uniform induction chemotherapy consisting of iHDAraC/VP-16. This chemotherapy alone is not assumed to prolong DFS, because even in studies using HDAraC the median survival does not exceed 6 to 7 months [20–22]. The optimal schedule of IL-2 administration still remains unsolved, but in most of the clinical trials intravenous IL-2 administration has been used. A prolongation of DFS by IL-2 consolidation therapy, however, has not been confirmed yet. The results of this pilot phase II study indicate that our approach of rIL-2 administration is feasible in AML patients with second remission and suggest a possible benefit for prolongation of DFS. Indeed, in 4/20 (20%) patients an inversion of remission duration could be achieved. However, since some of our patients relapsed before rIL-2 consolidation this may be the result of positive selection.

The side effects during rIL-2 therapy were moderate and manageable with a predominance of flu-like symptoms, nausea and slight hypotension as reported in other studies [23]. These toxicities occurred within 2–4 hours after the end of IL-2 infusion and lasted for about 2–4 hours as described for bolus infusion of rIL-2 [24]. Other side effects as malaise, erythema and arthralgia lasted up to 2 weeks after the rIL-2 course. Our impression is that rIL-2 following ABMT is associated with more severe side effects than in patients without ABMT. The occurrence of acute side effects seemed to be associated in time with the release of secondary cytokines as TNF-α and Il-6, which are known to be reponsible for severe side effects as fever, hypotension and capillary leak syndrome [23, 24]. In vitro, these secondarily induced cytokines have been reported to enhance activation of LAK cells and their possible antileukemic effect as well as affecting the expression of surface molecules responsible for cytotoxic cell target interactions as MHC antigens and adhesion molecules. The role of these secondary cytokines for the antileukemic effect of IL-2 in vivo in respect to direct antileukemic effect or to activation of cytotoxic cells and upregulation of surface molecules as MHC-antigens and adhesion molecules still has to be defined. The administration of rIL2 was associated with an increase of circulating LAK cells as described in other studies (data not shown) [23]. The study confirms the feasibility of immunotherapy with rIL-2 in the management of AML patients in 2nd CR and suggests a benefit for DFS, but randomized trials are required to ascertain its possible benefit. As a consequence from this experience we started a randomized trial with rIL-2 in 1st CR of advanced myelodysplastic syndrome and secondary AMLs [25].

Acknowledgements. Supported by the grant 01GA8802 of the Bundesministerium für Forschung und Technologie (BMFT) and Deutsche Krebshilfe grant W22/92.

References

1. McMillian AK, Goldstone AH, Linch DC, Gribben JG, Patterson KG, Richards JDM, Franklin I, Boughton BJ, Milligan DW, Leyland M, Hutchison RM, Newland AC (1990) High-dose chemotherapy and autologous bone marrow transplantation in acute myelocytic leukemia. Blood 67: 480–488
2. Horowitz MM, Gale RP, Sondel PM, Goldman JM, Kersey J, Kolb HJ, Rimm AA, Ringdén O, Rozman C, Speck B, Truirr RL, Zwaan FE, Bortin MM (1990) Graft-versus-leukemia reactions after bone marrow transplantation. Blood 75: 555–562
3. Slavin S, Ackerstein A, Naparsteck E, Or R, Weiss L (1990) The graft versus leukemia (GvL) phenomenon: is GvL separable from GVHD? Bone Marrow Transplant., 6: 155–161
4. Sullivan KM, Weiden PL, Storb R, Withersporn RP, Fefer A, Fisher L, Buckner CD, Anasetti C, Appelbaum FR, Badger C, Beatty P, Bensinger W, Berenson R, Bigelow C, Cheever MA, Clift R, Deeg HJ, Doney K, Greenberg P, Hansen JA, Hill R, Loughran T, Martin P, Neimann P (1989) Influence of acute and chronic graft-versus-host disease on relapse and survival after bone marrow transplantation from HLA-identical siblings as treatment of acute and chronic leukemia. Blood 73: 1720–1728
5. Reittie JE, Gottlieb D, Heslop HE, Leger O, Brexler HG, Hazlehurst G, Hoffbrand AV, and Brenner MK (1989) Endogenously generated activated killer cells circulate after autologous and allogeneic bone marrow transplantation but not after chemotherapy. Blood 73: 1351–1358
6. Jadus MR, Wepsic HT (1992): The role of cytokines in graft-versus-host reactions and disease. Bone Marrow Transplant., 10: 1–14
7. Foa R, Guarini A, Tos GA, Cardona S, Fierro GT, Meloni G, Tosti S, Mandelli F, Gavosto F (1991a) Peripheral blood and bone marrow immunophenotypic and functional modifications induced in acute leukemia patients treated with interleukin 2: Evidence of in vivo lymphokine activated killer cell generation. Cancer Res., 51: 964–968
8. Archimbaud E, Thomas X, Campos L, Fiere D, Dore JF (1992) Susceptibility of acute myelogenous blasts to lysis by lymphokine-activated killer (LAK) cells and its clinical relevance. Leukemia Res., 16: 673–680
9. Jahn B, Bergmann L, Fenchel K, Weidmann E, Schwulera U, Mitrou P.S. (1992) CD3+CD4+ T-cells as effective cells of autologous blast specific cytotoxicity in acute myelocytic leukemia. Ann. Haematol., 65 suppl.: 74 (abstr)
10. Foa R, Meloni G, Tosti S, Novarino A, Fenu S, Gavosto F, Mandelli F (1991b) Treatment of acute myeloid leukaemia patients with recombinant interleukin 2: a pilot study. Brit. J. Haematol., 77: 491–496
11. Gottlieb DJ, Brenner MK, Heslop HE, Bianchi ACM, Bello-Fernandez C, Mehta AB, Newland AC,, Galazka AR, Scott EM, Hoffbrand AV, Prentice HG (1989) A phase I clinical trial of recombinant interleukin 2 following high dose chemo-radiotherapy for haematological malignancy: applicability to the elimination of minimal residual disease. Brit. J. Cancer, 60: 610–615
12. Foa R (1993) Does interleukin-2 have a role in the management of acute leukemia? J. Clin. Oncol., 11: 1817–1825
13. Lim SH, Worman CP, Goldstone AH (1991b) Lymphocyte activation in patients with acute myelocytic leukemia evidence for the presence of myeloblast antigen? Cancer Immunol. Immunothe., 33: 417–420.
14. Fierro T, Liao XS, Lusso P, Bonferroni M, Matera L, Cesano A, Lista P, Arione R, Forni G, Foa R (1988) In vitro and in vivo susceptibility of human leucemic cells to lymphokine activated killer activity. Leuk., 2: 50–54
15. Hamon MD, Prentice HG, Gottlieb JD, MacDonald ID, Cunningham JM, Smith OP, Gilmore M, Gandhi L, Collis C (1993) Immunotherapy with interleukin-2 after ABMT in AML. Bone Marrow Transplant., 11: 399–401
16. Adler A, Albo V, Blatt J, Whiteside TL, Herberman RB (1989) Interleukin-2 induction of lymphokine-activated killer activity in the peripheral blood and bone marrow of acute leukemia patients: II. Feasibility of LAK generation in children with active disease and in remission. Blood 74: 1690–1697
17. Archimbaud E, Bailly M, Doré JF (1991) Inducibility of lymphokine activated killer (LAK) cells in patients with acute myelogenous leukaemia in complete remission and its clinical relevence. Briti. J. Haematol., 77: 328–334
18. Foa R, Fierro MT, Cesano A, Guarini A, Bonferroni M, Raspadori D, Miniero R, Lauria F, Gavosto F (1991c) Defective lymphokine activated killer cell generation and activity in acute leukemia patients with active disease. Blood 78: 1041–1046
19. Brieger J, Jahn B, Fenchel K, Appelhans H, Bergmann L, Mitrou PS (1992) Expression of transforming growth factor-β1 and interleukin-10 mRNA indicate immunosupressive potential of AML blasts. Ann. Haematol., 65 suppl: 40 (abstr)

20. Hines JD, Oken MM, Mazza JJ, Keller AM, Streeter RR, Glick JH (1984) High-dose cytosine arabinoside and m-AMSA is effective therapy in relapsed acute nonlymphocytic leukemia. J. Clin. Oncol., 2: 545–549
21. Zittoun R, Bury J, Stryckmanns P, Lowenberg B, Peetermans M, Rozendaal KY, Haanen C, Kerkhofs M, Jehn U, Willemze R (1985) Amsacrine with high-dose cytarabine in acute leukemias. Cancer Treat. Rep., 69: 1447–1448
22. Capiizzi RL, Davis R, Powell B, Cuttner J, Ellison RR, Cooper MR, Dillman R, Major WB, Dupre E, McIntyre OR (1988) Synergy between high-dose cytarabine and asparaginase in the treatment of adults with refractory and relapsed myelogenous leukemia – a cancer and leukemia group B study. J. Clin. Oncol., 6: 499–508
23. Bergmann L, Fenchel K, Enzinger HM, Weidmann E, Jahn B, Jonas D, Mitrou PS (1993) Daily alternating application of high dose interferon-alpha2b and interleukin-2 bolus infusion in metastatic renal cell carcinoma. Cancer, 72: 1733–1742
24. Weidmann E, Bergmann L, Stock J, Kirsten R, Mitrou PS (1992) Rapid cytokine release in cancer patients treated with interleukin-2. J. Immunother., 12: 123–131
25. Ganser A., Heil G., Kolbe K., Maschmeyer G., Fischer J.Th., Bergmann L., Mitrou P.S., Heit W., Heimpel H., Huber C., Hoelzer D. (1993) Aggressive chemotherapy combined with G-CSF and maintenance therapy with interleukin-2 for patients with advanced myelodysplastic syndrome, subacute or secondary acute myelocytic leukemia – initial results. Ann. Hematol., 66: 123–126

Acute Leukemias V
Experimental Approaches
and Management of Refractory Diseases
Hiddemann et al. (Eds.)

Interleukin-2 Postremission Therapy in Acute Myeloid Leukemia (AML): In Vitro and In Vivo Effects of a Five Day Continuous Infusion of IL-2 on Phenotype and Function of Peripheral Lymphocytes

H. S. P. Garritsen[1], C. Constantin[1], F. Griesinger[2], A. Kolkmeyer[1], R. Doornbos[3], B. G. de Grooth[3], J. Greve[3], B. Wörmann[2], and W. Hiddemann[2]

Abstract. In vitro studies have demonstrated the anti-leukemic effect of IL-2 stimulated cytotoxic lymphocytes on allogeneic leukemic blasts prompting clinical trials with IL-2 in vivo. We initiated a phase II study with IL-2 in 6 patients with acute myeloid leukemia. The patients were in second or third remission after successful salvage treatment for relapse. All patients had received a standardized first line treatment according to the protocol of the German AML cooperative group. Salvage treatment consisted of sequential high dosed cytosine-arabinoside and mitoxantrone (sHAM). the postremission IL-2 therapy consisted of continuous intravenous infusion of IL-2 in a dosis of 3×10^6 IU/m/day over 5 days, four weeks later the next cycle was given. Lymphocyte subsets in the peripheral blood and their IL-2 receptor expression of these patients were studied on day 0, 2 and 5 of the IL-2 cycle using multiparameter flow cytometry. 13 IL-2 cycles in 6 patients were analysed.

For functional studies (colony assay) peripheral blood lymphocytes (PBL) were isolated at day 0 of the IL-2 cycle and stimulated in vitro with 1000 IU/ml for 5 days. These activated cells were compared with their in vivo stimulated counterparts which were isolated at day 5 of the IL-2 cycle. Autologous leukemic blasts isolated at first relapse served as target cell in the colony assay (3 patients). If no autologous blasts were available or no growth of autologous blasts was observed the NK susceptible cell line K562 was used as target.

Immunophenotyping of PBL during IL-2 cycles showed a reversible decrease in CD4/CD8 ratios in 3 patients (day 0: mean 1.3 (0.3–2.4); day 2: mean 0.5 (0.2–0.8) and day 5: mean 1.6 (0.4–2.3)), in 1 patient an increase during IL-2 therapy was observed (day 0: 0.6, day 2: 0.9 and day 5: 0.3) and in 2 patients the data were not available.

The most significant change in lymphocyte subsets under IL-2 therapy was the consistent increase of the percentage of CD3+CD57+ cells on day 2 and a return to pre-therapeutical values at day 5 (day 0:mean 37% (10–63), day 2: 58% (31–79) and day 5: 39% (13–69). The relative number of cells expressing IL-2 receptors (P55) decreased at day 2 and increased at day 5 again (day 0: mean 8(1–21), day 2:2 (0–6) and day 5:18 (2–33).

In clonogenic assays the growth of leukemic colonies was inhibited by in vivo and in vitro IL-2 stimulated CD16 positive and gamma/delta T cell receptor expressing lymphocytes in 4 out of 6 patients. Consecutive treatment courses were monitored in two patients and showed a decrease of cytotoxic activity against K562.

We conclude that IL-2 therapy in AML patients leads to characteristic changes in the peripheral blood. Antileukemic activity was excerted in vivo and in vitro activated CD16+ NK cells and gamma/delta T cells.

[1] Dept. of Haematology/Oncology, University Hospital Münster, Münster, Germany
[2] Dept. of Haematology/Oncology, Georg August University, Göttingen, Germany
[3] Dept. of Applied Physics, University of Twente, Enschede, The Netherlands

Introduction

The prospects of AML patients after successful induction chemotherapy are still not satisfactory in terms of remission duration. 60–70% of all patients reach a complete remission, however only 15–40% are potentially cured. By using flow cytometry or detection of specific gene sequences by polymerase chain reaction (PCR) several researchers have demonstrated a population of residual blasts in complete remission bone marrows after intensive chemotherapy [1,2]. Therefore a continuous search for improvement of postremission therapy in AML is needed. The successful therapeutical application of interleukin-2 (IL-2) therapy in animal models of solid tumors and human solid tumors [3–7] has initiated basic research in the leukemia area [8–13]. Lotzova et al. [11] reported a defective NK cell functioning in active disease and they managed to restore the functional defect by in vitro IL-2 application. These in vitro studies have demonstrated an antileukemic effect of IL-2 stimulated cytotoxic lymphocytes (CTL) on allogeneic and autologous leukemic blasts prompting clinical trials with IL-2 in vivo [14,15]. We have investigated the in vivo effects of a five-day IL-2 postremission therapy in a total of 13 treatment courses in 6 AML patients in second complete remission (CR). The influence of IL-2 on immunophenotype and anti-leukemic capacities of peripheral blood lymphocytes was compared.

Patients, Material and Methods

6 patients (4 male, 2 female, mean age 54 years,range 37–66 years) were included in this study. All patients were in second or third remission after successful salvage treatment for relapse. All had been treated according to the protocols of the German Multicenter AML Study [16], using TAD9 (Thioguanine, Cytosine-Arabinoside and Daunorubicin) as induction chemotherapy, TAD9 or high dose cytosine-arabinoside and mitoxantrone (HAM) in the second part of the double induction protocol.

After successful treatment of their respective relapse with sequential high dose Cytosine-Arabinoside and Mitoxantrone (sHAM) an IL-2 postremission therapy was started.

IL-2 Therapy protocol. Four weeks after reaching CR a second bone marrow aspirate was taken to confirm continuous complete remission. The postremission therapy consisted of continuous intravenous infusion of IL-2 (Biotest Pharma, Dreieich, Germany) in a dose of 3 million IU/m/ day for 5 days. Four weeks later the next cycle of IL-2 therapy was applied. If side effects (grade 3 or 4 WHO) occurred during IL-2 application the IL-2 dose was reduced by 50%. The application of IL-2 was stopped when the patient suffered relapse, side effects (grade 4 WHO) even after 50% dose reduction, or an allogenic donor was identified for bone marrow transplantation.

Material

Isolation of the peripheral blood leukocytes. Blood of the AML patients was obtained by venipuncture on day 0, 2 and 5 of the IL-2 consolidation therapy. Heparine was used as anti-coagulant (150 USP sodium Heparine/10ml). Human leukocyte preparations were obtained by adding 190 ml of lysing buffer (8,29 g/l NH4 Cl, 0,0037 Na_2 EDTA, 1,00 g/l $KHCO_3$) to 10 ml of whole blood and incubating for 20 minutes at 40 °C. The (erythrocyte lysed) blood suspension was washed three times with phosphate buffered saline (PBS). Cell suspensions were adjusted to a concentration of 1×10^7 cells/ml in PBS containing 0,005% sodium azide and 1% serum albumine.

Immunofluorescence. 100 microliter of cell suspension was incubated with 20 microliter of pretitered monoclonal antibody for 30 minutes on ice. Subsequently cells were washed twice and resuspended in 1 ml standard buffer. Flow cytometric measurements (FACScan, BDIS, San José, CA, USA) were performed on the same day.

Monoclonal antibodies. The following monoclonal antibodies were used in this study: anti-CD3 (Leu4), anti-CD4 (Leu3), anti-CD8 (Leu2a), anti-CD16 (Leu11), anti-CD25, anti-CD57(Leu7).

All monoclonal antibodies were from BDIS (San José, CA, USA), and directly conjugated to either FITC or PerCP.

Colony Assays

Target cells. Autologous leukemic blasts of 3 patients in relapse obtained by Ficoll Hypaque density gradient isolation. The cells were frozen with 40% FCS and 10% DMSO and thawed just prior to the experiments.

A schematic representation is presented in Figure 1.

Effector cells. For in vitro analysis effector cells were isolated from peripheral blood prior to the start of the IL-2 cycle (day 0). Cells were stimulated in vitro with 1000 IU IL-2/ml in RPMI medium (Gibco) for five days. In vivo effector cells were isolated on day 5 of the IL-2 cycle by Ficoll Hypaque density gradient isolation.

Both in vitro and in vivo stimulated effector cells were separated with a home built cell sorter (department of Applied Physics, University of Twente, Enschede, The Netherlands) into T gamma/delta receptor expressing cell fraction, a CD16+ NK cell fraction and a fraction containing all cells.

Purity of all fraction was higher than 95%, viability was over 90% checked by microscopic evaluation. All preparation were done under sterile conditions.

Inhibition assay. Target and effector cells were incubated at a ratio effector to target ratio of 1:5 (100.000:500.000 with autologous blasts, 10.000:50.000 with K562 cells) in methylcellulose 0,9%, Iscove's Modified Dulbecco's Medium (IMDM, Gibco), Fetal Calf Serum (FCS) 30%, 10^{-5}M-Mercaptoethanol, 100U Granulocyte Macrophage-Colony Stimulating Factor (GM-CSF) and 100U Erythropoietin. The cells were incubated in Petri-dishes in 1 ml volume for 10–14 days at 37 C and 5% CO [17–19].

After 10 to 14 days colonies were evaluated on the basis of their morphology and growth characteristics. A cluster of cells was defined as a colony when it contained over 50 cells.

Results

Table 1 displays the CD4/CD8 ratio of the patients.

In patient 1,5 and 6 a clear shift towards higher relative percentage of CD8+ cells was observed (day 0: mean 1.3 (0.3–2.4); day 2: mean 0.5 (0.2–0.8) and day 5: mean 1.6 (0.4–2.3)), in patient 2 an increase during IL-2 therapy was

Table 1. CD4/CD8 ratio of peripheral blood lymphocytes before (day 0), during (day 2) and after (day 5) IL-2 treatment

Patient	# Il-2 cycle	day 0	day 2	day 5
1	1	2,4	0,6	2
	2	4,6	1	4,6
	3	3,1	1,2	4,2
	4	1,5	0,7	0,8
2	1	0,5	0,6	1,2
	2	0,6	0,9	0,3
	3	0,4	0,6	0,5
	4	0,4	1	0,5
	5	0,3	0,6	0,7
3	1	0,6	ND	3
4	1	1	1,3	ND
5	1	0,3	0,2	0,4
6	1	1,2	0,8	2,3

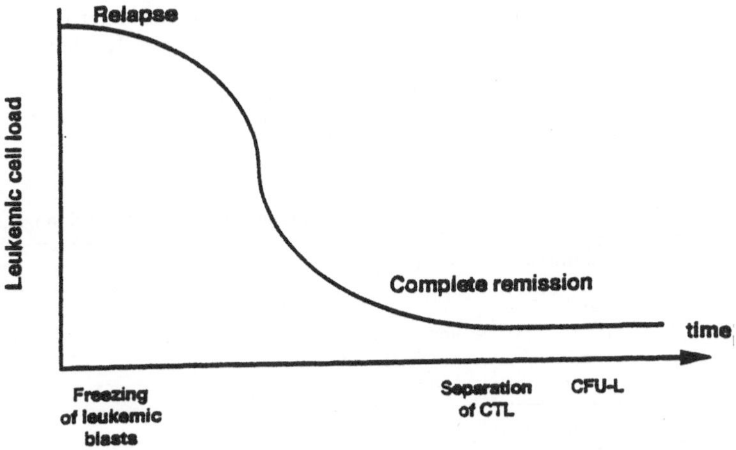

Fig. 1. Influence of cytotoxic cells on CFU-L in a patient with AML relapse. Schematic representation of the experimental design

observed (day 0: 0.6, day 2: 0.9 and day 5: 0.3). Patient 2 already had a high number of CD8+ cells compared to CD4+ cells before start of therapy. In 6 out of cycles the induced shift of CD4/CD8 ratio is completely restored at day 5 of the IL-2 cycle. In 3 patients however (patient 2 cycle 1 and 5, patient 3 cycle 1) changes in CD4/CD8 ratio remain present directly after IL-2 therapy.

Table 2 shows the results of changes in immunophenotypic CD3+ CD57+ cells during IL-2 treatment.

Table 2. Immunophenotyping of peripheral blood lymphocytes before (day 0), during (day 2) and after (day 5) IL-2 treatment (percentages) using the MAB combination anti-CD3 and anti-CD57

Patient	# Il-2 cycle	day 0	day 2	day 5
1	1	14	37	29
	2	14	42	19
	3	14	46	17
	4	10	39	27
2	1	59	70	54
	2	56	83	42
	3	58	68	69
	4	63	79	64
	5	16	65	58
3	1	56	ND	13
4	1	24	31	ND
5	1	57	73	50
6	1	42	60	23

Table 3. Expression of IL-2 (P-55) during IL-2 therapy

Patient	day 0	day 2	day 5
1	3,2	0,3	2,3
2	1	0	25
3	20,6	6,4	32,7
4	6,8	0	10,4

One can observe a shift towards more CD3+ CD57+ cells in all six patients (day 0: mean 37% (10–63), day 2: 58 % (31–79) and day 5: 39 % (13–69). The shift is reversible as can be seen at day 5 of the interleukin-2 cycle. In patients who received more than one cycle of IL-2 the effect was reproducible, even more distinct.

Table 3 displays the percentage of cells with express IL-2 receptors (CD25) during a therapy cycle of 4 patients. During therapy the number of cells positive for CD25 declines (day 0: mean 8 (1–21), day 2:2 (0–6) and day 5:18 (2–33).

Table 4 shows the results of the colony assays performed in four patients. In 3 patients autologous blasts from relapse were collected as autologous target cells, however only in one case (patient 3) autologous blasts displayed clonogenic growth after freezing and thawing. In the other patients it was necessary to use the NK-sensitive cell line for clonogenic assays. We observed different patterns of antileukemic effects. In some patients (patient 2) no inhibitory effects were observed by coincubating leukemic blasts with different IL-2 stimulated effector cell populations. In patient 1 only the in vitro stimulated CD16+ and g/d T effector fractions showed inhibitory effects. In patient 4 only the in vivo stimulated CD16+ and g/d T effector fractions showed moderate inhibitory effects. In one patient (patient 3) a strong inhibitory effect of IL-2 stimulated cells in vitro and in vivo can be seen (Target cells were autologous blasts).

Figure 2 displays the absolute numbers of colonies of patient 3. The inhibitory effects of autologous T-gamma/delta and CD16 positive NK cells after in vivo and in vitro IL-2 stimulation are also shown.

Table 4. Influence of in vivo and in vitro IL-2 stimulated lymphocytes on clonogenic outgrowth of CFU-L

Patient	control %*	total+vitro	vivo	CD16+vitro	vivo	g/d+vitro	vivo
1	100	93	89	37	103	21	103
2	100	102	105	91	98	93	90
3	100	6	22	0	17	0	0
4	100	80	69	100	89	142	68

*Control: without effector cells
+Total: all effector cells
Vitro = in vitro incubated with IL-2 for 5 days
Vivo = in vivo incubated with IL-2 for 5 days

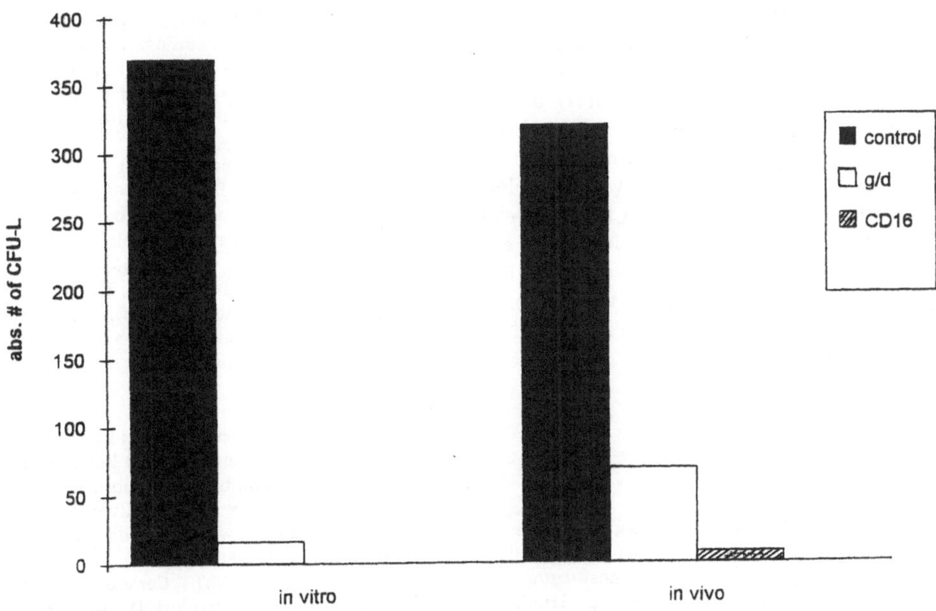

Fig. 2. CFU-L. Absolute count of leukemic colonies of patient 3 comparison of in vitro and in vivo simulation

Discussion

To elucidate the mechanisms which could help in an autologous antileukemic effect in AML patients by IL-2 we studied the immunophenotypic changes during cycles of continuous IL-2 infusions in patients after first relapse. It should be realized that this is a preliminary study with very limited number of patients. We found characteristic changes in lymphocyte distributions during IL-2 treatment. In 3 out of 4 evaluable patients there was a decrease in CD4/CD8 ratio. In patients who received multiple cycles of IL-2 this decrease in CD4/CD8 ratio was reproducible. The shifts in CD4/CD8 ratios cannot be explained by the increase of CD3+CD8+CD-57+ completely, there are also patients with an inversion of this ratio.

The relative number of CD3+CD57+ lymphocytes increased in the peripheral blood at day 2 of IL-2 therapy. Absolute numbers all decreased. IL-2 induces a lymphopenia, it is at this moment not known where peripheral lymphocytes are mobilised.

Lotzova et al. [14] studied the cytotoxic profile and distribution of lymphocyte subsets of a similar group of patients and similar IL-2 therapy (only 4 days continuous infusion of 1–1.25 million U/m2/day after IL-2 infusion). Phenotypic analysis demonstrated that CD3−, CD56+ NK cells were significantly increased by in vivo IL-2 treatment 34 to 47-fold in absolute numbers, while CD3−, CD56+ T cell subset remained low. However analyses were performed 5 days after IL-2 cycle.The reasons for the selective increase of CD3+CD57+ are not known. It could be an incompetence to respond to interleukin 2 by lack of receptors of this specific subset. At day 2 of the cycle there are very few cells expressing IL-2 receptors, but again this could also be caused by a specific blockade of the receptors by the large amount of IL-2 for the anti-CD25 receptor antibody. Perhaps the increase of CD3+CD57+ cells must be interpreted as response to IL-2. In healthy individuals CD3+CD57+ are also CD8+, there are almost none CD4+ CD57+ cells. This CD3+CD8+ CD57+subset is interesting because it has been associated with CMV infections [20] and are described as pre-cytotoxic T cells in long term bone-marrow transplanted patients [21].

The functional testing by means of colony assays of in vitro and in vivo stimulated lymphocytes shows divergent results. In some patients (e.g. patient 2) addition of IL-2 stimulated lymphocyte subset did not influence clonogenic outgrowth of CFU-L. In others (e.g. patient 3) addition of specific lymphocyte subsets had a strong inhibitory effect on clonogenic outgrowth of CFU-L. Patient 1 and 4 are examples of patients where either in vitro stimulated lymphocyte subset (patient 1) or the in vivo stimulated lymphocyte subset had an inhibitory effect on clonogenic outgrowth of CFU-L. In patient 3 there were autologous leukemic blasts available from his first relapse. The strong in vitro and in vivo inhibitory effects of his autologous IL-2 stimulated CD16 NK cells and gamma/delta T cells motivate us to continue the development of an adoptive immunotherapy in AML (Fig. 2).

References

1. Hagemeijer, A. and van der Plas, D.C.: Clinical relevance of cytogenetics in acute leukemia. In: Haematology and blood Transfusion. Acute leukemias II. Büchner, Schellong, Hiddemann, Ritter (Eds.). Springer Verlag, Berlin, Heidelberg 33 (1990) 23–30.
2. Delwel, R., van Gurp, R., Bot, F., Touw, I., Löwenberg, B.: Phenotyping of acute myelocytic leukemia (AML) progenitors: an approach for tracing minimal numbers of AML cells among normal bone marrow. Leukemia 2(12) (1988) 814–819.
3. Rosenberg, S.A., Spiess, P., Lafreniere, R.: A new approach to the adoptive immunotherapy of cancer with tumor-infiltrating lymphocytes. Science 233 (1986) 1318–1321.
4. Rosenberg, S.A., Lotze, M.T., Muul, L.M., Leitman, S., Chang, A.E., Ettinghausen, S.E., Matory, Y.L., et al.: Observations on the systematic administration of autologous lymphokine-activated killer cells and recombinant interleukin-2 to patients with metastatic cancer. N. Engl. J. Med., Vol. 313(23) (1985) 1485–1492.
5. Rosenberg, S.A., Lotze, M.T., Muul, L.M., Chang, A.E., Avis, F.P., Leitman, S., Marston Linehan, W., et al.: A progress report on the treatment of 157 patients with advanced cancer using lymphokine-activated killer cells and interleukin-2 or high-dose interleukin-2 alone. N. Engl. J. Med. 316(15) (1987) 889–897.
6. Topalian, S.L., Solomon, D., Avis, F.P., et al: Immunotherapy of patients with advanced cancer using tumor-infiltrating lymphocytes and recombinant interleukin-2: a pilot study. J. Clin. Oncol. 6 (1988) 839–843.
7. West, W.H., Tauer, K.W., Yannelli, J.R. Marshall, G.D., Orr, D.W., Thurman, G.B., Oldham, R.K.: Constant infusion recombinant interleukin-2 in adoptive immunotherapy of advanced cancer. N. Engl. J. Med. 316(15) (1987) 898–905.
8. Hakim, A.A.: Peripheral blood lymphocytes from patients with cancer lack interleukin-2 receptors. Cancer 61 (1988) 689–701.
9. Slavin, S., Eckerstein, A. and Weiss, L.: Adoptive Immunotherapy in conjugation with bone marrow transplantation – amplification of natural host defence mechanisms against cancer by recombinant IL-2. Nat. Immun. Cell Growth Regul. 7 (1988) 180–184.
10. Trentin, L., Pizzolo, G., Feruglio, C., Zambello, R., Masciarelli, M., Bulian, P., Agostini, C., et al.: Functional analysis of cytotoxic cells in patients with acute nonlymphoblastic leukemia in complete remission. Cancer 64 (1989) 667-672.
11. Lotzová, E., Savary, C., Herbermann, R.B.: Inhibition of clonogenic growth of fresh leukemia cells by unstimulated and IL-2 stimulated NK cells of normal donors. Leuk. Res. 11-12 (1987) 1059–1066.
12. Adler, A., Chervenick, P.A., Whiteside, T.L., Lotzová, E., Herberman, R.B.: Interleukin 2 induction of lymphokine-activated killer (LAK) activity in the peripheral blood and bone marrow of acute leukemia patients. I. Feasibility of LAK generation in adult patients with active disease and in remission. Blood 71 (1988) 709–716.
13. Foa, R., Fierro, M.T., Cesano, A., Guarini, A., Bonferroni, M., Raspadori, D., Miniero, R., Lauria, F. and Gavosto, F.: Defective lymphokine-activated killer cell generation and activity in acute leukemia patients with active disease. Blood 78–4 (1991)1041–1046.
14. Lotzová, E., Savary, C.A., Schachner, J.R., Huh, J.O. and McCredie, K.: Generation of cytotoxic NK cells in peripheral blood and bone marrow of patients with acute myelogenous leukemia after continuous infusion with recombinant interleukin-2. American Journal of Hematology 37 (1991) 88–99.
15. Anderson, P.M., Bach, F.H. and Ochoa, A.C.: Augmentation of cell number and LAK activity in peripheral blood mononuclear cells activated with anti-CD3 and interleukin-2. Cancer Immunology Immunotherapy 27 (1988) 82–88.
16. Büchner, Th., Urbanitz, D., Hiddemann, W., Rühl, H., Ludwig, W.D., Fischer, J., Aul, H.C., et al.: Intensified induction and consolidation with or without maintenance chemotherapy for acute myeloid leukemia (AML): two multi-center studies of the german AML Cooperative Group. J. Clin. Oncol. 3(12) (1985) 1583–1589.
17. Vellenga, E., Young, D.C., Wagner, K., Wiper, D., Ostapovicz, D. and Griffin, J.D.: The effects of GM-CSF and G-CSF in promoting growth of clonogenic cells in acute myeloblastic leukemia. Blood 69 (1987) 1771– 1776.
18. Rowley, S.D., Zühlsdorf, M., Brayne, H.G., et al.: CFU-GM content of bone marrow graft correlates with time to hematological reconstitution following autologous bone marrow transplantation with 4-hydroperoxy-cyclophosphamide- purged bone marrow. Blood 70 (1987) 271–276.
19. Krehmeier, C., Zühlsdorf, M., Büchner, Th. and Hiddemann, W.: Synergistic cytotoxicity of cytosine arabinoside and mitoxantrone for K562 and CFU-GM. In: Haematology and blood Transfusion, Acute leukemias II. Büchner, Th., Schellong, G.,

Hiddemann, W., Ritter, J. (Eds.). Springer Verlag, Berlin 33 (1990).

20. Gratama, J.W., Kluin-Nelemans, H.C., Langelaar, R.A., den Ottolander, G.J., Stijnen, T., D'Amaro, J., Torensma, R. and Tanke H.J.: Flow cytometric and morphologic studies of HNK1+ (Leu 7+) lymphocytes in relation to cytomegalovirus carrier status. Clin. Exp. Immunol. 74 (1988) 190–195.

21. Leroy, E., Madariaga, L., Ben Aribia, M., Mishal, Z., Theodorou, I., Rochant, H., Vernant, J-P. and Senik, A.: Abnormally expanded CD8+/Leu7+ lymphocytes persisting in long-term bone marrow-transplanted patients are resting pre-cytotoxic T-lymphocytes. Exp. Hematol. 18 (1990) 770–774.

Acute Leukemias V
Experimental Approaches
and Management of Refractory Diseases
Hiddemann et al. (Eds.)

Comparison of Immunological and Molecular Markers When Using Interleukin-2 (IL-2) Alone or in Combination with γ-Interferon (IFN-γ) in the Maintenance Therapy of Acute Myeloid Leukemia (AML)

A. Neubauer[1], O. Knigge, R. Zimmermann, D. Krahl[2], C. A. Schmidt, J. Oertel, and D. Huhn

Abstract. Since interleukin-2 (IL-2) has been shown to induce lysis of autologous AML blasts, maintenance therapy with IL-2 could be of value in AML. However, IL-2 normally is given at high doses, and side effects commonly occur. Low-dose regimens have been described [1]. Cytokines are capable of inducing other biological active mediators, and it is not known whether the *in-vivo* effects of low-dose IL-2 can be augmented by the addition of γ-IFN. We studied the biological effects of low-dose IL-2 alone or in combination with γ-interferon in the maintenance phase. AML patients were first treated using idarubicin and ara-C. 27 patients (25 *de novo*, 2 relapses) were enrolled in this study. Median age was 53y (range 21–81). 10/27 patients were investigated using standard cytogenetics, of which 6 were abnormal (4 of these 6 revealed del (5q). 13 (48%) patients entered CR. As maintenance treatment 4-week cycles of either low-dose IL-2 alone or IL-2 in combination with γ-IFN were alternated. Patients were randomized to start with IL-2 cycles, or with IL-2 + γ-IFN. After each cycle, patients were crossed over to the other arm. By this method, 23 immunological and 9 molecular markers of 13 cycles with IL-2 alone and of 14 cycles of IL-2 + γ-IFN could be compared. No side effects were observed. Immunological analysis using two-color flow cytometry showed activation of T-cells in single patients. No difference between cycles with IL-2 alone as compared to IL-2 plus IFN-γ was observed with regard to activation of T-cells. However, an increase of B-cells was demonstrated when using the combination treatment compared to IL-2 alone. Polymerase chain reaction using primers specific for various human cytokines and the respective receptors (IL-2; IL-2 receptor; IL4; IL6; IFN-γ; GM-CSF) revealed no correlation with treatment. In conclusion, maintenance with low-dose IL-2 seems to be safe and is well tolerated; the only difference observed between the two cycles was an increase of B-cells in the cycles with IL-2 plus IFN-γ as compared to IL-2 alone.

Introduction

Acute myeloid leukemia is a clonal proliferation of myeloid progenitor cells leading to outgrowth of the malignant clone which results in the impairment of normal bone marrow function.

In recent years, molecular biology has brought deep insights into the biology of this heterogenous disease: for instance, the translocation of the retinoic acid receptor alpha gene (RAR-alpha) into another gene termed PML results in a fusion gene PML-RAR-alpha. This molecular lesion is thought to cause AML FAB-M3. Other molecular aberrations frequently observed in AML include translocations involving transcription factors AML1-ETO1 (t [8;21]; AML-M2) and transcription factor CBFβ/PEBP2 (inv 16q; AML-M4Eo) [7]. However, except for

[1]Universitätsklinikum Rudolf Virchow, Freie Universität Berlin, Abteilung für Innere Medizin m.S. Hämatologie/Onkologie, 14050 Berlin, Germany
[2]Abteilung für Onkologie und Tumorimmunologie, Robert Rössle Klinik, Universitätsklinikum Rudolf Virchow, Germany

AML-M3, this knowledge has not yet lead to specific therapeutic strategies.

AML is normally treated using a combination of different drugs including cytosin-arabinoside (ara-C) and anthracyclines such as daunorubicin. It has been shown that more aggressive strategies in the induction therapy leads to higher complete remission (CR) rates, even in the elderly patients [5]. Furthermore, post-remission therapy in all patients is necessary to avoid early relapses.

Although recent chemotherapeutic regimens have resulted in complete remission rates up to 85% of AML in adults, most patients still die from a relapse of their disease. One strategy to prevent relapses is to administer maintenance therapy using combination chemotherapy [4].

Another option is the stimulation of immune competent cells in order to kill residual leukemic cells. A variety of immunotherapeutic strategies have been published, one of which being the administration of interleukin-2 (IL-2) in these patients. Normally, IL-2 is given at high doses of several million units intravenously. This often results in severe side effects. Other application regimens applicable on an outpatient basis have been published [1]. In order to augment the biological effects of IL-2, other cytokines may be given without increasing toxicity. One candidate is interferon-γ (IFN-γ), which *in-vitro* has been shown to increase sensitivity to IL-2 due to upregulation of the IL-2-receptor [6,12].

In the present study, IL-2 and IFN-γ were given on a outpatient basis and ex-vivo parameters such as expression of cytokine genes and activation of lymphocyte subsets were assessed. Treatment cycles consisted of either IL-2 alone or IFN-γ followed by IL-2.

An alternative to chemotherapy in the maintenance phase of treatment is immunotherapy, since AML-cells are subject to killing of immune competent cells. Different protocols use vaccination of patients with either allogeneic or autologous AML-cells. Another option is the application of biological active cytokines such as interleukin-2 (IL-2). Since IL-2 has been shown to induce lysis of autologous AML blasts, maintenance therapy with IL-2 could be of value in AML. However, IL-2 normally is given at high doses, and side effects commonly occur. Low-dose regimens have been described and applied in patients suffering from solid tumors [1].

Since cytokines are capable of inducing other biological active mediators, we sought to study the *in-vivo* effect of the combined treatment of two *in-vitro* synergizing cytokines, namely IL-2 and γ-interferon (IFN-γ). We studied the biological effects of low-dose IL-2 alone or in combination with IFN-γ in the maintenance phase. We chose a recently published induction regimen consisting of ara-C (200mg/m² × five days) and idarubicine, a novel and potent anthracycline (12mg/m² × three days) [2].

Patients, Materials and Methods

Patients: 27 patients suffering from *de novo* (N = 25) and first relapsed (N = 2) AML were treated using a combination chemotherapy consisting of idarubicin (IDA) and cytosin-arabinoside (ara-C) as described [2]. The clinical data of the 27 patients are presented in Table 1. After obtaining complete remission, patients eligible for further treatment were randomized in two arms:

arm I: treatment with cycles: A-B-A-B-A-B-A
arm II: treatment with cycles: B-A-B-A-B-A-B.

Cycle A consisted of: interleukin-2 (Proleukin, Eurocetus) monotherapy, 1×10^5 Cetus-Units/m², three times weekly for four weeks. Cycle B consisted of: IFN-γ (Polyferon, Rentschler), $1{,}5 \times 10^6$ IE/m² days 1 and 3, then start with IL-2 as in cycle A.

During the maintenance treatment, *in-vitro* studies were performed to study expression of different cytokines using reverse transcriptase polymerase chain reaction (RT-PCR). Furthermore, multi-parameter flow cytometry was used

Table 1. Clinical data of the 27 patients before chemotherapy

Age median (range)	53y (21–81)
Sex (m/f)	18/9
de novo AML	25
relapsed AML	2
Mo	3
M1	6
M2	14
M3; M3v	2
M5b	1
M6	1
Cytogenetics	
normal	4
abnormal*	6
not performed	17

*1 × t[15;17]; 1 × t[9;11]; 4 × del 5q

to determine the activation of immune competent cells during and after the treatment.

The study was approved by the ethical committee of the Freie Universität Berlin.

Multiparameter-flow cytometry: Flow cytometry was essentially performed as described using a FACScan flow cytometer (Becton Dickinson, Heidelberg) [11,14]. Dual color immunoflourescence was assesed using different combinations of: CD45 (pan-leukocyte); CD14 (monocyte); CD19 (B-cells); CD3 (T-cells); CD4 (T-helper); CD8 (T-suppressor); as "activation" markers, HLA-DR and CD25 (IL-2 receptor Ó-chain) were used. In addition, the following antigens specific for natural killer cells were determined: CD16; CD56; and CD57.

Reverse-transciptase polymerase chain reaction (RT-PCR): Extraction of RNA, and PCR were performed as described previously [9]. Primers specific for the following cytokines or receptors were used: interleukin-1β; IL-2; IL-2 receptor α chain; interleukin-4; interleukin 6; interleukin 7; TNF-α; GM-CSF; IFN-γ. Primers were either purchased from Clontech (Palo Alto, CA) or synthesized by TIB Mol Biol (Berlin). PCR was optimized for each primer pair. The sequence of the primers, and the conditions for PCR are provided upon request.

Statistical analysis: Data were stored in a database program on a personal computer. Statistics were performed using different tests and the CSS statistical program (StatSoft, Tulsa, OK).

Results

Treatment outcome after idarubicin and ara-C: 27 patients were prospectively treated in two institutions using idarubicin and ara-C in a conventional dosage as described [2]. Table 2 presents the response criteria of all 27 patients.

Table 2. Results of induction treatment by age

	age < 60	age ≥ 60	total
complete remission	9	4	13
partial response	3	4	7
no response	1	0	1
early death	4	2	6

Maintenance treatment with low-dose IL-2 and IFN-γ: Seven patients were eligible for randomization in the two maintenance treatment arms, four of which received arm A, and three arm B. A total amount of 27 cycles was given to these seven patients (N = 13 cycle A; N = 14 cycle B). The treatment was tolerated without serious side effects. In two cases, mild inflammation at the side of injection after s.c. application of IL-2 was observed. No systemic side effects such as fever, night sweats or weight gain or loss were observed in any patient.

Five of seven patients relapsed during the maintenance therapy. One patient relapsed five months after the termination of maintenance therapy, whereas one patient is in continous complete remission six months after the end of maintenance therapy. Blast cells of one patient originally lacking CD25 were positive at the time of relapse for expression of CD25.

With regard to the *in-vitro* determined "activation" parameters (coexpression of HLA-DR and CD25), "activation" of T-cells could be observed in single patients. However, this phenomenon was not observed in every patient. When the expression-PCR data, and the evaluation of the multiparameter-flow cytometric data were analysed according to the two different treatment arms, no significant differences were observed with respect to most parameters. However, the absolute, and relative number of B-cells were significantly higher in the treatment arm utilizing IFN-γ + IL-2 compared to the arm with IL-2 alone ($p = 0.008$; $p = 0.013$; Fig. 1).

Discussion

In this study, we sought to investigate *in-vitro* and *in-vivo* effects of either combined treatment with IL-2 and IFN-γ or IL-2 alone in patients suffering from AML in their first or second remission. The induction and consolidation consisted of ara-C in a conventional dosage and the new anthracycline idarubicin as published [2]. The data of induction and consolidation treatment were worse in this unselected group of AML-patients compared to other prospective studies [2,17,18]. This may be explained in part by the cytogenetic phenotype of the patients: of 10 patients investigated cytogenetically, 5 patients harbored an abnormality of either chromosome 5q (N = 4) or t(9;11)(N = 1), aberrations known to be associated with a poor prognosis (Table 1; 13).

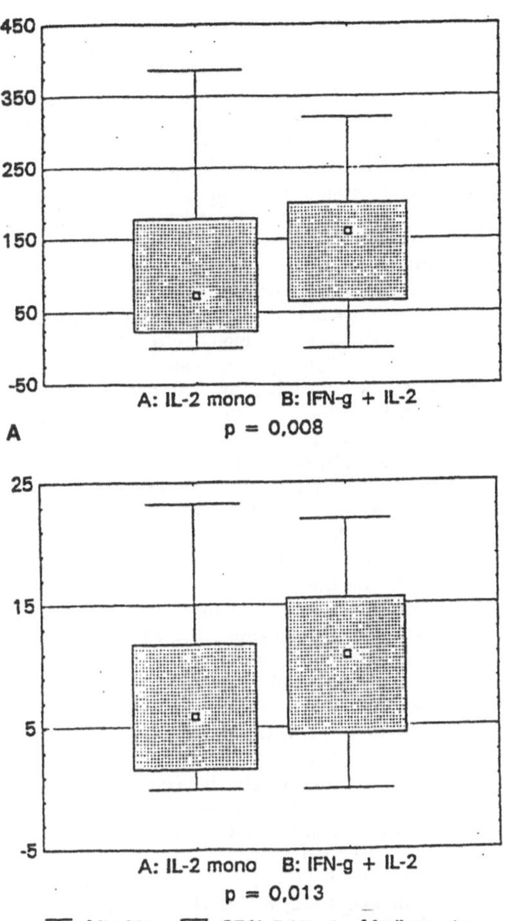

Fig. 1. Box blots displaying the absolute (A) and relative (B) number of B-cells of IL-2 given alone (*left*) or in combination with IFN-γ (*right*). Shown is the minimum and maximum, the 25–75% range, and the median value. The absolute and relative number of B-cells was higher when the combined therapy was given (p = 0.008 and 0.013)

Further, the median age in our study was higher compared to many other studies.

27 cycles consisting of IL-2 alone or in combination with IFN-γ- "priming" could be analysed. Our data show no augmentation of cellular activation after the combined cytokine treatment as compared to IL-2 alone. In detail, there was no significant difference regarding the activation of all subsets of T-cells, namely expression of the alpha chain of the IL-2-receptor (CD25), and coexpression of the DR-antigen on different subtypes of lymphocytes such as CD4- and CD8-positive T-cells. Thus, a "priming" effect of IFN-γ on T-cells with respect to upregulation of the IL-2-receptor as described *in-vitro* [3,6,16] could not be observed in our study. Several reasons could account for this phenomenon: first, the doses of the cytokines may be different from what has been described in the literature. It is unlikely that this is the case for the dose of IFN-γ, which was in the range of 120 μg corresponding to about 3×10^6 units. However, when comparing our dose of IL-2 to the doses reported in the literature, it is evident that even after converting cetus-units to international units the dose given in this trial was lower than others have used. There are, however, some reports where similar doses of IL-2 were used [15]. This trial used continous intravenous infusion over several weeks thus providing a permanent supply of IL-2; in contrast, we used subcutaneous injections three times per week for four weeks. The cumulative dosis in our trial was thus lower than the one reported by others within 90 days (2.2×10^6 Units/m² vs. 18×10^6 Units/m²).

The observed increase in the number of CD19-positive B-lymphocytes in the cycles containing IFN-γ as compared to the cycles providing IL-2 alone is interesting. IFN-γ has different effects on B-cells: it inhibits the growth accesory effects of IL-4 on B-cells; in contrast, together with anti-Ig antibodies, IFN-γ augments the proliferation of human, but not murine, B-cells. Since both the absolute, and relative number of B-cells increased during the cycles consisting of IFN-γ and IL-2, it may be speculated that these two cytokines augment the number of B-cells in humans.

In conclusion, the addition of IFN-γ to low-dose IL-2 in the maintenance treatment of AML does not augment the number of activated T-cells or NK-cells, but seems to increase the number of B-cells.

Acknowledgement. This study was supported by the Deutsche Krebsgesellschaft Berlin (A.N.).

References

1. Atzpodien J, Körfer A, Franks CR, Poliwoda H and Kirchner H (1990) Home therapy with recombinant interleukin-2 and interferon-α2b in advanced human malignancies. Lancet I: 1509–1512
2. Berman E, Heller G, Santorsa J, McKenzie S, Gee T, Kempin S, Gulati S, Andreeff M, Kolitz J, Gabrilove J, et al. (1991) Results of a randomized trial comparing idarubicin and cytosine arabinoside with

daunorubicin and cytosine arabinoside in adult patients with newly diagnosed acute myelogenous leukemia. Blood 77: 1666–1674
3. Brunda MJ, Tarnowski D and Davatelis V (1986) Interaction of recombinant interferons with recombinant interleukin-2: Differential effects on natural killer cell activity and interleukin-2 activated killer cells. Int. J. Cancer. 37: 787–793
4. Buchner T, Hiddemann W, Wormann B, Loffler H, Maschmeyer G, Hossfeld D, Ludwig WD, Nowrousian M, Aul C, Schaefer UW, et al. (1992) Longterm effects of prolonged maintenance and of very early intensification chemotherapy in AML: data from AMLCG. Leukemia 6 Suppl 2: 68–71
5. Buechner T and Hiddemann W (1990) Treatment strategies in acute myeloid leukemia (AML). Blut 60: 61–67
6. Herrmann F, Cannistra SA, Levine H and Griffin JD (1985) Expression of interleukin 2 receptors and binding of interleukin 2 by gamma interferon-induced human leukemic and normal monocytic cells. J. Exp. Med. 162: 1111–1116
7. Lu;P, Tarle SA, Hajra A, Claxton DF, Mariton P, Freedman M, Siciliano MJ and Collins FS (1993) Fusion between transcription factor CBFβ/PEBP2 and a myosin heavy chain in acute myeloid leukemia. Science 261: 1041–1044
8. Mertelsmann R, Thaler HT, To L, Gee TS, McKenzie S, Schauer P, Friedman A, Arlin Z, Cirrincione C and Clarkson B (1980) Morphological classification, response to therapy and survival in 263 patients with acute non lymphocytic leukemia. Blood 56: 773–781
9. Neubauer A, de Kant E, Rochlitz CR, Laser J, Zanetta AM, Gallardo J, Oertel J, Herrmann R and Huhn D (1993) Altered expression of the retinoblastoma susceptibility gene in chronic lymphocytic leukemia. Br. J. Haematol. 85: 498–503
10. Neubauer A, Dodge R, George SL, Davey FR, Silver RT, Schiffer CA, Mayer R, Ball ED, Wurster-Hill D, Bloomfield CD and Liu ET (1994) Prognostic importance of mutations in the ras protooncogenes in de novo acute myeloid leukemia. Blood in press:
11. Neubauer A, Serke S, Siegert W, Kroll W, Musch R and Huhn D (1989) A flow cytometric assay for cell proliferation using an anti-DNA-methyltransferase antibody. Br. J. Haematol. 72: 492–496
12. Prentice HG (1991) Mechanisms of cure in AML revealed by allogeneic bone marrow transplantation in first CR: Rationale for cytokine therapy and preliminary data review. Ann. Hematol. 62: A33
13. Schiffer CA, Lee EJ, Tomiyasu T, Wiernik PH and Testa JR (1989) Prognostic impact of cytogenetic abnormalities in patients with de novo acute nonlymphocytic leukemia. Blood 73: 263–270
14. Serke S, Neubauer A and Van Lessen A (1989) Binding of mitogenic plant lectins to human lymphocytes> Flow cytometric analysis. J. Immunol. Meth. 121: 231–235
15. Soiffer RJ, Murray C, Cochran K, Cameron C, Wang E, Schow PW, Daley JF and Ritz J (1992) Clinical and immunologic effects of prolonged infusion of low-dose recombinant interleukin-2 after autologous and T-cell-depleted allogeneic bone marrow transplantation. Blood 79: 517–526
16. Sosman JA, Hank JA and Sondel PM (1990) In vivo activation of lymphokine-activated killer activity with interleukin-2: Prospects for combination therapies. Sem. Oncol. 17: 22–30
17. Vogler WR, Velez-Garcia E, Weiner RS, Flaum MA, Bartolucci AA, Omura GA, Gerber MC and Banks PL (1992) A phase III trial comparing idarubicin and daunorubicin in combination with cytarabine in acute myelogenous leukemia: a Southeastern Cancer Study Group Study. J. Clin. Oncol. 10: 1103-1111
18. Wiernik PH, Banks PL, Case DC Jr, Arlin ZA, Periman PO, Todd MB, Ritch PS, Enck RE and Weitberg AB (1992) Cytarabine plus idarubicin or daunorubicin as induction and consolidation therapy for previously untreated adult patients with acute myeloid leukemia. Blood 79: 313–319

Acute Leukemias V
Experimental Approaches
and Management of Refractory Diseases
Hiddemann et al. (Eds.)

Immunological Response to IL-2 and α-IFN-Treatment After Autologous BMT in Patients with BCR-ABL-positive ALL

Hans Martin, Lothar Bergmann, Jochen Bruecher, Susanne Christ, Bernd Schneider, Barbara Wassmann, and Dieter Hoelzer

Introduction

Patients with Ph1+/BCR-ABL+ALL have an extremely poor prognosis after treatment with conventional chemotherapy [19, 31]. Bone marrow transplantation, however, offers a chance of cure for a proportion of these patients [1, 25]. Evidence from preclinical [9] and clinical studies at various institutions including our own [3, 4] suggests that maintenance immunotherapy with IL-2 may exert an additional "GvL"-like antileukemic effect after chemotherapy or autologous BMT in patients with *AML* [5, 6, 11, 15, 24, 28]. Less data are published on posttransplant therapy with IL-2 in patients with high risk *ALL* [5,10,24,30]. Alternatively, some patients with Ph1-pos ALL were reported to receive maintenance therapy with α-IFN [14, 16, 26, 27]. We combined these approaches and initiated a pilot phase II study for patients with BCR-ABL-positive ALL to receive sequential cycles of rIL-2 and α-rIFN after autologous BMT as part of an ongoing ABMT-program [23].

Patients and Methods

Patients. Patients with Ph1+/BCR-ABL+ ALL without histocompatible allogeneic bone marrow donor in complete remission were eligible for this study. Here we present data on 4 patients (median age 47,5 years) who were autografted in CR 1 (n=3) or in CR 2 (n=1). The 3 CR1-patients were referred to our center for ABMT after they received consolidation chemotherapy according to the high risk stratum of the German Multicenter ALL (04/89) trial at several participating hospitals (HD-AraC 1 g/m² × 8 doses and mitoxantrone 10 mg/m² × 4 doses) [18,20]. The fourth patient was referred for ABMT in second CR [12]. All patients gave written informed consent.

Autologous BMT. Autologous bone marrow was harvested within 2–4 weeks after completion of hematopoietic recovery following consolidation chemotherapy. The marrow was ficolled using a Cobe 2991 blood cell separator, followed by in vitro purging with a cocktail of mouse IgM antihuman B-lineage MoAbs directly coupled to immunomagnetic beads. The incubation was 30 min at 4 °C at a ratio beads : target B-cells of 40:1 (Dynabeads™ M450 CD10, CD19 and AB-4= anti HLA-DR [21]). Subsequently the beads were separated using a Baxter MaxSep™ device, followed by a second round of immunomagnetic beads incubation and MaxSep™ separation . The patients proceeded to conditioning with hyperfractionated TBI 14,4 Gy + CY 200 mg/m² and ABMT within 2 weeks [23].

Maintenance immunotherapy with rIL-2/α-IFN. The patients were scheduled to receive sequential cycles of rIL-2/α-rIFN after ABMT. The initial intention was to start rIL-2/α-rIFN after engraftment and independance of platelet transfusions. However, posttransplant hematopoietic reconstitution was delayed in all three CR1-patients, probably due to the intensity of chemotherapy prior to bone marrow harvest [22]. Eventually it

Dept. of Hematology, Johann-Wolfgang-Goethe-University Hospital, D-60590 Frankfurt/Main, Germany

was decided to start rIL-2/α-rIFN, while hematopoietic reconstitution was still incomplete (see Table 1). The treatment per cycle was α-rIFN 3×10^6 IU s.c. 3 × per week for 2 weeks, and rIL-2 (Proleukin®) at initially 9×10^6 IU/m² as 1-h-infusion on day 1–5 and 8–12. Due to major side effects in the first two patients, the dose of rIL-2 was reduced to 6×10^6 IU/m² in all further cycles.

Evaluation of lymphocyte subsets and NK-cell activity. Peripheral blood cells were analyzed during and after rIL-2/α-rIFN therapy on days 0, 8, 15, 22 and 28 of each treatment cycle. The following parameters were evaluated: absolute lymphocyte count/µl, T-cell subsets (CD3 CD4, CD8), IL-2-receptor alpha (TAC=CD25) and beta chain-(TU27) pos. cells, CD56+ NK cells, and in vitro cytotoxicity against Daudi- and K562-cells using ^{51}Cr-release. Cell phenotyping by flow cytometric analysis and ^{51}Cr-release cytotoxicity assays were described in detail elsewhere [2].

Results

Adherence to the treatment schedule. The posttransplant treatment with rIL-2/α-IFN was offered to 4 patients and all of them completed at least 1 cycle. However, patient #1 objected to proceed due to the side effects experienced during the first cycle and the longlasting previous hospitalisation [22]. Patient #4 postponed cycle 2 for similar reasons and eventually relapsed on d+160. Patients #2 completed three and patient #3 all four cycles (Table 1). A total of nine cycles were administered. Due to persisting low platelet counts it was not feasible to give continuous treatment with α-rIFN 3×10^6 IU s.c. 3 × weekly for 1 year as initially scheduled.

Table 1. Begin of rIL-2/α-IFN cycles (days after ABMT)

Pat	Age/sex/ status		Cycle 1	Cycle 2	Cycle 3	Cycle 4
# 1.	50/F	CR 1	d+165	–		
# 2.	45/M	CR 1	d+109	d+144	d+284	
# 3.	45/F	CR 1	d+155	d+208	d+272	d+321
# 4.	56/M	CR 2	d+ 95	–		

Side effects. Side effects were skin rush, fluid retention, fever as described in previous studies, and pleuritis (n=1) and streptococcal septicemia (n=1). Patient #3 had early posttransplant irreversible renal failure requiring chronic hemodialysis [29] and first objected but later agreed to start rIL-2/α-IFN. She tolerated this treatment reasonably well and completed all 4 scheduled cycles.

Response of lymphocyte subsets to rIL-2/α-IFN. The posttransplant counts for leukocytes, total lymphocytes and subsets were subnormal in all patients prior to rIL-2/α-IFN treatment. The three patients autografted in CR1 represent a homogenous group in respect of pretreatment and delayed posttransplant hematopoietic engraftment. Their mean response to rIL-2/α-IFN during the first cycle is shown in Table 2 and Figure 1. The numbers of lymphocytes, CD3+, CD4+, and CD8+ cells increased 2 to 3-fold on either day 8 or day 15. The peak response of CD25+, TU27+ and CD56+ (NK-cells) on day 8 or day 15 was 5 to-7-fold compared to pretreatment values.

Table 2. Immunological response during the first cycle of rIL-2/α-IFN BCR-ABL+ ALL patients autografted in CR 1 (mean ± SEM, n=3)

	day0	day8	day15	day22
Leukocytes	2033 ± 291	2350 ± 250	3500 ± 600	2650 ± 1050
Lymphocytes	835 ± 153	1731 ± 349	1842 ± 335	1521 ± 433
CD3+	676 ± 186	722 ± 44	1063 ± 662	1135 ± 525
CD3+DR	362 ± 78	626 ± 23	741 ± 304	557 ± 89
DR+	73 ± 26	693 ± 265	438 ± 242	147 ± 49
CD4+	145 ± 23	239 ± 74	343 ± 72	276 ± 135
CD8+	557 ± 125	1111 ± 9	988 ± 189	1095 ± 214
CD25+	54 ± 30	139 ± 69	164 ± 38	35 ± 20
TU27+	106 ± 21	821 ± 282	446 ± 156	279 ± 14
CD56+	104 ± 20	n.d.	558 ± 211	242 ± 22

n.d. = not done

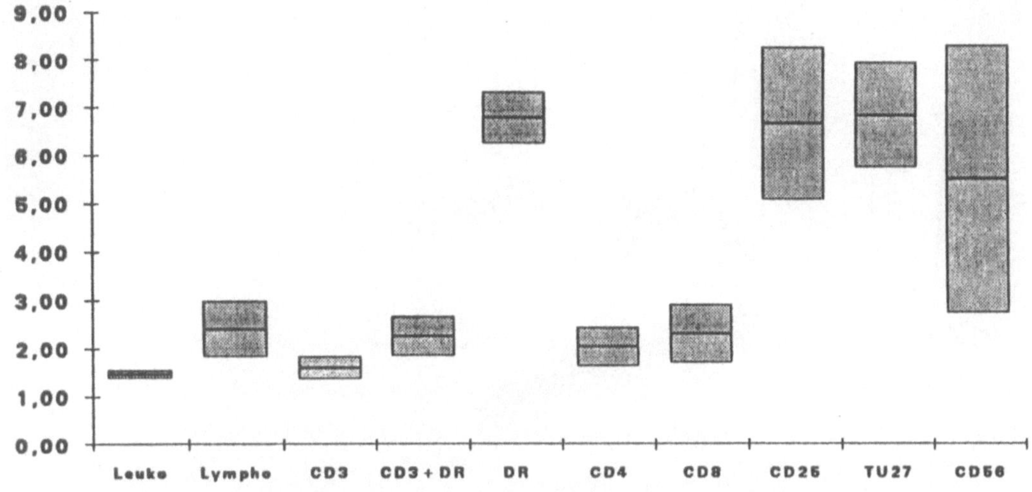

Fig. 1. Peak response during the first cycle of rIL-2/α-IFN. Ratio of peak values compared to pretreatment values (mean ± SEM, n = 3)

NK-cell function before and after rIL-2/α-IFN. The response of NK-cell function of the CR1-patients during the first treatment cycle as assessed by in vitro cytotoxicity chromium release assay at various effector:target cell ratios is shown in Figure 2 (Daudi) and Figure 3 (K562).

Discussion

Ph1+/BCR-ABL+ ALL is virtually incurable by conventional chemotherapy. A few reports on allografts in patients with Ph1+/BCR-ABL+ ALL leukemia suggest that alloBMT may results

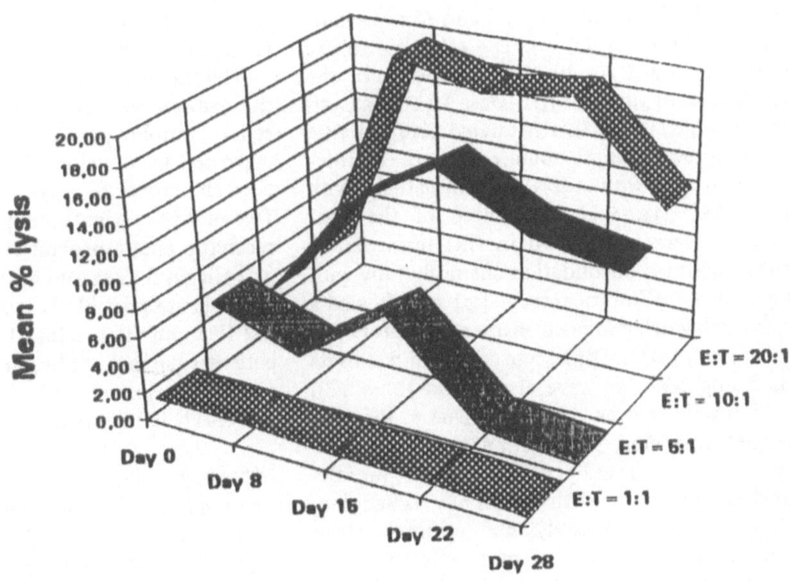

Fig. 2. Mean % lysis. DAUDI. In vitro cytotoxicity during rIL-2/α-IFN treatment in CR1 patients (n = 3)

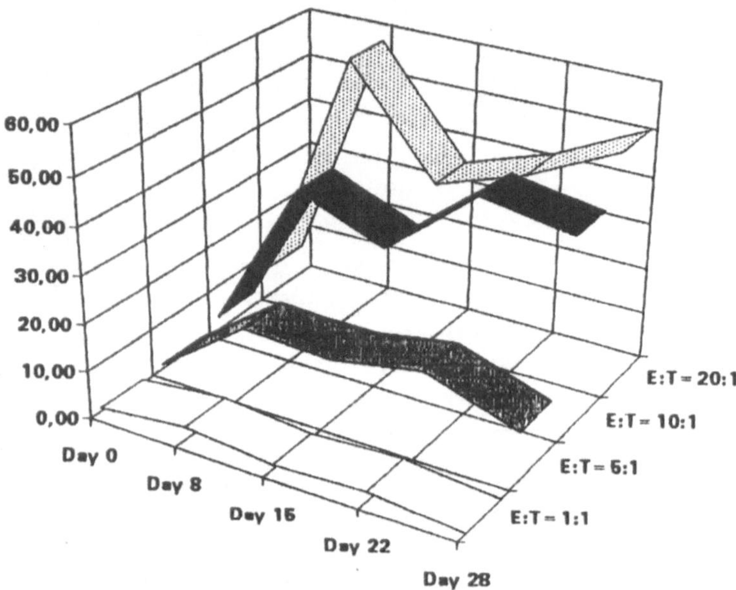

Fig. 3. Mean % lysis: K562. In vitro cytotoxicicty during rIL-2/α-IFN treatment in CR1 patients (n = 3)

in about 30–35 percent long-term disease free survival [1, 7, 13, 25]. Less results are published on autologous BMT [8, 13, 25]. We studied a combination of ABMT with posttransplant maintenance therapy with rIL-2/α-IFN in these patients. The rationale to use rIL-2 is based on the accumulating experience with IL-2 treatment in AML patients [3, 5, 15] and ALL-patients after ABMT [5, 10, 24, 30]. The rationale to use α-IFN is based on its effect to increase the expression of surface MHC-class I antigens and the synergism with IL-2 mediated LAK activity. In addition, there are some reports on maintenance therapy with α-IFN alone in patients with Ph+ ALL [14, 16, 26, 27]. Three of the four patients were autografted in CR1 immediately subsequent to consolidation chemotherapy with high dose AraC/mitoxantrone [17] and showed a remarkable delay in postransplant hematopoietic recovery [22]. Lymphocyte counts and subsets including NK-cells were also found to remain subnormal for a many months. Due to the prolonged cytopenia, the treatment with rIL-2/α-IFN was started about 3–4 months posttransplant, later than initially scheduled. This timing is possibly not optimal, since immunotherapy might be more effective early posttransplant when the possible burden of residual leukemic cells might be minimal.

The posttransplant therapy with rIL-2/α-IFN was feasible in these patients, but in our experience less well tolerated than in non-transplanted AML-patients [3]. Two of the 4 patients stopped the treatment after the first cycle. They might have been convinced to continue if the side effects were balanced by a proven clinical benefit and not only by a hypothetical benefit as in the setting of this study.

The therapy with rIL-2 and α-IFN stimulated the subnormal counts of immunocompetent cells. Lymphocytes and T-cell subsets were increased by a factor of 2–3, and NK-cells and NK-cell activity by a factor of 5–7, respectively. Two of three patients autografted in first CR and receiving posttransplant rIL-2/α-IFN remain in first CR on d+482 and d+510. However, at present it is not possible to assess the impact of rIL-2/α-IFN on the clinical outcome of these patients. Further studies are needed to evaluate an posttransplant antileukemic effect of rIL-2 and α-IFN in high risk ALL patients

Acknowledgements. We thank the colleagues participating in the German multicenter ALL trial for their cooperation. The patients studied in this paper were referred by OÄ Dr. Lengfelder, OÄ Dr. Weiss and Prof Hehlmann from Mannheim, OÄ Dr. Fuhr from Wiesbaden, OÄ

Dr. Eggeling and Prof. Hirschmann from Kassel and Prof. Brittinger from Essen.

This work was supported by the Deutsche Forschungsgemeinschaft (grant Ho 684/2-1).

References

1. Barrett AJ, Horowitz MM, Ash RC et al. (1992) Bone marrow transplantation for Philadelphia chromosome-positive acute lymphoblastic leukemia Blood 79: 3067–3070
2. Bergmann L, Fenchel K, Weidmann E et al. (1993) Daily alternating administration of high-dose alpha-2b-interferon and interleukin-2 bolus infusion in metastatic renal cell cancer. A phase II study Cancer 72: 1733–1742
3. Bergmann L, Heil G, Kolbe K et al. (1996) Interleukin-2 bolus infusion as consolidation therapy in 2nd remission of acute myelocytic leukemia. In: Hiddemann W and Büchner T (eds) Acute Leukemias V. Springer-Verlag, Berlin Heidelberg New York Tokyo
4. Bergmann L, Mitrou PS, and Hoelzer D. (1992) Interleukin-2 in the treatment of acute myelocytic leukemias -in vitro data and presentation of a clinical concept. In: Hiddemann W, Büchner T, Plunkett W, Keating M, Wörmann B, and Andreeff M (eds) Haematology and Blood Transfusion, Vol.34, Acute leukemias, Springer-Verlag, Berlin Heidelberg, New York Tokyo, pp 601–607
5. Blaise D, Attal M, Reiffers J et al. (1994) IL-2 in acute leukemia. Ann Hematol 68 Suppl. I: A11-abstr. 42
6. Blaise D, Stoppa AM, Olive D et al. (1991) Use of recombinant IL-2 (RU49637) after autologous bone marrow transplantation (BMT) in patients with hematological neoplasias: a phase 1 study. Bone Marrow Transplant 7 Suppl 2: 146
7. Blume KG, Schmidt GM, Chao NJ, and et al. (1990) Bone marrow transplantation for acute lymphoblastic leukemia. In: Gale RP and Hoelzer D (eds) Acute Lymphoblastic Leukemia. A. Liss, New York, pp 279–283
8. Carella AM, Pollicardo N, Pungolino E et al. (1993) Mobilization of cytogenetically 'normal' blood progenitors cells by intensive conventional chemotherapy for chronic myeloid and acute lymphoblastic leukemia Leuk Lymphoma 9: 477–483
9. Charak BS, Choudhary GD, Tefft M, and Mazumder A. (1992) Interleukin-2 in bone marrow transplantation: preclinical studies Bone Marrow Transplant 10: 103–111
10. Favrot MC, Negrier S, Michon J et al. (1994) Early and late intravenous interleukin-2 infusion after autologous bone marrow transplantation: report of multicentric french studies. In: Bergmann L and Mitrou PS (eds) Cytokines in Cancer Therapy. Karger, Basel, pp 156–167
11. Fefer A, Benyunes M, Higuchi C et al. (1993) Interleukin-2 +/- lymphocytes as consolidative immunotherapy after autologous bone marrow transplantation for hematologic malignancies Acta Haematol 89 Suppl 1: 2–7
12. Freund M, Diedrich H, Ganser A et al. (1992) Treatment of relapsed or refractory adult acute lymphoblastic leukemia Haemat Blood Transf 34: 472–480
13. Gehly GB, Bryant EM, Lee AM, Kidd PG, and Thomas ED. (1991) Chimeric BCR-abl messenger RNA as a marker for minimal residual disease in patients transplanted for Philadelphia chromosome-positive acute lymphoblastic leukemia. Blood 78: 458–465
14. Haas OA, Mor W, Gadner H, and Bartram CR. (1988) Treatment of Ph-positive acute lymphoblastic leukemia with a-interferon Leukemia 2: 555
15. Hamon MD, Prentice HG, Gottlieb DJ et al. (1993) Immunotherapy with interleukin 2 after ABMT in AML Bone Marrow Transplant 11: 399–401
16. Harousseau JL, Guilhot F, Fiére D, and Casassus P. (1994) Alpha interferon maintenance therapy in Philadelphia positive acute lymphoblastic leukemia. Ann Hematol 68 Suppl. I: A11-abstr. 41
17. Hoelzer D. (1991) High-dose chemotherapy in adult acute lymphoblastic leukemia Semin Hematol 28, Suppl.4: 84–89
18. Hoelzer D. (1993) Therapy of the newly diagnosed adult with acute lymphoblastic leukemia Hematol Oncol Clin North Am 7 No.1: 139–160
19. Hoelzer D. (1994) Treatment of acute lymphoblastic leukemia Semin Hematol 31: 1–15
20. Hoelzer D, Thiel E, Ludwig WD et al. (1992) The German multicentre trials for treatment of acute lymphoblastic leukemia in adults Leukemia 6 (Suppl.2): 175–177
21. Kvalheim G, Funderud S, Kvaloy S et al. (1988) Successful clinical use of an anti-HLA-DR monoclonal antibody for autologous bone marrow transplantation J Natl Cancer Inst 80: 1322–1325
22. Martin H, Bruecher J, Claudé R, Elsner S, Wassmann B, and Hoelzer D. (1993) Delayed and incomplete hematopoietic engraftment after autologous BMT is not due to immunomagnetic bead purging but due to previous intensive chemotherapy. Ann Hematol 67 suppl.: A80-abstr. 310
23. Martin H, Hoelzer D, Atta J, Elsner S, Claudé R, and Bruecher J. (1993) Autologous bone marrow transplantation in Ph'-positive/bcr-abl positive acute lymphoblastic leukemia. Blood 82 Suppl. 1: 167a-abstract 653
24. Meloni G, Foa R, Tosti S et al. (1992) Autologous bone marrow transplantation followed by interleukin-2 in children with advanced leukemia: a pilot study. Leukemia 6: 780–785
25. Miyamura K, Tanimoto M, Morishima Y et al. (1992) Detection of Philadelphia chromosome positive acute lymphoblastic leukemia by polymerase chain reaction: possible eradication of minimal residual disease by marrow transplantation. Blood 79: 1366–1370
26. Ochs J, Brecher ML, Mahoney D et al. (1991) Recombinant interferon alfa given before and in combination with standard chemotherapy in children with acute lymphoblastic leukemia in first

marrow relapse: a Pediatric Oncology Group pilot study. J Clin Oncol 9: 777–782
27. Ohyashiki K, Oyhashiki JH, Tauchi T et al. (1991) Treatment of Philadelphia chromosome-positive acute lymphoblastic leukemia: a pilot study which raises important questions. Leukemia 5: 611–614
28. Slavin S, Or R, Kapelushnik Y et al. (1992) Immunotherapy of minimal residual disease in conjunction with autologous and allogeneic bone marrow transplantation (BMT). Leukemia 6 Suppl 4: 164–166
29. Wassmann B, Bruecher J, Martin H et al. (1993) Reversible hemolysis and chronic renal failure following autologous bone marrow transplantation (ABMT) – a case of hemolytic uremic syndrome? Ann Hematol 67 suppl.: A133-abstr. 522
30. Weisdorf DJ, Anderson PM, Blazar BR, Uckun FM, Kersey JH, and Ramsay NK. (1993) Interleukin 2 immediately after autologous bone marrow transplantation for acute lymphoblastic leukemia—a phase I study Transplantation 55: 61–66
31. Westbrook CA, Hooberman AL, Spino C et al. (1992) Clinical significance of the BCR-ABL fusion gene in adult acute lymphoblastic leukemia: a Cancer and Leukemia Group B Study (8762). Blood 80: 2983–2990

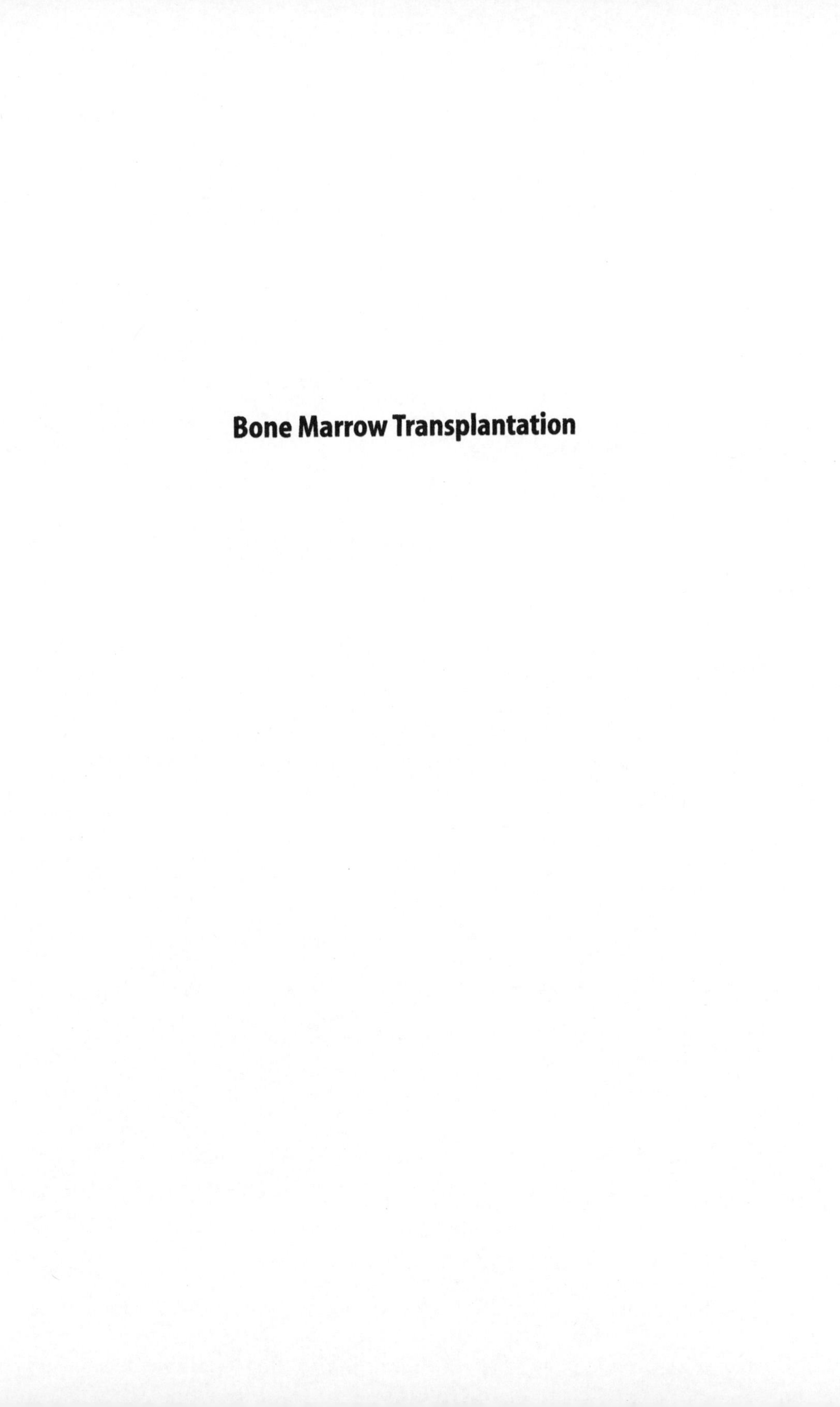

Bone Marrow Transplantation

Bone Marrow Transplantation

Acute Leukemias V
Experimental Approaches
and Management of Refractory Diseases
Hiddemann et al. (Eds.)

Conditioning Regimens for Bone Marrow and Peripheral Blood Stem Cell Transplantation

Angelo M. Carella

Introduction

Patients with acute leukemias or CML still have a poor prognosis when treated with standard dose chemotherapy alone. In view of this situation, myeloablative chemotherapy with bone marrow transplantation (BMT) or, more recently, autologous peripheral blood stem cell transplantation (ASCT), has become more and more an established methodology in the treatment of hematological neoplasias as well as some solid tumor types [Sheridan 1992, Brugger 1993].

The preparatory chemotherapeutic regimen administered prior to marrow or stem cell transplantation is of crucial importance with regard to treatment outcome. It is intended to effectively eradicate the malignant cell clones and, especially in allogeneic BMT, to immunosuppress the host to allow for rapid engraftment.

Over the past decade, a variety of pretransplant myeloablative and immunosuppressive regimens have been developed, each associated with a different spectrum of side effects and remission rates.

In a "Meet the Professor" session at the international symposium "Acute Leukemias V", Angelo M. Carella summarized the Genoa experience on conditioning regimens for bone marrow and peripheral blood stem cell transplantation.

Pretransplant Regimens in Acute Leukemias with TBI

Early conditioning regimens before bone marrow transplantation usually involved a combination of cyclophosphamide and total body irradiation. However, these protocols failed to be effective in eliminating all leukemic cells and resulted in considerable risk for graft failure in allogeneic BMT. Furthermore, a high incidence of side effects, e.g., pulmonary toxicity and infectious complications, was observed resulting in a 5–10% therapy-related mortality. The development of secondary cancer years after cure was significantly higher after treatment with TBI than after non-TBI-based regimens [Witherspoon 1989]. A reduction in irradiation-associated toxicity was achieved by lung shielding as well as by introduction of fractionated and hyperfractionated TBI.

Attempts to increase the irradiation dose intensity resulted in a decreased relapse incidence.

In AML in first complete remission, patients given cyclophosphamide and 15.75 Gy of fractionated total body irradiation showed a reduced relapse rate compared to those receiving cyclophosphamide and 12 Gy TBI. However, due to a corresponding increase in toxicity and transplant-related mortality no real improvement in leukemia-free survival was obtained [Clift 1991]. Advantages with regard to treatment

Department of Hematology and Bone Marrow Transplantation Unit, Ospedale San Martino, Genova, Italy outcome were achieved with novel protocols. Combinations of high-dose etoposide and fractionated TBI [Blume 1987] or high-dose cytosine arabinoside and TBI [Coccia 1988] led to reports of prolonged event-free survival.

Most recent data [Aversa 1993] revealed that the addition of Thiotepa to hyperfractionated TBI and Cyclophosphamide improves results for T-Cell depleted BMT in patients with advanced Leukemia.

Pretransplant Regimens without TBI: Busulfan + Cyclophosphamide

Santos et al. introduced the first pretransplant regimen without TBI, which included busulfan and cyclophosphamide. For AML, the combination of busulfan 4 mg/kg/d orally for 4 days and cyclophosphamide 50 mg/kg/d intravenously for four days was reported to result in long-term event-free survival similar to that observed with TBI-based regimens [Santos 1989, Geller 1989]. Similar efficacy but significantly lower toxicity was observed after application of busulfan as given above and cyclophosphamide for two days only [Tutschka 1989]. These data led to comparison of TBI-based regimens versus busulfan and cyclophosphamide in several prospective randomized studies. Blaise et al. reported on treatment of 101 patients with AML in first remission with either busulfan and cyclophosphamide (BU-CY) or cyclophosphamide and TBI (CY-TBI). Two-year disease-free survival was significantly better in patients receiving TBI versus those given busulfan ($p < 0.01$) [Blaise 1992]. On the other hand, Sayer et al. observed equivalent overall survival, disease-free survival, pulmonary complications and transplant-related mortality in 77 patients with AML in first remission treated with either BU-CY or CY-TBI [Sayer 1994]. The same results were obtained by Biggs et al. in 115 patients with CML in chronic phase [Biggs 1992].

In Seattle, a total of 142 patients with hematological neoplasias were prospectively randomized to receive either cyclophosphamide and TBI or busulfan and cyclophosphamide [Buckner, 1994]. Patient characteristics and toxicity are given in Table 1.

69 patients received CY-TBI, 73 patients were treated with BU-CY. Patient groups were comparable with regard to age, gender and pretreatment leukocyte count. The rate of acute graft versus host disease (grades 2–4) was slightly higher in the CY-TBI group, however, the mortality rate in both treatment arms was identical. Veno-occlusive disease was not observed, which may be due to prophylactic application of anticoagulants. Overall survival, relapse rate and event-free survival were identical in both groups.

Table 1. Comparison of cyclophosphamide and total body irradiation (CY-TBI) versus busulfan and cyclophosphamide (BU-CY) in patients with hematological malignancies

Parameter	CY-TBI	BU-CY
Patient Characteristics		
No. of patients	69	73
Sex (m:f)	43:26	46:27
Age (years)		
mean	37.1	38.6
range	6–54	7–55
standard deviation	10.3	10.3
pretherapeutic WBC ($\times 10^9$/l)		
mean	168.4	148.8
range	10–570	4–582
standard deviation	140.6	131.6
Acute GVHD grades 2–4		
day 20	31%	17%
day 50	48%	34%
Mortality		
total no. of deaths	14	15
Causes of death		
chronic GVHD	1	1
interstitial pneumonia	7	2
bacterial infection	0	1
fungal infection	2	6
liver failure	2	0
bronchiolitis obliterans	1	0
respiratory failure/ARDS	1	1
pulmonary fibrosis	0	1
leukemia	0	3

WBC white blood cell count
GVHD graft-versus-host disease
ARDS acute respiratory distress syndrome

In conclusion, the chemotherapeutic conditioning regimen without total body irradiation yielded results similar to the TBI-based protocol [Buckner, 1994].

Considerations in CML and High-Risk ALL

In chronic myelogenous leukemia and high-risk acute lymphoblastic leukemia, conventional chemotherapy remains unsatisfactory with regard to relapse rate and long-term survival. Allogeneic bone marrow transplantation without T-cell depletion is the only therapeutic strategy with a curative intent in both disorders. However, in the majority of cases, an HLA compatible donor cannot be identified.

The leukemic clones in CML and high-risk ALL are characterized by specific chromosomal aberrations suitable for cytogenetic or PCR analysis as given in Table 2.

However, normal stem cells also persist in the bone marrow in any stage of the disease, as demonstrated both by in vitro and in vivo studies [Singer 1980].

In CML, Philadelphia chromosome negative (Ph−) progenitor cells survived better than Philadelphia chromosome positive (Ph+) cells, when marrow from patients was established in long-term cultures [Coulombel 1983]. In purified populations from CML patients, Ph− cells can be clearly identified [Goldman 1990]. In theory, "normal" pluripotent hematopoietic stem cells are metabolically and mitotically more quiescent and less sensitive to chemotherapy than mature progenitor cells. Acute depopulation by chemotherapy generates messengers which stimulate the stem cells to repopulate the committed and maturing compartments [Juttner 1985]. Recent data have demonstrated, that intensive chemotherapy and subsequent application of hematopoietic growth factors allows for a proliferative advantage of residual normal progenitor cells and an overshoot in peripheral blood [Carella 1991, Sessarego 1992, Carella 1992, 1993, 1994].

Regarding these considerations, collection of normal pluripotent stem cells by leukapheresis from peripheral blood seems feasible in the early marrow reconstitution phase after intensive chemotherapy, even in hematologic neoplasias with bone marrow involvement. Subsequent myeloablative high-dose chemotherapy with peripheral blood stem cell support could allow an increase in dose intensity and drug efficacy.

Autologous Peripheral Blood Stem Cell Transplantation

Peripheral blood stem cell transplantation (ASCT) is a viable alternative to autologous BMT and offers various advantages including more rapid hematological recovery after high-dose chemotherapy [Sheridan 1992, Brugger 1993], autograft collection by leucapheresis with avoidance of general anesthesia and the chance of performing high-dose chemotherapy in patients with residual marrow disease, myelofibrosis or pelvic irradiation [Kessinger 1991, Carella 1991, Brugger 1994].

Since the first clinical application in 1986 [Körbling 1986], the technical principles of high-dose chemotherapy with autologous stem cell support have largely been standardized. In general, intensive standard chemotherapy with subsequent application of hematopoietic growth factors and leucapheresis of peripheral progenitor cells is given. In a second step, myeloablative chemotherapy with stem cell retransfusion is possible.

If this procedure is to be applied for CML and high-risk ALL, the chemotherapy protocols used for stem cell mobilization and high-dose therapy have to be adapted for treatment of both disorders.

Table 2. Chromosomal markers in adult CML and ALL suitable for PCS analysis

type of leukemia	chromosomal translocation	molecular target	DNA or RNA	Frequency
CML				
Ph-positive	t(9;22)(q34;q11)	bcr-abl	RNA	95%
ALL				
precursor B-ALL (80–85%)	t(9;22)(q34;q11)	bcr-abl	RNA	30–40%
	t(1;19)(q23;p13)	E2A-PBX1	RNA	5–8%
B-ALL (1–3%)	t(8;14)(q24;q32)	c-myc-Sμ	DNA	1%
T-ALL (15–20%)	tal deletion	tal	DNA	10–30%
	t(1;14)(p34;q11)	tal-TCRδ	DNA	1–3%
	t(10;14)(q24;q11)	TCL3-TCRδ	DNA	1–3%
	t(11;14)(p13;q11)	bcr-TCRδ	DNA	5–10%

Mobilizing Chemotherapy with Idarubicin, Cytarabine and Etoposide (ICE)

Initial chemotherapy in CML and high-risk ALL should cover several aspects, i.e., effective treatment of the underlying disease, induction of bone marrow hypoplasia and mobilization of sufficient numbers of peripheral blood progenitor cells for bone marrow reconstitution after subsequent high dose chemotherapy.

Carella and colleagues have chosen a regimen combining the novel anthracycline idarubicin with etoposide and intermediate dose cytarabine (ICE protocol, Table 3).

It allows for mobilization of stem cells by chemotherapy with three effective, non-cross-resistant cytotoxic agents demonstrating antitumor activity in CML and ALL.

Inclusion of the novel anthracycline idarubicin is based on a variety of preclinical and clinical advantages of this compound as compared to daunorubicin or doxorubicin: highly lipophilic behavior, oral bioavailability and penetration of the CNS. Due to its high lipophilicity, idarubicin and its active metabolite, idarubicinol, show strong DNA-binding and intranuclear concentration [Plumbridge 1978, Capranico 1987]. As compared to all other anthracyclines, idarubicin is less susceptible to P-glycoprotein-mediated drug transport (multidrug resistance) due to reduced cytoplasmic concentration of the compound [Berman 1992, Müller 1992, Gieseler 1994]. In randomized comparative trials, idarubicin showed a higher rate of complete remissions than daunorubicin, with more patients achieving CR after a single course of treatment [Berman 1991, Wiernik 1991].

Overall, 93 patients with hematologic neoplasias were treated with the ICE protocol for stem cell mobilisation in Genoa, the disease entities included chronic myelogenous leukemia (n=69, blastic phase: 35 patients, accelerated phase: 14 patients, chronic phase: 20 patients), acute lymphoblastic leukemia (n=16), acute myelogenous leukemia (n=4), Hodgkin's disease (n=2) and Non-Hodgkin's lymphoma (n=2, t(14;18), BCL2-positive). Leucapheresis procedures were initiated at white blood cell counts of 0.5 to 0.8×10^9/l and were completed successfully in all cases. Nucleated cells collected varied between 1.1 and 7.6×10^8/kg body weight [Carella 1992, 1993].

In CML, besides sufficiently allowing leucapheresis of peripheral blood progenitor cells, ICE chemotherapy effectively induced cytogenetic remissions (Table 4).

Table 3. ICE protocol as mobilizing chemotherapy followed by collection of peripheral blood progenitor cells

Idarubicin	8 mg/m²/d × 5	iv, bolus	days 1–5
Cytarabine	800 mg/m²/d × 5	iv, 2h-infusion	days 1–5
Etoposide, VP16	150 mg/m²/d × 3	iv, 2h-infusion	days 1–3

Table 4. Therapy of CML with ICE intensive chemotherapy followed by collection of peripheral blood hematopoietic progenitor cells

Response category	Patients: Total		Accelerated Phase		Chronic Phase	
Complete cytogenetic remission, CCyR	16	41%	4	22%	12	57%
Major cytogenetic remission, MCyR	7	18%	1	6%	4	19%
Minor cytogenetic remission, mCyR	3	8%	3	17%	2	10%
No cytogenetic remission, NCyR	13	33%	10	55%	3	14%
total	39		18		21	
Previous IFNα treatment	34		18		17	

CCyR = disappearance of all Ph+ metaphases
MCyR = ≥50% reduction in the proportion of Ph+ metaphases
mCyR = <50% reduction in the proportion of Ph+ metaphases
NCyR = 100% Ph+ metastases

Thirty-nine patients were cytogenetically analysed for persistance of Ph+ metaphases. Complete cytogenetic remission was achieved in 16 patients (41%), major cytogenetic remission in 7 patients (18%). Patients in chronic phase demonstrated significantly higher remission rates than patients in accelerated phase. Leucapheresis was performed up to ten times in each patient (median 3 times). The majority of initial leucapheresis specimens were cytogenetically Ph−, later specimens were increasingly positive for the Philadelphia chromosome. several patients showed Ph+ specimens after an interval of 6 to 12 months only.

Autologous Stem Cell Transplantation in CML

Leucapheresis specimens collected after ICE mobilizing chemotherapy were used for peripheral blood progenitor cell support after myeloablative high-dose chemotherapy, if stem cell preparations were cytogenetically determined to be Philadelphia chromosome negative.

As conditioning regimen before stem cell transplantation (SCT), patients with CML received either a combination of etoposide (VP16), cyclophosphamide and total body irradiation, or, more recently, idarubicin, etoposide (VP16) and TBI (IVT protocol, Table 5).

Due to its steep dose-response curve and reduced cardiotoxicity, idarubicin appears to be the anthracycline of choice for high-dose chemotherapy approaches [Casazza 1979, Carella 1990].

In a pilot study, 14 patients with chronic myelogenous leukemia were treated with myeloablative therapy and autologous Philadelphia chromosome negative blood progenitor cell transplantation. Ten patients were in chronic and 4 in accelerated phase, respectively. All patients showed Ph+ marrow as determined by cytogenetical methods. Nine patients received etoposide, cyclophosphamide and TBI as conditioning regimen, 5 patients were treated according to the IVT protocol. The median interval between therapy and neutrophil recovery to more than 1×10^9/l was 18 days (range 12–69 days), the median time to platelet recovery to more than 25×10^9/l was 54 days (range 10–240 days). Nine patients are alive and well, five patients are Philadelphia chromosome negative (at 4, 12, 16, 17 and 28 months after transplantation). 5 patients died, two had been transplanted in chronic phase, three in accelerated phase. Causes of death were graft failure (3 cases) and blast crisis (2 cases).

In view of these data, two prospectively randomized study at diagnosis or in early phase of CML were started in Genoa in collaboration with many worldwide teams, in order to evaluate the efficacy, toxicity and long-term outcome of autologous SCT in CML patients. The study flow chart is given in Figure 1 and 2, for high dose chemotherapy the IVT regimen will be used.

Autologous Stem Cell Transplantation in High-Risk ALL

In high risk ALL with defined chromosomal translocations or abnormalities, a similar approach with mobilizing and myeloablative chemotherapy courses was chosen in Genoa.

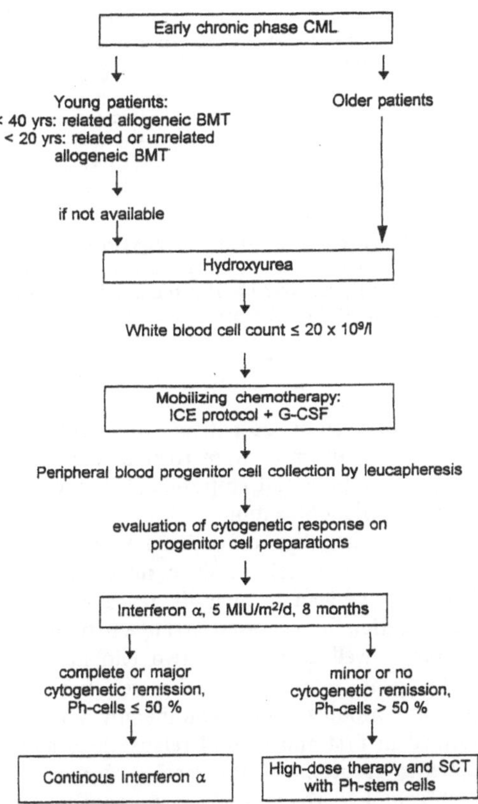

Fig. 1. Prospectively randomized study of autologous stem cell transplantation in chronic phase CML. ICE therapy for stem cell mobilisation, IVT chemotherapy as conditioning myeloablative regimen

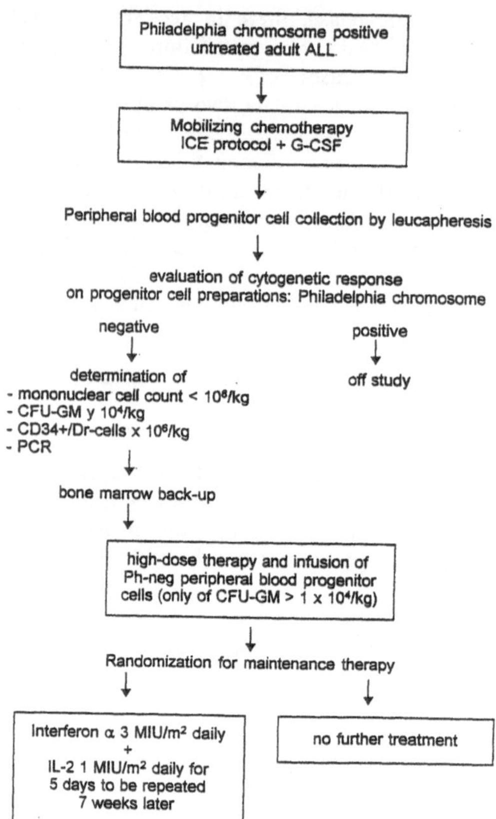

Fig. 2. Prospectively randomized study of autologous stem cell transplantation in untreated Philadelphia chromosome positive ALL. ICE therapy for stem cell mobilisation, IVT chemotherapy as conditioning myeloablative regimen

Table 5. IVT protocol as myeloablative conditioning regimen for autologous stem cell transplantation in CML and high-risk ALL

day	treatment	dose
−11	Idarubicin	30 mg/m²/d, iv, 3h-infusion
−7	VP 16	800 mg/m²/d, iv
−6	VP 16	800 mg/m²/d, iv
−2	TBI (single dose)	8.5 Gy (16–18 cGy/min)
0	retransfusion	Philadelphia chromosome negative peripheral blood progenitor cells
+8	G-CSF	5 μg/kg/d, until marrow reconstitution

Table 6. Cytogenetic remission rates after high-dose chemotherapy and ASCT in patients with acute lymphoblastic leukemia

Patients n	Cytogenetics at relapse	Cytogenetic remissions blood	Cytogenetic remissions bone marrow
10	t(9;22)	5/10	1/10
4	t(4;11)	3/4	1/4
2	t(8;14)	2/2	1/2
2	t(4;8)	2/2	2/2
2	igH+	2/2	1/2

In a pilot study, 20 patients with acute lymphoblastic leukemias were treated with idarubicin, cytarabine and etoposide (ICE protocol) for stem cell mobilization.

The median age of patients was 35 years (range 17–50 years), 13 were males and five females. Cytogenetic analysis revealed t(9;22) translocation in 10 cases, t(4;11) in 4 patients and t(8;14) as well as t(4;8) in two patients each. IgH+ gene rearrangements were seen in 2 patients. Mobilization chemotherapy was performed in first and second relapse in 9 and 6 patients, respectively, the median duration of first complete remission was 8 months. One patient had been refractory to first line chemotherapy, two patients presented with newly diagnosed ALL. Peripheral blood progenitor cell collection was possible in all patients studied. High-dose chemotherapy was performed subsequently.

As in CML, the conditioning regimens for stem cell transplantation (SCT) consisted of a combination of etoposide (VP16), cyclophosphamide and total body irradiation, or, more recently, idarubicin, etoposide (VP16) and TBI (IVT protocol, Table 5). Feasibility and tolerability of this form of treatment were clearly demonstrated.

Results with regard to cytogenetic remission rates in peripheral blood and bone marrow are given in Table 6.

Conclusions

Leukemic relapse and development of drug resistance remain significant factors limiting long-term survival in patients with CML and high-risk ALL. Increased dose intensity in myeloablative chemotherapy with marrow reconstitution by means of peripheral blood progenitors or bone marrow cells might result in improved treatment efficacy. Against this background, the choice of induction therapy and high-dose chemotherapy protocols is of major importance.

In Genoa, Carella and colleagues decided to treat patients with CML and high risk ALL with an anthracycline in combination with cytarabine and etoposide (ICE protocol). Idarubicin is a new anthracycline analogue that has shown less cardiotoxicity, advantageous pharmakokinetic properties and superior antileukemic effect as compared to other anthracyclines [Berman 1991, Wiernik 1991, Carella 1990].

Application of ICE chemotherapy allowed for sufficient collection of peripheral blood progenitor cells as well as high antineoplastic efficacy with tolerable, reversible side effects. For myeloablative conditioning treatment, a combination of idarubicin, etoposide and total body irradiation (IVT protocol) was applied. Excellent remission rates were achieved with good extrahematologic tolerance. Peripheral blood progenitor cell support led to rapid engraftment and reconstitution of bone marrow compartments. In conclusion, although the numbers of patients treated are small, the preliminary results of the Genoa pilot studies on combination chemotherapy protocols for CML and high-risk ALL are encouraging. As the data given above seem to indicate high effectiveness of early high-dose therapy and autologous stem cell transplantation in CML and high-risk AML, prospectively randomised studies on these treatment strategies have been designed and are currently open for patient recruitment.

References

1. Aversa F, Terenzi A,Carrotti A, Martelli MP, Latini P, Gambelunghe C, Martelli MF. Addition of thiotepa improves results in T-Cell depleted bone marrow transplant for advanced leukemia. Blood ASH 1993;Vol. 82 u. 10, suppl. 1
2. Berman E, Heller G, Santorsa JA, McKenzie S, Gee T et al. Results of a randomized trial comparing idarubicin and cytosine arabinoside with daunorubicin and cytosin arabinoside in adult patients with newly diagnosed acute myelogenous leukemia. Blood 1991; 77: 1666–1674.
3. Berman E, McBride M. Comparative cellular pharmacology of daunorubicin and idarubicin in human multidrug-resistant leukemia cells. Blood 1992;79: 3267–3273.
4. Biggs JC, Szer J, Czilley P, Atkinson K, Downs K, Dodds A, Concannon AJ, Avalos B, Tutschka P, Kapoor N, Bzodsky I, Topolsky D, Bulsva SI, Copelan EA. Treatment of chronic myeloid leukemia with allogeneic bone marrow transplantation after preparation with BuCy 2. Blood 1992;80: 1352–1357.
5. Blaise D, Maraninchi D, Archimbaud E, Reiffers J, Devergie A, Jouet JP, Milpied N, Attal M, Michallet M, Ifrah N, Kuentz M, Dauriac C, Bordigoni P, Gratecos N, Guilhot F, Guyotat D, Gouvernet J, Gluckman E. Allogeneic bone marrow transplantation for acute myeloid leukemia in first remission: a randomized trial of busulfan-cytoxan versus cytoxan-total body irradiation a preparative regimen. Blood 1991;79: 2578–2582.
6. Blume KG, Forman SJ, O'Donnell MR, Doroshow JH, Krance RA, Nademanee AP, Snyder DS, Schmidt GM, Fahey JL, Metter GE, Hill LR, Findley DO, Sniecinski IJ. Total body irradiation and high-dose etoposide: a new preparatory regimen for bone marrow transplantation in patients with advanced hematologic malignancies. Blood 1987; 69: 1015–1020.
7. Brugger W, Bross K, Glatt M, Weber F, Mertelsmann R, Kanz L. Mobilization of tumor cells and hematopoietic progenitor cells into peripheral blood of patients with solid tumors. Blood 1994;83: 636.
8. Brugger W, Birken R, Bertz H, Hecht T, Pressler K, Frisch J, Schulz G, Mertelsmann R, Kanz L. Peripheral blood progenitor cells mobilized by chemotherapy plus G-CSF accelerate both neutrophil and platelet recovery after high-dose VP-16, ifosfamide and cisplatin. Br J Hematol 1994;84: 402.
9. Buckner. Blood in press.1994.
10. Capranico G, Riva A, Tinelli S, Dasdia T, Zunino F. Markedly reduced levels of anthracycline-induced DNA strand breaks in resistant P388 leukemia cells and isolated nuclei. Cancer Res 1987;47: 3752–3756.
11. Carella AM, Podesta M, Frassoni F, Raffo MR, Pollicardo N. Collection of "normal" blood repopulating cells during early hemopietic recovery after intensive conventional chemotherapy in CML. Bone marrow Transplantation 1993;12: 267–271.
12. Carella AM, Podesta M, Pollicardo N, Pungolino E, Raffo MR, Ferrero MR, Belgumaschi. G, Rost V, Cazzola M, Saglio G, Frassoni F. Idarubicin-containing regimen and G-CSF are capable of recruiting CD34+/D2− cells with high proliferative potential which sustain Ph-negative polyclonal hematopotesis. Leukemia 1994;1: 212–213.
13. Carella AM, Pollicardo N, Raffo MR, Podesta M, Carlier P, Valbonesi M, Lercari G, Vitale V, Gallamini A. Intensive conventional chemotherapy can lead to a precocious overshoot of cytogenetically normal blood stem cells in chronic myeloid leukemia and acute lymphoblastic leukemia. Leukemia 1992;6(suppl.4): 120–123.
14. Carella AM, Gaozza E, Raffo MR, Carlier P, Frassoni F, Valbonesi M, Lercari G, Sessarego M, Defferrari R, Guerrasio A. Therapy of acute phase chronic myelogenous leukemia with intensive chemotherapy, blood cell autotransplant and cyclosporine A. Leukemia 1991;6: 517–521.

15. Carella AM, Berman E, Maraone MP, Ganzina F. Idarubicin in the treatment of acute leukemias. An overview of preclinical and clinical studies. Haematologica 1990;75: 159–169.
16. Casazza AM, Bertazolli G, Pratesi G. Antileukemic activity and cardiac toxicity of 4-demethoxy-daunorubicin. Proc Am Ass Cancer Res 1979;20: 16.
17. Clift RA, Buckner CD, Appelbaum FA, Bryant E, Bearman SI, Petersen FB, Fisher LD, Anasetti C, Beatty P, Bensinger WI, Doney K, Hill RS, McDonald GB, Martin P, Meyers J, Sanders J, Singer J, Stewart P, Sullivan KM, Witherspoon R, Storb R, Hansen JA, Thomas ED. Allogeneic marrow transplantation in patients with chronic myeloid leukemia in the chronic phase. A randomized trial of two irradiation regimens. Blood 1991;77: 1660–1665.
18. Coccia PF, Stranjord SE, Warkentin PI, Cheung NV, Gordon EM, Novak LJ, Shina DC, Herzig RH. High-dose cytosine arabinoside and fractionated total body irradiation: an improved preparative regimen for bone marrow transplantation of children with acute lymphoblastic leukemia in remission. Blood 1988;71: 888–893.
19. Coulombel L, Kalousek DK, Eaves CJ, Gupta CM, Eaves A. Long-term marrow culture reveals chromosomally normal hematopoietic progenitor cells in patients with Philadelphia chromosome-positive chronic myelogenous leukemia. N Engl J Med 1983;308: 1493–1498.
20. Geller RB, Saral R, Piantadosi S, Zahurak M, Vogelsang GB, Wingard JR, Ambinder RF, Beschorner WB, Braine HG, Burns WH, Hess AD, jones RJ, May WS, Rowley SD, Wagner JE, Yeager AM, Santos GW. Allogeneic bone marrow transplantation after high-dose busulfan and cyclophosphamide in patients with acute nonlymphocytic leukemia. Blood 1989;73: 2209–2218.
21. Gieseler F, Clark M, Wilms K. Cellular uptake of anthracyclines, intracellular distribution, DNA binding and topoisomerase II activity. Determinants for hematopoietic cell sensitivity in chemotherapy. Ann Hematol 1994;68(suppl.1): A24, abstract 95.
22. Goldman JM. Options for the management of chronic myeloid leukemia 1990. Leukemia and Lymphoma 1990;3: 159–164.
23. Juttner CA, To LB, Haylock DN, Branford A, Kimber RJ. Circulating autologous stem cells collected in very early remission from acute non-lymphoblastic leukemia produce prompt but incomplete hematopoietic reconstitution after high dose melphalan or supralethal chemoradiotherapy. Br J Hematol 1985;61: 739–744.
24. Kessinger A, Armitage JO. The evolving role of autologous peripheral stem cell transplantation following high-dose therapy for malignancies. Blood 1991;77: 211–213.
25. Körbling M, Dörken B, Ho AD. Autologous transplantation of blood-derived hematopoietic stem cells after myeloablative therapy in a patient with Burkitt's lymphoma. Blood 1986;72: 529–534.
26. Müller MR, Lennartz K, Boogen C, Nowrousian MR, Rajewski MF, Seeber S. Cytotoxicity of adriamycin, idarubicin, and vincristine in acute myeloid leukemia: chemosensitization by verapamil in relation to P-glycoprotein expression. Ann Hematol 1992;65: 206–212.
27. Plumbridge TW, Brown JR. Studies on the mode of interaction of 4′-epi-adriamycin and 4-demethoxy-daunomycin with DNA. Biochem Pharmacol 1978;27: 1881–1882.
28. Santos GW. Marrow transplantation in acute nonlymphocytic leukemia. Blood 1989;74: 901–908.
29. Sayer HG, Beelen DW, Quabeck K, Mohnke M, Oidtmann M, Schaefer UW. Comparison of high-dose busulfan and total body irradiation prior to allogeneic bone marrow transplantation. In: Büchner T, Hiddemann W, Wörmann B, Schellong G, Ritter J (eds) Acute Leukemias IV. Springer, Berlin Heidelberg New York, 1994, pp. 689–693.
30. Sessarego M, Fugazza G, Frassoni F, Defferrari R, Bruzzone R, Carella AM. Cytogenetic analysis of hematopoietic peripheral blood cells collected by leukapheresis after intensive chemotherapy in advanced phase Philadelphia-positive chronic myelogenous leukemia. Leukemia 1992;6: 715–719.
31. Sheridan WP, Begley CG, Juttner CA. Effect of peripheral blood progenitor cells mobilised by filgrastim (G-CSF) on platelet recovery after high-dose chemotherapy. Lancet 1992; 339: 640–644.
32. Singer JW, Arlin ZA, Najfeld V, Adamson JW, Kempin SJ, Clarkson BD, Fialkow PJ. Restoration of nonclonal hematopoiesis in chronic myelogenous leukemia following a chemotherapy induced loss of the Ph1+ chromosome. Blood 1980; 56: 356–360.
33. Tutschka PJ, Copelan EA, Kapoor N. Replacing total body irradiation with busulfan as conditioning of patients with leukemia for allogeneic marrow transplantation. Transplant Proc 1989; 21: 2952–2954.
34. Wiernik PH. New agents in the treatment of acute myeloid leukemia. Sem Hematol 1991; 28(suppl.4): 95–98.
35. Witherspoon RP, Fisher LD, Schoch G, Martin P, Sullivan KM, Sanders J, Deeg HJ, Doney K, Thomas D, Storb R, Thomas ED. Secondary cancers after bone marrow transplantation for leukemia or aplastic anemia. N Engl J Med 1989; 321: 784–789.

Acute Leukemias V
Experimental Approaches
and Management of Refractory Diseases
Hiddemann et al. (Eds.)

Influence of Different Conditioning Regimens on Stroma Precursors

K. Momotjuk, L. Gerasimova, V. Savchenko, S. Kulikov, L. Mendeleeva, and L. Lubimova

Introduction

Bone marrow transplantation (BMT) has become a widely acceptable treatment of various hematologic diseases, mostly leukemias. It is a well known fact that chemoradiotherapy applied before BMT sufficiently influence on hematopoietic microenvironment that plays a decisive role in hemopoiesis in vivo. The outgrowth of hematopoietic precursors is supported by direct cellular contact between stromal (endotelial cells, reticular/fibroblasts, monocyte/macrophages) and hematopoietic cells, and also by soluble factors, especially, GM-CSF, G-CSF, M-CSF, IL-3, IL-4 [1]. It may be questioned whether a relationship can be found between the in vitro outgrowth of hematopoietic precursor cells and different types of stromal cells. We estimated the influence of pre-BMT conditioning regimens on the growth characteristics of reticular cells/fibroblasts, assessed in as short-term bone marrow cultures, and of hematopoietic precursor cells, prior and after BMT .

Patients and Methods

20 patients transplanted for haemotological malignancies were studied from 1991 to 1993. 15 received allografts, 2 syngeneic grafts and 3 autografts. 15 patients were treated with Busulfan (BU) 4 mg/kg, days −7 to day −4, and Cyclophosphamide (CPH) 60 mg/kg, days −3 and −2 (all cases CML, ALL and 5 AML) and 5 with CPH 60 mg/kg, days −7 and −6 and fractionated total body irradiation (FTBI) 2′ × 2 Gy, days −4 to −2 (5 AML patients). All patients survived early post-BMT period, 5 have relapsed within 4 month after transplantation. 5 patients with AML and 1 with CML had graft-versus-host disease (GVHD) Methotrexate and Cyclosporin A were given as prophylaxis of acute GVHD to all patients with allogeneic BMT. All AML patients were treated with Daunorubicin and ARA-C during 10 months before BMT, ALL patients with Daunorubicin, Oncovin, Prednisone, ARA-C, Asparaginase, CPH, 6-mercaptopurine, Methotrexate during 20 months before BMT. Patients with CML were treated with BU during 15 months.

CFU-F and CFU-GM from bone marrow were assayed before conditioning, on week 3, 4, month 3, 6, 9. CFU-GM were assayed by the method reported by Pice and Robinson[4]. For CFU-F assay bone marrow aspirates were layered over Ficol-Hypaque gradient and after following centrifugation mononuclear cells were cultured in triplicate in 35mm plastic petri dishes at concentrations of 10^5 cells of medium, consisting of Alpha MEM supplemented with 5% fetal calf serum, 5% inactivated human serum AB (IV), 1% L-glutamine. Number of CFU-F and CFU-GM has been assessed in 10/5 myelocaryocytes.

Results

We did not divide patients according to the type of BMT. The dividement of the patients was performed according to the conditioning regimen

National Research Center for Hematology, Moscow, Russia

and type of leukemia. We used the bone marrow from 20 healthy donors for our assay in order to investigate the normal level of CFU-F. It was 21,3+/− 3,5.

The dynamics of CFU-F number in AML patients, treated with CHP and BU is shown in Fig. 1. There were no significant differences in initial level of CFU-F in this group (16,8+/−2,8). The number of CFU-F decreased up to the 3rd week after BMT and did not rise during the whole time of observation (up to 6 month). In the group of AML patients treated with CHP and FTBI (Fig. 2) initial level of CFU-F was 6,7+/−4,7. The level of CFU-F decreased critically at the 3rd week after BMT and state constantly during 3 months. In 2 cases (patient 1 and 2) CFU-F number increased at 6th month and contained 4-fold cell number compared to the initial level.

The group of ALL patients (Fig. 3), treated with CPH and BU (initial level 5,1+/−2,7) was the most heterogenous as regards early response to conditioning regimen. But there was a common trend of the CFU-F number reduction and

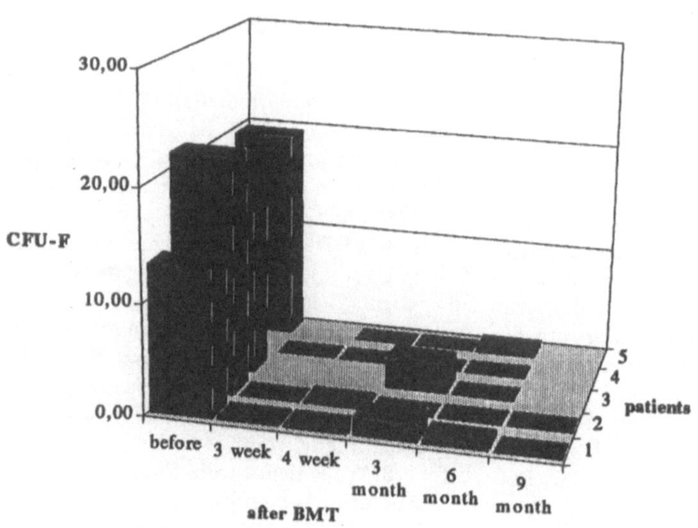

Fig. 1. Dynamics of CFU-F number in AML patients treated with CHP and BU

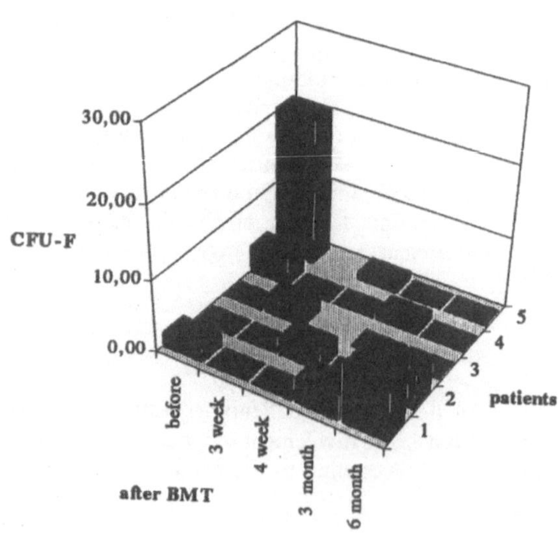

Fig. 2. Dynamics of CFU-F number in AML patients treated with CPH and TBI

their level was critically decreased to the 6th month after BMT. The initial level of CFU-F in CML patients (Fig. 4) was 4,9+/−2,7. CFU-F number ranged from 44% to 150% of initial level up to the 4th week after BMT. Alterations became maximum (CFU-F level 0, 0,9) at the 3rd month. The level increased up to 26% and 58% of initial one at the 6th month. At the end of the first year after BMT the level of fibroblast precursors was identical to the initial in 3 cases. There was no significant correlation between the number of CFU-F and CFU-GM in samples taken at the 3rd and the 4th month after transplantation (Fig. 5A,B).

Discussion

The bone marrow is composed of two types of cells, that is, the hematopoietic and the stromal cells [1]. In case of leukemia the proliferation and differentiation of myeloid precursors and their interactions with stromal cells are significantly disturbed [6]. AML is characterised by nearly normal level of fibroblastic precursors at the moment of initial diagnostics and in remission, but not early after the cytostatic treatment, when their number is significantly decreased [5].

In our study the initial level of CFU-F in 2 groups of AML patients was different and was

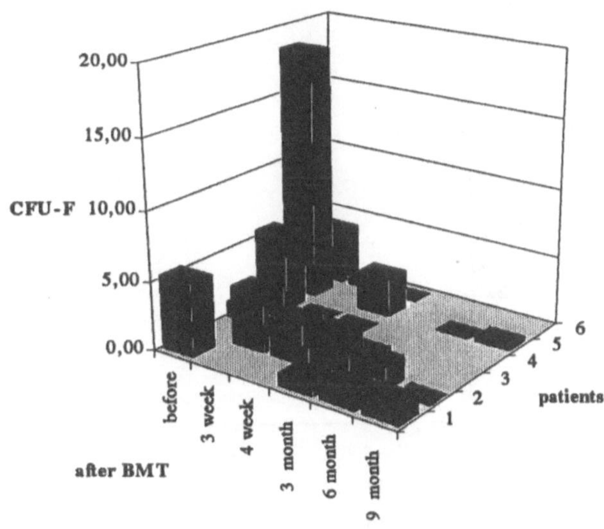

Fig. 3. Dynamics of CFU-F numbers in ALL patients treated with CHP and BU

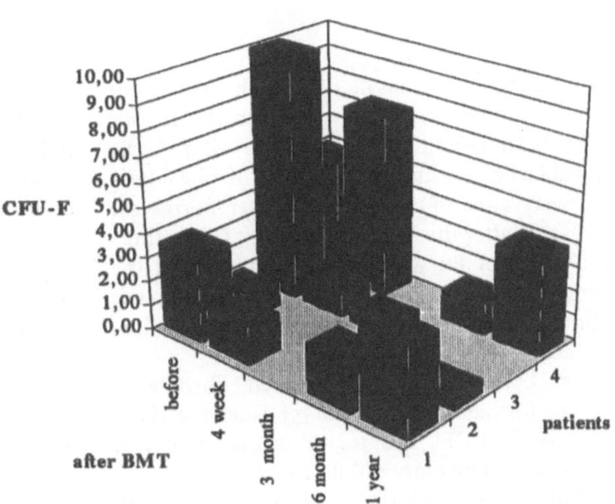

Fig. 4. Dynamics of CFU-F numbers in CML patients treated with CHP and BU

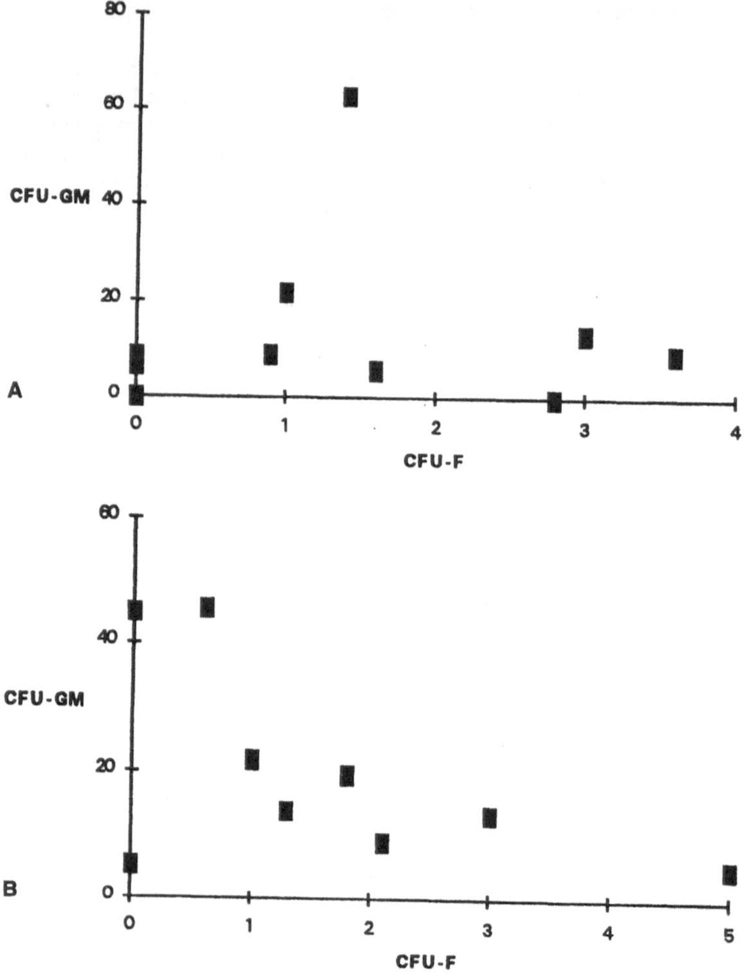

Fig. 5. Diagram showing the CFU-F outgrowth versus CFU-GV at different time after BMT (**A** – 3 months, **B** – 6 months)

not taken into account during the choice of BMT conditioning regimen. According to our data both conditioning regimens altered the fibroblastic precursors. The time of fibroblasts recovery after CPH + FTBI regimen correlated with that after the irradiation only [3]. The altering effect of Bu was more prolonged and the time of our observation (6 months) does not allow us to make any conclusions about the time of recovery.

In ALL patients the reduced fibroblastic colony formation was shown [5]. One case of the high level of CFU-F observed in this study can be explained by more cellularity of bone marrow samples obtained during harvesting. This group is the most heterogeneous in reaction to Busulfan containing regimen. But in all cases the reduction of CFU-F level was registered up to 9 month after BMT that may be due to the postponed influence of Bu.

The patients with AL, treated with autografting were also included in our study because the stromal compartment of hematopoiesis is not transplantable in humans and the host origin of the bone marrow fibroblasts is proved in all cases of allografts [10].

In the cases of untreated CML, the number of fibroblastic precursors was increased. All investigated patients recieved Busulfan before BMT, and showed the decreased level of CFU-F [7, 8].

The reduced CFU-F level up to the 6th month after BMT might be due to the conditioning regimen, which included BU. The recovery of the CFU-F number to initial level at the 1st year.

References

1. Emerson SG, Gale RP (1987) The regulation of hematopoiesis following bone marrow transplantation. Int J Cell Cloning 5: 432
2. Li S, Champlin R, Fitchen JH, Gale RP (1985) Abnormalities of myeloid progenitor cells after "successful" bone marrow transplantation. J Clin Invest 75: 234
3. Gualtieri RJ (1987) Consequences of extremely high doses of irradiation of bone marrow stromal cells and the release of hematopoietic growth factors. Exp Hematol 15: 952
4. Pice BL, Robinson WA (1970) Human bone marrow colony-growth in agar gel. J Cell Physiol 76: 77
5. Hirata H, Katsuno M, Kaneko S, Umemura T et al (1986) Clinical significance of human bone marrow stromal cell colonies in acute Leucemias. Leukemia Res.10: 1441
6. El-Khatib Y, Gidali J, Feher I et al (1991) Stromal cell growth and blast colony-forming cells in AML bone marrow. Leukemia Res 15: 1037
7. Nagao T, Casro-Malaspina H (1983) Characteristics and functions of fibroblasts colony forming cells in human bone marrow. Rincho Ketsuchi 24: 1455
8. Yonehure S, Nagao T, Arimoso S (1985) Increased growth and collagen synthesis of bone marrow fibroblast from patients with chronic myelocytic leucemia. Br J Haematol 61: 93
9. van den Berg H, Kluin RhM, Zwaan FE, Vossen GM (1989) Histopathology of bone marrow reconstitution after allogeneic bone marrow transplantation. Histopathology 15: 363
10. Agematsu K, Nakahori J (1991) Recipient origin of bone marrow-derived fibroblastic stromal cells during all periods following bone marrow transplantation in humans. Br J Haematol 79: 359
11. van den Berg, Maarten JD, van Tol et al (1992) Study of possible correlation between in vitro growth of bone marrow stromal and hematopoietic precursor cells early after bone marrow transplantation. Exp Hematol 20: 184

Acute Leukemias V
Experimental Approaches
and Management of Refractory Diseases
Hiddemann et al. (Eds.)

Autologous Bone Marrow Transplantation in Relapsing Acute Leukemias

C. Annaloro, A. Della Volpe, R. Mozzana, A. Oriani, E. Pozzoli, D. Soligo, E. Tagliaferri, and G. Lambertenghi Deliliers

Introduction

Second complete remission (CR) can be achieved in more than 50% of relapsing patients with acute myelogenous (AML) and lymphoblastic leukemia (ALL); however, in spite of this relatively favourable CR rate, only a scant proportion of these patients experience long-term disease-free survival [1,2]. Various strategies have been designed in order to improve the above figure. Allogeneic (BMT) and autologous bone marrow transplantation (ABMT) appear to be therapeutic choices which could offer a significant advantage in terms of event free survival (EFS) [3,4].

Information concerning BMT and ABMT in relapsing acute leukemias are mainly derived from observational studies, but comparisons with historical control groups are less difficult than in first CR series. This is because relapsing patients make up a rather homogeneous group characterized by an almost invariably negative outcome, which makes it unlikely that neglected prognostic factors may play a confounding role [1,5,6].

Some authors argue that relapsing disease is the most appropriate condition for BMT since its ability to prolong EFS after first CR is not such as to offer an advantage clearly outweighing the risk of transplant-related mortality [7]. On the other hand, the question should be raised as to whether the policy of performing BMT in this more advanced disease phase might not lead to a further increase in toxicity and a consequent reduction in the number of eligible patients [8]. For patients relapsing after BMT performed in first CR, a second myeloablative treatment followed by BMT has been investigated with encouraging results [9].

The results of most investigators show that ABMT can allow a substantial proportion of relapsing acute leukemia patients to achieve long-term EFS and, in this setting, ABMT compares favourably with BMT [10]. According to the majority of studies, the best figures can be achieved in AML rather than in ALL (although many series collect cases of both diseases) and, generally, no differences in outcome according to the site of relapse have been reported [11,12]. Most of the series are small, as well as being heterogeneous by diagnosis (either AML or ALL), disease phase (either first relapse or second remission) and previous treatment. However, since the expected long-term EFS after conventional chemotherapy is very low, the improved outcome of patients receiving ABMT can be partially attributed to ABMT itself.

There is still considerable debate about the best way of performing ABMT. No conclusive evidence has yet been found regarding the most effective conditioning regimen [3,4,7,13,14]. The timing of bone marrow (BM) harvesting is another matter of controversy, since some authors favour the collection of BM in all patients achieving first CR [15] but, in other trials, second CR BM has been harvested [3,4]: in the former case the matter is made more intriguing by the question as to which is of the best phase of the chemotherapy regimen for BM collection. In the latter case, the possibility of

Centro Trapianti di Midollo, University of Milan, 20122 Milano, Italy

achieving good quality second CR is uncertain, particularly in ALL where a substantial aliquot of residual leukemic cells can be documented in the majority of cases [2,16]. "Ex vivo" bone marrow purging can overcome this problem, but only at the expense of an increased risk of graft failure [17,18]. A further matter of disagreement concerns the best disease phase for submitting relapsing patients to ABMT. Although the reported results are generally rather scant, they seem to be better for patients in second CR than for those in early relapse; however, adopting the former policy leads to the exclusion of a substantial proportion of patients failing to achieve second CR, some of whom may have been cured by early ABMT [15]. Therefore, any comparisons between these two groups of patients should be made very cautiously, since the better results obtained in second CR patients is counterbalanced by the higher number of enrollments if ABMT is performed soon after relapse. On the other hand, the latter choice obviously requires BM pre-harvesting in all patients after the achievement of first CR.

The present study refers to a single-Institution series of acute leukemia patients (both AML and ALL), who underwent autologous BMT with unpurged bone marrow harvested during second or subsequent CR.

Materials and Methods

Over the last ten years, 25 patients with AML [8] and ALL [17] in second [19] or subsequent CR [6], have undergone ABMT in our Institution. Their essential characteristics are summarized in Tables 1, 2.

All of the AML patients were in second CR after hematological [7] or meningeal [1] relapse. The median interval between the last CR and ABMT was 6 months (range 1–21). The ALL patients were in second [11] or third CR [6], after hematological [9], hematological and CNS [1], and isolated CNS relapse [7]. The median interval between the last CR and ABMT was 3 months (range 1–6).

Table 1. Characteristics of 25 AL patients receiving ABMT

Sex (M/F)	17/8	
Median age	20 years	(range 10–53)
Adults	16	(5 AML, 11 ALL)
Children	9	(3 AML, 6 ALL)

Table 2. Disease status at ABMT

	2nd CR	3rd CR
Disease-phase (AML/ALL)	19 (8/11)	6 (0/6)
	CNS	Bone marrow
Site of previous relapse (AML/ALL)	8 (1/7)	17 (7/10)
	AML	ALL
Interval between last CR and ABMT	6 months (range 1–21 months)	3 months (range 1–6 months)

The patients had been referred to our Center by a number of different hematological Divisions in which they had been treated by various second line regimens.

In all but one patient, autologous BM had been harvested during the same disease-phase as that in which the autografting was performed. CR and relapse were defined according to conventional criteria, and the persistence of CR was assessed by means of BM aspiration and biopsy before both BM harvesting and ABMT.

The BM was collected, processed and cryopreserved according to routine techniques; with the only exception of one AML M3 female patient, whose second CR bone marrow was purged with maphosphamide, no "ex vivo" purging procedure was performed.

The conditioning regimen included Ara-C 3g/m^2/12 h on Days −9 and −8; CTX 60 mg/kg/day on Days −6 and −5; and TBI at a total dosage of 10 Gy, fractionated in 3 equal doses over Days −3, −2 and −1 (dose rate, 5 cGy/min).

The patients were treated in a laminar air flow room; antimicrobial prophylaxis and therapy, parenteral nutrition and transfusional support with irradiated blood products were given according to conventional criteria. Peripheral neutrophil and platelet levels of respectively >500/mm^3 and > 50000/mm^3 on two consecutive days without transfusions were selected as markers of successful engraftment. Toxicity was graded according to the WHO scoring system.

Survival was calculated from the day on which the ABMT was performed, and relapses and toxic deaths were selected as events. DFS and event-free survival (EFS) curves were calculated according to the life-table method and compared by means of the Lee-Desu logrank test.

Results

The median number of infused nucleated cells and CFU-GM were respectively 2.35×10^8/kg (0.75–9.4) and 10.8×10^4/kg (0.9–55.2).

Almost all of the patients experienced grade 2 or more nausea, vomiting and oropharyngeal mucositis; the frequency of diarrhea was the same, but was generally milder. No other significant forms of extra-hematologic toxicity were recorded; there was no case of hepatic venoocclusive disease. Persisting fever exceeding 38°, and requiring empirical antibiotic therapy occurred in 24 patients.

One AML patient died of lung hemorrhage before engraftment in the absence of any leukemic signs. One AML patient achieved peripheral neutrophil recovery but still needed periodic platelet transfusions six months after ABMT. Successful engraftment was demonstrable in the other 23 patients, median times to neutrophil and platelet recovery being respectively 22 (13–55) and 45 days (22–>180). Clinical observation was interrupted on 31/12/1993, when the median follow-up for censored patients was 44 months in AML (range 6–122) and 61 months in ALL (range 18–90). Two AML patients had relapsed 3 and 26 months after ABMT; eleven ALL patients had relapsed a median of 6 months after ABMT (range 3–48). Seven of these ALL patients had received ABMT in second, and 4 in third CR; 3 after isolated CNS relapse (2 hematological relapses 6 and 48 months after ABMT, and 1 meningeal relapse 15 months after ABMT), 1 after combined bone marrow and CNS relapse, and 7 after hematological relapse. None of the relapsing patients achieved a further remission. Five AML patients (including the one with previous CNS relapse) and 6 ALL patients (4 with previous CNS relapse) were still alive and leukemia-free. Clinical outcome is summarized in Table 3.

The median EFS for ALL patients was 11 months, while it had not been reached for the AML patients; the corresponding 5-year EFS chances were 32.9% and 60% respectively (Fig. 1, 2).

The median EFS of 10 ALL patients undergoing autografting after hematological relapse was 7 months, with a 5-year EFS chance of 20% (Fig. 3). If the 8 patients (7 ALL and 1 AML) who received ABMT after isolated CNS relapse are considered separately, median EFS had not been reached, and the 5-year EFS chance was 56.25% (Fig. 4).

Table 3. Present disease status

Follow-up	AML ALL CCR	Median 44 mo. Median 61 mo. Relapse	(range 6–122) (range 18–90) Early death
AML	5	2	1
ALL (all)	6	11	0
ALL/BM relapse	2	8	0
CNS relapse (1 AML, 7 ALL)	5	3	0

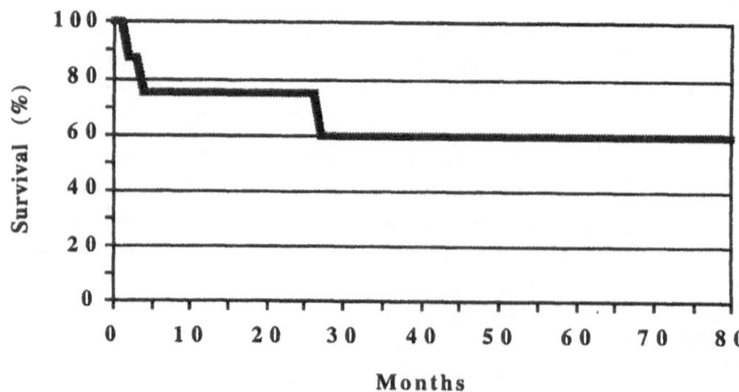

Fig. 1. EFS of AML patients autografted in 2nd CR

Fig. 2. EFS curve of ALL patients autografted in 2nd or 3rd CR

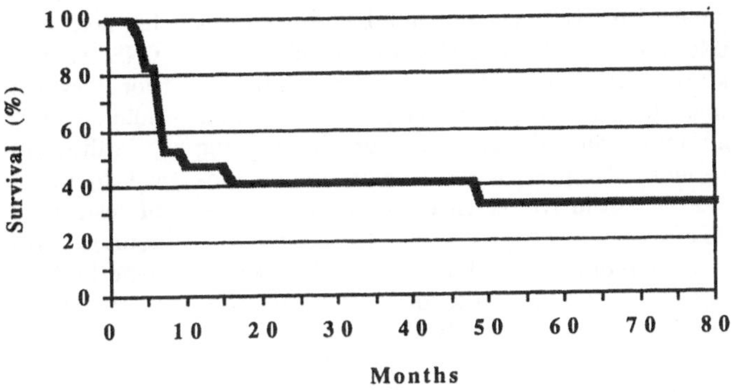

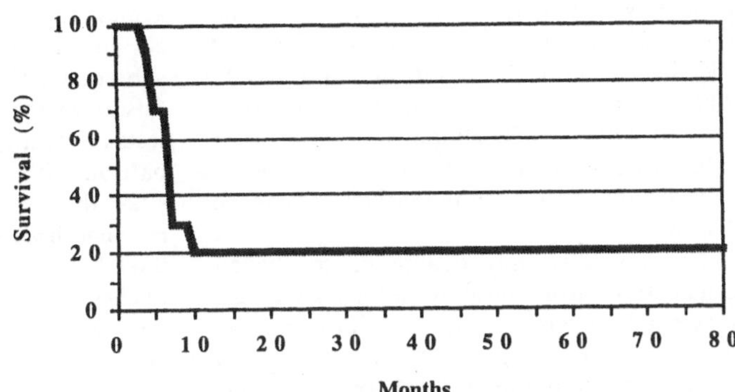

Fig. 3. EFS curve of ALL patients autografted after hematological relapse

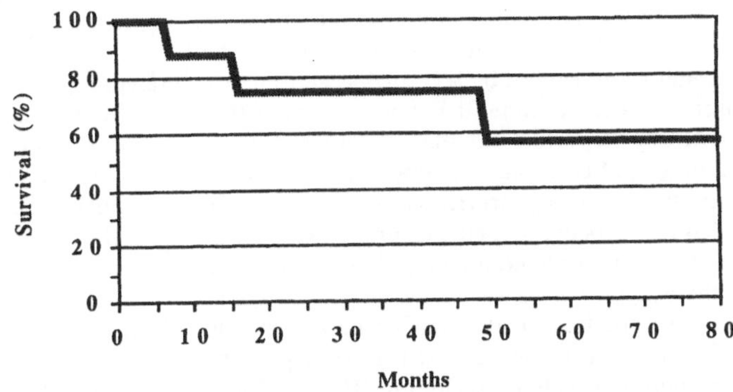

Fig. 4. EFS curve of patients autografted after isolated CNS relapse

Discussion

The present study concerns a small but not negligeable single-Institution series. The patients were homogeneous in many respects, including age (mostly adult), disease phase (all were in CR) and conditioning regimen; furthermore, they had received unpurged BM harvested in second or subsequent CR. On the other hand, they were heterogeneous and unselected in terms of diagnosis, previous chemotherapy (both induction and reinduction) and the time interval between the last CR and ABMT.

At first glance, the long-term EFS in AML is very encouraging, since it compares favourably with the best series of both ABMT and BMT performed in second CR [11,19]. There is no question that the present figure is superior to those reported in patients undergoing autografting in early relapse [3,4,15]; nevertheless any comparison is made difficult by the obvious selection bias of our series, which only represents a sample of AML patients achieving second CR in the referral centers, who account for an undetermined proportion of all relapsing patients. The present study can therefore provide no conclusive evidence concerning this specific issue.

On the other hand, long-term EFS in relapsing AML is a rather anecdotal event after conventional chemotherapy [1,6]. In spite of a high CR rate and a favourable median EFS, we were unable to find any long-term EFS case in a previous experience collecting relapsing AML patients who underwent an aggressive chemotherapeutic protocol including intensive post-CR therapy [20]. In terms of survival after ABMT, the observed advantage can be attributed to ABMT itself, although to an undetermined extent. The present study cannot help to solve the question about the real effectiveness of "ex vivo" purging.

Consequently, only qualitative conclusions can be drawn from the above results: good quality second CR can be achieved in AML after second line chemotherapy and "ex vivo" purging is not necessarily required. Furthermore, an aggressive conditioning regimen proved to be active in succesfully managing residual disease.

Quite different considerations come from an analysis of the data relating to ALL patients. The overall result cannot be regarded as satisfactory but, at the same time, it is no worse than that generally reported in the literature [21,22]. However, after a longer follow-up, we can confirm the results of a previous report suggesting a distinction between patients undergoing autografting after isolated meningeal relapse and the others [23].

Since the former group achieved a high rate of EFS, it can be speculated that an aggressive conditioning regimen including HD-Ara-C and TBI may play an ideal role in the management of residual extramedullary (primarily CNS) disease, which is characterized by its unfavourable location rather than by a huge mass [24]. The significance of the results is considerably increased when comparison is made with the very poor life expectancy of such ALL patients after conventional chemotherapy [25,26]. Isolated CNS relapse can therefore be proposed as a clearcut indication for autologous BMT provided that the "in vivo" purging effect of previous chemotherapy was successful in restricting failure to the CNS. The low rate of further CNS relapses in these patients provides additional evidence for the satisfactory activity of autologous BMT in this disease phase.

Although the comparison is made more difficult by the lack of distinction between the sites of relapse in many reports [16,21,22], our discouraging results in terms of EFS after hematological relapse are no worse than those reported in the literature, although the comparison is made more difficult by the lack of distinction between the sites of relapse in many reports [16,21,22]. The persistence of a high degree of residual disease in many ALL patients after the achievement of CR has been clearly demonstrated, and this is even more true after second or subsequent CR [16]. It can be speculated that this may simply reflect the greater availability of tests to identify residual disease in ALL in comparison with AML [2,10]. On the other hand, since the relationship between the amount of residual disease and the outcome of autologous BMT has been suggested [16], the limited effectiveness of conditioning regimens in managing poor quality CR can be indicated as the more obvious explanation for most of these failures. The possibility of inducing leukemic relapse through the infusion of pre-harvested bone marrow should not be overlooked. However, against this possibility, there is the limited effectiveness of "ex vivo" purging in reducing the relapse rate in ALL [11,27–29] and, furthemore, "ex vivo" purging in such an advanced disease phase can be expected to lead to the delayed engraftment of autologous bone marrow [18]. In conclusion, relapsing ALL cannot be indicated as a clearcut indication for ABMT.

References

1. Davis C. L., Rohatiner A.Z., Lim J., et al.: The management of recurrent acute myelogenous leukaemia at a single centre over a fifteen-year period. Br. J. Haem. 1993, 83: 404–411.
2. Hoelzer D.: Acute lymphoblastic leukemia – Progress in children, less in adults. New Engl. J. Med. 1993, 329: 1343–1344.
3. Petersen F. B., Lynch M.H.E., Clift R.A., et al.: Autologous marrow transplantation for patients with acute myeloid leukemia in untreated first relapse or in second complete remission. J. Clin. Onc. 1993, 11: 1353–1360.
4. Blume K.G., Kopecky K. J., Nenslee-Downey J.P., et al.: A prospective randomized comparison of Total Body Irradiation-Etoposide versus Busulfan-

Cyclophosphamide as preparatory regimens for bone marrow transplantation in patients with leukemia who were not in first remission: A Southwest Oncology Group Study. Blood 1993, 81: 2187–2193.

5. Hoelzer D., Gale R.B.: Acute lymphoblastic leukemia in adults: recent progress, future directions. Sem. Hemat. 1987, 24: 27–39.
6. Pavlovsky S., Fernandez I., Palau V., et al.: Combination of rubidazone and cytosine arabinoside in the treatment of first relapse in acute myelocytic leukemia. Ann. Oncol. 1991, 2: 441–442.
7. Linker C.A., Ries C.A., Damon L.A., et al.: Autologous bone marrow transplantation for acute myeloid leukemia using Busulfan plus Etoposide as a preparatory regimen. Blood 1993, 81: 311–318.
8. Foon K.A., Gale R.P.: Therapy of acute myelogenous leukemia. Blood Rev. 1992, 6: 15–25.
9. Wagner J.E., Vogelsang G.B., Zehnbauer B.A., et al.: Relapse of leukemia after bone marrow transplantation: effect of second myeloablative therapy. Bone Marrow Tranplant. 1992, 9: 205–209.
10. Vogler W.R.: Strategies in the treatment of acute myelogenous leukemia. Leukemia Research 1992, 16: 1141–1153.
11. Gale R.P., Horowitz M., Butturini A.: Autotransplants in acute leukaemia. Br. J. Haematol. 1991, 78: 135–137.
12. Vogler W.R., Berdel W.E., Olson A.C., et al.: Autologous bone marrow transplantation in acute leukemia with marrow purged with Alkyl-Lysophospholipid. Blood 1992, 80: 1423–1429.
13. Chao N.J., Stein A.S., Long G.D., et al.: Busulfan/Etoposide-Initial experience with a new preparatory regimen for autologous bone marrow transplantation in patients with acute nonlymphoblastic leukemia. Blood 1993, 81: 319–323.
14. Fyles G.M., Messner H.A., Lockwood G., et al.: Long-term results of bone marow transplantation for patients with AML, ALL and CML prepared with single dose total body irradiation of 500 cGy delivered with high dose rate. Bone Marrow Transplant. 1991, 8: 453–463.
15. Schiffman K., Clift R., Appelbaum F.R., et al.: Consequences of cryopreserving first remission autologous marrow for use after relapse in patients with acute myeloid leukemia. Bone Marrow Transplant. 1993, 11: 227–232.
16. Uckun F.M., Kersey J.H., Haake R., et al.: Pretransplantation burden of leukemic progenitor cells as a predictor of relapse after bone marrow transplantation for acute lymphoblastic leukemia. N. Eng. J. Med. 1993, 329: 1296–1301.
17. Robertson M.J., Soiffer R.J., Freedman A.S., et al.: Human bone marrow depleted of CD33-positive cells mediates delayed but durable reconstitution of hematopoiesis: clinical trial of MY9 monoclonal antibody-purged autografts for the treatment of acute myeloid leukemia. Blood 1992, 79: 2229–2236.
18. Rill D.R., Moen R.C., Buschle M., et al.: An approach for the analysis of relapse and marrow reconstitution after autologous marrow transplantation using retrovirus-mediated gene transfer. Blood 1992, 79: 2694–2700.
19. Gorin N.C., Labopin M., Meloni G., et al.: Autologous bone marow transplantation for acute myeloblastic leukemia in Europe: further evidence of the role of marrow purging by mafosfamide. European Co-operative Group for Bone Marrow Transplantation (EBMT). Leukemia 1991, 5: 896–904.
20. Lambertenghi-Deliliers G., Maiolo A.T., Annaloro C. et al.: Idarubicin in sequential combination with cytosine arabinoside in the treatment of relapsed and refractory patients with acute non lymphoblastic leukemia. Eur. J. Clin. Oncol. 23: 1041–1045, 1987.
21. Sallan S.E., Niemeyer C.M., Billett A.L. et al: Autologous bone marrow transplantation for acute lymphoblastic leukemia. J. Clin. Oncol. 1989, 7: 1594–1601.
22. Burnett A.K.: Autologous BMT for ALL. Bone Marrow Transplant. 1989, 4 (Suppl 3): 79–80.
23. Annaloro C., Mozzana R., Butti C., et al.: Results of autologous bone marrow transplantation (ABMT) in 20 ALL patients after a 5-year follow-up. Ann. Hematol. 65 (Suppl 1): A30, 1992.
24. Coccia P.F., Strandjord S.E., Warkentin P.I., et al.: High-dose cytosine arabinoside and fractioned total-body irradiation: an improved preparative regimen for bone marrow transplantation of children with acute lymphoblastic leukemia in remission. Blood 1988, 71: 888–893.
25. Rivera G.K., Mauer A.M.: Controversies in the management of childhood acute lymphoblastic leukemia: treatment intensification, CNS leukemia, and prognostic factors. Semin Hematol 1987, 24: 12–26.
26. Bleyer W.A., Poplack D.G.: Prophylaxis and treatment of leukemia in the central nervous system and other sanctuaries. Semin. Oncol. 1985, 12: 131–148.
27. Gilmore M.J.M.L., Hamon M.D., Prentice H.G. et al.: Failure of purged autologous bone marrow transplantation in high risk acute lymphoblastic leukemia in first complete remission. Bone Marrow Transplant. 1991, 8: 19–.26.
28. Simmonsson B., Burnett A.K., Prentice H.G., et al.: Autologous bone marrow transplantation with monoclonal antibody purged marrow for high risk acute lymphoblastic leukemia. Leukemia 1989, 3: 631–636.
29. Dicke K.A., Spinolo J.A.: High dose therapy and autologous bone marrow transplantation in acute leukemia: is purging necessary? Bone Marrow Transplant. 1989, 4 (suppl 1): 184–186.

Acute Leukemias V
Experimental Approaches
and Management of Refractory Diseases
Hiddemann et al. (Eds.)

Autologous Vs. Unrelated Donor Bone Marrow Transplantation for Acute Lymphoblastic Leukemia: Considerations and Logistics

Daniel Weisdorf

Introduction

Acute lymphoblastic leukemia frequently responds to conventional remission induction and maintenance therapy and leads to extended leukemia-free survival for the majority of children and a fraction of adults. However, high risk groups (e.g., those with extreme leukocytosis, Ph^1 positive, mature B-cell, older age) and those following a first relapse will surely develop recurrent leukemia and resultant shortened survival. Though matched sibling allogeneic bone marrow transplantation (BMT) can lead to extended disease control and prolonged survival for 30–50% of patients [1–5], those lacking a histocompatible related donor must seek other options.

Autologous BMT offers the advantage of rapid applicability for those in remission and relatively low transplant-associated morbidity. Unfortunately, it is often followed by leukemia relapse and only 20–40% of patients have been reported to enjoy extended leukemia-free survival after autotransplantation [7–15].

As another alternative, closely matched unrelated donor marrow transplantation has also been tested [16]. Unrelated donor (URD) BMT involves electronic searching of one of several international databases of volunteer donors, subsequent retrieval of blood samples from those donors for further histocompatibility testing and, finally, medical evaluation of the donor's fitness and willingness to donate marrow. This evaluation process can be time-consuming, costly and identifies a donor for only 30–50% of patients requiring transplantation. Additionally, URD BMT can be clinically complicated by increased risks of graft failure, graft-versus-host disease and secondary infection [16–17]. Conversely, the greater histoincompatibility between donor and recipient may enhance graft-versus-leukemia activity and thereby lower the risks of post-transplant relapse. The exaggerated morbidity and mortality accompanying URD transplantation may thus be counterbalanced by better protection against recurrent leukemia.

Timing of Transplantation

Autologous transplantation involves the aspiration and harvesting of sufficient numbers of benign hematopoietic progenitor and stem cells, possible ex vivo purging to deplete residual leukemia cells and then cryopreservation. After pretransplant anti-leukemia conditioning the cryopreserved marrow is reinfused. The clinical prerequisites for autologous marrow harvesting include a sufficiently cellular bone marrow in morphologic complete remission at a time when the patient's general physical condition is satisfactory to allow the anesthesia and harvest before initiation of the transplant course. However, recurrent acute lymphoblastic leukemia, especially if the relapse occurred following an intensive multi-drug consolidation and maintenance regimen is often multiply drug-resistant and durable complete remission may be hard to achieve. Such transient remissions or those accompanied by a hypocellular marrow can

Department of Medicine, University of Minnesota, Minneapolis, MN 55455, USA delay or prevent the successful completion of a marrow harvest. Often, in an attempt to allow marrow cellularity to increase and thus facilitate the harvest, anti-leukemic treatment is suspended. This strategy may leave patients at greater risk for early relapse before harvest and autotransplantation can be effected.

Unrelated donor marrow transplantation also presents logistical obstacles to the transplant, but most involve the identification of a suitable allogeneic donor. Even with the available multinational volunteer donor registries which include well over one million potential donors and with instantaneous electronic communication, the coordination of donor tissue type searching, donor contact and recall for additional histocompatibility testing can generate substantial delays.

Recognizing the high risks of leukemia relapse after autotransplantation and the delays inherent in searching for and identifying an unrelated donor, at the University of Minnesota Bone Marrow Transplantation Program we have established a dual option search strategy for BMT candidates with ALL. We allow only four months from the time of referral for identification of an unrelated donor. After four months, if no URD donor is identified, then patients in remission proceed promptly to autologous transplantation.

Exercising this policy, we evaluated 75 consecutive referrals of potential BMT candidates with ALL. Of these, 32 had related donors, thus had no search initiated. Eventually 10 proceeded to related sibling donor BMT. Forty-three others had no related donor and for 37 an unrelated donor search was initiated. The search was discontinued early for 20 of these patients because of persisting relapse or patient death, alternative therapy arranged at another institution or lack of third-party coverage for the costs of the URD search. For the others, the search process identified an unrelated donor for 17 patients after a median of 14 weeks (range 10–30 weeks) following initial referral. An additional 11 weeks median (range 6–16 weeks) were required from the time the donor was identified until transplant totaling 26 weeks median (range 17–42 weeks) between initial referral and eventual URD marrow transplantation. Six patients for whom an unrelated donor was identified did not proceed to transplantation because of either patient relapse or death while the search process was underway.

Within this time interval, of the 33 patients who had no search or had no URD identified, 13 received autotransplantation at the University of Minnesota. However, because of both the time required to achieve complete remission and to perform the (eventually unsuccessful) unrelated donor search, these 13 autotransplants took place at a median of 25 weeks following initial referral (range 6–42 weeks).

Therefore, these three transplant options (autologous, allogeneic related or unrelated donor) were effected at different times. For this group of 75 referred patients, 34 received a transplant. Ten underwent allogeneic related donor BMT at a median of 9 weeks following referral (range 4–28 weeks) while 11 URD transplants took place at a median of 26 weeks following referral and 13 autotransplants after a median of 25 weeks. While this search policy allows for consideration of both unrelated allogeneic and autologous transplantation, several criteria must be met for it to be of practical value for patients with ALL. 1) The unrelated donor search should be initiated while the patient is receiving remission induction therapy. 2) Third party payer approval of coverage for search and transplant costs need be prompt. 3) A suitable and consenting unrelated donor must be identified for a substantial number of the patients searched. Acceleration of the search process will certainly be required before greater numbers of patients with ALL can be treated with URD allogeneic transplantation.

Comparison of Unrelated Donor Versus Autologous Transplantation

Because of these time delays in donor searching and the availability of donors for only a fraction of patients, the comparison of clinical outcomes following unrelated donor vs. autologous transplantation is neither simple nor straightforward. Comparative clinical analysis must involve assessment of patient demographics (age, gender and gender match with the donor, histocompatibility with the donor and CMV serostatus). Additionally, critical leukemia characteristics include complete remission number, immunophenotype, karyotype, diagnostic leukocyte count, duration of first complete remission, extramedullary leukemia involvement and time from remission to transplant. Importantly, loss of potential BMT candidates because of persisting relapse (unresponsive leukemia) or complications of remission induction may differ in the brief interval before autotransplantation versus the longer interval required to find an unrelated donor. Appropriate comparison must consider this time bias and the differential loss of patients while plans for autotransplantation or unrelated donor searching are underway. Conventional statistical comparison of survival time, event-free survival and time to leukemia relapse after either autologous or unrelated donor transplantation may seriously under-estimate the pre-transplant selection bias inherent in any comparative series of these two transplant techniques.

Analytical Considerations

While reported experience with unrelated donor marrow transplantation for ALL is still limited, the above problems ought to be addressed in future reports. Matched case control analyses may allow valid comparisons, perhaps using data from large multi-center registries to address the problems cited above. Additionally, scientific reports should cite the number of patients referred for possible transplantation because the selection bias may be unequal with different forms of transplantation. One technique to aid standardization of data presentation could include reporting the duration of initial complete remission (for those transplanted in second complete remission) but, in addition reporting the time from remission until transplantation - the period in which differential relapse and removal from either transplant cohort may skew the composition of each group.

Summary

While the above considerations emphasize the difficulties in comparative analysis of unrelated donor vs. autologous marrow transplantation for patients with ALL, they also highlight issues which can allow interpretive commentary on the results of any given transplant series. The literature of marrow transplantation has most often assumed that the patients' risk period begins at day zero, the day of transplantation. For assessment of these alternative transplant techniques with their inherent delays and complexities preceding transplantation, it must be acknowledged that the patients' period of risk begins well before transplantation. Careful interpretation of post-transplant results should recognize these pretransplant hazards accordingly.

References

1. Brochstein JA, Kernan NA, Groshen S, Cirrincione C, Shank B, Emmanuel D, Laver J, O'Reilly RJ (1987) Allogeneic bone marrow transplantation after hyperfractionated total-body irradiation and cyclophosphamide in children with acute leukemia. N Engl J Med 317: 1618–1624
2. Dopfer R, Henze G, Bender-Götze H (1991) Allogeneic bone marrow transplantation for childhood acute lymphoblastic leukemia in second remission after intensive primary and relapse therapy according to the BFM- and CoALL-protocols: Results of the German Cooperative Study. Blood 78: 2780–2784
3. Horowitz MM, Messerer D, Hoelzer D, Gale RP, Neiss A, Atkinson K, Barrett AJ, Büchner T, Freund M, Heil G, Heit W, Hiddemann W, Kolb H-J, Löffler H, Marmont AM, Rimm AA, Rozman C, Sobocinski KA, Speck B, Thiel E, Weisdorf DJ, Zwaan FE, Bortin MM (1991) Chemotherapy compared with bone marrow transplantation for adults with acute lymphoblastic leukemia in first remission. Ann Int Med 115: 13–18
4. Weisdorf DJ, Woods WG, Nesbit ME Jr, Uckun F, Dusenbery K, Kim T, Haake R, Thomas W, Kersey JH, Ramsay NKC (1994) Allogeneic bone marrow transplantation for acute lymphoblastic leukaemia: Risk factors and clinical outcome. Brit J Haematol 86: 62–69
5. Chao NJ, Forman SJ, Schmidt GM, Snyder DS, Amylon MD, Konrad PN, Nademanee AP, O'Donnell MR, Parker PM, Stein AS, Smith E, Wong RM, Hoppe RT, Blume KG (1991) Allogeneic bone marrow transplantation for high-risk acute lymphoblastic leukemia during first complete remission. Blood 78: 1923–1927
6. Doney K, Fisher LD, Appelbaum FR, Buckner CD, Storb R, Singer J, Fefer A, Anasetti C, Beatty P, Bensinger W, Clift R, Hansen J, Hill R, Loughran TP Jr, Martin P, Petersen FB, Sanders J, Sullivan KM, Stewart P, Weiden P, Witherspoon R, Thomas ED (1991) Treatment of adult acute lymphoblastic leukemia with allogeneic bone marrow transplantation. Multivariate analysis of factors affecting acute graft-versus-host disease, relapse-free survival. Bone Marrow Transplantation 7: 453–459
7. Carey PJ, Proctor SJ, Taylor P, Hamilton PJ (1991) Autologous bone marrow transplantation for high-grade lymphoid malignancy using melphalan/irradiation conditioning without marrow purging or cryopreservation. The Northern Regional Bone Marrow Transplant Group. Blood 77: 1593–1598

8. Gorin NC, Aegerter P, Auvert B (1990) Autologous bone marrow transplantation for acute leukemia in remission: An analysis of 1322 cases. In Haematology and Blood Transfusion, vol. 33 Acute Leukemias II, ed Büchner T, Schellong G, Hiddemann W, Ritter J, pp 660–666. Berlin: Springer-Verlag
9. Kersey JH, Weisdorf D, Nesbit ME et al. (1987) Comparison of autologous and allogeneic bone marrow transplantation for treatment of high-risk refractory acute lymphoblastic leukemia. N Engl J Med 317: 461–467, 1987
10. Schmid H, Henze G, Schwerdtfeger R, Baumgarten E, Besserer A, Scheffler A, Serke S, Zingsem J, Siegert W (1993) Fractionated total body irradiation and high-dose VP-16 with purged autologous bone marrow rescue for children with high risk relapsed acute lymphoblastic leukemia. Bone Marrow Transplantation 12: 597–602
11. Soiffer RJ, Roy DC, Gonin R, Murray C, Anderson KC, Freedman AS, Rabinowe SN, Robertson MJ, Spector N, Pesek K, Mauch P, Nadler LM, Ritz J (1993) Monoclonal antibody-purged autologous bone marrow transplantation in adults with acute lymphoblastic leukemia at high risk of relapse. Bone Marrow Transplantation 12: 243–251
12. Uckun FM, Kersey JH, Haake R, Weisdorf D, Nesbit ME, Ramsay NKC (1993) Pretransplantation burden of leukemic progenitor cells as a predictor of relapse after bone marrow transplantation for acute lymphoblastic leukemia. N Engl J Med 329: 1296–1301
13. Weisdorf DJ (1994) Autologous bone marrow transplantation for acute lymphoblastic leukemia, in Atkinson K, ed. Clinical Bone Marrow Transplantation, Cambridge: Cambridge University Press
14. Uckun FM, Kersey JH, Haake R, Weisdorf D, Ramsay NKC (1992) Autologous bone marrow transplantation (BMT) in high risk remission B-lineage acute lymphoblastic leukemia using a cocktail of three monoclonal antibodies (BA-1/CD23, BA-2/CD9, BA-3/CD10) plus complement and 4-hydroperoxycyclophosphamide for *ex vivo* bone marrow purging. Blood 79: 1094–1104
15. Billett AL, Kornmehl E, Tarbell NJ, Weinstein HJ, Gelber RD, Ritz J, Sallan SE (1993) Autologous bone marrow transplantation after a long first remission for children with recurrent acute lymphoblastic leukemia. Blood 81: 1651–1657
16. Kernan NA, Bartsch G, Ash RC, Beatty PG, Champlin R, Filipovich A, Gajewski J, Hansen JA, Henslee-Downey J, McCullough J, McGlave P, Perkins HA, Phillips GL, Sanders J, Stroncek D, Thomas ED, Blume KG (1993) Analysis of 462 transplantations from unrelated donors facilitated by the national marrow donor program. N Engl J Med 328: 593–602
17. Bearman SI, Mori M, Beatty PG, Meyer WG, Buckner CD, Petersen FB, Sanders JE, Anasetti C, Martin P, Appelbaum FR, Hansen JA (1994) Comparison of morbidity and mortality after marrow transplantation from HLA-genotypically identical siblings and HLA-phenotypically identical unrelated donors. Bone Marrow Transplantation 13: 31–35

Acute Leukemias V
Experimental Approaches
and Management of Refractory Diseases
Hiddemann et al. (Eds.)

Comparison Between Allogeneic and Autologous Bone Marrow Transplantation for Childhood Acute Lymphoblastic Leukemia in Second Remission

P. Bordigoni, G. Leverger, A. Baruchel, H. Espérou-Bourdeau, Y. Perel, G. Michel, F. Bernaudin, C. Bergeron, G. Cornu, B. Lacour, G. Couillaud, B. Pautard, J. P. Dommergues, and J. L. Stephan for the Société d'Hématologie et d'Immunologie Pédiatrique (SHIP) France

Introduction

As a result of steady improvements in chemotherapy over the past 20 years, more than 70% of children with acute lymphoblastic leukemia (ALL) are cured with intensive induction regimens followed by maintenance therapy [1]. However, there is still a 30% therapeutic failure rate manifesting as disease recurrence, generally bone marrow relapses, early in the treatment period. In this context, several centers have reported the safety and efficacy of allogeneic or autologous bone marrow transplantation (BMT) or chemotherapy alone. The better results have been reported in patients who had BMT from a matched sibling donor as compared to those who did not have a matched sibling donor and received chemotherapy alone [2, 3, 4]. There have been few controlled studies comparing results of autologous and allogeneic BMT in similar patients by using the same preparative regimen [5, 6, 7, 8].

We now report data from a French prospective controlled survey comparing the results of autologous (ABMT) and allogeneic BMT (allo-BMT) in similar patients with ALL in second complete remission (CR2) after marrow relapse.

Methods and Patients

The study began in January 1990 and continued through October 1993. 134 children entered on RALL-90 protocol were reinduced with 4 or 5 courses of Vincristine, increasing doses of Methotrexate and L-Asparaginase Erwinia (Capizzi protocol). Bone marrow aspiration was performed on days 15 and 29 to determine remission status. Patients failing reinduction were offered different rescue chemotherapies. Children in remission were given an intensive consolidation (Table 1). Children who underwent ABMT were treated with 2 or 3 courses of continuation therapy, bone marrow being harvested after the 2nd course. Allo-BMT was scheduled after the intensification phase for all children who had either an HLA-compatible sibling, a matched unrelated donor (MUD) or a mismatched family donor.

This study was designed to compare the relative value of ABMT and allo-BMT with HLA-identical sibling donors and not to compare those groups of patients with transplantation from MUD or from mismatched family donors. Therefore, for children with marrow relapse before 18 months of first complete remission (CR1) the choice between an ABMT and transplantations using other than genotypically HLA-identical sibling was made by the individual participating institutions. 134 children (86 males and 39 females) between 9 months and 20 years of age (median : 7.8 years) entered the RALL-90 protocol. The majority had received primary therapy according to the current front-line FRALLE protocols (FRALLE 83-87-89) which included multiagent chemotherapy and CNS prophylaxis with high-dose Methotrexate, intrathecal medications and sometimes cranial irradiation in addition. Initial marrow relapse

Hopital d'Enfants, Unité de Transplantation Médullaire de Pédiatrie, 2, Rue du Morvan, 54511 Vandoeuvre-les-Nancy, France

Table 1. Treatment program (RALL-90)

REINDUCTION THERAPY

d1-8-15-22 (29)	**Vincristine** : 1.5 mg/m² I.V. - Weekly x 4-5 (maximum dose : 2.0 mg) **L-Asparaginase (Erwinia)** : 40 000 U/m² I.V. or I.M. (maximum dose : 40 000 U) **Methotrexate** : I.V. - weekly x 4-5 d2 : 80 mg/m² d16 : 160 mg/m² d9 : 120 mg/m² d23 (d30) : 200 mg/m²

INTENSIFICATION

d1 to 4 and d11 to 14	**Etoposide** : 100 mg/m²/d x 8 **Daunorubicine** : 10 mg/m²/d x 8 **Cytarabine** : 100 mg/m²/d x 8	Continuous I.V.
	Dexamethasone : 20 mg/m²/d I.V.	

CONTINUATION THERAPY

d1 to 5 →	**Dexamethasone** : 20 mg/m²/d
d1 to 5 →	**6-Thioguanine** : 100 mg/m²/d p.o.
d 1 and 8 →	**Vindesine** : 3 mg/m² I.V.
d1 →	**Cyclophosphamide** : 0.6 g/m² I.V.
d1 →	**Methotrexate** : 1 g/m² Continuous I.V. 36 h

IT CHEMOPROPHYLAXIS

Given on days 1 and 15 (induction), days 1 and 8 (intensification) and during each course of continuation therapy	**Methotrexate** **Hydrocortisone** **Cytarabine**

(isolated : 96 ; combined : 38 {testicular or CNS}) occured either while receiving chemotherapy (before 24 months : 76 ; after 24 months : 36) or after chemotherapy had been discontinued (22 patients).

Sustained complete remission was achieved in 98 out of 128 evaluable (76.5%) patients. Early toxic deaths occured in 3 (2.3%) patients. 27 patients (21%) failing induction were then offered rescue reinduction and 22 achieved CR2. Six patients were taken off the study due to an unacceptable toxicity. The second remission rate after one or two reinduction protocol(s) was 89.5% (120/128). Among those 120 patients, 50 were given an ABMT, 36 an allo-BMT. Moreover, 34 patients were not eligible for BMT for different reasons: relapses occuring after initial chemotherapy was stopped [11], very early 2nd relapse [14], others [4]. 5 children are waiting for a transplantation.

The characteristics of transplanted patients are summarized on Table 2.

Only 7 out of 50 children with ABMT had marrow treated in vitro and 27 were given recombinant interleukin 2 (IL2) after transplantation [9]. The median interval between ABMT and IL2 was 60 days (33–98). A continuous infusion of 12 millions U/m²/day of IL2 (Roussel-Uclaf) was administered over a first cycle of 5 days and then for 4 cycles of 2 days given every 2 weeks. No toxic death was recorded and all toxicities reversed on stopping IL2 infusion. 16 out of 27 patients (60%) received 100% of the planned dose.

35 patients in the allo-BMT group were given marrow either from HLA-genoidentical siblings (21 patients – 1 twin) (allo-id-BMT) of from MUD (9 patients) or from family mismatched donors (6 ps). One infant received hemopoietic stem cell transplant using HLA-matched sibling umbilical cord blood cells.

Graft-versus-host disease (GVHD) prophylaxis for allo-id BMT consisted of Cyclosporine (CyA) and Methotrexate (MTX) (16 patients) or

Table 2. Characteristics of the patients

CHARACTERISTICS		TRANSPLANT GROUP ALLOGENEIC [1] (N = 21)	AUTOLOGOUS (N = 50)	P VALUE
SEXE	Male	14	33	0.9
	Female	7	17	
AGE	≤ 10 yrs	16	40	0.90
	> 10 yrs	5	10	
LENGHT [2] OF CR1 (months)	≤ 18	8	12	0.48
	> 18	10	29	
	Off therapy [3]	3	9	
WBC AT DIAGNOSIS (x 10^9/l)	< 50	14	40	0.18
	≥ 50	7	8	
IMMUNE PHENOTYPE (%)	T cell	3	6	1
	Pre B cell	17	34	
EXTRA-MEDULLARY DISEASE	No	14	32	0.83
	Yes	7	18	
MARROW STATUS AT d15 (induction)	≤ 40 % (blast cells)	11	33	0.53
	> 40 %	4	6	
CR2 [4] POST 1st INDUCTION (%)	Yes	16	40	0,9
	No	5	10	
CYTARABINE DOSAGE [5] (g/m ^{2})	24	13	28	0.63
	< 24	6	17	

1 : HLA geno-identical BMT
2 : CR1 : 1st complete remission
3 : Off therapy relapses : > 6 months after cessation of therapy
4 : CR2 : 2nd complete remission
5 : In conditioning regimen

CyA(4 patients). It included CyA+MTX (6 patients), CyA+ATG (1 patient), CyA (1 patient) and in vitro T-cell depletion (anti CD7 plus anti CD2 monoclonal antibodies plus complement) (7 patients) for other children.

To prevent graft-failure, these latter received in addition, two monoclonal antibodies specific for the CD11a and CD2 infused from day −1 to +11 post BMT [10].

All patients received the same preparative regimen (TAM) as follows: fractionated TBI (200 cGy twice a day for 6 doses: 1 200 cGy) (48 out of 50 ABMT and 30 out of 36 allo-BMT) or single dose of TBI (1 000 cGy) (ABMT: 2; allo-BMT: 2) followed by cytarabine at a dose of 3gm/m² twice daily for 6 or 8 doses (18 to 24 gm/m²) for children less than 12 years old and for 4 doses (12 gm/m²) for children more than 12 years old. Preparation for patients less than 4 years old consisted of: AMBT (2 patients): Busulfan (Bu) 20 mg/kg, Etoposide 40 mg/kg, Cyclophosphamide (CPM) 120 mg/kg or Bu 16 mg/kg, Cytarabine 12 g/m², Melphalan 140 mg/m² (BAM); allo-id-BMT (6 patients): Bu 16 mg/kg, CPM 200 mg/kg (3 patients); BAM (2 patients) or Bu 16 mg/kg, Etoposide 720 mg/m^2, CPM 120 mg/kg (1 patient).

Statistical methods. Statistical evaluation of outcome after BMT was performed by actuarial life-table analysis according to the Kaplan-Meier method. Log-rank tests were used for comparison of subgroups. The Cox regression model was used for risk factor multivariate analysis.

Results

Disease free survival and relapses. All patients engrafted as shown by increasing peripheral cell counts. Table 3 summarized the results according to the

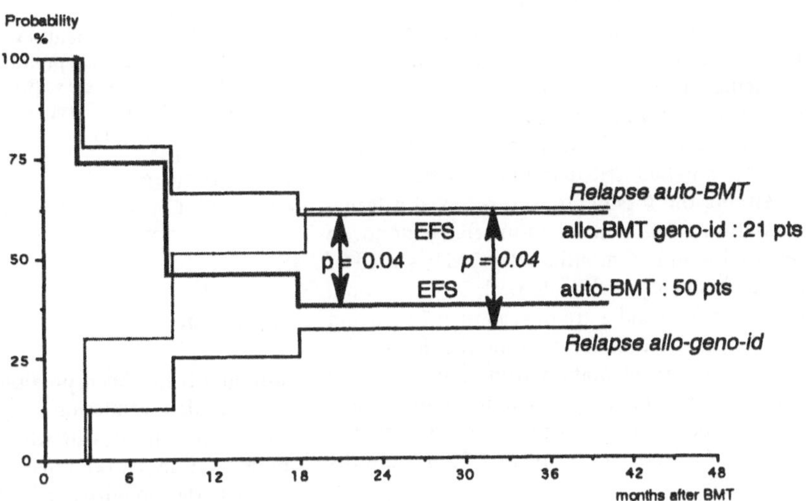

Fig. 1. Kaplan-Meier estimation of EFS and relapse after autologous and allogeneic BMT for childhood ALL in CR2 RALL 90

Table 3. Transplant results

		ALLOGENEIC			AUTOLOGOUS
		HLA MM	MUD	HLA id	
N° OF PATIENTS		6	9	21	50
GVHD	Acute ≥ II	3	6	60 %	NA
	Chronic	2	2/4	25 %	NA
RELAPSE RATE (% ± SE)		3/6 Med : 4 mo (2 - 27)	2/9 4 - 16 mo	Med : 7.8 mo (2 - 17) 27.8 ± 11.8	Med : 8 mo (3 - 12) 61.3 ± 7.7 (p = 0.04 vs HLA id)
	Marrow	3	2	4	24
	M + CNS	0	0	0	1
	M + Lymph nodes	0	0	0	1
	M + mediastinum	0	0	0	1
TRANSPLANT RELATED DEATHS		1/6 CGVHD	5/9 AGVHD : 3 Infection : 1 BLPD : 1	9.5 % AGVHD : 1 VOD : 1	6 % Infection : 1 Cardiac failure : 1 Leucoencephalopathy : 1
DFS (% ± SE) (3 yrs)		2/6	2/9	63.9 ± 11.5	36,5 ± 7,3 (p = 0.04 vs HLA id)
	Median (range) (months)	22	8 and 10	27 (2 - 48)	26 (7 - 50)

type of transplantation. Among the patients who received an ABMT the estimated chance (mean ± SE) of surviving without disease for 3 years was: 36.5 ± 7.3% (median: 26 months (7–50)). Among patients who received allo-id-BMT the chance was 63.9 ± 11.8% (median: 27 months (2–48))(p = 0.04). The estimated chances of relapse at 3 years were 61.3 ± 7.7% (median: 7.8 months (2–17)) in patients with ABMT and 27.8 ± 11.8% (median: 8 months (3–12)) in those with allo-id-BMT (p = 0.04).

The most common site of relapse was bone marrow alone: 24, or combined with the CNS: 1, or mediastinum: 1, or lymph node: 1 for ABMT group. For allo-id-BMT group, relapses were only in marrow. No CNS relapse occured in patients who had CNS disease before BMT.

Among the 9 patients who received a transplantation from a matched-unrelated donor, 2 relapsed 4 and 16 months after BMT, 5 died of non-leukemic causes (acute GVHD: 3, infection: 1 and BLPD: 1) and 2 are in sustained CR2 8 and 10 months post BMT. Among the 6 ps who received a transplantation from a mismatched family donor, 3 relapsed 2, 9 and 27 months post BMT, 1 died from transplant related toxicity (chronic GVHD) and 2 are in CR2 22 months after BMT.

Transplantation related mortality and morbidity. The overall incidence of acute GVHD was 75% (grade ≥ II: 60%). Chronic GVHD occured in 25% of evaluable patients (allo-id-BMT). 2 out of 21 (acute GVHD: 1; veno-occlusive disease: 1) patients with allo-id-BMT (9.5%) and 3 out of 50 with ABMT (6%) died from transplant-related toxicity (leucoencephalopathy: 1; infection: 1 and cardiac failure: 1).

Influence of prognostic factors on DFS and relapse rate. Table 4 shows the pre and post BMT factors examined for their influence on remission duration and leukemic mortality.

None of potential prognostic factors was found to be significant by Cox regression analysis whatever the type of transplant. It has to be mentioned that in the ABMT group neither the duration of CR1 nor the white blood cell count (WBC) at diagnosis had any significance. However, there is a trend towards a shorter relapse-free survival for patients with T immunephenotype or who failed to attain CR2 with the first reinduction chemotherapy.

Table 4. Factors tested in multivariant analysis

- White blood cell count at diagnosis (< 50 000 vs ≥ 50 000)
- Cytogenetic analysis at diagnosis (structural abnormalities vs normal)
- Immunophenotype at diagnosis (T lineage vs pre B)
- Patient age
- Patient sex
- Mediastinum (yes vs no)
- Marrow aspirate at d15 (reinduction) (< 40% blast cells vs ≥ 40%)
- Length of CR1 (< 18 months vs > 18 months)
- Extramedullary disease pretransplant
- Achieved CR2 after one vs two courses
- Cytarabine dosage in preparative regimen (24 g/m^2 vs < 24 g/m^2)
- Acute GVHD
- Chronic GVHD
- Post ABMT Interleukin 2 (yes vs no)

Discussion

Although it has been possible to achieve a second complete remission in 80–90% of patients who relapse in marrow while receiving chemotherapy [11, 12, 13, 14], most studies have reported that the majority of children eventually succumbed to the leukemia. If more intensive front-line therapies combined with CNS radiation therapy [11] could increase the survival rate remains to be determined. The most significant negative prognostic factors of outcome being length of CR1 less than 18 months, T-ALL and high white-cell count at diagnosis. A more favorable prognosis seems evident in children who develop a marrow relapse more than 6 months after cessation of therapy. However, in a recent POG study, the 4-year DFS was no more than 37% [15] without a stable plateau in the curves of DFS [11]. Currently, BMT from matched sibling donors is the best way to eradicate residual leukemic cells and is the treatment of choice for children with ALL in CR2 particularly for those who relapse in the marrow earlier than 6 months after discontinuation of therapy, or have T-cell disease, or very early (< 18 months) isolated extramedullary failures (Table 5) [16, 17, 18, 19, 20, 21]. Overall, the DFS rate for children transplanted in CR2 ranges from 52 to 64% with a relapse rate of 13 to 26% and a non-leukemic death rate of 16 to 23%. However, 75 to 85% of patients do not have an HLA-matched sibling. Attemps to expand the

Table 5. Allogeneic bone marrow transplantation in childhood ALL – Literature review

Center Author Ref	No Patients	Status at BMT	BMT regimen	HLA Status	DFS (%) (5 yrs)	Relapse rate (%)	% BMT mortality	Negative prognostic factors
SFGM [1] Bordigoni P [19-20]	106	CR2 CR3 Relapse	TAM [2]	Geno-id	61.8 ± 5	25.9 ± 5.8 Med : 12 mo (3 - 32)	16	CR3 (DFS + RR) no CGVHD (RR)
Bordigoni P [19-20]	58	CR2 CR3 Relapse	CPM + TBI	Geno-id	28.2 ± 8.1	51.2 ± 7.9 Med : 9 mo (4 - 18)	17.2	CR1 duration (DFS) (< 18 mo) WBC > 50 000/mm (RR) AGVHD ≥ 2 (DFS) no CGVHD (RR)
SEATTLE Sanders JE [17]	57	CR2	CPM + TBI	Geno-id	40	42	28	Any
MSKCC Brochstein JA [16]	31	CR2	FTBI + CPM	Geno-id	64	13	22	CR3-4
	12	CR3		Geno-id	42	25		
	16	CR4 + relapse		Geno-id	23	64		
BFM Dopfer R [18]	51	CR2	CPM + TBI TBI + VP16	Geno-id	52	NA	NA	Any
OMAYA Gordon BG [19]	30	CR2-3	FTBI + Ara-C	Geno-id	52 Med : 99 mo	18	36	NA
WISCONSIN Casper J [23]	54	CR1 (10) CR2 (19) > CR2 (25)	Ara-C + CPM + FTBI ± Bu T Cell Depletion	MUD	44 ± 7 Med : 16 mo (CR2 : 58)	NA	35	> CR2

1 : Société Française de greffe de moelle 2 : TAM = TBI + Ara-C (12-24 g/m^2) + Melphalan (140 mg/m^2)

applicability of allogeneic BMT, including the use of matched unrelated or family mismatched donors have met with mixed results [22, 23]. The use of ABMT allows the application of therapy of comparable intensity to a larger number of patients (Table 6) [24, 25, 26, 27, 28] . The rate of DFS clustered between 12 to 25% for children undergoing BMT in second or subsequent remissions. The most common cause of failure was relapse which occured in 60 to 80% of patients. The non-leukemic death rate ranged from 10 to 18% of patients. The most significant predictors of relapse were: duration of CR1 [24], white blood cell count at diagnosis [26], pre-transplantation burden of leukemic progenitor cells [27] and expression of CD3 surface antigen [26]. One recent report [24] (Table 6) showed very good results of ABMT for children in CR2 but after a 1st remission of at least 24 months.

In our study, 75% of children could be admitted to the BMT program. They were given the same reinduction chemotherapy and the same preparative regimen (TAM). No major differences in patients characteristics between the two groups were seen (Table 2). Early BMT related mortality was the same (ABMT: 6%; allo-id-BMT: 9.5%) and was remarkably low for such a high-risk group of patients. The probability of relapse for patients receiving ABMT was significantly higher than in the group that underwent allo-id-BMT. As a result, DFS at 3 years after BMT was significantly better for these latter. As reported by Billett et al [24], none of 11 patients who achieved remission-inversion after ABMT has had a subsequent relapse. Our results compare favorably with other reports of ABMT for childhood ALL after relapse, particularly for patients with CR1 lasting less than 18 months. We considered two possible features of our cytoreductive regimen to be of potential importance. The first is the additional chemotherapy given to maintain pre-BMT remission, which may produce a more complete eradication of residual leukemic progenitor cells. The second feature is the kind of preparative regimen, as demonstrated in a similar group of children receiving allo-BMT after either TAM regimen or the more conventional CPM and TBI regimen. Statistical analysis revealed that the former yielded better results in regard to DFS and relapse rate, particularly in patients whose CR1 lasted less than 18 months [20, 21]. Indeed, the

Table 6. Autologous bone marrow transplantation in childhood ALL – Literature review

Center Author Ref	No Patients	Status at BMT	Length of CR1 (med)	Marrow purging	BMT regimen	DFS (%)	Relapse rate (%)	% BMT mortality	Negative prognostic factors
SFGM									
Baruchel A. [28]	47	CR2	26 mo	Yes	TAM	23.3 at 5.5 yrs	64.8 med : 8 mo	12.7	CR1 length (± 18 mo) DFS =
DFCI									
Billett AL [24]	51	CR2-3	> 24 mo 38 mo (24 - 84)	Yes	VM26 + CPM + Ara-C (18 g/m²) + fTBI (14 Gy)	53 ± 7 Med : 39 (9 - 124)	39 Med : 8 mo (2 - 29)	9.8	Cell dose ≥ 10⁸ CR1 duration < 48 mo
MINNESOTA (adults + children)									
Uckun FM [26]	19 T-ALL	CR1 (5) CR2-3 (14)	NA	Yes	CPM or Ara-C + TBI	16 ± 8 at 2.5 yrs Med : 0.8 ± 0.3 yrs	74 Med : 72 d (37 - 1284)	15.7	CD3 expression
Uckun FM [27]	83	CR1 (11) CR2-3 (72)	15 mo (1 - 61)	Yes	Ara-C + sTBI VP16 + CPM + sTBI CPM + hfTBI	12 med : 40 mo (11 - 54)	83 at 2 yrs Med : 106 d (27 d - 25 mo)	18	CR1 duration < 18 mo WBC > 50 000/mm³ Leukemic progenitors cells before purge

Table 7. Comparison of autologous and allogeneic bone marrow transplantation for childhood ALL

Center Author Ref	No Patients	Status at BMT	BMT regimen	DFS (%)	Relapse rate (%)	% BMT mortality	Follow-up median	Negative prognostic factors
AIEOP								
Uderzo C [5]								
auto BMT	35	CR1 (12) CR2-3	Purge VCR + fTBI + CPM	49.9	47	8 - 4	24 mo	NA
Allo BMT	30	CR1 (4) CR2-3-Rel		56.5	30	17		
BARCELONA								
Ortega JJ [6]								
auto BMT	32	CR2	Purge fTBI + CPM ± Ara-C	28	69	5	22 mo	NA
Allo BMT	19	CR2		44	40	18	30 mo	
MINNESOTA (adults + children)								
Kersey J [7]								
auto BMT	45	CR1 (3) CR2-3-4	Purge CPM + fTBI	20	79 med : 3 mo	4	48 mo	
					p : 0.0005	p < 0.01		
Allo BMT	46	CR1 (9) CR2-3-4		27	56 med : 9 mo	26		No GVHD (RR) WBC > 50 000 Extramedullary disease
JENA								
Zintl F [8]								
auto BMT	15	CR1 (6) CR2-3	CPM + TBI Purge	43 (2.5 yrs)	54	66	NA	NA
Allo BMT	15	CR1 (2) CR2	CPM + TBI	58 (5 yrs)	28	13	NA	CR1 < 24 mo

primary reason for the recurrence of leukemia seems to be inefficient pretransplant radio-chemotherapy rather than inefficient purging of autografts [26].

Our results are somewhat different from those recently (Table 7) reported in four controlled studies [5, 6, 7, 8]. Indeed, in the study of the University of Minnesota [7], overall survival did not differ between the 2 groups, but the causes of failure are different. In the ABMT group, 79% of patients relapsed, in the allo-BMT group 56% relapsed and 26% died of transplant-related toxicity. In the Italian study, the results of allo-BMT are slightly but not significantly better than those of ABMT, the higher relapse rate observed in the latter group being compensated by the lower fatal toxicity. In the Spanish study, the disease free survival rates are similar but there was a significant difference in the relapse rate (46% vs 70% in allo-BMT vs ABMT). Direct comparisons between these studies and ours are difficult because the initial and reinduction chemotherapy programs are not known but probably different, moreover patients in CR1 are not included in our study. In total, we suppose our different results are essentially due to the lower relapse rate and to the decrease in incidence of deaths from toxicity in our allogeneic transplantation group. The lower relapse rate after BMT during the more recent years may be attributed to improvements of reinduction chemotherapy and better prevention of relapses after introduction of the TAM regimen, the increased experience with this treatment modality leading to a decrease of the transplantation-related toxicity.

We conclude that for this group of patients the results of ABMT are significantly worse than those of allo-id-BMT. Nevertheless, ABMT is a good alternative either to continuation chemotherapy or to allo-BMT using other sources of marrow, including partially HLA-matched family members or matched unrelated donors, for patients with pre-B ALL who relapse more than 12 months after front-line treatment, or who enter CR2 after the first reinduction chemotherapy. In this good-risk group, long-lasting CR2 and may be cure of the disease, can be achieved in about 40–45% of patients.

References

1. Niemeyer CM, Reiter A, Riehm H, Donnelly M, Gelber RD, Sallan SE (1991) Comparative results of two intensive treatment programs for childhood acute lymphoblastic leukemia: The Berlin-Frankfurt-Münster and Dana-Farber Cancer Institute protocols. Annals of Oncology 2: 745–749.
2. Johnson FL, Bayever E, August CS, et al (1981) A comparison of marrow transplantation with chemotherapy for children with acute lymphoblastic leukemia in second or subsequent remission. N Engl J Med 305: 856–851.
3. Bacigalupo A, Van Lint MT, Frassoni F, et al (1986) Allogeneic bone marrow transplantation versus chemotherapy for childhood acute lymphoblastic leukemia in second remission. Bone Marrow Transplantation 1: 75–80.
4. Torres A, Martinez F, Gomez P, et al (1989) Allogeneic bone marrow transplantation versus chemotherapy in the treatment of childhood acute lymphoblastic leukemia in second complete remission. Bone Marrow Transplantation 4: 609–612.
5. Uderzo C, Colleselli P, Dini G, et al (1991) An italian study comparing allogeneic and autologous bone marrow transplantation in childhood acute lymphoblastic leukemia using Vincristine, fractionated total body irradiation and Cyclophosphamide. Bone Marrow Transplantation 7: 15–19.
6. Ortega JJ, Olivé T, Diaz de Heredia C, Giralt J, Bastida P, Canals C, Garcia J (1993) Comparison between allogeneic and autologous BMT in children with ALL. Med and Pediatr Oncol 21: 557.
7. Kersey JH, Weisdorf D, Nesbit ME, Lebien TW, Woods WG, McGlave PB, Kim T, Vallera DA, Goldman AI, Bostrom B, Hurd D, Ramsay NKC (1987) Comparison of autologous and allogeneic bone marrow transplantation for treatment of high-risk refractory acute lymphoblastic leukemia. N Engl J Med 317: 461–467.
8. Zintl F, Hermann J, Fuchs D, Prager J, Reiners B, Müller A, Kob D, Goetz I, Metzner G (1990) Comparison of allogeneic and autologous bone marrow transplantation for treatment of acute lymphoblastic leukemia in childhood. Haematology and Blood Transfusion, vol 33, Acute Leukemias II. Edited by Büchner, Schellong, Hiddemann, Ritter. Springer-Verlag Berlin Heidelberg.
9. Baruchel A, Michel G, Bernaudin F, Lemerle S, Leblanc T, Bordigoni P, Vilmer E, Gauraud F, Leverger G, Rubie H, Demeocq F, Hartmann O, Benz E, Couillaud G, Souillet G, Brandely M, Schaison G (1991) Recombinant Interleukine-2 (IL-2) after autologous bone marrow transplantation (ABMT) in children with leukemia. Blood 78: 502 a.
10. Cavazzana-Calvo M, Stephan JL, Leblanc T, Milpied N, Bordigoni P, Vilmer E, Demeocq F, Le Deist F, Landman-Parker J, Blanche S, Wijdenes J, Fischer A. BMT from donors other than HLA identical for children with high risk leukemia using anti-LFA-1 and anti-CD2 antibodies. Proceedings of the 18th Annual Meeting of the European Group for Bone Marrow Transplantation. Stockholm, Sweden May 31-June 3, 1992.
11. Henze G, Fengler R, Hartmann R, Kornhuber B, Janka-Schaub G, Niethammer D, Riehm H (1991) Six year experience with a comprehensive approach to the treatment of recurrent childhood acute lymphoblastic leukemia (ALL-REZ BFM 85). A relapse study of the BFM group. Blood 78: 1166–1172.
12. Bührer C, Hartmann R, Fengler R, Dopfer R, Gadner H, Gerein V, Göbel U, Reiter A, Ritter J, Henze G (1993) Superior prognosis in combined compared to isolated bone marrow relapses in salvage therapy of childhood acute lymphoblastic leukemia. Med and Pediatr Oncol 21: 470–476.
13. Buchanan GR, Rivera GK, Boyett JM, Chauvenet AR, Crist WM, Vietti TJ (1988) Reinduction thera-

py in 297 children with acute lymphoblastic leukemia in first bone marrow relapse: A Pediatric Oncology Group study. Blood 72: 1286–1293.
14. Belasco JB, Luery N, Scher C (1990) Multiagent chemotherapy in relapsed acute lymphoblastic leukemia in children. Cancer 66: 2492–2499.
15. Sadowitz D, Smith SD, Shuster J, Wharam MD, Buchanan GR, Rivera GK (1993) Treatment of late bone marrow relapse in children with acute lymphoblastic leukemia: A Pediatric Oncology Group Study. Blood 81: 602–609.
16. Brochstein JA, Kernan NA, Groshen S, et al (1987) Allogeneic bone marrow transplantation after hyperfractionated total-body-irradiation and cyclophosphamide in children with acute leukemia. N Engl J Med 317: 1618–1624.
17. Sanders JE, Thomas ED, Buckner CD, et al (1987) Marrow transplantation in children with acute lymphoblastic leukemia in second remission. Blood 70: 324–326.
18. Dopfer R, Henze G, Bender-Götze C, Ebell W, Ehninger G, Friedrich W, Gadner H, Klingebiel T, Peters C, Riehm H, Suttorp M, Schmid H, Schmitz N, Siegert W, Stollmann-Giebbels B, Hartmann R, Niethammer D (1991) Allogeneic bone marrow transplantation for childhood acute lymphoblastic leukemia in second remission after intensive primary and relapse therapy according to the BFM- and CoALL-protocols: Results of the German Cooperative Study. Blood 78: 2780–2784.
19. Gordon BG, Warkentin PI, Strandjord SE, Abromowitch M, Bayever E, Harper JL, Coccia PF (1992) Allogeneic bone marrow transplantation (BMT) for children with acute leukemia: long term follow-up of patients prepared with high dose Cytosine-Arabinoside (ARA-C) and fractionated total body irradiation (fTBI). Blood 80: 337 a.
20. Bordigoni P, Gluckman E, Souillet G, et al (1989) Total body irradiation, high-dose Cytosine-Arabinoside and Melphalan (TAM) followed by allogeneic bone marrow transplantation for on-therapy relapsed acute lymphoblastic leukemia in childhood. Exp Hematol 17: 545.
21. Bordigoni P, Michel G (1994). Role of allogeneic bone marrow transplantation in childhood leukemias. In Hervé P, Riffle G, Justabot E, Dureau G, Bechtel P, Vuiton D eds. Organ transplantation and tissues grafting. Ed INSERM and John Libbey 1994. in press.
22. Kernan NA, Bartsch G, Ash RC, Beatty PG, Champlin R, Filipovich A, Gajewski J, Hansen JA, Henslee-Downey J, McCullough J, McGlave P, Perkins HA, Phillips GL, Sanders J, Stroncek D, Thomas ED, Blume KG (1993) Analysis of 462 transplantations from unrelated donors facilitated by the National Marrow Donor Program. N Engl J Med 328: 593–602.
23. Casper J, Camitta B, Baxter-Lowe LA, Bunin N, Ash R, Pietryga D, Garbrecht F, Murray K, Lawton C, Truitt R, Keever C, Flomenberg N (1993) Bone marrow transplantation for childhood acute lymphoblastic leukemia using unrelated donors. Blood 82: 170 a.
24. Billett AL, Kornmehl E, Tarbell NJ, Weinstein JH,Gelber RD, Ritz J, Sallan SE (1993) Autologous bone marrow transplantation after a long first remission for children with recurrent acute lymphoblastic leukemia. Blood 81: 1651–1657.
25. Billett AL, Sallan SE (1993) Autologous bone marrow transplantation in childhood acute lymphoid leukemia with use of purging. Am J Ped Hematol Oncol 15: 162–168.
26. Uckun FM, Ramsay NKC, Waddick KG, Jaszcz W, Chandan-Langlie M, Obuz V, Haake R, Gajl-Peczalska K, Kersey JH, Song CW (1991) In vitro and in vivo radiation resistance associated with CD3 surface antigen expression in T-lineage acute lymphoblastic leukemia. Blood 78: 2945–2955.
27. Uckun FM, Kersey JH, Haake R, Wesdorf D, Nesbit ME, Ramsay NKC (1993) Pretransplantation burden of leukemic progenitor cells as a predictor of relapse after bone marrow transplantation for acute lymphoblastic leukemia. N Engl J Med 329: 1296–1301.
28 Baruchel A, Leverger G, Bordigoni P, Demeocq F, Lemerle S, Bernaudin F, Perel Y, Hartman O, Michel G, Plouvier E, Souillet G, Vilmer E, LEblanc T, Vannier JP, Schaison G. Autologous bone marrow transplantation in complete remission after bone marrow relapse in children with acute lymphoblastic leukemia. Proceedings of the 18th Annual Meeting of the European Group for Bone Marrow Transplantation. Stockholm, Sweden May 31-June 3, 1992.

Acute Leukemias V
Experimental Approaches
and Management of Refractory Diseases
Hiddemann et al. (Eds.)

Comparison of Allogeneic and Autologous Bone Marrow Transplantation for Treatment of Childhood Acute Myeloblastic Leukemia (AML) in First Complete Remission

F. Zintl, J. Hermann, D. Fuchs, A. Müller, J. Füller, and H. Vogelsang

Introduction

The goal of treatment of acute myeloblastic leukemia (AML) in children is cure. Treatment results in AML have considerably improved during the last decade [5]. Remission induction therapy has become increasingly successful, and approximately 70 to 80% of children achieved complete remission (CR). However, despite consolidation, intensification and maintenance therapy, relapses have become, at least for a certain group of children, the limiting factor in the efforts to increase the event-free-survival rate.

Bone marrow transplantation from HLA identical sibling donors is a therapeutic option with promising results [2,3]. Allogeneic BMT is associated with a substantial treatment-related toxicity and only approximately 30% of all patients have a fully matched donor. Autologous BMT offers a way for a myeloablative therapy without the complications of allografting.

We report the results of a single institution study in which we compare allogeneic and autologous BMT in children with AML in first remission.

Patients and Methods

From November 1982 to February 1994 thirty-five out of 43 children with acute myeloblastic leukemia were transplanted in first remission. The diagnosis of the de novo AML was based on criteria of the French-American-British (FAB) cooperation group [4]. All patients given a diagnosis of AML received induction, consolidation and maintenance therapy according to the AML-1 [81] or AML-2 [87] protocol [5]. Fourteen children who had HLA-identical and MLC-negative sibling donors received allogeneic marrow transplants, twenty-one without a matched sibling donor received autologous unpurged marrow. Among the children who underwent transplantation during first remission, the median time from diagnosis to transplantation was 8 months (range, 3 to 14 months), for the allogeneic group, and 9 months (range, 5–18 months) for the autologous group. Marrow harvesting was performed just before transplantation.

Cytoreduction for BMT was similar for patients transplanted allogeneic or autologous (Table 1).

Bone marrow harvesting and processing were described elsewhere [6]. All patients were nursed in laminar air flow rooms and received total decontamination. Trimethoprim sulfamethoxazole therapy to prevent Pneumocystis carinii pneumonitis was given from day −14 to day +180. Prophylaxis for graft-versus-host disease (GVHD) consisted of MTX and prednisolone, since 1989 of cyclosporine A, MTX and prednisolone. As an equivalent for a missing GVLD the autografted children received post-transplant thioguanine and MTX for one year.

Indications for BMT in first remission were initial white blood cells above 20000/µl, FAB subtype M 4 to M 7, time to remission longer than 70 days, and AML as a second malignancy. Only one patient did not meet this requirements.

Disease free survival was calcutated by the Kaplan-Meier plots [7].

University of Jena, Department of Pediatrics, D-07745 Jena, Germany

Table 1. Conditioning regimens

	Allogeneic BMT No. of patients	Autologous BMT No. of patients
Total body irradiation (1 × 10 Gy) and cyclophosphamide (2 × 60 mg/kg)	6	–
Fractionated total body irradiation (6 × 2 Gy) and cyclophosphamide (2 × 60 mg/kg)	4	2
Busulfan (4 × 4 mg/kg and cyclophosphamide (4 × 50 mg/kg)	4	19

Table 2. Results of BMT

	Allogeneic BMT	Autologous BMT
No. of patients	14	21
Relapses after BMT	2(14%)	5 (24%)
CR after BMT	5–11 months	2–15 months
(median)	(8 months)	(7 months)
BMT related deaths	3 (21 %)	–
Survival after BMT	1–6 months	–
(median)	(2 months)	–
In CR after BMT	9 (64 %)	16 (76 %)
	11–137 months	12–70 months
(median)	(65 months)	(34 months)
pCCR rate	0.64 (SD = 0.13)	0.75 (SD = 0.10)

Results

Allogeneic BMT

Event free survival (EFS). Table 2 summarizes the results of transplantation according to the type of BMT.

Nine of 14 children remained alive at a median follow-up for the surviving patients of 65 months (range, 11 to 137 months). The estimated chance of surviving without disease for 10 years was 64 ± 13% (Fig. 1).

Engraftment. Leukocyte engraftment with an absolute leukocyte count ⩾1000/µl occurred at a median of 18 days (range, 8 to 25 days). The last substitution of platelets was on day 31 (range, 21 to 64 days).

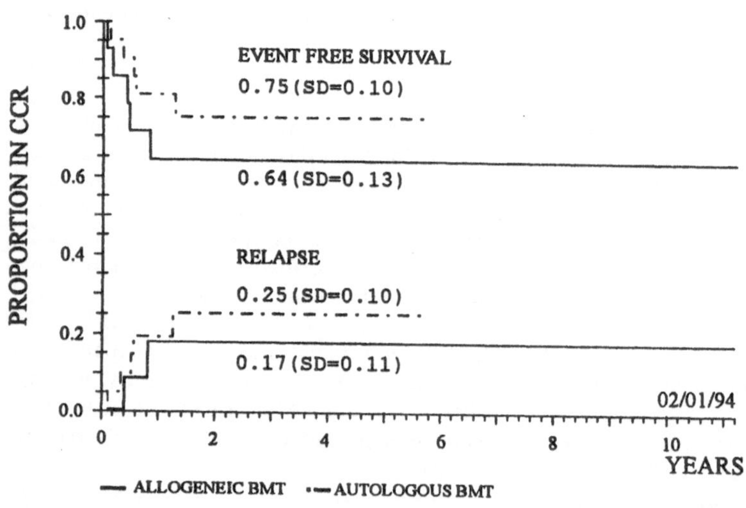

Fig. 1. Event free survival and incidence of relapse after allogeneic and autologous BMT of AML in 1st remission; allogeneic BMT: n = 14, 9 in CCR, 2 relapses; autologous BMT: n = 21, 16 in CCR, 5 relapses

BMT related mortality. Three patients died of transplantation-related complications including leukoencephalopathy [1], CMV-pneumonitis [1] and acute GVHD grade IV [1]. The median time to death was 2 months (range, 1 to 6 months) (Table 2).

Relapses. Two children relapsed (bone marrow) 5 and 11 months after allogeneic BMT (median 8 months) (Table 2). The estimate of the chances of relapse in 10 years after transplantation was 17±11% (Fig. 1).

Graft-versus-host-disease (GVHD). The overall incidence of acute GVHD (grade III or IV) was 14% (2/14 children). Chronic GVHD occurred in 6 children (43%). In this small group no relapse could be observed. Two of 6 children without chronic GVHD had bone marrow relapses.

Autologous BMT

Event free survival. The overall survival rate for 21 children after autologous transplantation was 75±10%. (16 of 21 patients. The median follow-up of the 16 children surviving in continuous complete remission was 34 months (range, 12 to 70 months).

Engraftment. An engraftment of leukocytes with a count⩾1000/μL occurred at a median of 16 days (range, 11 to 63 days). Platelets were substituted up to a median time of 41 days (range, 21 to 139 days).

BMT related mortality. None of 21 children died of transplantation-related complications.

Relapses. Five of 21 children relapsed. The only site of relapse was bone marrow. The median time to relapse was 7 months (range, 2 to 15 months) (Table 2). The estimate of the chances of relapse in the five years after transplantation was 25±11% (Fig. 1).

Discussion

In this report we gave an update of our results with allogeneic and autologous unpurged bone marrow transplantation in children with acute myeloblastic leukemia in first remission. Allogeneic and autologous bone marrow transplantation in AML in first remission is increasingly used as an option to improve the results of treatment of AML in adults and in children. Allogeneic BMT in adult patients with AML in first CR provides a superior outcome when directly compared with the results of autologous BMT [19]. Although there is a general acceptance for BMT in first CR for adults [8, 9] the indication for BMT in first CR in children is controversial [1]. The German AML-BFM Study Group defined two risk groups for AML in childhood [1]. According to the results of the study AML-BFM-83 the risk group I had an EFS of > 80% and the risk group II an EFS of < 45%.

For the low risk group neither autologous nor allogeneic BMT in first CR is recommended because of the low relapse rate.

In our study we compared the results of allogeneic and autologous BMT for 35 children. Children of both groups were qualified for BMT by initial leukocytes above 20000/μl, FAB subtype M 4 to M 7, delay of achieving a complete remission and AML as a second malignancy. The EFS for 14 children transplanted allogeneic is after more than 10 years 64 + 13%; for 21 children transplanted autologous after 6 years 75+10%. The relapse rate was higher in the autologous group (5/21=25%) than in the allogeneic group (2/14=14%). No toxic death was observed in the autologous transplanted children. 3 of 14 allografted children died of BMT related complications: Encephalopathy (1), acute GVHD IV (1), acute GVHD III with CMV pneumonitis (1).

After starting the autologous BMT program using fractionated TBI and cyclophosphamide in two children we changed this regimens to busulfan and cyclophosphamide without an increasing relapse rate or toxic complications.

In contrast to most other groups our autologous transplanted children received for one year thioguanine daily and MTX once weekly as an equivalent for a theoretically graft-versus-leukemia reaction in allografted patients.

Our pretransplant intervals between diagnosis and transplantation were median 8 and 9 months. Gorin [14] described a better outcome of ALL patients transplanted in first CR after an interval of more than 7 months. Patients with relapses in the autografted group were transplanted 7 months (range, 5–17), in the allografted group 3 and 8 months after diagnoses.

Current results show that 50–70% of young patients with AML who undergo allogeneic BMT experience prolonged DFS and may be cured [3, 2, 11, 12, 13].

This study was designed to compare the efficacy of the autologous BMT with the more traditional allogeneic BMT in children with AML in first CR with similar demographics and disease characteristics.

Bone marrow transplantation, whether allogeneic or autologous, is a safe procedure in children with an acceptable risk for complications. Allo- and autografting are both effective at maintaining remission but there is a trend towards a higher relapse rate in the autologous group. Our results strongly support our strategy to transplant children with high risk AML in first remission as an effective alternative therapy.

References

1. Creutzig U, Ritter J, Schellong G (1990) Identification of two risk groups in childhood acute myelogenous leukemia after therapy intensification in study AML-BFM-83 as compared with study AML-BFM-78: Blood 75: 1932–1940
2. Sanders JE, Thomas ED, Buckner CD et al. (1985) Marrow transplantation for children in first remission of acute nonlymphoblastic leukemia: an update. Blood 66: 460–462
3. Brochstein JA, Kernan NA, Groshen S et al. (1987) Allogeneic BMT after hyperfractionated TBI and cyclophosphamide in children with acute leukemia. N Engl J Med 317: 1618–1624
4. Bennett JM, Catovsky D, Daniel MT et al. (1985) Proposed revised criteria for the classification of acute myeloid leukemia. A report of the French-American-British Cooperative Group. Ann Intern Med 103: 620–625
5. Hermann J, Zintl F, Krause M et al. (1991) Therapie der akuten myeloischen Leukämie bei Kindern – Ergebnisse der multizentrischen Therapiestudie AML II/87. Kinderärztl. Praxis 59: 321–327
6. Zintl F (1988) Knochenmarktransplantation im Kindesalter, Teil I, Kinderärztl. Praxis 56: 259–264
7. Kaplan EL, Meier (1958) Nonparametric estimation from incomplete observations. J Am Stat Assoc 53: 457–462
8. Linker CA, Ries CA, Damon LE et al. (1993) Autologous bone marrow transplantation for acute myeloid leukemia using busulfan plus etoposide as a preparative regimen. Blood 81: 311–318
9. Chao NJ, Stein AS, Long GD et al. (1993) Busulfan/etoposide-initial experience with a new preparatory regimen for autologous bone marrow transplantation in patients with acute nonlymphoblastic leukemia. Blood 81: 319–323
10. Löwenberg B, van Putten WLJ, Verdonck LF et al. (1990) Autologous bone marrow transplantation in acute myeloid leukemia first remission: First Dutch prospective study. Haematology and Blood Transfusion, Acute Leukemias II, Eds. Büchner T, Schellong G, Hiddemann W, Ritter J. Springer-Verlag Berlin Heidelberg 33: 655–659
11. Bostrom B, Brunning R, McGlave P et al. (1985) Bone marrow transplantation for acute nonlymphocytic leukemia in first remission: analysis of prognostic factors. Blood 65: 1191–1196
12. Snyder DS, Chao NJ, Amylon MD et al. (1993) Fractionated total body irradiation and high-dose-etoposide as a preparatory regimen for bone marrow transplantation for 99 patients with acute leukemia in first complete remission. Blood 82: 2920–2928
13. Vowels M, Stevens M, Tiedemann K et al. (1992) Autologous and allogeneic bone marrow transplantation for childhood acute nonlymphoblastic leukemia. Transplantation Proceedings 24: 184–185
14. Gorin NC, Aegerter P, Auvert M (1990) Autologous bone marrow transplantation for acute leukemia in remission: An analysis of 1322 cases, Haematology and Blood Transfusion, Acute Leukemias II, Eds. Büchner T, Schellong G, Hiddemann W, Ritter J. Springer-Verlag Berlin Heidelberg 33: 660–666
15. Dahl GV, Kalwinsky K, Mirro J (1990) Allogeneic bone marrow transplantation in a program of intensive sequential chemotherapy for children and young adults with acute nonlymphocytic leukemia in first remission. J Clin Oncol 8: 295–303

Acute Leukemias V
Experimental Approaches
and Management of Refractory Diseases
Hiddemann et al. (Eds.)

Long-Term Results in Adult AML: Comparison of Postremission Chemotherapy vs. Autologous BMT vs. Allogeneic BMT

W. Helbig[1], R. Krahl[1], M. Kubel[1], H. Schwenke[1], M. Herold[2], F. Fiedler[3], A. Franke[4], V. Lakner[5], R. Rohrberg[6], D. Kämpfe[6], F. Strohbach[7], G. Schott[8], U. V. Grünhagen[9], N. Grobe[10], R. Pasold[11], M. Stauch[12], J. Fleischer[13], C. Klinkenstein[14], C. Boewer[15], J. Steglich[16], P. Richter[17], R. Pillkahn[18], R. Schubert[19], I. Rudorf[20], K. Eisengarten[21], and D. Morgenstern[22] for the East German Study Group (EGSG)

Abstract. From January 1985 to June 1991, three hundred adults aged 15 to 60 years with de novo acute myeloblastic leukemia (AML) were treated in two clinical studies. Induction chemotherapy consisted of thioguanine, cytosine arabinoside, daunorubicin, vincristine, and prednison (TAD-VP). The protocols AML '85 (using a dose of 45 mg/m^2 daunorubicin) and AML '89 (intensified by two linked obligatory courses of TAD-VP with an increased dose of 60 mg/m^2 daunorubicin) resulted in complete remission rates of 54.2% and 58.3%, respectively. All patients achieving complete remission received three courses of consolidation. Patients below 40 years with a HLA-identical sibling were offered bone marrow transplantation (BMT). Patients without HLA-identical sibling and those who refused transplantation were randomized to maintenance therapy given monthly for two years vs. three courses of intensification without any further antileukemic therapy vs. autologous BMT (ABMT) (age below 40 years).

After a median follow-up of more than 4 years in both studies, there is no advantage of maintenance therapy (n = 79) against intensification (n = 38) concerning to leukemia-free survival (LFS) (0.23 vs. 0.27). The LFS of patients who received only postremission chemotherapy is 0.16 at 5 years in AML '85 (n = 91) and 0.34 at 3 years in AML '89 (n = 77) (p = 0.046). Since the postremission chemotherapy was unchanged, the improvement of LFS might be due to a higher dose of daunorubicin or early intensification by means of "double" induction.

[1] Division of Hematology and Oncology, Department of Internal Medicine, University of Leipzig, 04103 Leipzig
[2] Department of Internal Medicine, Klinikum Erfurt, Erfurt
[3] Department of Internal Medicine, Stadtpark Klinikum Chemnitz, Chemnitz
[4] Department of Internal Medicine, University of Magdeburg, Magdeburg
[5] Department of Internal Medicine, University of Rostock, Rostock
[6] Department of Internal Medicine, Martin-Luther-University of Halle, Halle
[7] Department of Internal Medicine, Klinikum Berlin-Buch, Berlin-Buch
[8] Oncology Center, Klinikum Zwickau, Zwickau
[9] Department of Internal Medicine, Carl-Thiem-Klinikum Cottbus, Cottbus
[10] Department of Internal Medicine, Klinikum Neubrandenburg, Neubrandenburg
[11] Division of Internal Medicine, Klinikum Ernst von Bergmann, Potsdam
[12] Department of Internal Medicine, Friedrich-Schiller-University of Jena, Jena
[13] Department of Internal Medicine, Technical University of Dresden, Dresden
[14] Department of Internal Medicine, Klinikum Frankfurt/Oder, Frankfurt/Oder
[15] Division of Internal Medicine, St. Hedwig-Hedwig-Krankenhaus Berlin, Berlin
[16] I. Department of Internal Medicine, Krankenhaus Dresden-Friedrichstadt, Dresden-Friedrichstadt
[17] Städtisches Krankenhaus Zella-Mehlis, Zella-Mehlis
[18] I. Department of Internal Medicine, Klinikum der Stadt Gera, Gera
[19] Division of Hematology and Oncology, Klinikum Schwerin, Schwerin
[20] Department of Internal Medicine, Vogtland-Klinikum Plauen, Plauen
[21] Division of Internal Medicine, Städtisches Krankenhaus Meißen, Meißen
[22] Krankenhaus Zittau, Zittau

Comparing the different postremission treatment regimens, there is a trend of better LFS in BMT (n=12, 4-year LFS 0.75) (p=0.07) but no difference between ABMT (n=17, LFS 0.35) and chemotherapy (n=35, LFS 0.20) (not significant).

Introduction

Since 1985 the East German Study Group (EGSG) initiated clinically controlled studies to improve long-term results and to estimate the efficiency of different types of postremission therapy after three courses for consolidation of the complete remission (CR) followed by allogeneic bone marrow transplantation (BMT) from HLA-identical siblings or autologous BMT (ABMT) or by further three courses of consolidation without maintenance treatment or by maintenance treatment for 2 years, respectively.

Patients and Methods

Study population. Between January 1885 and December 1989, 181 consecutive adults (AML '85) and between January 1989 and June 1991, 153 consecutive patients (AML '89) with newly diagnosed untreated AML aged 15 to 60 years were registered in a multicenter prospective randomized trial (Table 1).

All patients achieving a complete remission after induction chemotherapy were treated with three courses of consolidation. Patients below 40 years with a HLA-identical sibling were offered marrow transplantation. Patients without HLA-identical sibling and those who refused transplantation were randomized to maintenance therapy given monthly for two years vs. three courses of intensification without any further antileukemic therapy vs. ABMT (age below 40 years).

Treatment protocol. Induction chemotherapy consisted of TAD-VP in both protocols, in AML '85: 1–3 courses of daunorubicin 45 mg/m² i.v. days 1–3, Ara-C 100 mg/m²/12h by i.v. bolus days 1–7, 6-thioguanine 100 mg/m²/12h p.o. days 1–7, vincristine 2 mg day 1 and predniso(lo)ne 60 mg/m² i.v. or. p.o. days 1–7; in AML '89: 2 obligatory courses of TAD-VP with increased dose of daunorubicin 60 mg/m² i.v. days 1–3 and start of the second course on day 21 if there was evidence of a beginning recovery of hematopoiesis and no life-threatening infections. If no complete remission was reached a renewed remission induction was started by means of cyclophosphamide 600 mg/m² i.v. days 1+10, vincristine 2 mg i.v. days 1+10, methotrexate 30 mg/m² i.v. days 2+5 and 6-mercaptopurine 60 mg/m² p.o. days 1–10 (COMM). Patients who failed to achieve a complete remission after TAD-VP and/or COMM were taken off study. All patients in complete remission were

Table 1. Clinical Characteristics of patients enrolled on the studies AML '85 and AML '89

Characteristic	AML '85	AML '89	p Value
No. of patients	181	153	
Median age, yr (range)	33 (15–60)	42 (15–60)	<0.001
Sex (M/F)	82/99	80/73	ns
FAB (%) M1	25.7	14.5	<0.01
M2	35.7	34.5	
M3	4.1	8.3	
M4	20.5	22.1	
M5	12.9	17.2	
M6	1.2	2.8	
M7		0.7	
MDS / secondary AML	10	8	
expired before or within 3 days from start of therapy	2	4	
not evaluable	1	9	
No studied	168	132	

FAB = French-American-British Cooperative Group Morphology

assigned to three courses of consolidation with DA administered at lower doses (daunorubicine 45 mg/m² i.v. days 1+2 and Ara-C 100 mg/m²/12h i.v. days 1–5). The intervals between induction and consolidation courses were kept as short as possible. Maintenance given monthly for two years consisted of rotating courses of MOM (methotrexate 7.5 mg/m² p.o. days 1–5, vincristine 2 mg i.v. day 1, and 6-mercaptopurine 60 mg/m² p.o. days 1–5), COT (cyclophosphamide 750 mg/m² i.v. day 1, vincristine 2 mg i.v. day 1, and 6-thioguanine 50 mg/m²/12h p.o. days 1–5) and DA. Patients randomized to intensification received further three courses of DA.

Transplantation. Marrow transplantation was performed as soon as possible after consolidation. If the intervall between consolidation and transplantation was greater then five weeks maintenance therapy was started as relapse prophylaxis. For ABMT the marrow was harvested by multiple aspirations from the posterior iliac crest during the phase of beginning hematological reconstitution after third course of consolidation. The cell suspension was depleted of red blood cells and immediately frozen (7.5% DMSO) without any other manipulation. The frozen bags were stored in liquid nitrogen. Marrow transplantation followed conditioning with busulfan (total dose of 16 mg/kg was administered orally in four divided daily doses over 4 days) and cyclophosphamide (60 mg/kg was given intravenously on each of the next 2 days). As prophylaxis for graft-versus-host disease recipients of allogeneic marrow received methotrexate, cyclosporine, and methylprednisolone.

Response criteria. Complete remission was defined as 5% or less blasts in a normocellular bone marrow with normal peripheral and differential counts [1]. Patients failing induction therapy were categorized as partial remission (PR) if hematological improvement was achieved (6% to 25% marrow blasts); non responders (NR) were defined as persistence of a marrow leukemic infiltrate of more than 25% during induction chemotherapy; early death (ED) means that patients died while receiving induction therapy including the aplastic phase before hematological reconstitution.

Statistical methods. Actual differences were analysed for statistical significance by the chi-square method. Survival was calculated from date of diagnosis, leukemia free survival (LFS) was considered from the time of complete remission until relapse or death, and probability of relapse were assessed from date of complete remission to relapse. Patients who were lost to follow up or alive at time of analysis were cencored. The LFS, relapse and survival curves were obtained by Kaplan-Meier product limit method[2] and statistical test of significance were performed by log-rank test[3].

Results

Induction therapy. The median age of patients in study AML '89 was higer than that in AML '85 ($p < 0.001$), because until October 1987 patients above 40 years were enrolled on a separate study. CR was achieved in 91 cases of 168 patients (54.2%) in AML '85 (Table 2), 11 after one induction course, 46 after two courses and 34 after three or more courses. In AML '89, the rate of CR was only a little improved and 77 of 132 patients (58,3%) achieved remission. The

Table 2. Results of induction therapy

	AML '85	AML '85 clinics treated		AML '89	AML '89 clinics treated	
	total	⩾ 10 pts	< 10 pts	total	⩾ 10 pts	< 10 pts
n	168	111	57	132	106	26
CR [%]	54.2	61.3	40.4[a]	58.3	62.3	42.3[b]
PR	11.3	8.1	17.5	6.8	7.5	3.8
NR	15.5	15.3	15.6	13.6	11.3	23.1
ED	19.0	15.3	26.3	21.2	18.9	30.8

CR = complete remission, PR = partial remission, NR = non responder, ED = early death, pts = patients
[a]chi-square test including CR, PR, NR, and ED $p < 0.01$, [b]$p < 0.05$

number of induction courses was significantly diminished compared to AML '85 ($p < 0.001$), 28 patients achieved CR after one course, 41 after two courses, and only 8 after three or more courses. The rate of ED did not increase by the intensification of the induction treatment.

Participants of the studies who treated more than 10 patients reached a higher rate of CR compared to those who treated a smaller number of patients: 61.3% versus 40.4% in AML85 ($p < 0.01$); 62.3% versus 42.3 in AML'89 ($p < 0.05$) (Table 2).

Postremission chemotherapy. In the study AML'85 the LFS for patients who received maintenance treatment is 0.16 versus 0.22 for the group without maintenance but with three courses of additional consolidation (not significant different = ns) after a median follow up of 59 months. The protocol AML '89 (median follow up of 39 months) has led to an improvement of LFS both for patients who were assigned to maintenance and for those who received intensification by three additional courses of consolidation (0.34 vs. 0.29, ns). Because there is no statistically different outcome concerning to maintenance or additional consolidation in both studies (Fig. 1) we took together the postremission chemotherapy results of each study to compare both in regard to long-term survival. Thus, LFS in the AML '89 study was improved ($p < 0.05$) from 0.16 at 5 years in the AML85 to 0.34 at 3 years in the AML '89 study (Fig. 2).

Comparison of chemotherapy and bone marrow transplantation. Due to the exclusion of relapsed patients before ABMT and BMT we used biometrics by "intention to treat" to compare (A)BMT with chemotherapy. There is a trend of better LFS in BMT ($p = 0.07$) but no difference between ABMT and chemotherapy (Fig. 3A). The Kaplan-Meier plot for relapses is complete conversely (Fig. 3B).

Because of an unusual long period from the end of consolidation to further postremission

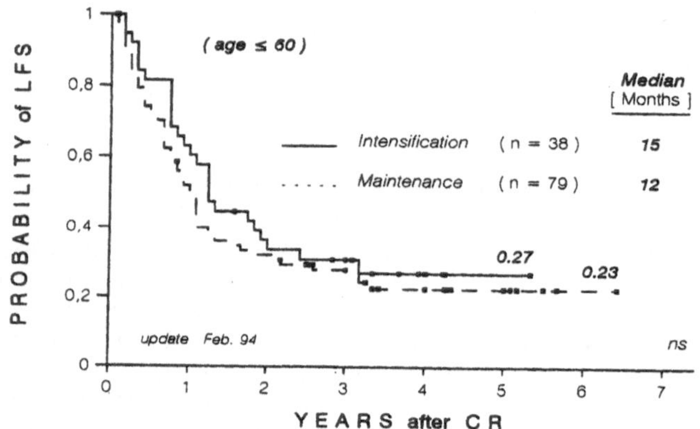

Fig. 1. Actuarial probability of LFS for patients ≤60 years who achieved a complete remission and received consolidation followed by maintenance or intensification without maintenance in sutdies AML '85 ad AML '89. Tick marks depict patients alive in continuous first complete remission

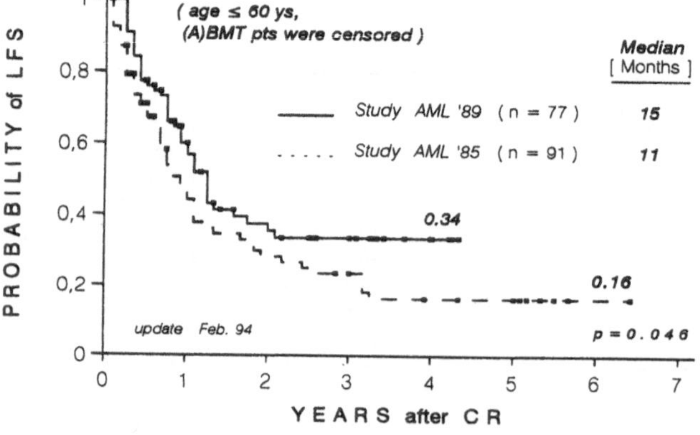

Fig. 2. Actuarial probability of LFS for patients ≤60 years who entered complete remission and received postremission chemotherapy in study AML '85 or AML '89. All patients grafted were censored at time of transplant

treatment (only one BMT center available) only 12 of 22 patients with a HLA-identical sibling were allografted (9 relapsed, 1 refused) and 17 of 27 randomized patients were autografted (9 relapsed, 1 refused), we excluded in another biometric calculation all relapses within the chemotherapy group until the median of the period between CR and transplantation to compare the actually grafted with nongrafted patients (Fig. 4A,B). Similar results could be obtained, e.g. BMT was superior to chemotherapy and no advantage of ABMT versus chemotherapy has been found.

In both studies 14 of 300 patients (4.7%) has been allografted and 18 (6.0%) autografted in first CR. Later, in a higher stage of AML further 4 patients (1.3%) received a BMT and 3 (1.0%) an ABMT.

Reflecting the overall survival of the total patients from both studies the long-term survival from the diagnosis up to more than 5 years could be improved only to 4% by (A)BMT (Fig. 5).

Discussion

The rate of CR over 50% corresponding to the international level could be only slightly increased by the higher doses of daunorubicin (60 mg/m² vs. 45 mg/m² daily) and by two linked induction courses, where at the rate of ED and NR did not increase. Since participants of both studies who treated more than 10 AML patients reached more CR than others, it seems to be important to develop sufficient own experiences especially with supportive care.

The postremission results of the nongrafted patients under chemotherapy could be improved markedly from 0.16 to 0.34 LFS after 5 or 3 years, respectively. Because the postremission chemotherapy was the same in both studies, the

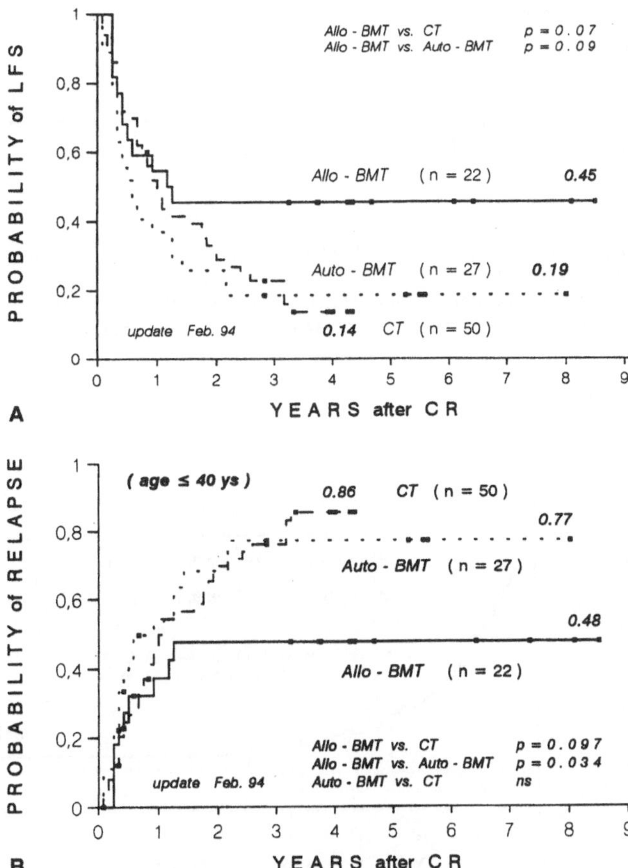

Fig. 3. Actuarial probability of LFS (**A**) and relapse (**B**) among patients ≤40 years allograftes or autografted in first remission received postremission chemotherapy in both studies n conformity with "intention to treat"

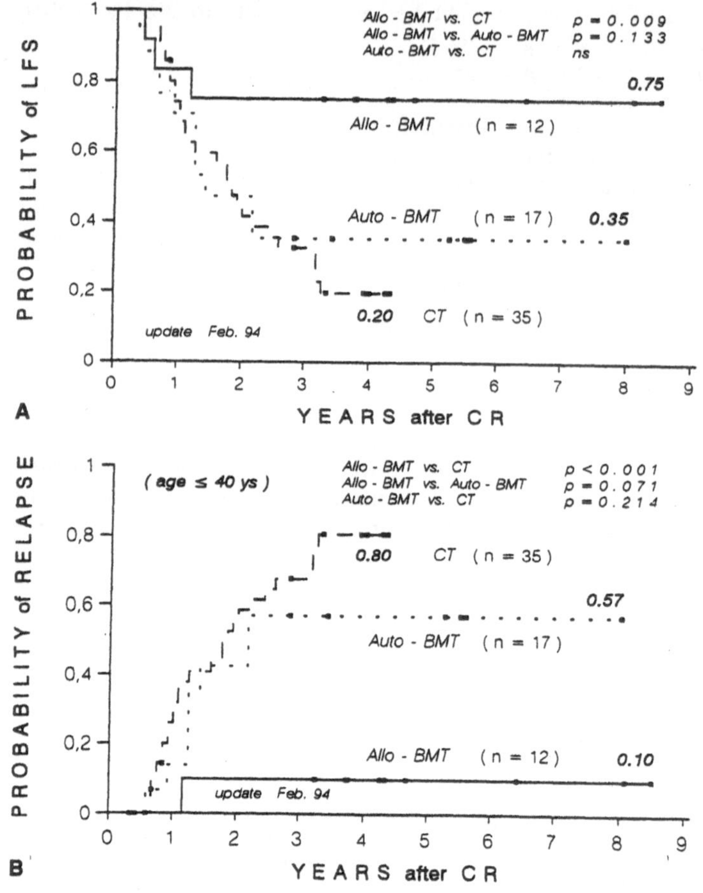

Fig. 4. Actuarial probability of LFS (A) and relapse (B) among all patients ≤40 who entered complete remission in studies AML '85 and AML '89, stratified by postremission treatment regimens received. In order to compare the different postremission treatment regimens, patients of chemotherapy group relapsed within 210 days (median period of time until transplant) were excluded from analysis

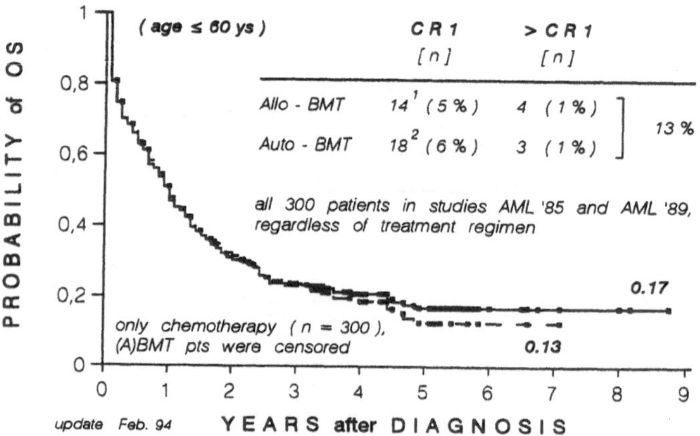

Fig. 5. Actuarial probability of overall survival (OS) for all patients in studies AML '85 and AML '89 represented first regardless of postremission treatment regimen, ie, including (A)BMT in first remission or higher stage of disease, and second without (A)BMT, ie, all patients grafted were censored at time of transplant (for the sake of clearness no tick marks). [1)] 2 patients above 40 years included. [2)] 1 patient above 40 years included

quality of CR after double induction with increased dose of daunorubicin might be responsible for this. No significant different results could be obtained if patients received postremission treatment by additional consolidation courses (intensification) or maintenance therapy.

It can be concluded that intensification of induction therapy might led to a higher quality of CR. That and further intensive postremission treatment by consolidation added by maintenance or additional consolidation seems to be the reason for better long-term results.

Allogeneic BMT for HLA-identical siblings is superior to chemotherapy but, at least in our hands, ABMT without purging similar to chemotherapy and no real improvement of AML management. Although allogeneic BMT improves the results of AML treatment for allografted patients, chemotherapy remains to be the basic management of AML.

References

1. Cheson BD et al: J Clin Oncol 8: 813–819, 1990
2. Kaplan EL, Meier P: Nonparametric estimation from incomplete observations. J Am Stat Assoc 53: 457–481, 1958
3. Mantel N: Evaluation of survival date and two rank order statistics arising in its consideration. Cancer Chemother Rep 50: 163–170, 1966

Acute Leukemias V
Experimental Approaches
and Management of Refractory Diseases
Hiddemann et al. (Eds.)

Allogeneic BMT in Patients with AML: Influence of the Prior Response to Induction Chemotherapy on Outcome After BMT

R. Arnold, D. Bunjes, B. Hertenstein, C. Duncker, J. Novotny, M. Stefanic, M. Theobald, G. Heil, M. Wiesneth, and H. Heimpel

Introduction

In chemotherapy treated patients the achievement of a complete remission is the prerequisite for cure. There is evidence that the kinetics of response is an important prognostic factor for the duration of remission. In patients undergoing allogeneic bone marrow transplantation supralethal radio/chemotherapy is given as conditioning regimen. Furthermore, an allogeneic graft versus leukaemia effect could be demonstrated. We analyzed whether primary responsiveness to chemotherapy influences the outcome after allogeneic bmt.

Patients and Methods

Patient characteristics. Between 11/1980 and 11/1993 eighty-five adult patients with newly diagnosed acute myeloid leukaemia (AML) underwent allogeneic bone marrow transplantation (BMT). The median age at BMT was 34 years (15–51 years). The diagnosis of AML was made by peripheral blood and bone marrow analysis including cytochemistry. Since 1985 all patients with AML have been classified according to the FAB classification. FAB M2 was the largest subgroup of AML transplanted (FAB M1 n=15), M2 n=29, M3 n=2, M4 n=19, M5 n=5, M6 n=2, unclassified n=13). Induction therapy of AML varied with time, but all patients received anthracyclines and Ara-C. 19 out of 85 patients received the TAD protocol [1] and 49 out of 85 patients the DAV protocol [2]. Of 85 patients 17 were treated according to other protocols. These patients were referred for BMT from other chemotherapy centres.

Response to induction chemotherapy. After induction chemotherapy 79 out of 85 patients achieved a first complete remission. Most of the patients (69 one of 79 patients) responded to first line therapy. 10 out of 79 patients, who failed first line therapy received a salvage protocol including high dose Ara-C and went into 1. CR. 6 out 85 patients treated failed salvage therapy and were evaluated as having refractory leukaemia. In patients with DAV as first line therapy the following kinetics of response was observed: 23 out 49 patients achieved 1. CR after the first course of the DAV protocol, 16 out of 49 patients responded after the second course of the DAV protocol. In 10 out of 49 patients data on the kinetics of response were missing or patients failed the DAV protocol.

Bone marrow transplantation. The conditioning regimen for patients transplanted in 1. CR (n=79) consisted mainly of total body irradiation (up to 1985 10 Gy TBI single dose, from 1985 onwards 12 Gy TBI fractionated in 6 doses) and 120 mg/kg bw cyclophosphamide (n=73). When cardiac contraindications against cyclophosphamide existed, melphalan (n=3) or VP-16 (n=2) were given instead. One further patient received busulfan and cyclophosphamide. The conditioning regimen for patients with refractory leukaemia (n=6) consisted mainly of TBI and

Departments of Internal Medicine III and Transfusion Medicine, University of Ulm, 89081 Ulm, Germany

VP-16 (n = 5) and busulfan and VP-16 in one patient.

Bone marrow donors were HLA identical siblings in 82 cases and HLA mismatched family members in three cases.

For gvhd prophylaxis in patients in 1. CR different regimen were used over time (methotrexate n = 9, cyclosporin A n = 1, ex vivo T-cell depletion n = 19), cyclosporin A plus methotrexate n = 26 and since 1990 combined in vivo/ex vivo T-cell depletion n = 24. All patients with refractory leukaemia received cyclosporin A plus methotrexate (n = 6).

Statistical methods. The probability of survival, probability of disease free survival (DFS), the probability of relapse and the probability of transplant related mortality were calculated by life table analysis according to Kaplan and Meier.

Results

Out of 85 patients 50 are alive, 35 are dead. The cause of death was transplant related mortality in 23 out of 35 patients. 16 of 85 patients relapsed after bmt. 11 out of 16 patients died due to leukaemic relapse, 5 of 16 patients are alive in 2. CR after radiation therapy (n = 1), reinduction chemotherapy and buffy coat therapy (n = 2) or after 2nd BMT (n = 2).

Analysis with regard to response and kinetics of response to induction chemotherapy revealed its influence on the rate of disease free survival after bmt (Table 1). The probability of DFS for AML patients transplanted in 1. CR is 0.45 with a median follow up of 35 (6–149) months (Fig. 1). Patients with an early response to induction therapy have a higher DFS (0.69) compared with patients with a late response (0.42) or a response to salvage therapy (0.15) (Fig. 2). Transplant related mortality was similar in all groups (Table 1).

Discussion

Allogeneic bone marrow transplantation for treatment of AML patients in 1. CR leads to a high rate of long terms survivors (54%). We found that the response and the kinetics of response to primary induction chemotherapy have a strong influence on long-term outcome after bmt. This presumably reflects the primary sensitivity of leukaemic sterm cells to cytotoxic drugs and/or the development of drug resistance during therapy. Both factors are also likely to influence the response to high-dose chemotherapy and radiation given as conditioning treatment. One can speculate if intensified conditioning regimens and/or immunotherapy after bmt can improve disease from survival (DFS) after BMT.

Table 1. Allogeneic BMT in newly diagnosed AML patients. Transplantation period 11/1980–11/1993

	all patients (group 1)	1. CR (group 2)	1. CR post DAV I (group 3)	1. CR post DAV II (group 4)	1. CR post salvage therapy (group 5)	refractory leukemia (group 6)
no of patients	85	79	23	16	10	6
age median + range	34(15–51)	34(15–51)	32(15–51)	41(15–51)	35(21–47)	49(25–51)
sex M/F	45/40	41/38	17/6	5/11	7/3	4/2
probability of survival	0.53	0.54	0.69	0.73	0.42	0.31
probability of transplant related mortality	0.31	0.32	0.24	0.21	0.11	0.17
probability of relapse	0.32	0.33	0.1	0.46	0.83	0.6
probability of disease free survival	0.47	0.45	0.69	0.42	0.15	0.33
median follow up post bmt (months)	33(5–149)	35(6–149)	35(13–85)	22(6–71)	47(12–109)	11(5–83)

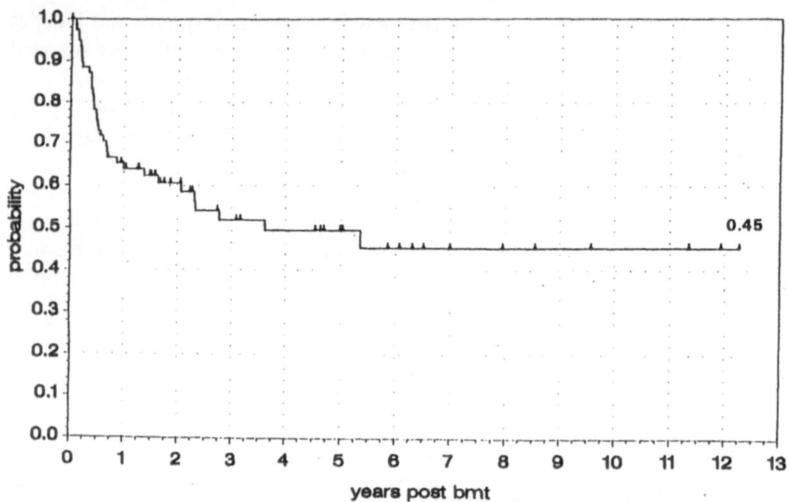

Fig. 1. AML: Allogeneic bmt in 1. CR (1980–11/1993) probability of disease free survival. Group 2:1. CR, n = 79

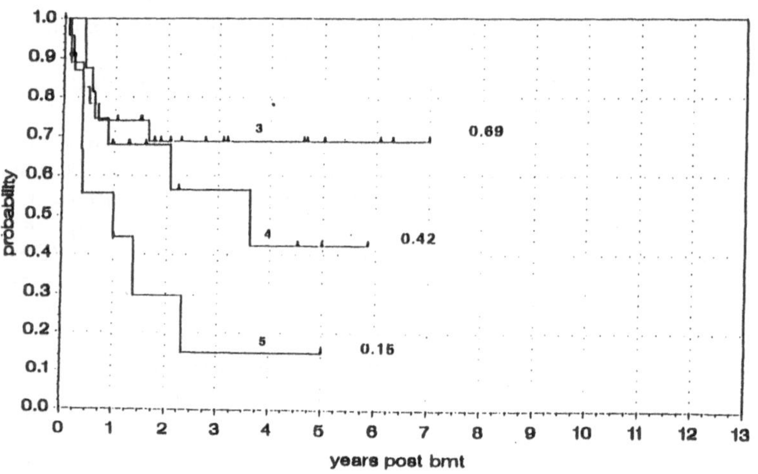

Fig. 2. AML: Allogeneic bmt in 1. CR (1980–11/1993) probability of disease free survival. Group 3:1. CR post DAV I, n = 23; Group 4:1. CR post DAV II, n = 16; Group 5:1. CR post salvage therapy, n = 10

References

1. Link H., Kurrle E., Frauer HM., Heil G., Heimpel H., Waller HD., Ostendorf P., Wilms K., Hoelzer D. (1986) TAD-induction therapy for 175 adults with acute myeloid leukaemia, followed by consolidation and maintenance therapy. Onkologie 9: 135–138
2. Kurrle E., Ehninger G., Freund M., Heil G., Hoelzer D., Link H., Mitrou PS., Öhl S., Queisser W., Schlimok G., Wandt H. (1988) A multicentre study on intensive induction and consolidation therapy in acute myelogenous leukaemia. Blut 56: 233–236

Acute Leukemias V
Experimental Approaches
and Management of Refractory Diseases
Hiddemann et al. (Eds.)

Donor Leukocyte Infusions (DLI) in the Treatment of AML Patients Relapsed After Allogeneic Bone Marrow Transplantation

V. Savchenko, L. Mendeleeva, L. Lubimova, H. Parovitchnikova, H. Gribanova, L. P. Poreshina, and M. Petrov

Introduction

High-dose chemoradiotherapy and allogeneic bone marrow transplantation (BMT) can cure some patients with acute leukemia and lymphoma. However, approximately 50% of patients relapse after BMT and constitute the group with unfavourable prognosis. Results of salvage chemotherapy in these patients are extremely poor [1], so new alternatives have emerged during the past decade in the field of immunotherapy. The efficacy of allogeneic BMT is usually associated with graft versus host disease (GVHD) and especially with graft versus leukemia (GVL) phenomenon that is carried out by donor's T-lymphocytes [2]. The absence of GVHD in syngeneic and autologous BMT, T-depletion in allogeneic BMT, more intensive GVHD prophylaxis lead to the higher leukemia relapse rate. It was revealed that induction of GVL effect may be independent of GVHD and can be mediated by cyclosporine A, interleukin-2 (IL-2), transfusion of donor's leukocytes [3, 4, 5]. Those approaches are being used in order to prevent or to treat leukemia relapse after bone marrow transplantation that is to say to prolong disease-free survival. The largest report concerning DLI in relapsed BMT patients comprises 82 cases (chronic myeloid leukemia, acute leukemias) and demonstrates encouraging results [6]. This article will briefly summarise our experience in the treatment of relapses after allogeneic BMT with donor's leukocytes infusions.

Patients and Methods

Two patients with acute myeloid leukemia underwent allogeneic BMT using HLA identical sibling donor and relapsed within 5 and 24 months. Both patients received cyclophosphamide and total body irradiation as conditioning therapy and were treated with methotrexate and cyclosporin A for GVHD prophylaxis. Both patients were monitored for chimaerism during and after BMT using erythrocytes markers by means of hemagglutinating test in low delutions.

At the time of relapse (12.3.93) patient No 1 had 70% blast cells in bone marrow aspirate, blastic infiltration in bone marrow biopsy, severe pancytopenia. No salvage chemotherapy was applied.

Patient No 2 had 92% of blasts in bone marrow at the time of relapse (21.4.93), hypoplasia with myelodisplastic features in b/m biopsy. She was treated with standard 7+3 (ara-c 100 mg/m^2 i.v. bid 1–7 days, daunorubicin 45 mg/m^2 i.v. 1–3 days). Complete remission was achieved within 1 month. There were no further chemotherapy. The patients characteristics are detailed in Table 1.

Donor leukocyte infusions were started at the time of relapse without prior treatment in Patient No 1 and after achievement of 2 CR in Patient No 2. Donor leukocytes were obtained by Blood Cell Separator Fenwall CS-3000. Mean collected leukocyte count was $12{,}1 \times 10^7$/kg. Leukocytes were infused within one hour.

National Research Center for Hematology, Moscow, Russia

Table 1. Characteristics and clinical course of two patients with AML

	Patient No 1	Patient No 2
Age (at diagnosis)	20 y	28 y
Sex	female	female
Blood group	O(I)Rh+	B(III)Rh+
Prior illness	AML	AML
FAB subtype	M2	M2
Induction chemotherapy	7+3	7+3
Response to induction	CR	CR
Disease status at BMT	1st CR	1 st CR
Time of BMT	3.11.92	26.4.91
Donor sex	male	male
Donor blood group	O(I) Rh –	O(I)Rh+
GVHD after BMT	none	skin (Grade I)
Interval BMT to relapse	130 days	24 months
Salvage chemotherapy	none	7+3
Leukocyte infusions	No 8	No 6
GVHD after leukocyte infusions	none	none
Complications	none	none
Outcome	Alive, 2 CR > 10 months	Alive, 2 CR > 8 months

Interleukin-2 was added during the 3rd, 4th, and 5th procedures as 48-hours infusion started 2 hours before DLI at dose 6 U/m² per day. The first two DLI were done with two weeks interval, the following were performed and continued to be applied with two months interval. In all cases bone marrow aspirate was studied in conjunction with bone marrow biopsy.

Results

Two AML patients in relapse after allogeneic bone marrow transplantation received donor leukocyte infusions. One of them was treated with chemotherapy (1 course 7+3) before DLI. Information concerning DLI in each patient is reflected in Table 2.

At the time of relapse the chimaeric erythrocytes in patient No 1 constituted 20% (3 months after BMT the percent was 53). She achieved complete remission after second DLI. It was proved by normal peripheral blood analysis, bone marrow aspirate. The most impressive picture was observed in the bone marrow biopsy as it showed the disappearance of blastic methaplasia, moderately hypoplastic bone marrow with focuses of small lymphocyte infiltration. CR is maintained for 10 months. What is worth of note that the rate of chimaeric erythrocytes now is 82% (more than after BMT) and continues to grow. It is interesting that in patient No 2 the chimaeric erythrocytes in relapse were 100% of donor type, and till now the patient demonstrates 100% red cells chimaerism.

There were no graft versus host disease (GVHD) symptoms in any case during the first months of treatment. In one patient mild signs of GVHD (stomatitis, conjuctivitis, skin dryness) developed 6 months after the beginning of DLI. No special treatment was applied.

Discussion

Residual disease after bone marrow transplantation quite frequently becomes the cause of

Table 2. Course of treatment with donor leukocyte infusions

		Patient No 1		Patient No 2	
No of procedure	Time to next DLI	leuk × 10^7/kg	b/m blasts before DLI	leuk × 10^7/kg	b/m blasts before DLI
1.	2 weeks	8,1	70%	7,5	2,5%
2.	2 weeks	9,75	–	23,8	–
3.*	2 months	11,9	2,3%	26,2	2,8%
4.*	2 months	20,4	–	9,8	–
5.*	2 months	10,3	3,1%	21,7	1,2%
6.	2 months	15,3	–	13,4	2,5%
7.	2 months	12,8	1,9%	–	–
8.	2 months	19,7	2,2%	–	–

DLI combined with IL-2

leukemia relapse but also can persist in a balanced state due to immune mechanisms that keep control over malignant cell proliferation. The existence of immune-mediated anti-leukemic activity after allogeneic BMT was first described in mice at the end of fifties [7] and now is summarized by the term "graft versus leukemia" effect. GVL is probably supported by cellular (CD-4+ cytotoxic T-lymphocytes directed to antigens of minor complex of histocompartibility, natural killer cells) and humoral (cytokines, e.g. IL-2 generating LAK cells) effectors, and can be induced by those factors without GVHD [2,4,5].

The cases described in this report clearly demonstrate such a possibility. We induced a pure graft versus leukemia effect in patient No 1 as no salvage chemotherapy was applied for AML relapse after allogeneic BMT. DLI were started at time of advanced disease when bone marrow was totally expanded by leukemic clone. Though there was some evidence of remaining donor hematopoiesis (20% of chimaeric erythrocytes) it was difficult to interpret as red cells are late markers. The infused donor leukocytes produced a direct cytotoxic effect towards the leukemic cells. IL-2 did not play a crucial role as CR was achieved before it was used. But we suggest that it can enchance the further development of immune control over residual malignant cells. We can also speculate that the remaining donors lymphocytes promoted cytotoxic effect by "teaching" infused donor cells. The additional explanation may be that buffy coat containing hematopoietic progenitors supported the graft, and perhaps small lymphocyte infiltrates seen in bone marrow biopsy at time of remission registration are donor progenitors colonizing the host bone marrow. Constantly growing chimaerism (82%) is a further confirmation to the fact that repeated DLI supported the graft. It should be emphasized that the schedule of DLI in our report differs from the others as we use them in maintaining regimen. This approach can provide a constant influence of donor leukocytes towards the residual leukemic population. There were no problems with GVHD complications.

The second case is not so convincing in the demonstration of pure GVL effect because CR in patient No 2 was attained after chemotherapy. But complete remission is still maintained for a long period of time without any treatment, and we have an evidence that the graft continues to function normally.

From our point of view our observation contributes to all other reports that describe new biological approaches in the treatment of hematologic malignancies and provide new perspectives in the field of immunotherapy.

References

1. Mortimer J., Blinder M.A., Schulman S et al. Relapse of Acute Leukemia after Bone marrow transplantation: Natural History and Results of Subsequent Therapy. J.Clin.Oncol. 1989, 7 pp 50–57
2. Jiang Y.-Z., Cullis J.O., Kanfer E.J. et al. T cell and NR cell Mediated Graft-versus-leukemia Reactivity Following Donor Buffy Coat Transfusion to Treat Relapse after Bone Marrow Transplantation for Chronic Myeloid Leukemia. Bone Marrow Trans. 1993, 11 pp 133–138
3. Szer J., Grigg A.P., Phillips G.L., Sheridian W.P. Donor Leucocyte Infusions after Chemotherapy for Patients Realpsing with Acute Leukaemia Following Allogeneic BMT. Bone Marrow Trans. 1993, 7 pp 109–111
4. Klingemann H.-G., Phillips G.L. Immunotherapy after Bone Marrow Transplantation. Bone Marrow Trans. 1991, 8 pp 73–81
5. Fefer A., Beneynes M., Higuchi C. et al. Interleukin-2+Lymphocytes as Consolidative Immunotherapy after Autologous Bone Marrow Transplantation for Hematologic Malignancies. Acta Haematologica 1993, 89 (suppl.1) pp2–7
6. Kolb H.J., de Witte T., Mittermuller J. et al. Graft-versus-leukemia Effect of Donor Buffy Coat Transfusions on Recurrent Leukemia after Bone marrow Transplantation. Blood 1993 82 (suppl.1) 241a, No 840
7. Barnes D.V.H., Loutit J.F. Treatment of Murine Leukemia with X-ray and Homologus Bone Marrow: II. Br.J.Haematol. 1957, 3 pp 241–252

Acute Leukemias V
Experimental Approaches
and Management of Refractory Diseases
Hiddemann et al. (Eds.)

Recombinant Human Erythropoietin After Bone Marrow Transplantation – A Placebo Controlled Trial

H. Link, M. A. Boogaerts, A. Fauser, R. Or, J. Reiffers, N. C. Gorin, A. Carella, F. Mandelli, S. Burdach, A. Ferrant, W. Linkesch, S. Tura, A. Bacigalupo, F. Schindel, and H. Heinrichs

Introduction

Several historically controlled studies [1,3,5] and one small open prospective randomized trial [4] showed an acceleration of erythropoietic reconstitution after allogeneic bone marrow transplantation (BMT). Some authors claimed a stimulatory effect on thrombopoiesis after BMT [2,4]. This double-blind, placebo-controlled randomized trial was conceived to analyze the impact of rHu EPO on regeneration of erythropoiesis after allogeneic or autologous bone marrow transplantation.

Aim of the Trial

The effects of recombinant human Erythropoietin on regeneration of erythropoiesis after allogeneic or autologous bone marrow transplantation should be evaluated.

Recombinant human Erythropoietin. rHu EPO was expressed by murine cells (mouse C-127) by Behringwerke AG Marburg, Germany. The specific activity was 1.2×10^5 IU/mg of glycoprotein as measured in an in vivo assay according to WHO-standard.

Dosage. 150 IU rHu EPO per kg body weight or placebo were given as 24h continous i.v. infusion from day 1 after BMT until independence from erythrocyte transfusions for 7 days or until day 42. Intravenous ambulatory or s.c. application for a maximum of seven days after hospital discharge was allowed.

Study design. This was a randomized placebo-controlled double-blind study in 17 BMT centers with 329 patients.

The randomization was performed per each center and stratified for allogeneic or autologous BMT and none/minor or major blood group

Table 1. Patients – Allogeneic BMT

	rHu EPO	Placebo
All patients	106	109
Sex		
male	61	71
female	45	38
Age (years)		
Median (range)	31 (4–55)	31 (1–55)
ABO mismatch		
none/minor	84	86
major/total	22	23

Table 2. Diagnosis – Allogeneic BMT

	rHu EPO	Placebo
CML	38	36
AML	29	33
ALL	23	16
NHL	1	6
HD	1	1
MDS	5	6
SAA	7	9
other	2	2

Department of Haematology and Oncology, Medizinische Hochschule Hannover, Germany for a European Study Group

Table 3. Patients – Autologous BMT

	rHu EPO	Placebo
All patients	57	57
Sex	29	31
male		
female	28	26
Age (years)		
Median (range)	35 (3–55)	33 (5–56)
Purging		
Cytostatics	9	9
MAB	3	2

Table 4. Diagnoses – Autologous BMT

	rHu EPO	Placebo
AML	20	13
ALL	4	2
CML	0	2
NHL	18	25
HD	12	13
other	3	2

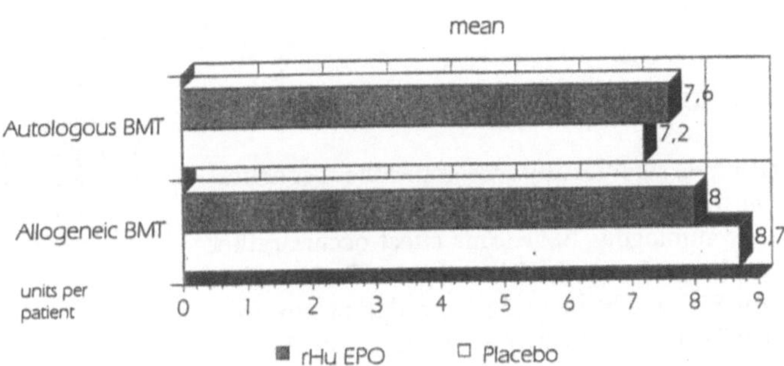

Fig. 1. Erythrocyte transfusions after allogeneic and autologous BMT between day 0 and day 41

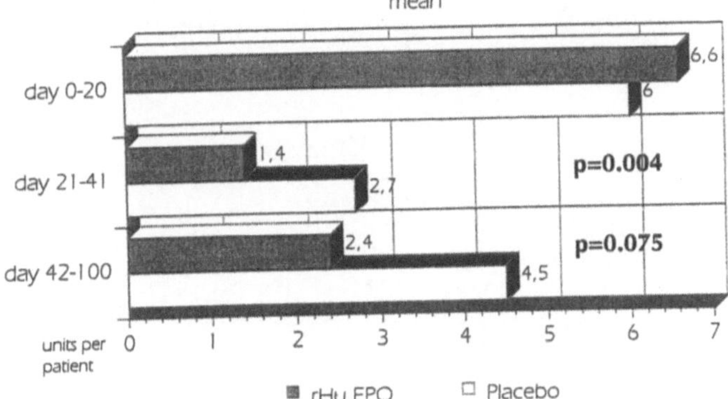

Fig. 2. Erythrocyte transfusions after allogeneic BMT during different time intervals

(ABO) incompatibility between donor and recipient.

Study objective. It should be shown that rHu EPO reduces the time period of erythrocyte transfusion dependence after allogeneic or autologous BMT.

Primary endpoint. Time to reach independence from erythrocyte transfusions, which was defined as follows:

- Day after last erythrocyte transfusion and Hb nadir >9 g/dl followed by 7 consecutive Hb values above this nadir

or

- Hb nadir after last transfusion < 9 g/dl followed by 7 consecutive days with Hb values > 9 g/dl.

Results

The median time to transfusion independence was 19 days with rHu EPO and 27 days with placebo ($p < 0.003$ by log rank test). The median amount of erythrocyte transfusions was significantly reduced with rHu EPO between days 21 and 42 (see Figure 2). After autologous BMT, rHu EPO did not influence the time to transfusion independence or the amount of erythrocyte transfusions. There was no relevant difference in side effects between all rHu EPO or all placebo treated patients.

Conclusions

rHu EPO significantly accelerates the reconstitution of erythropoiesis after allogeneic but not after autologous BMT. This effect occurs rather late beyond day 20 following BMT. Therefore rHu EPO might be given from day 14 onwards. rHu EPO is not effective after autologous BMT.

References

1. Link H, Brune T, Hübner G, et al. Effect of recombinant human erythropoietin after bone marrow transplantation. Ann Hematol. 1993, 67: 169–179.
2. Locatelli F, Zecca M, Beguin Y, et al. Accelerated erythroid repopulation with no stem-cell competition effect in children treated with recombinant human erythropoietin after allogeneic bone marrow transplantation. Br J Haematol 1993; 84: 752–754.
3. Mitus AJ, Antin JH, Rutherford CJ, et al. Significant reduction in homologous red cell transfusion requirements with the use of recombinant human erythropoietin in allogeneic bone marrow transplantation. Blood 1992, 80, (Suppl. 1) 330a
4. Stegmann JL, Lopez J, Otero JM, et al. Erythropoietin treatment in allogeneic BMT accelerates erythroid reconstitution: results of a prospective controlled randomized trial. Bone Marrow Transplant. 1992, 10: 541–546.
5. Vannucchi AM et al. Stimulation or erythroid engraftment by recombinant human erythropoietin ABO-compatible, HLA-identical, allogeneic bone marrow transplant patients. Leukemia 1992, 6: 215–219.

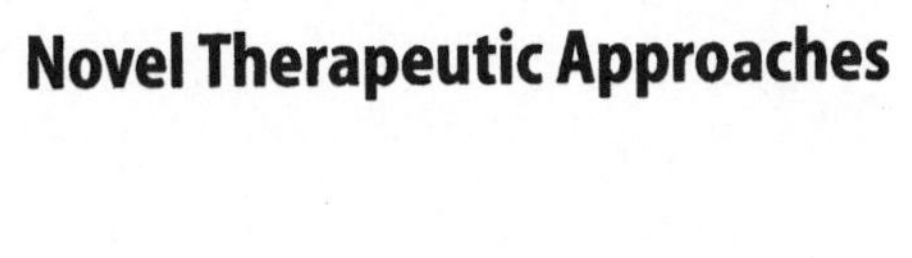

Novel Therapeutic Approaches

Acute Leukemias V
Experimental Approaches
and Management of Refractory Diseases
Hiddemann et al. (Eds.)

Combination of rhSCF + rhG-SCF, But Not rhG-CSF Alone Potentiate the Mobilization of Hematopoietic Stem Cells with Increased Repopulating Ability into Peripheral Blood of Mice

N. J. Drize[1], J. L. Chertkov[1], and A. R. Zander[2]

Introduction

The early hematopoietic progenitor including cells capable for long-term maintenance of hematopoiesis circulates in low amount in peripheral blood during steady-state conditions [1–4]. However, these progenitors were found to belong to one of more mature category in the hierarchy of hematopoietic stem cells (HSC). Indeed, in competitive repopulation assays the progeny of peripheral blood HSC is rapidly replaced by the progeny of bone marrow stem cells [5,6]. During last decade it was repeatedly demonstrated that some hematopoietic cytokines affect not only survival, proliferation and differentiation of hematopoietic cells, but also capable to mobilize HSC into circulation [7–11]. Such ability of cytokines is studying very intensively both in experimental and clinical conditions because mobilized HSC can be used itself or in combination with bone marrow cells as a source of progenitors for transplantation [12]. Among cytokines capable to mobilize HSC into circulation the most attention are payed now on SCF and its combination with other growth factors, especially G-CSF [7,13,14]. Inspite of the cytokine-mobilized HSC (usually after intensive course of chemotherapy in the period of regeneration of hematopoiesis) are now used in patients, a lot of questions has no answer. Up to now it is obscure if peripheral blood progenitors are mobilized from bone marrow by pharmacological doses of cytokines or their expansion in bone marrow and/or peripheral blood take place. For G-CSF it was shown that more probable mechanism is HSC mobilization [7,15]. The data about similar effect of G-CSF plus SCF combination was not published; meanwhile, SCF in combination with other cytokines produces in vitro more strong effect on HSC proliferation than G-CSF alone [14,16]. We have no data about the optimal time of peripheral blood HSC (pbHSC) collection: is it necessary to collect pbHSC during their highest concentration or later in the cytokine course when pbHSC level is not so high, but quality of progenitors possibly better, for example because of enrichment of population by more immature members of HSC compartment? Here these questions were addressed on murine system with use of rhG-CSF and rhSCF.

Material and Methods

Mice and spleen colony assay. Twelve- 25 weeks old CBF1 (CBA/Lac × C57Bl/6)F1 female mice were used. Recipients in the spleen colony-forming (CFU-S) assay were exposed to 1200 cGy ^{137}Cs irradiation (the dose rate 18 cGy/min, IPK irradiator). The dose was delivered into equal fractions, given 3 h apart. Irradiated mice were injected i.v. with 3 to 6×10^4 marrow, or 1 to 10×10^6 blood nucleated cells within several hours after the irradiation. Macroscopic colonies number was counted 8 or 11 days later

[1] Dept. of Hematological Oncology and Bone Marrow Transplantation, Hematological Research Center, Moscow, 125167 Russia
[2] Universitat Hamburg, Universitats-Krankenhaus Eppendorf, II Medizinische Klinik, Abt. Onkologie/Hämatologie, 20246 Hamburg, Germany

[17]. To assess the self-renewal capacity of CFU-S (spleen repopulating ability/SRA/), the spleens of mice that had been irradiated and injected 11 days earlier (CFU-S-11), were excised, colony number was scored and single-cell suspension of spleen cells was injected into irradiated secondary recipients (0.1–0.2 colony per mouse). The number of daughter colonies were counted 8 days later and the number of colonies generated per one CFU-S-11 was calculated. Proliferative activity of CFU-S-11 was determined by hydroxyurea (HU) suicide. Cells were incubated in RPMI 1640 media (Flow) supplemented with 5% Fetal Calf Serum (FCS) (Vector, Russia) for 2 hours at 37 °C with and without 1 mg/ml HU (Serva), washed trice with Hanks' balanced salt solution (HBSS) and injected into irradiated recipients [18].

Long-term bone marrow culture (LTBMC) and limiting dilution analysis. The Dexter method[19] of LTBMC was used with some modifications. Briefly, the content of one femur were flushed into a 25-cm^2 tissue culture flask (Flow) containing 10 ml of Fisher's medium supplemented with 2 mM L-glutamine, 14% horse serum (Vector, Russia), 7% FCS (Vector, Russia), 10^{-6} M hydrocortisone sodium succinate (Sigma). The cultures were placed in 33°C, 5% CO_2 incubator. Half of the medium was replaced weekly with the same volume of fresh medium. Three to 4 weeks after confluent adherent cell layer formation, the cultures were irradiated (30 Gy) and recharged with either 2 to 3×10^6 peripheral blood mononuclears or with 1/100 femur equivalent bone marrow cells in fresh medium. Peripheral blood cells was drawn with 50 u/ml heparin, and mononuclear cells was separated by centrifugation over Hystopaque (density 1.083 g/ml) (Sigma) for 30 min, 450 g, and washed 3 times with HBSS. In 5 weeks (peripheral blood cells) or 6 weeks (bone marrow cells) the adherent layers were scrapped of with a cell scrapper and after repeated pipetting cells from each flask were injected into lethally irradiated syngeneic mice for CFU-S-8 assay. In peripheral blood cultures the number of CFU-S-8 in non-adherent fraction was also detected weekly.

Limiting dilution of the cell populations was assayed for the presence or absence of cells responsible for the long-term generation of CFU-S-8 in LTBMC [20]. Such cells should be distributed among samples in a Poisson fashion. The concentration (N) of primitive hematopoietic stem cells (P-HSC/LTC-IC/) in the sample can then be expressed as $N = -\ln Po/x$, where Po is the proportion of samples (flasks) devoid of CFU-S-8, and x is the number of cells in the sample[21]. Proliferative activity of bone marrow LTC-IC was studied by HU suicide.

rhSCF and rhG-CSF. rhSCF (Amgen) and rhG-CSF (Neupogen 48, Amgen) were used. The cytokines were diluted in saline with 0.1% BSA and injected s.c. at 24 hour interval to yield the treatment levels of 250 μg/kg/d for rhG-CSF and 34 μg/kg/d for rhSCF for 10 or 17 days. Part of control mice was injected with vehicle (PBS+0.1% BSA). The results were the same as in non-injected control. All data of both control groups were pooled. Twenty hours after the last injection heparinized peripheral blood was collected under light ether anesthesia from orbital plexus in sterile conditions. Bone marrow was collected from femora by sterile punction through knee joint by 22 gauge needle. Some mice were sacrificed and femoral bone marrow was flushed out and resuspended in HBSS; spleens of these mice were homogenized by glass homogenizer in HBSS. The cell suspensions were diluted and injected into lethally irradiated mice or explanted on irradiated adherent cell layer of LTBMC. Peripheral blood and marrow cellularity was determined, differential cell count carried out on May Grunwald Giemsa stained smears. One month after last injection of cytokine all mice were sacrificed for study the peripheral blood, bone marrow and spleen cells. The single blood donation had no influence on the hematopoiesis one month later and the results obtained on mice with and without blood loss were pooled.

Results

CFU-S analysis. Cytokine treatment induced very strong mobilization of CFU-S into circulation (Fig. 1). After 10-day-course the content of CFU-S-11 in peripheral blood was increased 93-fold and 169-fold following rhG-CSF and rhG-CSF + rhSCF, respectively. The less pronounced effect was observed after 6 and 17-day-course. Simultaneously with observed augmentation of CFU-S-11 in peripheral blood, in the bone marrow the 1.5–3-fold depletion of CFU-S-11 number was detected. One month following last cytokine injection the content of CFU-S-11 both in

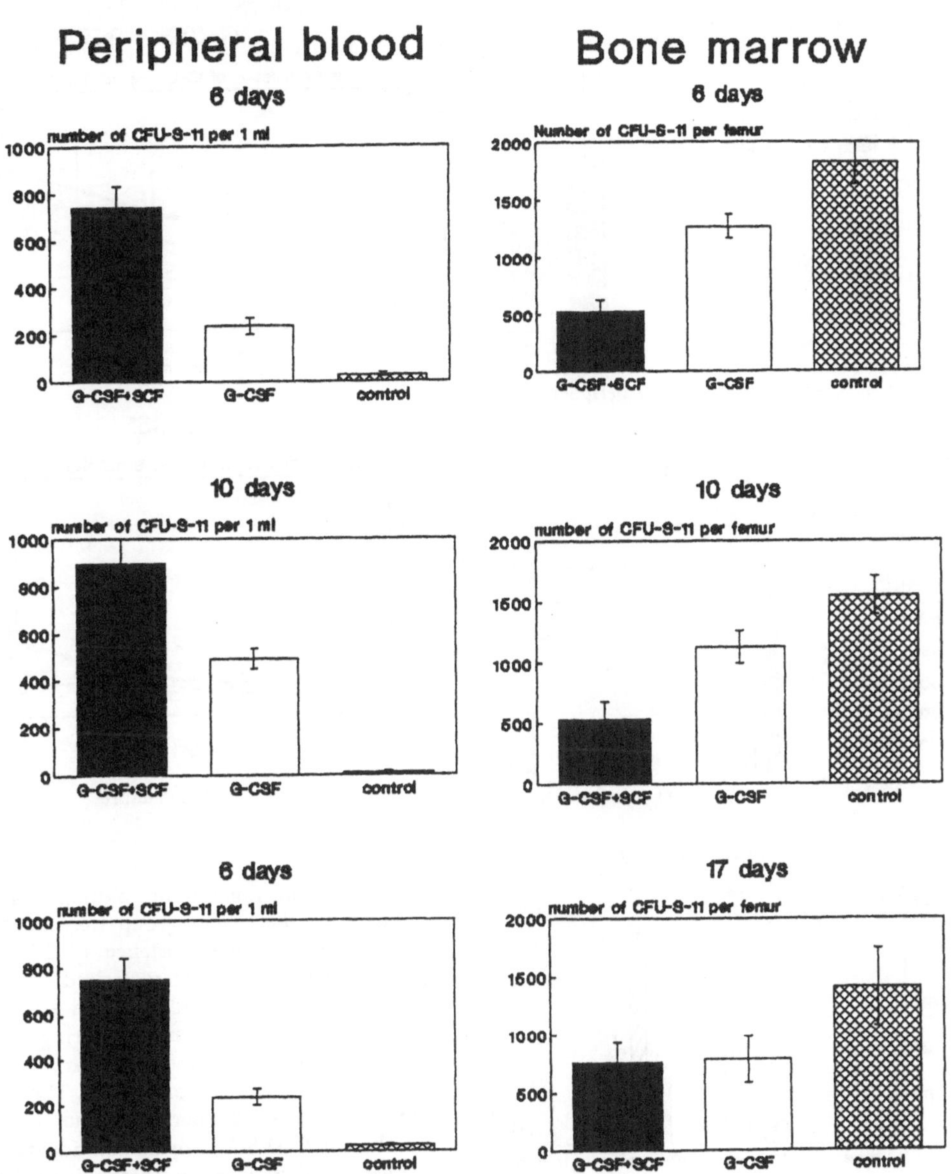

Fig. 1. CFU-S-11 in cytokine treated mice

peripheral blood and bone marrow was normalized (data not shown).

After 10- and 17-day-course of cytokine treatment the significant increase of proliferative activity of mobilized in peripheral blood CFU-S-11, as measured by HU suicide was observed; the effect of cytokine combination was more expressed than effect of rhG-CSF alone, however the differences were not significant (Fig. 2). In the bone marrow of cytokine treated animals as well as in control mice the suicide level of CFU-S-11 was less than 10% in all groups (data not shown).

Self-renewal capacity of CFU-S-11 was measured as SRA (number of daughter CFU-S-8 per 11 day spleen colony). It was demonstrated that both cytokine administration schedules strongly increase SRA of CFU-S-11 in peripheral blood. This response was higher following cytokine combination and 17-day-course (Fig. 3). One

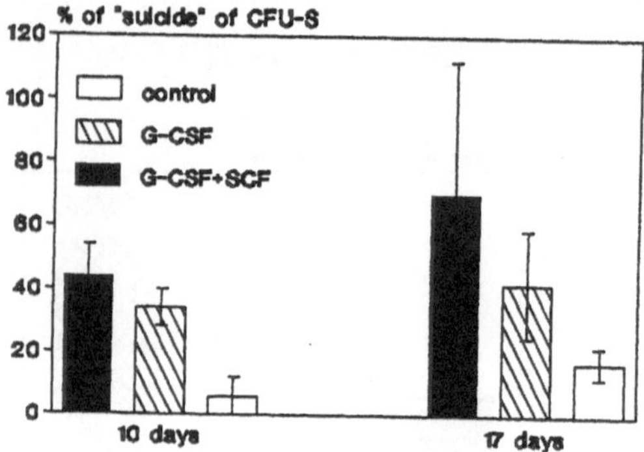

Fig. 2. Proliferation of CFU-S-8 in peripheral blood

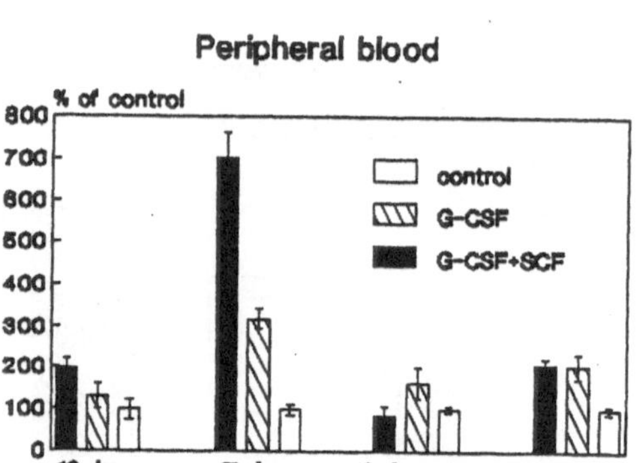

Fig. 3. Self-renewal capacity of CFU-S-8

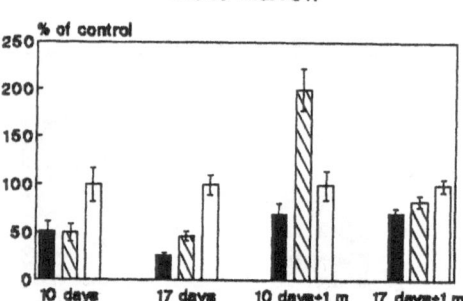

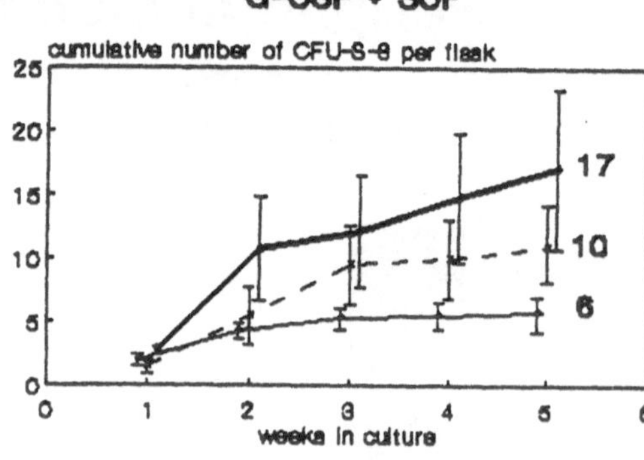

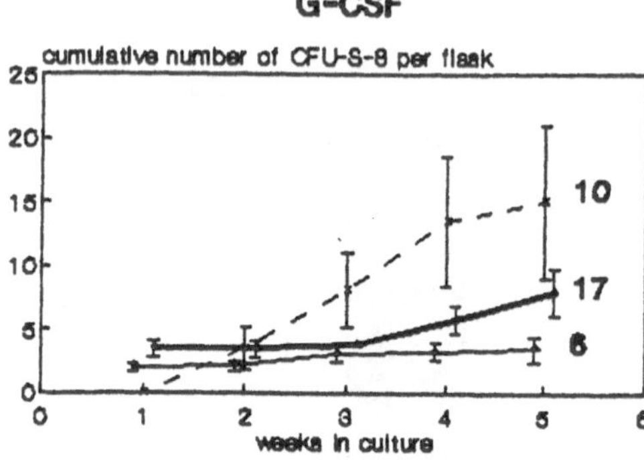

Fig. 4. CFU-S-8 in long-term culture

month following cytokine administration the SRA was normal. Cytokines decreased SRA in bone marrow, more significantly after 17-day-course of cytokines combination. This index was normalized after one month, apart from the observed overshot after 10 days course of rhG-CSF administration.

LTC-IC in peripheral blood and bone marrow. The number of peripheral blood mononucleares is not enough for full range limiting dilution analysis (usually 3–4 flasks per group were used) and because of that the existence of LTC-IC in peripheral blood was characterised by mature cells and CFU-S-8 production in suspension fraction of long-term culture during 5 weeks after seeding $2–3 \times 10^6$ mononuclears on irradiated adherent cell layer of LTBMC. The 5-week-old cultures were sacrificed and the total number of CFU-S-8 both in non-adherent and adherent cell fraction was determined. LTC-IC were not detected in peripheral blood of normal mice. Cytokines mobilize LTC-IC in peripheral blood. During 5 weeks of culture continuous production of non-adherent CFU-S-8 was observed (Fig. 4). The effect of cytokines combination was significantly higher than rhG-CSF alone. The number of adherent CFU-S-8 was maximal in cultures seeded with peripheral blood mononuclears from mice treated by 17-day-course of cytokine combination (Fig. 5).

The number of LTC-IC in bone marrow of cytokine treated mice was determined by limiting dilution analysis (Fig. 6). Both schedules of

Fig. 5. Number of CFU-S-8 in 5-week-old culture

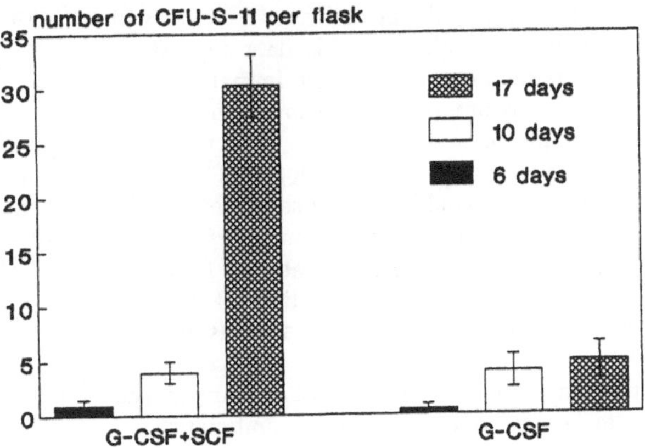

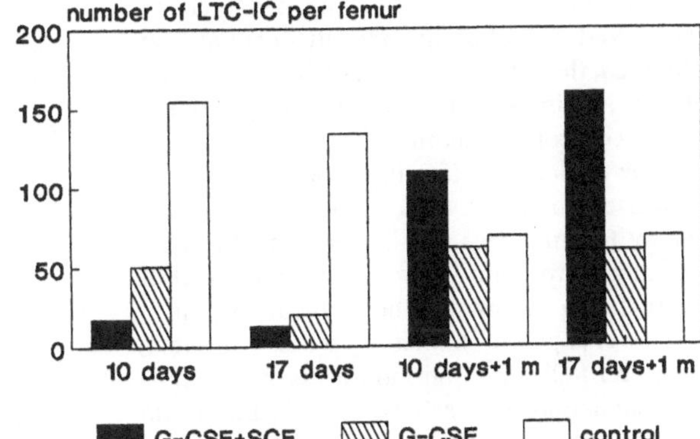

Fig. 6. LTC-IC bone marrow of cytokine treated mice

cytokine administration induced sharp decrease of LTC-IC. This effect was more expressed after combination of growth factors as compared to rhG-CSF alone; 17-day-course induced more dramatic response than 6 and10-day-course. Proliferation of bone marrow LTC-IC after cytokine treatment was not revealed by HU suicide (data not shown). The content of LTC-IC in bone marrow one month following rhG-CSF treatment was normal, however, after rhG-CSF+rhSCF course the rebound overshot of LTC-IC was shown.

Discussion

Here the high increase of CFU-S content in peripheral blood of animals treated with G-CSF and G-CSF + SCF was confirmed; it was also shown the appearence of LTC-IC in circulation. The effect of growth factor combination was more expressed than rhG-CSF alone. The increase of circulating progenitors was accompanied by decrease of CFU-S and LTC-IC number in bone marrow. This effect was higher from cytokine combination and was proportional to longevity of the course. Simultaneously, the high increase of CFU-S content in spleen has been observed, what was described earlier[16]. These results suggest the mobilization of progenitors into circulation rather than their expansion by cytokine treatment. The lack of CFU-S-11 and LTC-IC proliferation in the bone marrow immediately after cytokine course also supports but of course do not proves this conclusion.

The population of mobilized HSC differ from steady-state pbHSC not only quantitatively but also by progenitor characteristics. The more primitive HSC, LTC-IC, appear in circulation following cytokine administration. The age structure of mobilized progenitor population differs from normal bone marrow HSC compartment. In particular, mobilized CFU-S-11 are characterized by higher proliferative activity and spleen repopulating ability, as compare with bone marrow CFU-S-11. This data suggest the selective mobilization of more immature CFU-S-11 by cytokines. If the cells capable to maintain long-term hematopoiesis are also mobilized selectively, the peripheral blood of cytokine treated donors could be better source of HSC for transplantation than normal bone marrow cells.

The results demonstrated at first time that pbHSC collected in different time of cytokine course can be characterized by various proliferative potential and the peak of HSC concentration and maximal SRA is not in coincidence. After 10-day-course of cytokine combination the number of CFU-S-11 in peripheral blood was increased 169-fold, while augmentation of their SRA was only two-fold; following 17-day-course the 30-fold level of peripheral CFU-S-11 has been observed, though the increase of SRA was 7-fold. Hence, in clinical setting the time of peripheral blood cell collection must be determined not only by the level of HSC, in particular high proliferative potential cells, LTC-IC and blast colony forming cells, but by their quality also. The most important index in this case could be the replating potential of these precursor cells.

The changes of hematopoiesis were short-term and following one month essentially normal hematopoiesis recovered. It is important that the content of LTC-IC in bone marrow was significantly increased one month after last injection of cytokine combination. The incapacity to regeneration of LTC-IC in the bone marrow during many months after sublethal irradiation of mice was observed[22]. The difference of the results could not be explained by reverse migration of LTC-IC from spleen into bone marrow, first of all, because one month following 10- and especially 17-day-course of G-CSF+SCF the bone marrow content of LTC-IC was 1.5–2 times higher than in control animals. This data suggest that the amplification of early progenitors was induced by triggering the resting progenitor cells into proliferation.

References

1. Metcalf D, Moore MAS: Haemopoietic cells. North Holland, Publishing Company, Amsterdam-London, 1971
2. Barnes DWH, Loutit JF: Haemopoietic stem cells in the peripheral blood. Lancet ii:1138, 1967
3. Goodman JW, Hodgson GS: Evidence for stem cells in the peripheral blood. Blood 19:702, 1962
4. Fliedner TM, Steinbach KH: Repopulating potential of hematopoietic precursor cells. Blood Cells 14:393, 1988
5. Micklem HS, Anderson N, Ross E: Limited potential of circulating hemopoietic stem cells. Nature 256: 41, 1975
6. Chertkov JL, Gurevitch OA, Udalov GA: Self-maintenance ability of circulating hemopoietic stem cells. Exp Hematol 18: 90, 1982
7. Gordon MY: Physiological mechanisms in BMT and haemopoiesis – revisited. Bone Marrow Transplantation 11:193, 1993
8. Molineux D, Migdalska A, Szmitkowski M, Zsebo K, Dexter TM: The effect on hematopoiesis of recombinant stem cell factor (ligand for c-kit) administered in vivo to mice either alone or in combination with granulocyte colony-stimulating factor. Blood 78: 961, 1991
9. Drize NJ, Gan OI, Zander AR: Effect of recombinant human granulocyte colony-stimulating factor treatment of mice on spleen colony-forming unit number and self-renewal capacity. Exp Hematol 21: 1269, 1993
10. Goodnough LT, Anderson KC, Kurtz S, Lane TA, Pisciotto PT, Sayers MH, Silberstein LE: Indication and guidelines for the use of hematopoietic growth factors. Transfusion 33: 944, 1993
11. McNiece IK, Briddell RA, Hartley CA, Smith KA, Andrews RG: Stem cell factor enchances in vivo effects of granulocyte colony stimulating factor for stimulating mobilization of peripheral blood progenitor cells. Stem cells 11 (supl): 36, 1993
12. Zander AR, Lyding J, Bielack S: Transplantation with blood stem cells. Blood Cells 17: 301, 1991
13. Briddell R, Hartley C, Stoney G, McNiece I: SCF synergize with G-CSF in vivo to mobilizmurine peripheral blood progenitor cells with enchanced engraftment potential. Exp Hematol 21: 1150, 1993
14. Bodine DM, Seidel NE, Zsebo KM, Orlic D: In vivo administration of stem cell factor to mice increases the absolute number of pluripotent hematopoietic stem cells. Blood 82: 445, 1993
15. Tavassoli M: Expansion of blood stem cell pool or mobilization of its marrow counterpart? Exp Hematol 21: 1205, 1993
16. Drize NJ, Chertkov JL, Zander AR: Hematopoietic stem cell mobilization into peripheral blood of mice by combination of recombinant rat stem cell factor (rhSCF) and recombinant human granulocyte colony-stimulating factor (rhG-CSF). Manuscript in preparation
17. Till JE, McCulloch EA: A direct measurement of the radiation sensitivity of normal mouse bone marrow cells. Rad Res 14: 213, 1961
18. Chertkov JL, Drize NJ: Cells forming spleen colonies at 7 or 11 days after injection have different proliferation rates. Cell Tissue Kinet 17: 247, 1984

19. Dexter TM, Allen TD, Lajtha LG: Conditions controlling the proliferation of hemopoietic stem cells in vivo. J Cell Physiol 91: 335, 1977
20. Deryugina EI, Drize NJ, Olovnikova NI, Sadovnikova EYu, Chertkov JL: Primitive hemopoietic stem cell: Origin during the ontogenesis, proliferative activity and proliferative potential. Ontogenes 22: 125, 1991
21. Breivik H Hematopoietic stem cell content of murine bone marrow, spleen and blood. Limiting dilution analysis of diffusion chamber culture. J Cell Physiol 78: 73, 1971
22. Deryugina EI, Drize NJ, Chertkov JL: Long-term culture inititating cells do not regenerate after irradiation. Bull Exp Biol Med 7: 96, 1987

Acute Leukemias V
Experimental Approaches
and Management of Refractory Diseases
Hiddemann et al. (Eds.)

High-dose Therapy and Autografting with Mobilized Peripheral Blood Progenitor Cells in Patients with Malignant Lymphoma

R. Haas, H. Goldschmidt, R. Möhle, S. Frühauf, S. Hohaus, B. Witt, U. Mende, M. Flentje, M. Wannenmacher, and W. Hunstein

Abstract. In this report we present the data of 100 patients who were autografted with peripheral blood progenitor cells (PBPC) following high-dose conditioning therapy. Fifty-six patients were male and 44 were female with a median age of 36 years (range 19–58). Thirty-five patients had Hodgkin's disease and 65 non-Hodgkin lymphoma (NHL). PBPC were collected either following the administration of recombinant human GM-CSF or G-CSF during steady-state hematopoiesis or during cytokine-enhanced recovery after cytotoxic chemotherapy. Seven patients were autografted using PBPC harvested post-chemotherapy without cytokine support. At the time of PBPC mobilization 21 patients had bone marrow involvement by histopathological examination. The high-dose preparatory regimens were either BEAM (BCNU, etoposide, cytosine arabinoside, melphalan), CBV (cyclophosphamide, BCNU, etoposide), or a combination of total body irradiation (TBI) and cyclophosphamide. In 92 patients hematological reconstitution was evaluable. The median time to reach a neutrophil count $\geq 0.5 \times 10^9$/l was 14 days (range 9–69) and an unsubstituted platelet count $> 20 \times 10^9$/l was observed after a median of 12 days (range 6–205). Seven patients died of transplant-related toxicity. Twenty-seven patients relapsed or had further tumor progression after a median time of 5 months (range 1 – 49) post-transplantation. With a median follow-up of 14 months (range 1–64), 66 patients are alive in unmaintained remission. There is no evidence for late graft failure. These data reflect the ability of blood-derived hematopoietic progenitor cells to restore long-term hematopoiesis after myeloablative therapy without additional bone marrow support.

Introduction

Peripheral blood progenitor cells (PBPC) for the support of high-dose therapy were first used in patients considered to be not eligible for bone marrow harvesting [1]. This included patients with hypocellular or fibrotic marrow due to previous irradiation, bone marrow infiltration with tumor cells or metastatic lesions at the sites of harvest [2]. An earlier concern was related to the restorative capacity of PBPC. Data from animal studies suggested that blood predominantly contains lineage-committed progenitor cells lacking the ability to support long-term hematopoiesis after myeloablative therapy [3]. When hematopoietic growth factors were introduced for PBPC mobilization, it was speculated that cytokines may induce an accelerated consumption of more primitive stem cells [4]. Clinical trials then demonstrated the capacity of cytokine-mobilized PBPC to restore marrow function following high-dose therapy. This was also true for regimens with total body irradiation (TBI) which are considered myeloablative [5, 6]. The study presented here includes 100 patients who were autografted with PBPC during the last 5 years in our institution. In 93 patients cytokines were part of the mobilization

Department of Internal Medicine V, University of Heidelberg, Germany
Department of Radiology, University of Heidelberg, Germany

regimen. The patients had different hematological malignancies and were entered into the transplant protocol at different stages of their disease. Our report contains data on the transplant-related toxicity, the duration of hematological recovery, and event-free survival (EFS).

Material and Methods

Patients. Between October 1988 and March 1994, one hundred patients were included into the study. Their median age was 36 years (range 19 – 58). There were 56 males and 44 females. Thirty-five patients had Hodgkin's disease and 65 had non-Hodgkin lymphoma (NHL). According to the working formulation, 40 patients had low- or intermediate-grade and 25 patients had high-grade NHL. At the time of mobilization, 21 patients had bone marrow involvement by histopathological examination. Prior to high-dose therapy, 64 patients were in complete remission (CR), 30 in partial remission (PR) and 6 had progressive disease. The patient characteristics are shown in Table 1.

Patients were treated in the Departments of Internal Medicine V and Radiology, University of Heidelberg. Informed consent was obtained in each patient before therapy. The study was conducted under the guidelines of the Joint Ethical Committee of the University of Heidelberg. The cut-off date of this report is May 5th, 1994.

Table 1. Patient characteristics

Patients	100
Age	36 [19–58)
Males / Females	56/44
Hodgkin's disease	35
non-Hodgkin lymphoma	65
low- /intermediate-grade	40
high-grade	25
Bone marrow involvement at the time of PBPC collection	21

Peripheral blood progenitor cell collection and cryopreservation. PBPC collection was performed with a Fenwal CS 3000 (Baxter Deutschland GmbH, Munich, Germany). Usually, a total of 10 l blood per apheresis was processed at a flow rate of 50 to 70 ml/min. The apheresis product was mixed with the same volume of minimal essential medium (MEM) containing 20% dimethylsulfoxide (DMSO). The final cell suspension was transferred into freezing bags (DELMED Inc., New Brunswick, NJ, USA) and frozen to −100 °C with a computer-controlled cyropreservation device (Cryoson DV-6, Cryoson Deutschland GmbH, Germany). The frozen cells were transferred into the liquid phase of nitrogen and stored at −196 °C.

In 7 patients, PBPC harvesting was performed during hematological recovery following chemotherapy-induced marrow aplasia. Sixteen patients were treated with recombinant human GM-CSF (250 ug/kg/day, continuous i.v. infusion; Behringwerke AG, Marburg, Germany). The cytokine was administered either during steady-state hematopoiesis or started 24 hours post-chemotherapy to increase the number of circulating progenitor cells. Six patients received GM-CSF and IL-3 sequentially following high-dose cytosine arabinoside/ mitoxantrone. IL-3 and GM-CSF were made available by Sandoz AG, Nuremberg, Germany. Twenty-four hours after chemotherapy, patients received IL-3 (5 ug/kg per day sc) for 6 days. Then GM-CSF (5 ug/kg per day s.c.) was given until PBPC collection was completed. More recently, recombinant human G-CSF (R-metHuG-CSF, filgrastim, Amgen, Thousand Oaks, CA, USA, 300 ug/day sc) has been used during steady-state hematopoiesis as well as after cytotoxic therapy in a group of 71 patients. The mobilization regimens are detailed for the different patient groups in Table 2.

Table 2. Mobilization schemes

	no factor post-chemo	GM-CSF steady-state	IL-3/GM-CSF post-chemo	post-chemo	G-CSF steady state	post-chemo
Hodgkin's disease	6	4	9	–	1	15
high-grade NHL	–	2	–	6	3	14
low-grade NHL	1	1	–	–	–	38

High-dose conditioning regimens and intensive care post-transplant. High-dose regimens consisted of the CBV protocol (cyclophosphamide, 6.8 g/m²; BCNU, 450 mg/m²; etoposide, 1,600 mg/m²; 34 patients), the BEAM regimen (BCNU, 300 mg/m²; etoposide, 1,200 mg/m²; cytosine arabinoside, 800 mg/m²; melphalan, 140 mg/m²; 18 patients) or a combination of cyclophosphamide (200 mg/kg) with hyperfractionated total body irradiation (14.4 Gy; 47 patients). In one patient with progressive Hodgkin's disease PBPC were used to support high-dose cytosine arabinoside/mitoxantrone. The distribution of the conditioning regimens is detailed in Table 3. The patients were treated in reverse isolation. Antibiotic combination therapy was given for fever > 38.5 °C and amphothericin-B was added for documented fungal infection or persistent fever. A platelet count of $> 20 \times 10^9$/l was maintained by HLA-A/B-matched platelet transfusions and packed red cells were given when the hemoglobin was below 8 g/dl.

Clonogenic assay for hematopoietic progenitor cells. The concentration of hematopoietic progenitor cells in the leukapheresis products and in peripheral blood was assessed using a semisolid clonogenic culture assay as previously described [6]. Since January 1991, a commercially available culture system (Terry Fox Laboratories, Vancouver, Canada) was used.

Immunofluorescence staining and flow cytometry. For dual color immunofluorescence analysis, 1×10^6 mononuclear cells of the leukapheresis products were incubated for 30 min at 4 °C with the fluorescein (FITC)-conjugated monoclonal antibody (moAb) HPCA-2 (CD34, Becton-Dickinson, Heidelberg). 10,000 cells were acquired and analyzed using a Becton-Dickinson FACScan with a 2-W argon ion laser as light source. Excitation was at 488 nm and fluorescence was measured at 530 nm (FITC) and 588 nm (PE). Fluorescence (FL) intensities were recorded at photomultiplier tube settings of 518 V (FITC) and 527 V (PE) and logarithmically amplified. An example of a CD34+ cell measurement is given in Fig. 1.

Table 3. Preparatory regimes

	Cyclophosphamide and TBI	CBV	BEAM
Hodgkin's disease*	–	34	–
high-grade NHL	9	–	16
low-grade NHL	38	–	2

* In one patient with Hodgkin's disease PBPC were used to support high-dose cytosine arabinoside/mitoxantrone

Statistics. Event-free survival (EFS) was calculated from the day of PBPC autografting using Kaplan and Meier's method. We regarded as events: death including toxic death, relapse for patients autografted in PR/CR, and disease progression for patients known to progress.

Results

Mobilization and collection of peripheral blood progenitor cells. The patient group presented here is heterogeneous with respect to diagnosis and history of

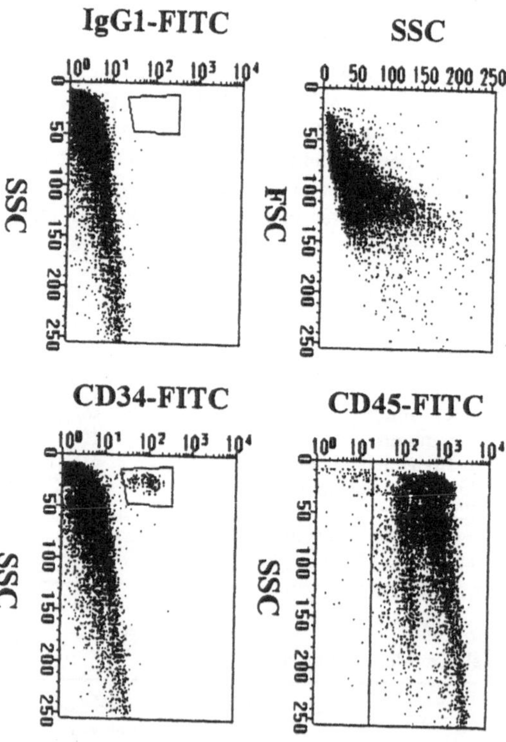

Fig. 1. Assessment of CD34+ cells in leukapheresis products. Only CD34+ cells with low side scatter characteristics (SSC) are considered. The pan-leucocyte antigen CD45 serves to discriminate between white blood cells and erythrocytes or debris

disease. The patients have in common that PBPC were used instead of bone marrow to support high-dose conditioning therapy. To characterize the autograft, the number of total nucleated cells (TNC) and colony-forming units granulocyte-macrophage (CFU-GM) is available in 95 patients. With a median of 5 (range 1–11) leukaphereses, an average (mean $\pm$ SEM) of $0.75 \pm 0.06 \times 10^9$/kg TNC and $19.56 \pm 2.29 \times 10^4$ CFU-GM/kg could be harvested (Fig. 2).

Direct immunofluorescence analysis was used in 77 patients to determine the number of autografted CD34+cells which accounted for an average of $6.03 \pm 0.53 \times 10^6$/kg. Based on 72 paired samples a correlation could be demonstrated between CFU-GM and CD34+ cells ($R = 0.74$, $p < 0.001$). The mobilizing efficacy of the different regimens cannot be addressed, since some mobilization regimens were only used for a specific indication making a valid comparison impossible.

Hematological reconstitution following high-dose therapy and PBPC autografting. Following high-dose conditioning therapy, all patients were autografted using mobilized PBPC without additional bone marrow or cytokine support. Four patients with toxic death were not evaluable for hematological reconstitution. Two patients were excluded since early relapse and tumor progression may have interferred with engraftment, and for two patients the data are not available. The reconstitution data are therefore based on a total of 92 patients (Fig. 3). A white blood count (WBC) of $\geq 1.0 \times 10^9$/l was achieved within 7–45 days (median 12). An absolute neutrophil count (ANC) of $\geq 0.5 \times 10^9$/l was reached as early as 9 days post-grafting with a latest recovery after 69 days (median 14 days). Platelet counts $\geq 20 \times 10^9$ were observed after a median of 12 days (range 6 –205). For 77 patients, the quantity of CD34+ cells in the autografts is known. It could be shown that autografts containing $\geq 2.5 \times 10^6$ CD34+cells/kg allowed platelet recovery ($> 20.0. \times 10^9$/l) within 14 days in the majority of patients (Fig. 4). There was no significant difference in the time of recovery between patients receiving TBI and patients receiving high-dose chemotherapy alone.

Follow-up post-transplantation. Of the 100 patients autografted, 4 patients died of early transplant-related death, i.e. one patient of cardiac failure, one of pulmonary edema, one of BCNU-related pneumonitis and one due to toxoplasmic encephalitis. Three patients developed late complications. There was one patient with lethal BCNU-pneumopathy, one suffering from hepatic coma and one patient with multi-organ failure due to vasculitis of unknown etiology.

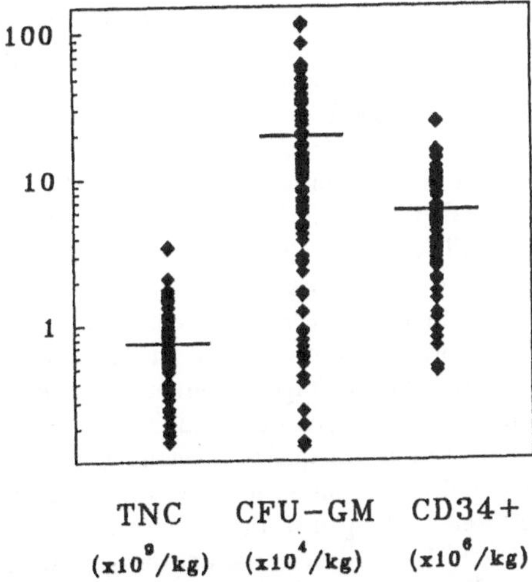

Fig. 2. Number of total nucleated cells (TNC) and colony-forming units granulocyte-macrophage per kg bodyweight contained within the autografts of 95 patients. The quantity of CD34+cells transplanted is available for 77 patients

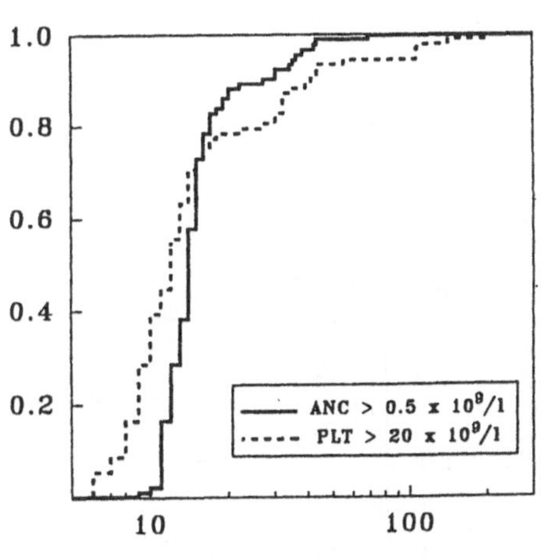

Fig. 3. Cumulative frequency of hematological reconstitution. The analysis is based on 92 patients

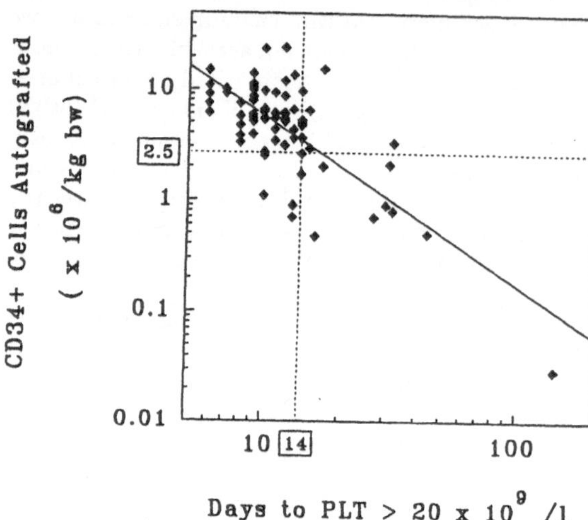

Fig. 4. A number of 2.5×10^6 CD34+ cells/kg is a minimum requirement for rapid platelet recovery within 14 days post-transplantation

Accordingly, the treatment-related mortality rate is 7%. At the cut-off date of this report, 66 patients are alive in unmaintained remission. The median follow-up for the patients in remission is 14 months (range 1–64). Relapse or tumor progression were observed in 27 patients after a median time of 5 months (range 1–49). Of these patients 9 are alive following standard-dose chemotherapy or palliative regimens. Patients with high-grade NHL relapsed as early as 1 month post-transplantation. On the other hand, 2 patients with Hodgkin's disease relapsed late, 3 and 4 years following PBPC autografting. As shown in Fig. 5, the probability of event-free survival is 31% for high-grade NHL after 26 months and 86% for low-grade NHL after 46 months. The difference reflects the nature of the respective histological subtypes. For patients with Hodgkin's disease, the probability of EFS was calculated as 35% after 64 months.

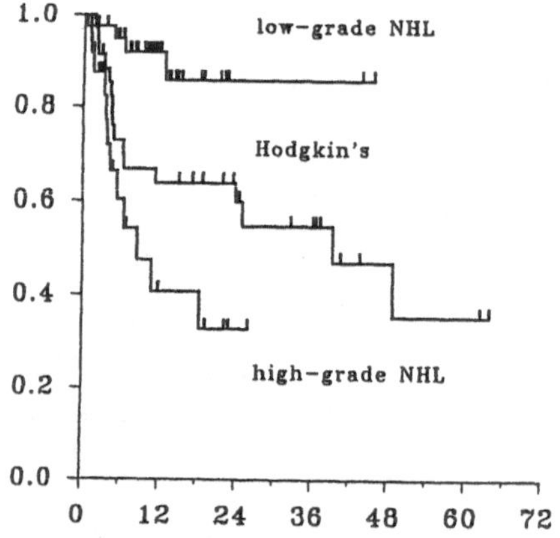

Fig. 5. Probability of event-free survival in 100 patients with malignant lymphoma autografted with mobilized PBPC following high-dose therapy

Discussion

We report on 100 patients who were autografted with mobilized blood-derived hematopoietic progenitor cells following high-dose conditioning therapy. The patients differ with respect to diagnosis, disease status, the amount of previous cytotoxic therapy and the type of high-dose conditioning therapy. The use of PBPC for the support of dose-escalated cytotoxic chemotherapy is the common denominator. The results show that blood-derived hematopoietic progenitor cells collected after cytotoxic chemotherapy, cytokine administration or cytokine-supported chemotherapy allow complete and sustained hematological reconstitution after myeloablative therapy. With a longest follow-up of 5 years, no late graft failure was observed.

An important question relates to the transplantation-associated toxicity, which has to be outweighted against the potential therapeutic benefit. Usually, bacterial and fungal infections are the major complications encountered during the period of neutropenia. Therefore, it is of note that only one patient died of an infection with Toxoplasma gondii. The other transplant-related deaths were due to toxic organ failure.

There were no obvious patient characteristics associated with an increased risk of mortality. The rate of toxic deaths is 7% and comparable with data from other centers [7].

The number of CD34+ cells in the autografts is known for 77 patients. A threshold became evident indicating that a minimum of 2.5×10^6 CD34+ cells/kg bodyweight are necessary to obtain an unsubstituted platelet count $> 20 \times 10^9$/l within 14 days [8]. The conditioning regimens had no influence on the time of recovery indicating that homing and seeding of hematopoietic progenitor cells within the marrow microenvironment are not dependent on total body irradiation.

Another issue relates to event-free survival and relapse. With a median follow-up of 14 months, 66% of our patients are alive in unmaintained remission, while there were 27 patients who relapsed or further progressed after a median of 5 months post-transplantation. Early relapses within the first three months post-transplantation were predominantly observed in patients with high-grade non-Hodgkin lymphoma. The results are different for patients with low- and intermediate-grade NHL of whom only two relapsed 4 and 12 months following PBPC autografting. Prospective studies would be needed to demonstrate the therapeutic benefit of PBPC-supported high-dose therapy particularly for these histological subtypes of lymphoma. Since June 1992, we have performed involved-field irradiation post-grafting in 5 patients. The local radiotherapy included previous bulk manifestations. The efficacy of the CBV protocol compared with conventional chemotherapy in patients with Hodgkin's disease is disappointing, although the patients included into the transplant protocol had suffered from chemosensitive relapse and are considered to have poor prognostic features [9]. The late relapses of which one occurred 4 years following autografting are of particular concern. They show the obvious inability of the preparatory regimen of eradicating tumor cells with relapse-inducing capacity.

Another aspect relates to the origin of relapse since blood-derived autografts may harbor tumor cells. As we have shown more recently, patients with low-grade NHL autografted with leukapheresis products which contain PCR-detectable t(14;18)-positive cells may turn negative after a follow-up between 9 and 16 months [10]. These data suggest that potentially contaminating tumor cells may not be sustained in vivo following their transplantation. However, gene-marking studies would be necessary to address this issue prospectively.

We propose high-dose therapy for chemosensitive patients at an early time during their disease course when the tumor burden is low, drug resistance unlikely and hematopoiesis not compromized by previous cytotoxic therapy. Moreover, the treatment failures clearly mark the limitations of the high-dose regimens and argue for new therapeutic strategies.

Acknowledgements. We thank the nursing staff of the Department of Internal Medicine for their outstanding care of these patients. We are grateful to Kirsten Flentje, Evi Holdermann, Magdalena Volk, and Margit Pförsich for excellent technical assistance, and Ulla Scheidler for expert secretarial help.

References

1. Körbling M, Dörken B, Ho A, Pezzutto A, Hunstein W, Fliedner TM (1986) Autologous transplantation of blood-derived hemopoietic stem cells after myeloablative therapy in a patient with Burkitt's lymphoma. Blood 67: 529
2. Kessinger A, Armitage JO (1991) The evolving role of autologous peripheral stem cell transplantation following high-dose therapy for malignancies. Blood 2: 211
3. Micklem HS, Anderson N, Ross E (1975) Limited potential of circulating stem cells. Nature 256: 41
4. Socinski MA, Cannistra SA, Elias A, Antman KH, Schnipper L, Griffin JD (1988) Granulocyte-macrophage colony stimulating factor expands the circulating haemopoietic progenitor cell compartment in man. The Lancet I: 1194
5. Siena S, Bregni M, Brando B, Belli N, Ravagnani F, Gandola L, Stern AC, Lansdorp PM, Bonadonna G, Gianni AM (1991) Flow cytometry for clinical estimation of circulating hematopoietic progenitors for autologous transplantation in cancer patients. Blood 77: 400
6. Haas R, Ho AD, Bredthauer U, Cayeux S, Egerer G, Knauf W, Hunstein W (1990) Successful autologous transplantation of blood stem cells mobilized with recombinant human granulocyte-macrophage colony-stimulating factor. Exp Hematol 18: 94
7. Stewart FM (1993) Indications and relative indications for stem cell transplantation in non-Hodgkin's lymphoma. Leukemia 7: 1091
8. Haas R, Möhle R, Frühauf S, Goldschmidt S, Witt B, Flentje M, Wannenmacher M, Hunstein W (1994) Patient characteristics associated with successful mobilizing and autografting of peripheral

blood progenitor cells in malignant lymphoma. Blood, in press
9. Bierman PJ, Armitage JO (1993) Role of autotransplantation in Hodgkin's disease. Hematol Oncol Clin North Am 7: 591
10. Haas R, Moos M, Karcher A, Möhle R, Witt B, Goldschmidt H, Frühauf S, Flentje M, Wannenmacher M, Hunstein W (1994) Sequential high-dose therapy with peripheral blood progenitor cell support in low-grade non-Hodgkin lymphoma. J Clin Oncol, in press

Acute Leukemias V
Experimental Approaches
and Management of Refractory Diseases
Hiddemann et al. (Eds.)

Cord Blood Banking for Hematopoietic Stem Cell Transplantation

E. Gluckman

Abstract. The number of umbilical cord blood cells transplantation is increasing worldwide. The results are comparable to allogeneic bone marrow transplantation in a large variety of hematological diseases curable by bone marrow transplantation. The incidence of GVH has been so far limited. The advantages of using cord blood are related to the high number of hematopoietic progenitors in circulation at birth and to the relative immaturity of the immunological reactivity of the new-born. A European cord blood bank project is described in order to obtain related or unrelated, matched or partially mismatched hematopoietic stem cell transplant for treating patients without a bone marrow donor.

Introduction

Following the work of Boyse and Broxmeyer [1], and the first report of a successful transplant in a patient with Fanconi's anemia by means of umbilical cord blood from an HLA-identical sibling [2] several authors have shown that a single human umbilical cord blood sample collected at birth contains enough progenitor/stem cells to reconstitute hematopoiesis following a myeloablative conditioning regimen in children or in adults [3–6].

The clinical experience with this approach is still limited but preliminary results have shown a good engraftment with no or limited graft versus host disease (GVH) in several patients transplanted with a matched sibling donor. The longest follow-up, now at 5 years, shows a permanent engraftment with complete donor chimerism.

Due to the relative immaturity of the immune system in the new-born, it was thought that these cells would give less graft versus host disease (GVH) than adult bone marrow cells. There are some in-vitro data which seem to confirm this hypothesis and also several partially family mismatched transplants have been successful. As it appears that the use of matched unrelated adult bone marrow donors gives an increased rate of severe GVH, there is some hope that the use of neonate hematopoietic stem cells would decrease the frequency of this complication.

The other advantage is the unlimited supply of cord blood collection leading to the possi bility to select rare haplotypes, or to limit the number of samples of frequent haplotypes. The safety of the product is better because during the period of storage, it is easy to control the number of hematopoietic stem cells and check the absence of any infectious or genetic transmissible disease. The immediate availibility of stored HLA typed hematopoietic stem cells diminishes the delay between the bone marrow donor search request, which averages currently 2 to 6 months in marrow donor registries, to few days.

Clinical Results

A recent study from the international cord blood transplant registry has collected 26 cases

Bone Marrow Transplant Unit, Hôpital Saint-Louis, Paris, France of cord blood transplants in 26 children [7]. Their age varied from 1.3 to 16 years; 17 had malignant disease and 9 a non malignant disorder; 19 sibling donor recipient pairs were HLA identical and 7 were HLA non identical at 1 antigen (n=3), 2 antigens (n=1) or 3 antigens (n=3). The median recipient weight was 19 kg (range 10.3–45.5 kg). The median volume of cord blood collected was 100ml (range: 44–282 ml) with a median number of nucleated cells of 4.0 $\times 10^7$/kg (range: 1.0–16.0 $\times 10^7$/kg) and a median number of CFU-GM of 2.42 $\times 10^4$/kg (range: 0.23–25.6 $\times 10^4$/kg). The median time to recovery was 23.5 days for neutrophils (ANC $\geqslant$ 500/μl, range: 12–46 days) and 44.5 days for platelets ($\geqslant$ 50,000/μl, range: 15–105 days).

The median time to recovery did not correlate with the numbers of nucleated cells or CFU-GM. Donor cell engraftment was confirmed in 18 patients, including 4 of 6 evaluable recipients of HLA non identical cord blood cell transplants. Four patients failed to engraft, 2 died too early and 2 are yet to be evaluated for donor chimerism. Grade 2–4 GVHD was observed in only 1 of 19 evaluable patients, occurring in a recipient of an HLA 3 antigen mismatched transplant. Chronic GVH was observed in only 1 of 18 patients with donor engraftment surviving for more than 100 days and occurred in a recipient of an HLA 1 antigen mismatched transplant. The median time of survival for the 17 cord blood transplants currently alive is 1.9 years (range: 0.2–4.9). Causes of death were hepatic veno-occlusive disease (n=1), interstitial pneumonia (no2), relapse (no2), intracerebral hemorrhage (n=1) and graft failure (n=3).

These data demonstrate that umbilical cord blood is a source of hematopoietic stem cells which can be used for allogeneic bone marrow transplantation with low GVHD potential in children and in adults with matched and closely matched related donors. More recent preliminary results have been announced on 2 successful matched unrelated cord blood transplants by the New York cord blood bank team.

Rationale for Establishing a Cord Blood Bank

Engraftment potential. It has been shown that cord blood is enriched with immature hematopoietic stem cells which differ from adult stem cells by their high proliferative and differentiating capability [8–11].

Several studies have shown that one single cord blood collection contained enough hematopoietic stem cells to reconstitute the marrow of an adult as well as a child. This point is currently under study because the quantification of the minimum number of stem cells necessary for a complete allogeneic engraftment is not known and the techniques of measure are not standardized. Studies are also performed for improving the yield of stem cells: purification by various gradients and enrichment of CD34+ cells by incubation with magnetic beads or columns with a monoclonal anti CD34+ antibody. The methods of cryopreservation are well known. It has been shown that cord blood cells can be kept in DMSO and liquid nitrogen for periods of more than 10 years as it has been shown for bone marrow cells.

The advantage of using cord blood as a source of stem cells are obvious: the supply is unlimited and there is a possibility to increase the recruitment of donors from ethnic minorities which are poorly represented in large marrow donors registries. The other advantage is the rapidity of the search process speeding the delay between the initiation of a search and the transplant, because cord blood can be immediately used as the number of progenitors stem cells and the HLA typing are known in advance. Histocompatibility testing would be speeded up by directly testing small aliquots of donated cord blood by newly developed HLA matching techniques. An European cord blood bank project of collecting 20000 samples in several European countries is currently planned. Similar projects are developing in other parts of the world, mostly in the USA and more recently in Asia [12].

Immunological reactivity of cord blood cells. One of the major and still partially unsolved problems of allogeneic bone marrow tranplant is graft versus host disease (GVH). There is now convincing evidence that cytotoxic T cells and NK cells of donor origin, together with cytokines and especially tumor necrosis factor (TNF) may play an important role in acute GVH. Despite the use of HLA identical donors and the development of new immunosuppressive agents, its incidence is still frequent with an incidence of 30% with matched sibling marrow tranplants and 75% with matched unrelated marrow transplants. So far, GVH has been limited or absent in the small number of children transplanted with cord blood, the majority had received a matched sibling transplant and it is well known that the incidence and severity of GVH is reduced in this age group. Of note, 7 patients received a cord blood transplant from a sibling with 1, 2 or 3 HLA mismatches without any major GVH. On the other hand, the new-born baby seems to be the best donor, because it is known that the incidence of GVH increases with donor age and exposition to viral infections or immunisation by blood transfusions or pregnancies. In vitro studies have shown that new-born lymphocytes present in cord blood were functionally immature with a large proportion of naive T cells and increased helper-suppressor activity [13,14].

The phenotypic of cord blood lymphocytes appears to be immature with a smaller percentage of T cells, the majority of T cells express the TCR-alpha/beta, it contains small proportion of CD38+ cells and CD37+ cells. If the CD3-8+ cells were substracted from the total percentage of CD8+, the CD4/CD8 ratio was slightly higher than that seen in adult blood. Most T cells were of naive phenotype expressing the CD45RA phenotype [15]. Two major differences between cord and post natal blood samples were found. First, in the cord blood>99% of T cells strongly express the CD38 antigen while in the post natal blood CD38 expression on T cells was heterogeneous. Second, in the cord blood CD45RO+ T cells were seen as well as double negative populations CD45RO−, RA− which exhibit unique features of functional and phenotypic immaturity. This observation emphasizes some advantages of cord blood transplantation. During bone marrow transplantation T cell reconstitution is slow with IL-2 deficiency and poor T cell function which is a predisposing factor for GVH. By contrast, in the cord blood both immature and umprimed T cells, dominantly CD4+ are rich in IL-2 secreting populations, and after cord blood transplant GVH may diminish rather than increase. In addition, the cord blood precursors might also be further purified by eliminating CD45RA+ unprimed T cells while retaining CD45RA− immature T cells and hematopoietic progenitor cells. A novel population of NK progenitor cells was recently isolated from cord blood being CD34–, lin–, NK+ and NK–, CD7+. These cells were shown to be functionally immature when freshly isolated, but became cytotoxic after in vitro culture in IL-2:/PHA/PHA-CM [16]. Neonatal lymphocytes have been reported to be defective in IFN-gama and in IL-4 production, but not in IL-2 production. Recently, Clerici et al detected a defect in IL-2 production which is selective for response to recall antigens and to self APC processed alloantigens but not to stronger stimuli such as allo or PHA stimulation further supporting a deficiency in HLA self-restricted Th that is dependent on functional APC responses [17–19]. A recent study has shown that T cells do not constitutively express perforin in contrast to adult peripheral blood T cells. Cord blood T lymphocytes would be defective in the ability to exert T cell-mediated cytotoxicity at least via the perforin lytic pathway. Lack of effector cytotoxic T cells might reduce the relative risk of acute GVHD after cord blood transplantation. Therefore, the cytotoxic function of cord blood cells appears first and foremost to be dependent on NK cells. Because of their lower perforin content, when compared to adult NK cells, cord blood NK cells could display a reduced MHC unrestricted cytotoxicity.

Strategy for Establishing a Bank of Cryopreserved Cord Blood

The advantages of establishing a bank of cryo preserved umbilical cord blood seems well established according to in vivo and in vitro results described in this article. It has been clearly shown that these cells can be used in HLA identical or partially mismatched family transplants as well as in matched unrelated situations. More clinical data are obviously required in order to evaluate the overall results. For this purpose an international cord blood transplant registry has been set up in order to collect all new cases and attempt to study the role of the number of cells, the degree of HLA matching on survival, engraftment, GVH and leukemic relapse.

It has been shown that cord blood transplantation can be successful in a large variety of malignant and non malignant hematological disorders. It remains to be demonstrated that the number of cells is sufficient for an adult transplant.

The European cord blood bank group is planning to establish a European cord blood bank for use in matched or partially mismatched transplants. A number of 20000 cryopreserved cord blood bank collected in 2 years seems to be a possible objective. A similar effort is being made in other countries, mostly in the USA [11] and also in Asia.

Working groups are currently discussing and establishing guidelines for:

1. Standardisation of the procedure of collection, volume depletion, cryopreservation and thawing of cord blood.
2. Comparison and standardisation of various criteria for assessing quantification of hematopoietic progenitors, detection of genetic or infectious transmissible diseases.
3. Determination of the criteria for donor selection and methods of HLA typing.
4. Establishment of a computer network for data collection and exchange.
5. Establishment of ethical and legal guidelines for informed consent, infectious disease screening and data protection.

References

1. Broxmeyer HE, Douglas GW, Hangoc G et al: Proc. Natl. Acad. Sci. USA 1989; 86: 3828–3832.
2. Gluckman E, Broxmeyer HE, Auerbach AD et al: N. Engl. J. Med. 1989; 321: 1174–1178.
3. Hows JM, Marsh JCW, Bradley BA et al: The Lancet. 1992; 340: 73–76.
4. Broxmeyer HE, Hangoc G, Cooper S et al: Proc. Natl. Acad. Sci. USA. 1992; 89: 4109–4113.
5. Thierry D, Hervatin F, Traineau R et al: Bone Marrow Transpl. 1992; 9 sup 1: 101–104.
6. Wagner JE, Broxmeyer HE, Byrd RL et al: Blood. 1992; 79: 1874.
7. Wagner JE, Kerman NA, Broxmeyer HE, Gluckman E et al: Allogeneic umbilical cord blood transplantation. Report of results in 26 patients. Abstract submitted ASH meeting December 1993.
8. Brossard Y, Van Nifterik J, De Lachaux V et al: Nouv Rev Fr Hematol. 1990; 32: 427–429.
9. Gluckman E, Devergie A, Thierry D et al: Bone Marrow Transpl. 1992; Vol 9 sup 1: 114–117.
10. Broxmeyer HE, Kurtzburg J, Gluckman E et al: Umbilical cord blood hematopoietic stem and repopulating cells in human clinical transplantation. Blood Cells 1991; 17: 313–329.
11. Rubinstein P, Rosenfeld RE, Adamson JW, Stevens CE. Stored placental blood for unrelated bone marrow reconstitution. Blood 1993; 81: 1679–1690.
12. Gluckman E, Wagner J, Hows J, Kernan N, Bradley B. Cord blood banking for hematopoietic stem cell transplantation: An international cord blood transplant registry. Bone Marrow Transpl. 1993; 11: 199–200.
13. Rabian-Herzog C, Lesage S, Gluckman E. Bone Marrow Transplant. 1992; Vol 9 Sup 1: 64–67.
14. Deacock S, Schwarer AP, Batchelor JR et al: Transplantation. 1992; 53: 1128–1134.
15. Harris DT, Schumacher MJ, Locascio J et al: Phenotypic and functional immaturity of human umbilical cord blood T lymphocytes. Proc. Natl. Acad. Sci. USA. 1992; 89: 10006–10010.
16. Cicuttini FM, Martin M, Petrie HT, Boyd AW. A novel population of natural killer progenitor cells isolated from human umbilical cord blood. The J. of Immunol. 1993; 151: 29–37.
17. Clerici M, Deplama L, Roilides E, Baker R, Shearer GM. Analysis of T Helper and Antigen- presenting cell functions in cord blood and peripheral blood leukocytes from healthy children of different ages. J. of Clin. Invest. 1993; 91: 2829–2836.
18. Haynes BF, Denning SM, Singer KH, Kurtzberg J. Ontogeny of T cell precursors: a model for the initial stages of human development. Immunol. Today 1989; 10: 87.
19. Philips JH, Hori T, Nagler A, Bhat N, Spits H, Lanier L. Ontogeny of human natural killer cells mediate cytolytic function and express cytoplasmic CD3ed proteins. J. Exp. Med. 1992; 172: 1409.

Acute Leukemias V
Experimental Approaches
and Management of Refractory Diseases
Hiddemann et al. (Eds.)

Molecular Basis for Retinoic Acid Effects in Acute Promyelocytic Leukemia

C. Chomienne

Abstract. All-trans retinoic acid, one of the active metabolites of vitamin A, is known to specifically induce fresh human promyelocytic leukemic cells (AML3) to differentiate in vitro to mature functional granulocytes which loose their self-renewal potency and spontaneously die. These results were confirmed in vivo: AML3 patients treated with oral all-trans RA alone achieve complete remission. Two distinct classes of proteins directly interact with RA: nuclear receptors (RARs and RXRs) and specific cytoplasmic proteins (CRABP). The retinoic receptor alpha (RAR α) gene located on chromosome 17, is rearranged through the t(15;17) translocation observed in these cells and fused to a newly identified gene, PLM, localized on chromosome 15. The specificity of the PML/RAR fusion protein and RA sensitivity of the APL leukemia points to a close relationship between the leukemogenesis and the therapeutic efficacy. We show that multiple parameters among which feature the normal RA binding proteins (RARα and CRABP) and the effective retinoid concentration, play a crucial role in the efficacy of RA therapy in these patients.

Retinoic Acid-induced Differentiation of Acute Promyelocytic Leukemia

In vitro differentiation of acute promyelocytic leukemic cells with retinoids. Structure function relationship fod-ifferent existing retinoid molecules have been studied in myeloid leukemic cell lines. All-trans and 13-cis forms are equally effective in the HL-60 and U-937 cells (Chomienne, 1986). Other compounds are either more or like the ethyl ester (Tigason®) less effective (Chomienne, 1986) than the naturally occurring isomers.

Though retinoids have been shown to alter leukemic cell growth (Douer, 1982), only AML3 cells (Bennett, 1976) are successfully induced to differentiate in vitro (Imaizumi, 1987; Chomienne, 1989). Morphologically, the modifications of the promyelocytic leukemic cells during the differentiation induced by all-trans RA are variable from one sample to another as are often the promyelocytic leukemic cells before treatment. After 5 days incubation with RA however, all leukemic cells have a smaller cell volume, a low nucleus cytoplasm ratio, disappearance of nucleoli if initially present.

The respiratory burst function is acquired rapidly (50% of the cell population is NBT positive after 3 days in culture with RA and 100% by day 7). These differentiated leukemic cells can no longer produce leukemic clones in soft agar and significant decrease of the BCL2 protein in these cells strongly suggest that, at least in vitro, the elimination of the leukemic clone may be in part due to programmed cell death.

We observed that of the three identified isomers, the all-trans and 9-cis retinoids are equally effective on AML3 cell differentiation and viable cell count. The 13-cis isomer, however induces an equivalent effect at only high concentration (10^{-6} M). We have also studied the effects of the major metabolites of RA: 4-oxo-13 cis and 4-oxo-all trans RA which both induce differentiation of AML3 cells (Chomienne, 1990).

Laboratoire de Biologie Cellulaire Hématopoïétique, Institut d'Hématologie, Hôpital Saint Louis, Paris, France

In vivo differentiation of APL with retinoids. The first available retinoid for in vivo use of RA treatment in acute leukemias was the 13-*cis* isomer. In AML3 patients refractory to conventional chemotherapy, at a 45 to 100mg/m² daily dose, little to no efficacy was observed (Hoffman, 1988; Flynn 1983). The original experience of Huang and coll (Huang, 1988) with all-*trans*-RA in 24 AML3 patients treated with a daily dose of 45 mg/m² was striking: 23 patients obtained complete remission and coagulation disorders were rapidly corrected. Our own experience corroborates their data: In first relapse AML3 patients, 26 out 28 patients achieved complete remission (CR) (Castaigne, 1990; Degos, 1990). These data were rapidly corroborated by different groups (Warrel, 1991; Chen, 1991; Warrel, 1992). In an recent European Multicenter Trial, 80 de novo patients with no initial increase in the WBC were treated with retinoic acid alone or conventional chemotherapy followed by chemotherapy consolidation. CR rate was of 74 % in the RA group versus 43 % in the chemotherapy group. Though the number of early deaths was identical in both groups, the percentage of disease free survival was significantly greater with RA (Fenaux, 1993).

The complete remission is obtained via a differentiation mechanism. An intermediate population expressing both mature (CD16) and immature (CD33) markers is detected during the 3rd and 4th week of treatment by cell surface immunophenotyping (Warrel, 1991). In situ hybridization with a chromosome 17 probe (Warrel, 1991) and DNA polymorphism studies (Fearon 1986; Elliott; 1992), confirmed the relationship between the clinical response and the maturation of the leukemic clone. After 30 to 45 days of treatment, normal myeloid cells have replaced the leukemic differentiated cells and the remission is polyclonal (Elliott, 1992).

Coagulation disorders, when present, were rapidly controlled. The bleeding diathesis was recently attributed to a more general activation of fibrinolysis, with a minor DIC. Four patients investigated eight days after treatment with ATRA had a normalization of the fibrinolytic disorder but persistance of DIC (Dombre, 1993).

The complete remission is achieved without any signs of aplasia. Most patient were treated on an out-patient basis and few (25%) patients needed antibiotics and transfusions (Warrel, 1992). ATRA therapy is well tolerated and minor inconvenience (namely dryness of skin and mucosae, transient bone pain, increases of triglycerides and transaminases) is easily overcome by creams, eyedrops or analgesics.

The major side-effect is the occurrence of a hyperleucocytosis (WBC > 10 to 100 10^9/ml) and the "RA syndrome" (fever, respiratory distress, pulmonary infiltrates, pleural effusions and impaired myocardial function) (Frankel, 1992).

Length of complete remission was noted to be short if all-trans RA alone or low dose chemotherapy were given as maintenance therapy (4–47 months) (Huang, 1988; Warrel, 1991). Recent results suggest that consolidation therapy with conventional (daunorubicin and cytosine arabinoside) chemotherapy not only provides long disease free complete remissions (Warrel 1992; Fenaux, 1993) but that these remissions may be longer than when induction chemotherapy consisted of only chemotherapy.

Hypotheses for the Molecular Basis of APL Leukemogenesis

Through the t(15;17) translocation (Larson, 1984) these APL leukemic cells harbour PML/RARα fusion transcripts and to a lesser extent the reciprocal RARα/PML transcripts (Chomienne, 1992; Longo, 1990). The transcripts are variable in sizes depending on the breakpoint localization on the PML gene, each AML3 patient being characterized by a specific fusion transcript. These transcripts are not easily detectable on Northern blots (poor cellular samples and weak expression of the messenger RNA) but can now be observed in all AML3 cases by reverse transcriptase polymerase chain reaction (Castaigne, 1992; Miller, 1992). So far, these different types of fusion transcripts do not allow to discriminate between different AML3 subtypes, or for a specific outcome or response to RA.

PML-RARα inhibits the transactivation of RARE myeloid specific reporter genes (either spontaneously or in the presence of RA) (de Thé, 1991; Rousselot 1992). In normal hematopoietic cells retinoids enhance granulocytic differentiation (Van Bockstaele, 1992; Sakashita, 1993). Our results on total bone marrow mononucleated cells shows a significant increase of CFU-G in the presence of retinoids (Gratas, 1993). It is to be noted however that the effect is strictly dose-related. A stimulatory effect is observed at low < 10^{-9} to 10^{-7} M concentration. At higher concentrations, a true inhibitory effect is observed. A similar effect is observed whatever the retinoid used, whether all-trans, 9-cis, or 13-cis. The same granulocytic enhancement is observed on purified $CD34^+$ cells.

The specific differential expression of RARα and RXRα genes in myeloid cells determined to the granulocytic pathway further stresses the role of retinoids on granulocytic maturation. In hematopoietic cells (HL-60) PML/RAR inhibits RA-mediated transactivation (Rousselot, 1994). However it already appears that PML/RAR blocks the RA-mediated granulocytic differentiation or the vitamin D3 mediated monocytic differentiation of HL-60 cells (Rousselot, 1994) or U 937 cells (Pelicci, 1993) and that on its own, the truncated RARα protein, has no repressor effect in transactivation assays. The inhibition is observed at low doses of retinoids.

The PLZF RARα which originates from t(11;17) leukemias breaks the RARα gene in the second intron as for t(15;17) (Chen, 1992). Like PML-RARα we have shown that PLZF RARα inhibits the transactivation of RARE- myeloid specific reporter genes (Chen, 1994). Thus alteration of RA's physiological differentiation pathway by the t(15;17) or t(11;17) translocations may result in the leukemogenesis of these leukemias.

Hypotheses for the Molecular Basis of RA's Efficacy in APL Cells

Retinoic acid's effect in a cell is closely related to the retinoic acid receptors and cytoplasmic binding proteins present in the cell and to the concentration of the active metabolite arriving in the nucleus. The same rules seem to be required in APL cells. The mechanism(s) through which RA induces leukemic cell differentiation have not been elucidated though many effects consecutive to RA action have been observed at different levels of the cell. Monitoring RA's efficacy and side effects during prolonged RA therapy has suggested that RA's outcome and biological consequences in tissues other than hematopoietic must be considered.

Presence of the PML/RAR. In the presence of high concentrations of ATRA, PML/RARα can activate RA-inducible reporter genes (Rousselot, 1992; Pelicci, 1993) and restores RA-mediated differentiation in PML/RAR transfected HL-60 cells. This is in agreement with the structural conservation of the ligand binding domain in the PML/RARα protein and its identical binding affinity for all-trans RA compared to RARα (Nervi, 1992), though it is not yet known how the tridimensional structure of the abnormal protein affects the stability of the RA binding in the cell. This may imply that the PML/RARα protein could be responsible both for the oncogenic effect and RA responsiveness of AML3 cells.

Presence of the normal RARα gene. Another explanation which need not be exclusive is that RA-efficacy may be linked to the normal remaining RARα gene. Various data implicate RARα in normal granulocytic differentiation: RARα is highly expressed in normal differentiated granulocytes (Chomienne, 1991) and in the myeloid tissue by in situ hybridization (Guidez personal communication). On normal myeloid progenitor cells, all-trans RA increases granulocytic differentiation (Douer, 1992; Gratas, 1993). This has led us to postulate that RA and its receptor may play a role in normal granulocytic differentiation. In AML3 cells, we noted a significant increase of the normal RARa gene expression after treatment with all-trans RA. This appears as an early event of RA and forwards an explanation for the paradoxical effect of all-trans RA in this disease. The level of expression of RARa gene was correlated to the concentration of all-trans RA used (Rousselot, 1992). RARa is known to form heterodimers both RXRa and PML, PML/RARa (Kastner, 1992). It is not yet known how the equilibrium between these different proteins affect transactivation and differentiation in AML3 cells.

Levels of all-trans RA concentrations: a prerequisite for RA sensitivity of AML3 cells and secondary resistance to ATRA. Pharmacological studies of all-trans RA in AML3 patients have brought forward interesting data. The plasma concentration of all-trans RA achieved in AML3 patients was within the in vitro differentiating concentrations; time to peak concentration of all-trans RA was between 60 and 120 minutes (median: 90 minutes) after ingestion, with maximum concentrations between 0.03 μg/ml and 2.5 μg/ml (median 0.4 μg/ml), median AUC 630 ng.h/ml. These concentrations were within the in vitro differentiating concentration range of all-trans RA for these patients' cells. Interpatient variations were linked to an increased clearance rate and to the leukemic cell burden (Lefebvre,1991;

Muindi, 1992). The great interpatient variability observed suggests that intracellular concentration determinations may prove essential in the pharmacological studies of all-trans RA in AML3 patients undergoing RA therapy. A significant decrease of the area under the curve is found very early after onset of ATRA treatment (Muindi, 1992).

Little is known about the exact physiological outcome of all-trans RA in normal or AML3 patients. Different enzymes are implicated in the conversion of the exogenous Vitamin A to retinoic acid and its various metabolites. These enzymes depend on the presence of cytochrome P450, NAD and certain cellular binding proteins such as CRABP which have been recently shown to act as substrate for retinoic acid metabolism (Cornic, 1992). RA induces P450 metabolism and AML3 cells of patients after RA therapy may be linked to increased RA catabolism show reduced ATRA sensitivity of AML3 cells in vitro (Delva, 1993).

The quantity of CRABP detected is related to the length of ATRA therapy and decreases very slowly (months) after withdrawal of ATRA. These data strongly suggest a metabolism cause for the resistance of ATRA in relapse patients and the failure of continuous ATRA therapy as maintenance therapy is related to an hypercatabolytic state. Drugs that reduce P450 activity or binding to CRABP may circumvent resistance to ATRA. Revision of the schedule, dose and length of ATRA therapy in the induction treatment of AML3 may prevent the induction of this "salvage" cascade and therefore the induction of resistance.

Cytokines. Differentiation of leukemic cells by retinoids is enhanced by the addition of cytokines (Peck, 1991). We have shown that AML3 cells express and secrete cytokines such as TNFa, IL-6, IL-8, IL-1β. Absence of TNFα or presence of IL-3, G or GM-CSF significantly reduced the efficacy of all-trans RA to differentiate AML3 cells (Dubois, 1994). Interestingly these cytokines are implicated in leucocyte activation and may related to the APL-ATRA syndrome.

Conclusion

Terminal differentiation of acute myeloid leukemic cells has opened both new perspectives on the understanding of leukemogenesis, and new possibilities of therapies in malignancy. To date, in vitro and in vivo differentiation of acute promyelocytic leukemic cells with all-trans RA is the first model of differentiation therapy. The monitoring of ATRA efficacy in AML3 patients requires a thorough knowledge of the proteins. The parallel studies on the role of the PML/-RARα product on the blockage of myeloid differentiation and of the normal RARα in normal and leukemic differentiation will provide the necessary elements. Biodisponibility, cellular uptake and metabolism of all-trans RA in AML3 cells along with the determination of the presence, quantity and affinity of the different RA binding proteins.

References

1. Alcalay, M., Zangrilli, D., Pandolfi, PP., Longo, L., Mencarelli, A., Giacomucci, A., Rocchi, M., Biondi, A., Rambaldi, A., Lo Coco, F., Diverio, D., Donti, E., Grignani, F., and Pelicci, PG. (1991): Proc. Natl. Inst . Acad . Sc., 88: 1977.
2. Ballerini, P., Balitrand, N., Huang, ME., Krawice, I., Castaigne, S., Fenaux, P., Tiollais, P., Dejean, A., Degos, L., and de Thé, H. (1990): Leukemia., 4: 802.
3. Bennett, JM., Catovsky, D., Daniel, MT., Flandrin, G., Galton, DAG., Gralnick, HR., and Sultan, C. (1976): Br .J. Haematol., 33: 451.
4. Biondi, A., Rambaldi, A., Pandolfi, PP., Rossi V., Guidici, G., Alcalay, M., Lo Coco, F., Diverio, D., Pogliani, EM., Lanzi, EM., Mandelli, F., Masera, G., Barbui, T., and Pelicci, PG. (1992): Blood, 80: 492–497.
5. Borrow, J., Goddard, AD., Sheer, D., and Solomon, E. (1990): Science, 249: 1577.
6. Borrow, J., Goddart, AD., and Gibbon, B. (1992): Brit. Jour. Haematol., 82: 529–540.
7. Bradley, EC., Ruscetti, FW., Steinberg, H., Paradise, C., and Blaine, K. (1983): J. Natl. Cancer Inst.,71: 1189.
8. Breitman, TR., Collins, SJ., and Keene, BR. (1981): Blood, 57: 1000.
9. Castaigne, S., Chomienne, C., Daniel, MT., Berger, R., Fenaux, P., and Degos, L. (1990): Blood, 76: 1704.
10. Castaigne, S., Balitrand, N., de The, H., Dejean, A., Degos, L., and Chomienne, C. (1992): Blood, 79: 3110–3115.
11. Chen, Z., Chen, SJ., Tong, JH., Zhu, YJ., Huang, ME., Wang, WC., Wu, Y., Sun, GL., Wang, ZY., Larsen, CJ., and Berger, R. (1991): Leukemia, 5: 288.
12. Chen, ZX., Xue, YQ., Zhang, R., Tao, RF., Xia, XM., Li, C., Wang, W., Zu, WY., Yao, XZ., and Ling, BJ. (1991): Blood, 78: 1413.
13. Chen, Z., Brand, N., Chen, A., Chen, SJ., Tong, JH., Wang, ZY., Waxman, S., and Zelent, A. (1993): EMBO, 12: 1161–1167.

14. Chen, Z., Guidez, F., Rousselot, P., Agadir, A., Chen, SJ., Wang, ZY., Degos, L., Waxman, S., Zelent, A., and Chomienne, C. (in press 1994): PNAS .
15. Chen, SJ., Chen, Z., Chen, A., Tong, JH., Dong, S., Wang, ZY., Waxman, S., and Zelent, A. (1992): Oncogene, 7: 1223–1232.
16. Chomienne, C., Balitrand, N., and Abita, JP. (1986): Leuk Res, 10: 1079.
17. Chomienne, C., Balitrand, N., Cost, H., Degos, L., Abita, JP.(1986): Leuk Res, 10: 1301.
18. Chomienne, C., Ballerini, P., Balitrand, N., Amar, M., Bernard, JF., Boivin, P., Daniel, MT., Berger, R., Castaigne, S., and Degos, L.(1989): Lancet, 1: 746.
19. Chomienne, C., Ballerini, P., Balitrand, N., Daniel, MT., Fenaux, P., Castaigne, S., and Degos, L. (1990). Blood , 76: 1710. Chomienne, C.,
20. Chomienne, C., Ballerini, P., Balitrand, N., Krawice, I., Fenaux, P., Castaigne, S., de Thé, H., and Degos, L. (1991): ICI , 88: 210.
21. Cornic, M., Delva, L., Balitrand, N., Guidez, F., and Chomienne, C. (1992): Cancer Res., 52: 3329.
22. Dalton, WT., Ahearn, MJ., Mc Credie, KB., Freireich, EJ., Stass, SA., and Trujillo, JM. (1988): Blood, 71: 242–247.
23. Degos, L., Chomienne, C., Daniel, MT., Berger, R., Dombret, H., Fenaux, P., and Castaigne, S. (1990): Lancet., 336: 1440.
24. Delva, L., Cornic, M., Guidez, F., Balitrand, N., Castaigne, S., Fenaux, P., Delmer, A., Teillet, F., Degos, L., and Chomienne, C. (1993): Blood, 82: 2175–2181.
25. Dombret, H., Scrobohacci, ML., Ghorra, P., Zini, JM., Daniel, MT., Castaigne, S., and Degos, L. (1993): Leukemia, 7: 2.
26. Douer, D., and Koeffler, HP. (1982): Exp. Cell. Res., 138: 193.
27. Douer, D., and Koeffler HP. (1982): J. Clin. Invest.., 69: 277.
28. Dubois, C., Schlageter, MH., de Gentile, A., Guidez, F., Balitrand, N., Toubert, ME., Krawice, I., Fenaux, P., Castaigne, S., Najean, Y., Degos, L., Chomienne, C. Blood (in press 1994).
29. Elliott, S., Taylor, K., White, S., Rodwell, R., Marlton, P., Meagher, D., Wiley, J., Taylor, D., Wright, S., and Timms, P.(1992): Blood.8: 1916.
30. Fearon, ER., Burke, PJ., Schiffer, CA., Zehnbauer, BA., and Vogelstein, B. (1986): N. Engl. J. Med., 315: 15.
31. Fenaux, P., Castaigne, S., Dombret, H., Chomienne, C., Duarte, M., Archimbaud, E., Lamy, T., Tibeghien, P., Tilly, H., Dufour, P., Cransac, M., Guerci, A., Sadoun, A., and Degos, L. (1993): Blood, 80: 2176.
32. Frankel S, Weiss M, Warrel RP (1992): Ann. Int. Med. , 117: 292.
33. Goddard, AD., Borrow, J., Freemont, PS., and Salomon, E. (1991): Science, 254: 1371–1374.
34. Gratas, C., Menot, ML., Dresch, C., and Chomienne, C. (1993): Leukemia, 7: 1156–1162.
35. Grignani, F., Ferrucci, Testa, U., Giampaoio, T., Fagioli, M., Alcalay, M., Mencarelli, A., Peschle, C., Nicoletti, L., and Pelicci, PG. (1993): Cell, 74: 423–431.
36. Guidez, F., Huang, W., Tong, JH., Dubois, C., Balitrand, N., Waxman, S., Michaux, JL., Martiat, P., Degos, L., Chen, Z., and Chomienne, C. (1994). Leukemia, 8: 312–317.
37. Huang, ME., Ye, YI., Chen, SR., Chai, JR., Lu, JX., Zhoa, L., Gu, LJ., and Wang, ZY. (1988): Blood, 72: 567.
38. Kakizuka, A., Miller, WH., Umesono, K., Warrel, RP., Frankel, SR., Murry, VVVS., Dmistrovsky, E., and Evans, R. (1991): Cell, 66: 663.
39. Kastner, P., Perez, A., Lutz, Y., Rochette-Egly, C., Gaub, MP., Durand, B., Lanotte, M., Berger, R., and Chambon, P. (1992): EMBO J, 11: 629.
40. Larson, RA., Kondo, K., Vardiman, JW., Butler, AE., Golomb, HM., and Rowley, D. (1984): Am. J. Med., 76: 827.
41. Lefebvre, P., Thomas, G., Gourmel, B., Dreux, C., Castaigne, S., and Chomienne, C. (1991): Leukemia, 5: 1054.
42. Leroy, P., Nakshatri, H., and Chambon, P. (1991): Pro. Natl. Acad. Sci. USA, 88: 10138–10142.
43. Lo Coco, F., Diverio, D., Pandolfi, PP., Biondi, A., Rossi, V., Avvisati, G., Rambaldi, A., Arcese, W., Petti, MC., and Meloni, G. (1992): Lancet, 340: 1437.
44. Longo, L., Dionti, E., Mencarelli, A., Avanzi, G., Pegoraro, L., Alimena, G., Tabilio, A., Venti, G., Grignani, F., and Pelicci, PG. (1990): Oncogene, 5: 1557.
45. Longo, L., Pandolfi, PP., Biondi, A., and Rambaldi, A. (1990): J. Exp. Med., 172: 1571.
46. Matsuoka, A., Miyamura, K., Emi, N., Tahara, T., Tanimoto, Naoe, T., Ohno, R., Kakizuka, A., Evans, R., and Saito, H. (1993): Leukemia, 7: 1151–1155.
47. Miller, WH., Kakizuka, A., Frankel, SR., Warrel, RP., Levine, K., Arlin, Z., Evans, R., and Dmitrovsky, E. (): PNAS, 89: 2694–8.
48. Miller, WH., Warrel, RP., Frankel, SR., Jakubowski, A., Gabrilove, JL., Muindi, J., and Dmitrovsky, E. (1990): J. Natl. Cancer. Inst., 82: 1932.
49. Miller, WHJ., Kakizuka, A., Frankel, SR., Warrell, RP., DeBlasio, A., Levine, K., Evans, R., and Dmitovsky, E. (1992): PNAS., 89: 2694– 2698.
50. Muindi, J., Frankel, SR., Miller, WH., Jakubowski, A., Scheinberg, DA., Young, CW., and Dimitrovsky, E. (1992): Blood, 79: 299.
51. Muindi, J., Frankel, SR., Huselton, C., Degrazia, F., Garland, WA., Yong, CW., and Warrel, RP. (1992): Cancer Res., 52: 2138.
52. Nervi, C., Poindexter, C., Grignani, F., Pandolfi, PP., Lo Coco, F., Avvisati, G., Pelicci PG., and Jetten, AM. (1992): Cancer Res., 52: 3687.
53. Pandolfi, P., Alcalay, M., Fagioli, M., Zangrilli, D., Mencarelli, A., Diverio D, Biondi A, Lo Coco F, Rambaldi, A., Grignanin, F., Rochette-Egly, C., Gaube, M., Chambon, P., and Pelicci PG. (1992): EMBO, 11: 1397–1407.
54. Peck, R., Bollag, W. (1991): Eur. Jour. Cancer, 27, 53–57.
55. Rousselot, P., Hardas, B., Castaigne, S., Dejean, A., de Thé, H., Degos, L., Farzaneh, F., and Chomienne, C. (1994): Oncongene, 9: 545–551.

56. Sakashita, A., Kizaki, M., Pakkala, S., Schiller, G., Tsuruoka, N., Tomasaki, R., Cameron, JF., Dawson, and Koeffler, HP. (1993): Blood, 81: 1009.
57. de Thé, H., Chomienne, C., Lanotte, M., and Dejean, A. (1990): Nature, 347: 558.
58. de Thé, H., Lavau, C., Marchio, A., Chomienne, C., Degos, L., and Dejean, A. (1991): Cell, 66: 675.
59. Van Bockstaele, DR., Lenjou, M., Snoeck, HW., Lardon, F., Stryckmans, P., and Peetermans, ME. (1993): Ann. Hematol ., 66: 61–66.
60. Warrell, RP., Frankel, SR., Miller, WH., Scheinberg, DA., Itri, IM., Hittelman, WN., Vyas, R., Andreeff, M., Tafuri, A., Jakubowski, A., Gabrilove, J., Gordon, MS., and Dimitrovsky, E. (1991): New. Engl. J. Med., 324: 1385.
61. Warrell, RP., de Thé, H., Wang, ZY., and Degos, L. (1993): New. Eng. J. Med., 329: 177–189.

Acute Leukemias V
Experimental Approaches
and Management of Refractory Diseases
Hiddemann et al. (Eds.)

Acute Promyelocytic Leukemia: Advantage of A-Trans Retinoic Acid (ATRA) over Conventional Chemotherapy

E. Lengfelder[1], M. Simon[1], D. Haase[2], F. Hild[2], and R. Hehlmann[1]

Introduction

Acute promyelocytic leukemia (APL) is characterized by the typical morphology of blast cells [1,2], the specific translocation t(15;17) [18], which fuses the PML gene to the retinoic acid receptor- α gene [8,15], and a coagulopath which frequently causes fatal bleeding [23].

In the past, conventional chemotherapy consisting of anthracycline and cytosine-arabinoside induced complete remission rates of 50–80% [6,7,10,14,17,20,21]. The availiability of the vitamin A precursor, "all-trans retinoic acid (ATRA)" has changed treatment and prognosis of APL profoundly.

In contrast to chemotherapy, which induces complete remission by a transient bone marrow aplasia, ATRA selectively induces differentiation of promyelocytic blasts to mature neutrophiles [3,5,9,19,24]. By this way remission rates of about 90% in newly diagnosed and first relapsing APL cases have been achieved [3,4,11,12,19,24,25]. Advantages of ATRA therapy are rapid improvement of coagulopathy and avoidance of bone marrow aplasia. A rapid increase in white blood cells during ATRA treatment occurring in approximately 25% is associated with a high early mortality rate and requires immediate cytoreduction by chemotherapy [11,12,13].

We describe here the results of ATRA treatment in 4 patients with newly diagnosed APL in comparison to a historical control group of 3 patients treated with chemotherapy, thereby demonstrating characteristic aspects of the different therapy modalities.

Patients and Methods

Patients. Seven patients with APL were newly diagnosed between 1989 and 1993. The initial characteristics of the patients are listed in Table 1. Six patients had AML FAB M3, one patient was categorized as a microgranular FAB

Table 1. Initial characteristics of the APL patients

Therapy	Patients	Sex/Age (y)	WBC $10^6/l$	Platelets ($10^6/l$)	Karyotype
ATRA	1	M/54	800	124000	t(15;17)(q22;q21)
	2	M/40	1400	8000	15q+, i(17q−)
	3	M/53	800	77000	normal
	4	M/55	1900	3000	15q+, i(17q−)
Chemotherapy	5	M/24	1100	92000	not performed
	6	F/47	600	31000	not performed
	7*	M/28	50000	16000	t(15;17) (q22;21)

*microgranular FAB M 3 variant; M, male, F, Female; WBC, white blood cell count; y, years

[1] III. Med Klinik, Klinikum Mannheim, Universität Heidelberg, Germany
[2] Institut für Humangenetik, Arbeitsgruppe für Tumorzytogenetik, Universität zu Lübeck, Germany

M3 variant. Peroxidase reaction was strongly positive and HLA-DR expression of blast cells was negative in all patients. Coagulation parameters indicated coagulopathy in all cases. No patient had clinical bleeding.

Therapy. Induction therapy consisted of ATRA in the four patients with diagnosis after December, 1 of 1991 and of cytosine arabinoside/anthracycline-based chemotherapy regimens in the three patients, which were diagnosed before this date (see Table 2).

ATRA. ATRA dosage was 45 mg/sqm/day p.o. One patient with rapidly increasing white blood cells was treated with additional chemotherapy (cytosine arabinoside and daunorubicin, AD) to prevent hyperleukocytosis. In all cases ATRA was given continuously until complete remission was obtained. All patients were further treated with three courses of an intensive consolidation chemotherapy (see Table 2).

Chemotherapy. Patients received one course of an intensive chemotherapy (cytosine arabinoside/daunorubicin with or without thioguanine, AD or TAD). If a complete remission was not achieved, a second cycle was given within three weeks. All patients were treated with intensive consolidation chemotherapy (see Table 2).

Chemotherapy Regimens

TAD: Cytosine arabinoside (ara-C) 100 mg/m²/day i.v. (continuous infusion), day 1 and 2, ara-C 100mg/m²/day/12h i.v., day 3 through 8, daunorubicin 60 mg/sqm/day i.v., day 3 through 5, thioguanine 100 mg/m²/day /12h p.o., day 3 through 9.
AD: Ara-C 100 mg/m²/day i.v. (continuous infusion), day 1 through 7, daunorubicin 60 mg/m²/day i.v., day 1 through 3.
HAM: Ara-C3 g/m²/day /12h i.v., day 1 through 3, mitoxantron 10 mg/m²/day i.v., day 3 through 5.
HAD: Ara-C 1 g/m²/day /12h i.v., day 1 through 4, daunorubicin 45 mg/m²/day i.v., day 1 through 3.

Coagulopathy

The treatment of coagulopathy consisted of intensive platelet support to maintain the platelet count above 20.000/μl and on support of fresh frozen plasma. All patients received 15.000 IE heparin per day until significant coagulopathy had disappeared.

Results

In all patients complete remissions were obtained. The results are summarized in Table 2.

In the ATRA group the mean duration of leukopenia (white blood cell count < 1000/μl), of coagulopathy and of the time required to complete remission was considerably shorter than in the chemotherapy group. During treatment with ATRA the improvement of coagulopathy was generally the first sign of clinical response. Two patients developed a thrombocytosis with platelet counts between 850×10^9/l and 1300×10^9/l with a maximum on day 29 and 40 of ATRA treatment. After an initial increase a transient decrease of the white blood cell count (WBC) to levels that were below normal occurred in all patients in the third or fourth week of ATRA treatment. No toxic side effects of ATRA were observed.

In the chemotherapy group, one therapy cycle was required for complete remission in one patient and two cycles in two patients. After the first course the bone marrow showed 50% blast cells without hypoplasia of the marrow in both patients. In one of these patients a prolonged persistence of blasts (20% on day 21 after the second course) was observed. By day 39 the blasts had disappeared without further chemotherapy. In the second patient a complete remission was obtained by day 31 after the second course. Since no early bone marrow control was done, a persistence of marrow blasts could not be proven in this patient.

Adverse effects of chemotherapy included mucositis, fever and infection (WHO grades 2–4). One patient of the chemotherapy group died of a severe mycosis due to aplasia after consolidation therapy.

Discussion

Both treatment strategies – ATRA and conventional chemotherapy – were successful in remission induction in our APL patients. A clear advantage of ATRA was the rapid improvement of coagulopathy which disappeared after a mean of 9 days compared to 25 days in the chemotherapy group. The risk of fatal hemorrhage was

Table 2. Treatment results

Patient	Remission ATRA	Induction CT	Duration of Leukopenia	Duration of Coagulopathy	Time to CR	Adverse Effects	Consolidation Chemotherapy	Survival
		No. of cycles	(days)	(days)	(days)		No. of cycles	(months)
1	yes	0	1	10	31	no	3 (AD, HAD)	24+cyt. rem.
2	yes	0	0	7	39	no	3 (AD, HAD)	9+cyt. rem.
3	yes	0	10	3	48	no	3 (AD, HAD)	4+
4	yes	1	3	15	33	increase of WBC	2 (AD, HAD)	23+cyt. rem.
			mean 3,5	mean 9	mean 38			
						WHO-grade		
5	no	2	46	24	60	4	1 (HAD)	26+
6	no	2	33	28	59	2	1 (HAM)	death in cons.
7	no	1	10	23	26	3	1 (TAD)	45+total (41 after allo BMT)
			mean 30	mean 25	mean 48			

Abbreviations: CT, chemotherapy; CR, complete Remission;; cyt rem., cytogenetic remission; cons., consolidation; allo. BMT, allogenic bone marrow transplantation
*White blood cells<1000/μl

reduced substantially. Our data are in agreement with observations of others, who report an improvement of coagulopathy after a few days of treatment with ATRA [3,4,11,12,19,24].

Further, ATRA reduced the risk of infection by shortening the duration of leukopenia. The mean time to reach white blood cell counts > 1000/μl was 3,5 days during ATRA treatment compared to 30 days in the chemotherapy group. In the recently published French/European APL trial a WBC of > 1000/μl was reached after a mean of 16+8 days in the ATRA group vs. 26+4 days in the chemotherapy group [12].

The mean time to complete remission was 38 days in our ATRA patients compared to 48 days in the patients with chemotherapy. This agrees well with the 38 to 53 days to complete remission reported for ATRA patients in the literature [3,4,12,19,24]. Two of our chemotherapy patients required two therapy courses and reached complete remission after 59 and 60 days. In one of these patients a prolonged persistence of marrow blasts for more than 21 days after the second course was observed. Recent chemotherapy studies [16,22] demonstrated, that some APL patients showed a long persistence of marrow blasts necessitating a second chemotherapy cycle more frequently than in other AML subtypes. These patients did not develop bone marrow hypoplasia and obtained complete remissions 6 to 8 weeks after start of chemotherapy by a slow disappearance of the blast cells [16,22], as shown in the one of our patients.

An additional advantage of ATRA was the reduction of chemotherapy - related adverse effects. ATRA was well tolerated in all patients. In the one patient with rapid increase in WBC the "ATRA-syndrome" was successfully prevented by an immediate cytotoxic therapy as has been recommended also by others [11,12,13].

Because of the brief duration of remission after ATRA therapy alone [3,4,19,24], our patients received intensive consolidation chemotherapy. The cytogenetic remissions of the three patients, documented after consolidation chemotherapy, confirm the effectiveness of this treatment strategy. Our results agree well with the favourable results of the recently published French/European APL trial reporting an event free survival of 79% after 12 months [12]. This study also demonstrated a significant advantage in event free survival of ATRA followed by intensive chemotherapy vs. chemotherapy alone. This seems also comfirmed by our results, where the only death occurred in the chemotherapy group [12].

We could demonstrate a clear advantage of ATRA compared to conventional chemotherapy, because the duration of coagulopathy and of leukopenia as well as the time to complete remission are clearly shorter. Furthermore, the toxic side effects of chemotherapy are avoided and event free survival seems to be longer. Thus, ATRA reduces important risks in remission induction of APL - bleeding and infection.

References

1. Bennett JM, Catovsky D, Daniel MT, Flandrin G, Galton D, Gralnick HR, Sultan C: Proposals for the classification of acute leukemias. Br J Haematol 33: 451, 1976.
2. Bennett JM, Catovsky D, Daniel MT, Flandrin G, Galton D, Gralnick HR, Sultan C: A variant form of hypergranular promyelocytic leukemia. Br J Haematol 44: 169, 1980.
3. Castaigne S, Chomienne C, Daniele MT, Ballerini P, Berger R, Fenaux P, Degos L: All-trans retinoic acid as a differentiation therapy for acute promyelocytic leukemia. I. Clinical results. Blood 76: 1704, 1990.
4. Chen ZX, Xue JQ, Zhang R, Tao RF, Xia XM, Li C, Wang W, Zu WY, Yao XZ, Ling BJ: A clinical and experimental study on all trans retinoic acid-treated acute promyelocytic leukemia patients. Blood 78: 1413, 1991.
5. Chomienne C, Ballerini P, Balitrand N, Daniele MT, Fenaux P, Castaigne S, Degos L: All-trans retinoic acid in acute promyelocytic leukemias. II.In vitro studies: Structure-function relationship: Blood 76: 1710, 1990.
6. Cordonnier C, Vernant JP, Brun B, Gouault M, Kuentz M, Bierling P, Imbert M, Jouault H, Mannoni P, Reyes F, Dreyfus B, Rochant M: Acute promyelocytic leukemia in 57 previously untreated patients. Cancer 55: 18, 1985.
7. Cunningham I, Gee TS, Reich LM, Kempin SJ, Naval AN, Clarkson BD: Acute promyelocytic leukemia: Treatment results during a decade at memorial hospital. Blood 73: 1116, 1989.
8. De The H, Chomienne C, Lanotte M, Degos L, Dejean A: The t(15; 17) translocation of acute promyelocytic leukemia fuses the retinoic acid receptor-α gene to a novel transcribed locus. Nature 347: 558, 1990.
9. Elliott S, Taylor K, White S, Rodwell R, Marlton P, Meagher D, Wiley J, Taylor D, Wright S, Timms P: Proof of differentiation mode of action of all-trans retinoic acid in acute promyelocytic leukemia using X-linked clonal analysis. Blood 79: 1916, 1992.
10. Fenaux P, Tertia G, Castaigne S, Tilly H, Leverger G, Guy H, Bordessoule D, Leblay R, Le Gall E,

Comblat Ph, Tchernia G, Bauters F, Marty M: A randomized trial of amsacrine and rubidazone in 39 patients with acute promyelocytic leukemia. J Clin Oncol 9: 1556, 1991.
11. Fenaux P, Castaigne S, Dombret H, Achimbaud E, Duarte M, Morel P, Lamy T, Tilly H, Guerci A, Maloisel F, Bordessoule D, Sadoun A, Tibereghien P, Fegueux N, Daniele MT, Chomienne C, Degos L: All-trans retinoic acid followed by intensive chemotherapy gives a high remission rate and may prolong remissions in newly diagnosed acute promyelocytic leukemia: A pilot study on 26 cases. Blood 80: 2176, 1992.
12. Fenaux P, Le Deley MC, Castaigne S, Archimbaud E, Chomienne C, Link H, Guerci A, Duarte M, Daniele MT, Bowen D, Huebner G, Bauters F, Fegueux N, Fey M, Sanz M, Lowenberg B, Maloisel F, Auzanneau G, Sadoun A, Gardin C, Bastion Y, Ganser A, Jacky E. Dombret H, Chastang C, Degos L: and the European APL 91 Group: Effect of all-trans retinoic acid in newly diagnosed acute promyelocytic leukemia. Results of a multicenter randomized trial. Blood 82: 3241, 1993.
13. Frankel SR, Eardley A, Lauwers G, Weiss M, Warrell RP: The retinoic acid syndrome in acute promyelocytic leukemia. Ann Intern Med 117: 292, 1992.
14. Hoyle CF, Swirsky DM, Freedman L, Hayhoe FG: Beneficial effect of heparin in the management of patients with APL. Br J Haematol 68: 283, 1987.
15. Kakizuka A, Miller, Jr, WH, Umesono K, Warrell, Jr, RP, Frankel SR, Murty VS, Dimitrovsky E, Evans RE: Chromosomal translocation t(15;17) in human acute promyelocytic leukemia fuses RAR-α with a novel putative transcription factor, PML. Cell 66: 663, 1991.
16. Kantarjian H, Keating MJ, McCredie KB, Beran M, Walters R, Dalton, Jr, WT, Hittleman W, Freireich EJ: A characterisctic pattern of leukemic cell differentiation without cytoreduction during remission induction in acute promyelocytic leukemia. J Clin Oncol 3: 793, 1986.
17. Kantarjian H, Keating MJ, Walters RS, Estey EH, McCredie KB, Smith TL, Dalton WT, Cork A, Trujillo JM, Freireich EJ: Acute promyelocytic leukemia. M.D. Anderson Hospital Experience. Am J Med 80: 789, 1986.
18. Larson RA, Kondo K, Vardiman JW, Butler AE, Golomb HM, Rowley JD: Evidence for a 15;17 translocation in every patient with acute promyelocytic leukemia. Am J Med 76: 827, 1984.
19, Meng-er H, Yu-chen YS, Shu-rong C, Jin-ren C, Jia-xiang L, Lin Z, Long-jun G, Zhen-yi W: Use of all-trans retinoic acid in the treatment of acute promyelocytic leukemia. Blood 72: 567, 1988.
20. Rodeghiero F, Avvisati G, Castaman G, Barbui T, Mandelli F: Early deaths and anti-hemorrhagic treatments in acute promyelocytic leukemia. A GIMEMA retrospective study in 268 consecutive patients. Blood 75: 2112, 1990.
21. Sanz MA, Jarque I, Martin G, Lorenzo I, Martinez J, Rafecas J, Pastor E, Sayas MJ, Sanz G, Gomis F: Acute promyelocytic leukemia. Therapy results and prognostic factors. Cancer 61: 7, 1988.
22. Stone RM, Maguire M, Goldberg MA, Antin JH, Rosenthal DS, Mayer RJ: Complete remission in acute promyelocytic leukemia despite persistence of abnormal bone marrow promyelocytes during induction therapy: Experience in 34 patients. Blood 71: 690, 1988.
23. Tallman S, Kwaan HC: Reassessing the hemostatic disorder associated with acute promyelocytic leukemia. Blood 79: 543, 1992.
24. Warrell, Jr, RP, Frankel SR, Miller WH, Scheinberg DA, Itri LM, Hittelman WL, Vyas R, Andreeff N, Tafuri A, Jakubowski A, Gabrilowe J, Gordon MS, Dimithrowsky E: Differentiation therapy of acute promyelocytic leukemia with tretinoin (all-trans retinoic acid). N Engl J Med 324: 1385, 1991.
25. Warrell, Jr, RP, Frankel SR, Miller WH, Eardley A, Dimitrowsky A: All-trans retinoic acid for remission induction of acute promyelocytic leukemia: Results of the New York study. Blood 80, No 10, suppl., 360 A, abstr No 1430, 1992.

Acute Leukemias V
Experimental Approaches
and Management of Refractory Diseases
Hiddemann et al. (Eds.)

Studies of 2-Chlorodeoxyadenosine (Cladribine) at St. Jude Children's Research Hospital

Victor M. Santana, William R. Crom, and Raymond L. Blakle

Introduction

2-Chloro-2′-deoxyadenosine (2-Cd Cladribine) was first synthesized in the early 1970's but did not undergo wide clinical testing until the last decade. This purine analogue has shown potent oncolytic activity in a variety of adult lymphoid malignancies; in fact, many investigators regarded it as an antilymphocyte drug exclusively [1–3]. Such perceptions grew from observations that lymphocytes contain unusually high concentrations of deoxycytidine kinase, the enzyme primarily (but not solely) responsible for the first step in phosphorylation of 2-CdA, whereas peripheral granulocytes have low concentrations of the kinase. To the contrary, results of in vitro studies indicate that the purine analogue is rapidly phosphorylated by both myeloid cell lines and leukemic blasts from patients with acute myeloid leukemia (AML), and that human cell lines of myeloid origin, as well as human peripheral monocytes, are quite sensitive to this agent [4–6]. 2-CdA is also toxic to cell lines derived from solid tumors, although higher concentrations are needed to produce this effect. We were sufficiently encouraged by these findings to undertake, in 1987, a research program focusing on 2-CdA in pediatric patients. Here we review noteworthy progress in the laboratory and clinical development of this agent and suggest possible applications for the future.

Preclinical Information

The concentration of 2-CdA that causes 50% inhibition of replicating T-lymphoblastic, B-lymphoblastic, or myeloid lines is 5 to 340 nM, depending on the cell line but not the cell lineage [4,5]. Resting human lymphocytes and monocytes (both normal and malignant) are killed by such concentrations of 2-CdA, but extensive cell kill requires several days [7,8]. 2-CdA is also toxic to cell lines derived from solid tumors [9,11].

2-CdA is much more stable metabolically than its parent compound, 2-deoxyadenosine, because it is a poor substrate for adenosine deaminase, the enzyme that catalyzes the first step in the catabolism of 2′-deoxyadenosine [4,9]. The purine analogue is rapidly taken up and phosphorylated by hematopoietic cell lines, and by the peripheral blasts of patients with AML or acute lymphoblastic leukemia (ALL) [12]. Phosphorylation to the 5-monophosphate is carried out by deoxycytidine kinase, and the toxicity of the drug for cells of different origin was initially proposed to correlate with the ratio of deoxycytidine kinase to deoxynucleotidase activity [7]. In a subsequent study of established hematopoietic cell lines, however, there was little correlation between the steady-state intracellular concentration of 2-CdA triphosphate (CldATP) and sensitivity to the drug [5]. Similarly, there was no obvious correlation between the clinical responses of pediatric AML and ALL patients to 2-CdA and the capacity of

Departments of Hematology-Oncology, Pharmacokinetics, and Molecular Pharmacology, St. Jude Children's Research Hospital, Memphis, Tennessee, USA

their leukemic cells to form the triphosphate of 2-CdA *in vitro* [12]. The mono- and triphosphate forms of 2-CdA accumulate in lymphoblastic and myeloid cell lines to concentrations of 0.4 – 27 μM within 3 hours [5,12]. Little is known about the metabolism of 2-CdA, except that 2-chloroadenine has been identified in the plasma of patients treated with the analogue. In pediatric patients, 2-CdA appears to be cleared from the kidneys as unchanged drug [13]. The monophosphate is cleared from leukemic cells in vitro with a half-life of 0.56–3.3 hours (mean, 1.3 hours); the triphosphate has a half life of 0.85–20 hours (mean, 2.5 hours) [12].

2-CdA specifically inhibits DNA synthesis, both in cultured cells and in the organs of treated mice [4,14]. Consistent with these observations, the nucleoside was found to arrest cells in culture at the G_1-S interface [14]. The triphosphate of 2-CdA is a potent inhibitor of human ribonucleotide reductase, and the consequent drop in the pool of one of more of the deoxyribonucleoside triphosphates required for DNA synthesis may be one mechanism by which the growth of replicating cells is inhibited [15–17]. However, because the synthesis of DNA in replicating cells exposed to 2-CdA decreases so rapidly, other important, more direct effects seem likely [15]. One of these is the effect of CldATP on DNA polymerases. The purine analogue is incorporated into DNA by polymerases α or β into positions normally occupied by dAMP [15–19]. The most significant effect of the incorporation of CldAMP into the growing DNA chain seems to be on the subsequent addition of nucleotides [18,19]. Addition of a single CldAMP residue to the primer by DNA polymerase β decreases the rate constant for the addition of the next nucleotide to 2–7% of that after dAMP addition, and further extension is negligible. Consecutive additions of 2-CdA residues by polymerase α progressively decrease the rate of subsequent chain extension, and after five consecutive additions, extension virtually stops. Thus, chain termination due to CldAMP incorporation into DNA may account for a major part of the cytotoxicity produced by 2-CdA.

Much less is known about the mechanism by which 2-CdA kills quiescent (G_0) cells. When normal human lymphocytes or monocytes are incubated with the drug at 0.1–100 μM 2-CdA, DNA strand breaks begin to accumulate as early as 4 hours, and shortly thereafter the rate of RNA synthesis begins to decrease [8,20]. By 8 hours intracellular concentrations of NAD decrease, by 24 hours ATP levels drop significantly, and by 48 hours the cells show a marked loss of viability. At longer intervals (1–5 days) the unrepaired DNA damage triggers programmed cell death (apoptosis), as indicated by the cleavage of DNA into nucleosome-sized multimers [21,22]. This sequence of events has been interpreted to indicate inhibition of DNA repair by 2-CdA. Some evidence indicates that in the DNA of quiescent lymphocytes, single-strand breaks are continually being induced and repaired [23,24]. Although this view has been challenged, the increase in strand breaks seen in resting cells treated with 2-CdA may well reflect the inhibition of DNA repair [25]. Since the accumulation of strand breaks and their repair is associated with the poly(ADP)ribosylation of nuclear proteins at the expense of NAD, the depleted levels of NAD and ATP in quiescent cells treated with 2-CdA may relate to this process.

2-CdA substantially prolongs the survival of mice inoculated with L1210 leukemia, and in some instances eradicates the disease entirely [4,14]. 2-Bromodeoxyadenosine produces similar effects in leukemia-bearing mice, and in a more extensive investigation the compound yielded a 58% cure rate in leukemic mice [26]. Yet, the therapeutic effects of these two nucleosides are highly schedule dependent, such that cures are noted only when the drug is administered at an optimal dose every 3 hours on days 1, 4, and 7 or days 1, 5, and 9 (total of 24 injections).

Clinical Studies

Phase I, acute leukemia. Our phase I study in children with relapsed acute leukemia began in 1987 and was completed in 1990 with 31 patients enrolled [6]. Because of the schedule dependency of the drug in murine models, a continuous intravenous 120-hour infusion was selected as the clinical schedule. Myelosuppression was dose-limiting. At the highest dose level tested (10.7 mg/m²/day × 5), three of seven patients developed fatal systemic bacterial or fungal infections. Definite clinical responses were noted in three of 12 patients with AML who received the drug at doses ⩾5.2 mg/m²/day, with all patients (both ALL and AML) showing some evidence of oncolytic effects. No systemic renal, hepatic or neurologic toxicities were identified in this group of patients with relapsed or refractory acute leukemia.

Phase I, solid tumors. In 1991 we began a phase I trial in children with recurrent solid tumors, starting at a dose of 7.0 mg/m²/day, or 80% of the maximal tolerated dose (MTD) in children with leukemia. To date, three children (two with neuroblastoma, one with a sarcoma) have been treated. Dose-limiting toxicity has not been reached, and the trial continues to accrue patients.

Phase II, relapsed acute leukemia. In view of the encouraging results observed in our phase I acute leukemia study, we performed a pilot study for children with acute leukemia in first or subsequent relapse [27]. Twenty-four patients with either AML (n=17) or ALL (n=7) were given continuous infusions of 2-CdA for 5 days at the MTD determined in our phase I trial, 8.9 mg/m²/day. Eight (47%) of the 17 patients with AML had a complete hematologic remission, four after a single infusion. Two others had partial remissions. Of seven patients with ALL who received 2-CdA, one had a complete response. In another child, the drug eradicated leukemic blasts from the cerebrospinal fluid (CSF).

Phase II, previously untreated patients. To assess the effects of 2-CdA against newly diagnosed AML, we began a trial in 1991 in which 22 consecutive patients received a single 120-hour infusion of 2-CDA – before the introduction of standard remission induction therapy [28]. Six patients (27%) had complete hematologic remissions by a median of 21 days after treatment with the nucleoside (range, 14–33 days). Seven others had partial responses, yielding a total response rate of 59% (95% confidence interval = 36% to 79%). The times to recovery of neutrophil counts $\geq$ 500/mm³ and platelet counts $\geq 50 \times 10^3$/mm³ ranged from 17 to 31 days and from 0 to 28 days, respectively. The drug also eliminated leukemic blasts from the CSF in four of six patients tested. Severe but reversible myelosuppression and thrombocytopenia were noted in all patients. There were no unusual infections due to opportunistic infections, although a single child developed fatal disseminated aspergillosis. It may be important that lymphocytopenia developed in 17 of 22 patients, persisting in nine until the time of bone marrow transplantation. Mucositis, a common complication of anthracycline therapy, was not observed, nor were hepatic or neurologic toxicities.

Since 1993, a second course of 2-CdA has been administered to patients who have had an initial reponse to the drug. To date, 10 additional patients have received this modified induction regimen, six of whom achieved a complete response (Fig. 1, columns 2 and 3).

Thus, as predicted from *in vitro* models, added drug exposure may allow greater accumulation of DNA strand breaks and improve the clinical reponse rate. These preliminary results also suggest a higher response rate in patients with the M0-M2 subtypes of AML, although analysis of larger numbers of patients is needed to substantiate this trend.

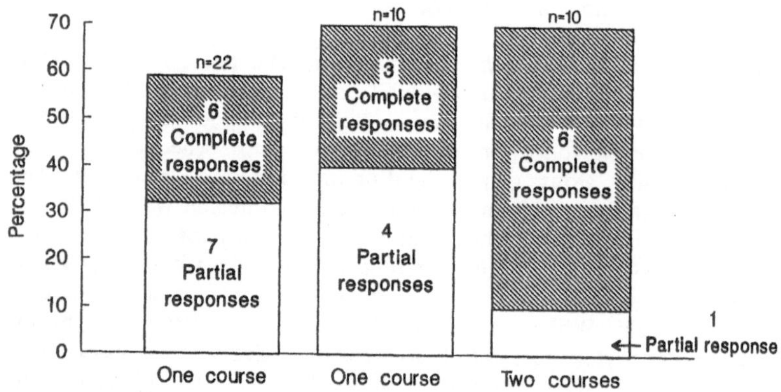

Fig. 1. Response rates of 2-CdA in de novo AML. Twenty-two patients received only a single course of 2-CdA (column 1); ten additional patients received two courses. The second and third columns depict the responses after the initial and subsequent courses in that subset of patients

Pharmacokinetics

The pharmacokinetics of 2-CdA have been studied in a relatively small number of patients. The data obtained thus far suggest that disposition of the drug is relatively slow. Plasma concentrations persist for several hours after drug administration, in contrast to the rapid elimination of other nucleoside analogues such as cytarabine. These findings are consistent with the resistance of 2-CdA to catabolism by adenosine deaminase. Our group has studied 25 children with acute leukemia treated with a 120-hour intravenous infusion of 8.9 mg/m²/day [13]. The mean (SD) clearance, normalized to body surface area in these 25 patients, was 39.4 (12.4) l/hr/m², with clearance ranging from 14.4 to 55.5 L/hr/m². When normalized to body weight, the mean (SD) clearance was 1.44 (0.62) L/hr/kg and ranged from 0.31 to 2.43 L/hr/kg. The steady-state plasma concentration of 2-CdA ranged from 23.2 to 84.5 nM, with a mean (SD) of 37.7 (17.3) nM and a median of 29.6 nM. The half-life of the terminal phase ($t_{1/2}$ β) for 22 patients who had plasma concentrations measured for at least 12 hours after the end of the infusion was 19.7 (3.4) hours, ranging from 14.3 to 25.8 hours. 2-CdA appeared to distribute into a relatively large volume at steady state. In these children, the steady-state volume of distribution ranged from 32.0 to 799 L/m², with a mean (SD) of 356 (225) L/m² and a median of 323 L/m².

The measured mean renal clearance was 51.0% of total systemic clearance in seven patients, but the percentage of total clearance accounted for by renal clearance ranged from 11.0% to 85.1%. The fate of the remainder of the drug is unknown, as no metabolites have been identified in urine or plasma. One possibility is that residual amounts of 2-CdA bind to tissues or intracellular sites. Additional work is needed to determine the role and importance of nonrenal clearance mechanisms.

Concentrations of 2-CdA were also measured in the CSF of 10 patients, on either day 4 or day 5 of the 5-day infusion. The mean (SD) CSF to plasma concentration ratio was 18.2% (10.0), with concentrations ranging from 1.68 to 14.75 nM. Higher ratios were achieved on day 5 than on day 4 (22.7% vs 7.6%). These values are similar to the limited findings in adults (CSF concentrations of 2.2 to 24.7 nM at drug doses of 0.1, 0.15, and 0.2 mg/kg/day given by continuous intravenous infusion to three patients) [29]. Transfer of 2-CdA into the CSF may be a "membrane-limited" process rather than a "flow-limited" one, which suggests that the amount of drug reaching the CSF is directly related to the length of time a concentration gradient is maintained between the plasma and the CSF.

Taken together, these results suggest a potential role for systemic 2-CdA therapy in the treatment of primary malignancies of the central nervous system, as well as for meningeal leukemia. However, much more work is needed to identify the factors (plasma concentration, length of exposure, etc.) that influence the amount of drug reaching the central nervous system.

Conclusions

The unique mechanism of action of 2-CdA, including its activity against resting as well as dividing cells, and its limited toxicity profile make it an attractive drug for further study in pediatric cancer patients. Future clinical challenges will be to identify the tumor types for which 2-CdA is especially effective, to develop other schedules of administration that could produce fewer side effects with equally good or better therapeutic results, and perhaps most important, to devise drug combinations that would enhance the clinical utility of this novel compound.

Supported in part by grant CA 20180 from the National Cancer Institute, by Orphan Products Development grant FD-R-000349 from the Food and Drug Administration, and by the American Lebanese Syrian Associated Charities (ALSAC).

References

1. Piro LD, Carrera CJ, Beutler E, Carson DA. 2-Chlorodeoxyadenosine, an effective new agent for the treatment of chronic lymphocytic leukemia. Blood 72: 1069, 1988.
2. Carson DA, Wasson DB, Taetle R, Yu A. Specific toxicity of 2-chloroadenosine toward resting and proliferating human lymphocytes. Blood 62: 737, 1983.
3. Hickish T, Serafinowski P, Cunningham D, Oza D, Dorland E, Judson I, Millar BC, Lister TA, Roldan A. 2′-Chlorodeoxyadenosine: evaluation of a novel predominantly lymphocyte selective agent in lymphoid malignancies. Br J Cancer 67: 139, 1993.
4. Carson DA, Wasson DB, Kaye J, Ullman B, Martin DW Jr, Robins RK, Montgomery JA. Deoxycytidine

kinase-mediated toxicity of deoxyadenosine analogs toward malignant human lymphoblasts in vitro and toward murine L1210 leukemia in vivo. Proc Natl Acad Sci USA 77: 6865, 1980.

5. Avery TL, Rehg JE, Lumm WC, Harwood FC, Santana VM, Blakely RL. Biochemical pharmacology of 2-CDA in malignant human hematopoietic cell lines and therapeutic efects of 2-bromodeoxyadenosine in drug combinations in mice. Cancer Res 49: 4972, 1989.
6. Santana VM, Mirro J Jr, Harwood FC, Cherrie J, Schell M, Kalwinsky D, Blakley RL. A phase I clinical trial of 2-CDA in pediatric patients with acute leukemias. J Clin Oncol 9: 416, 1991.
7. Carson DA, Wasson DB, Taetle R, Yu A. Specific toxicity of 2-chlorodeoxyadenosine toward resting and proliferating human lymphocytes. Blood 62: 737–743, 1983.
8. Carrera CJ, Terai C, Lotz M, Curd JG, Piro LD, Beutler E, Carson DA. Potent toxicity of 2-chlorodeoxyadenosine toward human monocytes in vitro and in vivo. A novel approach to immunosuppressive therapy. J Clin Invest 86: 1480–1488, 1990.
9. Bennett LL Jr, Chang C-H, Allan PW, Adamson JJ, Rose LM, Brockman RW, Secrist JA III, Shortnacy A, Montgomery JA. Metabolism and metabolic effects of halopurine nucleosides in tumor cells in culture. Nucleosides Nucleotides 4: 107–116, 1985.
10. Hirota Y, Yoshioka A, Tanaka S, Wantanabe K, Otani T, Minowada J, Matsuda A, Veda T, Wataya Y. Imbalance of deoxyribonucleoside triphosphates, DNA double-strand breaks, and cell death caused by 2-chlorodeoxyadenosine in mouse FM3A cells. Cancer Res 49: 915–919, 1989.
11. Parsons PG, Bowman EPW, Blakley RL. Selective toxicity of deoxyadenosine analogues in human melanoma cell lines. Biochem Pharmacol 35: 4025–4029, 1986.
12. Santana VM, Mirro J Jr, Harwood FC, Cherrie J, Schell M, Kalwinsky D, Blakley RL. A phase I clinical trial of 2-chlorodeoxyadenosine in pediatric patients with acute leukemias. J Clin Oncol 9: 416–422, 1991.
13. Kearns CM, Blakley RL, Santana VM, Crom WR. Pharmacokinetics of cladrabine 2-chlorodeoxyadenosine) in children with acute leukemia. Cancer Res 54: 1235–1239, 1994.
14. Huang M-C, Ashmun RA, Avery TL, Kuehl K, Blakley RL. Effects of cytotoxicity of 2-chloro-2′-deoxyadenosine on cell growth, clonogenicity, DNA synthesis, and cell cycle kinetics. Cancer Res 46: 2362–2368, 1986.
15. Griffig J, Koob R, Blakley RL. Mechanisms of inhibition of DNA synthesis of 2-chlorodeoxyadenosine in human lymphoblastic cells. Cancer Res 49: 6923–6928, 1989.
16. Parker WB, Bapat AR, Shen JX, Townsend AJ, Cheng Y-C. Interaction of 2-halogenated dATP analogs (F, Cl, and Br) with human DNA polymerases, DNA primase, and ribonucleotide reductase. Mol Pharmacol 34: 485–491, 1988.
17. Parker WB, Shaddix SC, Chang C-H, White EL, Rose LM, Brockman RW, Shortnacy AT, Montgomery JA, Secrist JA III, Bennett LL Jr. Effects of 2-chloro-9-(2-deoxy-2-fluoro-β-D-arabinofuranosyl)adenine on K562 cellular metabolism and the inhibition of human ribonucleotide reductase and DNA polymerases by its triphosphate. Cancer Res 51: 2386–2394, 1988.
18. Hentosh P, Koob R, Blakley RL. Incorporation of 2-halogeno-2′-deoxyadenosine 5′-triphosphates into DNA during replication by human polymerases α and β. J Biol Chem 265: 4033–4040, 1990.
19. Chunduru SK, Appleman JR, Blakley RL. Activity of human DNA polymerases α and β with 2-chloro-2′-deoxyadenosine 5′-triphosphate as a substrate and quantitative effects of incorporation on chain extension. Arch Biochem Biophys 302: 19–30, 1993.
20. Seto S, Carrera CJ, Kubota M, Wasson DB, Carson DA. Mechanisms of deoxyadenosine and 2-chlorodeoxyadenosine toxicity to nondividing human lymphocytes. J Clin Invest 75: 377–383, 1985.
21. Carrera CJ, Piro LD, Saven A, Beutler E, Terai C, Carson DA. 2-Chlorodeoxyadenosine chemotherapy triggers programmed cell death in normal and malignant lymphocytes. In Harkness RA (ed): Purine and Pyrimidine Metabolism in Man. VII. New York, NY, Plenum, p 15, 1991.
22. Robertson LE, Chubb S, Meyn RE, Story M, Ford R, Hittleman WN, Plunkett W. Induction of apoptotic cell death in chronic lymphocytic leukemia by 2-chloro-2′-deoxyadenosine and 9-β-D-arabinosyl-2-fluoroadenine. Blood 81: 143–150, 1993.
23. Johnstone AP, Williams GT. Role of DNA breaks and ADP-ribosyl transferase in eukaryotic differentiation demonstrated in human lymphocytes. Nature 300: 368–370, 1982.
24. Greer WL, Kaplan JG. Early nuclear events in lymphocyte proliferation. The role of DNA strand break repair and ADP ribosylation. Expl Cell Res 166: 399–415, 1986.
25. Jostes R, Reese JA, Cleaver JE, Molero M, Morgan WF. Quiescent human lymphocytes do not contain DNA strand breaks detectable by alkaline elution. Expl Cell Res 182: 513–520, 1989.
26. Huang M-C, Avery TL, Blakley RL, Secrist JA III, Montgomery JA. Improved synthesis and antitumor activity of 2-bromo-2′-deoxyadenosine. J Med Chem 27: 800–802, 1984.
27. Santana WM, Mirro J Jr, Kearns C, Schell MJ, Crom W, Blakley RL 2-Chlorodeoxyadenosine produces a high rate of complete hematologic remission in relapsed acute myeloid leukemia. J Clin Oncol 10: 364, 1992.
28. Santana VM, Hurwitz C, Blakley RL, Crom WR, Luo XL, Roberts WM, Ribeiro R, Mahmoud H, Krance RA. Complete hematologic remissions induced by 2-chlorodeoxyadenosine in children with newly diagnosed acute myeloid leukemia. Blood (in press).
29. Saven A, Kawasaki H, Carrera CJ, Waltz T, Copeland B, Zyroff J, Kosty M, Carson DA, Beutler E, Piro LD. 2-Chlorodeoxyadenosine dose escalation in nonhematologic malignancies. J Clin Oncol 11: 671–678, 1993.

Acute Leukemias V
Experimental Approaches
and Management of Refractory Diseases
Hiddemann et al. (Eds.)

The Role of 2-Chlorodeoxyadenosine (2-CDA) in the Treatment of Lymphoid Malignancies; Preliminary Observations

T. Urasiński*, I. Jankowska-Kurek, and E. Zuk

Introduction

2-chlorodeoxyadenosine (2-CDA) is a relatively new purine analogue selectively active against both resting and dividing lymphoid cells. The compound has been synthetized by Kazimierczuk et al. in 1984 [1,2]. Its mode of action remains the subject of current investigations. Laboratory data suggest that 2-CDA inhibits DNA synthesis in human lymphoblastic cells [3]. It has been shown by Petzer et al. that 2-CDA produces a marked inhibition of myeloid progenitor and lymphocyte colony-forming cells in a dose dependent manner [4]. Cross-resistance studies reveal a correlation between 2-CDA and the alkylator nitrogen mustard but no correlation between 2-CDA and doxorubicin, vincristin nor cytosine arabinoside [5].

Clinical data suggest that 2-CDA seems to be a drug of choice in the treatment of hairy-cell leukemia (HCL) and other lymphoid, as well as myeloid malignancies [6,7]. Most of clinical trials with 2-CDA have been conducted in adults; experiences in children are still limited [7,8]. This report is to summarize our preliminary observations on the role of 2-CDA in the treatment of various lymphoid malignancies.

Patients and Methods

The study comprised 8 patients (5 males and 3 females) aged 16–59 years (median 46 years), treated with 2-CDA since February, 1992. They were diagnosed as having: hairy-cell leukemia (HCL) – 3 patients, chronic lymphocytic leukemia (CLL) – 3 patients, and acute lymphoblastic leukemia (ALL) – 2 patients. Two of them – 1 patient with HCL and 1 patient with CLL were previously untreated, while the rest were non-responders or at relapse. Clinical characteristics of patients is given in Table 1.

2-CDA was given as a continuous infusion in the dose of 0.1–0.15 mg/kg/day for seven days, either alone or in combination with other agents (bleomycin, methylprednisolon). Observation was closed on November, 1993. The follow-up time was within the range of 3–20 months (median 8 months). Details of treatment are given in Table 2.

Results

Clinical remission, lasting from 2 to 19 months (median 5 months) was achieved in 6 patients: 3 with HCL and 3 with CLL. This could be proven

Table 1. Clinical characteristics of patients

Patient	Age	Sex	Diagnosis
1	49	F	relapsed HCL
2	46	F	relapsed HCL
3	42	M	HCL
4	46	M	refractory CLL
5	59	M	CLL
6	59	F	relapsed CLL
7	16	M	refractory ALL
8	42	M	refractory ALL

I Pediatric Department* and Clinic of Hematology, Pomeranian Medical Academy, 71–344 Szczecin-Poland

Table 2. Treatment results and its side effect

Patient	Treatment	Clinical remission	Follow-up	Histology	Side effects
1	2CDA/ 7 days	YES	5 mo.	PR	leukopenia trombocytopenia HZV infection
2	2CDA/ 7 days	YES	19 mo.	CR	leukopenia
3	2CDA/ 7 days	YES	4 mo.	no remission	leukopenia pneumonia
4	2CDA/ 7 days	YES	2 mo.	not evaluated	none
5	2CDA/ 7 days	YES	5 mo.	not evaluated	none
6	2CDA/ 7 days	YES	7 mo.	PR	leukopenia
7	2CDA/y days + bleomycin	NO	1 mo.	no remission	leukopenia
8	2CDA/ 7 days + methylprednisolon	NO	1 mo.	no remission	pancytopenia septicaemia death

by histology only in 3 cases: complete remission was observed in 1 patient with HCL, partial remission in 1 patient with HCL and in 1 with CLL. There was no histologic remission in third patient with HCL; bone marrow samples, obtained by trephine biopsy revealed persistent infiltrates of leukemic cells. Two patients with relapsed ALL did not respond to 2-CDA. Two patients were not histologically evaluated.

One of ALL patients, who did not respond to 2-CDA became pancytopenic and died of sepsis within 6 weeks from therapy. Leukopenia was the most common side effect, seen in 5 of 8 patients. This was complicated by infectious episodes in 3 cases (septicaemia, pneumonia, HZV infection). Trombocytopenia was observed in one patient. One patient developed maculo-papular rash on the skin of his face and chest. Results of treatment and its side effects are presented in Table 2.

Discussion

Management of lymphoid malignancies has changed during last two decades. The introduction of new drugs has significantly improved prognosis for patients with hairy cell leukemia and other lympho-proliferative disorders. One of this drugs: 2-chlorodeoxyadenosine (2-CDA) appears like a very promising compound in patients with hairy cell leukemia, chronic lymphocytic leukemia and low grade lymphomas [6, 9, 10]. The overall response rate in patients with HCL reaches 95% and the complete remission rate 82%. 2-CDA remains an experimental therapy, but its higher response rate and ease of administration may make it the first line treatment of choice [11]. Our observations seem to confirm this opinion; 2 of our patients with HCL, both with relapsed disease responded clinically to 2-CDA. Moreover, one of them has entered complete hematologic remission, lasting 19 months.

Nucleoside analogs are also of value in the treatment of chronic lymphocytic leukemia. Juliusson et al demonstrated that a total response rate of 67% could be achieved with limited toxicity in 18 patients with CLL [12]. Similar results were reported by Kay et al. They also noted that histology and prior therapy history did not seem to correlate with responses [13]. In our observation all 3 patients with CLL, including 1 with refractory and 1 with relapse d disease responded to 2-CDA.

This is not surprising that 2 patients with refractory ALL did not respond to 2-CDA. Refractory or relapsed all is still a disease of poor prognosis, even in children. Santana et al. demonstrated that the oncolytic response to 2-CDA is dose-dependent and that continuous infusion is necessary to maintain the desired plasma concentration [8]. Two reported patients were given continuous infusion of 2-CDA in standard doses of 0.15mg/kg/day, which could be not sufficient to produce a clinical response.

Most of reports underline a relatively low toxicity of 2-CDA. Even at higher doses a prohibitive nonhematologic toxicity does not occur [8]. Myelosuppression with leukopenia and trombocytopenia are the most common side effects [4, 12, 13]. This always carry a risk of overwhelming infections. The major reported morbidity associated with the use of 2-CDA are infections associated with neutropenia [14]. One of reported patients died of septicaemia, but his death could not be directly related to myelosuppressive effect of 2-CDA; he died in the phase of progressive disease. We also observed a case of HZV infection. Opportunistic infections seen in patients with lymphoid malignancies are probably related to the hypo-gammaglobulinaemia a T-cell immunodeficiency, which can be aggravated by the nucleoside analogs.

It seems to us that our preliminary observations confirm the opinion that 2-CDA is of clinical value in the treatment of HLC and CLL at different stages of disease.

References

1. Kazimierczuk Z, Cottom HB, Revankar GR, et al. Synthesis of 2'-deoxynucleosides via a novel direct Sereospecific sodium salt glycosylation procedure. J Am Chem Soc 1984, 106, 6379 -6382.
2. Kazimierczuk Z, Ilgo J, Hildebrand Z, et al. Synthesis and cytotoxicity of deoxyadenosine analogues: isomer distribution in the salt glycosylation of 2,6- disubstituted purines. J Med Chem 1990, 33, 1683–1687.
3. Griffig J, Koob R, Blakley RL. Mechanism of inhibition of DNA synthesis by 2-chlorodeoxyadenosine in human lymphoblastic cells. Cancer Res, 1989, 49, 6923–6928.
4. Petzer AL, Bilgeri R, Zilian U, et al. Inhibitory effect of 2-chlorodeoxyadenosine on granulocytic, erythroid, and T lymphocytic colony growth. Blood, 1991, 78, 2583–2587.
5. Nagourney RA, Evans SS, Messenger JC, et al. 2-chlorodeoxyadenosine activity and cross resistance pattern in primary cultures of human hematologic neoplasms. Br J Cancer, 1993, 67, 10–14.
6. Robak T, Grieb P. 2-chlorodeoksyadenozyna (2-CDA) – nowy lek przeciwnowotworowy i immunosupresyjny. Acta Haematol Pol, 1992, 23, 141–148.
7. Santana VM, Mirro J, Kearns C, et al. 2-chlorodeoxyadenosine produces a high rate of complete hematologic remission in relapsed acute myeloid leukemia. J Clin Oncol, 1992, 10, 364–370.
8. Santana VM, Mirro J, Harwood FC, et al. A phase I clinical trial of 2-chlorodeoxyadenosine in pediatric patients with acute leukemia. J Clin Oncol, 1991, 9, 415–422.
9. Robak T. Nowe analogi deoksyadenozyny w leczeniu nowotworów ukladu chlonnego. Przegl Lek, 1992, 49, 355–358
10. Castaigne S. 2-chlorodeoxyadenosine in haematological malignancies. Nouv Rev Fr Hematol, 1993, 35, 13–14.
11. Jaijesimi IA, Kantarjian HM, Estey EH. Advances in therapy for hairy cell leukemia. Cancer 1993, 72, 5–16.
12. Juliusson G, Liliemark J. High complete remission rate from 2-chloro-2'-deoksyadenosine in previous- ly treated patients with B-cell chronic lymphocytic leukemia: response predicted by rapid decrease of blood lymphocyte count. J Clin Oncol, 1993, 11, 679–689.
13. Kay AC, Saven A, Carrera CJ et al. 2-chlorodeoxyadenosine treatment of low-grade lymphomas. J Clin Oncol, 1992, 10, 371–377.
14. Keating MJ, O'Brien S, Kantarjian H, et al. Nucleoside analogs in treatment of chronic lymphocytic leukemia. Leuk Lymphoma, 1993, 10 suppl, 139–145.

Acute Leukemias V
Experimental Approaches
and Management of Refractory Diseases
Hiddemann et al. (Eds.)

Cytarabine Ocfosfate, a New Oral Ara-C Analogue, in the Treatment of Acute Leukemia and Myelodysplastic Syndromes

Ryuzo Ohno and YNK-01 Study Group

Abstract. Cytarabine ocfosfate (1-β-D-arabinofuranosylcytosine-5′-stearyl-phosphate, YNK-01) is a prodrug of Ara-C, and is slowly converted to Ara-C in the liver, releasing Ara-C into the blood over a prolonged period. It is resistant to both cytidine deaminase and phosphodiesterase. Its activity does not depend on the administration schedule and route, and unlike Ara-C, single administration is as effective as daily administration. YNK-01 is the first commercially available oral derivative of Ara-C in Japan. Phase I studies by single or 5-day consecutive oral administration revealed dose-dependent plasma levels of Ara-C, and the dose-limiting toxicities were thrombocytopenia and gastrointestinal side effects. Five daily oral administrations of 100 mg of YNK-01 gave continuous plasma Ara-C levels at around 1 ng/ml on day 1, and 2 to 4 ng/ml on day 5, plasma Ara-C was detected up to day 7. A phase II study with oral daily administration of 100–450 mg resulted in 2 CR (3%) and 10 PR (18%) in 58 evaluable patients with previously-treated AML, acute leukemia from MDS, CML-BC, hypoplastic acute leukemia or ALL, and 2 CR (4%), 6 GR (13%) and 5 PR (11%) in 45 evaluable patients with RAEB, RAEB-T and CMMoL. Major toxic effects were myelosuppression and gastrointestinal toxicity, including anorexia (35%), nausea/vomiting (19%), diarrhea (9%), malaise (18%), and elevation of GOT/GPT (9%), LDH (6%) and ALP (4%).

In spite of such disadvantages as unpredictable absorption due to nausea/vomiting, this newly developed orally administrable Ara-C analogue will be useful for leukemia, to which low-dose Ara-C is indicated, such as MDS and acute leukemia in elderly patients.

Introduction

1-β-D-arabinofuranosylcytosine (cytarabine) is one of the most effective drugs for the treatment of acute myeloid leukemia (AML) [1, 2]. Since cytarabine is rapidly deaminated to an inactive metabolite in vivo, a great deal of effort has been devoted to converting cytarabine into a compound which resists cytidine deaminase or is slowly metabolized to cytarabine. Recently, a series of phosphorylated cytarabine analogues were synthesized [3]. The derivatives having a long alkyl group on the phosphate moiety of 1-β-D-arabinofuranosylcytosine-5′-monophosphate were found to be effective against L1210 leukemia in mice. 1-β-D-arabinofuranosylcytosine-5′-stearylphosphate (cytarabine ocfosfate, YNK-01) (Fig. 1) having stearylphosphate as alkyl group, exhibited the most potent antitumor activity, and was proved to be slowly converted to cytarabine in the liver, releasing cytarabine into the blood over a prolonged period [4].

Phase I clinical and pharmacokinetic study of YNK-01 by single or 5-day consecutive oral administration revealed dose-dependent plasma levels of cytarabine, and the does-limiting toxicities were thrombocytopenia and gastrointestinal side effects [5]. In this paper the results of the phase II study of YNK-01 for patients with

Department of Medicine III, Hamamatsu University School of Medicine, Hamamatsu 431-31, Japan

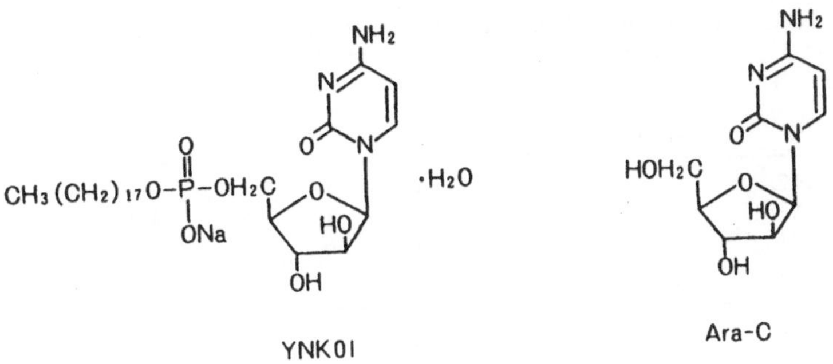

Fig 1. Cytarabine ocfosfate (YNK-01) and cytarabine

acute leukemia [6] and myelodysplastic syndromes [MDS) [7] in a multicenter study are summarized.

Patients and Methods

Patients with refractory AML, refractory acute lymphoblastic leukemia (ALL), blast crisis of chronic myeloid leukemia (CML-BC), acute leukemia which had derived from proven MDS (MDS-AL), hypoplastic acute leukemia, and MDS with more than 5% blasts in the bone marrow were entered to this study from 35 hospitals throughout Japan. Cytarabine ocfosfate (YNK-01) was supplied by Yamasa Shoyu CO. Ltd. and Nihon Kayaku CO. Ltd. in capsules containing 25, 50 or 100 mg of fosteabine. The drug was given orally after meals two or three times daily for 14 to 28 days until leukopenia (<1,500/cmm) or thrombocytopenia (<30,000/cmm) appeared.

The response for acute leukemia was evaluated by the standard criteria. The response for MDS was evaluated by the scoring method [7]; complete remission (CR) if the total points came to 75 or more with less than 5% blasts in the bone marrow, good response (GR) if the points came to 50 or more, partial response (PR) if 25 to 49 points were scored, and minor response (MR) if there was a score of 10 to 24. The response should be sustained for at least 4 weeks for CR and GR, and at least 2 weeks for PR.

Results

Fifty-eight patients with acute leukemia and 62 patients with MDS were evaluated for response. Patients' age ranged from 18 to 88 years with a median of 62 years. Among patients with acute leukemia, there were 23 AML, 17 MDS-AL, 9 CML-BC, 5 ALL and 4 hypoplastic leukemia. Starting daily doses were 100 mg in 14, 150 to 20 mg in 23, 200 to 300 mg in 16, and 400 to 450 mg in 5 cases. Among patients with MDS, there were 18 refractory anemia with excess of blasts (RAEB), 23 RAEB in transformation (RAEB-T) and 4 chronic myelomonocytic leukemia (CMMoL). Starting daily doses were 25 mg in one patient, 50 mg in 2, 100 mg in 22, 150 mg in one, 200 mg in 28, 300 mg in 7 and 600 mg in 1 case.

The treatment results for acute leukemia are shown in Table 1. Among 58 evaluable patients,

Table 1. Treatment result of YNK-01 in acute leukemia

Diagnosis	No. of cases	Response			CR	CR+PR
		CR	PR	MR		
AML	23	2	1	20	9%	13%
MDS-AML	17		5	12	0%	29%
Hypoplastic Leukemia	4		1	3	0%	25%
CML-BC	9		2	7	0%	22%
ALL	5		1	4	0%	20%
Total	58	2	10	46	3%	21%

Table 2. Treatment result of YNK-01 in myelodysplastic syndromes

Type	No. of cases	Response				Rate
		CR	GR	PR	MR	(CR+GR+PR)
RAEB	18	1	1	2	4	29%
RAEB-T	23	1	4	3	3	35%
CMMoL	4	0	1	0	1	25%
Total	45	2	6	5	8	27%

2 (3%) achieved CR and 10 (17%) obtained PR. CR was obtained only in AML. Days required to reach PR were 49±31 (mean±standard deviation) days, and to CR were 50±19 days. PR lasted for 31±28 days, and CR for 46±44 days. CR was obtained in patients receiving more than 200 mg/day, while PR was reached with doses from 100 to 450 mg/day.

The treatment results for MDS are shown in Table 2. Among 45 evaluable patients, 2 (4%) achieved CR, 6 (13%) GR, 5 (11%) PR and 8 (18%) MR. Days required to reach PR, GR and CR were 29±27, 70±45 and 87±22 days, respectively, PR, GR and CR lasted for 80±58, 110±61 and 208±202 days respectively. CR was obtained in patients receiving 150 or 200 mg/day, while GR and PR was reached with 100 mg/day.

Myelosuppression was observed commonly. The nadir of myelosuppression was reached around 3 weeks after the start of therapy and returned to the pretreatment levels 2 to 4 weeks after the cessation of therapy. Anemia was mostly macrocytic in nature. Other toxicities included nausea/vomiting in 19%, anorexia in 35%, and diarrhea in 9%, mild elevation of GPT in 9% and mild elevation of LDH in 6%, although direct correlation to YNK-01 of the latter two was not clear. GI toxicities were not entirely dose-dependent in all patients. However, they were apparently dose-dependent in individual patients, because they became milder when the daily dose of YNK-01 was reduced.

Discussion

Since YNK-01 exerts its antitumor activity by both parenteral and oral administration, and the minimal effective dose after oral administration was only about twice that obtained with intraperitoneal injection in mice [8], it has been introduced clinically as an oral form. A phase I study was performed by a single or by 5-day administration, and revealed that the dose-limiting toxicities were thrombocytopenia and gastrointestinal side effects [5]. Maximal tolerated dose was 900 mg for the 5-day administration. The pharmacokinetic study in the single oral administration of 800 mg of YNK-01 demonstrated that the cytarabine derived from it reached its maximal plasma level of 3.4 ng/ml 24 hours after the administration, and that the plasma half life of cytarabine was 20.9 hours. In the 5-day oral administration (300 mg), the cytarabine concentrations were maintained at levels ranging from 1 to 5 ng/ml during and until 2 days after the administration [5]. These results indicated that the blood levels of cytarabine after oral administration of YNK-01 might correspond to the blood levels of cytarabine achieved by low-dose (15 to 20 mg/day) continuous infusion of cytarabine.

The effect of YNK-01 in acute leukemia and MDS was observed when it was given at a dosage of 100 to 450 mg for more than 14 days. Long-term daily use of YNK-01, however, may not be advisable, because of the development of macrocytic anemia. Therefore, for such acute leukemia as in elderly patients who require no cure-oriented therapy, YNK-01 may be useful, if it is given at starting doses of 200 to 300 mg for around 2 to 3 weeks, and then restarted after the recovery of myelosuppression with an interval of 2 to 3 weeks. And also for fairly slowly progressive disease like MDS, YNK-01 may be useful, if it is given at starting doses of 100 to 200 mg for around 2 to 3 weeks, and then restarted after the recovery of myelosuppression with an interval of 2 to 3 weeks.

A disadvantage or oral forms of drugs is the unpredictable absorption in any individual patient. Although the pharmacokinetic study of YNK-01 in the phase I study showed a dose-dependent plasma level [5], actual absorption apparently would have varied in individual patients, since 20% of the patients vomited and

9% had diarrhea after the oral intake of YNK-01. Besides, the drug is supplied in capsules, the blood levels of the active form, cytarabine, would vary according to the body surface area of individual patients. In spite of these disadvantages, YNK-01 will be a useful drug in the treatment of certain types of malignancies including MDS and acute leukemia in elderly patients, to which continuous infusion or twice a day injections of low-dose cytarabine are sometimes indicated, and for which hospitalization is not necessarily required.

References

1. Champlin R, Gale PR: Acute myelogenous leukemia, Recent advance in therapy. Blood 1987; 69: 1551–1562.
2. Ohno R: Current progress in the treatment of adult acute leukemia in Japan. Jpn J Clin Oncol 1993; 22: 85–97.
3. Saneyoshi M, Morozumi M, Kodama K et al. Synthetic nucleosides and nucleotides. XVI. Synthesis and biological evaluations of a series of 1-β-D-arabinofuranosylcytosine 5′-alkyl or aryl-phosphates. Chem Pharm bull 1980; 28: 2915–2923.
4. Kodama K, Morozumi M, Saitoh K et al. Antitumor activity and pharmacology of 1-β-D-arabinofuranosylcytosine-5′-stearylphosphate: an orally active derivative of 1-β-D-arabinofuranosylcytosine. Jpn J Cancer Res 1989; 80: 679-685.
5. Fukuoka M, Miyazaki T, Yoshida Y et al. Phase I study of YNK-01 (1-β-D-arabinofuranosylcytosine-5′-stearylphosphate), Gan-to-Kagakuryouhou 1990; 17: 2213-2219.
6. Tatsumi N, Yamada K, Ohshima T et al. Phase II study of YNK-01 (1-β-D-arabinofuranosylcytosine5′-stearylphosphate) on hematological malignancies, Gan-to-Kagakuryouhou 1990; 17: 2387–2395.
7. Ohno R, Tatsumi N, Hirano M et al. Treatment of myelodysplastic syndromes with orally administered1-β-D-arabinofuranosylcytosine-5′-stearylphosphate. Oncol 1991; 48: 451–53.
8. Hori K, Tsuruo T, Naganuma K et al. Antitumor effects and pharmacology of orally administered N^4-palmitoyl-1-β-D-arabinofuranosylcytosine in mice. Cancer Res 1984; 44: 172–177.

Acute Leukemias V
Experimental Approaches
and Management of Refractory Diseases
Hiddemann et al. (Eds.)

Tumor Immunotherapy by IL-2 and IL-2 Gene Transfected Cells

A. Lindemann, F. M. Rosenthal, A. Mackensen, H. Veelken, P. Kulmburg, M. Lahn, and R. Mertelsmann

Introduction

Tumortherapy is based on a variety of treatment modalities. Directly operating cytoreductive approaches are designed to work either locally like surgery or radiotherapy, or systemically like cytotoxic drugs. Other ways of treatment are going to exploit the interaction of tumor and host. They are designed to block the host supply of hormones and growth factors the tumor relies on, to inhibit angiogenesis, or to recruit the intrinsic host defense system. The latter is translated into practice by immunotherapy that has made considerable progress recently. Aside from using monoclonal antibodies against tumor associated antigens (TAA) to mediate tumor cytotoxic effects, various approaches to recruit cytotoxic lymphocytes have been worked out.

Immunotherapy with IL-2

The availability of cytokines like IL-2 made it possible to modulate the function of immunocompetent cells and to induce cytotoxic lymphocytes capable to kill tumor cells in vitro. High dose IL-2 and IL-2 induced $CD3^-CD56^+$ NK cells, so called lymphokine activated killer (LAK) cells induced tumor regressions in various mouse tumor models. In humans this therapy was found to be active in selected tumor types especially renal cell carcinoma and malignant melanoma. About 15% of these patients responded with partial remissions, however, complete remissions were not but occassionally observed [1–4]. The limited efficacy of high-dose IL-2 therapy may be due to the fact that cytotoxic T-lymphocytes (CTL) are not readily induced but may even be inhibited in their function [5].

The appropriate recruitment of CTL, however, may be of major importance since TAA recognized by CTL have been identified and shown to be involved in tumor regression in mice and humans [6–8]. An adoptive transfer of these cells in mice has been shown to specifically protect from challenge with specific tumor and may also mediate regression of the established neoplasms [9,10]. In patients bearing tumors however, the malignant cells generally grow although TAA specific CTL are circulating in the peripheral blood [11]. Thus, it is a major question, how to recruit or induce autoreactive CTL specific for TAA and capable to kill tumor cells.

Since it is well known from in vitro experiments that low concentrations of IL-2 may preferentially stimulate CTL while the continuous presence of high concentrations induces IL-2 receptor downmodulation and unresponsiveness of T cells [12], we decided to use very low amounts of IL-2 for immunotherapy. Indeed we found that once daily subcutaneous (s.c.) administration of IL-2 ($1{,}8 \times 10^5$–$4{,}5 \times 10^6$ IU/m^2; Fig. 1) had stimulatory effects on T cell number and function as shown by cytokine release, surface marker expression and DTH responses as reported previously [13,14]. Intermittant administration, designed to prevent tolerance induction was found to be most appropriate for T cell activation. The specific role of scheduling of IL-2

Department Medicine I, Hematology and Oncology, University of Freiburg, Germany

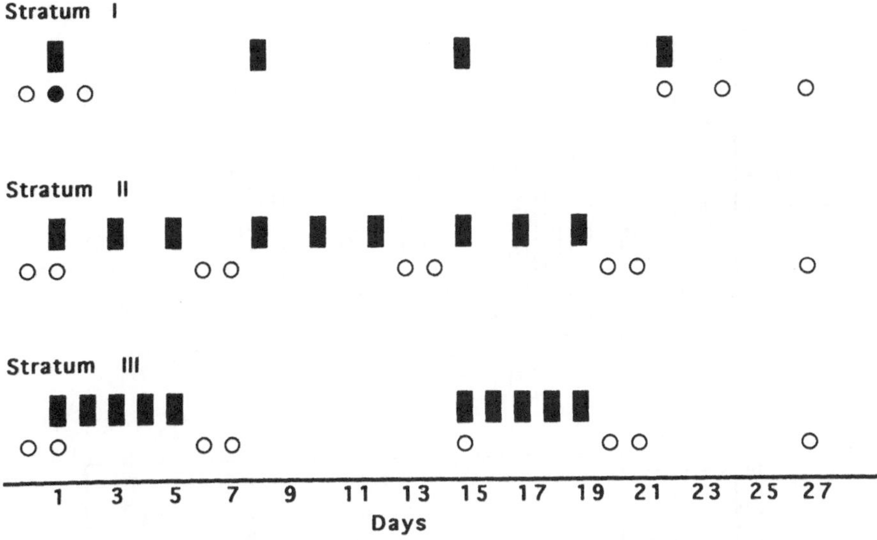

Fig. 1. Time frame of diagnostic procedures (open circle) and therapy (black rectangle) in strata I,II and III. A single dose of IL-2 was administered daily, once weekly, 4 doses (stratum I); thrice weekly every other day, 9 doses (stratum II); 5 times weekly every other week (stratum III). Three dose levels of IL-2 (A,B,C) were administered: 0.18, 0.9, and 4.5 MIU/m² resulting in 9 treatment groups (IA, IB, IC, IIA,...IIIC). Serum collections for cytokine and soluble receptor assays were done as indicated (open circle: once daily before start of therapy; hatched circle: every 8 hours)

is exemplified by the cytokine profile that differed considerably in patients treated thrice weekly every other day (Stratum II) from those treated sequentially for 5 days every other week (Fig. 1). While cytokine levels didn't increase in the third week of therapy in Stratum II or even decreased (sCD8, neopterin) despite continuation of therapy, some sort of priming was observed for sCD8 and Neopterin in patients treated according to Stratum III (Fig. 2). Only sTNF-RI levels exhibited an opposite profile in these patients. However, despite considerable activation of immunocompetent cells, this approach did not result in an improvement of therapeutic efficacy [13].

This outcome might be explained by the most recent model of T cell activation that describes the requirement of at least two signals for activation [15]. The first signal is provided by the T cell receptor (TCR) which binds the appropriate MHC presented peptide. The second signal for naive T cells is mediated by costimulatory molecules such as CD28 binding to CD80 (B7) on the target cell. For antigen specific CTL precusors

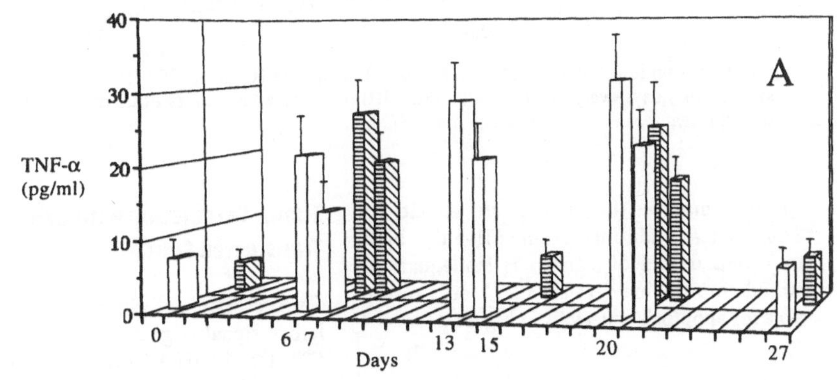

Fig. 2A

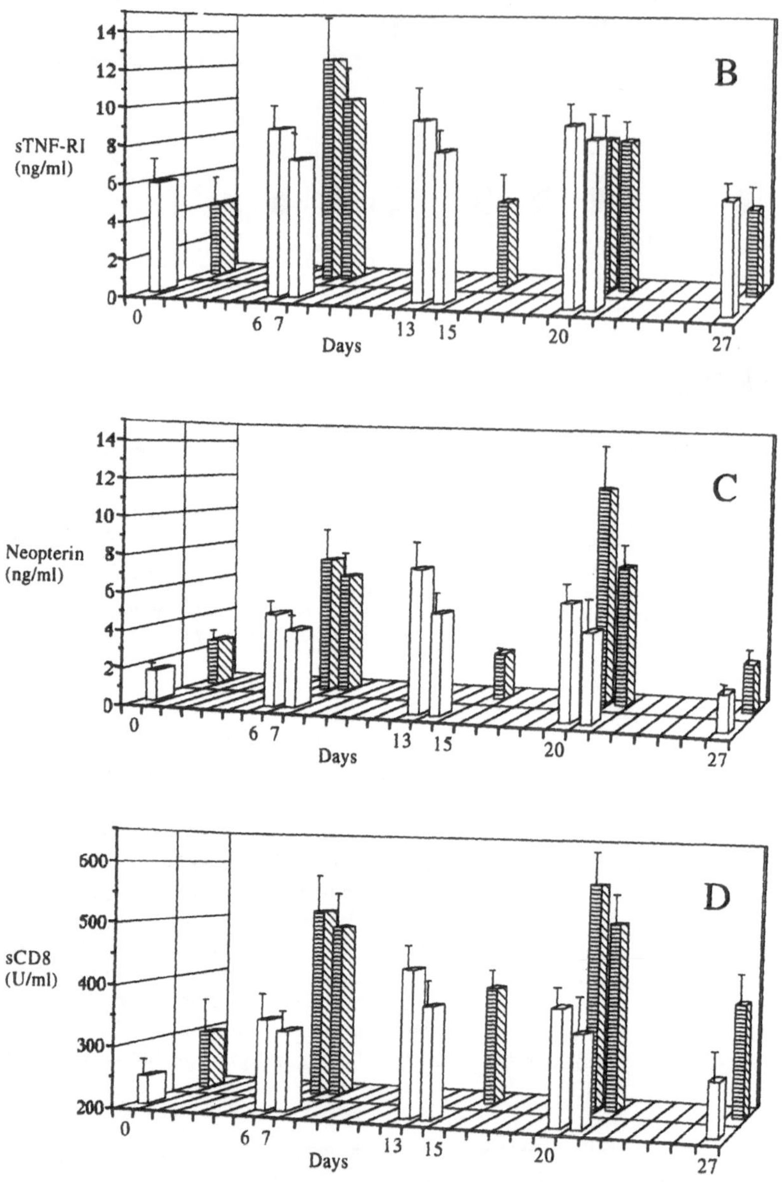

Fig. 2A–D. Serum levels of TNF-α (A), sTNF-RI (B), neopterin (C), and sCD8 (D) at 4.5 MIU/m² IL-2 administered daily for 5 days every other week (stratum III) or thrice weekly every other day for 3 weeks (stratum II). Values represent means of at least 4 patients ± SEM

(p) IL-2 may be the appropriate second hit. Thus, systemic administration of IL-2 that binds to T cells devoid of signal 1 is inadequate for stimulation and may even render T cells susceptible for apoptosis especially at higher doses.

Tumor Vaccination with Gene Transfected Cells

For successful activation of T cells, the costimulatory signal (signal 2) has to be provided to a CTL that binds a TAA (signal 1) on the tumor

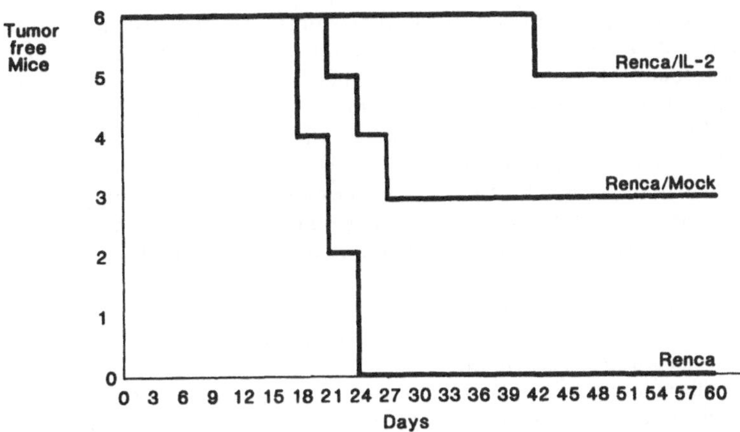

Fig. 3. Growth of Renca tumors in Balb/c mice after inocculation of 10^5 parental tumor cells in three animals (Renca) compared to a similar number of cells transfected with an IL-2 gene (Renca/IL-2; 24 000IU IL-2/10^6 cells/24h) or a mock construct in six mice each

cells itself or on a professional antigen presenting cell (APC). In order to meet these requirements Leder et al. and several other groups have transfected tumor cells with genes for T cell stimulatory molecules like IL-2, IL-4, IL-7, B7 and others [16–18]. These transfected tumor cells were found to be rejected and capable to induce tumor specific immunity. Immunized animals rejected later inocculated parental tumor cells by means of tumor specific CTL. However, the outcome of these studies was found to be highly dependent on the tumor model and the molecules transfected. In a lot of cases the effects could be mimicked by just using irradiated tumor cells for immunization [19,20].

We studied the CMS5-fibrosarcoma that was transfected by electroporation with an IL-2 gene to produce 400 IU IL-2/10^6 cells/24h. By inocculating 125.000 or 250.000 cells 0/3 and 1/3 mice, respectively developed a late occuring tumor, while all animals inocculated with parental malignant cells formed rapidly growing neoplasms. Since a higher amount of IL-2 at the vaccination site may even be more effective, we looked for a technique to achieve a more potent expression of the gene of interest. This was possible by using the receptor mediated gene transfer (RMGT) described by Cotton et al. [21]. It is based on inactivated adeno virus particles being linked by polylysine to a tranferrin ligand and the DNA of interest. The transfected DNA enters the nucleus at up to 50 copies, therefore expression is very high. However, due to an episomal localization expression is transient and decreases generally within 1–3 weeks down to base line levels.

Murine fibroblasts and renal cell carcinoma cells of the murine Renca tumor produced up to 50.000 IU of IL-2/10^6 cells/24h after receptor mediated IL-2 gene transfer with a decrease of expression down to 1.000 U on day 7. The IL-2 transfected Renca cells induced a major protection in mice with 5/6 rejecting the inoculum of malignant cells, while all animals treated with parental tumor cells developed rapidly growing tumors (Fig. 3). Mock transfected cells also mediated a certain degree of protection, probably due to the induction of neo-antigens by the transfection construct.

Interestingly some of these tumor models also work, when IL-2 is provided in a paracrine mode by bystander cells. Transfected fibroblasts admixed with tumor cells are highly effective in the M3 melanoma model with respect to rejection and induction of specific immunity as evidenced from studies by the group of Cotton et al. (personal communication). Bystander fibroblasts as a source of IL-2 that have also been studied by Lotze et al. [22] are more suitable in the clinical setting since transfection of primary human tumor cells is difficult and highly variable due to profound differences in the susceptibility of individual tumors.

Given the fact that induction of anti-tumor immunity has been demonstrated by different groups in mouse tumor models, we set off to develop a phase I clinical protocol. It is designed to use autologous tumor cells admixed with IL-2 transfected autologous or allogeneic fibroblasts as a source of IL-2. The cells will be mixed and irradiated with 100 Gy before being injected s.c. three times at 2 week intervals and as a boost one month later (Fig. 4). Tumor cells are prepared from renal cell carcinoma or melanoma biopsies as single cell suspensions. About 10^6–10^7 cells are generated per gram of tumor tissue and used after first passage for vaccination. Having worked up more than 50 tumor specimens, about 40% were found to generate enough cells for vaccination.

Fibroblasts are prepared from skin biopsies with 5×10^5 cells being released from $1cm^2$. The cells grow in culture with a doubling time of 4.3 days to more than 10^{11} cells within 10 weeks [23]. While preparation of fibroblasts is easily achieved, stable transfection of these primary cells by physical methods is of very low efficacy. Therefore we are currently using a transfected human fibroblast cell line as a paracrine source of IL-2 until transfection of autologous fibro blasts is feasible. So far three patients have been vaccinated according to this approach without systemic toxicity. Therapeutic effects and specific immune responses are currently analysed.

Prospects

So far the role of tumor vaccination in humans remains to be defined. The major issue concerns efficient stimulation of autoreactive CTLs in the tumor bearing host capable to exert tumor specific cytolytic effects. It is unknown whether these cells have to be induced at the tumor or vaccination site in contact with viable tumor cells or whether antigen presentation via professional APCs in the lymphnode is essential to produce Th_1 cells as a prerequisite for efficient CTL generation. In the latter case it might be advantageous to use professional APCs in the vaccine as suggested by work of Levitzky et al. [24].

Another aspect relates to the tumor mass as a parameter of response. From the mouse model it is quite clear that tumor immunotherapy is more likely to be efficient the smaller the tumor is [25]. Elegant studies by Riethmüller et al. [26] have substantiated this notion by demonstrating therapeutic effects of a complement binding monoclonal antibody directed against an epithelial antigen on colon carcinoma cells. In the situation of minimal residual disease (MRD) an improvement of overall survival was shown in this randomised study. Thus, MRD or the adjuvant situation is probably the setting of choice for immunotherapy.

Finally it has to be considered that standard vaccination with tumor lysates was shown to be most effective after previous cytotoxic treatment [27]. Whether this might be due to elimination of suppressor T cells or rather due to a shift in the ratio of Th1/Th2 helper T cells remains to be defined. The use of short term cyclosporine to induce GvHD like symptoms and perhaps graft versus tumor effects points the same direction. A means to provide minimal residual disease and a permissive environment for autoreactive T cells is chemotherapy. Thus, a favorable setting for tumor vaccination may be after high dose chemotherapy with or without peripheral

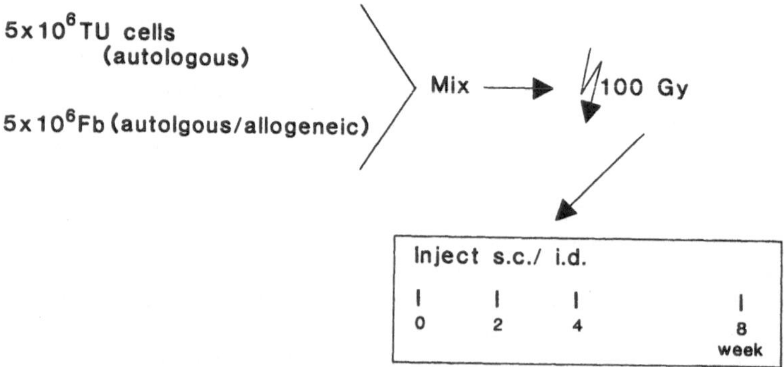

Fig. 4. Schedule for vaccination with irradiated autologous tumor cells and IL-2 gene transfected fibroblasts. Cells are injected subcutanuously (s.c.) while a minor proportion is given intradermally (i.d.) to monitor specific delayed type hypersensitivity reactions

blood stem cell transplantation to achieve maximal tumor reduction on the one hand and an immunological environment that allows optimal induction and expansion of autoreactive CTL with tumor specificity on the other hand. The feasibility of this approach will be tested in the near future.

References

1. Lindemann, A., Herrmann, F., Oster, W., and Mertelsmann, R.: Lymphokine activated killer cells, Blut 59: 1–10, 1989.
2. Lindemann, A., Höffken, K., Schmidt, R.E., Diehl, V., Kloke, O., Gamm, H., Hayungs, J., Oster, W., Böhm, M., Kolitz, E., Franks, C.R., Herrmann, F., and Mertelsmann, R.: A phase II study of low-dose cyclophosphamide and recombinant human interleukin-2 in metastatic renal cell carcinoma and malignant melanoma. Cancer Immunol. Immunother. 28: 275–281, 1989.
3. Veelken, H., Rosenthal, F.M., Schneller, F., von Schilling, C., Guettler, I.C., Herrmann, F., Mertelsmann, R., and Lindemann, A.: Combination of interleukin-2 and interferon- α in renal cell carcinoma and malignant melanoma a phase II clinical trial. Biotech. Therap. 3: 1–14, 1992.
4. Rosenberg, S.A., Lotze, M.T., Muul, L.M., Chang, A.E., Avis, F.P., Leitman, S., Linehan, W.M., Robertson, C.N., Lee, R.E., Rubin, J.T., Seipp, C.A. Simpson, C.G., and White D.E.: A progress report on the treatment of 157 patients with advanced cancer using lymphokine-activated killer cells and interleukin-2 or high-dose interleukin-2 alone. N. Engl. J. Med. 316: 889–897, 1987.
5. Wiebke, E.A., Rosenberg, S.A. Lotze, M.T.: Acute immunologic effects of interleukin-2 therapy in cancer patients: decreased delayed type hypersensitivity response and decreased proliferative response to soluble antigens. J. Clin. Oncol. 6: 1440–1449, 1988.
6. De Plaen, E., Lurquin, A., Van Pel, B., Mariamé, J.P., Szikora, R., Wölfel, T., Sibille C., Chomez, P., and Boon, T.: Tum-variants of mouse mastocytoma P815.IX. Cloning of the gene of tum-antigen P91A and identification of the tum-mutation. Proc. Natl. Acad. Sci USA. 85: 2274–2280, 1988.
7. van der Bruggen, Traversari, C., Chomez, P., Lurquin, C., de Plaen, E., van den Eynde, B., Knuth, A., Boon, T.: Gene encoding an antigen recognized by cytolytic T lymphocytes on a human melanoma. Science 254: 1643–1647, 1991.
8. Mackensen, A., Carcelain, G., Viel, S., Raynal, M.C., Michalaki, H., Triebel, F., Bosq, J., and Hercend, Th.: Direct evidence to support the immunosurveillance concept in a human regressive melanoma. J. Clin. Invest., 1994 in press
9. Greenberg, P.D., Klarner, J.P., Kern, D.E., and Cheever, M.A. Prog. Exp. Tumor Res. 32: 104–127, 1988.
10. Kast, W.M., Offringa, R., Peters, P.J., Voordouw, A.C., Meloen, R.H. van der Eb, A. J. Melief, C.J.M.: Eradication of Adenovirus E1-induced tumors by E1A-specific cytotoxic T Lymphocytes. Cell 59: 603–614, 1989.
11. Knuth, A., Wölfel, T., Klehmann, E., Boon, T., and Meyer zum Büschenfelde, K.-H.: Cytolytic T-cell clones against an autologous human melanoma: specificity study and definition of three antigens by immunoselection. Proc. Natl. Acad. Sci. USA: 86: 2804–2810, 1989.
12. Cantrell, D.A., Smith, A.: The transient expression of interleukin-2 receptors. Consequences for T cell growth. J. Exp. Med. 158: 1895–1905, 1988.
13. Lindemann, A., Brossart, P., Höffken, K., Flaβhove, M., Voliotis, D., Diehl, V., Hecker, G., Wagner, H., Mertelsmann, R.: Immunomodulatory effects of ultra-low-dose interleukin-2 in cancer patients: a phase-1B study. Cancer Immunol. Immunother. 37: 307–315, 1993.
14. Lindemann, A., Brossart, P., Höffken, K., Flasshove, M., Voliotis, D., Diehl, V., Kulmburg, P.,Wagner, H., and Mertelsmann, R.: Serum cytokine levels in cancer patients treated with different schedules of ultra-low-dose interleukin-2. J. of Immunother. 15: 225–230, 1994.
15. Janeway, Ch.A., and Bottomly, K.: Signals and signs for lymphocyte responses. Cell 76: 275–285, 1994.
16. Tepper, R.I., Pattengale, P.K. and Leder, Ph.: Murine interleukin-4 displays potent anti-tumor activity in vivo. Cell 57: 503–512, 1989.
17. Hock, H., Dorsch, M., Diamantstein, T., and Blankenstein, Th.: Interleukin 7 induces CD4+ T cell-dependent tumor rejection. J. Exp. Med. 174: 1291–1298, 1991.
18. Chen, L., Ashe, S., Brady, W.A., Hellström, I., Hellström, K.E., Ledbetter, J.A., McGowan, P., and Linsley, P.S.: Costimulation of antitumor immunity by the B7 conterreceptor for the T lymphocyte molecules CD28 and CTLA-4. Cell 71: 1093, 1992.
19. Dranoff, G., Jaffee, E., Lazenby, A., Golumber, P., Levitsky, H., Brose, K., Jackson, V., Hamada, H, Pardoll, D, and Mulligan, R.C.: Vaccination with irradiated tumor cells engineered to secrete murine granulocyte-macrophage colony-stimulating factor stimulates potent, specific, and long-lasting anti-tumor immunity. Proc. Natl. Acad. Sci. USA. 90: 3539–3543, 1993.
20. Chen, L., McGowan, P., Ashe, St., Jonston, J., Li, Y., Hellström, I., and Hellström, K.E.: Tumor immunogenicity determines the effect of B7 costimulation on T cell-mediated tumor immunity. J. Exp. Med. 179: 523–532, 1994.
21. Cotton, M., Wagner, E., Birnstiel, M.L.: Recceptor-mediated transport of DNA into eukaryotic cells. Meth. Enzymol. 217: 618–644, 1993.
22. Tahara, H., Zeh, H.J. 3rd, Storkus, W.J., Pappo, I., Watkins, S.C., Gubler, U., Wolf S.F., Robbins, P.D., Lotze, M.T.: Fibroblasts genetically engineered to secrete interleukin-12 can suppress tumor growth and induce antitumor immunity to a murine melanoma in vivo. Cancer Res. 54: 182–189, 1994.

23. Veelken, H., Jesuiter, H., Rosenthal, F.M., Mackensen, A., Kulmburg, Pl. Schultze, J., Wagner, E., Mertelsmann, R., and Lindemann, A.: Primary fibroblasts form human adults as target cells for ex vivo transfection and gene therapy. Human Gene Therapy, in press.
24. Huang, A.Y.C., Golumbek, P., Jaffee, E.M., Ahmadzadeh, M., Pardoll D.M., and Levitsky, H.: Host bone marrow derived cells, not tumor cells, present MHC closs I restricted tumor antigens in priming of antitumor immune response. J. of Cell. Biochem. Suppl. 18D, V168, 1994.
25. Golumbek, P.T., Lazenby, A.J., Levitsky, H.I., Jaffee, L.M., Karasuyama, H., Baker, M., and Pardoll, D.M.: Treatment of established renal cancer by tumor cells engineered to secrete interleukin-4. Science 254: 713–716. 1991.
26. Riethmüller, G., Schneider-Gädicke, E., Schlimck, G., Schmiegel, W., Raab, R., Höffken, K., Gruber R., Pichlmaier, H., Hirche, H., Pichlmayr, R., Buggisch, P., Witte, J.: Randomised trial of monoclonal antibody for adjuvant therapy of resected Dukes`C colorectal carcinoma. The Lancet 343: 1177–1183, 1994.
27. Berd, D., Mastrangelo, M.J.: Effect of low dose cyclophosphamide on the immune system of cancer patients: reduction of T suppressor function without depletion of the $CD8^+$ subset. Cancer Res. 47: 3317–3322, 1987.

Acute Leukemias V
Experimental Approaches
and Management of Refractory Diseases
Hiddemann et al. (Eds.)

Myeloid Differentiation Mediated Through New Potent Retinoids and Vitamin D_3 Analogs

E. Elstner[1], M. I. Dawson[2], S. de Vos[1], S. Pakkala[1], L. Binderup[3], W. Okamura[4], M. Uskokovic[5], and H. P. Koeffler[1]

Abstract. A focus of our investigations is to identify and study the biological activities and mechanism of action of novel vitamin D_3 analogs and retinoids. Our model system is clonal proliferation and differentiation of hematopoietic cells *in vitro*. All-*trans*-retinoic acid and 9-*cis*-retinoic acid are naturally occurring ligands of the nuclear retinoic receptors (RARs). In concert with binding of ligand, these receptors form heterodimers with the retinoic X receptor (RXR), and transactivate RAR/RXR-responsive genes. Synthetic ligands to the RAR and RXR receptors have been developed that selectively bind and activate RAR/RXR (TTAB) and RXR/RXR dimers (SR11217). We investigated the effect of these ligands either alone or in combination on clonal growth and differentiation of leukemic promyelocitic cell line HL-60 and AML blasts from patients. TTAB inhibited 50% clonal growth at an effective dose (ED50) of 5×10^{-9} M for HL-60 and 8×10^{-8} M for AML blasts. SR11217 at 9×10^{-6} M was necessary to achieve an ED_{50} for HL-60 cells and an ED_{50} for AML blasts was not reached. Combinations of both ligands showed no synergistic effects. Parameters of differentiation were also examined. Results paralleled those of clonal growth, showing that ligands selective for RXR-homodimers have little effect on either induction of differentiation or inhibition of clonal growth of leukemic cells. The differentiative and antiproliferative effects of retinoids on hematopoietic cells are mainly induced through RAR/RXR heterodimers, and development of therapeutic analogs should focus on this category of retinoids.

A variety of vitamin D_3 analogs were also analysed. The 1,25-dihydroxy-20-epi-vitamin D_3 [1,25$(OH)_2D_3$-20-epi-D_3] showed extraordinary activity; at 10^{-11} M, it inhibited clonal growth of 87% of HL-60 myeloblasts, 60% of S-LB1 (HTLV-1 immortalized human T-lymphocyte cell line) and 50% of leukemic clonogenic cells (CFU-L) obtained from patients with AML. Neither 1,25$(OH)_2D_3$ nor 1,25$(OH)_2$-20-epi-D_3 affected clonal proliferation of a HTLV-1 immortalized human T lymphocyte cell line (Ab-VDR), having non-functional 1,25$(OH)_2D_3$ cellular receptors (VDR). The activity of 1,25 $(OH)_2$-20-epi-D_3 to induce differentiation of HL-60 cells as measured by generation of superoxide and nonspecific esterase production, paralleled its antiproliferative activities. In contrast, this analog stimulated CFU-GM growth from normal human bone marrow. This analog appears to generate biological responses via the classical VDR pathway. Future studies should be directed to the identification of new compounds with greater differentiating abilities and less toxicity and to combined use of differentiating agents.

[1] Division of Hematology/Oncology, Cedars-Sinai Medical Center, UCLA, Los Angeles, Ca, USA
[2] Bio-Organic Chemistry Laboratory, SRI International, Menlo Park, Ca 94025, USA
[3] Department of Biology, Leo Pharmaceutical Products, Ballerup, Denmark
[4] Department of Chemistry, UC Riverside, Riverside, Ca 92521, USA
[5] Hoffman-LaRoche, Nutley New Jersey 07110, USA

Introduction

Conventional chemotherapy of hematologic malignancies is associated with severe complications. The successful treatment of acute promyelocytic leukemia (APL) with all-trans retinoic acid (ATRA) showed that triggering malignant promyelocytes towards terminally differentiated, non-dividing cells provided an effective method of inducing a remission without life-threatening side-effects [1–3]. In addition to retinoids, other ligands of the steroid-thyroid receptor superfamily, such as members of the vitamin D_3 family, also have cytodifferentiating actions in model system. A focus of our study is to identify and study the biological activities and mechanism of action of novel vitamin D_3 analogs and retinoids. Our model system is clonal proliferation and differentiation of hematopoietic cells *in vitro*.

Retinoids. Play a critical role in hematopoesis. Selective vitamin A (retinol, Fig. 1) deficiency induces anemia in humans and rats that is reversible by readministering retinol [4–6]. Retinol and its aldehyde derivative, retinal (Fig. 1) are relatively poor inducers of differentiation and inhibitors of proliferation of leukemic cells [7–8]. Oxidation of the polar terminus of these two retinoids to a carboxyl group yields ATRA, whereas oxidation and isomerization about the double bond adjacent to this group provides 13-*cis*-retinoic acid (13-*cis*-RA). Each of these retinoids is an effective modulator of hematopoiesis, being capable of inducing 50% of HL-60 cells to differentiate (ED_{50}) at 10^{-7} M [7]. Among the naturally occurring retinoids, ATRA has been considered to have the most potent affect on hematopoiesis. Incorporation of the double bonds of the side-chain into aromatic rings such as those of TTAB (Fig. 1) enhances the capacity of a retinoid to induce differentiation of HL-60 and other leukemic cells [8].

Cellular responsiveness to retinoids is conferred through two distinct classes of nuclear receptors, the retinoic acid receptors (RARs) and the retinoic X receptors (RXRs). The ATRA binds to RARs, but apparently does not bind RXRs [9]. The 9-*cis*-retinoic acid (9-*cis*-RA) (Fig. 1), a naturally occurring retinoic acid double-bond isomer, appears to be the ligand for RXR. For example, 9-*cis*-RA in conjunction with RXR transactivates a target gene up to 40 times more efficiently than does ATRA [10–11]. It also binds efficiently to RAR. Studies suggest that 9-*cis*-RA may be slightly more potent than ATRA in inhibiting the proliferation and inducing the differentiation of leukemic cells, as well as stimulating the clonal growth of normal myeloid committed stem cells *in vitro* [12–13]. For effective DNA binding and transactivation, the RARs must heterodimerize with RXRs [14–20]. In addition, RXRs form homodimers that have response element specificities that are distinct from those of RAR/RXR heterodimers [21]. This suggests that the two pathway of retinoic response could activate distinct sets of genes. Therefore, retinoids that selectively bind and activate either RAR/RXR or RXR/RXR could have a unique range and potency of action on hematopoietic cells.

Recently, retinoids have been synthesized that can selectively activate RXR homodimers, but do not necessarily affect RAR/RXR heterodimers [22]. The 4-[2-Methyl-1-(5,6,7,8-tetrahydro-5,5,8,8-tetramethyl-2-nap htalenyl)-1-propen-1-yl] benzoic acid (SR11217) is one of the more potent RXR/RXR-binding analogs

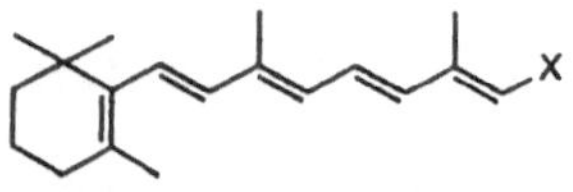

X

1 all-*trans*-retinoic acid X = CO_2H
2 retinol X = CH_2OH
3 retinal X = CHO

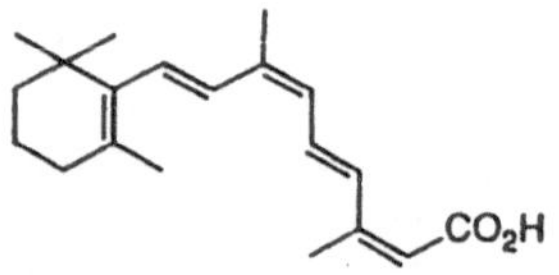

CO_2H

4 9-*cis*-retinoic acid

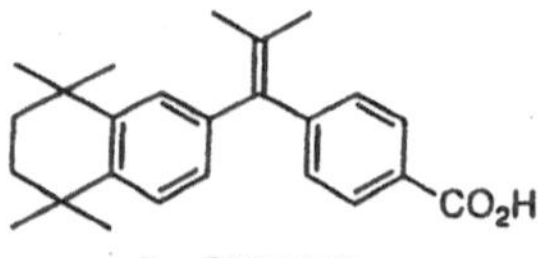

CO_2H

5 SR11217

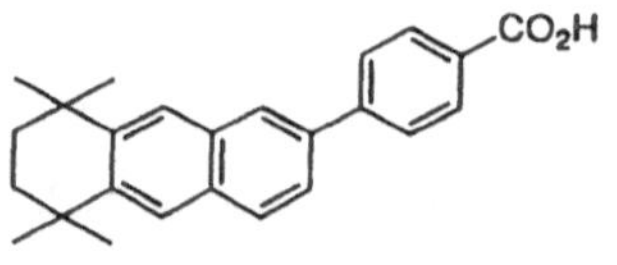

CO_2H

6 TTAB

Fig. 1. Structures of all-*trans*-retinoic acid, 9-*cis*-retinoic acid, TTAB and SR112117

(Fig. 1). This analog now allows us to define if myeloid leukemic differentiation is specifically induced by either the RXR homodimer or RAR/RXR heterodimer response pathway. This question is of strategical importance in the development of therapeutic analogs.

Vitamin D_3 analogs. The 1,25-dihydroxyvitamin D_3 [1,25$(OH)_2D_3$] is the physiologically active vitamin D_3 compound which is capable of regulating many genes that are critical for development and cellular differentiation. This biological response is mediated by binding to nuclear receptors for 1,25$(OH)_2D_3$ (VDR) [23–24], which belong to the same steroid-thyroid receptor superfamily as retinoids [25] and act as ligand-dependent transcription factors that bind to specific DNA sequences [26–27]. The 1,25$(OH)_2D_3$ induces differentiation of AML cell lines and inhibits their proliferation *in vitro*; but in contrast to retinoids, the leukemic cells are triggered towards macrophage-like cells [28–31]. The inhibition of leukemic cell growth by either 1,25$(OH)_2D_3$ or 1a$(OH)D_3$ has also been demonstrated *in vivo* in mice challenged with syngeneic leukemic cells [32–33]. Several small studies of oral administration of 1,25$(OH)_2D_3$ to myelodysplastic patients resulted in hypercalcemia before concentrations necessary for an antileukemic activity could be achieved [34–36]. Therefore, the research focus has been directed at finding new vitamin D_3 analogs with a more favorable therapeutic profile. In the present study, we have analyzed a variety of 1,25$(OH)_2D_3$ analogs *in vitro*.

The 1,25$(OH)_2$-20-epi-D_3 (code name IE and also known as MC1288), belongs to a new series of vitamin D_3 analogs, characterized by an inversion of the steriochemistry at carbon 20 [37]. It showed extraordinary activities in inhibition of clonal growth of HL-60 myeloblastic leukemic cells and leukemic myeloid clonogenic cells (CFU-L) from patients with AML. In contrast, analog IE stimulated growth of granulocyte-macrophage colony forming units (CFU-GM) from normal human bone marrow. In order to gain insights into the remarkable antileukemic activities of analog IE, we examined its ability to affect the clonal growth of a hematopoietic cell line having no functional VDR and also examined its ability to enter HL-60 cells and interact with a transfected vitamin D_3 response element (VDRE) attached upstream of a TK promoter-driven reporter gene [(chloramphenicol acetyl transferase (CAT)].

Material and Methods

Cells. The following cell lines were used in this study: HL-60 cells are late myeloblasts established from a patient with M-2 leukemia [38]. These cells express both RARs and RXRs [12, 14]. The S-LB1 is a HTLV-1 immortalized human T-lymphocyte line from a normal individual [39]; and Ab-VDR is a HTLV-1 immortalized human T-lymphocyte cell line established from a patient with vitamin D-resistant rickets type II (these cells have undetectable 1,25$(OH)_2D_3$ cellular receptors [40]. The cells were grown in tissue culture flasks in alpha-medium (Flow Laboratories, Inc., McLean, VA) with 10% fetal calf serum (FCS; Irvine Scientific, Santa Ana, CA) and 1% penicillin/streptomycin (Sigma Chemical Co., St. Louis, MO). Bone marrow was obtained from five healthy volunteers and peripheral blood blast cells were drawn from six patients with AML (M1, M1, M2,M2, M2, M5a), after their informed consent. The percentage of circulating blast cells was more than 98%.

Retinoids. The 4-(5,6,7,8-tetrahydro-5,5,8,8-tetramethyl-2-anthracenyl) benzoic acid (TTAB, SR3961) and 4-[2-methyl-1-(5,6,7,8-tetrahydro-5,5,8,8-tetramethyl-2-nap hthalenyl)propen-1-yl] benzoic acid (SR11217) and were prepared as previously described [41, 42]. Each analog was dissolved in absolute ethanol at 10^{-3} mol/l to create a stock solution that was then stored at −20 °C. Dilutions of the stock solution were made in alpha medium without FCS. The maximum concentration of ethanol in the culture (0.1%) did not influence either cellular growth or differentiation.

Vitamin D_3 analogs. The code names of the twelve analogs of vitamin D_3 employed in this study are shown on the Table 1. The 1,25$(OH)_2D_3$ (code name, C), analog Ro25-6760, analogs EO and V were synthesized at Hoffman-LaRoche, Nutley, NJ, USA; analog IE (also known as MC1288) and analog IC (also known as EB1089) were produced at the Departments of Biology and Chemical Research, Leo Pharmaceutical Products, Denmark; and analogs HF, HJ, HH, HL, HQ, and HR were provided by Drs. W. H. Okamura, K. R. Muralidharan, A. Craig and M. Curtin at UC Riverside. The compounds were dissolved in absolute ethanol at 10^{-3} mol/l, stored in aliquots at −20 °C and protected from light. For *in vitro* use, analogs were diluted in IMDM.

Table 1. Effect of vitamin D_3 analogs on cellular proliferation and differentiation of HL-60 cells

Chemical name of analogs	Brief name	Inhibition of Clonal growth	NBT	NAE
		$ED_{50}(\times 10^{-9}$mol/L)		
$1\alpha,25(OH)_2D_3$	C	16	37	70
$1\alpha,25(OH)_2$-20-epi-D_3	IE*	0.006	5.8	1.2
(22S)-1,25-$(OH)_2$-22,23-diene-D_3	HQ	11	60	ND
(22R)-1,25-$(OH)_2$-22,23-diene-D_3	HR	5.2	50	ND
$1\alpha,25$-$(OH)_2$-pre-D_3-9,14,19,19,19,d_5	HF	22	86	ND
$1\beta,25$-$(OH)_2$-3-epi-D_3	HH	NR	NR	ND
$1\alpha,25$-$(OH)_2$-3-epi-D_3	HJ	NR	NR	ND
$1\beta,25(OH)_2D_3$	HL	NR	NR	ND
1,25$(OH)_2$-24a,26a,27a-tri-homo-22,24-diene-D_3 IC*	0.23	3.0	5.5	
1,25$(OH)_2$-16ene-23yne-19-nor-26,27,F_6-D_3	RO 25-6760	0.5	4.0	5.0
1,25$(OH)_2$-16ene-23yne-26,27-F_6-D_3	EO	0.2	1.3	1.0
1,25$(OH)_2$-16ene-23yne-D_3	V	4.0	12.0	16.0

Abbreviation: NBT – nitroblue tetrazolium; NAE – non specific esterase; ED_{50} represents effective dose achieving 50% response
NR – ED_{50} was not reached; ND – none done; Standard deviation was less than 10% in all cases
*code names by Leo Pharmaceutical Prod. are MC 1288 for (IE) and EB 1089 (for IC)

Colony formation assay in soft agar and in methylcellulose. Human cell lines and normal bone marrow cells (NBMC) from 5 volunteers were cultured in a two-layer soft agar system as previously described [31]. For CFU-GM of NBMCs, we added 5×10^{-5}mol/l b-mercaptoethanol (Sigma, St. Louis, MO). As a source of CSF for CFU-GM, 200 pM of human recombinant GM-CSF was used (generous gift from S. Clark, Genetics Institute, Boston, MA). The circulating clonogenic blast cells from 5 AML patients (CFU-L) were cultured in IMDM, 20% FCS, 10% PHA-LCM and 10^{-4} mol/l b-mercaptoethanol in a final concentration of 0.8% methylcellulose (Mithocel MC 4000 cP, Fluka AG, Buchs SG). Cell concentrations were 2×10^3/plate for leukemic cell lines and 1×10^5 for NBMC and AML blasts. After 10 days of incubation at 37 °C in a humidified atmosphere containing 5% CO_2 in air, colonies were counted.

Studies of induction of differentiation. Differentiation of HL-60 was assessed by ability of cells to produce superoxide as measured by reduction of nitroblue tetrazolium (NBT) and to stain with α-naphthyl acetate esterase (NAE) (Sigma, St. Louis, MO). The cells were grown in liquid culture with alpha-medium, 10% FCS for six days in a humidified atmosphere, 5% CO_2 at 37 °C. The differentiation of AML blasts by morphology was studied using cells from suspension culture and from CFU-L. Cells were cytocentrifuged onto microscope-slides and slides were stained with Diff-Quik Set (Baxter).

Transfection and assay of CAT (chloramphenicol acetyl transferase) activity. The HL-60 cells were grown in alpha-medium with 5% FCS and 1% penicillin/streptomycin. After washing in serum-free medium, 2.5×10^7 cells were transfected by electroporation with 35 μg of pBL-CAT2-VDRE plasmid [43–44]. The reporter consists of synthesized complementary sequences comprising human osteocalcin gene between −509 and −489 (3 repeats) fused to pB-CAT2 expression vector containing thymidine kinase promotor. The cells were cultured with vitamin D_3 compounds, IE (20-epi-vitamin D_3) and C [$1,25(OH)_2D_3$] at 10^{-11} to 10^{-7} M for 48 hours in serum-free conditions, harvested, and CAT lysates prepared. CAT activity was assayed by thin layer chromatography and autoradio graphy.

Results

Effects of retinoids on clonal proliferation and differentiation of HL-60 cells. Dose-response effects of RAR/RXR-specific retinoid (TTAB) and RXR/RXR-specific retinoid (SR11217) on the clonogenic proliferation of HL-60 leukemic promyelocytes are shown on Figs. 2A and 2B. TTAB is a potent inhibitor of clonal proliferation of HL-60 cells, causing a 50% inhibition of clonal growth (ED_{50}) of HL-60 cells at about 2×10^{-9} M (Fig. 2A). In contrast, SR11217 is nearly 1000-fold less potent, with an ED_{50} of about 2.5×10^{-6} M (Fig. 2A). We looked for possible synergy between the two analogs (Fig. 2A, 2B). TTAB at either 10^{-11} or 10^{-10} M alone or with increasing concentrations of SR11217 (10^{-11}–10^{-5} M) had no effect on HL-60 clonal growth (Fig. 2A). TTAB (10^{-9} M) in the presence of high concentrations of SR11217 (5×10^{-7}–7.5×10^{-6} M) inhibited clonal growth of HL-60 cells in either an additive or less than additive fashion (Fig. 2B).

The HL-60 cells differentiate toward granulocytes when cultured in the presence of retinoids. A marker of cellular differentiation is the production of superoxide, which can be measured by the ability to reduce NBT. Using this as a marker, we examined the ability of the retinoids to induce differentiation of HL-60 cells (Fig. 3). The TTAB induced differentiation with a half-maximal effect of about 1×10^{-9} M. In contrast, SR11217 had little effect on the ability to induce differentiation of HL-60 cells, with only a small effect observed at 10^{-6} M (Fig. 3). TTAB at either 10^{-10} M (Fig. 4) or 10^{-11} M (data not shown), and with different concentrations of SR11217 (10^{-11} – 10^{-6} M), had either no effect or was less than additive in inducing HL-60 cells to reduce NBT.

Effect of retinoids on clonal proliferation of leukemic human myeloid clonogenic cells (CFU-L) and on differentiation of leukemic cells. We studied the effect of SR11217 alone and in the combination with TTAB (10^{-8} to 10^{-6} M) on the CFU-L from 3 patients with AML (Fig. 4). TTAB inhibited proliferation of clonogenic leukemic cells with an ED_{50} of about 8×10^{-8} M. SR11217 alone showed no inhibitory effect at 10^{-8} – 10^{-7} M and only 15% inhibition at 10^{-6} M. In combination with TTAB (10^{-9} M), SR11217 inhibited the CFU-L with an ED_{50} of about 5×10^{-6} M. TTAB induced differentiation of AML blasts in suspension culture and from

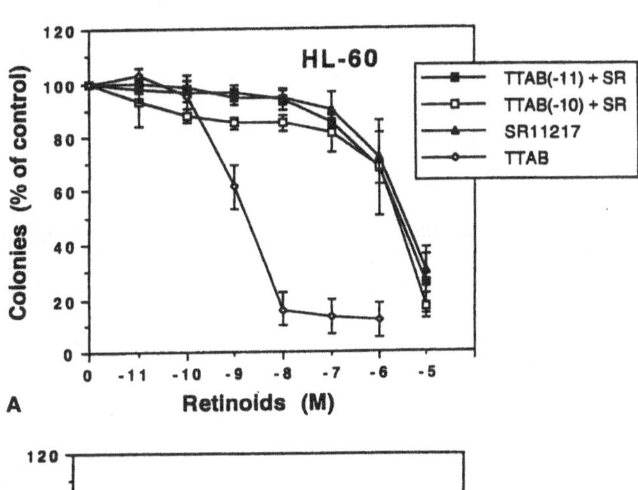

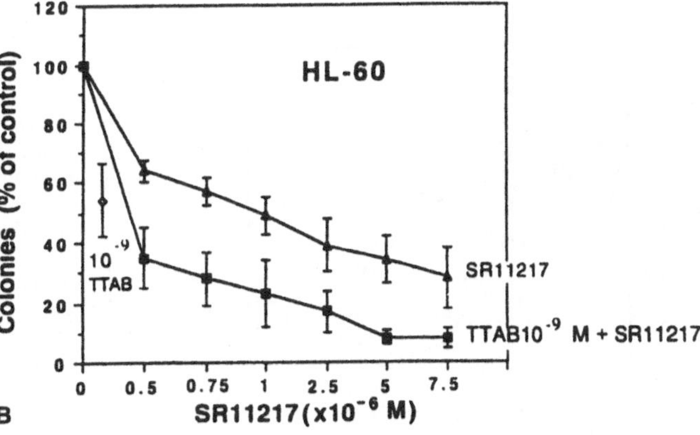

Fig. 2. Effect of retinoids on clonal proliferation of HL-60. Results are expressed as a percent of control plates not exposed to retinoid. Panel A: Each point represents mean ± SD of five experiments with triplicate plates for each point. SR11217, (▲); TTAB, (◇); TTAB 10^{-11} M + SR11217, (■); TTAB 10^{-10} M + SR11217, (□). Panel B: Each point represents mean of three experiments. SR11217, (▲); TTAB 10^{-9} M + SR11217, (■); and 10^{-9} M TTAB alone, (◇)

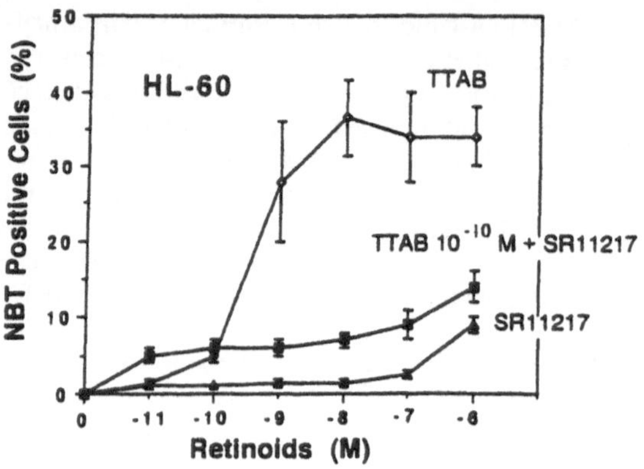

Fig. 3. Effect of retinoids on differentiation of HL-60 cells. Results are expressed as a percent of HL-60 cells that reduces NBT. Each point represents the mean of three experiments

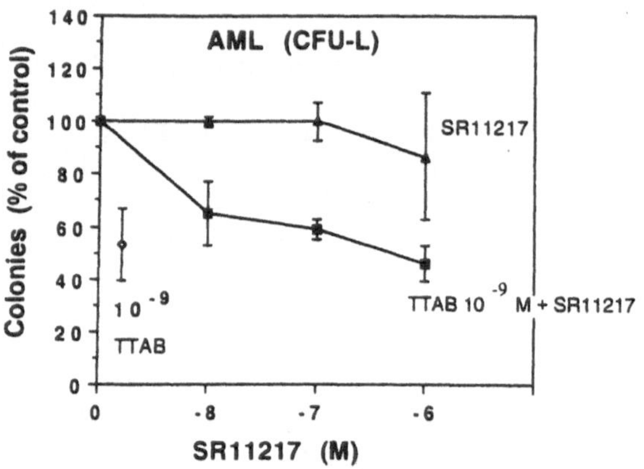

Fig. 4. Effect of retinoids on clonal proliferation of AML cells. Results are expressed as a percent of control plates not exposed to retinoid. Results represent the mean clonal growth of 3 AML patients with triplicate plates for each point

CFU-L in methylcellulose to band forms as well as granulocytes. No differentiation was observed in cultures either without retinoids or with SR11217 alone.

Effect of Vitamin D_3 anologs on clonal growth of HL-60 cells. Previous studies have shown that $1,25(OH)_2D_3$ could inhibit the clonal proliferation of HL-60 cells [28, 29, 31]. We examined the effect of novel vitamin D_3 analogs to inhibit the clonal proliferation of myeloid leukemic cell line HL-60 in soft agar (Fig. 5).

Concentrations that inhibited 50% growth (ED_{50}) are shown on Table 1. Seven analogs (C,

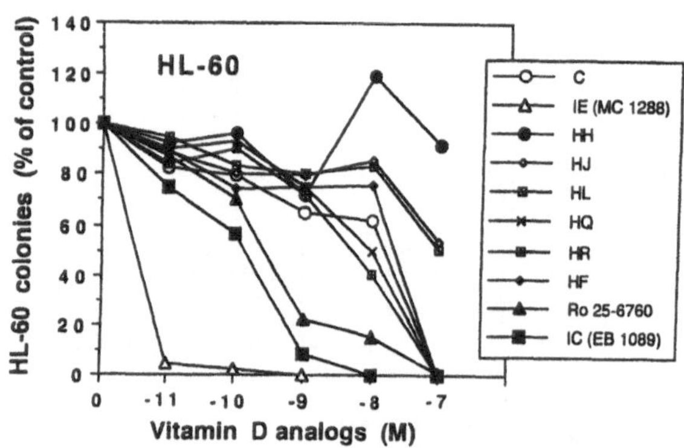

Fig. 5. Effect of vitamin D_3 compounds on clonal proliferation of HL-60 cells. Results are expressed as a percentage of control plates containing no vitamin D_3 compounds. Each point represents a mean of at least three independent experiments with triplicate dishes. Control cultures contained 245 ± 28 (mean ± SD) colonies. SD is not placed on figure for simplicity of reading the graph

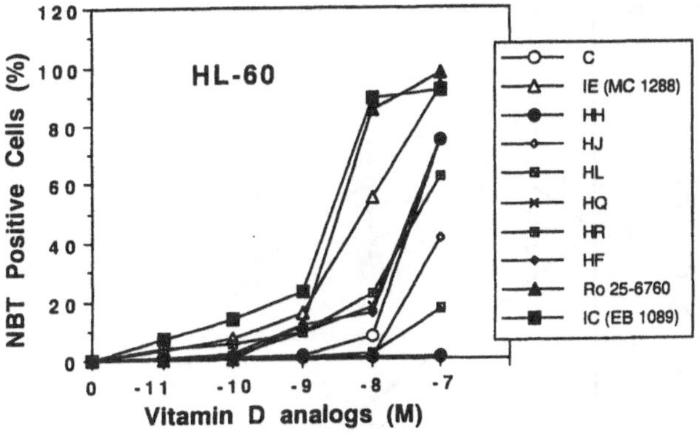

Fig. 6. Effect of vitamin D_3 analogs on differentiation of HL-60 cells as measured by reduction of nitroblue tetrazolium (NBT). Results are expressed as a percentage of HL-60 cells that reduced NBT. Each point represents a mean of at least three independent experiments. Control cells had less than 1% NBT-positive cells. The SD is not placed on figure for simplicity of reading the graph

IE, HQ, HR, HF, IC, Ro 25-6760) inhibited clonogenic proliferation of HL-60 cells in a dose-dependent fashion; the remaining three analogs (HH, HJ, HQ) had little affect on the clonal growth of HL-60 cells. The reference compound $1,25(OH)_2D_3$ (C), achieved a 50% inhibition of clonal growth at 1.6×10^{-8} M. The most potent analog was IE ($1,25(OH)_2$-20-epi-D_3), having an ED_{50} of about 6×10^{-12} M (1% colony formation at 1×10^{-11} M). Therefore, an alteration of stereochemistry at carbon 20 increased potency over 2,600-fold. The rank order of vitamin D_3 analogs from most to least potent in terms of clonal growth was IE≫IC = Ro25-6760 > HR > HQ > C > HF > HL = HJ > HH.

Effect of vitamin D_3 analogs on differentiation of HL-60 cells. The HL-60 cells are able to differentiate toward monocytes/macrophages when cultured in the presence of $1,25(OH)_2D_3$ [28–29]. The Ro25-6760 had nearly the same activity as IC with an ED_{50} for NBT reduction of 3×10^{-9} M (Fig. 6) and an ED_{50} induction of NSE of 5×10^{-9} M (Fig. 7). Compound IE has an ED_{50} of 5.8×10^{-9} M for NBT reduction and 1.2×10^{-9} M for induction of NAE (Table 1, Fig. 6, 7). The $1,25(OH)_2D_3$ was a weaker inducer of differentiation of HL-60 cells, with the ED_{50} for NBT and NAE of 20×10^{-9} M and 7×10^{-8} M, respectively (Table 1, Fig. 6, 7).

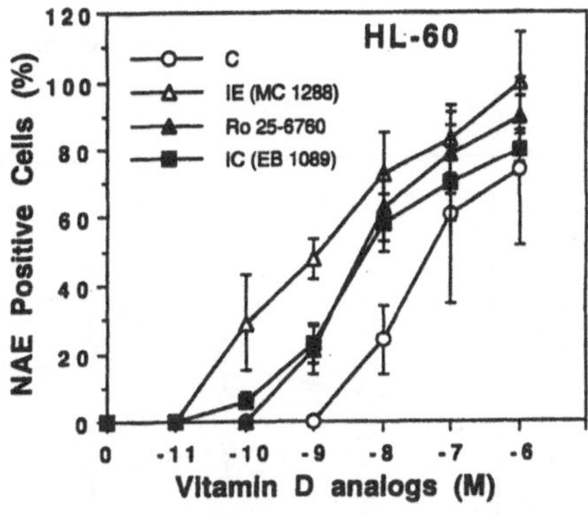

Fig. 7. Effect of vitamin D_3 analogs on differentiation of HL-60 cells. Results are expressed as percentage of HL-60 cells that developed NAE activity. Each point represents a mean of at least three independent experiments. Control cells had less than 1% NAE-positive cells. The SD is not placed on figure for simplicity of reading the graph

Effect of $1,25(OH)_2D_3$ (C) and 20-epi-$1,25(OH)_2D_3$ (IE) on clonal proliferation of T-lymphocyte cell lines S-LB1 and Ab-VDR. We have used HTLV-I immortalized T-lymphocytes from a normal individual (S-LB1) as well as from a patient with vitamin D-resistant rickets type II (Ab-VDR). Cells of this latter individual has non-functional vitamin D_3 receptors [40].The 20-epi-$1,25(OH)_2D_3$ (IE) had a strong inhibitory effect on clonogenic growth of S-LB1 cell line with an ED_{50} of 3.5×10^{-11} M (Fig. 8). The $1,25(OH)_2D_3$ slightly stimulated the clonal growth of S-LB1 cells at 10^{-11} – 10^{-10} M and inhibited the clonal proliferation at 10^{-10} –10^{-7} M, with an ED_{50} of 6×10^{-9} M. Neither 20-epi-$1,25(OH)_2D_3$ (IE) nor $1,25(OH)_2D_3$ (C) (10^{-11}–10^{-7} M) effected growth of VDR-defective Ab-VDR cells (Fig.8).

Effect of $1,25(OH)_2D_3$ (C) and 20-epi-$1,25(OH)_2D_3$ (IE) on clonal proliferation of normal (CFU-GM) and leukemic (CFU-L) human myeloid clonogenic cells. The normal committed myeloid stem cells, CFU-GM, were stimulated in their clonal growth by $1,25(OH)_2D_3$ (C) and 20-epi-$1,25(OH)_2D_3$ (IE) at 10^{-10} M to 10^{-8} M, with peak enhancement of growth at 10^{-9} M (Fig. 9). At 10^{-7} M, both compounds

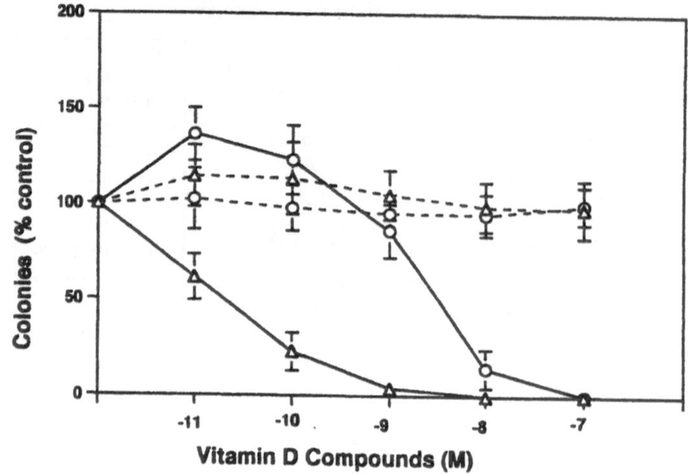

Fig. 8. Effect of 1,25$(OH)_2$-20epi-D_3 (IE) (---) and 1,25$(OH)_2D_3$ (C) (-○-) on clonal proliferation of T-lymphocyte cell line, S-LB1 (-) and Ab-VDR (---). Control cultures contained 453 ± 30 (mean ± SD) colonies for S-LB1 and 528 ± 42 colonies for Ab-VDR. The Ab-VDR cells have nonfunctional VDR

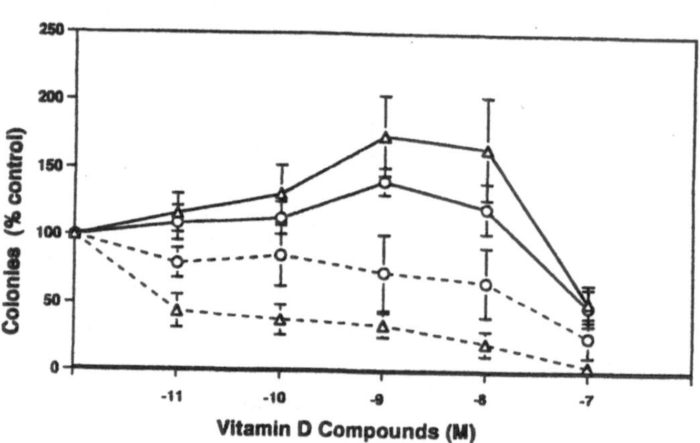

Fig. 9. Effect of 1,25$(OH)_2$-20epi-D_3 (IE) (---) and 1,25$(OH)_2D_3$ (C) (-○-) on clonal proliferation of leukemic clonogenic cells (CFU-L) from 4 patients with AML (---), and from 5 normal volunteers on myeloid clonogenic cells (CFU-GM) (-). Control cultures contained 262 ± 32 (mean ± SD) colonies for CFU-L and 89 ± 16 colonies for CFU-GM

inhibited clonal growth of CFU-GM. Further experiments examined the effects of C and IE on the clonal growth of CFU-L from individuals with acute myeloid leukemia. Both compounds (10^{-11} to 10^{-7} M) inhibited the proliferation of CFU-L with a 50% inhibition of clonogenic cells at about 10^{-11} M for 20-epi-1,25$(OH)_2D_3$ (IE) and 5×10^{-8} M for 1,25$(OH)_2D_3$ (C).

Effect of compound IE on transcriptional activation. The vitamin D response element (VDRE) was placed in front of a minimal thymidine kinase promoter of the reporter gene CAT. This construct was transfected into HL-60 cells. In the absence of either 1,25$(OH)_2D_3$ (C) or 20-epi-1,25$(OH)_2D_3$ (IE), almost no CAT activity was detectable (Fig. 10A, 10B). Both C and IE increased CAT activity in a dose-response manner. At 10^{-7} M, both increased CAT activity nearly 16-fold as compared to cells transfected with reporter vector in the absence of vitamin D_3 compounds (Fig. 10A, 10B).

Discussion

This study examines the effects of several novel retinoids and vitamin D_3 analogs on differentiation and proliferation of myeloid leukemic cells *in vitro*. Retinoids bind RAR and/or RXR, vitamin D_3 analogs bind VDR. Both RAR and VDR bind RXR. In the presence of 9-*cis*-retinoic acid, RXR can form either RAR/RXR heterodimers [15] or RXR-RXR homodimers. These ligand-receptor complexes can have specificities for different response elements that result in activating distinct sets of genes. We previously showed that 9-*cis*-retinoic acid was slightly more potent

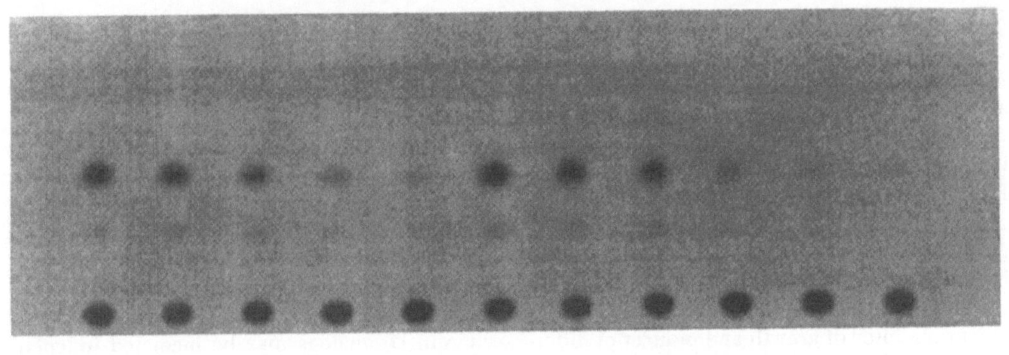

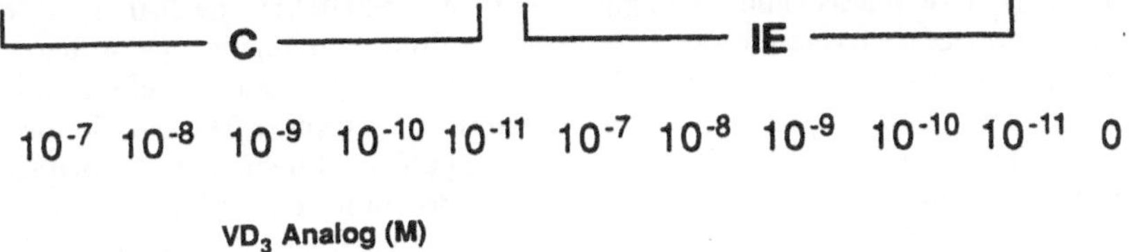

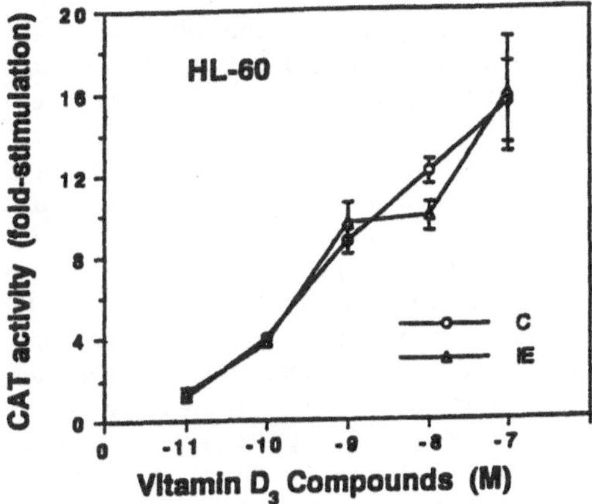

Fig. 10A,B. Effect of 1,25$(OH)_2$-20epi-D_3 (IE) and 1,25$(OH)_2D_3$ (C) on transcriptional activation as measured by CAT assay using transient transfection system in HL-60 cells

than all-*trans* retinoic acid in inhibiting the proliferation and inducing the differentiation of both myeloid leukemia cell lines and fresh acute promyelocytic leukemia cells [12, 13]. This slight increase in activity, however, is unlikely to have resulted from activation of a unique set of myeloid differentiation genes that relied on RXR/RXR homodimerization. Indeed, we show here that RXR/RXR-specific retinoids such as SR11217 [12] have very little ability to induce differentiation of HL-60 cells. In contrast, the RAR/RXR-specific retinoid TTAB [22] is a potent inducer of differentiation of these cells. The RAR/RXR-specific ligand TTAB was approximately 1000-fold more potent than the RXR/RXR-specific ligand SR11217 at inhibiting the proliferation and inducing the differentiation of HL-60 cells. We also examined the effect of these two retinoids on fresh leukemic cells from patients and noted similar effects; therefore, their actions do not appear to be cell type specific to only HL-60 cells. The results suggest that genes with RXR/RXR-specific response elements are not pivotal to myeloid differentiation. Therefore, 9-*cis*-retinoic acid probably does not attain its enhanced potency for induction of leukemic differentiation as compared to either all-*trans* retinoic acid or TTAB, by forming complexes with RXR/RXR homodimers. Indirect evidence of the importance of RARa in differentiation of myeloid cells is that alteration of the gene, by fusion with PML gene, inhibits differentiation in patients with APL. Future experiments that attempt to develop retinoids that enhance differentiation and inhibit proliferation of leukemic cells, as well as probably other types of cancer cells, should focus on RAR/RXR-binding analogs, rather than those that bind to RXR/RXR.

The 20-epi-1,25(OH)$_2$D$_3$ belongs to the new group of vitamin D$_3$ analogs, characterized by an inverted steriochemistry at carbon 20 in the side-chain. A prior study showed that IE was a potent inhibitor of growth and inducer of differentiation of U937 monoblasts and strongly modulated activation of cytokine-mediated T-lymphocytes; and in addition, IE exerted calcemic effects in rats comparable to those of 1,25(OH)$_2$D$_3$ [37]. In our study, we examined the biological profiles of eight analogs of 1,25(OH)$_2$D$_3$ and indentified that 1,25(OH)$_2$-20-epi-D$_3$ (IE) is the most potent modulator of clonal growth and cellular differentiation of HL-60 cells that has been reported to date. The 1,25(OH)$_2$-epi-20-D$_3$ (IE) was at least 2,600-fold more potent than 1,25(OH)$_2$D$_3$ (C) in inhibition of clonal growth of HL-60 cells. In addition, IE was approximately 5,000-fold more effective than 1,25(OH)$_2$D$_3$ (C) in preventing clonal proliferation of leukemic cells from patients with acute myelogenous leukemia. For reasons that are unclear, 1,25(OH)$_2$-20-epi-D$_3$ (IE) was only 6–9-fold more active than 1,25(OH)$_2$D$_3$ (C) in the induction of differentiation of HL-60. We have observed that other vitamin D$_3$ analogs also inhibited proliferation more effectively than it fostered cellular differentiation [45–46]. In contrast to the effect on leukemic cells, 1,25(OH)$_2$-20-epi-D$_3$ (IE, 10^{-10}–10^{-8} M) slightly stimulated (1.3- to 1.7-fold) the clonal growth of normal human myeloid committed stem cells (CFU-GM).

The identification of 1,25(OH)$_2$D$_3$ receptors in activated T and B lymphocytes from normal individuals [47–48] has suggested that immunoregulatory processes may be modulated by 1,25(OH)$_2$D$_3$ and vitamin D$_3$ analogs. Analogous to the potent immunosuppressive agent cyclosporin A, 1,25(OH)$_2$D$_3$ has been shown to inhibit the proliferation of activated T-lymphocytes [49–50]. The 20-epi analogs of 1,25(OH)$_2$D$_3$ have been shown to inhibit cytokine-mediated T lymphocyte activation [37]. The cell line S-LB1 was established by HTLV-1 infection of T lymphocytes from a normal individual [39].The present studies showed that the 1,25(OH)$_2$-20-epi-D$_3$ (IE) was 100-fold more potent that 1,25(OH)$_2$D$_3$ (C) in inhibition of clonal growth of the S-LB1 cell line suggesting that 1,25(OH)$_2$-20-epi-D$_3$ (IE) probably deserves further investigation as an immunsuppressive agent.

The alteration of stereochemistry at carbon 20 on the side chain, is the only difference between 1,25(OH)$_2$D$_3$ (C) and 1,25(OH)$_2$-20-epi-D$_3$ (IE). Why this change at carbon 20 enhances the antiproliferative and differentiation effects on leukemic cells *in vitro* is unclear. Recently, evidence has accumulated that some effects of vitamin D$_3$ analogs may be mediated independent of 1,25(OH)$_2$D$_3$ nuclear receptors. One series of our experiment suggest that 1,25(OH)$_2$-20-epi-D$_3$ (IE) mediates its effects through the vitamin D$_3$ receptor. The T-cell line Ab-VDR from a patient with vitamin D dependent rickets type II do not have functional vitamin D$_3$ receptors [40]. Clonal growth of these cells were unaffected by high concentrations (10^{-7} M) of either 1,25(OH)$_2$-20-epi-D$_3$ (IE) or 1,25(OH)$_2$D$_3$ (C). In contrast, the matched control, S-LB1 cells (HTLV-1 transformed T-cells from a normal individual) having functional vitamin D$_3$ receptors, were markedly inhibitedy 1,25(OH)$_2$-20-epi-D$_3$ (IE) suggesting that 1,25(OH)$_2$-20-epi-D$_3$ (IE) is not mediating its effects through a non-1,25(OH)$_2$D$_3$ receptor mechanism.

Potentially, 20-epi-1,25(OH)$_2$D$_3$ (IE) might have either a higher affinity for the vitamin D$_3$ nuclear receptors or the ligand/receptor complex might interact more efficiently with the VDRE to modulate gene expression. To pursue these possibilities, a reporter gene containing the VDRE was transfected into HL-60 cells. The cells were cultured in media containing different concentrations of either 1,25(OH)$_2$-20-epi-D$_3$ (IE) or 1,25(OH)$_2$D$_3$ (C) and reporter gene activities were measured. These two analogs had nearly identical activities, strongly suggesting that the difference between 1,25(OH)$_2$-20-epi-D$_3$ (IE) and 1,25(OH)$_2$D$_3$ (C) can not be ascribed to differential abilities to enter the cells or bind to VDR and then to VDRE and transactive a target gene. Potentially, the 1,25(OH)$_2$-20-epi-D$_3$/VDR complex may interact with a different groups of VDREs than those bound by the 1,25(OH)$_2$D$_3$ /VDR complex; the testing of this possibility will have to await the identification of appropriate target genes that control myeloid differentiation.

In the current studies, we have shown that 1,25(OH)$_2$-20-epi-D$_3$ (IE) is amongst the most potent vitamin D$_3$ analogs as a modulator of induction of differentiation and inhibition of clonal proliferation of leukemic cells without inhibition of normal myeloid clonal growth. Future studies should be directed to the identification of new retinoids and vitamin D_3 compounds with greater differentiating ability and less toxicity, and to the combined use of differentiating agents which act through different pathways.

Acknowledgements. Support by NIH-CA-42710, NIH-CA43277 and the Parker Hughes Fund are gratefully acknowledged. Elena Elstner and Sven de Vos are supported in part by grant aid for science research from DFG.

References

1. Huang M, Ye Y, Chen S, Chai J, Lu J, Xhoa L, Gu L, Wang Z: Use of all-*trans*-retinoic acid in the treatment of the acute promielocytic leukemia. Blood 72: 567, 1988.
2. Castaigne S, Chomienne C, daniel MT, Ballerini P, Berger R, Fenaux P, Degos L: All-*trans*-retinoic acid as a differentiation therapy for acute promyelocytic leukemia: 1 Clinical results. Blood 76: 1704, 1990
3. Warrell RP, Frankel SR, Miller WH Jr, Scheinberg DA, Itri LM, Hittelman WN, Vyas R, Andreeff M, Tafuri A, Jakubowski A, Gabrilove J, Gordon MS, Dmitrovsky E: Differentiation therapy of acute promyelocytic leukemia with tretinoin (all-trans-retinoic acid). N Engl J Med 324: 1385, 1991.
4. Wollbach SB, Howe PR: Tissue changes following deprivation of fat soluble A vitamin J Exp Med 42: 753, 1925.
5. Hodges RE, Sauberlich HE, Canham JE, Wallace DL, Rucker RB, Mejia LA, Mohanram M: Hematopoietic studies in vitamin A deficiency. Am J Clin Nutr 31: 876, 1978.
6. Meja LA, Hodges RE, Rucker RB: Clinicial signs of anemia in vitamin A-deficient rats. Am J Clin Nutr 32: 1439, 1979.
7. Douer D, Koeffler HP: Retinoic acid enhances colony-stimulating factor-induced clonal growth of normal human myeloid progenitor cells *in vitro*. Exp Cell Res 138: 193-198, 1982.
8. Tobler A, Dawson MI, Koeffler HP: Retinoids; structure-function relationship in normal and leukemic hematopoiesis *in vitro*. J Clin Invest 78: 303, 1986.
9. Mangelsdorf DJ, Ong ES, Dyck JA, Evans RM: A nuclear receptor that identifies a novel retinoic acid response pathway. Nature 345: 224, 1990.
10. Levin AA, Sturzenbecker LJ, Kazmer S, Bosakowski T, Huselton C, Allenby G, Speck J, Kratzeisen C, Rosenberger M, Lovey A, Grippo JF: 9-*cis* retinoic acid steroisomer binds and activates the nuclear receptor RXRa. Nature 355: 359, 1992.
11. Heyman RA, Mangelsdorf DF, Dyck Ja, Stein RB, Eichele G, Evans RM, Thaller C: 9-*cis* retinoic acid is a high affinity ligand for the retinoid X receptor. Cell 68: 397, 1992.
12. Sakashita A, Kizaki M, Pakkala S, Schiller G, Tsuruoka N, Tomosaki R, Dawson M, Cameron J, Koeffler HP: 9-*cis*-retinoic acid: effect on normal and leukemic hematopoiesis *in vitro*. Blood 81: 1009–16, 1993.
13. Kizaki M, Ikeda Y, Tanosaki R, Nakajima H, Morikawa M, Sakashita A, Koeffler HP: Effects of novel retinoic acid compound, 9-*cis*-retinoic acid, on proliferation, differentiation and expression of RARa, RXRa RNA by HL-60 cells. Blood 82: 3592–3599, 1993.
14. Yu VC, Delsert C, Andersen B, Hollway JM, Devary OV, Naar AM, Kim SY, Boutin JM, Glass CK, Rosenfeld MG: RXR beta: a coregulator that enhances binding of retinoic acid, thyroid hormone, and vitamin D receptors to their cognate response elements. Cell 67: 1251–66, 1991.
15. Zhang XK, Hoffmann B, Tran PB, Graupner G, Pfahl M: retinoid X receptor is an auxiliary protein for thyroid hormone and retinoic acid receptors. Nature 355: 441–6, 1992.
16. Leid M, Kastner P, Lyons R, Nakshatri H, Saunders M, Zacharewski T, Chen JY, Staub A, Garnier JM, Mader S: Purification, cloning, and RXR identity of the HeLa cell factor with Which RAR or TR teterodimerizes to bind target sequences efficiently. Cell 68: 377–95, 1992.
17. Kliewer SA, Umesono K, Mangelsdorf DJ, Evans RM: Retinoid X receptor is an auxiliary protein for thyroid hormone and retinoic acid receptor. Nature 355: 441–6, 1992.
18. Bugge TH, Pohl J, Lonnoy O, Stunnenberg HG: RXR alpha, a promiscuous partner of retinoic acid and thyroid hormone receptors. EMBO 11: 1409–18, 1992.
19. Marks MS, Hallenbeck PL, Nagata T, Segars JH, Appella E, Nikodem VM, Ozato K: H-2RIIBR (RXR beta) heterodimerization provides a mechanism for combinatorial diversity in the regulation of retinoic acid and thyroid hormone responsive genes. EMBO 11:1419–35, 1992.
20. Hermann T, Hoffmann B, Zhang XK, Tran P, Pfahl M: Heterodimeric receptor complexes determine 3,5,3′-triiodothyronine and retinoic signaling specificities. Mol Endocrin 6: 1153–62, 1992.
21. Zhang XK, Lehmann J, Hoffmann B, Dawson MI, Cameron J, Graupner G, Hermann T, Tran P, Pfahl M: Homodimer formation of retinoid X receptor induced by 9-*cis* retinoic acid. Nature 358;587–91, 1992.
22. Lehmann JM, Jong L, Fanjul A, Cameron JF, Lu XP, Haefner P, Dawson MI, Pfahl M: Retinoids selective for retinoid X receptor response pathways. Science 258: 1944–1946, 1993.
23. Minghetti PP, Norman AW: 1,2(OH)o_2-Vitamin D3 receptors: gene regulation and genetic circuity. FASEB J 2: 3043–3053, 1988.
24. DeLuca HF, Krisinger J, Darwish H: The vitamin D system. Kidney Int 38: S3–S8, 1990.

25. Baker AR, McDonnell DP, Hughes M, Crisp TM, Mangelsdorf DJ, Haussler MR, Pike JW, Shine J, O'Malley BW: Cloning and expression of full-length cDNA encoding human vitamin D receptor. Proc natl Acad Sci USA 85, 3294–3298, 1988.
26. Evans RM: The steroid and thyroid hormone receptor superfamily. Science 240,889–895, 1988.
27. Beato M: Gene regulation by steroid hormones. Cell 56, 335–344, 1989.
28. Mangelsdorf DJ, Koeffler HP, Donaldson CA, Pike JW, Haussler MR: 1,25-dihydroxyvitamin D_3 induced differentiation in a human promyelocytic leukemia cell line (HL-60): receptor-mediated maturation to macrophage-like cells. J Cell Biol 98: 391–398, 1994.
29. Tanaka H, Abe C, Miyaura T, Kuribayashi K, Kondo K, Nishii Y, Suda T: 1-alpha,25-dihydroxy-cholecalciferol and a human myeloid leukemia cell line (HL-60). The presence of a cytosol receptor and induction of differentiation. Biochem J 204: 713–719, 1982.
30. Abe E, Miyaura C, Sakagami H, Takeda M, Kondo K, Yamazaki T, Yoshiki S, Suda T: Differentiation of mouse myeloid leukemia cell induced by 1, alpha 25 dihydroxyvitamin D_3. Proc Natl Acad Sci USA 78: 4990–4994, 1981.
31. Munker R, Norman A, Koeffler HP: Vitamin D compounds: Effect on clonal proliferation and differentiation of human myeloid cells. J. Clin. Invest. 78: 474–480, 1986.
32. Honma Y, Hozumi M, Abe E, Konno K, Fukushima M, Hata S, Nishii Y, DeLuca HF, Suda T: 1,25-dihydroxyvitamin D3 and 1 alpha-hydroxy-vitamin D_3 prolongs survival time of mice inoculated with myeloid leukemic cells. Proc Natl Acad Sci USA 80: 201–204, 1987.
33. Zhou JY, Norman AW, Chen DL, Sun GW, Uskokovic M, HP Koeffler: 1,25(OH)2-16ene-23ene-vitamin D3 prolongs survival time of leukemic mice. Proc Natl Acad Sci USA 87: 3929–3933, 1990
34. Koeffler HP, Hirji K, Itri L, Southern California Leukemic Group: 1,25-dihydroxyvitamin D_3: *in vivo* and *in vitro* effects on human preleukemic and leukemic cells. Cancer Treat Rep 69: 1399–1407, 1985.
35. Mehta AB, Kumaran TO, Marsh GW: Treatment of advanced myelodysplastic syndrome with alfacalcidol [letter]. Lancet. 2: 761–762, 1984.
36. Richard C, Mazo E, Cuadrado MA, Iriondo A, Bello C, Gandarillas M, Zubizarreta A: Treatment of myelodysplastic syndrome with 1,25-dihydrovitamin D3. Am J Hematol. 23: 175-178, 1986.
37. Binderup L, Latini S, Binderup C, Calverley M, Hansen K: 20-epi-vitamin D_3 analogues: a novel class of potent regulators of cell growth and immune responses. Biochem Pharmacol 42: 1569–1575, 1991.
38. Collins SJ, Gallo RC, Gallagher RE: Continuous growth of human myeloid leukemic cells in suspension culture, Nature 270: 347– 349, 1977.
39. Koeffler HP, Chen ISY, Golde D: Characterization of a novel HTLV-infected cell line. Blood 64: 482–490, 1984.
40. Koeffler HP, Bishop JE, Reichel H, Singer F, Nagler A, Tobler A, Walka M, Norman AW: Lymphocyte cell lines from vitamin D-dependent rickets type II show functional defects in the 1α,25-dihydroxyvitamin D_3 receptor. Molecular and Cellular Endocrinology 70: 1-11, 1990.
41. Dawson MI, Hobbs PO, Derdzinski KA, Chao W, Fenking G, Loew GH, Jetten AM, Napoli JL, Williams JB, Sani BR, Willer Jr, Schiff LJ: Effect of structural modifications in the C-7-C11 region of the retinoid skeleton on biological activity in a series of aromatic retinoids. J Med Chem.32: 1504–17, 1989.
42. Maignan J, Lang G, Malle G, Restle S, Shroot B: (CIRD). Nouveux derives bicycliques aromatiques, leur procede de preparation et leur utilization en medicine humaine et veterinaire et en cosmetique. French Patent 2, 601, 670 (January 22, 1988).
43. Luckow B, Schuetz G: Cat constructions with multiple unique restriction sites for the functional analysis of eukaryotic promotors and regulatory elements. Nucleic Acids Research 15: 5490, 1987.
44. Ozono K, Liao J, Kerner SA, Scott RA, Pike JW: Vitamin D-responsive element in the human osteocalcin gene. J Biol Chem 265: 2181–2188, 1990.
45. Koeffler HP, Amatruda T, Ikekawa N, Kobayashi Y, DeLuca HF: Induction of macrophage differentiation of human normal and leukemic myeloid stem cells by 1,25-dihydroxyvitamin D_3 and its fluorinated analogs. Cancer Res. 44: 5624, 1984.
46. Provvedini DM, Mandagas SC: 1α, 25-Dhydroxy-vitamin D_3 receptor distribution and effects in subpopulation of normal human T lymphocytes. J Clin Endocrinol Metab 68: 774–779, 1989.
47. Koizumi T, Nakao Y, Nakagawa T, Katakami Y, Fujita T: Effect of 1α,25-dihydroxyvitamin D_3 on cytokine-induced thymocyte proliferation. Cell Immunol 96: 455–461, 1985.
48. Gupta S, Fass D, Shimizu M, Vayuvegula B: Potentiation of immunosuppressive effects of cyclosporin A by 1α,25-dihydroxyvitamin D_3. Cell Immunol. 121: 290–297, 1989.
49. Tobler A, Gasson J, Reichel H, Norman AW, Koeffler HP: Granulocyte-macrophage colony-stimulating factor. J Clin Invest 79: 1700-1705, 1987.
50. Reichel H, Koeffler HP, Barbers R, Norman AW: Regulation of 1,25-dihydroxyvitamin D_3 production by cultured alveolar macrophages from normal human donors and from patients with pulmonary sarcoidosis. J Clin Endocrinol Metab 65: 1201–1209, 1987.

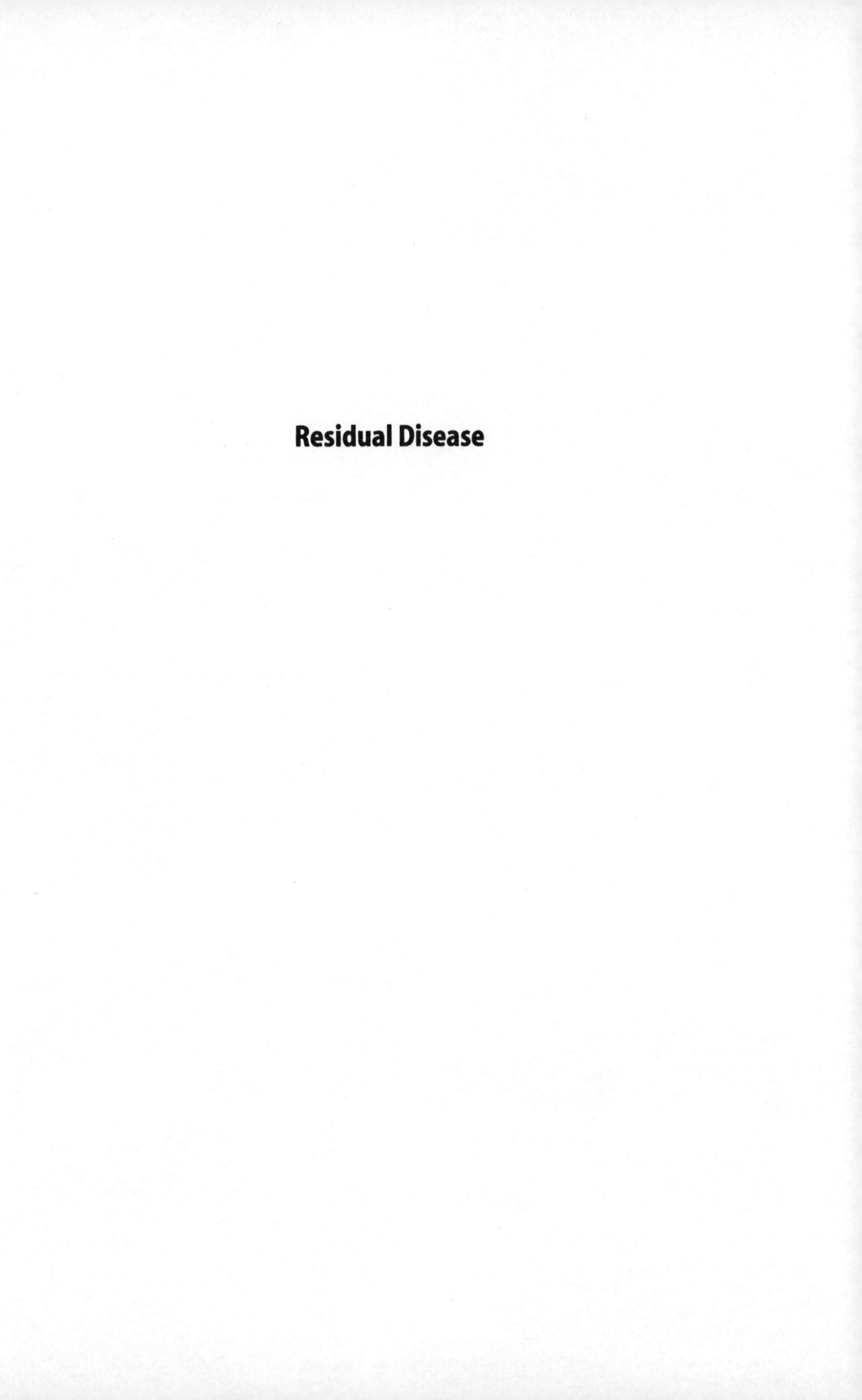

Residual Disease

Acute Leukemias V
Experimental Approaches
and Management of Refractory Diseases
Hiddemann et al. (Eds.)

Functional Assays for Human AML Cells by Transplantation into SCID Mice

Tsvee Lapidot[1], Christian Sirard[1], Josef Vormoor[1], Trang Hoang[4], Julio Caceres-Cortes[4], Mark Minden[2], Bruce Paterson[3], Michael A. Caligiuri[5], and John E. Dick[1]

Human hematopoiesis is tightly regulated, but genetic alterations in stem cells can perturb the developmental program resulting in a clonal outgrowth of one or more lineages [1, 2, 3]. In AML, the impaired differentiation program results in the excess production of leukemic blasts, the vast majority of which have limited proliferative capacity [4]. As a result, rare sub-populations of leukemic cells with extensive proliferative and self-renewal capacity must maintain the leukemic clone [5, 6]. Efforts to characterize these leukemic stem cells have focused on the development of in vitro colony assays (eg. AML-CFU) and/or liquid cultures [6, 7]. However, the progenitors detected in these assays have very limited proliferative and replating potential [8] making it difficult to establish a link with the human disease.

Numerous attempts have been made to establish an in vivo model of human myeloid leukemia in immunodeficient nude mice [9, 10, 11]. Unfortunately, the AML cells grew locally as solid tumors at the site of injection, atypical of the human disease. The recent success in transplanting normal human hematopoietic cells [12, 13] and acute lymphoid leukemia (ALL) [14] into immunodeficient SCID mice suggested a novel strategy to develop an assay for leukemic stem cells. Although pre-B ALL cells obtained directly from patients in relapse readily proliferate in SCID mice [15], primary AML cells did not engraft SCID mice following IV injection [16, 17, 18] perhaps because of their unique growth factor requirements. AML-CFU are highly dependent on cytokines for proliferation and some of these growth factors are species-specific (eg. GM-CSF, IL-3) [7]. Implantation of AML cells from a small sample of patients into the peritoneum or under the renal capsule of SCID mice resulted in the local growth of leukemic cells, but their dissemination to the bone marrow was poor and limited to a few patients even after long periods of time [16, 17]. The close inter-cellular contact following implantation presumably permits the outgrowth of those samples where autocrine or paracrine growth stimulation occurs. Implantation of AML cells into human fetal bone chips previously implanted into SCID mice resulted only in local growth of palpable tumors uncharacteristic of the original disease [19]. Based on the success of establishing multilineage human hematopoiesis in SCID mice by cytokine stimulation of primitive normal bone marrow cells with kit ligand and PIXY321 (human IL3 and GMCSF fusion protein) [13], we developed an AML model in SCID mice that permits high levels of leukemic cell proliferation with biological properties and morphology similar to the original patients [20].

AML cells, directly obtained from patients at diagnosis, were transplanted into immunodeficient SCID mice and stimulated in vivo with human cytokines. The leukemic cells homed to the murine bone marrow and rapidly

[1] Department of Genetics, Research Institute, Hospital for Sick Children, Toronto, and
[2] Department of Molecular and Medical Genetics, University of Toronto
[3] Department of Medicine, and Department of Oncologic Pathology, Princess Margaret Hospital, Toronto
[4] Clinical Research Institute, Montreal, Quebec
[5] Department of Medicine, Roswell Park Cancer Institute, Buffalo, New York

proliferated in response to cytokine treatment resulting in a pattern of dissemination and leukemic cell morphology that was similar to the original patients. We have now examined a large number of samples (n = 17) obtained from patients with newly diagnosed AML of different FAB subtypes (M1, M2, M4) for their ability to proliferate in SCID mice. The cell source was either bone marrow or PBL obtained fresh or from banked frozen samples and all transplanted mice were treated with growth factors for the entire length of the experiment (30–45 days). AML cells from all of the FAB subtypes (16 of 17 patients) engrafted SCID mice to high levels, indicating high reproducibility of the transplant system.

In contrast to AML-M1 and M2, some mice transplanted with AML-M4 cells became sick or died as early as 10–20 days post-transplant with dissemination of leukemic blasts to the liver, lungs, spleen, and kidney. Clinically, leukemic blasts from AML patients with the monocytic subtypes AML-M4 and M5 disseminate more extensively to extramedullary sites than those from patients with AML-M1/M2 suggesting that the SCID-LEUKEMIA model may allow for the analysis of biological differences between different AML subtypes.

AML-CFU were present in mice transplanted with 11 of 11 donor samples regardless of the FAB classification. Leukemic cells, before and after transplantation into SCID mice, were plated at limiting dilution in methylcellulose assays to compare the frequency of AML-CFU. The assay was linear and similar frequencies were obtained from the patient sample and the mouse bone marrow. Interestingly, the response in culture of AML-CFU from the patient and the transplanted mouse for IL-3 and MGF was identical, indicating that neither the murine environment nor exogenous cytokine treatment selected for clones with altered responses to growth factors.

The establishment of human AML in SCID mice and the significant expansion of AML colony-forming progenitors (AML-CFU) over at least 45 days post-transplant indicated that immature leukemic stem cells could be assayed in SCID mice. Engraftment of AML-M1 cells was linear with respect to the transplanted cell dose, providing the foundation for a quantitative assay of the leukemic stem cell that can initiate AML in SCID mice.

Quantitative limiting dilution analysis demonstrated that the frequency of leukemic stem cells in the peripheral blood (PBL) of four newly diagnosed AML-M1 patients was 1 in 250,000 cells. Characterization of the leukemic stem cells indicated that AML cells enriched for $CD34^{+}CD38^{-}$ cells engrafted SCID mice, while $CD34^{-}$ $CD38^{+}$ cells that in vitro give rise to large numbers of AML-CFU did not.

Our data provide the first biological identification of an AML stem cell that can initiate human leukemia in SCID mice, the *S*CID *L*EUKEMIA-*I*NITIATING *C*ELL or SL-IC. The SL-IC can engraft the bone marrow of SCID mice following IV injection, proliferate extensively producing large numbers of AML-CFU in response to cytokine treatment and develop a cellular morphology similar to the original donor leukemia. The frequency of SL-IC in the PBL of AML-M1 patients is between 1000–2500 fold lower than the frequency of AML-CFU. Based on the low proliferative capacity of AML-CFU in vitro [6], even with maximal growth factor stimulation, it is likely that their maintenance in SCID mice for over 45 days post-transplant is due to the proliferation and differentiation of SL-IC. Thus, the murine bone marrow can provide a microenvironment for the long-term maintenance of SL-IC, in contrast to liquid cultures of AML which have a short lifespan. In addition, long-term cultures of AML cells on stromal layers usually results in the proliferation of normal human progenitors rather than AML cells [21, 22], suggesting that in vitro the human stroma is not sufficient to support leukemic stem cells.

The availability of an assay for SL-IC provides an important tool for purification and characterization of the leukemic stem cell. The experiments presented here indicate that SL-IC express CD34 on their cell surface. Future experiments can focus on other cell surface markers (eg. KIT, THY) and phenotypic properties (eg. up-take of Rhodamine 123). It will be interesting to determine if differences between normal stem cells and SL-IC can be found to enable purging of AML cells for autologous transplantation. Purification strategies combined with new methods to create cDNA libraries from single cells [23] could permit molecular characterization of genes expressed in SL-IC compared to normal stem cells and more differentiated AML-CFU. These studies should help address the relationship between SL-IC and the target cell for leukemic transformation that maintains the disease in patients. Finally, the establishment of a

SCID-LEUKEMIA model that replicates many features of human AML provides an important tool to understand the cellular and molecular processes that govern the transformation and progression of leukemic stem cells and to test the efficacy of new therapeutic strategies in vivo.

References

1. C. Sawyers, C. Denny, O. Witte, Cell 64, 337 (1991).
2. E. Fearon, P. Burke, C. Schiffer, B. Zehnbauer, B. Vogelstein, N. Eng. J. Med. 315, 15 (1986).
3. M. Keinänen, J. Griffin, C. Bloomfield, J. Machnicki, A. de la Chapelle, N. Eng. J. Med. 318, 1153 (1988).
4. H. Grier, C. Civin, Acute and chronic myeloproliferative disorders and myelodysplasia. D. Nathan, F. Oski, Eds., Hematology of infancy and childhood (W.B. Saunders Company, Philadelphia, 1993), vol. 2.
5. E. McCulloch, Blood 62, 1 (1983).
6. J. Griffin, B. Löwenberg, Blood 68, 1185 (1986).
7. B. Löwenberg, I. Touw, Blood 81, 281 (1993).
8. E. McCulloch, C. Izaguirre, L. Chang, S. Smith, LJ, J. Cell Physiol. Suppl. 1, 103 (1982).
9. J. Fogh, J. M. Fogh, T. Orfeo, J. Natl. Cancer. Inst. 59, 221 (1977).
10. C. R. Franks, D. Bishop, F. R. Balkwill, R. T. D. Oliver, W. G. Spector, Br. J. Cancer 35, 697 (1977).
11. R. D. Clutterbuck, et al., Leuk. Res. 9, 1511 (1985).
12. S. Kamel-Reid, J. E. Dick, Science 242, 1706 (1988).
13. T. Lapidot, et al., Science 255, 1137 (1992).
14. S. Kamel-Reid, et al., Science 246, 1597 (1989).
15. S. Kamel-Reid, et al., Blood 78, 2973 (1991).
16. A. Cesano, et al., Oncogene 7, 827 (1992).
17. C. Sawyers, M. Gishizky, S. Quan, D. Golde, O. Witte, Blood 79, 2089 (1992).
18. C. De Lord, et al., Exp. Hematol. 19, 991 (1991).
19. Namikawa
20. T. Lapidot , et al. Nature 367: 645–648, 1994
21. L. Coulombel, C. Eaves, D. Kalousek, C. Gupta, A. Eaves, J. Clin. Invest. 75, 961 (1985).
22. R. Schiró, et al., Blut 61, 267 (1990).
23. G. Brady, M. Barbara, N. Iscove, Meth. Molec. Cell. Biol. 2, 17 (1990).

Acute Leukemias V
Experimental Approaches
and Management of Refractory Diseases
Hiddemann et al. (Eds.)

Cytogenetics and Clonal Evolution in Childhood Acute Lymphoblastic Leukemia (ALL)

J. Harbott[1], I. Reinisch-Becker[1], J. Ritterbach[1], W.-D. Ludwig[2], A. Reiter[3], and F. Lampert[1]

Introduction

Clonal evolution which becomes visible by karyotypic changes is a well-known phenomenon in malignancies, and especially in solid tumors it is described as an indicator for strong cell proliferation and the grade of malignancy [1,2]. Also in chronic myelogeneous leukemia (CML) secondary chromosomal abnormalities were found during the follow-up of the disease. Specially the i(17q) and a second Philadelphia chromosome are considered as markers for a poor prognosis, sometimes predicting a blast crisis [3–5].

In acute lymphoblastic leukemia (ALL), however, clonal evolution is not as well investigated, because most of the patients achieve remission very early and a cytogenetic analysis during this period seems to be not meaningful because of the low percentage of blast cells [6–8]. In this type of leukemia two groups of clonal evolution have to be distinguished: In the first group those patients are comprised who show at diagnosis either two different cell clones or more than one chromosomal aberration in only one clone, especially those with one of the subgroup specific aberrations like t(9;22) or t(8;14) together with a secondary change. The second group includes patients showing a karyotypic switch between diagnosis and relapse.

Materials and Methods

Bone marrow samples, mostly received by mail (80–90%), were prepared directly or incubated in RPMI 1640+20% FCS (10^6 cells/ml) for a 24 h culture. The cell suspension was then brought to hypotonic solution (KCl, 30 min.) and fixed in methanol-acetic acid (3:1). After being washed several times, the cells were dropped on a cold wet slide to spread the metaphases. G-banding followed a trypsin pretreatment (10–15 sec.) after air drying 3–5 days later. Karyotyping was done according to the Third International Workshop on leukemia 1980 [9] and the ISCN 1985 and 1991 [10,11].

Results

To evaluate clonal evolution at diagnosis of ALL the karyotype of 504 children with chromosomal aberrations were compared (Table 1). About two thirds of them showed only one chromosomal aberration (n = 320; 63.5%), whereas secondary

Table 1. Different types of cell clones at diagnosis (504 patients)

Aberr. Clones	Type of aberration	No of patients
1	46,XY,t(A;B)	320
1	46,XY,t(A;B),t(C;D)	164
2	46,XY,t(A;B)/46,XY,t(A;B),t(C;D)	18
2	46,XY,t(A;B),t(C;D)/46,XY,t(A;B),t(E;F)	1
3	46,XY,t(A;B),t(C;D)/46,XY,t(A;B),t(E;F)/46,XY,t(E;F),t(G;H)	1

[1] Children's Univ. Hospital, 35385 Gießen, Germany
[2] Robert-Rössle Klinik, Dept. of Oncology/ Molecular Biology, 13125 Berlin, Germany
[3] Dept. of Pediatrics, Hannover Medical School, 30625 Hannover, Germany

changes or more than one cell clone were found in only 184 (36.5%). In the vast majority of the latter (n = 164) only one cell clone with one additional abnormality could be detected, whereas two or more clones were only found in 20.

For the comparison of the involved chromosomes only those patients were evaluated who showed more than one cell clone or one of the subgroup specific aberrations to identify the secondary change unequivocally. In karyotypes of 106 children used for this analysis nearly all chromosomes were found to be involved in secondary chromosomal aberrations, but especially the chromosomes #1, and also #6, #7, and #9 were more often found than others. This is due to the fact, that the appearance of secondary changes are not quite random. Abnormalities of chromosome 1, for example, is very often found in combination with a t(8;14) and also in hyperdiploid karyotypes with more than 50 chromosomes where always the long arm is involved in different aberrations. Other combinations were the chromosome #9 with t(1;19) and chromosome #6 with the different changes of chromosome #14 [der(14)(q11)] in T-cell ALL. Secondary changes involving #7 were found as i(7q) with t(4;11) or partial monosomy 7 with t(9;22).

For the evaluation of clonal evolution at relapse the number of patients is smaller. 87 children were analyzed successfully at diagnosis and at relapse. Forty of them, however, had to be excluded, because in one or both cytogenetic analyses only a normal karyotype was detected, indicating that the aberrant clone had been missed. Of the remaining 47 children a clonal evolution was found in 20 (42.5%) (Table 2). Most of them (n = 14) showed only one clone with a single secondary abnormality. In two patients this type was detected together with the original clone, whereas in two others a new secondary change appeared. The remaining two patients of this group expressed a completely new karyotype.

In 10 out of the 20 children with clonal evolution the chromosomes #1 or #7 were involved in the secondary abnormalities, whereas other chromosomes were found less frequently. The breakpoints of chromosomes 1 differed in all five patients and were spread all over the chromosome (Table 3). In the other five patients, however, always a duplication of the long arm was detected with a large consensus region (7q11–7q36).

To evaluate the clinical relevance of clonal evolution at diagnosis a life-table analysis by Kaplan-Meier was performed of the children with and without secondary changes at diagnosis who were all treated uniformly by the therapy protocol ALL-BFM-90. Both groups showed nearly the same result: an EFS of 0.77 and 0.75, respectively. A similar result was found when the children with and without clonal evolution at relapse were compared. Because of the low number of patients no life-table analysis was performed, but the comparison of remission duration and the survival after relapse showed no difference. In both groups only three children were still alive.

If, however, only patients with chromosome 1 and 7 abnormalities were compared, the results were completely different: The mean period of remission (18.1 vs 7.3 months) and the mean survival time after relapse (15.2 vs 2.9) were much shorter for patients with secondary aberrations of chromosome 7. All five children with this abnormality died whereas two of the other group are still alive.

To test the clinical meaning of distinct chromosomal aberrations as secondary changes the frequency of chromosome 1 aberrations in 46 children with hyperdiploid karyotype >50 at diagnosis was evaluated (Fig. 1). An abnormality

Table 2. Different types of cell clones at relapse (20 patients with clonal evolution)

	Type of aberration	No of patients
diagnosis: relapse:	46,XY,t(A;B) 46,XY,t(A;B),t(C;D)	14
diagnosis: relapse:	46,XY,t(A;B) 46,XY,t(A;B)/46,XY, t(A;B),t(C;D)	2
diagnosis relapse:	46,XY,t(A;B),t(C;D) 46,XY,t(A;B),t(E;F)	2
diagnosis: relapse:	46,XY,t(A;B) 46,XY,t(C;D)	2

Table 3. Abnormalities of chromosomes #1 and #7 at relapse

Chromosome 1	Chromosome 7
inv(1)(p36q32)	dirdup(7)(q11q36)
del(1)(p34)	dirdup(7)(q11q36)
der(1p)	i(7q)
del(1)(q25)	i(7q)
der(1q)	+7

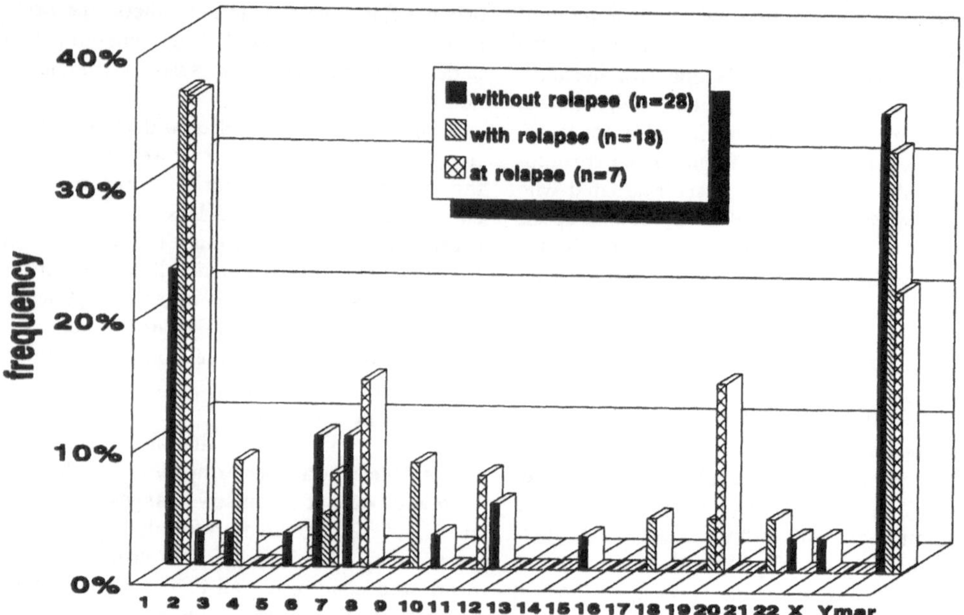

Fig. 1. Frequency of secondary aberrations in children with hyperdiploid karyotype >50. The incidence of chromosome 1 aberrations is much higher in patients with relapse

of the long arm of chromosome 1 was the most frequent secondary change in this group. Comparing the outcome of these patients a pronounced difference was detected: The incidence of chromosome 1 aberrations in children who relapsed was much higher as compared to those who were still in CCR at the time of evaluation (36 vs 22.5%). Also in the bone marrow of the 7 patients only analyzed at relapse a very high percentage of this type of abnormality was found (35.7%).

Discussion

Clonal evolution in solid tumors and chronic leukemias is described as an indicator for poor prognosis. In ALL, however, this phenomenon is not as well investigated, because most of the patients achieve CCR very early and cytogenetic analysis is only performed at diagnosis and relapse.

The cytogenetic analysis of 504 children with ALL at diagnosis showed a clonal evolution in only 1/3 of the patients and also at relapse the frequency of karyotypic changes compared to the first analysis was only slightly higher (42.5%). In spite of all secondary changes which occurred during remission in the residual pathological cell clone, the original chromosomal abnormality remained detectable in the bone marrow of nearly all the patients. This makes those chromosomal aberrations which are detectable by molecular techniques a good tool for the identification of minimal residual disease. Only two patients showed a completely new karyotype indicating a secondary malignancy. The clinical features, however, especially the immunophenotype remained completely the same in both children (c-ALL).

The chromosomes which were involved in secondary changes most frequently, were chromosomes 1 and 7 as well at diagnosis as at relapse [8,12]. This is due to the fact that secondary changes are not completely random, but were often found in combinations with subgroup specific abnormalities. If these combinations may have a clinical relevance regarding prognosis as sometimes described [13–15] is not yet clear, because of the small number of patients. It might be remarkable, however, that all aberrations of chromosome 7 at relapse included a duplication of nearly the whole long arm (7q11–7q36), the region where the gene for multiple drug resistance (MDR-1) is located [16].

The clinical meaning of secondary chromosomal changes at diagnosis and at relapse is not yet clear. The comparison of all patients with and without clonal evolution shows completely no difference in outcome for both groups. Some of these abnormalities, however, may indicate a poorer prognosis in combination with one of the subgroup specific abnormalities (chr.1 in hyperdiploids > 50), but more patients treated by the same protocol and longer follow-up times are needed.

References

1. Collard JG, van de Poll M, Scheffer A, Roos E, Hopman AHN, Geurts van Kessel AHM, van Dongen JJM (1987) Genetic control of invasion and metastasis. Cancer Res 47: 6666–6670
2. Sandberg AA (1990): The chromosomes in human cancer and leukemia. Elsevier Science Publishers B.V., New York, Amsterdam, Oxford
3. Cervantes F, Rozman M, Rosell J, Urbano-Ispizua A, Montserrat E, Rozman C (1990) A study of prognostic factors in blast crisis of Philadelphia chromosome-positive chronic myelogenous leukaemia. Br J Haematol 76: 27–32
4. Haus O, Noworolska A, Laskowski M, Kuliszkiewicz-Janus M, Kozlowska J, Harlozinska-Szmyrka A, Jagielski J, Kotlarek-Haus S (1990) Prognostic significance of secondary cytogenetic changes and nonspecific cross-reacting antigen (NCA) in patients with Ph-positive chronic myeloid leukemia. Exp Mol Pathol 52: 235–242
5. Guilhot F, Tanzer J (1991) Prognosis of chronic myelocytic leukemia. Presse Med 20: 171–175
6. Zuelzer WW, Inoue S, Thompson RI, Ottenbreit MJ (1976) Long-term cytogenetic studies in acute leukemia of children; the nature of relapse. Am J Hematol 1: 143–190
7. Abshire TC, Buchanan GR, Jackson JF, Shuster JJ, Brock B, Head D, Behm F, Crist WM, Link M, Borowitz M, Pullen DJ (1992) Morphologic, immunologic and cytogenetic studies in children with acute lymphoblastic leukemia at diagnosis and relapse: A Pediatric Oncology Group study. Leukemia 6: 357–362
8. Heerema NA, Palmer CG, Weetman R, Bertolone S (1992) Cytogenetic analysis in relapsed childhood acute lymphoblastic leukemia. Leukemia 6: 185–192
9. Third International Workshop on Chromosomes in Leukemia 1980 (1981) Clinical significance of chromosomal abnormalities in acute lymphoblastic leukemia. Cancer Genet Cytogenet 4: 111–137
10. ISCN (1985): An international system for human cytogenetic nomenclature. Karger, Basel,
11. ISCN (1991): Guidelines for cancer cytogenetics, supplement to an international system for human cytogenetic nomenclature. S. Karger, Basel,
12. Mamaeva SE, Mamaeva NN, Jartseva NM, Belyaeva LV, Scherbakova EG (1983) Complete or partial trisomy for the long arm of chromosome 1 in patients with various hematologic malignancies. Hum Genet 63: 107–112
13. Russo C, Carroll AJ, Kohler S, Borowitz MJ, Amylon MD, Homans A, Kedar A, Shuster JJ, Land VJ, Crist WM, Pullen DJ, Link MP (1991) Philadelphia chromosome and monosomy 7 in childhood acute lymphoblastic leukemia: A Pediatric Oncology Group study. Blood 77: 1050–1056
14. Petkovic I, Nakic M, Tiefenbach A, Konja J, Kastelan M, Rajic L, Feminic-Kes R (1987) Marker chromosome $1q^{+}$ in acute lymphoblastic leukemia. Cancer Genet Cytogenet 24: 251–255
15. Morris CM, Fitzgerald PH, Neville M, Wyld P, Beard M (1984) Does multisomy of chromosome 1q confer a proliferative advantage in B-cell acute lymphoblastic leukemia? Cancer 54: 48–53
16. Callen DF, Baker E, Simmers RN, Seshadri R, Roninson IB (1987) Localization of the human multiple drug resistance gene, MDR1, to 7q21.1. Hum Genet 77: 142–144

Acute Leukemias V
Experimental Approaches
and Management of Refractory Diseases
Hiddemann et al. (Eds.)

Molecular Biology of Acute Lymphoblastic Leukemia: Implications for Detection of Minimal Residual Disease

A. Beishuizen[1], E. R. van Wering[2], T. M. Breit[1], K. Hählen[2,3], H. Hooijkaas[1], and J. J. M. van Dongen[1]

Abstract. Acute lymphoblastic leukemias (ALL) are characterized by high frequencies of clonal chromosome aberrations (ploidy aberrations and translocations) as well as by clonal rearrangements of immunoglobulin (Ig) and T-cell receptor (TcR) genes. These two types of clonal molecular characteristics can be used as leukemia-specific markers for detection of minimal residual disease (MRD) by use of polymerase chain reaction (PCR) technology.

In case of chromosome aberrations, this concerns translocations which result in fusion genes and fusion transcripts, such as in t(9;22), t(1;19), and t(4;11) in precursor B-ALL, or aberrations with site-specific breakpoints such as *tal*-1 deletions in T-ALL. In fact, any precisely identifiable breakpoint fusion region of a chromosome aberration can be used as PCR target for MRD detection during follow-up of leukemia patients. So far such breakpoint fusion regions can be identified in 15–20% of childhood ALL and 25–30% of adult ALL.

Junctional regions of rearranged Ig and TcR genes represent the second type of MRD-PCR target, which can be precisely identified in ~80% of precursor B-ALL and in >90% of T-ALL. This especially concerns the junctional regions of rearranged Ig heavy chain (IgH), TcR-γ, and TcR-δ genes. In contrast to chromosome aberrations, the junctional regions of Ig and TcR genes might not remain stable during the disease course, because of continuing rearrangement processes and subsequent subclone formation. These continuing rearrangements are extensive in IgH genes, resulting in the presence of subclones in 30–40% of precursor B-ALL at diagnosis and changes in rearrangement patterns at relapse in 40% of the cases. Continuing rearrangement processes also cause changes in TcR-γ and TcR-δ gene rearrangement patterns at relapse in 10–20% of T-ALL and 35–45% of precursor B-ALL. This heterogeneity in Ig/TcR gene rearrangement patterns at diagnosis and relapse might hamper PCR-mediated MRD detection. However in 75–90% of ALL cases, at least one IgH, TcR-γ, or TcR-δ allele remains stable at relapse. Therefore, two or more junctional regions of different Ig/TcR genes should be monitored for optimal MRD detection during follow-up of ALL patients.

Well-designed prospective studies on large series of ALL patients have to demonstrate the clinical impact of MRD detection.

Introduction

Approximately 80–85% of childhood leukemias and approximately 7% of adult leukemias represent ALL with an incidence of 3–4 per 100,000 children and, 1–2 per 100,000 adults, respectively. Despite major improvements in ALL treatment during the last two decades, 20–30% of children with ALL and 60–75% of adult ALL patients relapse [1–7]. Apparently, the current treatment protocols are not capable of killing all leukemic cells in these patients, although the far majority reach complete remission according to

[1] Dept. of Immunology, Erasmus University/University Hospital, Rotterdam
[2] Dutch Childhood Leukemia Study Group, The Hague
[3] Division of Hematology/Oncology, Dept. of Pediatrics, Sophia Children's Hospital, Rotterdam, The Netherlands

cytomorphological criteria. Since the detection limit of cytomorphological techniques is not lower than 1–5% leukemic cells, it is obvious that such techniques can only provide superficial information about the effectiveness of leukemia treatment. Techniques with a higher sensitivity to detect MRD are needed to obtain better insight in the reduction of tumor mass during induction treatment and further eradication of the leukemic cells during maintenance treatment (Fig. 1).

During the last decade several methods for detection of MRD have been developed and evaluated, such as cytogenetics, cell culture systems, immunological marker analysis, fluorescence in situ hybridization, and molecular-biological techniques [8–18]. In most studies, the detection limits of these techniques are 1–5% malignant cells. However, depending on the immunophenotype and the genotype of the leukemia, immunological marker analysis and the PCR technique are able to detect lower frequencies of leukemic cells, as low as 10^{-4} to 10^{-5} (10 to 1 leukemic cells per 100,000 normal cells) (Fig. 1) [9,10,15,19–21].

In the PCR technique leukemia-specific nucleotide sequences are used as targets for MRD detection, such as junctional regions of rearranged Ig and TcR genes as well as breakpoint fusion regions of chromosome aberrations.

Ig and TcR Gene Rearrangement Processes

Ig and TcR gene complexes consist of multiple variable (V), diversity (D), and joining (J) gene segments, combinations which code for the variable protein domains of the antigen-specific receptors [16].

The rearrangement processes in Ig and TcR genes during early lymphoid differentiation result in specific combinations of V, (D,) and J gene segments, thereby deleting all intervening sequences. These gene rearrangements are mediated via recombination signal sequences (RSS), -generally heptamer-nonamer sequences, which flank the V, (D,) and J gene segments [16,22,23].

The many possible different combinations of V, (D,) and J gene segments form the so-called combinatorial diversity. This diversity is drastically increased by random deletion and insertion of nucleotides at the junctions of the rearranging gene segments, which together form the junctional diversity. The junctional regions are different in each lymphocyte, even in unrelated lymphocytes which have rearranged the same V, (D,) and J gene segments [16,22,23].

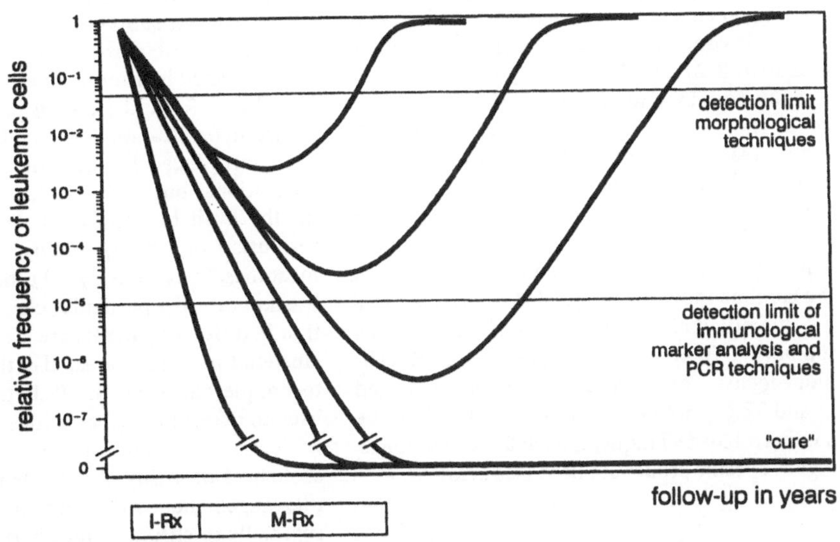

Fig. 1. Diagram of putative relative frequencies of ALL cells in blood and bone marrow during treatment and development of relapse. The detection limit of cytomorphological techniques as well as the detection limit of immunological marker analysis and PCR techniques are indicated. I-Rx = induction treatment; M-Rx = maintenance treatment

Table 1. Frequencies of Ig and TcR gene rearrangements and deletions in precursor B-ALL and T-ALL[a]

	IgH		Igκ		Igλ	TcR-β	TcR-γ	TcR-δ	
	R	D	R	D	R	R	R	R	D
Precursor-B-ALL (n=108)	96%	3%	29%	50%	21%	36%	57%	50%	40%
T-ALL (n=138)	20%	0%	0%	0%	0%	90%	93%	70%	25%
TOTAL ALL[b]	81%	2%	23%	40%	17%	47%	64%	54%	37%

Abbreviations: R, one or both alleles rearranged; D, both alleles deleted or one allele deleted with the other in germline configuration

[a]Beishuizen, Breit, Van Dongen, unpublished results

[b]Estimated frequencies, based on the fact that in children precursor B-ALL and T-ALL represent 80–85% and 15–20% of ALL, respectively and that in adults precursor B-ALL and T-ALL represent 75–80% and 20–25% of ALL, respectively

Therefore, junctional regions are "fingerprint-like" sequences, which can be used for identification of lymphocytes [20]. The combined combinatorial and junctional diversity not only guarantees the enormous diversity of antigen-specific receptors of normal lymphocytes, but also represents an unique diagnostic identification system for "immature" and "mature" clonal lymphoproliferative diseases, such as ALL and other lymphoid leukemias and lymphomas [24].

The far majority of both B-lineage ALL (i.e. precursor B-ALL) and T-lineage ALL (T-ALL) indeed have rearranged Ig and TcR genes, respectively [24–27]. Also cross-lineage gene rearrangements occur in high frequencies. This especially concerns TcR gene rearrangements in precursor B-ALL (Table 1) [24,25,27].

Southern blot and PCR analysis of Ig and TcR genes allow the detection of clonal Ig and TcR gene rearrangements. Application of the Southern blot technique is based on detection of clonal changes in length of restriction fragments due to clonal rearrangements of V, (D,) and J gene segments and therefore takes advantage of the combinatorial diversity. This technique has a detection limit of ~5%, i.e. ~5 clonal cells between 100 normal (polyclonal) cells [16]. The PCR technique focusses on junctional region of rearranged Ig and TcR genes and is more sensitive than the Southern blot technique, especially if junctional-region-specific probes are used (see below).

Chromosome Aberrations

Like other malignancies, ALL can be regarded as an acquired genetic disease, which is caused by alterations in the structure or expression of critical genes. In particular, derangements of genes which normally control growth and differentiation of early lymphoid cells are thought to play a role in the development of ALL, such as protooncogenes, tumor suppressor genes, transcription factors, and especially Ig and TcR genes. The latter is illustrated by the fact that chromosome breakpoints in ALL often involve chromosome bands, which contain Ig or TcR genes: 14q32 (IgH gene), 2p12 (Ig κ gene), 22q11 (Ig λ gene), 14q11 (TcR-α/δ gene complex), 7q35 (TcR-β gene), and 7p15 (TcR-γ gene). Several chromosome aberrations in ALL appear to be associated with particular subtypes [28–30].

So far, most chromosome aberrations have been detected by routine microscopic cytogenetics (G and R band staining patterns). Recently *in situ* hybridization and flow karyotyping have been introduced for detection of chromosome aberrations, but their application is dependent on the availability of suitable probes and the resolution of scatter/staining patterns of chromosomes, respectively. Futhermore, if the breakpoints of a particular chromosome aberration in different patients are well-defined and/or clustered in a small area, also the Southern blot technique and even the PCR technique can be used to detect these aberrations (see below).

Several studies indicate that RSS-like sequences probably play a role in aberrant gene rearrangements in lymphoid malignancies, especially in chromosome aberrations involving Ig and TcR genes. In T-ALL the TcR-α/δ locus in band 14q11 is frequently involved, such as in t(10;14)(q24;q11) and t(1;14)(p34;q11) [31–33]. In the latter aberration the *tal*-1 gene on chromosome 1 is translocated to the TcR-δ gene. Studies on this translocation have lead to the discovery of site-specific (sub-microscopic) deletions of ~90 kb in the *sil* gene/*tal*-1 gene region on chromosome 1 [31,32]. These so-called *tal*-1 gene deletions are reported to occur in 10–30% of T-ALL [32,34–42]. So far five types of *tal*-1 deletions have been described, all of which represent rearrangements occurring via RSS-like sequences [37,39,40]. All five types of *tal*-1 deletions appear to use the same 5′ heptamer RSS, located between the first and second *sil* exons, but different 3′ heptamer-nonamer RSS, which are located in the 5′ part of the *tal*-1 locus. This results in the deletion of all coding *sil* exons and places the coding *tal*-1 exons under direct control of the *sil* gene regulatory elements. The fusion regions of the breakpoints in all five types of *tal*-1 deletions show random deletion and insertion of nucleotides. Therefore, these fusion regions are different in each patient and resemble junctional regions of rearranged Ig and TcR genes [42–44].

Detection of MRD by Use of the PCR Technique

Basic principles of PCR-mediated MRD detection. The PCR technique allows selective amplification of a particular DNA segment or mRNA (after reverse transcription into cDNA) [45–47]. If the target DNA or mRNA sequences are tumor-specific, it is possible to detect a few malignant cells in between many normal cells. Theoretically the detection limit of the PCR technique is approximately 10^{-6}, if a DNA segment is used as PCR target. This is based on the assumption that one cell contains ~10 pg DNA and that one PCR tube can contain maximally 10 µg DNA. This detection limit can indeed be reached, but generally varies between 10^{-4} and 10^{-6}, dependent on the type of tumor-specific PCR target [15,19,20,48, 49]. In the initial PCR studies on the detection of MRD, well-defined chromosome translocations were used as tumor-specific markers [48–51]. However, it is also possible to detect MRD by use of PCR-mediated amplification of junctional regions of rearranged Ig and TcR genes [20,52–59]. Because the PCR technique is highly sensitive, all possible precautionary measures should be taken to prevent cross-contamination of PCR products between patient samples in PCR-mediated MRD studies [47,60].

Chromosome aberrations as leukemia-specific PCR targets for MRD detection. In the initial MRD-PCR studies, t(14;18)(q32;q21) and t(9;22)(q34;q11) were used as PCR targets [48–51]. For this purpose oligonucleotide primers were designed to recognize sequences at opposite sides of the breakpoint fusion region so that the PCR product contained the tumor-specific fusion sequences. In routinely performed MRD-PCR analysis, the PCR products should not exceed ~2 kilobases (kb) [46,47]. Therefore, PCR-mediated amplification of DNA sequences can only be used for chromosome aberrations in which the breakpoints of different patients cluster in a small area (total breakpoint area: <2 kb), such as in t(14;18) where the *bcl*-2 gene is juxtaposed to one of the J gene segments of the IgH genes [61,62]. Other examples are the T-ALL-associated aberrations t(1;14)(p34;q11), t(10;14)(q24;q11) and the *tal*-1 deletions [31–33].

In most translocations, the breakpoints are spread over much larger areas than 2 kb. This implies that the precise breakpoint recombination area has to be determined for each individual patient, which is a laborious and time-consuming effort [63]. However, in several leukemias it has been found that, as a consequence of the translocation, a new leukemia-specific fusion gene has been created, which is transcribed into a leukemia-specific fusion mRNA. This fusion mRNA can be used as target for the MRD-PCR analysis after reverse transcription into cDNA (Table 2). Examples are: *bcr-abl* mRNA in case of t(9;22) [64–66], *E2A-Pbx1* mRNA in most cases of t(1;19) [67–69], and the recently discovered *MLL/ALL-AF4* mRNA in null ALL with t(4;11)(q21–q23) (Table 2) [70–78].

An advantage of using specific chromosome translocations as tumor-specific markers is their stability during the disease course. However, only 20–25% of childhood ALL and 30–35% of adult ALL, have a specific, microscopically detectable chromosome translocation and in a part of these aberrations the precise breakpoints are not (yet) known [30,36,79,80].

One should be aware that PCR products obtained via leukemia-specific fusion mRNA are not patient-specific. Therefore, false-positive results due to cross-contamination of PCR products between samples from different patients are difficult to recognize. This is in contrast to the PCR products obtained from breakpoint fusion regions of *tal*-1 deletions, which can be identified by use of patient-specific oligonucleotide probes [42–44].

Table 2. PCR techniques for MRD detection in ALL patients

PCR analysis of junctional regions of Ig or TcR genes[a]		PCR analysis of chromosome aberrations[b]		
Ig or TcR gene	Frequency of applicability[c]	Aberration	Frequency of applicability[c]	Target (mRNA or DNA)
Precursor-B-ALL				
IgH: V-D-J	80%	t(9;22)(q34;q11)	adult: 30–35% childhood: 5–8%	bcr-abl (mRNA)
TcR-γ: Vγ-Jγ	55%			
TcR-δ: Vδ2-Dδ3 or Dδ2-Dδ3	40%	t(1;19)(q23;p13)	5–8%	*E2A-Pbxl* (mRNA)
		t(4;11)(q21; q 23)	~ 3%	*ALL-AF4* (mRNA)
T-ALL				
IgH: V-D-J	15%?	deletion in TAL-1 gene	10–30%	del (*tal-1*) (DNA)
TcR-γ: Vγ-Jγ	90%	t(1;14)(p34;q11)	1–3%	*tal-1*-TcR-δ (DNA)
TcR-δ: Vδ-Jδ, Dδ-Jδ or Vδ-Dδ	50%	t(10;14)(q24;q11)	1–3%	*tcl-3*-TcR-δ (DNA)

[a]The detection limit of PCR analysis of junctional regions of rearranged Ig and TcR genes varies from 10^{-3} to 10^{-6} and is dependent on "normal background" and the size of the junctional region
[b]The detection limit of PCR analysis of chromosome aberrations is 10^{-4} to 10^{-6}
[c]The indicated percentages represent frequencies within the precursor B-ALL and T-ALL groups

Junctional regions as leukemia-specific PCR targets for MRD detection. As indicated above, junctional regions of rearranged Ig and TcR genes are "fingerprint-like" sequences which are assumed to be different in each lymphocyte and therefore also in each ALL. Based on this assumption, it has been suggested that Ig and TcR gene junctional regions can be used as targets for MRD-PCR analysis, using V, (D), and J gene-specific oligonucleotides as primers (Table 2) [52–54,56–59]. The choice of primers is dependent on the type of Ig or TcR gene as well as the rearranged gene segments. It may be possible to design general primers, which recognize (virtually) all V or J gene segments of a particular Ig or TcR gene complex, or specific primers, which recognize individual V or J gene segments or families of V or J gene segments [52–54,81,82].

An advantage of using IgH, TcR-γ, and TcR-δ junctional regions as targets for the MRD-PCR technique is the fact that the IgH gene complex contains only six V_H families and six J_H gene segments (Fig. 2) and the fact that the TcR-γ and TcR-δ genes contain only a few V, (D), and J gene segments [16,83–89], whereas the junctional regions of most complete V-(D-)J rearrangements are large [57,58,82,88–91]. This implies that only a restricted number of oligonucleotide primers is needed, while the junctional regions will differ extensively between the leukemias. In principle, also PCR analysis of junctional regions of rearranged Ig light chain, TcR-α, and TcR-β genes may be applicable for detection of MRD. However, especially PCR analysis of TcR-α and TcR-β genes at the DNA level needs many different oligonucleotide primers.

In ~80% of precursor B-ALL, IgH gene rearrangements can be detected by PCR analysis with V_H and J_H primers [92], suggesting that in the remaining cases only incompletely rearranged (D-J_H), germline, or deleted IgH genes occur (Table 2). In principle Vγ and Jγ primers detect each TcR-γ gene rearrangement, whereas ~80% of TcR-δ gene rearrangements in precursor B-ALL and ~70% of TcR-δ gene rearrangements in T-ALL can be identified by PCR analysis (Table 2) [27].

The obtained junctional region PCR products can be analysed in a dot blot or Southern blot by use of a leukemia-specific junctional region probe in order to discriminate between the leukemia-derived junctional regions and junctional regions from normal cells which have rearranged the same (or comparable) V and J gene segments as the leukemic cells. For each leukemia one should determine at diagnosis which junctional region(s) can be used as targets for the MRD-PCR analysis during follow-up and which primers are optimal for this purpose (Table 2). Also the leukemia-specific junctional region probes have to be designed for each individual patient at initial diagnosis [20,21,52–59].

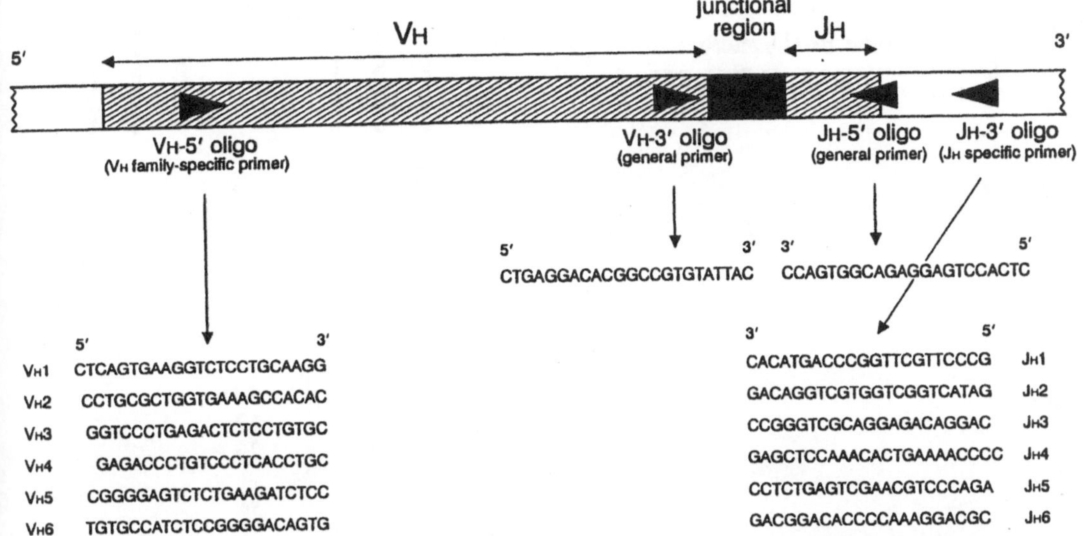

Fig. 2. Schematic diagram of a V_H gene segment joined to a J_H gene segment via a fictitious junctional region, which consists of D_H-derived nucleotides and randomly inserted nucleotides. The approximate position of the V_H-family-specific primers, V_H consensus primer, J_H consensus primer, and J_H specific primers are indicated with arrows. The presented oligonucleotides can be used as primers for the PCR-mediated amplification of the junctional regions of rearranged IgH genes [52,81,83]

Pitfalls of MRD-PCR Analysis of Junctional Regions

From the above described data, it can be concluded that PCR-mediated amplification of junctional regions for detection of MRD is a sensitive technique, which can be applied in the majority of ALL. However, one should realize that this technique has several pitfalls (Table 3).

Occurrence of oligoclonality. A necessary condition for the MRD-PCR technique is the stability of the leukemia-specific junctional region during follow-up. However, in 30–40% of precursor B-ALL at diagnosis multiple IgH gene rearrangements are found (Fig. 3A) [26,93–96]. These are probably caused by continuing rearrangement processes, which lead to subclone formation (bi-/oligoclonality) [26,94]. Such subclone formation at diagnosis appeared to be rare at the TcR-γ and TcR-δ gene level in T-ALL and in cross-lineage TcR gene rearrangements in precursor B-ALL [24,27,97].

Occurrence of clonal evolution. Changes in Ig and TcR gene rearrangement patterns at relapse is also an important pitfall in PCR analysis of

Table 3. Limitations and pitfalls of MRD-PCR analysis of junctional regions

1. Occurrence of oligoclonality at Ig or TcR gene level (e.g. IgH gene level in precursor B-ALL).
   Consequence: false-negative results.
2. Occurrence of clonal evolution at Ig or TcR gene level.
   Consequence: false-negative results.
3. Background of normal cells with the same rearranged gene segments as the leukemic cells. (e.g. Vδ1-Jδ1 rearrangements and VγI-Jγ2.3 rearrangements occur in 0.1–5% and a large part of normal blood T-lymphocytes, respectively).
   Consequence: lower sensitivity of the PCR technique and high dependence on the specificity of the junctional region probe for detection of leukemia-specific PCR products.
4. Type of rearrangement and size of junctional region (e.g. complete Vδ-Jδ rearrangements have large junctional regions, but Dδ-Dδ rearrangements have short junctional regions).
   Consequence: size of junctional region influences the sensitivity of the MRD-PCR technique.
5. Hybridization conditions, washing stringency and exposure time influence the specificity and sensitivity of the MRD-PCR technique.
   Consequence: careful evaluation of the conditions for each patient and use of positive and negative control samples in various dilutions is necessary.

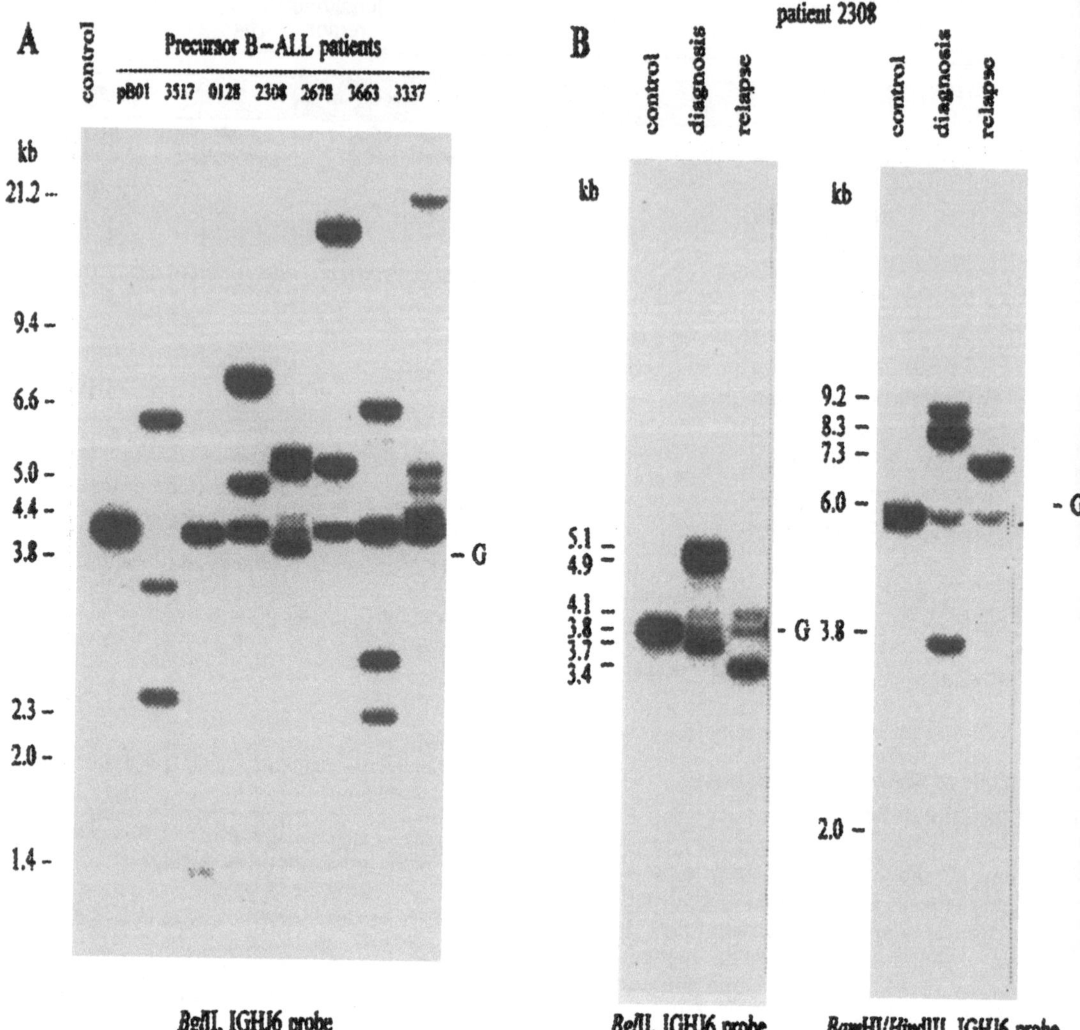

Fig. 3. Southern blot analysis of IgH genes in several precursor B-ALL patients at diagnosis (**A**) and one precursor B-ALL patient (2308) at diagnosis and subsequent relapse (**B**). Control DNA and DNA from precursor B-ALL patients were digested with *Bgl*II and in case of patient 2308 also with *Bam*HI/*Hind*III, size fractioned, and blotted onto nylon membrane filters, which were hybridized with the ^{32}P-labeled IGHJ6 probe. (**A**) In five of the here presented patients, more than two rearranged IgH gene bands were observed. The multiple IgH gene bands differed in density in most cases. With cytogenetic analysis we could exclude the presence of more than two chromosomes 14. (**B**) In patient 2308, three distinct and one weak rearranged band, were seen at diagnosis in both digests, whereas only one distinct and one weak rearranged band were detected at relapse. The weak band at diagnosis was probably identical to the weak band at relapse, but all other bands differed in size in both digests, indicating that clonal evolution had occurred in this precursor B-ALL patient at relapse

junctional regions for MRD detection. In 40 children with ALL, we compared the Ig and TcR gene rearrangement patterns at diagnosis and relapse. An example is shown in Figure 3B. In Table 4, we summarized the data concerning the changes and stability of IgH, TcR-γ, and TcR-δ gene rearrangements at relapse [97]. This table shows that changes in IgH gene rearrangement patterns at relapse occur at high frequency in precursor B-ALL, especially when subclone formation is already present at diagnosis [97]. Changes in TcR-γ and TcR-δ gene rearrange-

Table 4. Changes in IgH, TcR-γ and TcR-δ gene rearrangement patterns in 40 childhood ALL at relapse[a]

	Changes in rearrangement patterns at relapse			Stability of at least one major rearranged band (allele)		
	IgH	TcR-γ	TcR-δ	IgH	TcR-γ and/or TcR-δ	IgH, TcR-γ and/or TcR-δ
precursor B-ALL with monoclonal IgH genes at diagnosis (n = 22)	19% (4/21)[b]	29% (4/14)	40% (8/20)	90% (19/21)[b]	72% (13/18)[c]	91% (20/22)
precursor B-ALL with bi-/oligoclonal IgH genes at diagnosis (n = 8)	100% (8/8)	50% (2/4)	57% (4/7)	38% (3/8)[d]	63% (5/8)	75% (6/8)
T-ALL (n = 10)	50% (2/4)	20% (2/10)	10% (1/10)	100% (4/4)	90% (9/10)	90% (9/10)

[a] The frequencies only concern ALL with IgH, TcR-γ and/or TcR-δ gene rearrangements. If no IgH, TcR-γ or TcR-δ gene rearrangement was found at diagnosis, the ALL was excluded from the calculations (all 40 ALL were extensively tested for the occurrence of IgH, TcR-γ, and TcR-δ gene rearrangements). "New" rearrangements at relapse in genes which were in germline configuration or deleted at diagnosis were also not included in the calculations, because such rearrangements could not have been used for prospective MRD-PCR studies

[b] One patient was excluded from the calculations because both IgH alleles were deleted at diagnosis and at relapse

[c] Two patients were excluded from the calculations because of germline TcR-γ genes and biallelic TcR-δ gene deletions at diagnosis

[d] In two additional bi-/oligoclonal cases, a rearranged band at relapse was identical to a weak rearranged band at diagnosis, suggesting selection of a minor subclone

ments at relapse are found in both precursor B-ALL and T-ALL, but generally concern only one allele [97]. It should be emphasized that Table 4 focusses on changes and stability of gene rearrangements which already existed at diagnosis, i.e. "new" rearrangements at relapse in genes which were in germline configuration or deleted at diagnosis were not included in the calculations, because such rearrangements could not have been used for prospective MRD-PCR studies.

Figure 4 shows the changes and stability of rearranged Ig and TcR gene bands (alleles) and their relation to the remission duration in the 40 childhood ALL cases. Changes in at least one of the three major MRD-PCR targets (IgH, TcR-γ, and TcR-δ) were found in 40% [9/22] of the monoclonal precursor B-ALL after remission duration of at least 18 months (Fig. 4A). All [8/8] bi-/oligoclonal precursor B-ALL showed changes at relapse in IgH, TcR-γ, and/or TcR-δ genes, which were already found after a short remission duration of at least 6 months (Fig. 4B). In 30% of T-ALL, changes in IgH, TcR-γ, and/or TcR-δ gene rearrangement patterns occurred after a remission duration of at least 14 months (Fig. 4C). Despite the high frequency of immunogenotypic changes, at least one major IgH, TcR-γ and/or TcR-δ rearranged band (allele) remained stable in 75–90% of precursor B-ALL and 90% of T-ALL (Fig. 4 and Table 4).

Several reports indicate that changes in IgH gene rearrangements at relapse do not necessarily imply that the complete sequence of the junctional regions has changed [98,99]. For example, V_H replacements in completely rearranged IgH genes generally do not affect the original V-D-J_H junctional regions, and also the D-J_H junctional regions will generally remain stable in subclones, which rearranged different V_H gene segments to an identical D-J_H precursor [100].

Our childhood ALL study indicates that IgH genes represent optimal targets for MRD detection in monoclonal precursor B-ALL, but it might be valuable to monitor the TcR-γ and/or TcR-δ gene rearrangements as well, especially in cases with germline or deleted IgH genes on one or both alleles. In T-ALL the TcR-γ and TcR-δ genes represent optimal MRD-PCR targets [97]. However, in bi-/oligoclonal precursor B-ALL (30–40% of the total group of precursor B-ALL), it will be difficult to estimate which minor or major IgH gene band (allele) will remain stable, especially in cases with more than two sub-

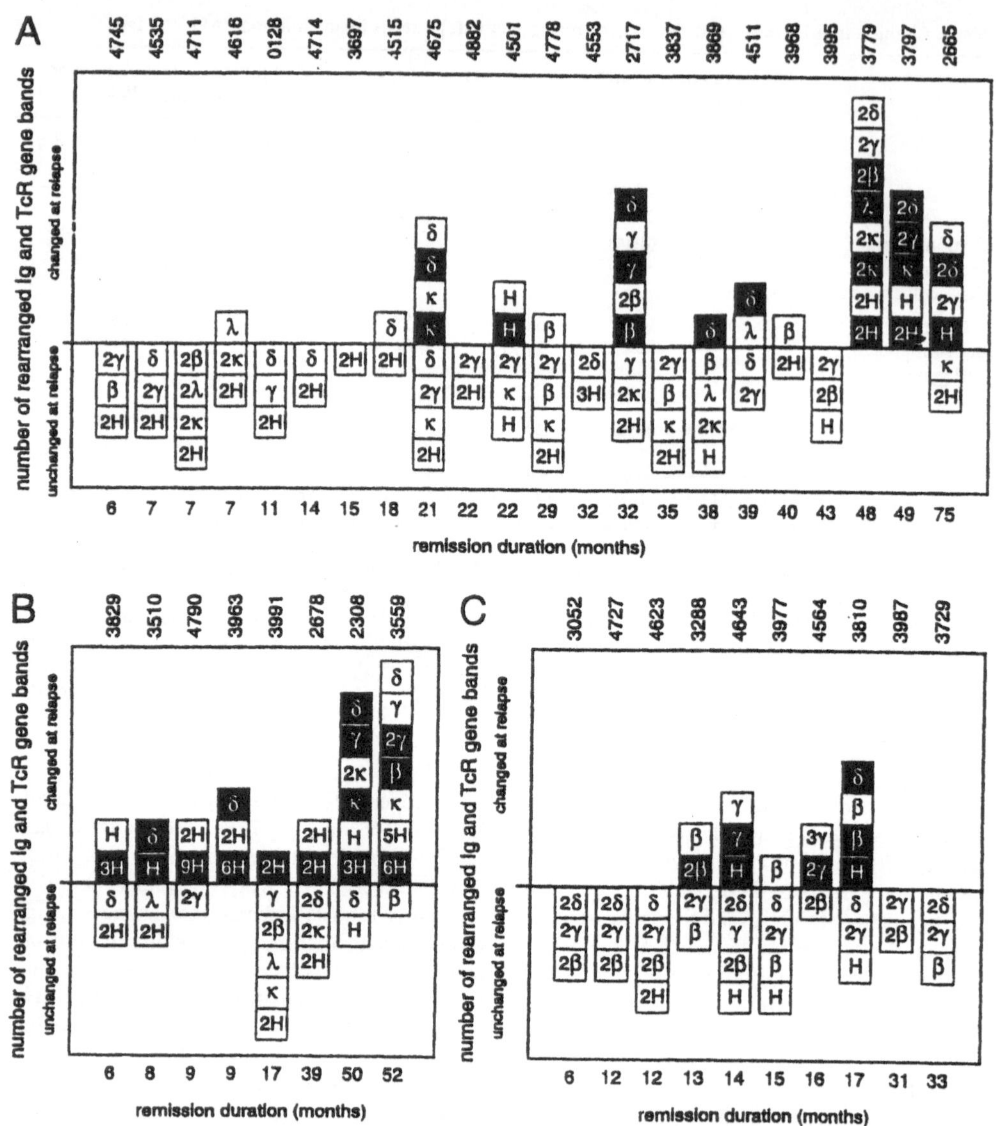

Fig. 4. Changes in Ig and TcR gene rearrangement patterns at relapse and their relation with remission duration. Each bar summarizes the Ig and TcR gene configuration per patient, who are numbered according to the registry of the Dutch Childhood Leukemia Study Group. The letter codes in the boxes of each bar indicate the presence (open boxes) or loss (black boxes) of rearranged Ig and TcR gene bands at relapse (H, IgH; κ, Igκ; λ, Igλ; β, TcR-β; γ, TcR-γ; δ, TcR-δ); the numbers indicate the sum of rearranged bands. The changes at relapse are shown above the horizontal line (black boxes: loss of rearranged bands; open boxes: "new" rearranged bands), whereas the stable rearrangements are shown underneath. **A**, 22 monoclonal precursor B-ALL (remission duration 6–75 months), **B**, eight bi-/oligoclonal precursor B-ALL (remission duration 6–52 months), and **C**, 10 T-ALL (remission duration 6–53 months). Detailed information concerning the changes in Ig and TcR gene configuration at relapse are given in reference 97

clones. This implies that in these leukemias the MRD-PCR monitoring should not be restricted to IgH genes, but that TcR-γ and TcR-δ gene rearrangements should be monitored as well. Two recently published PCR studies, describing changes and stability of IgH, TcR-γ, and TcR-δ gene rearrangements at relapse in ALL, subscribed to these findings [101,102]. Therefore, we conclude that MRD detection in ALL patients by PCR techniques needs monitoring of two or more junctional regions of IgH, TcR-γ, and/or TcR-δ genes in order to prevent false negative results [97].

The chance of changes in rearrangement patterns appears to increase with time (Fig. 4). This implies that in case of early relapse generally no changes will be found. This might be important for the choice of PCR targets in MRD-PCR studies in adult ALL patients, because in adult ALL remission duration is essentially shorter than in childhood ALL.

Background of normal cells. The sensitivity of the PCR technique and the specificity of the junctional region probe for detection of leukemia-specific PCR products is highly dependent on the background of normal cells with the same rearranged gene segments as the leukemic cells. This concerns for instance Vδ1-Jδ1 rearrangements and VγI-Jγ2.3 rearrangements which occur in 0.1–5% and a large part of normal blood T-lymphocytes, respectively [82]. This may result in lower sensitivity and specificity of the junctional region MRD-PCR technique.

Type of rearrangement and size of the junctional region. It should be emphasized that the detection limit of the MRD-PCR technique is related to the size of the junctional region. Junctional regions of complete Vδ-Jδ rearrangements are three to four times larger than Vγ-Jγ junctional regions [27,57,82], implying that TcR-δ junctional regions are more suitable targets for MRD-PCR analysis [27,82]. However, TcR-δ gene rearrangements may be incomplete, such as Vδ-Dδ and Dδ-Dδ rearrangements, which have relatively short junctional regions [27,82,103]. Incomplete TcR-δ gene rearrangements with short junctional regions are especially found in precursor B-ALL, e.g. Vδ2-Dδ3 and Dδ2-Dδ3 [27,90,103–106]. This may result in detection limits which are 10^{-3} to 10^{-4}. In case of short junctional regions, it may theoretically happen that normal cells occur which have junctional regions that are identical to those in leukemic cells.

Technical influences on the MRD-PCR technique. Finally, it should be emphasized that the specificity and sensitivity of the junctional region MRD-PCR technique is influenced by the hybridization conditions, washing stringency and film exposure time of the junctional region specific probe. These should be carefully determined to obtain reproducible results.

PCR Analysis for MRD Detection in Childhood ALL

So far the MRD-PCR studies are restricted to retrospective studies or short-term prospective follow-up studies on limited numbers of patients. Most investigators use junctional regions of rearranged Ig and TcR genes as PCR targets [55,58,59,92,107–112]. Analysis of cell samples from ALL patients who developed a relapse, indicate that relapse during treatment might be predicted by persisting PCR positivity, often at a high level (e.g. 10^{-2} or 10^{-3}), or by an increase of PCR positivity over a period up to 12 months before cytomorphological relapse [55,58,59,92, 107,111]. Several research groups concluded that PCR detection of high levels of residual disease at the end of induction therapy identifies patients at increased risk for relapse during therapy [108–111]. Furthermore, they concluded that absence of detectable MRD at the end of chemotherapy is not sufficient to assure that the patient is cured, indicating that after treatment frequent serial monitoring is required for the early prediction of relapse [108–111]. In a small prospective study of twenty children followed for 7 to 30 months, Cavé et al. found progressive decrease of the tumor load and no detectable blasts within 6 months. In three patients who developed BM relapse slower kinetics of decrease were found [112]. They concluded that the kinetics of blast decrease in the first months of treatment may be of prognostic value [112].

Conclusion

PCR analysis of chromosomal aberrations and junctional regions of antigen specific receptors is valuable for the detection of MRD in ALL. However, one should realize that each MRD-PCR target has its own limitations and pitfalls.

MRD-PCR analysis using chromosome aberrations has the advantage that these aberrations are most probably directly related to the oncogenic event and therefore represent stable tumor-specific markers. The first limitation of this technique is the fact that in only 15–20% of childhood ALL and in 25–30% of adult ALL, chromosome aberrations with well-defined breakpoints have been found so far. The second limitation is the fact that in many translocations the PCR target is a fusion mRNA, which is not patient-specific and therefore might cause false positive results due to cross-contamination between patient samples.

MRD-PCR analysis using junctional regions of rearranged Ig and TcR genes seems to be a promising technique, which can be applied in the majority of ALL. Despite the relatively high frequency of changes in Ig and TcR gene rearrangement patterns, which might cause false negative results (due to subclone formation and clonal evolution), at least one major IgH, TcR-γ, and/or TcR-δ rearranged band (allele) remained stable in the majority [75–90%] of ALL. Still, the size of the junctional region will influence the detection limit of the PCR technique. This especially concerns incomplete TcR-δ gene rearrangements, which represent the most frequent TcR-δ rearrangements in precursor B-ALL.

Prospective studies on large groups of ALL patients using several PCR targets in parallel are needed to evaluate which target is most efficient and reliable for each patient group. In the future, the MRD-PCR target of choice will probably depend on the presence of a chromosome aberration with well-defined breakpoints and the presence of a rearranged Ig and/or TcR gene, as well as on the chance of changes in Ig/TcR gene rearrangement patterns. The origin of the cell sample (BM, PB, or cerebrospinal fluid), its volume, and its cellularity will influence the choice as well.

Acknowledgements. We are grateful to Prof. Dr. R. Benner for his continuous support, to M-A.J. Verhoeven, I.L.M. Wolvers-Tettero, and E.J. Mol for their technical assistance, to T.M. van Os for his assistance in the preparation of the figures, and to A.D. Korpershoek for her secretarial support.

This work was financially supported by the Dutch Cancer Foundation (Nederlandse Kankerbestrijding, Koningin Wilhelmina Fonds), grant IKR 89-09 and the Stichting Ank van Vlissingenfonds, The Netherlands.

References

1. Riehm H, Gadner H, Henze G, et al (1990) Results and significance of six randomized trials in four consecutive ALL-BFM studies. Haematol Blood Transfusion 33: 439–450
2. Veerman AJP, Hählen K, Kamps WA, et al (1990) Dutch childhood leukemia study group: Early results of study ALL VI (1984–1988). Hematol Blood Transfusion 33: 473–477
3. Ellison RR, Mick R, Cuttner J, et al (1991) The effects of postinduction intensification treatment with cytarabine and daunorubicin in adult acute lymphocytic leukemia: A prospective randomized clinical trial by cancer and leukemia group B. J Clin Oncol 9: 2002–2015
4. Rivera GK, Pinkel D, Simone JV, Hancock ML, Crist WM (1993) Treatment of acute lymphoblastic leukemia. N Engl J Med 329: 1289–1295.
5. Hoelzer DF (1993) Therapy of the newly diagnosed adult with acute lymphoblastic leukemia. Hematol Oncol Clin North Am 7: 139–160
6. Hoelzer DF (1993) Acute lymphoblastic leukemia-progress in children, less in adults. N Engl J Med 329: 1343–1344
7. Pui C-H, Crist WM (1994) Biology and treatment of acute lymphoblastic leukemia. J Pediatr 124: 491–503
8. Sonta S, Sandberg AA (1977) Chromosomes and causation of human cancer and leukemia: XXVIII. Value of detailed chromosome studies on large numbers of cells in CML. Am J Hematol 3: 121–126
9. Van Dongen JJM, Hooijkaas H, Hählen K, et al. Detection of minimal residual disease in TdT positive T cell malignancies by double immunofluorescence staining. In: Löwenberg B, Hagenbeek A (eds) (1984) Minimal residual disease in acute leukemia. M Nijhoff Publishers, The Hague 67–81
10. Van Dongen JJM, Hooijkaas H, Adriaansen HJ, Hählen K, Van Zanen GE. Detection of minimal residual acute lymphoblastic leukemia by immunological marker analysis: Possibilities and limitations. In: Hagenbeek A, Löwenberg B (eds) (1986) Minimal residual disease in acute leukemia 1986. M Nijhoff Publishers, Dordrecht 113–133
11. Wright JJ, Poplack DG, Bakhshi A, et al (1987) Gene rearrangements as markers of clonal variation and minimal residual disease in acute lymphoblastic leukemia. J Clin Oncol 5: 735–741
12. Estrov Z, Freedman MH (1988) Growth requirements for human acute lymphoblastic leukemia cells: Refinement of a clonogenic assay. Cancer Res 48: 5901–5907
13. Hittelman WN, Tigaud J-D, Estey E, Vadhan-Raj S (1990) Premature chromosome condensation in the study of minimal residual disease. Bone Marrow Transplantation 6: 9–13
14. Campana D, Coustan-Smith E, Janossy G (1990) The immunologic detection of minimal residual disease in acute leukemia. Blood 76: 163–171
15. Bartram CR, Yokota S, Hansen-Hagge TE, Janssen JWG (1990) Detection of minimal residual leukemia by polymerase chain reactions. Bone Marrow Transplantation 6s: 4–8
16. Van Dongen JJM, Wolvers-Tettero ILM (1991) Analysis of immunoglobulin and T cell receptor genes. Part I: Basic and technical aspects. Clin Chim Acta 198: 1–91

17. Anastasi J, Thangavelu M, Vardiman JW, et al (1991) Interphase cytogenetic analysis detects minimal residual disease in a case of acute lymphoblastic leukemia and resolves the question of origin of relapse after allogeneic bone marrow transplantation. Blood 77: 1087–1091
18. Heerema NA, Argyropoulos G, Weetman R, Tricot G, Secker-Walker LM (1993) Interphase in situ hybridization reveals minimal residual disease in early remission and return of the diagnostic clone in karyotypically normal relapse of acute lymphoblastic leukemia. Leukemia 7: 537–543
19. Campana D, Yokota S, Coustan-Smith E, Hansen-Hagge TE, Janossy G, Bartram CR (1990) The detection of residual acute lymphoblastic leukemia cells with immunologic methods and polymerase chain reaction: A comparative study. Leukemia 4: 609–614
20. Van Dongen JJM, Breit TM, Adriaansen HJ, Beishuizen A, Hooijkaas H (1992) Detection of minimal residual disease in acute leukemia by immunological marker analysis and polymerase chain reaction. Leukemia 6S1: 74–85
21. Bartram CR (1993) Detection of minimal residual leukemia by the polymerase chain reaction: potential implications for therapy. Clin Chim Acta 217: 75–83
22. Hesse JE, Lieber MR, Mizuuchi K, Gellert M (1989) V(D)J recombination: a functional definition of the joining signals. Genes Dev 3: 1053–1061
23. Schatz DG, Oettinger MA, Schlissel MS (1992) V(D)J recombination: molecular biology and regulation. Annu Rev Immunol 10: 359–383
24. Van Dongen JJM, Wolvers-Tettero ILM (1991) Analysis of immunoglobulin and T cell receptor genes. Part II: Possibilities and limitations in the diagnosis and management of lymphoproliferative diseases and related disorders. Clin Chim Acta 198: 93–174
25. Felix CA, Poplack DG, Reaman GH, et al (1990) Characterization of immunoglobulin and T-cell receptor gene patterns in B-cell precursor acute lymphoblastic leukemia of childhood. J Clin Oncol 8: 431–442
26. Beishuizen A, Hählen K, Hagemeijer A, et al (1991) Multiple rearranged immunoglobulin genes in childhood acute lymphoblastic leukemia of precursor-B-cell origin. Leukemia 5: 657–667
27. Breit TM, Wolvers-Tettero ILM, Beishuizen A, Verhoeven M-AJ, Van Wering ER, Van Dongen JJM (1993). Southern blot patterns, frequencies, and junctional diversity of T-cell receptor- δ gene rearrangements in acute lymphoblastic leukemia. Blood 82: 3063–3074
28. Pui C-H, Williams DL, Roberson, et al (1988) Correlation of karyotype and immunophenotype in childhood acute lymphoblastic leukemia. J Clin Oncol 6: 56–61
29. Pui C-H, Crist WM, Look AT (1990) Biology and clinical significance of cytogenetic abnormalities in childhood acute lymphoblastic leukemia. Blood 76: 1449–1463
30. Raimondi SC (1993) Current status of cytogenetic research in childhood acute lymphoblastic leukemia. Blood 81: 2237–2251
31. Chen Q, Cheng J-T, Tsai L-H, et al (1990) The tal gene undergoes chromosome translocation in T cell leukemia and potentially encodes a helix-loop-helix protein. EMBO J 9: 415–424
32. Brown L, Cheng J-T, Chen Q, et al (1990) Site-specific recombination of the tal-1 gene is a common occurrence in human T cell leukemia. EMBO J 9: 3343–3351
33. Kagan J, Finger LR, Besa E, Croce CM (1990) Detection of minimal residual disease in leukemic patients with the t(10;14)(q24;q11) chromosomal translocation. Cancer Res 50:5240–5244
34. Aplan PD, Lombardi DP, Ginsberg AM, Cossman J, Bertness VL, Kirsch IR (1990). Disruption of the human SCL locus by "illegitimate" V-(D)-J recombinase activity. Science 250: 1426–1429
35. Aplan PD, Lombardi DP, Kirsch IR (1991) Structural characterization of SIL, a gene frequently disrupted in T-cell acute lymphoblastic leukemia. Mol Cell Biol 11: 5462–5469
36. Jonsson OG, Kitchens RL, Baer RJ, Buchanan GR, Smith RG (1991) Rearrangements of the tal-1 locus as clonal markers for T cell acute lymphoblastic leukemia. J Clin Invest 87: 2029–2035
37. Bernard O, Lecointe N, Jonveaux P, et al (1991) Two site-specific deletions and t(1;14) translocation restricted to human T-cell acute leukemias disrupt the 5′ part of the tal-1 gene. Oncogene 6: 1477–1488
38. Macintyre EA, Smit L, Ritz J, Kirsch IR, Strominger JL (1992) Disruption of the SCL locus in T-lymphoid malignancies correlates with commitment to the T-cell receptor αβ lineage. Blood 80: 1511–1520
39. Breit TM, Mol EJ, Wolvers-Tettero ILM, Ludwig W-D, Van Wering ER, Van Dongen JJM (1993). Site-specific deletions involving the tal-1 and sil genes are restricted to cells of the T-cell receptor αβ lineage: T-cell receptor δ gene deletion mechanism affects multiple genes. J Exp Med 177: 965–977
40. Bash RO, Crist WM, Shuster JJ, et al (1993) Clinical features and outcome of T-cell acute lymphoblastic leukemia in childhood with respect to alterations at the *TAL1* locus: a Pediatric Oncology Group study. Blood 81: 2110–2117
41. Borkhardt A, Repp R, Harbott J, et al (1992) Frequency and DNA sequence of tal-1 rearrangement in children with T-cell acute lymphoblastic leukemia. Ann Hematol 64: 305–308.
42. Breit TM, Beishuizen A, Ludwig WD, (1993) tal-1 deletions in T-ALL as target for detection of minimal residual disease by PCR techniques. Leukemia 7: 2004–2011
43. Kikuchi A, Hayashi Y, Kobayashi S, et al (1993) Clinical significance of TAL1 gene alteration in childhood T-cell acute lymphoblastic leukemia and lymphoma. Leukemia 7: 933–938
44. Janssen JWG, Ludwig W-D, Sterry W, Bartram CR (1993) SIL-TAL1 deletion in T-cell acute lymphoblastic leukemia. Leukemia 7: 1204–1210

45. Todd JA, Bell JI, McDevitt HO (1987) HLA-DQ_β gene contributes to susceptibility and resistance to insulin-dependent diabetes mellitus. Nature 329: 599–604
46. Erlich HA, Gelfand DH, Saiki RK (1988) Specific DNA amplification. Nature 331: 461–462
47. White TJ, Arnheim N, Erlich HA (1989) The polymerase chain reaction. Trends Genet 5: 185–189
48. Lee M-S, Chang K-S, Cabanillas F, Freireich EJ, Trujillo JM, Stass SA (1987). Detection of minimal residual cells carrying the t(14;18) by DNA sequence amplification. Science 237: 175–178
49. Crescenzi M, Seto M, Herzig GP, Weiss PD, Griffith RC, Korsmeyer SJ (1988) Thermostable DNA polymerase chain amplification of t(14;18) chromosome breakpoints and detection of minimal residual disease. Proc Natl Acad Sci USA 85: 4869–4873
50. Morgan GJ, Janssen JWG, Guo A-P, et al (1989) Polymerase chain reaction for detection of residual leukaemia. Lancet i: 928–929
51. Gabert J, Lafage M, Maraninchi D, Thuret I, Carcassonne Y, Mannoni P (1989) Detection of residual *bcr/abl* translocation by polymerase chain reaction in chronic myeloid leukaemia patients after bone-marrow transplantation. Lancet ii: 1125–1128
52. Yamada M, Hudson S, Tournay O, et al (1989) Detection of minimal disease in hematopoietic malignancies of the B-cell lineage by using third-complementarity-determining region (CDR-III)-specific probes. Proc Natl Acad Sci USA 86: 5123–5127
53. D'Auriol L, Macintyre E, Galibert F, Sigaux F (1989) In vitro amplification of T cell γ gene rearrangements: A new tool for the assessment of minimal residual disease in acute lymphoblastic leukemias. Leukemia 3: 155–158
54. Hansen-Hagge TE, Yokota S, Bartram CR (1989) Detection of minimal residual disease in acute lymphoblastic leukemia by in vitro amplification of rearranged T-cell receptor δ chain sequences. Blood 74: 1762–1767
55. Yamada M, Wasserman R, Lange B, Reichard BA, Womer RB, Rovera G (1990) Minimal residual disease in childhood B-lineage lymphoblastic leukemia: Persistence of leukemic cells during the first 18 months of treatment. N Engl J Med 323: 448–455
56. Jonsson OG, Kitchens RL, Scott FC, Smith RG (1990) Detection of minimal residual disease in acute lymphoblastic leukemia using immunoglobulin hypervariable region specific oligonucleotide probes. Blood 76: 2072–2079
57. Macintyre EA, D'Auriol L, Duparc N, Leverger G, Galibert F, Sigaux F (1990) Use of oligonucleotide probes directed against T cell antigen receptor gamma delta variable-(diversity)-joining junctional sequences as a general method for detecting minimal residual disease in acute lymphoblastic leukemias. J Clin Invest 86: 2125–2135
58. Neale GAM, Menarguez J, Kitchingman GR, et al (1991) Detection of minimal residual disease in T-cell acute lymphoblastic leukemia using polymerase chain reaction predicts impending relapse. Blood 78: 739–747
59. Yokota S, Hansen-Hagge TE, Ludwig W-D, et al (1991) Use of polymerase chain reactions to monitor minimal residual disease in acute lymphoblastic leukemia patients. Blood 77: 331–339
60. Kwok S, Higuchi R (1989) Avoiding false positives with PCR. Nature 339: 237–238
61. Bakhshi A, Wright JJ, Graninger W, et al (1987) Mechanism of the t(14;18) chromosomal translocation: Structural analysis of both derivative 14 and 18 reciprocal partners. Proc Natl Acad Sci USA 84: 2396–2400
62. Cotter F, Price C, Zucca E, Young BD (1990) Direct sequence analysis of the $14q^+$ and $18q^-$ chromosome junctions in follicular lymphoma. Blood 76: 131–135
63. Hermans A, Heisterkamp N, Von Lindern M, et al (1987) Unique fusion of *bcr* and *c-abl* genes in Philadelphia chromosome positive acute lymphoblastic leukemia. Cell 51: 33–40
64. Blennerhassett GT, Furth ME, Anderson A, et al (1988) Clinical evaluation of a DNA probe assay for the Philadelphia (Ph1) translocation in chronic myelogenous leukemia. Leukemia 2: 648–657
65. Hermans A, Selleri L, Gow J, Wiedemann L, Grosveld G (1989) Molecular analysis of the Philadelphia translocation in chronic myelogenous and acute lymphocytic leukemia. Cancer Cells 7: 21–26
66. Maurer J, Janssen JWG, Thiel E, et al (1991) Detection of chimeric BCR-ABL genes in acute lymphoblastic leukemia by the polymerase chain reaction. Lancet 337: 1055–8
67. Kamps MP, Murre C, Sun X, Baltimore D (1990) A new homeobox gene contributes the DNA binding domain of the t(1;19) translocation protein in pre-B ALL. Cell 60: 547–555
68. Kamps MP, Look AT, Baltimore D (1991) The human t(1;19) translocation in pre-B ALL produces multiple nuclear E2A-Pbx1 fusion proteins with differing transforming potentials. Genes Develop 5: 358–368
69. Hunger SP, Galili N, Carroll AJ, Crist WM, Link MP, Cleary ML (1991) The t(1;19)(q23;p13) results in consistent fusion of *E2A* and *PBX1* coding sequences in acute lymphoblastic leukemias. Blood 77: 687–693
70. Chen C-S, Medberry PS, Arthur DC, Kersey JH (1991) Breakpoint clustering in t(4;11)(q21;q23) acute leukemia. Blood 78: 2498–2504
71. Cimino G, Moir DT, Canaani O, et al (1991) Cloning of ALL-1, the locus involved in leukemias with the t(4;11)(q21;q23), t(9;11)(p22;q23), and t(11;19)(q23;p13) chromosome translocations. Cancer Res 51: 6712–6714
72. Tkachuk DC, Kohler S, Cleary ML (1992) Involvement of a homolog of drosophila trithorax by 11q23 chromosomal translocations in acute leukemias. Cell 71: 691–700
73. Gu Y, Nakamura T, Alder H, et al (1992) The t(4;11) chromosome translocation of human acute

leukemias fuses the ALL-1 gene, related to drosophila trithorax, to the AF-4 gene. Cell 71: 701–708
74. Gu Y, Cimino G, Alder H, et al (1992) The (4;11)(q21;q23) chromosome translocations in acute leukemias involve the VDJ recombinase. Proc Natl Acad Sci USA 89: 10464–10468
75. Biondi A, Rambaldi A, Rossi V, et al (1993) Detection of ALL-1/AF4 fusion transcript by reverse transcription-polymerase chain reaction for diagnosis and monitoring of acute leukemias with the t(4;11) translocation. Blood 82;2943–2947
76. Downing JR, Head DR, Raimondi SC, et al (1994). The der(11)-encoded MLL/AF-4 fusion transcript is consistently detected in t(4;11)(q21;q23)-containing acute lymphoblastic leukemia. Blood 83: 330–335
77. Griessinger F, Elfers H, Ludwig W-D, et al (1994) Detection of *HRX-FEL* fusion transcripts in pre-pre-B-ALL with and without cytogenetic demonstration of t(4;11). Leukemia 8: 542–548
78. Borkhardt A, Repp R, Haupt E, et al (1994) Molecular analysis of MLL-1/AF4 recombination in infant acute lymphoblastic leukemia. Leukemia 8: 549–553
79. Ahuja H, Cline MJ (1988) Genetic and cytogenetic changes in acute lymphoblastic leukemia. Med Oncol Tumor Pharmacother 5: 211–222
80. Boehm T, Rabbitts TH (1989) A chromosomal basis of lymphoid malignancy in man. Eur J Biochem 185: 1–17
81. Deane M, Norton JD (1990). Immunoglobulin heavy chain variable region family usage is independent of tumor cell phenotype in human B lineage leukemias. Eur J Immunol 20: 2209–2217.
82. Breit TM, Wolvers-Tettero ILM, Hählen K, Van Wering ER, Van Dongen JJM (1991). Extensive junctional diversity of γδ T-cell receptors expressed by T-cell acute lymphoblastic leukemias: Implications for the detection of minimal residual disease. Leukemia 5: 1076–1086
83. Ravetch JV, Siebenlist U, Korsmeyer S, Waldmann T, Leder P (1981) Structure of the human immunoglobulin μ locus: characterization of embryonic and rearranged J and D genes. Cell 27: 583–591
84. Kodaira M, Kinashi T, Umemura I, et al (1986) Organization and evolution of variable region genes of the human immunoglobulin heavy chain. J Mol Biol 190: 529–541
85. Berman JE, Mellis SJ, Pollock R, et al (1988) Content and organisation of the human Ig V_H locus: definition of three new V_H families and linkage to the Ig C_H locus. EMBO J 7: 727–738
86. Lefranc M-P (1988) The human T-cell rearranging gamma (TRG) genes and the gamma T-cell receptor. Biochimie 70: 901–908
87. Takihara Y, Tkachuk D, Michalopoulos E, et al (1988) Sequence and organization of the diversity, joining, and constant region genes of the human T-cell δ-chain locus. Proc Natl Acad Sci USA 85: 6097–6101
88. Loh EY, Cwirla S, Serafini AT, Phillips JH, Lanier LL (1988) Human T-cell-receptor δ chain: Genomic organization, diversity, and expression in populations of cells. Proc Natl Acad Sci USA 85: 9714–9718
89. Takihara Y, Reimann J, Michalopoulos E, Ciccone E, Moretta L, Mak TW (1989) Diversity and structure of human T cell receptor δ chain genes in peripheral blood γ/δ-bearing T lymphocytes. J Exp Med 169: 393–405
90. Macintyre E, D'Auriol L, Amesland F, et al (1989) Analysis of junctional diversity in the preferential Vδ1-$Jδ_1$ rearrangement of fresh T-acute lymphoblastic leukemia cells by in vitro gene amplification and direct sequencing. Blood 74: 2053–2061
91. Yamada M, Wasserman R, Reichert BA, Shane S, Caton AJ, Rovera G (1991) Preferential utilization of specific immunoglobulin heavy chain diversity and joining segments in adult human peripheral blood lymphocytes. J Exp Med 173: 395–407
92. Nizet Y, Martiat P, Vaerman JL, et al (1991) Follow-up of residual disease (MRD) in B lineage acute leukemias using a simplified PCR strategy: evolution of MRD rather than its detection is correlated with clinical outcome. Br J Haematol 79: 205–210
93. Kitchingman GR, Mirro J, Stass S, et al (1986) Biologic and prognostic significance of the presence of more than two μ heavy-chain genes in childhood acute lymphoblastic leukemia of B precursor cell origin. Blood 67: 698–703
94. Bird J, Galili N, Link M, Stites D, Sklar J (1988) Continuing rearrangement but abscence of somatic hypermutation in immunoglobulin genes of human B cell precursor leukemia. J Exp Med 168: 229–245
95. Katz F, Ball L, Gibbons B, Chessells J (1989) The use of DNA probes to monitor minimal residual disease in childhood acute lymphoblastic leukemia. Br J Haematol 73: 173–180
96. Beishuizen A, Hählen K, Van Wering ER, Van Dongen JJM (1991) Detection of minimal residual disease in childhood leukemia with the polymerase chain reaction. New Engl J Med 324: 772–773
97. Beishuizen A, Verhoeven M-AJ, Van Wering ER, Hählen K, Hooijkaas H, Van Dongen JJM (1994) Analysis of immunoglobulin and T-cell receptor genes in 40 childhood acute lymphoblastic leukemias at diagnosis and subsequent relapse: Implications for the detection of minimal residual disease by polymerase chain reaction analysis. Blood 83: 2238–2247
98. Wasserman R, Yamada M, Ito Y, et al (1992) V_H gene rearrangement events can modify the immunoglobulin heavy chain during progression of B-lineage acute lymphoblastic leukemia. Blood 79: 223–228
99. Steenbergen EJ, Verhagen OJHM, Van Leeuwen EF, Von dem Borne AEGKr, Van der Schoot CE. (1993) Distinct ongoing Ig heavy chain rearrangement processes in childhood B-precursor acute lymphoblastic leukemia. Blood 82: 581–589
100. Rovera G, Wasserman R, Yamada M (1991) Detection of minimal residual disease in

childhood leukemia with the polymerase chain reaction. New Enl J Med 324: 774
101. Taylor JJ, Rowe D, Kylefjord H, et al (1994) Characterisation of non-concordance in the T-cell receptor γ chain genes at presentation and clinical relapse in acute lymphoblastic leukemia. Leukemia 8: 60–66
102. Steward CG, Goulden NJ, Katz F, et al (1994) A polymerase chain reaction study of the stability of Ig heavy-chain and T-cell receptor δ gene rearrangements between presentation and relapse of childhood B-lineage acute lymphoblastic leukemia. Blood 83: 1355–1362
103. Yokota S, Hansen-Hagge TE, Bartram CR (1991) T-cell receptor δ gene recombination in common acute lymphoblastic leukemia: Preferential usage of Vδ2 and frequent involvement of the Jα cluster. Blood 77: 141–148
104. Loiseau P, Guglielmi P, Le Paslier D, et al (1989) Rearrangements of the T cell receptor δ gene in T acute lymphoblastic leukemia cells are distinct from those occurring in B lineage acute lymphoblastic leukemia and preferentially involve one Vδ gene segment. J Immunol 142: 3305–3311
105. Biondi A, Di Celle PF, Rossi V, et al (1990) High prevalence of T-cell receptor Vδ2-(D)-Dδ3 or Dδ1/2-Dδ3 rearrangements in B-precursor acute lymphoblastic leukemias. Blood 75: 1834–1840
106. Yano T, Pullman A, Andrade R, et al (1991) A common Vδ2-Dδ2-Dδ3 T cell receptor gene rearrangement in precursor B acute lymphoblastic leukaemia. Brit J Haematol 79: 44–49
107. Biondi A, Yokota S, Hansen-Hagge TE, et al (1992) Minimal residual disease in childhood acute lymphoblastic leukemia: Analysis of patients in continuous complete remission or with consecutive relapse. Leukemia 6: 282–288.
108. Wasserman R, Galili N, Ito Y, et al (1992)Residual disease at the end of induction therapy as a predictor of relapse during therapy in childhood B-lineage acute lymphoblastic leukemia. J Clin Oncol 10: 1879–1888
109. Ito Y, Wasserman R, Galili N, et al (1993) Molecular residual disease status at the end of chemotherapy fails to predict subsequent relapse in children with B-lineage acute lymphoblastic leukemia. J Clin Oncol 11: 546–553
110. Potter MN, Steward CG, Oakhill A (1993) The significance of detection of minimal residual disease in childhood acute lymphoblastic leukaemia. Br J Haematol 83: 412–418
111. Brisco MJ, Condon J, Hughes E, et al (1994) Outcome prediction in childhood acute lymphoblastic leukaemia by molecular quantification of residual disease at the end of induction. Lancet 343: 196–200.
112. Cavé H, Guidal C, Rohrlich P, et al (1994) Prospective monitoring and quantitation of residual blasts in childhood acute lymphoblastic leukemia by polymerase chain reaction study of δ and γ T-cell receptor genes. Blood 83: 1892–1902

Acute Leukemias V
Experimental Approaches
and Management of Refractory Diseases
Hiddemann et al. (Eds.)

Detection of AML1/ETO-Rearrangements in Acute Myeloid Leukemia with a Translocation t(8;21)

Ulrich Jaeger[1], Rajko Kusec[1], and Oskar A. Haas[2]

Chromosomal Translocation t(8;21) in AML

The chromosomal translocation t(8;21)(q22;q22) is the cytogenetic hallmark of a distinct class of acute myeloid leukemias (AML) which are predominantly of the FAB-M2 subtype [1]. Approximately 25% of adult and 50% of childhood M2-leukemias possess this reciprocal translocation. Patients with a t(8;21) respond well to chemotherapy and have a favourable clinical outcome with high long-term survival rates[2]. Therefore, it seems important to identify these patients at diagnosis and to monitor their response to treatment.

The t(8;21) juxtaposes the *AML1* gene on chromosome 21 with the *ETO/MTG8* gene on chromosome 8[3,4]. *AML1* is a DNA-binding protein with homology to the Drosophila gene runt[5], while *ETO/MTG8* is a putative zinc-finger protein with proline-rich regions reminiscent of a transcription factor[6]. The t(8;21) creates a fusion RNA which comes off the derivative (der) 8 chromosome. The fusion mRNA is translated into a chimeric *AML1/ETO* protein which retains DNA-binding properties and interacts with other proteins[5]. Thus, it is likely that the fusion protein plays a key role in the neoplastic transformation of the t(8;21)-carrying cells.

AML1/ETO RT-PCR

The chromosomal breakpoints are clustered within single introns of both the *AML1* and *ETO* genes resulting in a constant junction of the same 5′ *AML1* and 3′ *ETO* exons on the fusion mRNA of all t(8;21)-leukemias[7]. Reverse transcription polymerase chain reaction (RT-PCR) assays can reliably detect all cytogenetically proven 8;21 translocations (Fig.1) [8–12].

We have used a semi-quantitative two-step approach with a sensitivity of 1 in 10^3 in the first- and 1 in 10^5 in the second step for identification and monitoring of patients with t(8;21)-positive myeloid neoplasias[12]. The *AML1/ETO*-rearrangement was found in M2-leukemias, but also in AMLs of other FAB-types like M1,M4, or MDS progressing into acute leukemia[13] (Table 1). Patients with karyotypes other than t(8;21) as well as normal individuals are PCR-negative.

RT-PCR recognized all of 17 cytogenetically characterized t(8;21)-leukemias and helped clarifying complex karyotypes[14]. In addition, two-step PCR identified a few additional *AML1/ETO*-rearrangements in patients who had low blast cell counts.

PCR-Monitoring

Since patients with a t(8;21) can easily be identified at diagnosis, it seemed feasable to use the *AML1/ETO* RT-PCR for monitoring during and after therapy. Patients with acute leukemia tested positive in the first-step reaction in their bone marrow at diagnosis, while some of the MDS-patients were only detected by two-step

[1] Department of Medicine I, Division of Hematology, University of Vienna, A-1090 Vienna, Austria
[2] CCRI, St.Anna Children's Hospital, A-1090 Vienna, Austria

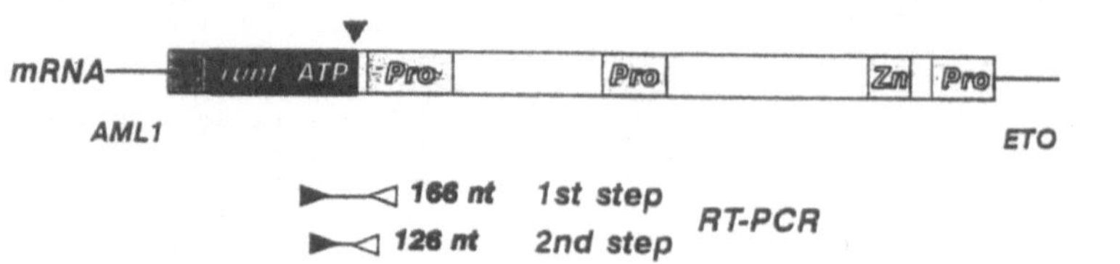

Fig. 1. AML1/ETO fusion RNA

Table 1. AML1/ETO OCR and FAB-classification

FAB	PCR+	%
M1	2	10
M2	13	65
M4	1	5
MDS	4	20
Total	20	100

PCR. Successful induction chemotherapy in patients with AML resulted in a reduction from first- to second-step positivity. The same effect was seen in patients who were treated with autologous bone marrow transplantation. None of the patients became PCR-negative during induction or consolidation therapy despite reaching a complete hematological remission.

Persistence of *AML1/ETO*-Positive Cells in Remission Blood Samples

We therefore tested patients who had been in long-term remission for up to 5 years. An *AML1/ETO* fusion RNA was detected in peripheral blood MNCs of all patients treated with chemotherapy or autologous marrow transplantation. Only allogeneic bone marrow transplantation resulted in PCR-negativity. These data are in accordance with the observations made by several other groups (Table 2).

Concluding Remarks

The *AML1/ETO* RT-PCR can identify virtually all patients with a t(8;21) at diagnosis and helps to resolve problems in the assessment of complex translocations. However, the value of this PCR-assay for clinical monitoring is limited

Table 2. Persistence of circulating AML1/ETO-positive cells in continuous complete remission

Number of Pts.	CCR	Reference
1		Nucifora et al., ref.8
1		Downing et al., ref.9
1		Kozu et al., ref. 10
3	1–5 yrs.	Chang et al., ref.11
7	1–5 yrs.	Kusec et al., ref. 12
4	-8 yrs	Nucifora et al., ref.15
17		

because *AML1/ETO*-positive cells even persist in patients with long-term remissions.

This raises interesting questions as to the leukemogenic potential of the t(8;21). Possibly, additional oncogenic events are required[16]. The persistence of *AML1/ETO*-positive cells suggests that this rearrangement is at least able to prolong the survival of these cells. A similar example is known from B cells where the t(14;18) protects the cells from apoptotic death[17]. Interestingly, long-term survivors after chemotherapy for follicular lymphoma can have circulating t(14;18) cells[18]. It is also possible that the t(8,21) resides in cells which have lost their original leukemic phenotype as well as their proliferative potential. The resolution of these questions will give further insights into the biology of acute leukemias and the role of the t(8;21).

References

1. Rowley JD. Recurring chromosomal abnormalities in leukemia and lymphoma. Semin Hematol 1990;27: 122–136.
2. Tashiro S, Kyo T, Tanaka K, Oguma N, Hashimoto T, Dohy H, Kamada N. The progonostic value of cytogenetic analyses in patients with acute nonlymphocytic leukemia treated with the same intensive chemotherapy. Cancer 1992; 70: 2809–2815.

3. Miyoshi H, Shimizu K, Kozu T, Maseki N, Kaneko Y, Ohki M: t(8;21) breakpoints on chromosome 21 in acute myeloid leukemia are clustered within a limited region of a single gene, AML1. Proc Natl Acad Sci USA 1991;88: 10431–10434.
4. Erickson P, Gao J, Chang KS, Look T, Raimondi S, Lasher R, Trujillo J, Rowley J, Drabkin H: Identification of breakpoints in t(8;21) acute myelogenous leukemia and isolation of a fusion transcript, AML1/ETO,with similarity to drosophila segmentation gene, runt. Blood 1992;80: 1825–1831.
5. Meyers S, Downing JR, Hiebert S: Identification of AML-1 and the (8;21) translocation protein (AML1/ETO) as sequence-specific DNA-binding proteins: the runt homology domain is required for DNA binding and protein-protein interactions. Mol Cell Biol 1993;13: 6336–6345.
6. Miyoshi H, Kozu T, Shimizu K, Enomoto K, Maseki N, Kaneko Y, Kamada N, Ohki M: The t(8;21) translocation in acute myeloid leukemia results in production of an AML1-MTG8 fusion transcript. EMBO J 1993;12: 2715–2721.
7. Shimizu K, Miyoshi H, Kozu T, Nagata J, Enomoto K, Maseki M, Kaneko Y, Ohki M. Consistent disruption of the AML1 gene occurs within a single intron in the (8;21) chromosomal translocation 1992;52: 6945–6948.
8. Nucifora G, Birn DJ, Erickson P, Gao J, LeBeau MM, Drabkin HA, Rowley JD. Detection of DNA rearrangements in the AML1 and ETO Loci and of an AML1/ETO fusion mRNA in patients with t(8;21) acute myeloid leukemia. Blood 1993;81: 883–888.
9. Downing JR, Head DR, Curcio-Brint AM, Hulshof MG, Motroni TA, Raimondi SA, Carroll AJ, Drabkin HA. An AML1/ETO fusion transcript in consistently detected by RNA-based polymerase chain reaction in acute myelogenous leukemia containing the (8;21)(q22;q22)translocation. Blood 1993;81: 2860–2865.
10. Kozu T, Miyoshi H, Shimizu K, Maseki N, Kaneko Y, Asou H, Kamada N, Ohki M. Junctions of the AML1/MTG8(ETo) fusion are constant in t(8;21) acute myeloid leukemia detected by reverse transcription polymerase chain reaction. Blood 1993;-82: 1270–1276.
11. Chang KS, Fan YH, Stass SA, Estey EH, Wang G, Trujillo JM, Erickson P, Drabkin H. Expression of AML1-ETO fusion transcripts and detection of minimal residual disease in t(8;21)-positive acute myeloid leukemia. Oncogene 1993;8: 983–988.
12. Kusec R, Laczika K, Knöbl P, Friedl J, Greinix H, Kalhs P, Linkesch W, Schwarzinger I, Mitterbauer G, Purtscher B, Haas OA, Lechner K, Jaeger U: AML1/ETO fusion mRNA can be detected in remission blood samples of all patients with t(8;21) acute myeloid leukemia after chemotherapy or autologous bone marrow transplantation. Leukemia 1994; 8: 735–739.
13. Kwong YL, Ching LM, Liu HW, Lee CP, Pollock A, Chan LC: 8;21 translocation and multilineage involvement. Am J Hematol 1993;43: 212–216.
14. Maruyama F, Yang P, Stass SA, Cork A, Freireich EJ, Lee M-S, Chang K-S. Detection of the AML1/-ETO fusion transcript in the t(8;21) masked translocation in acute myelogenous leukemia. Canc Res 1993;53; 4449–4451.
15. Nucifora G, Larson RA, Rowley JD: Persistence of the 8;21 translocation in patients with acute myeloid leukemia type M2 in long-term remission. Blood 1993;82: 712–715.
16. Sakurai M,Oshimura M, Kakti S, Sandberg AA. 8–21 translocation and missing sex chromosomes in acute leukemia. Lancet 1974 2: 227–228.
17. McDonnell TJ, Deane N, Platt FM, Nunez G, Jaeger U, McKearn JP, Korsmeyer SJ: bcl-2-immunoglobulin transgenic mice demonstrate extended B cell survival and follicular lymphoproliferation. Cell 1989;57: 79–88.
18. Price CGA, Meerabux J, Murtagh S, Cotter FE, Rohatiner AZS, Young BD, Lister TA. The significance of circulating cells carrying t(14;18) in long-term remission from follicular lymphoma. J Clin Oncology 1991;9: 1527–1532.

Acute Leukemias V
Experimental Approaches
and Management of Refractory Diseases
Hiddemann et al. (Eds.)

Mastocytosis in AML-M2 with t(8;21) – a New Characteristic Association

Dietrich Kämpfe[1], Werner Helbig[2], Robert Rohrberg[1], Janina Boguslawska-Jaworska[3], and Oskar A. Haas[4]

Abstract. We present four cases with hematologic malignancies characterized by a t(8;21) and systemic mast cell disease (SMCD). The patients consisted of a 51 year old man with AML-M2 and two 55 and 75 year old women with AML-M5b and AML-M4, respectively. The fourth patient was a twelve year old girl with refractory anemia and excess of blasts in transfomation to AML-M2 (RAEB-T). In all patients mastocytosis persisted during complete remission and, in the girl, even after allogeneic bone marrow transplantation (BMT). Based on these findings and a review of the literature, we suggest that SMCD is a rare, but rather unique biological feature of leukemias with a t(8;21). The pathogenetic significance and the specific association between AML with t(8;21) and increased mast cells deserves further investigation in order to determine whether these mast cells also harbor a t(8;21) or rather represent a benign reactive cell population.

Introduction

Many morphologic subtypes of solid tumors and hematologic neoplasms have specific chromosome abnormalities which determine the biological and prognostic features of the respective diseases. For example, the t(8;21)(q22;q22) occurs in 40% to 60% of AML-M2 and, at a lower frequency, in AML-M1, AML-M4 and RAEB-T [1,2]. It prevails in younger patients in whom long-lasting remissions are achieved in most instances. Typical biological features of this disease are the presence of auer-rods, the occurrence of solid tumor-like deposits and, occasionally, BM eosinophilia [1–3]. Moreover, they may sometimes show a pronounced differentiation of the myeloid cell lineage which can make it difficult to morphologically distinguish them from CML and/or MDS [2]. Unique immunophenotypic features of these leukemias include the atypical expression of the B-cell antigen CD19 and the natural killer cell antigen CD56 together with myeloid markers [4]. Amongst the cases with a t(8;21) which were cytogenetically identified in our laboratories within the last ten years we have found four with a concurrent SMCD. Although the association of SMCD and malignant hematologic disorders is well documented, only few reports of cytogenetic studies in such cases exist. We therefore describe the case histories of four such patients .

Case Reports

The first patient is a 50 year old man. At the time of diagnosis, hemoglobin was 7,4 g/l, WBC 12,6 G/l (with 74 % blasts) and platelets were 3 G/l. His BM was hypercellular with 74% POX-positive myeloid blasts and pathologic promyelocytes and Auer rods consistent with the diagnosis of AML-M2. Complete remission was achieved only after the third cycle of poly-

[1]Dept. Int. Med., Div. Haematol., Martin-Luther-Univ., Halle, Germany
[2]Dept. Int. Med., Univ. Leipzig, Germany
[3]Med. Acad., Dept. Pediatrics, Wroclaw, Poland
[4]CCRI, St. Anna Children's Hospital, Vienna, Austria

chemotherapy four months later. Relapse occurred 17 months thereafter and was again successfully treated. Currently, the patient remains in second remission 32 months after diagnosis. Cytogenetic analysis was perormed only during relapse and revealed two clones, 46,XY,t(8;21)(q22;q22) and 45, Xo,t(8;21)(q22;q22). BM mastocytosis was evident during the whole course of the disease. Moreover, infiltration of the liver with mastocytes was confirmed in a biopsy which was performed during remission because of continuing hepatomegaly and pathological laboratory values.

The second patient was a 75 year old woman. At diagnosis, her hemoglobin was 89 g/l, WBC 20,8 G/l with 35% blasts and platelets were 4 G/l. Her BM was hypercellular with 75% blast cells, 40% of which were POX- and 60% esterase-positive. According to the FAB-criteria, AML-M4 without BM eosinophilia was diagnosed. Complete hematologic remission was achieved with induction therapy and continued for four months. At that time, a paravertebral tumor, most likely a myelosarcoma, developed and led to paralysis of both legs. Subsequently the patient died because of pneumonia. Cytogenetic analysis was performed at diagnosis and revealed a t(8;21)(q22;q22) in 22 metaphases. In addition, clonal evolution was observed with monosomy 11 in four, a pseudotetraploid karyotype in two and complex changes in another metaphase. BM mastocytosis was already noted at diagnosis and persisted during the whole course of the disease.

The third patient is a 55 year old woman. At diagnosis, hemoglobin was 113 g/l, WBC 6,1 G/l with 14% blasts and platelets were 6 G/l. Her BM was hypercellular with 55% POX-positive blasts, consistent with the diagnosis AML-M2. Seven months after diagnosis she remains in complete remission. Cytogenetic analysis revealed a t(8;21)(q22;q22) as the sole abnormality in 7 of 15 metaphases. In addition, a 45,Xo karyotype was seen in two and trisomy 4 in one metaphase. The remaining 5 metaphases were normal. BM mastocytosis was present in all BM smears obtained during the course of the disease.

The fourth patient is a 9 1/2 year old girl. RBC was 1,30 T/l, WBC 13,6 G/l with 27% blasts and platelets were 23 G/l. The BM smear revealed reduced erythropoiesis, only few small megakaryocytes, hyperplasia of granulopoietic precursors with decreased granulation and many mast cells. Auer rods were seen in most blast cells as well as in promyelocytes. Two weeks after diagnosis blast cells had increased from 20% to 32%. Refractory anemia with excess of blasts in transformation (RAEB-T) to AML-M2 was diagnosed. Induction therapy was initiated according to the BFM-83 protocol followed by consolidation therapy. Complete remission was achieved after three months of intensive treatment. Six months later, allogeneic BMT from her sister was performed. Two years after diagnosis, the girl remains in complete remission, but thrombocytopenia is still evident. Cytogenetic studies revealed two clones, one with a t(8;21)(q22;q22) and a second with an additional del(5q)(q13q23). Mastocytosis persisted during remission and even after BMT [5].

Discussion

Mast cells derive from hematopoietic stem cells [6]. Therefore, SMCD may be regarded as a myeloproliferative disorder in which mast cells proliferate and accumulate in a variety of organs, including the BM, liver spleen, lymph nodes and/or skin [7–10]. It has been estimated that 4% to 10% of patients with SMCD develop AML at some stage of their illness [9,10]. Conversely, in AML, mastocytosis is only found occasionally. Reports of cytogenetic studies of such cases are rare and have revealed no consistent picture [11]. In the context of our findings it is worth noting that in only one patient with AML and SMCD a t(8;21) was described [12].

Our observation of SMCD in four cases of AML with a t(8;21) suggests a specific biologic relationship. Since the significance of the increased mast cells in this type of leukemia is not yet known, one of the first steps to elucidate their pathogenetic role is to analyse whether these cells also harbor a t(8;21) and, thus, perhaps belong to the neoplastic cell population. Alternatively, they could represent a concomitant benign cell population. Whether the growth and development of these mast cells are triggered by specific cytokines released by the leukemic cells or, whether mastocytes release growth factors which stimulate the leukemic cell populations also remains to be investigated. In any case, the benign or malignant nature and the pathogenetic role of the mast cells in leukemias bearing a t(8,21) is of utmost clinical importance, since their persistence during complete hematologic remission and even after allogeneic BMT, which was noted in all cases reported so far, indicates their prolonged survival and pronounced resistance to chemotherapy [5,13].

Acknowledgement. This work was supported by the "Österreichische Kinderkrebshilfe".

References

1. Groupe Franáais de Cytogénétique Hématologique (1990) Acute myelogenous leukemia with an 8;21 translocation. A report on 148 cases from the Groupe Franáais de Cytogénétique Hématologique. Cancer Genet Cytogenet 44: 169–179
2. Swirsky DM, Li YS, Matthews JG, Flemans RJ, Rees JK, Hayhoe FG (1984) 8;21 translocation in acute granulocytic leukaemia: cytological, cytochemical and clinical features. Brit J Haematol 56: 199–213
3. Ishibashi T, Kimura H, Abe R, Matsuda S, Uchida T, Kariyone S (1986) Involvement of eosinophils in leukemia: cytogenetic study of eosinophilic colonies from acute myelogenous leukemia associated with translocation (8;21). Cancer Genet Cytogenet 22: 189–194
4. Kita K, Shirakawa S, Kamada N, the Japanese Cooperative Group of Leukemia-Lymphoma (1994) Cellular characteristics of acute myeloblastic leukemia associated with t(8;21)(q22;q22). Leuk Lymphoma 13: 229–234
5. Födinger M, Fritsch G, Winkler K, et al (1994) Origin of human mast cells: Development from transplanted hemopoietic stem cells after allogeneic bone marrow transplantation. (submitted):
6. Valent P, Sillaber C, Bettelheim P (1991) The growth and differentiation of mast cells. Prog Growth Factor Res 3: 27–41
7. Metcalfe DD (1991) The liver, spleen, and lymph nodes in mastocytosis. J Invest Dermatol 96: 45S–46S
8. Metcalfe DD (1991) Classification and diagnosis of mastocytosis: current status. J Invest Dermatol 96: 2S–4S
9. Travis WD, Li CY, Yam LT, Bergstralh EJ, Swee RG (1988) Significance of systemic mast cell disease with associated hematologic disorders. Cancer 62: 965–972
10. Lawrence JB, Friedman BS, Travis WD, Chinchilli VM, Metcalfe DD, Gralnick HR (1991) Hematologic manifestations of systemic mast cell disease: a prospective study of laboratory and morphologic features and their relation to prognosis. Am J Med 91: 612–624
11. Swolin B, Rodjer S, Roupe G (1987) Cytogenetic studies and in vitro colony growth in patients with mastocytosis. Blood 70: 1928–1932
12. Wong KF, Chan JK, Chan JC, Kwong YL, Ma SK, Chow TC (1991) Concurrent acute myeloid leukemia and systemic mastocytosis. Am J Hematol 38: 243–244
13. Ronnov-Jessen D, Lovgreen Nielsen P, Horn T (1991) Persistence of systemic mastocytosis after allogeneic bone marrow transplantation in spite of complete remission of the associated myelodysplastic syndrome. Bone Marrow Transplant 8: 413–415

Acute Leukemias V
Experimental Approaches
and Management of Refractory Diseases
Hiddemann et al. (Eds.)

Acute Myeloid Leukemia with Translocation (8;21). Cytomorphology, Dysplasia and Prognostic Factors in 41 Cases

T. Haferlach, J. M. Bennett, H. Löffler, W. Gassmann, J. Andersen, N. Tuzuner, P. A. Cassileth, C. Fonatsch, B. Schlegelberger, E. Thiel, W.-D. Ludwig, M. C. Sauerland, A. Heinecke, and Th. Büchner for AML Cooperative Group and ECOG

Abstract. The translocation t(8;21) is the single most common structural aberration in acute myeloid leukemia (AML). Excellent response rates and a better relapse-free survival were noted. We analyzed specific morphologic and cytochemical features including dysplasia and prognostic factors in forty-one patients with AML t(8;21). They all underwent aggressive chemotherapy in two cooperative study groups (AMLCG-85 and ECOG 3489/P-C486). Five patients were classified as AML M1 and 36 as AML M2 according to the FAB criteria. Auer rods could be detected in 28 patients but in only 16 were these "thin and elongated" as has been described as typical for t(8;21). The absence of Auer rods had no prognostic impact. Peroxidase was strongly positive in 100% of myeloid blasts in 22/40 cases. Golgi-zone associated non-specific esterase was detected in seven out of 25 available bone marrow smears. Dysgranulopoiesis was detected in 37/41 patients (90%), five of these patients additionally had dyserythropoiesis (12%). In six cases (12%), dysmegakaryopoiesis was seen in combination with dysgranulopoiesis. Only one patient had trilineage dysplasia. Dysplastic features had no influence on prognosis. In 24/41 patients additional cytogenetic abnormalities could be detected. Twelve male (48%) and four female (25%) had a loss of a sex chromosome. This was correlated with a better disease-free survival ($p=0.04$). The CR rate to chemotherapy was 90%. Resistance to induction chemotherapy was not observed. The early death rate was 10%. Disease-free survival of the complete responders was 60% after three years. The event-free survival rate was 53%. Because of the favorable disease-free survival rate with standard chemotherapy, one should speculate, whether allogeneic bone marrow transplantation is necessary for patients with AML t(8;21) in first complete remission.

Introduction

The translocation t(8;21) (q22;q22) is the single most common structural rearrangement in acute myeloid leukemia (AML) found in 7%–18% of all patients and in one-third among karyotypically abnormal M2 cases according to the French-American-British classification [1,2]. It is often accompanied by the loss of a sex chromosome or by other cytogenetic abnormalities [3–7].

The typical case of AML with t(8;21) shows large myeloblasts with an abundant cytoplasma and a frequently eccentric nucleus like that of a normal promyelocyte. Often in these blasts only a single, large Auer rod with tapered ends is observed. In a small number of cases Chediak-like granules are seen suggesting abnormal fusion of azur granules, and eosinophiles are increased [5,6]. Thus, this morphologic picture is so characteristic that it can be used to predict the results of the cytogenetic analysis [5].

Patients with AML t(8;21) are suggested to have a better prognosis than those suffering from other more common types of AML. Excellent response rates and a better relapse-free survival were noted compared to the other types of AML in some studies [1,4,7,8].

University Hospital II, Chemnitzstr. 33, 24116 Kiel, Germany

However, it is difficult to compare data in collected small series with heterogenous groups of patients that had been treated in various trials and countries with different chemotherapy protocols. We analyzed the results of two current prospective studies treating AML adult patients with aggressive chemotherapy. Prognostic factors and treatment outcome as well as several cytomorphologic aspects in AML t(8;21) were studied.

Patients and Methods

Forty-one patients with AML t(8;21) have been treated between 1985 and 1993 according to protocols of two cooperative study groups (AMLCG-85 and ECOG 3489/P-C486). The treatment schedules have been published elsewhere [9-11]. They are similar and included thioguanine, Ara-C, daunorubicin, and mitoxantrone. Some clinical data are summarized in Table 1.

We (T Haferlach, JM Bennett) retrospectively examined bone marrow slides and blood samples of patients who showed the translocation t(8;21) in cytogenetical analysis. Cytological examination included Wright-Giemsa (ECOG) or Pappenheim (AMLCG) stain and the following cytochemical reactions according to standard procedures: myeloperoxidase (POX), naphtyl-acetate esterase (NSE) and naphtol-AS-D-chloroacetate-esterase (CAE) staining.

Table 1. Clinical and morphological data of 41 patients with AML and t(8;21)

	number	% of patients
Male	25	61
Female	16	39
Age, median 38		
20–40	25	61
41–60	11	27
>60	5	12
ECOG	21	51
AMLCG	20	49
FAB type		
M1	5	12
M2	36	88
Auer rods		
no	13	32
yes	28	68
"typical"	16/28	39
Dysgranulopoiesis	37	90
Dyserythropoiesis	5	12
Dysmegakaryopoiesis	6	15
Trilineage- dysplasia	1	2

Results

Cytomorphology data: Five patients were classified as AML M1 and 36 as AML M2 according to the FAB criteria [2]. Auer rods could be detected in 28 of 41 patients. However, despite our knowledge of the karyotype, we were not able to detect Auer rods in the other 13 patients using Wright-Giemsa, Pappenheim or POX staining. Just in 16 of the 28 patients Auer rods were "thin and elongated" as has been described as typical for t(8;21) [5]. In addition, four patients with Auer rods had Chediak-like granules, another three patients showed Chediak-like granules but no Auer rods.

The percentage of blasts (type I, II, and III combined) [12] differed between 33 and 100% (median 71%). Seven patients had a blast count of 30–50%, fourteen had 51–70% and in 20 patients the percentage of blasts was greater than 70%. Erythropoiesis was decreased to 0–16% (median 3%), megakaryocytes were rare. All of the blasts were peroxidase positive in 22 out of 40 cases (in one patient no POX stain was available). In nine cases peroxidase activity could be demonstrated in more than 70% of the blasts and in six cases the percentage was between 20% and 70%. Two cases had only 5% or 10% POX positive blasts, respectively. Golgi-zone associated non-specific esterase (NSE) was detected in seven out of 25 available bone marrow smears [13]. This type of esterase positivity is clearly different from the diffuse esterase of monocytes and monoblasts in AML M4 and M5 [6].

Dysplasia was analyzed according to standard criteria [12]. Dysgranulopoiesis was detected in 37/41 patients (90%), five of these patients additionally had dyserythropoiesis (12%). In six cases (12%) dysmegakaryopoiesis was seen in combination with dysgranulopoiesis. Only one patient had trilineage dysplasia.

Cytogenetic data: In 24/41 patients with the translocation (8;21) additional cytogenetic abnormalities could be detected: 12 male (48%) and four female (25%) had a loss of a sex chromosome. In contrast to others [1,4,6,7] the loss of the sex chromosome was correlated with a better dis-

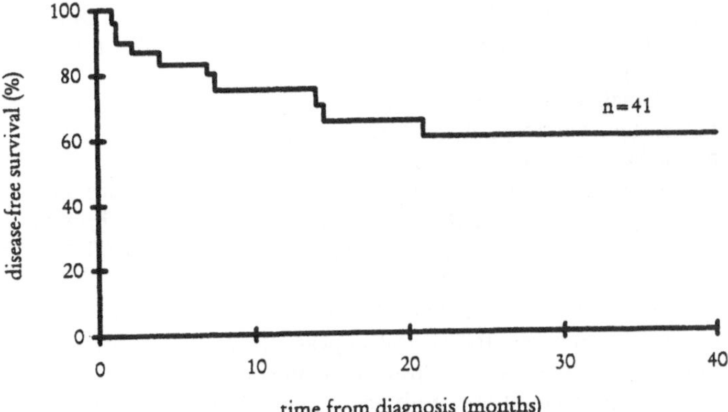

Fig. 1. Disease-free survival of patients with AML and t(8,21)

ease-free survival (p=0.04) in our cohort. Further cytogenetic abnormalities were deletion of chromosome 9 in six cases, one patient with t(3;19), one case with inv(13) and one case with trisomy 8. No systematic data on molecular biology are available.

Treatment results and survival: The patients were treated according to ECOG protocol 3489 or P-C486 or according to AMLCG protocols [9–11]. The complete remission rate of both study groups combined was 90% in 41 patients with AML and t(8;21). Resistance to induction chemotherapy was not observed. The early death rate was 10% with three patients dying of infections and one lethal bleeding episode. Another two patients in this cohort of 41 patients died during the procedure of allogeneic bone marrow transplantation (BMT) in the ECOG trial. One patient died at day 12 after BMT due to veno-occlusive disease and infection and one patient at day 22 of veno-occlusive disease.

Allogeneic bone marrow transplantation (BMT) was done in seven patients in first complete remission. In another eight patients autologous bone marrow transplantation (ABMT) was done as a part of the protocol in the ECOG trial in first CR. Patients who underwent allogeneic or autologous bone marrow translantation were not censored in the disease-free survival plot. The BMT was given in first CR as part of the two ECOG protocols. PC486 was a phase II trial verifying the feasibility of ABMT in a large coop group, and 3489 randomized between chemotherapy and BMT. Patients who relapsed or died after CR are considered to be treatment failures regardless of whether they got BMT or not.

Disease-free survival of the complete responders was 60% after three years (Fig. 1). The respective event-free survival rate was 53%.

After relapse three patients died without achieving a further remission and four patients reached a second complete remission in the AMLCG trial. Data for second CR are not available in the ECOG trial (Table 2).

Table 2. Treatment results

	number	% of patients
CR	37	90
Early death	4	10
Relapses	7	17
Second CR	4	57
BMT:		
Autologous	8	19
Allogeneic	7	17

Discussion

The acute myeloid leukemia with a reciprocal translocation between chromosomes 8 and 21 has been reported to show a specific morphological appearance in bone marrow smears and peripheral blood. Large myeloblasts with abundant cytoplasm containing one tapered, thin and elongated Auer rod, Chediak-like granules and increased eosinophiles seemed to be sufficient to predict this translocation [5]. Most of the cases were classified as FAB M2.

Translocation (8;21) has been reported to be a favorable prognostic indicator in patients with AML by most groups [1,4,7,8,14–17,26].

Some other studies however failed to confirm the superior prognosis of this translocation [6,18–20].

The main objective of our study was to investigate the cytomorphological aspects and the prognostic impact of this AML subtype in a homogeneous cohort of patients. All patients were treated in a standardized way within multicenter trials of the ECOG and the AMLCG.

We confirmed again that AML with t(8;21) usually has the morphology of the FAB subtype M2 [6,21]. However, the typical appearance of some of the blasts with one "thin and elongated" Auer rod [5] has only been observed in 39% of all forty-one cases in our study. One may predict the translocation, if the bone marrow smears show these typical abnormalities, but "normal" AML M2 or M1 without Auer rods may carry the translocation as well. The lack of typical Auer rods or no Auer rods demonstrable had no influence on the prognosis in our cohort. With the detection of a AML1/ETO-fusion gene new means for diagnosis and follow up are available [22–24].

Dysplasia especially in the granulopoiesis but also in the erythropoiesis and megakaryopoiesis was seen [12]. But dysplastic features did not have any influence on complete remission rate or prognosis.

The remarkable aspects of our forty-one patients with AML and t(8;21) were a high CR rate with 90% and a favorable disease-free survival at 3 years with 60%. This is equivalent to the high response rate in AML M4Eo [25]. The disease-free survival rate of AML t(8;21) is the most favorable of all AML subgroups. Early death rate was 10% in this cohort and is comparable with other FAB subtypes [25].

Loss of the sex chromosome was found in 48% of the male and in 25% of the female patients and was a predictor of good prognosis. This is in contrast to other studies [1,7,26,27].

In conclusion, AML with t(8;21) is a favorable subtype of AML with a high complete remission rate and disease-free survival. Neither the "typical" or "atypical" cytomorphology nor the incidence of dysplasia did influence the prognosis. The additional loss of the sex chromosome had a better prognosis in our cohort. Because of favorable disease-free survival rates with standard chemotherapy, one should speculate, whether allogeneic bone marrow transplantation is necessary for patients in first complete remission. Our results again underline the major clinical importance of cytomorphology and chromosomal status in AML.

References

1. Fourth International Workshop on Chromosomes in Leukemia 1982 (1984) Translocation (8;21) (q22;q22) in acute nonlymphocytic leukemia. Cancer Genet Cytogenet 11: 284–287
2. Bennett JM, Catovsky D, Daniel MT, Flandrin G, Galton AG, Gralnick HR, Sultan C (1985) Proposed revised criteria for the classification of acute myeloid leukemia. Ann Intern Med 103: 620–629
3. Trujillo JM, Cork A, Ahearn MJ, Youness EL, McCredie KB (1979) Hematologic and cytologic characterization of 8/21 translocation acute granulocytic leukemia. Blood 53: 695–706
4. Second International Workshop on Chromosomes in Leukemia (1980). Cancer Genet Cytogenet 2: 311
5. Berger R, Bernheim A, Daniel M-T, Valensi F, Sigaux F, Flandrin G (1982) Cytologic characterization and significance of normal karyotypes in t(8;21) acute myeloblastic leukemia. Blood 59: 171–178
6. Swirsky DM, Li YS, Matthews JG, Flemans RJ, Rees JK, Hayhoe FGJ (1984) 8;21 translocation in acute granulocytic leukemia: cytological, cytochemical and clinical features. Br J Haematol 56: 199–213
7. Keating MJ, Cork A, Broach Y, Smith T, Walters RS, McCredie KB, Trujillo J, Freireich EJ (1987) Toward a clinically relevant cytogenetic classification of acute myelogenous leukemia. Leuk Res 11: 119–133
8. Schiffer CA, Lee EJ, Tomiyasu T, Wiernik PH, Testa JR (1989) Prognostic impact of cytogenetic abnormalities in patients with de novo acute nonlymphocytic leukemia. Blood 73: 263–270
9. Büchner T, Urbanitz D, Hiddemann W, Rühl H, Ludwig W-D, Fischer J, Aul HC, Vaupel HA, Kuse R, Zeile G, Nowrousian MR, König HJ, Walter M, Wendt FC, Sodomann H, Hossfeld DK, von Paleske A, Löffler H, Gassmann W, Hellriegel K-P, Fülle HH, Lunscken Ch, Emmerich B, Pralle H, Pees HW, Pfreundschuh M, Bartels H, Koeppen K-M, Schwerdtfeger R, Donhuijsen-Ant R, Mainzer K, Bonfert B, Köppler H, Zurborn K-H, Ranft K, Thiel E, Heinecke A (1985) Intensified induction and consolidation with or without maintenance chemotherapy for acute myeloid leukemia (AML): two multicenter studies of the German AML Cooperative Group. J Clin Oncol 3: 1583–1589
10. Cassileth PA, Harrington DP, Hines JD, Oken MM, Mazza JJ, McGlave P, Bennett JM, O'Connell MJ (1988) Maintenance chemotherapy prolongs remission duration in adult non-lymphocytic leukemia. J Clin Oncol 6: 583–587
11. Cassileth PA, Andersen J, Lazarus HM, Colvin OM, Bennett JM, Stadtmauer EA, Kaizer H, Weiner RS, Edelstein M, Oken MM (1993) Autologous bone marrow transplantation in acute myeloid leukemia in first remission. J Clin Oncol 11: 314–319

12. Goasguen JE, Matsuo T, Cox C, Bennett JM (1992) Evaluation of the dysmyelopoiesis in 336 patients with de novo acute myeloid leukemia: major importance of dysgranulopoiesis for remission and survival. Leukemia 6: 520–525
13. Löffler H (1990) Morphology, immunology, cytochemistry, and cytogenetics and the classification of subtypes in AML. Haematol. and Blood Transfusion 33: 239–242
14. Yunis JJ, Lobell M, Arnesen MA, Oken MM, Mayer MG, Rydell RE, Brunning RD (1988) Refined chromosome study helps define prognostic subgroups in most patients with primary myelodysplastic syndrome and acute myelogenous leukaemia. Br J Haematol 68: 189–194
15. Palka G, Calabrese G, Fioritoni G, Stuppia L, Guanciali Franchi P, Marino M, Antonucci A, Spandano A, Torlontano G (1992) Cytogenetic survey of 80 patients with acute nonlymphocytic leukemia. Cancer Genet Cytogenet 59: 45–50
16. Marosi C, Käller U, Koller-Weber E, Schwarzinger I, Schneider B, Jäger U, Vahls P, Nowotny H, Pirc-Danoewinata H, Steger G, Kreiner G, Wagner B, Lechner K, Lutz D, Bettelheim P, Haas OA (1992) Prognostic impact of karyotype and immunologic phenotype in 125 adult patients with de novo AML. Cancer Genet Cytogenet 61: 14–25
17. Trujillo JM, Cork A, Hart JS, George SL, Freireich EJ (1974) Clinical implications of aneuploid cytogenetic profiles in adult acute leukemia. Cancer 33: 824–834
18. Fenaux P, Preudhomme C, Lay JL, Morel P, Beuscart R, Bauters F (1989) Cytogenetics and their prognostic value in de novo acute myeloid leukaemia: a report on 283 cases. Br J Haematol 73: 61–67
19. Pui C-H, Raimondi SC, Crist WM (1993) Clinical significance of cytogenetics in acute leukemia. XIIth meeting of the International Society of Haematology. Vienna, Abstract N. 55
20. Berger R, Bernheim A, Ochoa-Noguera ME, Daniel M-T, Valensi F, Sigaux F, Flandrin G, Boiron M (1987a) Prognostic significance of chromosomal abnormalities in acute nonlymphocytic leukemia: a study of 343 patients. Cancer Genet Cytogenet 28: 293–299
21. Davey DD, Patil SR, Echternacht H, Fatemi C, Dick FR (1989) 8;21 translocation in acute nonlymphocytic leukemia. Occurence in M1 and M2 FAB subtypes. Am J Clin Pathol 92: 172–176
22. Downing JR, Head DR, Curcio-Brint AM, Hulshof MG, Motroni TA, Raimondi SC, Carroll AJ, Drabkin HA, Willman C, Theil KS, Civin CI, Erickson P (1993) An AML1/ETO fusion transcript is consistently detected by RNA-based polymerase chain reaction in acute myelogous leukemia containing the (8;21)(q22;q22) translocation. Blood 81: 2860–2865
23. Maseki N, Miyoshi H, Shimizu K, Homma C, Ohki M, Sakurai M, Kaneko Y (1993) The 8;21 chromosome translocation in acute myeloid leukemia is always detectable by molecular analysis using AML1. Blood 81: 1573–1579
24. Nucifora G, Birn DJ, Erickson P, Gao J, LeBeau MM, Drabkin HA, Rowley JD (1993) Detection of DNA rearrangements in the AML1 and ETO loci and of an AML1/ETO fusion mRNA in patients with t(8;21) acute myeloid leukemia. Blood 81: 883–888
25. Haferlach T, Gassmann W, Löffler H, Jürgensen C, Noak J, Ludwig W-D, Thiel E, Haase D, Fonatsch C, Bücher R, Schlegelberger B, Nowrousian MR, Lengfelder E, Eimermacher H, Weh HJ, Braumann D, Maschmeyer G, Koch P, Heinecke A, Sauerland MC, Büchner Th (1993) Clinical aspects of acute myeloid leukemias of the FAB types M3 and M4Eo. Ann Hematol 66: 165–170
26. Weh HJ, Kuse R, Hoffmann R, Seeger D, Suciu S, Kabisch H, Ritter J, Hossfeld DK (1988) Prognostic significance of chromosome analysis in de novo acute myeloid leukemia (AML). Blut 56: 19–26
27. Berger R, Flandrin G, Bernheim A, Le Concial M, Vecchione D, Pacot A, Derré J, Daniel M-T, Valensi F, Sigaux F, Ochoa-Noguera ME (1987b) Cytogenetic studies on 519 consecutive de novo acute nonlymphocytic leukemias. Cancer Genet Cytogenet 29: 9–21

Acute Leukemias V
Experimental Approaches
and Management of Refractory Diseases
Hiddemann et al. (Eds.)

Simultaneous Occurrence of t(8;21) and del(5q) in Myeloid Neoplasms

Katharina Clodi[1], Alexander Gaiger[2], Christine Peters[1], Janina Boguslawska-Jaworska[3], Ulrich Jäger[2], and Oskar A. Haas[1]

Abstract. The translocation t(8;21)(q22;q22) and the deletion of the long arm of chromosome 5, del(5q), are two acquired chromosome abnormalities which characterize distinct biological entities of hematologic neoplasms. We have observed two patients, a 9 year old girl with refractory anemia with excess of blasts in transformation (RAEB-T) overting to M2-AML and a 50 year old woman with refractory anemia with excess of blasts (RAEB) in whom both abnormalities concurred in the same cell clone. After chemotherapy the girl underwent a successful allogeneic bone marrow transplantation (BMT) from her sister and has remained in complete remission two years after diagnosis. The other patient received only erythrocyte transfusions and has been in stable condition for three years. In addition, a 33 year old man with a complex translocation t(5;8;21)(q13;q13;q11) is presented for comparison. His hematologic findings and clinical course was similar to that of other patients with a t(8;21). We conclude that in cases with two specific karyotype changes the biological features typically associated with one or the other chromosome abnormality may dominate the phenotype. It remains unclear whether the clinical and hematological appearance of the disease is determined by the abnormality which occurs first or by the one which predominates.

Introduction

Acquired chromosome abnormalities are found in 50–80% of patients with acute myeloid leukemia (AML) and myelodysplastic syndromes (MDS). Many of the primary abnormalities are considered to be causative events in leukemogenesis and are therefore specifically associated with distinct biological as well as morphological entities. Whereas most of these entities are already well defined, the significance of the rare simultaneous coexistence of two of these abnormalities within the same cell population still has to be established. Therefore, we present two patients with simultaneous occurrence of a t(8;21) and a del(5q).

The t(8;21) is one of the most common abnormalities in AML. It occurs identified in 40 to 60% of AML-M2 and, at a lower frequency, in AML-M1, AML-M4 and RAEB-T [1]. It prevails in younger patients in whom long-lasting remissions are achieved in most instances. One of the unique biological features of leukemias with a t(8;21) is the occasional development of myelosarcoma. Neoplastic cells typically show a large number of Auer rods, occasionally a "CML-like" maturation of the granulocytic cell lineage and eosinophilia [1]. Unique immunophenotypic features of these leukemias include the atypical expression of the B-cell antigen CD19 and the natural killer cell antigen CD56 [2,3] together with myeloid markers.

Deletion of the long arm of chromosome 5, del(5q), as the sole karyotype abnormality is typically found in elderly women with chronic refractory macrocytic anemia, left-shifted myelopoiesis, normal or elevated platelet counts and small megakaryocytes with non-lobulated nuclei [4]. The clinical course of the disease is mild and progression to acute leukemia is rare. On the other hand, deletions of the long arm of

[1]Children's Cancer Research Institute (CCRI), St.Anna Children's Hospital, A-1090 Vienna, Austria
[2]University Medical Clinic, Dept.of Hematology, Vienna, Austria
[3]Medical Academy, Dept.of Pediatrics, Wroclaw, Poland

chromosome 5 with varying breakpoints are also found in complex karyotype changes of secondary MDS and AML with an unfavorable prognosis.

Case Reports

A 9 1/2 year old girl was admitted to hospital still in good clinical condition because of increased fatigue and loss of appetite. RBC was 1,30 T/l, WBC 13,6 G/l and platelets were 23 G/l. The differential count showed a left-shifted granulopoiesis and 27% blasts. The bone marrow (BM) smear revealed reduced erythropoiesis, only few small megakaryocytes, hyperplasia of granulopoietic precursors with decreased granulation and many mast cells. Auer rods were seen in most blast cells as well as in promyelocytes. Two weeks after diagnosis blast cells had increased from 20% to 32%. The diagnosis according to the French-American-British (FAB) classification was RAEB-T with transition to AML-M2. Cytogenetic studies of the BM revealed two clones, one with a t(8;21)(q22;q22) and a second with an additional del(5q)(q13q23) (Fig. 1). Induction therapy was initiated according to the BFM-83 protocol followed by consolidation therapy. Complete remission was achieved after three months of intensive treatment. Six months later, allogeneic bone marrow transplantation from her sister was performed. Two years after diagnosis, the girl is in continuing complete remission, but thrombocytopenia is still evident.

The second patient was a 51 year old woman. With the exception of splenomegaly the physical examination revealed no pathological findings. She had a hyperchromic anemia (RBC 2,11 T/l) with slight anisocytosis, poikilocytosis and polychromasy of erythrocytes as well as a moderate number of macrocytes and target cells, leukopenia (WBC 3,6 G/l) with a left-shifted differential count and anisocytosis of thrombocytes whose number was within normal range (153 G/l). The BM was hypercellular with a hypoplastic, left-shifted and dysplastic erythropoiesis. Myelopoiesis was increased, left-shifted and dysplastic with up to 10% blasts, some of which had basophilic granula. Megakaryocytes were small and mostly nonlobulated. These findings led to the diagnosis RAEB. Cytogenetic studies revealed a clone with the following abnormal karyotype: 46,XX,t(8;21)(q22;q22), del(5)(q13q31), t(X;20) (q13;q13) (Fig. 1). It is of interest to note that the patient did not require cytostatic treatment. With supportive measures she has remained in stable condition for three years.

The third patient, a 33 year old man was admitted to hospital because of fever, tonsillopharyngitis and hepatomegaly. RBC was 4,02 T/l, WBC 19,6 G/l and platelets were 145 G/l. His

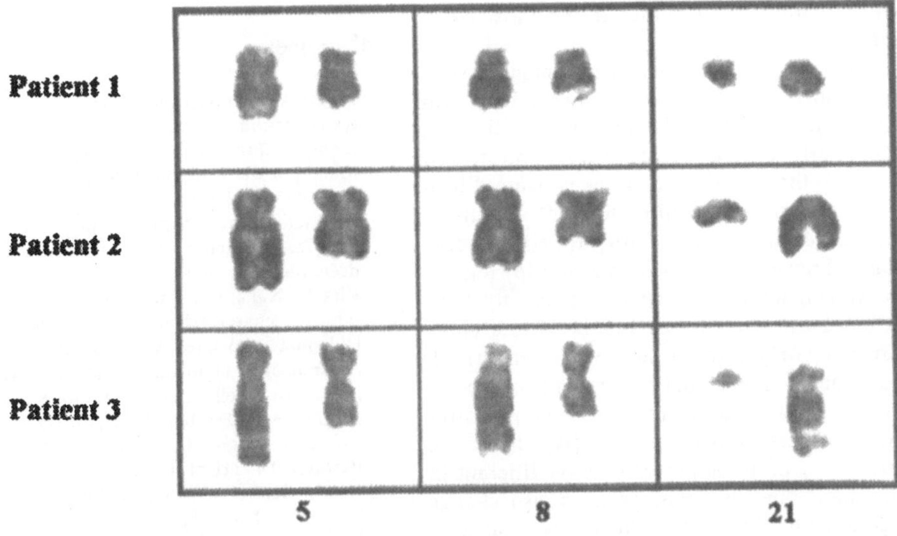

Fig. 1. Partial karyotypes of three patients with a t(8;21) and a chromosome 5 abnormality. The normal homologs are on the left, the abnormal on the right

BM was hypercellular with 47% myelomonocytic blasts which contained only few Auer rods. AML-M4 without eosinophilia was diagnosed. Cytogenetic analysis revealed a complex translocation t(5;8;21) (q13;q22;q22) (Fig. 1). Six months after initiation of chemotherapy the patient relapsed. After a second chemotherapy-induced remisson which lasted for another three years, the patient recently relapsed with a RAEB-T.

Discussion

The coexistence of two primary chromosome abnormalities in the same leukemic clone is a rather rare and yet unexplained cytogenetic phenomenon which challenges the current concepts of their specificity. To-date the following combinations have been reported in the literature: t(9;22) with either inv(16) [5,6], t(15;17) [7–9], t(8;21) [10–12] or del(5q) [13], t(15;17) with inv(16) [14], t(8;21) with t(15;17) [15], t(8;21) with del(5q)[16,17] as well as t(8;21) with del(5q) and inv(16) [18]. Xue et al. [12] suggested several possible explanations for these rather unusual cytogenetic findings: (1) seemingly identical cytogenetic abnormalities may differ at the molecular level, (2) two specific abnormalities may occur simultaneously by chance alone, (3) one of them may occur as a secondary change during clonal evolution or (4) they may not be related to leukemogenesis at all. Based on the few cases available it is not possible at present to assess which of these possibilities is the most likely one.

With regard to clincial management it is of importance to know which abnormality will determine the biological behavior of the disease, particularly in cases such as t(8;21) and del(5q) in which the two abnormalities indicate different prognosis or require different treatment approaches. In two cases with a t(8;21) the additional abnormalities, t(9;22) and inv(16) together with del(5q), respectively, seem to have occurred as secondary events, because a clone displaying only a t(8;21) was also present [11,18]. However, in another patient with a t(8;21) combined with a t(15;17), only the t(15;17)-positive clone persisted during relapse [15]. Thus, the chronology of development may be different in each individual, but may perhaps also change depending on the combination of the abnormalities. In contrast to the three AML cases with a t(8;21) and del(5q) reported previously [16–18], our two patients were diagnosed as MDS. In neoplasms with a t(8;21) this is a rather uncommon form of initial presentation. Furthermore, a del(5q) is also an extremely rare abnormality in childhood hematologic malignancies. The cytogenetic findings in the younger patient suggest that the t(8;21) was the primary and important event. This notion is further supported by the fast progression to AML. Despite the presence of several karyotype abnormalities, the benign clinical course in the second patient was typical for cases with a del(5q) syndrome. Unfortunately, we were unable to determine the pattern of cytogenetic evolution in this case. Although the third patient with a complex translocation t(5;8;21) had a clinical course resembling that of patients with a t(8;21), it should be pointed out that he was diagnosed as MDS at relapse.

In summary, we believe that in hematological neoplasms with two specific chromosome abnormalities peculiarities of the biological features and a clinical course typical of either abnormality can be observed. However, such modified disease patterns may vary individually depending on the prevailing abnormality. Molecular genetic and in situ hybridization studies may help to further elucidate their pathogenetic significance.

Acknowledgement. This work was supported by the “Österreichische Kinderkrebshilfe”.

References

1. (1990) Acute myelogenous leukemia with an 8; 21 translocation. A report on 148 cases from the Groupe Francais de Cytogenetique Hematologique. Cancer Genet Cytogenet 44: 169–179
2. Hurwitz CA, Raimondi SC, Head D, et al (1992) Distinctive immunophenotypic features of t(8; 21)(q22; q22) acute myeloblastic leukemia in children. Blood 80: 3182–3188
3. Kita K, Nakase K, Miwa H, et al (1992) Phenotypical characteristics of acute myelocytic leukemia associated with the t(8; 21)(q22; q22) chromosomal abnormality: frequent expression of immature B-cell antigen CD19 together with stem cell antigen CD34. Blood 80: 470–477
4. van den Berghe H, Vermaelen C, Meccuci C, Barbieri D, Tricot G (1985) The 5q- anomaly. Cancer Genet Cytogenet 17: 189–255
5. Mecucci C, Noens L, Aventin A, Testoni N, van den Berghe H (1988) Philadelphia positive acute myelomonocytic leukemia with inversion of chromosome 16 and eosinobasophils. Am J Hematol 27: 69–71

6. Li YS, Hayhoe FGJ (1989) A case of Ph-positive acute non-lymphocytic leukemia with inv(16). Chong Hua I Hsnech Tsa Chik 69: 119–120
7. Lai JL, Fenaux P, Zandecki M, et al (1987) Promyelocytic blast crisis of Philadelphia-positive thrombocythemia with translocations (9;22) and (15;17). Cancer Genet Cytogenet 29: 311–314
8. Hogge DM, Misawa S, Schiffer CA, Testa JR (1984) Promyelocytic blast crisis in chronic granulocytic leukemai with 15;17 tranlocation. Leuk Res 8: 1019–1023
9. Berger R, Bernheim A, Daniel MT, Flandrin G (1983) t(15;17) in a promyelocytic form of chronic myeloid leukemia blastic crisis. Cancer Genet Cytogenet 8: 149–152
10. Francesconi D, Pasquali F (1978) 8/21 translocation, loss of the Y chromosome and Philadelphias chromosome. Br J Haematol 38: 149–150
11. Dallorso S, Sessarego M, Garre ML, Haupt R, Pasino M, Sansone R (1990) Secondary acute promyelocytic leukemia with t(8; 21) and t(9; 22) at onset and loss of the Philadelphia chromosome at relapse. Cancer Genet Cytogenet 47: 41–46
12. Xue YQ, Guo Y, Lu DR, et al (1991) A case of basophilic leukemia bearing simultaneous translocations t(8;21) and t(9;22). Cancer Genet Cytogenet 51: 215–221
13. Dastugue N, Demur C, Pris F, et al (1988) Association of the Philadelphia chromosome and 5q- in secondary blood disorder. Cancer Genet Cytogenet 30: 253–259
14. Moir DJ, Pearson J, Buckle VJ (1984) Acute promyelocytic transformations in a case of acute myelomonocytic leukemia. Cancer Genet Cytogenet 12: 359–364
15. Charrin C, Ritouet D, Campos L, et al (1992) Association of t(15; 17) and t(8; 21) in the initial phase of an acute promyelocytic leukemia. Cancer Genet Cytogenet 58: 177–180
16. Prigogina EL, Fleischman EW, Puchkova GP, et al (1986) Chromosomes in acute nonlymphocytic leukemia. Hum Genet 73: 137–146
17. Bernstein R, Pinto MR, Morcom G, et al (1982) Karyotype analysis in acute nonlymphocytic leukemia (ANLL): comparison with ethnic group, age, morphology, and survival. Cancer Genet Cytogenet 6: 187–199
18. Battaglia D, Dube I, Pinkerton P, Senn J (1989) Acquisition of additional primary chromosome abnormalities in the course of karyotype evolution in a case of FAB-M2 acute leukemia. Cancer Genet Cytogenet 40: 105–110

Acute Leukemias V
Experimental Approaches
and Management of Refractory Diseases
Hiddemann et al. (Eds.)

Detection of MLL/AF4 Recombination by PCR Technique

A. Borkhardt, R. Repp, J. Hammermann, S. Brettreich, R. Gossen, E. Haupt, J. Harbott, and F. Lampert

Introduction

The molecular analysis of chromosomal translocations occurring in human leukemias revealed the existence of newly formed fusion genes. The balanced translocation between chromosomes 4 and 11, for instance, results in a new MLL/AF4 gene as the AF4 gene at chromosomal region 4q21 is juxtaposed next to the part of the MLL gene (also called ALL-1 or HRX gene) located on chromosome 11q23 [1].

As patients with an acute lymphoblastic leukemia (ALL) and a t(4;11) usually have a poor response to conventional chemotherapy [2] it is considered to stratify these patients into a high-risk-group in the new German multicenter ALL-therapy study (ALL-BFM 94) in childhood [3]. A rapid and sensitive diagnostic screening procedure for assessment of a t(4,11) in patients with ALL, therefore, could be a powerful tool to stratify these patients in different prognostic and therapeutic subgroups.

Using the RT-PCR technique, here we describe a <PCR-assay which is able to detect 1 leukemic cell with an MLL/AF4 rearrangement among 100.000 normal cells. The high sensitivity of the PCR technique makes our assay also suitable to monitor minimal residual disease in patients with leukemia and a t(4;11).

Methods

RNA was purified according to a single-step protocol by Chromczynski and Sacchi [4]. The RNA was denatured at 70 °C for 5 min and, subsequently, the cDNA synthesis was performed at 37 °C for 60 min in a total volume of 20 µl using random hexamer primers (Boehringer, Mannheim, Germany). To increase the specifity of the amplified products and the sensitivity of detection we applied a two step protocol: 1 µl of the first round PCR-product was subjected to the second PCR reaction using an internal (nested) primer set. The PCR amplification contained 2 µl from the total of 20 µl cDNA, 4 pmol of each 5′ and 3′ primer in the first PCR round and 20 pmol of each 5′ and 3′ primer in the second PCR round.

We used the following primers for the detection of the MLL/AF4 transcript: MLL extern, upstream, 5′-CTGAATCCAAACAGGCCACCA CTC-3′, MLL intern, upstream, 5′-GGTCTCCCA GCCAGCACTGGTC-3′, AF4 extern, downstream 5′-GTCACTGAGCTGAAGGTCGTCTTC-3′, AF4 intern, downstream 5′-AGCATGGAT-GACGTTCCTTGCTGA3-3′. To check the integrity of the isolated RNA and the correct cDNA synthesis the normal nonrearranged AF4 gene was also amplified by AF4 primers (AF4 extern, upstream 5′-ACCTACTCCAAT-GAAGTCCATTGTG-3′, AF4 intern, upstream 5′- GAAGAGATTCTGAAGGAAATGACCC-3′, AF4 extern, downstream 5′-GTCACTGAGCT-GAAGGTCGTCTTC, AF4 intern, downstream 5′-AGCATGGATGACGTTCCTTGCTGA-3′). For amplification, cyclic reactions were performed in a thermal cycler (biomed, Theres, Germany). Each cycle consisted of denaturation at 94 °C for 60 s, primer annealing at 60 °C for 90 s, and

Children's University Hospital, Feulgenstr. 12, 35385 Gießen, Germany polymerization at 72 °C and twenty-five amplification cycles were performed in the first or second PCR run, respectively. In the last cycle of each run the polymerization was extended to 20 min.

In each PCR run negative controls were included in which cDNA had been replaced by sterile water. Messenger RNA from the HL60 promyelocytic cell line was used as a second negative control for MLL-1/AF4 expression. As a positive control template we amplified cDNA from the MV411 cell line (DSM, Braunschweig, Germany) which bears a t(4;11) [5]. After PCR amplification 10 μl aliquots were run on a 2.0% agarose gel. Gels were stained with ethidium bromide and photographed using an UV-transilluminator.

Moreover, the PCR product obtained was also sequenced by the chain termination method [6] (Fig. 1).

Results and Discussion

We evaluated the sensitivity of our nested PCR assay by amplification of the MLL/AF4 rearrangement from the MV411 cell line mixed with an increasing amount of HL60 cells. Our PCR assay was shown to be able to detect one MLL/AF4 rearranged cell per 100.000 unrearranged cells.

Such a level of sensitivity is several orders of magnitude above that of other techniques, such as cytogenetics, morphological evaluation of bone marrow smears or Southern blotting. Therefore, regarding sensitivity, our protocol fulfils the requirements needed for looking at minimal residual disease in patients with MLL/AF4 recombination. Such an analysis is currently under progress in adults and children who were positive for the MLL/AF4 recombination at diagnosis (Janssen et al., manuscript in preparation).

Life-table analysis performed on patients with ALL have consistently identified the t(4;11) as a bad prognostic indicator [2]. As the t(4;11) has been associated with early progenitor B-cell ALL [7] we started a diagnostic screening procedure for all children with pre-pre-B-ALL at diagnosis using this PCR assay.

As published previously, we examined 10 cases of pre-pre-B ALL and 5 of them revealed a positive MLL/AF4 recombination [8]. The amplified PCR products differed in size from 380–670 basepairs indicating alternatively spliced hybrid mRNA transcripts. By DNA

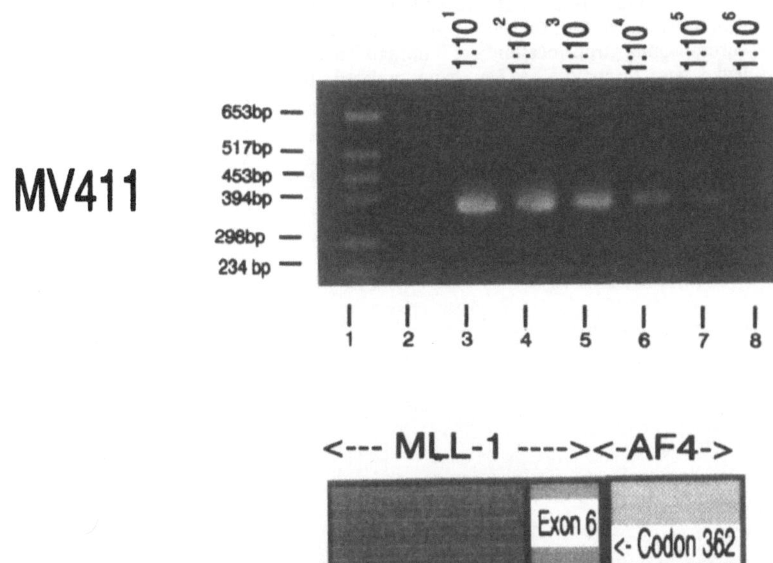

Fig. 1. Amplification of MLL-AF4 fusion mRNA in the MV411 cell line mixed with an increasing amount of HL60 cells. By DNA-sequencing we found a fusion between MLL exon 6 and codon 362 of the AF4 gene. Nucleotide positions were taken from Gene Bank Accession Number L04731 for MLL and L13773 for AF4

Table 1. Infant patients with pre-pre-B ALL and an MLL/AF4 recombination as detected by RT-PCR

Patient No	Sex	Age (months)	MLL-AF4 fusion transcript
1	f	1	exon 7 – codon 348
			exon 8 – codon 348
2	m	2	exon 7 – codon 362
			exon 8 – codon 362
3	f	6	exon 6 – codon 362
4	f	11	exon 6 – codon 362
5	f	11	exon 6 – codon 362

sequencing we determined furthermore the exact fusion pattern between the MLL gene and the AF4 gene. These results are summarized in Table 1.

Taken together, the RT-PCR assay presented here will provide a rapid and sensitive method to diagnose a substantial part of patients with high-risk leukemia and to monitor minimal residual disease in such patients under intensive treatment protocols. Moreover, we were able to demonstrate different molecular subtypes of t(4;11).

References

1. Gu Y, Nakamura T, Alder H, Prasad R, Canaani O, Cimino G, Croce CM, Canaani E (1992) The t(4;11) chromosome translocation of human acute leukemias fuses the ALL-1 gene, related to Drosophila trithorax, to the AF4 gene. Cell 71: 701–708
2. Pui C H, Frankel LS, Carroll AJ, Raimondi SC, Shuster JJ, Head DR, Crist WM, Land VJ, Pullen D J, Steuber CP, Behm FG, Borowitz MJ (1991) Clinical characteristics and treatment outcome of childhood acute lymphoblastic leukemia with the t(4;11)(q21;q23): A collaborative study of 40 cases. Blood 77: 440–447
3. Riehm H (1993) Studie zur Behandlung von Kindern und Jugendlichen mit akuter lymphoblastischer Leukämie (Non-B-ALL) ALL-BFM 94. pers communication
4. Chromczynski P, Sacchi N (1987) Single-step method of RNA isolation by guanidium thiocyanate-phenol-chloroform extraction. Anal Biochem 162: 156–159
5. Lange B, Valtieri M, Santoli D, Caracciolo D, Mavilio F, Gemperlein I, Griffin C, Emanuel B, Finan J, Nowell P, Rovera G (1987) Growth factor requirements of childhood acute leukemia: establishment of GM-CSF dependent cell lines. Blood 70: 192–198
6. Sanger F, Nicklen S, Coulson AR (1977) DNA seequencing with chain terminating inhibitors. Proc Natl Acad Sci USA 74: 5463–5467
7. Pui CH (1992) Acute leukemias with the t(4;11)(q21;q23). Leuk Lymphoma 7: 173–179
8. Borkhardt A, Repp R, Haupt E, Brettreich S, Buchen U, Gossen R, Lampert F (1994) Molecular Analysis of MLL-1/AF4 recombination in infant acute lymphoblastic leukemia. Leukemia 8: 549–553

Acute Leukemias V
Experimental Approaches
and Management of Refractory Diseases
Hiddemann et al. (Eds.)

Detection of Different 11q23 Chromosomal Abnormalities by Multiplex-PCR Using Automatic Fluorescence-Based DNA-Fragment Analysis

R. Repp, A. Borkhardt, E. Haupt, R. Gossen, S. Schlieben, I. Reinisch-Becker, J. Harbott, and F. Lampert

Introduction

Abnormalities at chromosome 11q23 can be found in many different kinds of leukemia. At the molecular level, a gene named MLL is involved in all these translocations. The 5'-region of this gene is fused to the 3'-part of different translocation partner genes resulting in transcription of a hybrid mRNA [1]. Most 11q23 abnormalities are clinically relevant. Patients bearing a translocation t(4;11), for example, have a very poor prognosis [2]. For this reason, routine diagnositic techniques are required. Conventional karyotyping, however, is rather time consuming and does only provide sufficient results in about 60% of the bone marrow specimens examined. Based on the PCR, much more sensitive assays became available during the last years. Usually, these techniques enable a sufficient analysis in more than 90% of the samples. However, an increasing number of detectable chromosomal translocations and a limited amount of patient's material require a restriction of the number of PCR-assays to be performed from each sample. Multiplex-PCR using several primers in a single PCR-reaction tube may overcome some of these problems and enable the detection of different chromosomal translocations by a single PCR-reaction. Translocations involving the q23 region of chromosome 11 seem to be an ideal target for this procedure, because acute leukemias of different lineages have similar MLL gene fusion sites at 11q23. For this reason, a combination an MLL specific primer with 3 other primers, each specific for a possible translocation partner gene, may enable the detection of 3 different 11q23 abnormalities by a single assay.

We have used a nested primer pair spanning a 3'-terminal region of exon 5 within the MLL gene and three nested primer pairs each located within one of the three possible translocation partner genes at chromosome 4, 9, and 19, respectively. A visable band after agarose gel analysis of the PCR-product clearly demonstrated the presence or absence of one of these three 11q23 abnormalities. However, a molecular heterogeneity at the 11q23 breakpoint can result in variable sizes of the PCR-products and prevent an exact definition of the translocation partner of the MLL gene simply by agarose gel analysis. To overcome these difficulties, we added three different fluorescent-labels to the 5'-end of the PCR primers specific for chromosome 4, 9, or 19, respectively. By using the Genescan-software on the automatic DNA-sequencer 373A (applied biosystems, Foster City, California) the translocation partners of the MLL gene were identified by their characteristic fluorescence and the molecular breakpoints were determined by an automatic size calculation of each PCR-product.

Materials and Methods

We used the cell lines MV4-11 and Mono-Mac 6 for amplification of the molecular equivalents of a t(4;11) or a t(9;11), respectively. These cell lines were kindly provided by H. Drexler (DSM, Braunschweig, Germany). As a positive control

Children's Hospital, University of Giessen, D-35392 Giessen, Germany

for amplification of the MLL/ENL rearrangement, the molecular equivalent of t(11;19), we used a bone marrow sample from a patient with a secondary AMl and a t(11;19). Mononuclear bone marrow cells from this patient were harvested after centrifugation over a Ficoll-Hypaque gradient. Cells grown in tissue culture suspension were used directly. Total RNA was purified by a single step method [3]. The RNA was denatured at 70 °C for 5 min and, subsequently, the cDNA synthesis was carried out at 37 °C for 60 min in a total volume of 20 µl using random hexamer primers (Boehringer, Mannheim, Germany).

PCR-primers were synthesized on an Applied Biosystems oligonucleotide synthesizer (abi, Foster City, California, USA) and purified by high performance liquid chromatography (HPLC). The PCR primers sequences were chosen based on published sequence data [4–6].

To improve sensitivity and specificity we performed a two step semi-nested PCR protocol using the synthetic oligonucleotide primers as shown in Table 1. After an initial melting step (5 min at 94 °C) the enzyme was added and 35 amplification cycles of 60 s at 94 °C, 120 s at 60 °C, and 120 s at 74 °C were carried out in 50 µl final volume containing 4 pmol of each primer during the first round of the nested PCR. One microliter of the first round product was subjected to the second round of PCR. This differed from the first round of PCR by the number of cycles which was reduced to 25, and the amount of primer (20 pmol). PCR-cycling was performed in a bio-med Thermocycler 60 (bio-med, Theres, Germany) using a GeneAmp kit (Perkin Elmer, Überlingen, Germany). PCR products were analyzed on a 2% agarose gel and visualized by ethidium bromide staining. One microliter of the final PCR product was diluted with 9 µl of sterile water. A master mix corresponding to 0,5 µl Genescan standard (Genescan $2500TM_{Rox}$, Applied Biosystems, Foster City, California, USA) and 2,5 µl formamide per sample was prepared. One µl of the diluted PCR product was added to 3 µl of this mastermix. The samples were heated to 90 °C for 2 min and quenched on ice for 3 min. Three µl of each sample were subjected to electrophoresis over a 6% polyacrylamide gel in an automatic DNA-sequencer 373A (Applied Biosystems, Foster City, California, USA). Gels were analysed using the "Genescan"-software.

Results

Our seminested-PCR assay was able to detect all three chromosomal translocations t(4;11), t(9;11), and t(11;19), respectively, as shown in Figure 1.

The sensitivity was higher than 100 cells bearing the translocation in the amount of 100000 cells used for RNA preparation (data not shown). Even though, the PCR-products obtained from these translocation were clearly different in size (Fig. 1) agarose gel analysis cannot be considered sufficient for a discrimination between the three translocation partner genes of MLL. In case of t(4;11) it is well proven that a variable number of MLL gene exons can be found within the hybrid mRNA generated by the gene translocation. This fact will lead to variable sizes of the PCR-products generated by our assay. In case of t(11;19) and t(9;11) the existence of variable splicing sites also can be assumed (Borkhardt et al., unpublished) but, so far, they have not yet been characterized in detail. For this reason the fluorescence-labeled PCR-products were subjected to genescan analysis. By this procedure each of the three translocations was clearly identifiable by a characteristic fluorescence color signal. As expected, it was blue in case of t(4;11), yellow in case of t(9;11), and green in case of a t(11;19) (Fig. 2). Furthermore, genes-

Table 1. Primer sequences used in the multiplex-PCR assay

Primer	Nucleotide sequence (5′–3′)	5′-dye label color in gene scan analysis
MLL, extern,sense	CCTGAATCCAAACAGGCCACCACT	–
MLL,intern, sense	GGTCTCCCAGCCAGCACTGGTC	–
AF4,antisense	AGCATGGATGACGTTCCTTGCTGA	FAM, blue
AF9. antisense	CGTGATGTAGGGGTGAAGAAGCAG	TAMRA, yellow
ENL,antisense	CCACGAAGTGCTGGATGTCACAT	JOE, green

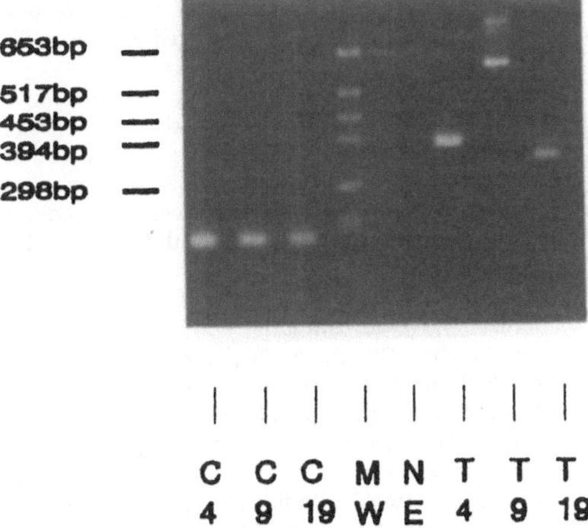

Fig. 1. Agarose gel analysis of the PCR-products. MW = molecular weight marker, NE negative control, T4-T19 = products of multiplex PCR to detect the translocations t(4,11), t(9;11), and t(11;19), C4-C19 = control amplification of the AF4 gene to ensure sufficient RNA quality

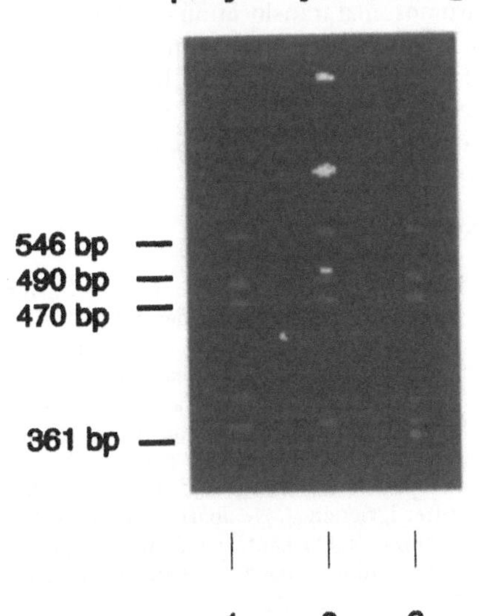

Fig. 2. Genescan analysis of fusion sites of the translocations t(4;11), t(9;11), and t(11;19) as amplified by multiplex PCR. Lane 1, MLL/AF4 rearrangement (blue), Lane 2 MLL/AF9 rearrangement (yellow), Lane 3 MLL/ENL rearrangement (green). Note the different spliced transcripts in Lane 2. The internal size marker is dye-labelled with Rox (red). (Color prints may be ordered directly from the authors)

can analysis produces an exact size calculation of each PCR-product. This enables a determination of the molecular subtypes of the chromosomal breakpoints if the possible different splicing variants are known.

Discussion

Chromosomal translocations involving 11q23 are most frequently found in infant's acute leukemias of an immature subtype (e.g. pre-pre-B-ALL). In case of the translocation t(4;11), especially, it is well established that these patients have a very poor prognosis [7]. For this reason, they will be considered to be stratified into the "high risk group" of the new German multicenter therapy study for childhood acute lymphoblastic leukemia (ALL-BFM94) [8]. Prior drawing therapeutic consequences, however, a sufficient diagnostic procedure is required to obtain exact results within a short time. For this purpose, PCR-based techniques display several advantages as compared to other conventional methods, such as karyotyping or Southern-blotting: their sensitivity is higher, sufficient results are obtained in a higher number of samples, and they are less time consuming. PCR-based techniques, on the other hand, usually only allow the detection of a single chromosomal translocation, whereas conventional cytogenetics or Southern-blotting can detect more than one translocation at the same time [9]. A reasonable compromise to overcome this disadvantage of PCR may be the use of several primers in a single reaction tube, each specific for one of the different translocations to be detected (multiplex-PCR). 11q23 abnormalities are an ideal target for this procedure because the MLL specific primer can maintained in combination with different other primers located on the possible translocation partner genes to detect several chromosomal transolcations involving 11q23 by one PCR-reaction. In multiplex-PCR, however, each of the different target translocations can be the reason for a visible band on the final agarose gel. Identification of the different chromosomal rearangements is usually achieved by placing the PCR-primers in a way that generates characteristic sizes of PCR-products from each of the translocations to be detected. In case of 11q23 abnormalities, however, this may be difficult due to the usage of alternative exons of MLL combined with variable splicing sites of the partner genes at chromosome 4, 9 and 19. Our assay simply allows the identification of the specific chromosomal translocation by different colors of the corresponding PCR product. After cloning of other 11q23 translocations like the t(6;11) [10] these rearrangements can also be included in such a 11q23 multiplex PCR approach.

References

1. Corral J, Forster A, Thompson S, Lampert F, Kaneko Y, Slater R, van der Schoot CE, Ludwig WD, Pocock C, Cotter F, Rabbitts TH (1993) Acute leukaemias of different lineages have similar MLL gene fusions encoding related chimeric proteins resulting from chromosomal translocation. Proc Natl Acad Sci USA 90: 8538–8542
2. Lampert F, Harbott J, Ludwig WD, Bartram CR, Ritter J, Gerein V, Neidhart M, Mertens R, Graf N, Riehm H (1987) Acute leukemia with chromosome translocation (4;11): 7 new patients and analysis of 71 cases. Blut 54: 325–335
3. Chromczynski P, Sacchi N (1987) Single-step method of RNA isolation by guanidium thiocyanate-phenol-chloroform extraction. Anal Biochem 162: 156–159
4. Iida S, Seto M, Yamamoto K, Komatsu H, Tojo A, Asano S, Kamada N, Ariyoshi Y, Takahashi T, Ueda R (1993) MLLT3 gene on chromosome 9p22 involved in t(9;11) leukemia encodes a serine/proline rich protein homologous to MLLT1 on 19p13. Oncogene 8: 3085–3092
5. Gu Y, Nakamura T, Alder H, Prasad R, Canaani O, Cimino G, Croce CM, Canaani E (1992) The t(4;11) chromosome translocation of human acute leukemias fuses the ALL-1 gene, related to Drosophila trithorax, to the AF4 gene. Cell 71: 701–708
6. Nakamura T, Alder H, Gu Y, Prasad R, Canaani O, Kamada N, Gale RP, Lange B, Crist WM, Nowell PC, Croce CM, Canaani E (1993) Genes on chromosomes 4, 9, and 19 involved in 11p23 abnormalities in acute leukemia share sequence homology and/or common motifs. Proc Natl Acad Sci USA 90: 4631–4635
7. Pui CH, Frankel LS, Carroll AJ, Raimondi SC, Shuster JJ, Head, DR, Crist WM, Land VJ, Pullen DJ, Steuber CP, Behm FG, Borowitz MJ (1991) Clinical characteristics and treatment outcome of childhood acute lymphoblastic leukemia with the t(4;11) (q21;q23): A collaborative study of 40 cases. Blood 77: 440–447
8. Riehm H (1993) Studie zur Behandlung von Kindern mit akuter lymphoblastischer Leukämie (Non-B-ALL) ALL-BFM 94. pers communication
9. Thirman MJ, Gill HJ, Burnett RC, Mbangkollo D, McCabe NR, Kobayashi H, Ziemin-van der Poel S, Kaneko Y, Morgan R, Sandberg AA, Chaganti RSK, Larson RA, Le Beau MM, Diaz MO, Rowley JD (1993) Rearrangements of the MLL gene in acute lymphoblastic and acute myeloid leukemias with 11q23 chromosomal translocations. N Engl J Med 329: 909–914
10. Prasad R, Gu Y, Alder H, Nakamura T, Canaani O, Saito H, Huebner K, Gale RP, Nowell PC, Kuriyama K, Miyazaki Y, Croce CM, Canaani E (1993) Cloning of the ALL-1 fusion partner, the AF6 gene, involved in acute myeloid leukemias with t(1;6) chromosome translocation. Cancer Res 53: 5624–5628

Acute Leukemias V
Experimental Approaches
and Management of Refractory Diseases
Hiddemann et al. (Eds.)

Designing Probe Sets for the Detection of Chromosome Abnormalities in Acute Myeloid Leukemia Using Fluorescence In Situ Hybridization

K. Fischer[1], C. Scholl[1], G. Cabot[1], M. Moos[1], R. Schlenk[1], P. Theobald[1], R. Haas[1], M. Bentz[2], P. Lichter[2], and H. Döhner[1]

Introduction

In recent years, the karyotype as a prognostic factor in acute myeloid leukemia (AML) has gained considerable interest. Clonal chromosome aberrations are identified in 50–60% of patients with AML (for review see [1]). The most frequent numerical abnormalities are trisomy 8 (+8), monosomy 7 (-7) and nullisomy Y, and the most frequent structural aberrations are t(15;17), t(8;21), abnormalities of band 16q22 (abnl 16q22), deletions of the long arm of chromosomes 5 [del(5q)] and 7 [del(7q)], translocations involving band 11q23 [t(9;11) and others], del(9q), del(11q), del(12p), and del(20q). The frequency of these chromosome aberrations varies from approximately 10% (+8) to less than 1% [del(12p)] with conventional cytogenetic analysis.

Retrospective and prospective clinical studies have shown that the karyotype in patients with AML is associated with significant differences in the complete remission (CR) rates and the survival times (for review see [1,2,3]). The possibility to identify risk-groups based on the karyotype opens the new perspective of selecting risk-adapted therapies [4].

G-banding analysis, however, may be technically difficult due to reduced cell viability after transport to the central reference laboratory, the complexity of the karyotype or the low in vitro proliferative activity of the leukemic cells. Improvements in fluorescence in situ hybridization (ISH) techniques have provided an approach alternative to G-banding analysis. Using specific DNA-probes, chromosome abnormalities cannot only be detected in metaphase cells but also in interphase nuclei (*interphase cytogenetics*) [5]. We have designed a DNA probe set that allows the detection of some of the most frequent numerical and structural chromosome aberrations in AML.

Patients and Methods

So far, 14 patients with de novo AML (age 16–59) were studied by G-banding analysis and by fluorescence ISH. G-banding analysis was performed as previously described [6].

For the detection of numerical abnormalities the following probes are currently used: D7Z1 (-7), D8Z1 (+8), D11Z1 (+11), DYZ3 (−Y) (all centromere specific probes; Oncor Sciences, Gaithersburg, MD); 22/1 (+22) [7]; and cosmid clone c518 mapping to 21q22.3 (+21) (generously provided by Dr. K. Klinger, Integrated Genetics, Framingham, MA). For the detection of structural chromosome abnormalities the following probes are used: yeast artificial chromosome (YAC)-clone yPR411 containing FMS encoding sequences (5q−) (generously provided by Dr. Brownstein, St. Louis, MO), a cosmid pool mapping to chromosome band 7q22 (7q−) (provided by Dr. K. Klinger), YAC-clone 13HH4 spanning a 440-kb region on band 11q23 including the MLL gene [t(9;11) and variants; provided by Dr. B. Young, London], and a cosmid pool recognizing the p53 tumor suppressor gene

[1] Medizinische Klinik und Poliklinik V, Universität Heidelberg, 69115 Heidelberg, Germany
[2] Organisation Komplexer Genome, Deutsches Krebsforschungszentrum, 69120 Heidelberg, Germany

(17p−) (provided by Dr. A. Poustka, Heidelberg). The probes were labeled by nick translation with biotin-16-dUTP or digoxigenin-11-dUTP (Boehringer Mannheim). Fluorescence ISH was performed as described [8–9]. Fluorescence signals were enumerated in 200 to 400 interphase cells. Slides were viewed on a microscope (Axioskop, Zeiss, Oberkochen) equipped for epifluorescence and illustrations were produced using a cooled charged coupled device (CCD) camera (KAPPA, Gleichen).

Results

The cut-off level for each probe was derived from hybridization experiments of five probands. A trisomy was diagnosed if patients exhibited highly significant (mean+3 standard deviations) percentages of cells with three fluorescence signals. For the detection of monosomies or deletions, dual-color hybridization using two probes of similar complexity was performed as previously described [9].

So far, 14 patients with de novo AML were investigated. The comparison between the results of G-banding analysis and fluorescence ISH is shown in Table 1. In four patients (nos. 3,4,10,12) no adequate metaphases were found on G-banding analysis: In one of these patients (no. 3) trisomy 8 was detected by ISH, the other three patients showed no clonal aberrations regarding the regions investigated. Three patients (nos. 2,8,11) had a normal karyotype on G-banding analysis and by ISH. Seven patients had clonal abnormalities by G-banding: One of these patients (no. 5) had a t(9;11) and trisomy 8 that was also detected by ISH. Another patient (no. 14) had loss of 17p11-pter on G-banding and a p53 deletion by ISH. In three patients (nos. 1,7,13), who exhibited a complex karyotype that could not be completely analyzed on G-banding, we could characterize the clone by ISH: these three patients had either 5q− (Fig. 1) or 7q. Two patients (nos. 6 and 9) had clonal aberrations on G-banding that could not be detected by the probe set.

Table 1. Comparison of the results obtained by G-banding analysis and by fluorescence ISH (FISH)

Pt.No.	G-banding	FISH
1	Complex [not completely evaluable]	5q−,+8,+11,+21,+22
2	46,XX	−*
3	No metaphases	+8
4	No metaphases	−
5	46,XX,t(9;11)(p22;q23)[18] 47,XX,+8,t(9;11)(p22;q23)[2]	+8,t(11q23)**
6	46,XY,ins(2;3)(p22;q21q26)	−
7	46,XY,del(7)(q11q36),complex	7q−
8	46,XX	−
9	46,XX,del(9)(p13), der(10)t(10;11)(q22;q12), add(11)(q11),−14,+mar	−
10	No metaphases	−
11	46,XX	−
12	No metaphases	−
13	3p−,5q−,−7,complex [not completely evaluable]	5q−,+21
14	46,XY,del(9q)(q12q22), −17,+der(17)t(11;17)(q13;p11)	del(p53),+11q**

*no clonal aberration found
**pts 5 and 14 had three signals with YAC clone 13HH4; using this clone only, the diagnosis of the t(11q23) and the partial trisomy 11 (+11q) cannot be made by ISH alone, but only with knowledge of the G-banded karyotype

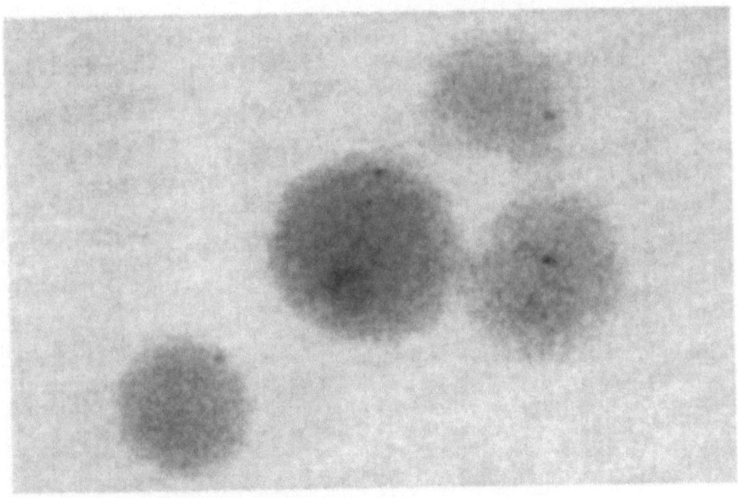

Fig. 1. Hybridization of interphase cells from patient 1 with YAC clone yPR411 recognizing the FMS gene: Note only one fluorescence signal in all cells indicating the FMS gene deletion. On G-banding analysis the patient exhibited a complex karyotype that could not be completely evaluated

Conclusions and Perspectives

We have designed a DNA probe set that allows the detection of some of the most frequent numerical (-7, +8, +11, +21, +22, -Y) and structural [del(5q), del(7q), t(11q23)] chromosome aberrations in AML. In a pilot phase, 14 patients with de novo AML were investigated with this probe set at initial presentation: In one patient without adequate metaphases trisomy 8 was detected by ISH. In three other patients who exhibited a complex karyotype that could not be completely evaluated on G-banding, we could characterize the clone by fluorescence ISH. These preliminary experiments indicate that fluorescence ISH using a disease-specific DNA probe set may become a valuable adjunct to conventional banding analysis for the rapid and reliable identification of clonal chromosome aberrations. This DNA probe set is currently being investigated in a multicenter AML treatment trial evaluating different postremission therapies that are stratified according to the karyotype.

Another potential application for this DNA probe sets is the monitoring of the remission status and the detection of minimal residual disease. However, for the detection of less than 3% to 5% malignant cells by ISH more complex probe sets have to be used. This is due to the occurrence of false positive cells in a frequency comparable to that of residual tumor cells. To increase the sensitivity of detection two or more probes that serve as mutual internal controls can be combined in a multi-color multi-probe ISH [10]. The sensitivity can be further increased by hybridizing cell fractions enriched for the malignant cells (e.g. CD34 positive cells). In comparison to polymerase chain reaction (PCR) based diagnostic tests, detection of residual disease by fluorescence ISH may be less sensitive and more time consuming. However, it allows the quantification of the malignant clone and the detection of chromosome abnormalities for which no PCR assays are available.

Acknowledgement. This work was supported by a grant (Do 436/3-1) from the Deutsche Forschungs-gemeinschaft.

References

1. Bloomfield CD and de la Chapelle A: Chromosome abnormalities in acute nonlymphocytic leukemia: Clinical and biologic significance. Semin Oncol 14: 372-378, 1987.
2. Fourth International Workshop on Chromosomes in Leukemia, 1982: Clinical significance of chromosomal abnormalities in acute nonlymphoblastic leukemia. Cancer Genet Cytogenet 11: 332-350, 1984.

3. Arthur DC, Berger R, Golomb HM, Swansbury GJ, Reeves BR, Alimena G, van den Berghe H, Bloomfield CD, de la Chapelle A, Dewald GW, Garson OM, Hagemeijer A, Kaneko Y, Mitelman F, Pierre RV, Ruutu T, Sakurai M, Lawler SD and Rowley JD: The clinical significance of karyotype in acute myelogenous leukemia. Cancer Genet Cytogenet 40: 203, 1989.
4. Bloomfield CD: Prognostic factors for selecting curative therapy for adult myeloid leukemia. Leukemia 6(Suppl 4): 65–67, 1992.
5. Cremer T, Landegent J, Brückner A, Scholl HP, Schardin M, Hager HD, Devilee P, Pearson P, van der Ploeg M: Detection of chromosome aberrations in the human interphase nucleus by visualization of specific target DNAs with radioactive and non-radioactive in situ hybridization techniques: Diagnosis of trisomy 18 with probe L1.84. Hum Genet 74: 346–352, 1986.
6. Döhner H, Arthur DC, Ball ED, Sobol RE, Davey FR, Lawrence D, Gordon L, Patil SR, Surana RB, Testa JR, Verma RS, Schiffer CA, Wurster-Hill DH, Bloomfield CD: Trisomy 13 – A new recurring chromosome abnormality in acute leukemia. Blood 76: 1614–1621, 1990.
7. McDermid HE, Duncan AMV, Higgins MJ, Hamerton JL, Rector E, Brasch KR, White BN: Isolation and characterization of an α-satellite repeated sequence from human chromosome 22. Chromosoma 94: 228–234, 1986.
8. Lichter P and Cremer T: Chromosome analysis by non-isotopic in situ hybridization. In: Rooney DE, Czepulkowski BH (eds.). Human Cytogenetics. Oxford University Press, New York 1: 157–192, 1992.
9. Stilgenbauer S, Döhner H, Bulgay-Mörschel M, Weitz S, Bentz M, Lichter P: Retinoblastoma gene deletion in chronic lymphoid leukemias: A combined metaphase and interphase cytogenetic study. Blood 81: 2118–2124, 1993.
10. Bentz M, Cabot G, Moos M, Speicher MR, Ganser A, Lichter P, Döhner H: Detection of chimeric bcr-abl genes on bone marrow samples and blood smears in chronic myeloid and acute lymphoblastic leukemia by in situ hybridization. Blood April 1994, in press.

Acute Leukemias V
Experimental Approaches
and Management of Refractory Diseases
Hiddemann et al. (Eds.)

The Amplification of the Wilms Tumor Gene (wt-1) mRNA Using the Polymerase Chain Reaction Technique (PCR) May Enable Sensitive Detection of Small Blast Populations in AML

J. Brieger, E. Weidmann, K. Fenchel, P. S. Mitrou, L. Bergmann, and D. Hoelzer

Abstract. Leukemic cells from 52 patients with AML were examined for the expression of wt-1 mRNA. Blast cells were isolated from bone marrow or peripheral blood. Total RNA was extracted and wt-1 transcription was studied via RT-PCR. Mononuclear cells and bone marrow from healthy persons were used as controls. Cell surface antigens were determined using FACS-analysis. In dilution experiments the detection limit was assessed as 1 out of 10000 cells. Wilms' tumor mRNA was detectable in 41 out of 52 cases of AML (79%). None of the 13 controls expressed wt-1. After chemotherapy, six out of eleven patients in complete remission (CR) lost wt-1 expression completely. The remaining five patients expressed wt-1 mRNA at the same or a lower level. The significance of wt-1 persistance for desease free survival will have to be defined.

No relation of wt-1 expression to FAB, age, sex or phenotype was found. Further experiments for later evaluation of the value of the Wilms' tumor gene as a prognostic factor are in progress. Our data show that expression of wt-1 mRNA is widely spread in akute AML blast cells. Our observations suggest that analysis of wt-1 gene-expression via PCR may be a sensitive technique for the detection of residual blast cells following chemotherapy of AML.

Introduction

The detection of small blast populations in leukemias may be important after chemotherapy or autologous bone marrow transplantation. Various translocations have been considered as genetic markers for different types of acute myelocytic leukemia (AML), but all have the disadvantage only accompanying restricted groups of AML-subtypes. Moreover, the sensitivity of the common detection systems is not always satisfying [1,2]. Recently the Wilms' tumor gene (wt-1), a tumor suppressor gene, was isolated [3,4]. The Wilms' tumor Gene (wt-1) is generally expressed in the fetal kidneys, gonads, spleen and in Wilms' Tumors, a tumor of the kidneys. The gene encodes a zinc finger DNA binding protein, that functions as a transcriptional suppressor of different growth and differentiation related genes, as insulin like growth factor-2 (IGF-2)[5] or platelet-derived growth factor α-chain (PGF)[6]. Moreover wt-1 is homologue to the early growth response genes 1 and 2 (EGR1,-2)[7,8,9], two other growth related genes. Additionally, PGF-gene expression can be upregulated by the wt-1 gene product [10]. Recently, a crossregulating activity with the tumor suppressor gene p53 was described [11], a gene widely involved in carcinogenesis [12] and discussed to be related to hematopoetical disorders [13,14]. Different deletions and point mutations in this gene have been detected in the tumor as well as in the germline of the same patients. Therefore, it seems likely that the mutated wt-1 gene product is involved in carcinogenesis [15,16]. Recently the expression of wt-1 exclusively in blasts with immature phenotypes of the myeloid lineage has been demonstrated [17,18].

This study was designed to obtain evidence for the hypothesis that the wt-1 gene might be

Dept. of Internal Medicine, Div. of Hematology and Oncology, J.W.Goethe University, Frankfurt/M., Germany

useful as a marker for the detection of blast cells using the highly sensitive PCR-technique. For this purpose we established a RT-PCR assay and evaluated the quote of wt-1 gene expression in untreated acute leukemias (AL), in complete remission (CR), healthy persons and in leukemia derived cell lines. Patients with untreated AL and three cell lines expressed high levels of wt-1 mRNA, whereas wt-1 expression was undetectable or reduced in bone marrow cells of AML patients in complete remission.

Materials and Methods

Samples. Fifty-two patients with previously untreated AML, 11 patients in CR, 13 healthy persons and 4 myeloid leukemia derived cell lines (Hel 921.7, HL 60, KG 1, K 562) were examined in this study (Table 1). For this purpose bone marrow (BM) or peripheral blood mononuclear cells (PBMNC), containing 35–95% blast cells, were recovered from heparinized BM aspirated at time of diagnosis or heparinized PB. After density gradient sedimentation using Ficoll-Hypaque, the cells were washed twice with phosphate buffered saline (PBS) and used for phenotyping or RNA extraction.

Leukemias were classified using the morphological and cytochemical criteria of the French-American-British (FAB) classification [19].

Table 1. Patients characteristics

Patients	n	wt-1+	%
Controls	13	0	0
AML, total	52	41	79
AML, de novo	45	36	80
M0	1	1	100
M1	4	4	100
M2	16	11	69
M3	4	4	100
M4	13	11	85
M5	5	3	60
M6	1	1	100
undefined	1	1	100
AML, following MDS	7	5	71
M1	1	1	100
M2	2	1	50
M5	1	0	0
undefined	3	3	100
age >60 years*	16	14	88
age <60 years*	33	24	73

* patients' median age: 51 years (range 21–75)

PCR. Aliquots of 5 μg total RNA were reverse transcribed and used for amplification with wt-1 specific oligonucleotides, according to published sequences [20]. Conditions of amplification were: 35 cycles of amplification starting with 5 min. at 94°C before adding the enzyme. The cycles were initiated by denaturating the DNA at 94°C for 30 sec., followed by an annealing reaction for 30 sec. at 64°C and extending at 72°C for 45 sec. After the last cycle, we applied a final extension reaction at 72°C for 7 min. The amplification products (857bp) were separated by electrophoresis on an 1% ethidium bromide stained agarosegel and classified in not amplified(–), weakly(+), moderately(++) and strongly amplified(+++).

Southern blot. Electrophoresed PCR products were blotted on uncharged nylon membran and hybridized with an wt-1 specific biotinylated oligonucleotide. Chemoluminescent detection of the hybridisation product was performed according to manufactors` instructions (Tropix, Bedford, MA).

Immunofluorescence analysis. Mononuclear cells were stained by double color direct immunofluorescence (phycoerythrin (PE) and fluorescein-isothiocyanate labeled (FITC)) with a series of monoclonal antibodies (MoAbs) and studied immediately. Detection was gated primarily on the subpopulation of malignant cells by forward and side scatter and by exclusion of normal lymphocyte populations via CD3 labeling. Analysis of phenotypical characteristics was performed using a FACScan flow cytometer and the Lysys II software (Becton-Dickinson, Heidelberg, FRG). The following MoAbs. were used: CD19 (Leu 12), CD34 (HPCA-2), CD2 (Leu 5), CD7 (Leu 9), CD33 (LeuM9). Antibodies were purchased from Becton-Dickinson. Controls were performed with unstained cells and non-reactive antibodies (MsIgG and MsIgM). Double fluorescence analysis was performed with CD7/CD33 MoAbs. Leukemias were defined as positive in cases expressing more than 20% of the studied antigen [21].

Blast cells from 6 representative patients were sorted using FACSort (Becton-Dickinson, Heidelberg, FRG) to 95–100% purity and wt-1 expression was studied.

Detection limit of wt-1 analysis via RT-PCR. Total RNA isolated from the wt-1 positive cell line Hel and from a healthy person was used in experiments evaluating the sensitivity of the technique. For this purpose 10^6 cells, containing 10, 100, 1000, 10000, 100000, 500000 wt-1 positive Hel-cells and corresponding amounts of wt-1 negative PBMNCs were mixed. Total RNA was extracted, reverse transcribed and amplified. The amplification products were separated on an agarose gel and stained with ethidium bromide. Finally the gel was blotted and hybridized with wt-1 specific oligonucleotides.

Results

After reverse transcription of total cellular RNA, isolated from 52 patients with AML, four leukemia derived cell lines and 13 healthy controls, wt-1 specific transcripts were amplified by PCR. After separation on an agarose gel, southern blot analysis was performed to confirm the specificity of the amplification. A representative gel and the corresponding southern blot are documented in Figure 1.

In none of the 13 examined healthy controls a signal was obtained. 41 out of 52 AMLs (79%) were wt-1 postive (Table 2). Three out of four leukemia derived cell lines expressed wt-1 mRNA; only the line HL 60 was wt-1 negative. No relation to FAB-subtype or age of the patient could be demonstrated (Table 1). No correlation of wt-1 expression to any predominance of cell surface antigens was detectable.

In order to analyze possible changes of wt-1 expression in patients with newly diagnosed acute leukemias and after reaching of CR, the ethidium bromide stained PCR-products were classified in not amplified to strongly amplified. In complete remission six patients out of eleven lost wt-1 expression completely and in two cases reduced signals were detectable. In two patients no altered wt-1 levels were detectable.

The achievement of remissions was so far independent of wt-1 expression (Table 2).

The detection limit of the described PCR-assay was evaluated as one wt-1 positive cell out of 10000 wt-1 negative cells, as documented in Figure 2.

Table 2. Expression of wt-1 in relation to response

	wt-1+patients at diagnosis (n)	%
AML, de novo	36/45	80
CR	21/29	72
NR	14/16	88
AML following MDS	5/7	71
CR	0/1	–
NR	5/6	83
Healthy controls	0/13	0

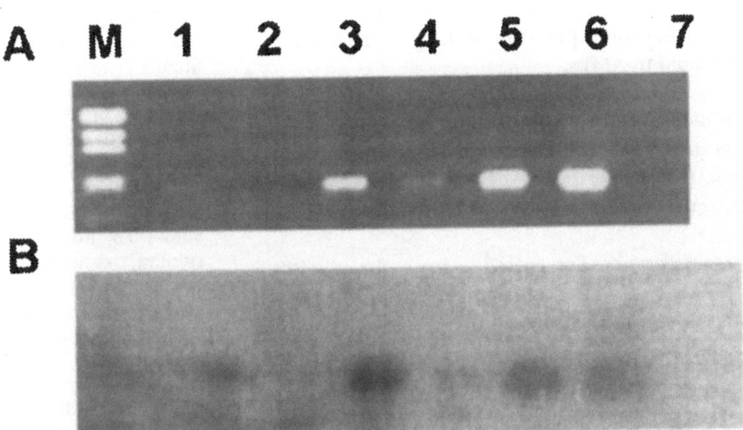

Fig. 1. Expression of wt-1 specific mRNA in acute myelocytic blast cells. jhnA: Ethidium bromide stained agarose gel; B: Corresponding southern blot M: Marker, Hind/Eco-digested Lambda DNA. 1: positive control; 2: negative control; 3–7: AMLs

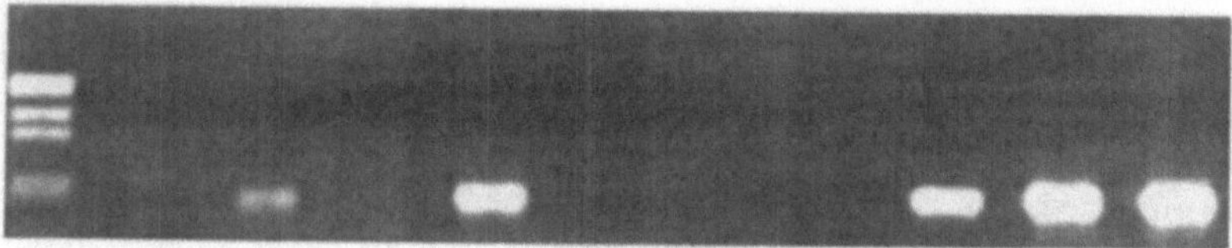

Fig. 2. Dilution series of blast cells to define the detection limit. M: Marker, Hind/Eco-digested Lambda DNA. 1: negative control. 2: positive control. 3: undiluted Hel 921.7 cells (wt-1 negative). 4: undiluted blast cells (wt-1 positive). 5: 10 blasts/10^6cells; 6: 100/10^6; 7: 1000/10^6; 8: 10000/10^6; 9: 100000/10^6; 10: 500000/10^6

Discussion

This study was designed to evaluate if the tumor suppresor gene wt-1 may serve as a genetic marker for the detection of blast cells. For this purpose we established a sensitive PCR assay and determined the frequency of wt-1 expression in leukemia derived cell lines and in untreated acute myelogenous leukemias or after achieving of CR, respectively.

We found that the wt-1 gene is widely expressed in acute myelogenous leukemias (about 80%), but not in healthy persons. Moreover, in complete remission the gene's expression is often reduced. As three out of four examined cell lines were positive, too, we suggest that the Wilms' tumor gene could be related to blast cells and therefore to the development of acute myelogenous leukemias. The presence of wt-1 was not correlated to FAB-subtype or phenotypical characteristics of the leukemias. The independency of the gene's expression from the differentiation of blast cells may suggest again, that the expression of the gene is generally related to AMLs.

The established PCR assay has a sensitivity of one positive cell out of 10000 negative cells. All together, the PCR facilitated detection of wt-1 gene transcripts might be a suitable technique for the detection of leukemic blast cells.

Acknowledgement. Supported by the grant 01GA8802 of the Bundesministerium für Forschung und Technik (BMFT) and Deutsche Krebshilfe grant W22/92.

References

1. Maseki N, Miyoshi H, Shimizu K, Homma C, Ohki M, Sakurai M, Kaneko Y. The 8;21 Chromosome translocation in acute myeloid leukemia is always detectable by molekular analysis using AML1. Blood 1993;81: 1573–1579.
2. van Dongen JJM, Breit TM, Adriaansen HJ, Beishuizen A, Hooijkaas H. Detection of minimal residual disease in acute leukemia by immunological marker analysis and polymerase chain reaction. Leukemia 1992;Suppl 1: 47–59.
3. Call KM, Glaser T, Ito CY, Buckler AJ, Pelletier J, Haber DA, Rose EA, Kral A, Yeger H, Lewis WH, Jones C, Housman DE. Isolation and characterization of a zinc finger polypeptide gene at the human chromosome 11 Wilms' tumor locus. Cell 1990;60: 509–520.
4. Gessler M, Poustka A, Cavenee W, Neve RL, Orkin SH, Bruns GAP. Homozygous deletion in Wilms' tumors of a zinc-finger gene identified by chromosome jumping. Nature 1990;343: 774–778.
5. Drummond IA, Madden SL, Rohwer-Nutter P, Bell GI, Sukhatme VP, Rauscher FJ 3d. Repression of the insulin-like growth factor II gene by the Wilms' tumor suppressor wt-1. Science 1992;257: 674–678.
6. Gashler AL, Bonthron DT, Madden SL, Rauscher FJ 3d, Collins T, Sukhatme VP. Human platelet-derived growth factor A chain is transcriptionally repressed by the Wilms tumor suppressor WT1. PNAS 1992;89: 10984–10988.
7. Sukhatme VP, Cao X, Chang LC, Tsai-Moris C-H, Stamenkovich D, Ferreira PCP, Cohen DR, Edwards SA, Shows TB, Curran T, Le Beau MM, Adamson ED. A zinc finger-encoding gene coregulated with c-fos during growth and differentiation, and after cellular depolarization. Cell 1988;53: 37–43.
8. Joseph LJ, Le Beau MM, Jamieson GA, Acharya S, Shows TB, Rowley JD, Sukhatme VP. Molekular cloning, sequencing, and mapping of EGR2, a human early growth response gene encoding a protein with 'zinc-binding finger' structure. PNAS 1988;85: 7164–7168.
9. Madden SL, Cook DM, Morris JF, Gashler A, Sukhatme VP, Rauscher 3d FJ. Transcriptional repression mediated by the WT-1 Wilms' tumor gene product. Science 1991;253: 1550–1553.
10. Wang ZY, Qiu QQ, Deuel TF. The Wilms' tumor gene product wt-1 activates or suppresses transcription through separate functional domains. J Biol Chem 1993;268(13): 9172–9175.

11. Maheswaran S, Park S, Bernard A, Morris JF, Rauscher 3d FJ, Hill DE, Haber DA. Physical and functional interaction between WT-1 and p53 proteins. PNAS 1993;90: 5100–5104.
12. Nigro JM, Baker SJ, Preisinger AC, Jessup JM, Hostetter R, Cleary K, Bigner SH, Davidson N, Baylin S, Devilee P, Glover T, Collins FS, Weston A, Modali R, Harris CC, Vogelstein B. Mutations in the p53 gene occur in diverse human tumour types. Nature 1989;342: 705-708.
13. Ahuja H, Bar-Eli M, Advani SH, Benchimol S, Cline MJ. Alterations in the p53 gene and the clonal evolution of the blast crisis of chronic myelocytic leukemia. PNAS 1989;86: 6783–6787.
14. Sugimoto K, Toyoshima H, Sakai R, Miyagawa K, Hagiwara K, Hirai H, Ishikawa F, Takaku F. Mutations of the p53 gene in lymphoid leukemia. Blood 1991;77: 1153–1156.
15. Haber DA, Buckler AJ, Glaser T, Call KM, Pelletier J, Sohn RL, Douglass EC, Housman DE. An internal delation within an 11p13 zinc finger gene contributes to the development of Wilms' tumor. Cell 1990;61: 1257–1269.
16. Coppes MJ, Liefers GJ, Paul P, Yeger H, Williams BR. Homozygous somatic wt-1 point mutations in sporadic unilateral Wilms tumor. PNAS 1993;90: 1416–1419.
17. Miwa H, Beran M, Saunders GF. Expression of the Wilms' tumor gene (wt-1) in human leukemias. Leukemia 1992;6: 405–409.
18. Tatsushi M, Ahuja H, Kubota T, Kubonishi I, Koeffler HP, Miyoshi I. Expression of the Wilms' tumor gene, wt-1, in human leukemia cells. Leukemia 1993;7: 970–977.
19. Bennet JM, Catovsky D, Daniel MT, Flandrin G, Galton DAG, Gralnick HR, Sultan C. Proposed revised criteria for the classification of acute myeloid leukemia. A report of the French-American-British Cooperative Group. Br J Haematol 1976;33: 451–458.
20. Brenner B, Wildhardt G, Schneider S, Royer-Pokora B. RNA polymerase chain reaction detects different levels of four alternatively spliced wt-1 transcripts in Wilms' tumors. Oncogene 1992;7: 1431–1433.
21. Fenchel K, Bergmann L, Christ S, Weidmann E, Brieger J, Mitrou PS, Hoelzer D. Prognostic value of simultaneous expression of CD7 and CD33 on leukemic blasts of patients with CD54+ blasts. Blood 1993;82: 122a, Suppl.1.

Acute Leukemias V
Experimental Approaches
and Management of Refractory Diseases
Hiddemann et al. (Eds.)

Distribution of Cells with a "Stem Cell Like" Immunophenotype in Acute Leukemia

Bernhard Wörmann[1], Doris Grove[1], Michael Falk[1], Stefan Könemann[1], Yvonne Markloff[1], Silvia Toepker[2], Axel Heyll[3], Carlo Aul[3], Jörg Ritter[4], Thomas Büchner[5], Wolfgang Hiddemann[1], Leon W. M. M. Terstappen[2], and Frank Griesinger[1]

Introduction

The differentiation of human pluripotent progenitor cells to the functional effector cells in the peripheral blood is accompanied by the sequential acquisition and loss of characteristic cell surface molecules. Stem cells are identified by function [1, 2] and by immunophenotype. They express a 110–115 kD cell surface molecule, classified as CD34 [3; 4]. The compartment of CD34 positive progenitor cells can be further subdivided based on coexpression of other, lineage-restricted and lineage-nonrestricted cell surface antigens such as CD38, HLA-DR [5], stem cell factor receptor (c-kit) [6], CD45 RA [7], CD19 [8], CD33 [9] and cytoplasmatic myeloperoxidase [10].

50–80% of patients with newly diagnosed acute myeloid leukemia (AML) or acute lymphoblastic leukemia (ALL) express CD34 on the leukemic blasts. Correlation of CD34 positivity in AML with other cell biological or clinical parameters have shown an association between a more immature morphological phenotype, expression of the multidrug resistance protein (MDR-1) [11], previous exposure to myelotoxic drugs [12], and clonal karyotypic abnormalities, i.e. –5, 5q–, –7, 7q–, complex karyotypic abnormalities [13; 14]. The prognostic significance of CD34 positivity is controversial. While some authors have observed an unfavorable prognosis with lower complete remission rates and shorter remission durations [15], others could not reproduce these findings in more intensive therapy protocols [16]. In ALL, CD34 positivity was more frequently observed in pre pre B ALL, followed by pre B ALL and T ALL. Among patients with B lineage ALL, CD34 expression was associated with hyperdiploidy, absence of central nervous system leukemia, low LDH and expression of CD10 [17]. Novel therapeutic strategies increasingly depend on discrimination of normal and leukemic progenitors. Postremission stratification based on persistence of minimal residual disease must include monitoring of the leukemic stem cell population. Myeloablative therapy with autologous stem cell transplantation also depends on the isolation of progenitor cell without malignant transformed stem cells. Gene therapeutic manipulation of either normal stem cells inducing a more chemotherapy-resistant phenotype or as part of causal therapies rely on reproducible methods for discrimination of both compartments.

In this study we have analyzed the composite immunophenotype of hematopoietic stem cells in bone marrow aspirates of 231 bone marrow aspirates from patients with newly diagnosed AML, and from 37 bone marrow aspirates of patients with newly diagnosed ALL. Samples were analyzed by multiparameter flow cytometry with three color immunofluorescence using directly conjugated monoclonal antibodies against CD34, CD38 and HLA-DR [18, 19, 20].

[1] University of Göttingen, Dept. of Hematology/Oncology, Göttingen, Germany
[2] Becton Dickinson Immunocytometry Systems San José, CA, USA
[3] University Hospital, Dept. of Internal Medicine, Düsseldorf, Germany
[4] University Hospital, Dept. of Pediatrics, Münster, Germany
[5] University Hospital, Dept. of Internal Medicine A, Münster, Germany

Patients, Material and Methods

Patients. Bone marrow aspirates from 231 patients with newly diagnosed AML were included in the study. They are part of a multicenter study for characterization of minimal residual disease in hematological complete remission. Patients were admitted to the Departments of Internal Medicine at the Universities of Münster, Düsseldorf or Göttingen, Germany. Diagnosis was based on light microscopical examination of Pappenheim-stained slides and cytochemical reaction with PAS, myeloperoxidase and esterase. Classification was performed according to the criteria of the FAB group [21]. Patients with a history of exposure to cancerogenic agents (radiation, benzene, cytostatic drugs) or antecedent hematological disorder were classified as secondary acute leukemia.

215 patients were treated according to the protocols of the German multicenter AML cooperative group (Coordinator: Prof. Dr. Th. Büchner). Patients received an induction course with thioguanine, Ara-C and daunorubicine for 9 days (TAD9) [22]. Patients under the age of 60 received a mandatory second induction course with high dose Ara-C and mitoxantrone (HAM). Patients above the age of 60 received a second induction course only when bone marrow aspiration on day 16 revealed $\geqslant 5$ % leukemic blasts. Patients treated after 1991 at the University Hospitals of Münster or Göttingen were randomized to priming with granulocyte macrophage colony stimulating factor (GM-CSF).

Evaluation of therapy response was based on the recommendation by the NIH [23]. Evaluation of the cause of death was performed either on autopsy, if performed, or on review of the patients charts.

31 children and 6 adults with acute lymphoblastic leukemia were included in the study. Diagnosis was also based on light microscopical evaluation of bone marrow aspirates by standard procedures. Immunological subclassification was based on two- and three-color immunofluorescence with monoclonal antibodies against CD1, CD2, CD3, CD4, CD5, CD7, CD8, CD10, CD15, CD19, CD20, CD22, CDw65, sIgM, sIgK, sIgL and HLA-DR. Children were treated according to the protocols of the German BFM study group, adults according to the protocols of the ALL-BMFT protocol. Definition of therapy response was also based on the criteria of the NIH group [21].

Cell preparation. Bone marrow aspirates were prepared for flow cytometric analysis using erythrocyte lysis. One volume of bone marrow was diluted with 14 volumes of the lysing solution (10^{-4} M EDTA, 10^{-3} M $KHCO_3$, 0.17 M NH_4Cl in H_2O (pH 7.3)) and gently mixed. Cells were lysed for 3 to 5 minutes at room temperature, and then centrifuged at $200 \times g$ for 5 minutes at room temperature. The pellet was resuspended in a volume of RPMI 1640 (Whittaker, Alkersville, MD) 14 times larger than the original bone marrow volume and centrifuged at 200 g for 5 minutes at 4 °C. This washing step was repeated twice and the cells were finally resuspended in phosphate buffered saline (PBS) containing 1 % bovine serum albumin and 20 mM Hepes (pH 7.3). The cell concentration was adjusted to 1×10^7 cells/ml. 20µl of the monoclonal antibody conjugated to PE at titer concentration was added to 100 µl of cell suspension, 10 minutes later the next two monoclonal antibodies conjugated to FITC and Biot/Streptavidin PerCP were added. After an additional 5 minutes of incubation on ice, the cells were washed once with 2 ml of the PBS solution at 4 °C. The pellet of the immunofluorescence labeled cells was resuspended in 1 ml of 0.5% paraformaldehyde in PBS. In the control experiments cells were incubated with fluorescence labeled isotype controls. Instrument set up samples included an unstained sample, and samples stained with CD3 FITC, CD4 PE and CD8 Biotin/Streptavidin PerCP. The following combinations of monoclonal antibodies were used for characterization of leukemic cells at diagnosis and at follow-up. In the recent analyses the indirect staining was substituted by directly PerCP-conjugated antibodies. All antibodies were obtained from Becton Dickinson Immunocytometry Systems (BDIS), San José, CA, USA.

Immunophenotyping. Flow cytometric analysis was performed on a FACScan (BDIS). Data acquisition was performed using the FACScan Research Software (BDIS). The instrument setup was standardized using T lymphocytes as reference. This was achieved by gating on the fluorescence intensity of CD3 positive lymphocytes followed an adjustment of the light scatter detectors to locate the CD3 positive lymphocytes in a standard position in the correlative display of forward light scatter and orthogonal light scatter. The fluorescence detectors were adjusted using a tight scatter gate, obtained from the light scatter of the CD3 positive lymphocytes, followed by adjustment of the three fluorescence detectors of an unstained samole. Adjustment of the cross over of fluorescence signals of FITC, PE and PerCP into other than the assigned detectors was obtained by compensation of samples stained with single fluorochromes. The forward light scatter and orthogonal light scatter signals and the two fluorescence signals were determined for each cell and data of 30000 events were stored in listmode data files.

The analysis of the five dimensional data was performed with the PAINT-A-GatePlus Software (BDIS). This program transforms the orthogonal light scatter parameter according to a polynomial function which increases the resolution between cell populations in orthogonal light scatter and permits the identification of multiple cell populations in the multidimensional data space.

Statistical analysis. Comparison of incidences in the different subgroups was performed by Fishers exact test.

Results

Acute Myeloid Leukemia

Heterogeneity. 231 bone marrow aspirates were classified according to the composite expression of CD34 and CD38. Two characteristic examples are shown in Figure 1. Differentiation is accompanied by acquisition of CD38 and sequential loss of CD34. Figure 1A shows a characteristic example of the bone marrow aspirate of a patient with newly diagnosed acute myeloid leukemia. In all maturation stages of the normal hematopoietic progenitors, leukemic cells can be found. A second example is given in Figure 1B. There is also a heterogeneity within the population of CD38 positive leukemic blasts with a CD34 high and a CD34 dim blast population. However, the percentage of CD34+/CD8− cells is not superior to that of normal bone marrow aspirate. Based on the maturation pathway of a normal hematopoietic progenitor we have classified AML aspirates in 5 groups:

group 1: CD34+/CD38−
group 2: CD34+/CD38+
group 3: CD34(+)/CD38+
group 4: CD34−/CD38+
group 5: CD34−/CD38−

Distribution. The distribution of CD34/CD38 coexpression was analyzed in 180 bone marrow aspirates of patients with newly diagnosed and 51 aspirates of patients with secondary acute myeloid leukemia. Results are summarized in Table 1.

Classification was based on the most immature cell population. Cells were classified in group 1, it at least 5 % of the leukemic blasts had the most immature phenotype, see Figure 1A.

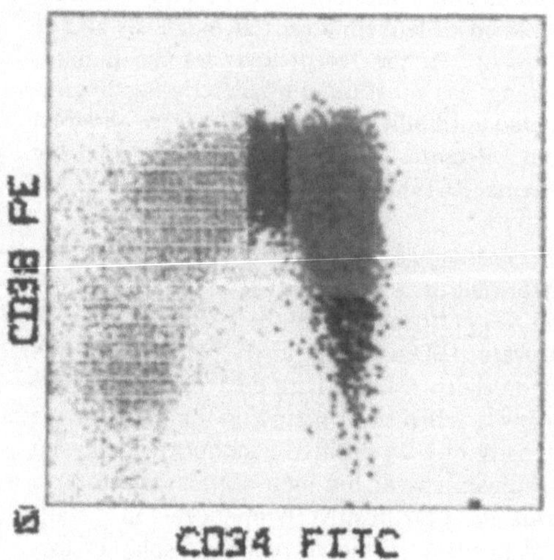

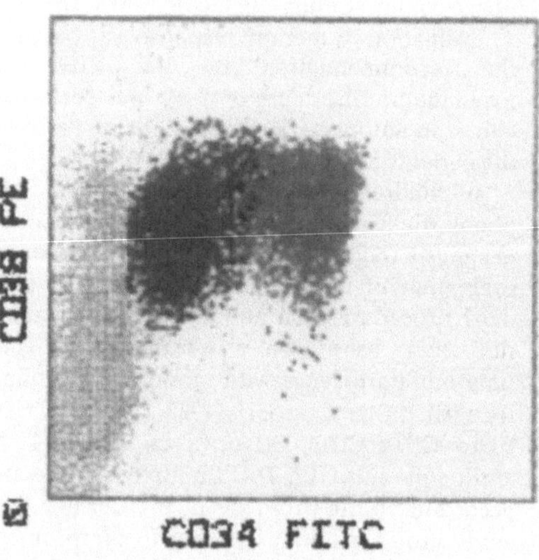

Fig. 1a,b. Continuous differentiation along the pathway of normal hematopoietic progenitors. **a** Example 1: 'stem cell' like immunophenotype. **b** Example 2: 'committed progenitor' phenotype

Table 1. Distribution of CD34 subpopulations in 231 patients with de novo and secondary AML

		total	1	2	3	4	5	unclassifiable
	n	231	84	46	9	18	40	4
de novo	n	180	64	36	30	14	34	2
	%	100	36	20	17	8	19	1
secondary	n	51	20	10	9	4	6	2
	%	100	39	20	18	8	12	4

The example in Figure 1B was classified in group 2. Only 4 bone marrow aspirates were not classifiable within this scheme.

The percentage of patients with a very immature immunophenotype of leukemic blasts was higher in secondary than in de novo AML, however this difference was statistically not significant ($p=0.2$).

Prognosis. 215 patients were treated according to the protocols of the German multicenter trial. Results are summarized in Table 2. The lowest CR rate was observed in the patient group with blasts presenting the most immature immunophenotype. It was about equal in the 4 other groups. Results also show that the rate of nonresponders was not significantly different between the groups. The lower CR rate in patients with CD34+/CD38 leukemic blasts was mainly due to a significantly higher rate of early death (ED). A more detailed analysis of the causes of ED is given in Table 3. The CR rate for patients with the very immature immunophenotype was even lower in the group of patients with secondary acute leukemia, treated according to the standard protocol. It is also lower in the second most immature group, while it is unexpectedly high in patients with a more mature immunophenotype.

Table 2A. Prognostic siginificance of the immunophenotype of AML blasts according to the coexpression of CD34 and CD38 in de novo AML

		total	1	2	3	4	5	unclassifiable
	n	180						
valuable		172	60	36	28	13	33	2
CR	n	121	35	28	22	11	24	1
	%	70	58	78	79	85	73	50
NR	n	18	7	4	3	0	3	1
	%	10	12	11	11	0	9	50
ED	n	33	18	4	3	2	6	0
	%	19	30	11	11	15	18	0

Table 2B. Prognostic siginificance of the immunophenotype of AML blasts according to the coexpression of CD34 and CD38 in secondary AML

		total	1	2	3	4	5	unclassifiable
	n	51						
valuable	43	17	9	8	4	3	2	
CR	n	25	5	4	7	4	3	2
	%	58	58	29	44	100	100	100
NR	n	10	8	2	0	0	0	0
	%	10	12	11	11	0	0	0
ED	n	8	4	1	3	0	0	0
	%	19	24	11	38	0	0	0

Table 3. Causes of Early Death in patients with newly diagnosed AML, classified according to the CD34/CD38 immunophenotype

	total	1	2	3	4	5	unclassifiable
n	41	22	7	4	2	6	0
Infection	18	7	1	3	2	5	0
Bleeding	14	7	5	1	0	1	0
cardiac insufficiency	7	6	1	0	0	0	0
other	2	2	0	0	0	0	0

Acute Lymphoblastic Leukemia

Distribution. The composite immunophenotyping of acute lymphoblastic leukemia is characterized by a great homogeneity of the blast population. In all of the 37 patients the composite coexpression of CD34, CD38 and HLA-DR followed the differentiation pathway of normal hematopoietic progenitors. Distribution of patients with different immunophenotypic subtypes of ALL are given in Table 4. Acute lymphoblastic leukemia, independent of the immunological subtype, is characterized by a very low population of CD34+/CD38− blasts. Only in rare cases is the incidence of this subpopulation higher than in normal bone marrow aspirate. The majority of CD34 positive leukemic blasts in B lineage ALL coexpress CD38 and HLA-DR while in T lineage ALL they are only CD38 positive.

Discussion

Treatment of acute leukemia has made significant progress during the last 10 to 20 years, however in the past 10 years improvement of remission rates and long-term cures have stalled. Treatment of patients in large multicenter trials with standardized therapy protocols have allowed identification of prognostic factors. Some entities have a dismal prognosis, including children with ALL and t4;11, adults with ALL and t9;22, adults with secondary AML. Improvements focus on intensification of post remission therapy, myeloablative therapy with retransfusion of autologous stem cells and gene therapeutic manipulation. A central role will be played by the successful discrimination of normal and progenitor cells. Strategies include isolation of CD34 positive normal progenitor cells. Since CD34 expression on leukemic blasts is a common phenomenon in AML and ALL, analysis of subpopulation becomes increasingly relevant. The functionally most immature population of pluripotent stem cells is characterized by expression of CD34, lack of CD38, lack of HLA-DR and lack of lineage restricted surface antigens [24]. In this study we have analyzed the composite phenotype of leukemic progenitors and as a basis for discrimination of normal and leukemic stem cells.

The results show a significant difference between AML and ALL. While one third of patients with AML have blasts with the most immature "stem cell like" phenotype, this population is very infrequent in ALL irrespective of the immunological subtype. AML is also characterized by a more inhomogeneous phenotype with frequent detection of several subpopulations with transition from one phase to the other. ALL in contrast is quite homogeneous and presence of more than one subpopulation is an exception. The phenomenon of a "stem cell like" immunophenotype is almost unique to acute myeloid leukemia. On the positive side, this may allow isolation of CD34+/CD38− progenitor cells in bone marrow aspirates from patients with ALL without contamination of leukemic progenitors. This hypothesis has to be confirmed by sorting experiments analysing the progenitor cell compartment by genetic and functional methods.

Blasts in acute myeloid leukemia are characterized by a very immature phenotype with ability to differentiation in vivo. The correlation to other clinical parameters and prognostic factors have identified a higher incidence of "stem cell like" blasts in patients with secondary leukemia, however with no statistically significant difference. This conclusion differs from a previously reported analysis from our group [25]. The higher number of analysed cases is the most likely explanation for this discrepancy, rather than a shift in the biology of AML over the past two to three years. Patients with CD34 positive blasts don't have a statistically significantly lower CR

Table 4. Stem cell like immunophenotype in ALL

subtype	CD34+, CD38–, HLA-DR –	CD34+, CD38+, HLA-DR^{+}	CD34 –, CD38+, HLA-DR+	CD34–, CD38+, HLA-DR –
c-ALL (n = 25)				
1	0,1	20	11	34
3	<0,01	65	2	21
5	0,01	0,1	94	4
6	0,1	32	38	30
7	<0,01	21	24	23
9	<0,01	11	68	16
10	0,1	40	46	7
11	0,03	7	41	34
12	<0,01	58	6	20
13	0,1	42	10	24
15	0,2	23	7	6
16	0,03	9	8	37
17	<0,01	20	2	10
18	<0,01	14	12	44
21	0,1	75	1	4
22	0,2	2	1	5
25	0,02	56	2	9
26	<0,01	47	14	7
28	<0,01	81	1	2
31	<0,01	10	5	6
34	0,03	28	18	3
40	<0,01	39	46	5
41	0,1	90	1,2	2
43	0,1	75	1,7	3
44	0,02	30	49	6
pre pre B ALL (n = 6)				
2	<0,01	2	71	4
4	0,01	1	51	43
14	0,2	79	2	3
33	1	81	7	6
36	<0,01	1	72	6
42	0,03	66	14	9
T lineage ALL (n = 6)				
8	0,01	0,3	2	64
27	<0,01	0,5	0,8	50
30	<0,01	10	8	47
19	0,1	1	2	39
20	0,01	0,1	3	60
35	<0,01	0,2	0,6	97

rate in the German multicenter trial [16]. However, patients with a stem cell like immunophenotype had a remission rate of only 52 %, while the other groups had CR rates between 70 and 80 %. The surprising observation was that patients with a stem cell like immunophenotype have a higher ED rate. Our initial hypothesis postulated that the higher risk for lethal outcome early in the course of chemotherapy was due to a prolonged phase of bone marrow aplasia, potentially as a result of an underlying, previously unrecognized myelodysplastic disorder. However, detailed analysis of the causes of death did not confirm this hypothesis. In contrast, there was a strikingly high incidence of bleedings early after diagnosis. A potential explanation for this finding is that the megakaryocytes and platelets in these patients are involved in the leukemic process leading to a functional defect. An alternative explanation would be a higher organ infiltration rate with secondary bleedings due to local endothelial damage. The first hypothesis can be tested performing detailed platelet function tests in the different subsets, grouped by CD34/CD38 coexpression.

Our study shows that the immunophenotype of hematopoietic progenitors is well conserved on leukemic blasts in both AML and ALL. This preservation is in marked contrast with the extreme heterogeneity in the expression of lineage restricted and associated antigens. They offer a basis for isolation and discrimination of normal hematopoietic progenitors. Methods will probably have to be different for AML and ALL. Specifically in AML the current repertoire of monoclonal antibodies doesn't seem to be able to discriminate normal and leukemic stem cells. While there is no leukemia-typic immunophenotype, individualized characterization of the composite antigenic profile with highly sensitive methods can provide a basis for identification and manipulation of the leukemic stem cell.

Summary

Discrimination of hematopoietic stem cells from leukemic progenitors is one of the prerequisites for improvements in myeloablative therapy with autologous stem cell retransfusion and in development of gene therapy. We have analysed the stem cell associated immunophenotype in bone marrow aspirates from patients with newly diagnosed acute myeloid and acute lymphoblastic leukemia. The composite immunophenotype with regulated coexpression of CD34, CD38 and HLA-DR was conserved in all but 4 of 231 bone marrow aspirates from patients with newly diagnosed acute myeloid leukemia and in all of 37 bone marrow aspirates of patients with acute lymphoblastic leukemia. Leukemic samples in AML were very heterogenous with sequential maturation, while the blast population was homogenous in ALL. 84 (36 %) of AML samples had ≥ 5% blasts with a stem cell like immunophenotype, while none of the ALL samples contained this blast population. AML patients with a stem cell like immunophenotype had a lower CR rate, due to a high incidence of early deaths. We conclude that the composite immunophenotype of hematopoietic stem cells is well conserved in acute leukemia. The population of CD34+/CD38− cells may be used in ALL for discrimination of normal hematopoietic progenitors, while this compartment is likely to contain leukemic progenitors in AML.

Acknowledgement. Supported in part by the German Cancer Society.

References

1. Till JE, McCollough EA: Direct measurement of the radiation sensitivity of normal mouse bone marrow cells. Radiat. Res. 14: 213, 1961
2. Dick JE, Lapidot T, Pflumio F: Transplantation of normal and leukemic human bone marrow into immune-deficient mice: Development of animal models for human hematopoieses. Immunol. Rev. 124: 25–43, 1991
3. Civin CI, Strauss LC, Brovall C, Fackler MJ, Schwartz JF, Shaper JH: Antigenetic analysis of hematopoieses: III. A hematopoietic progenitor cell surface antigen defined by a monoclonal antibody raised against KG-1a cells. J. Immunol. 133: 157, 1984
4. Molgaard HV, Spurr NK, Greaves MF: The hemopoietic stem cell antigen, CD34, is encoded by a gene located on chromosome 1. Leukemia 3: 773–776, 1989
5. Terstappen LWMM, Loken MR: Myeloid cell differentiation in normal bone marrow and acute myeloid leukemia assessed by multi-dimensional flow cytometry. Analytical Cellular Pathol. 2: 229–240, 1990
6. Strobl H, Takimoto M, Majdic O, Hücker P, Knapp W: Antigenic analysis of human haemopoietic progenitor cells expressing the growth factor receptor c-kit. Br. J. Haematol. 82: 287, 1992
7. Lansdorp PM, Sutherland HJ, Eaves CJ: Selective expression of CD45 isoforms on functional subpopulations of CD34+ hematopoietic cells from human bone marrow. J. Exp. Hematol. 172: 363, 1990
8. Loken MR, Shah VO, Dattilio KL, Civin CI: Flow cytometric analysis of human bone marrow. II Normal B lymphocyte development. Blood 70: 1316–1324, 1987
9. Huang S, Terstappen LWMM: Lymphoid and myeloid differentiation of single human $CD34^+$, HLA-DR+, CD38− hematopoietic stem cells. Blood 83: 1515–1526, 1993
10. Strobl H, Takimoto M, Majdic O, Fritsch G, Schenecker C, Höcker P, Knapp W: Myeloperoxidase expression in $CD34^+$ normal human hematopoietic cells. Blood 82: 2069–2078, 1993
11. Ball ED, Lawrence D, Malnar M, Ciminielli N, Mayer R, Wurster-Hill D, Davey FR, Bloomfield CD: Correlation of CD34 and multi-drug resistance P170 with FAB and cytogenetics but not prognosis in acute myeloid leukemia (AML). Blood 76 Suppl. 1: 252a (abstract 999), 1990

12. Borowitz MJ, Gockerman JO, Moore JO, Civin CI, Page SO, Robertson J, Bigner SH: Clinicopathologic and cytogenetic features of CD34 (My10) positive acute nonlymphocytic leukemia. Am. J. Clin. Pathol. 91: 265–270, 1989
13. Fagioli F, Cuneo A, Carli MG, Bardi A, Piva N, Previati R, Rigolin GM, Ferrari L, Spanedda R, Castoldi G: Chromosome aberrations in CD34 positive acute myeloid leukemia. Cancer Genet. Cytogenet. 71: 119–124, 1993
14. Myint H and Lucie NP: The prognostic significance of the CD34 antigen in acute myeloid leukaemia: Leukemia and Lymphoma 7: 425–429, 1992
15. Geller RB, Zahurak M, Hurwitz CA, Burke PJ, Karp JE, Piantdosi S, Civin CI: Prognostic importance of immunophenotyping in adults with acute myelocytic leukemia: the significance of stem cell glycoprotein CD34 (my10). Br. J. Haematol. 76: 340–347, 1990
16. Sperling C, Seibt-Jung H, Gassmann W, Komischke B, Sauerland C, Hiddemann W, Löffler H, Böchner T, Thiel E, Ludwig WD: Immunophenotype of acute myeloid leukemia: Correlation with morphological characteristics and therapy response. In: Ludwig WD, Thiel E (Eds.): Recent Results in Cancer Research. Recent advances in cell biology of acute leukemia – impact on clinical diagnosis and therapy. Springer Verlag, Berlin: 382–392, 1993
17. Pui CH, Hancock ML, Head DR, Rivera GK, Look T, Sandlund JT, Behm FG: Clinical Significance of CD34 expression in childhood acute lymphoblastic leukemia. Blood 82: 889–894, 1993
18. Terstappen LWMM, Huang S, Safford M, Lansdorp PM, Loken MR: Sequential generations of hematopoetic colonies derived from single nonlineage-committed CD34+ CD38– progenitor cells. Blood 77: 1218–1227, 1991
19. Terstappen LWMM, Huang S, Safford M, Lansdrop PM, Loken MR: Sequential generations of hematopoietic colonies derived from single non lineage committed progenitor cells. Blood, 1991
20. Wörmann B, Grove D, Unterhalt M, Toepker S, Aul C, Heyll A, Büchner Th, Hiddemann W, Terstappen LWMM: Characterization of CD34+/CD38– acute myeloid leukemia. Blood 82: 121a (Abstract), 1993
21. Bennett J: Morphologic, immunologic and cytogenetic (MIC) working classification of the acute myeloid leukaemias. Brit. J. Haemat. 1988, 68: 487–494
22 Büchner Th: Akute myeloische Leukämie. Internist 34: 511 – 517, 1993
23. Cheson BD, Cassileth PA, Head DR, Schiffer CA, Bennett JM, Bloomfield CD, Brunning R, Gale RP, Grever MR, Keating MJ, Sawitsky A, Stass S, Weinstein H, Woods WG: Report of the National Cancer Institute – sponsored workshop on definitions of diagnosis and response in acute myeloid leukemia. J. Clin. Onc. 8: 813–818, 1990
24. Huang S, Terstappen LWMM: Formation of haematopoietic microenvironment and haematopoietic stem cells from single human bone marrow stem cells. Nature 360: 745–749, 1992
25. Terstappen LWMM, Safford M, Unterhalt M, Könemann S, Zurlutter K, Piechotka K, Drescher M, Aul C, Büchner Th, Hiddemann W, Wörmann B: Flow cytometric characterization of acute myeloid leukemia. IV. Comparison to the differentiation pathway of normal hematopoietic progenitor cells. Leukemia 6: 993–1000, 1992

Acute Leukemias V
Experimental Approaches
and Management of Refractory Diseases
Hiddemann et al. (Eds.)

Expression of Human Endogenous Retroviral (HERV) Sequences in Hematological Disorders

M. Simon, P. Kister, C. Leib-Mösch, G. Papakonstantinou, M. Schenk, W. Seifarth, and R. Hehlmann

Introduction

The human genome contains a number of retroviral elements (*Human Endogenous Retroviruses, HERVs*) that are related to sequences found in infectious mammalian retroviruses. Some estimates account 0.5% of the genome to HERVs (Brack-Werner et al., 1989). Including highly repetitive retroelements and nonviral retroposons like LINE1, SINE and THE-1 elements, the portion of DNA generated by retrotransposition is estimated to constitute at least 5–10% of the human genome (Baltimore, 1985). Full length HERVs have the same basic structure as the integrated proviral form of infectious retroviruses: LTR-*gag-pol-env*-LTR. However, most HERVs are truncated and defective in these genes, or they contain multiple termination signals, thus lacking long open reading frames (for review see Leib-Mösch et al., 1990). Besides these retroviral elements, solitary LTRs have been described that may have been generated by recombination of full-length proviruses (Leib-Mösch et al., 1993). Most HERVs are considered to be replication defective and, to date, no infectious HERV has been recovered. However, HERV transcripts have been recently found associated with the formation of retrovirus-like particles (Löwer et al., 1993).

The target sites of HERV insertions are generally very flexible, but not completely random, and may have physiologic or pathogenic implications (Wilkinson et al., 1994): (i) Genomic integration can result in insertional mutagenesis of the affected gene; (ii) integrated retroelements may predispose to recombinational events with other retroelements (*hot spots*); (iii) the transcriptional regulatory sequences within the LTRs may control transcription of adjacent genes; (iv) in murine models, ERVs have been activated by environmental factors (UV radiation, nucleotide analogues, etc.); (v) retroelements have contributed to the evolutionary genetic diversity by gene duplication mediated by recombination events. Transcripts of HERVs have been shown in many human cell lines and various neoplastic and non-neoplastic tissues. Furthermore, antigens related with structural viral proteins as well as reactive antibodies have been detected by immunological methods in human sera and tissues (for review: Larssen et al., 1989).

The **HERV-K** family of human retroviral elements is related to the B-type mouse mammary tumor virus MMTV (Ono, 1986; Ono et al., 1986) and comprises about 50 copies of full-length proviruses per haploid human genome. Members of this family contain long ORFs within their *gag*, *pol*, and *env* genes. There is evidence that some HERV-K elements encode a functional protease (Müller-Lantzsch et al., 1993), and may be able to generate retrovirus-like particles in teratocarcinoma cell lines (Boller et al., 1993; Löwer et al., 1993a,b).

ERV3 (HERV-R) is a single copy full-length element and has been mapped to chromosome 7 (O'Connell et al., 1984). Genomic Southern hybridization under lowered stringency conditions suggests the presence of 10–15 related elements in the human genome. The *env* region of ERV3 contains a 1.9 kb ORF, comprising the sur-

III. Med. Klinik, Klinikum Mannheim, Universität Heidelberg, D-68305 Mannheim

face glycoprotein domain and most of the transmembrane domain, *p15E* (Cohen et al., 1985).

To address the question whether transcription of HERV-K or ERV3 sequences is associated with particular hematological disorders, we screened 24 RNA samples by RT-PCR, using primers derived from ORFs in HERV-K *gag, pol, env* and ERV3 *env p15E* genes. Additional samples were investigated for ERV3 *env* transcripts by Northern blotting.

Material and Methods

Purification of blood leukocytes and bone marrow cells. Peripheral blood or bone marrow aspirations were treated with 3 volumes of red blood cell lysis buffer (155 mM NH_4Cl/10 mM NH_4CO_3/0.1 mM EDTA). Nucleated cells were pelleted by centrifugation, washed in lysis buffer, resuspended in phosphate buffered saline, lysed in guanidine isothiocyanate buffer (4 M guanidine isothiocyanate/0.5% sarcosyl/25 mM sodium acetate pH 6/0.1 M mercaptoethanol), and stored at −70 °C for further analysis.

RNA extraction. The guanidine isothiocyanate preparations were separated by ultracentrifugation on a CsCl gradient (5.7 M CsCl in 25 mM sodium acetate pH 6) for at least 30 h at 174.000 g, 20 °C, allowing parallel extraction of total cellular RNA and DNA. The pelleted RNA was resuspended in DEPC-treated water, quantitated and analyzed for purity in a UV spectrometer, precipitated in ethanol, and stored at −70 °C.

Northern blot. Samples of 15µg of total cellular RNA were run on a gel of 1% agarose/0.66 M formaldehyde in MOPS buffer (0.2 M MOPS/ 0.05 M sodium acetate/0.01 M EDTA), generally at 23 V for 18 hours. The gel was blotted to Zetaprobe membranes (BioRad), and hybridized in 0.5 M NaH_2PO_4/7% SDS/1 mM EDTA at 60 °C. Washing stringency was 1 mM EDTA/40 mM NaH_2PO_4/1% SDS at 60°C. The filters were first probed for β-actin to assess integrity of RNA. Then, without stripping the probe, the filters were rehybridized to vector-free ERV3 *env* probe (1.7 kb HindIII-PstI fragment: O'Connell et al., 1984) that had been ^{32}P-labeled by a nick translation kit (Pharmacia).

Reverse transcription and PCR. Samples of 10 g of total RNA were treated with 10 U DNAse for 30 min. at 37 °C, followed by phenol/chloroform extraction. The cDNA first strand synthesis was primed with random oligonucleotides according to the protocol of the supplier (Stratagene). 5 µl of the reaction products were used for PCR. PCR buffer was 50 mM KCl, 10 mM Tris/HCl pH 8.3, 1.5 mM $MgCl_2$, 0.01% gelatin, 250 µM of each dNTP, 2 mM of each primer and 2.5 U Taq DNA polymerase in 100 µl reactions. The primers for HERV-K10 *gag, pol, env* genes are described elsewhere (Kister et al., in preparation); the primers for ERV3 *env p15E* were chosen to yield a fragment spanning the nucleotides 2103 to 2470 of the published sequence (Cohen et al., 1985). The reaction conditions were 1 min. 94 °C, 2 min. 55 °C, 3 min. 72 °C, 35 cycles. All amplifications were done with co-amplification of β-actin (0.2 mM of each primer). Amplification products were visualized after electrophoresis in 1% agarose by ethidium bromide staining. The gel was blotted to Zetaprobe membranes. Amplification products were confirmed by high stringency hybridization to fragments that have been amplified from human genomic DNA and verified by sequencing (Kister et al., in preparation).

Results and Discussion

Transcription of HERV-K-related sequences. Transcription of HERV-K-related sequences recently has been found in some cell lines and tissues by RT-PCR or Northern blotting, including peripheral blood cells of healthy individuals (Medstrand et al., 1992), various normal tissues (Medstrand and Blomberg, 1993), leukocytes of normal donors and leukemic (CML, AML) patients (Brodsky et al., 1993), and teratocarcinoma cell lines (Boller et al. 1993; Löwer et al., 1993a,b). Furthermore, transcription of solitary HERV-K LTR has been detected in human placenta and various human tumor cells including peripheral white blood cells and bone marrow of leukemic patients (Leib-Mösch et al., 1993; Simon et al., 1994).

Here we report a RT-PCR analysis for transcription of HERV-K10 *pol, gag, env* genes in RNA samples of 22 various hematological disorders (10 acute myelogenous leukemias AML, 6 myelodysplastic syndromes MDS, 3 myeloproliferative syndromes MPS, 3 acute lymphoblastic leukemias ALL) and RNA samples of 2 bone marrow controls. In all samples the specific amplification product of the three genes could be shown (HERV-K pol: Figure 1; HERV-K *env*: Figure 2; HERV-K *gag*: not shown). In some cases the signals in the ethidium bromide gel were very faint and almost invisible, but consecutive hybridization confirmed the presence of an amplification product in each case (Fig. 2). Although we cannot completely rule out preparational artifacts accounting for this heterogeneous level of amplification products, the relatively uniform signal of the co-amplified β-actin favors the idea that these variations in signal density are due to different levels of gene expression in the respective patients. Comparable variations in the amount of the amplified product have also been found in other primary tissues (Kister et al., in preparation). No disease-specific pattern emerged from these quantitative variations. Heterogeneous expression of HERV sequences, independent of underlying disease, has also been reported in studies that were based on the more quantitative Northern blot analysis: Kato et al. (1988) found largely varying levels of ERV3 transcription in different tissues, Krieg et al. (1992) reported expression of several classes of ERVs in lymphocytes of patients with autoimmune muscle diseases, occurring at a quite heterogeneous level; interestingly, the expression of several classes of ERV seemed to be coordinately regulated.

Amplification of HERV-K *env* sequences sometimes resulted in an additional minor product of smaller size (Fig. 2B). The five patients exhibiting this additional band were UPNs 117 (polycythemia vera), 270 (AML secondary to MDS), 290 (MDS of RAEB-t subtype), 310 (MDS of CMML subtype), and 324 (AML secondary to MDS). An overrepresentation of MDS or secondary AML is evident. Further characterization of this amplification product and a possible specific link to MDS is the object of ongoing studies.

Transcription of ERV3 has been studied by Northern blotting in a large spectrum of normal and pathologic tissues and cell lines (Kato et al., 1988). The transcripts were found to be expressed at different levels in different tissues. Highest transcription levels were found in placenta, but choriocarcinoma was characterized by complete absence of the respective transcripts (Kato et al. 1988; Cohen et al. 1988). Relatively high transcription levels have been reported for a monocytic leukemia cell line. But there was no evidence of disease- or tissue-specific transcription patterns. Recently, expression of ERV3 *env* has been shown to parallel the differentiation from placental cytotrophoblast to syncytiotrophoblast cells (Boyd et al., 1993).

For evaluation of ERV3 *env* transcription in hematological disorders we assayed RNA extracted from blood or bone marrow. 16 samples of total RNA (4 AML, 5 CML, 2 MPS, 3 CLL, 1 ALL, 1 healthy control person) were separated by agarose gel electrophoresis, blotted to nylon membranes and hybridized to a genomic 1.7 kb fragment of ERV3 *env*. In a diffuse background, some distinct bands corresponding to 1.5 kb, 1.8 kb and 3.7 kb transcripts, respectively, could be discerned (Fig. 3). The expression pattern did not correlate with specific disease entities. A 3.7 kb transcript has been reported by Kato et al. (1988), too.

For RT-PCR analysis we chose the *p15E* region of the ERV3 *env* gene. There is some evidence that the *env*-encoded transmembrane protein *p15E* of certain animal retroviruses

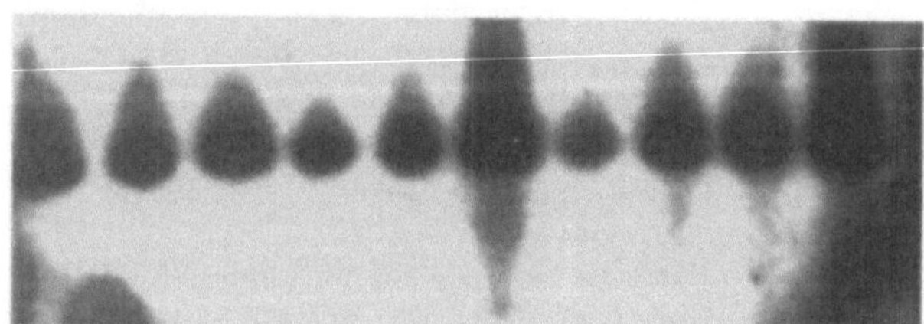

Fig. 1. RT-PCR amplification of HERV-K pol sequences in RNA samples from hematological disorders. Hybridization with a cloned genomic fragment from the pol region. (UPN = unique patient number. Lanes: 256 AML, 258 AML, 270 secondary AML, 290 MDS-RAEBt, 299 MDS-RAS, 310 MDS-CMML, 312 B-ALL, 315 B-ALL, 319 AML, 324 secondary AML)

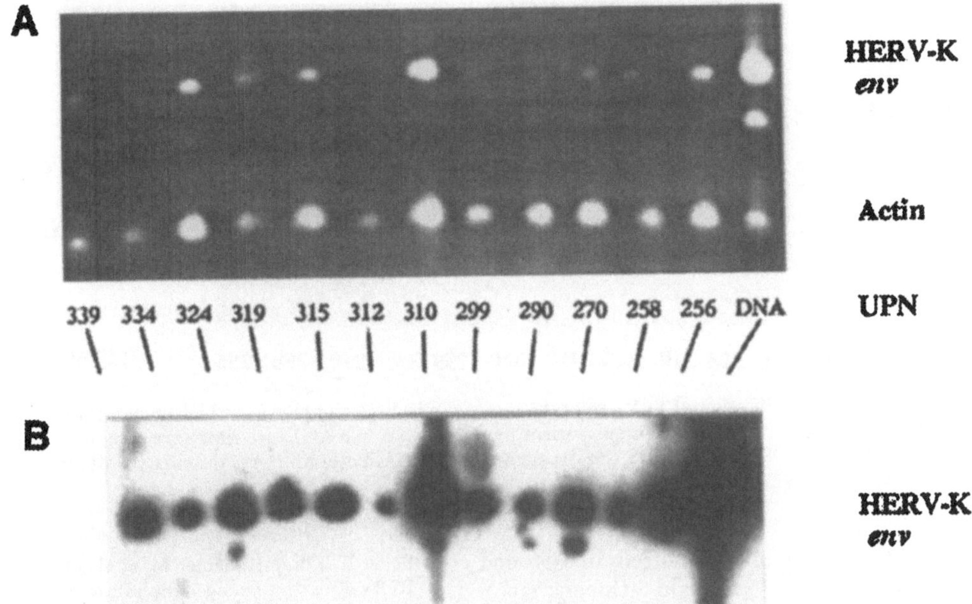

Fig. 2A,B. RT-PCR amplification of HERV-K env sequences in RNA samples from hematological disorders. Co-amplification of β-actin. **A** Ethidium bromide gel. **B** Hybridization with a cloned genomic fragment from the env region. (UPN = unique patient number. Lanes: 256 AML, 258 AML, 270 secondary AML, 290 MDS-RAEBt, 299 MDS-RAS, 310 MDS-CMML, 312 B-ALL, 315 B-ALL, 319 AML, 324 secondary AML, 334 AML, 339 secondary AML, DNA control)

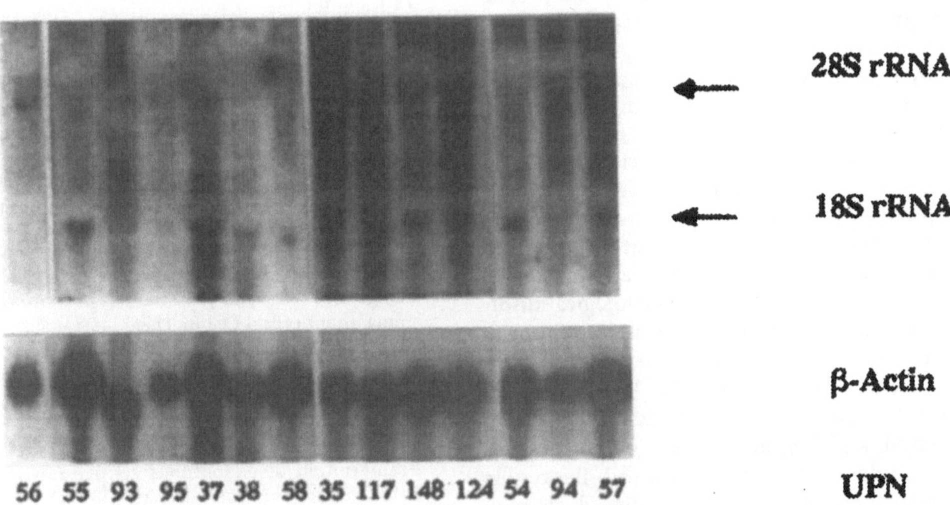

Fig. 3. Northern blot of 15 μg of total cellular RNA. Upper part: hybridization to a genomic ERV3 env fragment. The arrows indicate specific transcripts. Lower part: control hybridization to β-actin. (UPN = unique patient number. Lanes: 35 CLL, 37 AML, 38 AML, 54 CML, 55 CML, 56 c-ALL, 57 AML, 58 AML, 93 CML, 94 CML, 95 CML, 117 polycythemia vera, 124 control, 148 polycythemia vera)

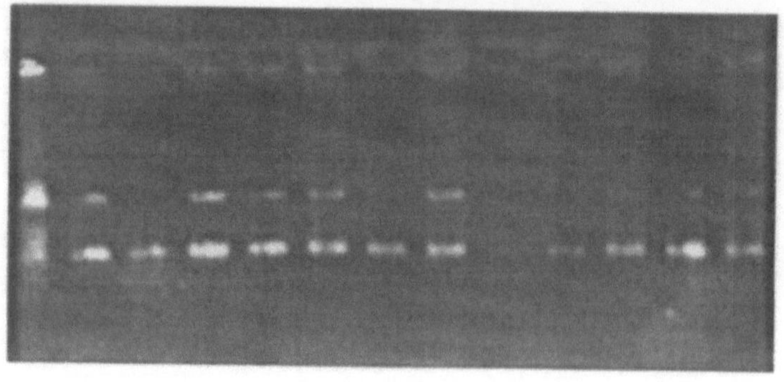

Fig. 4. RT-PCR amplification of ERV3 env p15E sequences in RNA samples from hematological disorders. co-amplification of β-actin (UPN = unique patient number. Lanes: 256 AML, 258 AML, 270 secondary AML, 290 MDS-RAEBt, 299 MDS-RAS, 310 MDS-CMML, 312 B-ALL, 315 B-ALL, 319 AML, 324 secondary AML, 334 AML, 339 secondary AML, DNA control)

exerts immunosuppressive effects *in vivo* and *in vitro* (for review: Krieg and Steinberg, 1990). In a recent study, all RNA samples tested showed transcription of an evolutionarily conserved transmembrane region. But the transcripts exhibited highly variable sequences that were related to ERV9 (Lindeskog et al., 1993).

Analyzing the same 24 RNA samples as described above for HERV-K expression, we found amplification products in all RNA samples. In contrast to the heterogeneous signal levels in HERV-K transcription, agarose gel analysis of the ERV3 *p15* amplification products revealed a relatively uniform signal intensity in all samples, with the exception of three cases showing an almost invisible specific signal: one case of MDS RAEB-t; MDS-RAS; AML FAB M5, respectively (Fig. 4).

Together, our results show that the examined endogenous retroviral sequences are transcribed in a constitutive way in all hematological disorders as well as in healthy controls. However, in the case of HERV-K-related sequences, transcription seems to occur at variable levels. Since no disease- or tissue-specific transcription pattern emerged, a pathogenetic impact on hematological disorders is not evident. Instead, the results support the concept of a basic physiologic role, e.g. in cellular growth control or metabolism.

References

1. Baltimore D. Retroviruses and retrotransposons: The role of reverse transcription in shaping the eukaryotic genome. Cell 1985; 40: 481.
2. Boller K, König H, Sauter M, et al. Evidence that HERV-K is the endogenous retrovirus sequence that codes for the human teratocarcinoma-derived retrovirus HDTV. Virology 1993; 196: 349–353.
3. Boyd MT, Bax CMR, Bax BE, et al. The human endogenous retrovirus ERV-3 is upregulated in differentiating placental trophoblast cells. Virology 1993; 196: 905–909.
4. Brack-Werner R, Leib-Mösch C, Werner T et al. Human endogenous retrovirus-like sequences. In "Modern trends in human leukemia VIII" 1989 (R.Neth, Ed.),pp. 464–467, Springer Verlag Berlin, Heidelberg, New York.
5. Brodsky I, Foley B, Haines D, et al. Expression of HERV-K proviruses in human leukocytes. Blood 1993; 81: 2369–2374.
6. Cohen M, Powers M, O'Connell C, and Kato N. Nucleotide sequence of the env gene from the human provirus ERV3 and isolation and characterization of an ERV3-specific cDNA. Virology 1985; 147: 449–458.
7. Cohen M, Kato N, Larsson E. ERV3 human endogenous provirus mRNAs are expressed in normal and malignant tissues and cells, but not in choriocarcinoma tumor cells. J Cell Biochem 1988; 36: 121–128.
8. Kato N, Larsson E, Cohen M. Absence of expression of a human endogenous retrovirus is correlated with choriocarcinoma. Int J Cancer 1988; 41: 380–385.
9. Kister P, Schenk M, Papakonstantinou G, et al. Transcription of endogenous retrovirus (HERV-K10) related elements detected by RT-PCR in normal and neoplastic human tissues. (in preparation).
10. Krieg AM and Steinberg AD. Retroviruses and autoimmunity. J Autoimmunity 1990; 3: 137.
11. Krieg AM, Gourley MF, Klinman DM, et al. Heterogeneous expression and coordinate regulation of endogenous retroviral sequences in human peripheral blood mononuclear cells. AIDS Res Hum Retroviruses 1992; 8: 1991–1998.

12. Larssen E, Kato N, Cohen M. Human endogenous proviruses. Curr Top Microbiol Immunol 1989; 148: 115–132.
13. Leib-Mösch C, Brack-Werner R, Werner T, et al. Endogenous retroviral elements in human DNA. Cancer Res 1990; 50: 5636s–5642s.
14. Leib-Mösch C, Haltmeier M, Werner T, et al. Genomic distribution and transcription of solitary HERV-K LTRs. Genomics 1993; 18: 261–269.
15. Lindeskog M, Medstrand P, Blomberg J. Sequence variation of human endogenous retrovirus ERV9-related elements in an env region corresponding to an immunosuppressive peptide: transcription in normal and neoplastic cells. J Virol 1993; 67: 1122–1126.
16. Löwer R, Boller K, Hasenmaier B, et al. Identification of human endogenous retroviruses with complex mRNA expression and particle formation. Proc Natl Acad Sci USA 1993a; 90: 4480–4484.
17. Löwer R, Löwer J, Tondera-Koch C, and Kurth R. A general method for the identification of transcribed retrovirus sequences (R-U5 PCR) reveals the expression of the human endogenous retrovirus loci HERV-H and HERV-K in teratocarcinoma cells. Virology 1993b; 192: 501–511.
18. Medstrand P and Blomberg J. Characterization of novel reverse transcriptase encoding human endogenous retroviral sequences similar to type A and type B retroviruses: Differential transcription in normal human tissues. J Virol 1993; 67: 6778–6787.
19. Medstrand P, Lindeskog M, Blomberg J. Expression of human endogenous retroviral sequences in peripheral blood mononuclear cells of healthy individuals. J Gen Virol 1992; 73: 2463–2466.
20. Müller-Lantzsch N, Sauter M, Weiskircher A, et al. Human endogenous retroviral element K10 (HERV-K10) encodes a full-length gag homologous 73-kDa protein and a functional protease. AIDS Res Hum Retroviruses 1993; 4: 343–350.
21. O'Connell C, O'Brien S, Nash WG, and Cohen M. ERV-3, a full-length human endogenous provirus: chromosomal localization and evolutionary relationships. Virology 1984; 138: 225–235.
22. Ono M. Molecular cloning and long terminal repeat sequences of human endogenous retrovirus genes related to types A and B retrovirus genes. J Virol 1986; 58: 937–944.
23. Ono M, Yasunaga T, Miyata T, Ushikubo H. Nucleotide sequence of human endogenous retrovirus genome related to the mouse mammary tumor virus genome. J Virol 1986; 60: 589–598.
24. Simon M, Haltmeier M, Papakonstantinou G, et al. Transcription of HERV-K-related LTRs in human placenta and leukemic cells. Leukemia 1994 (in print).
25. Wilkinson DA, Mager DL, and Leong JAC. Endogenous human retroviruses. In "The Retroviridae", vol.3, ed. J.Levy; Plenum Press, New York, 1994.

Acute Leukemias V
Experimental Approaches
and Management of Refractory Diseases
Hiddemann et al. (Eds.)

DNA-Analysis by Flow-Cytometry of up to Nine Year Old Methanol/Acetic Acid Fixed Samples of Childhood Acute Lymphoblastic Leukemia (ALL)

Konstantinos Romanakis[1], Anthi Argyriou-Tirita[2], Heinrich Zankl[1], and Oskar A. Haas[2]

Abstract. According to cytogenetic abnormalities, several prognostically important groups can be distinguished in childhood acute lymphoblastic leukemia (ALL). However, owing to the technical difficulties in obtaining a sufficient and representative number of analysable metaphases, additional techniques are required for substitution or for confirmation of cytogenetic findings. One of these alternatives using a fast and technically simple method is the determination of gross quantitative deviations of the DNA content by flow-cytometry. Although the best results are obtained with fresh material, in many instances the analysis of material previously used for cytogenetic analysis may be of interest. We have therefore adopted a DAPI-staining technique for flow-cytometric analysis of methanol/acetic acid fixed samples. We have used this method to measure 44 methanol/acetic acid fixed samples which had been stored in -20 °C for a period ranging from several months to nine years. Cytogenetically the samples comprised hypo-, pseudo- and hyperdiploid cases as well as some in which no results could be obtained. We detected 29 abnormal samples with 34 aneuploid clones. Six of them were hypo- (DNA-index (DI) 0.57–0.82) and 28 hyperdiploid (DI 1.04–1.92). Four samples contained a hypo- as well as a hyperdiploid clone, and one case two hyperdiploid clones. Twenty out of 28 hyperdiploid clones were also detected with cytogenetic analysis, whereas no hypodiploid clones were found. The variant of coefficiency (CV) of the measurements ranged from 1,40 to 4,20% (median $2.8 \pm 0.62\%$).

Based on these results, we conclude that flow cytometric DNA-analysis of methanol/acetic acid fixed material is feasible with nearly the same accuracy as with fresh material and that the quality of the analysis is not dependent on the duration of storage.

Introduction

Childhood ALL is a heterogeneous group of diseases characterized by distinct patterns of acquired karyotype abnormalities [1,2]. Since the prognosis of these entities differ significantly, cytogenetic data gain increasing importance for stratification of therapy. For example, cases with a DNA-index > 1.16 have an extremely low risk of failing therapy and may therefore be spared the toxic effects of more intensive treatment [3]. Unfortunately, cytogenetic analysis of ALL is particularly difficult and therefore the results are not always conclusive. On the other hand, flow-cytometric evaluation of the relative DNA content and ploidy level is a technically simple and fast technique. It has been proven to be very useful for delineation of cases with gross quantitative deviations of the DNA-content and can therefore also be used to monitor the accuracy of some of the cytogenetic results [3,4].

Although DNA flow-cytometry reveals the best results when carried out with fresh or ethanol fixed cell samples, at times there exists material which has been prepared for other purposes, such as paraffin-embedded tissue or methanol/acetic acid fixed material. We have

[1] Department of Human Biology and Human Genetics, University of Kaiserslautern, Kaiserslautern, Germany
[2] Children's Cancer Research Institute (CCRI), St. Anna Children's Hospital, Vienna, Austria

therefore adopted a DAPI-staining technique for analysis of residual material from cytogenetic analysis, and have evaluated our method by analysing 44 stored samples. The quality of measurement was compared with established staining methods and the results were correlated with the cytogenetic data.

Material and Methods

Patients. For our studies we have selected methanol/acetic acid fixed bone marrow (BM) and peripheral blood (PB) samples of 44 children with various immunologic subtypes of ALL which in most instances were obtained at diagnosis. The samples had been previously used for cytogenetic analysis and the remains had been stored in −20 °C for several months to nine years.

Flow cytometry. For analysis of the DNA content, the methanol/acetic acid fixed cell pellets were treated according to two different methods. The first was a slight modification of the method described by Otto [5]. Methanol/acetic acid fixed cells were resuspended in a solution containing 3 g citric acid and 0.5ml Tween 20 in 100ml distilled H_2O (CT) and incubated for 20 minutes at room temperature with slow agitation on a shaker board. Cell clumps were removed by passing the cells through a 30mm nylon mesh. The material was centrifuged at 1200 rpm for 8 minutes. The supernantant was discarded and the cell pellet was resuspended in 70% ethanol. After two hours at −20 °C the material was again centrifuged and the pellet resuspended in 0,3 ml CT solution for 10 minutes at room temperature. The cells were stained with 2ml of a solution consisting of 4 g $Na_2HPO_4 \times 2H_2O$, 1 g citric acid and 0,2 mg 4.6-diamino-2-phenylindole-2 hydrochloride (DAPI, Sigma Chemical Co., St Louis) per 100 ml distilled H_2O for one hour at room temperature.

Alternatively, 0,5ml of the methanol/acetic acid fixed cell suspension was resuspended directly in 0,5ml pepsin/HCl solution (0,5% pepsin (Sigma, P 7000) in 0,03M HCl, pH 1,5–1,7) and incubated for 10 minutes at room temperature. After the incubation, nuclei were passed through a 30mm nylon mesh to remove cell clumps and centrifuged at 1 200 rpm for 8 minutes. The supernatant was discarded and the pellet stained as described above.

The samples were analysed with a PAS III flow cytometer (Partec, Münster, Germany), which was equipped with a 100W mercury arc lamp HBO 100/2 (Osram, Germany). The filter combination used was a KG1, BG 38 and UG1 excitation filter, a dichroic mirror TK 420 and a CG 435 barrier filter. To assure the functionality of the flow cytometer, fresh samples from Ficoll-separated peripheral blood lymphocytes from healthy donors were analyzed (CV 0.7–1.00%). The linearity of the flow cytometer was tested with red trout erythrocytes (Partec) which comprise 2c, 4c, and 8c nuclei. The usual measuring rate was about 150–200 nuclei/sec and at least 10 000 nuclei were analysed and plotted.

For generation of histograms the "Multicycle" cell cycle analysis program (Phoenix Flow System, San Diego, CA) was used. This program provides excellent fits of histograms and allows the substraction of the background as well as the elimination of cell clumps. For description of the histograms, the criteria established by Hiddemann et al were applied [6]. A sample with only one Go/1 peak located at the diploid level was assigned a DI of 1,0. DNA aneuploidy was defined as the presence of one or more additional peaks. The DI of the aneuploid peaks was defined by the ratio of the mean channel number of the Go/1 peak of the aneuploid to the Go/1 peak of the diploid cell population. DI below 1,0 were considered hypodiploid; above 1,0 as hyperdiploid.

Results and Discussion

The results of the measurements are summarized in Table 1. Representative histograms of different samples are shown in Figure 1.

Table 1. Summary of results obtained by flow-cytometric analysis of 44 methanol/acetic acid fixed samples of childhood ALL

	DI 0.57–0.82	DI 1	DI 1.04–1.92	Overall
Samples	6*	15	28*	44
Clones	6		28	34
Range of CV (%)	2.80–3.80	1.4–3.8	1.7–4.2	1.4–4.2
Median of CV (%)	2.90	2.65	2.90	2.80
SD	0.36	0.57	0.70	0.62

*includes 4 cases with both a hypo- and a hyperdiploid clone as well as one case with two hyperdiploid clones

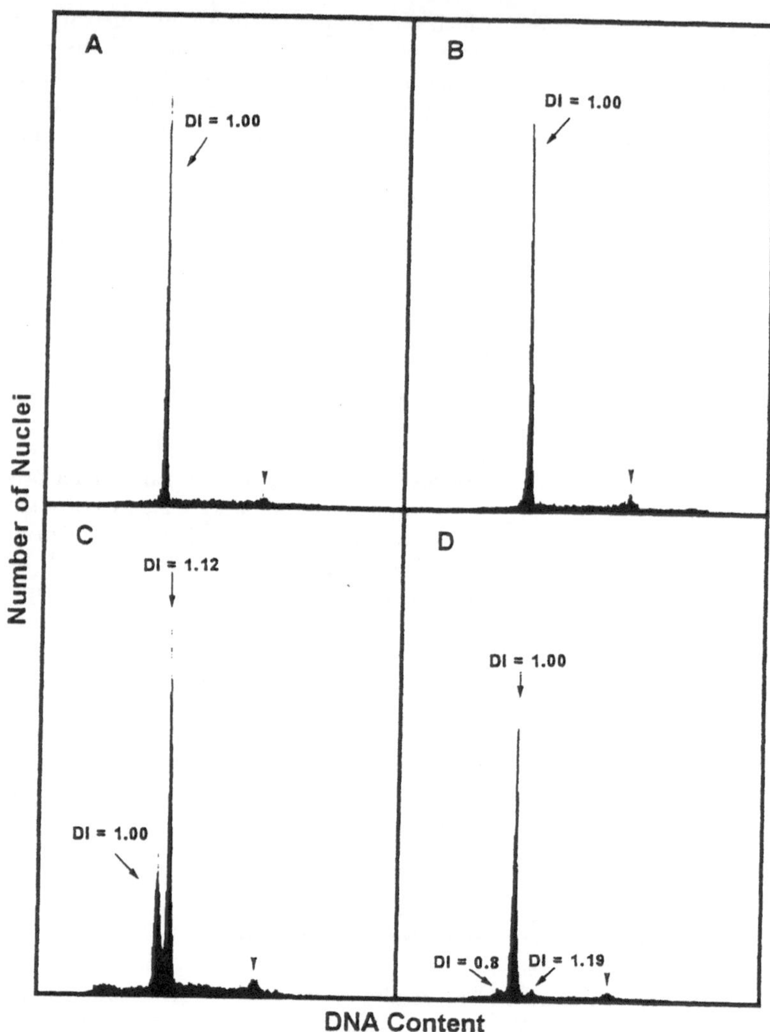

Fig. 1. Representative examples of our DNA-measurements. The individual diploid and aneuploid peaks are indicated by the long arrows, whereas the short arrows point to the respective G2/M populations. (**A**) A fresh ethanol-fixed sample is compared with the same material after cultivation and methanol/acetic acid fixation (**B**) (CV 1.1 versus 1.32, respectively). (**C**) A methanol/acetic acid fixed hyperdiploid sample which had been stored for eight years in $-20\,^{\circ}\mathrm{C}$ prior to DNA-analysis. (**D**) A sample which had been stored for nine months prior to DNA-analysis with small hypo- and hyperdiploid clones exemplifying the resolution of the method

The cases included in this study represent a random compilation of cytogenetic heterogeneous samples which were selected according to the availability of stored methanol/acetic acid fixed material. DNA-analysis revealed 29 abnormal samples with 34 aneuploid clones. Six of them were hypo- (DI 0.57–0.82) and 28 hyperdiploid (DI 1.04-1.92). Four samples contained a hypo- as well as a hyperdiploid clone, and in one case two hyperdiploid clones. Cytogenetic analysis had previously revealed 20 of the 28 hyperdiploid clones, whereas all six hypodiploid clones could not be detected. This discrepancy can be explained by the well known problems encountered with cytogenetic analysis, namely the low mitotic activity of ALL-blasts and/ or the lack of analysable metaphases. Moreover, three of the six hypodiploid and two of the 28 hyperdiploid clones were below 30%. (Data not shown. For representative example see Fig. 1D).

The pathogenetic significance of such small subpopulations remains to be investigated.

The variant of coefficiency of the measurements obtained with our method ranged from 1,40 to 4,20 (median 2.8 ± 0.62) which is superior to that reported in a previously published similar study [7]. It also represents a better value than that generally obtained with fresh samples when measured with a laser flowcytometer. Interestingly, the duration of storage of the fixed samples which ranged from several months to nine years did not influence the quality of the measurements. Admixture of diploid control cells which is commonly used for calibration and comparison with aneuploid populations was not necessary, since residual diploid cells which were still present in all analyzed samples served as a standard. Another advantage of our technique is the small number of cells required (10^5 minimum, 10^4 analysed).

In summary, determination of the DNA-content of methanol/acetic acid fixed material with our modified DAPI-staining method is feasible with almost the same accuracy as that obtained with fresh material irrespective of the duration of storage.

Acknowledgements. This work was supported by the "Österreichische Kinderkrebshilfe".

References

1. Pui CH, Crist WM, Look T (1990): Biology and clinical significance of cytogenetic abnormalities in childhood acute lymphoblastic leukemia. Blood 76: 1449–1463.
2. Raimondi SC (1993): Current status of cytogenetic research in childhood acute lymphoblastic leukemia. Blood 81: 2237–2251.
3. Trueworthy R, Shuster J, Look T, Crist W, Borowitz M, Carroll A, Frankel L, Harris M, Wagner H, Haggard M, Mosijczuk A, Pullen J, Steuber P, Land V (1992): Ploidy of lymphoblasts is the strongest predictor of treatment outcome in B-progenitor cell acute lymphoblastic leukemia of childhood: A Pediatric Oncology Group Study. J Clin Oncol 10: 606–613.
4. Hiddemann W, Harbott J, Haas OA, Budde M, Büchner Th, Lampert F (1987): Nachweis von Aberrationen des Karyotypes bei Kindern mit akuten Leukämien: eine vergleichende Analyse von Zytogenetik und Durchflußzytophotometrie. Klin Pädiat 199: 161–164.
5. Otto F (1990): DAPI staining of fixed cells for high resolution flow cytometry of nuclear DNA. Methods in Cell Biology 33: 105–110.
6. Hiddemann W, Schumann J, Andreeff M, Barlogie B, Hermann CJ, Leif RC, Mayall BH, Murphy RF, Sandberg AA (1984): Convention on nomenclature for DNA cytometry. Cytometry 5: 445–446.
7. Lowery MC, Bull RM, Sciotto CG (1993): Identification of hyperdiploidy in fixed cells from pediatric acute lymphoblastic leukemia cases using flow cytometry and cytogenetic analysis. Cancer Genet Cytogenet 67: 136–140.

Acute Leukemias V
Experimental Approaches
and Management of Refractory Diseases
Hiddemann et al. (Eds.)

Biological Entities in Acute Myelogenous Leukemia According to Morphological, Cytogenetic and Immunological Criteria: Data of Study AML-BFM-87

U. Creutzig[1], J. Ritter[1], J. Harbott[2], M. Zimmermann[1], H. Löffler[3], S. Schwartz[4], F. Lampert[2], and W.-D. Ludwig[5]

Introduction

The clinical implication of cell surface marker expression has been less well established in acute myeloid leukemia (AML) compared with acute lymphoblastic leukemia (ALL). Diagnosis of AML is largely based on morphology and cytochemistry for the differentiation between AML and ALL and for the subclassification according to the FAB criteria [3,4]. Immunophenotyping is required for diagnosis of the minimal differentiated acute myeloid leukemia (M0) [2] and the acute megakaryoblastic leukemia (M7) [5], which cannot be identified with sufficient certainty by morphological criteria.

Another approach to secure diagnosis of AML and FAB subtypes is karyotyping. Since new cytogenetic findings could be correlated with specific morphologic features, the morphologic, immunologic, and cytogenetic (MIC) group [25] has defined specific morphologic-cytogenetic entities, e.g. the subtype M2 with t(8;21), and the myelomonocytic variant with abnormal eosinophils (M4Eo) and inv(16), but only a few entities showing associations with FAB types and specific chromosomal abnormalities have been found so far [22].

Information on the influence on prognosis of other factors such as age and leucocyte count (WBC) and FAB type in children and adults with AML has been controversial. Analysis of our previous study AML-BFM-83 revealed specific morphological features for the individual FAB groups, e.g. the presence of Auer rods or eosinophils to be predictive for a favourable outcome [8]. Another approach to identify prognostic factors has been the characterization of surface antigen expression of AML blasts. In some studies in adults and children prognostic significance of surface antigens associated with myeloid or lymphoid differentiation or progenitor cells was seen [1,9,11,18,20,24]. In contrast, predominantly pediatric AML studies did not find any associations between prognosis and the expression of myeloid as well as lymphoid associated surface antigens [19,26].

For this study we investigated in 269 children of study AML-BFM-87 the relationships of surface marker expression, morphology according to the FAB classification and karyotyping. In addition, the prognostic value of immunophenotyping was compared with that of other prognostic features.

Patients and Methods

Patients. 309 previously untreated children with AML less than 17 years of age were enrolled in the cooperative study AML-BFM-87 between December 1986 and October 1992. Informed consent was obtained from all patients.

[1]University Children's Hospital, 48129 Münster, FRG
[2]University Children's Hospital, 35385 Gießen, FRG
[3]Department of Internal Medicine University of Kiel, 24116 Kiel, FRG
[4]Department of Hematology/Oncology, University Clinic Steglitz, 12203 Berlin, FRG
[5]Robert-Rössle-Clinic, Department of Medical Oncology and Applied Molecular Biology, Free University of Berlin, 13125 Berlin-Buch, FRG

Diagnosis was based on Pappenheim stained bone marrow and blood smears with additional cytochemical reactions. Morphological subtypes of AML were determined according to the French-American-British-(FAB) classification of AML [3,4].

Treatment. The details of the AML-BFM-87 protocol have been published [7]. In summary therapy started with an 8-day induction with ADE (cytosine arabinoside, daunorubicin, etoposide) followed by consolidation therapy with 7 different drugs, followed by two blocks of late intensification with high dose Ara-C and VP-16, and maintenance therapy with daily thioguanine and Ara-C every 4 weeks for 4 days until a total duration of therapy of 18 months. The effect of cranial irradiation was tested prospectively during the first 2 1/2 years of the study.

Immunologic marker analysis. Immunophenotyping was performed centrally at the University Hospital Steglitz in Berlin by W.-D. Ludwig and S. Schwartz. Mononuclear cells were isolated by standard Ficoll-Hypaque density gradient centrifugation from pretreatment heparinized bone marrow samples and stained with a panel of monoclonal antibodies (MoAbs) by indirect immunofluorescence (IF) assays as previously described [21]. Cells were evaluated for IF by epifluorescence Zeiss microscope or by flow cytometry (FACScan; Becton Dickinson). Coexpression of lymphoid-associated-antigens was assessed by double marker analysis using "forward" and "side scatter" properties to gate on the blast population.

The following panel of commercially available MoAbs were used: Progenitor-associated: CD34 (MY10); HLA-DR; panmyeloid-associated: CD13 (My7), CD33 (My9), CDw65 (VIM-2); monocyte/granulocyte-associated: CD14 (UCHM1), CD15 (VIM-C6); erythroid lineage associated: glycophorin A, megakaryocytic lineage associated: CD41 (J15), CD61 (Y2/51) ; T-lineage associated: CD2 (OKT11), CD4 (Leu-3a), CD7 (Leu-9); B-lineage associated: CD10 (J5), CD19 (HD37). For detection of terminal deoxynucleotidyl-transferase (TdT) immunological methods with IF techniques were used.

Due to the limited quantity of cells available not all of the listed MoAbs were tested in every patient. The criterion for marker positivity was expression by ≥ 20% of leukemic cells or intranuclear detection of terminal deoxynucleotidyl transferase (TdT) in ≥ 5% of cells.

Cytogenetics. Central karyotyping was performed in Gießen by J. Harbott and F. Lampert according to the Third International Workshop on Leukemia 1980 [13,14,27].

Statistical analysis. Relationships of marker reactivity to patient characteristics and cytogenetic results and response to treatment were determined by the Fisher's exact test or Chi-square test.

Variables assessing outcome included response-rate (rate of patients achieving complete remission, CR), and event-free survival (EFS). EFS calculation started from time of diagnosis until first event (relapse or death of any cause) or censoring (date of last follow up). Survival curves, standard errors (SE) and tests for differences in EFS between subgroups were calculated with standard methods [15,16,23]. Cox regression [6] was used for multivariate analysis. All tests were descriptive and explorative. Calculations were performed with SAS (SAS Institute, Cary, NC) on a 486 IBM compatible PC.

Follow-up data were actualized as of August 1, 1993.

Definitions

Sensitivity: The likelihood for correct association (= definitely positive) to a particular morphological subtype

$$= \frac{\text{number of FAB Mx patients with the MoAb combination (specific karyotype)}}{\text{all FAB Mx patients tested for MoAb combination (with aberrations)}}$$

Specificity: The likelihood for precise elimination (= definitely negative) of other morphological subgroups

$$= \frac{\text{number of non-FAB Mx patients without the MoAb combination (specific karyotype)}}{\text{all non-FAB Mx patients tested for MoAbs combination (with aberrations)}}$$

Predictive value (pv): Probability of finding an FAB type associated MoAb combination (or chromosome aberration)

$$= \frac{\text{number of FAB Mx patients with the MoAb combination (specific karyotype)}}{\text{all AML patients with the MoAb combination (specific karyotype)}}$$

Results

Patient characteristics and overall results in patients with immunophenotypic data are shown in Table 1.

Kaplan-Meier estimation for EFS and EFI was in the same range for patients with immunophenotypic data as compared to the total group of 309 patients (EFS (SE): .35 (.05); EFI (SE): .47 (.06).

Immunophenotypic analysis: The percentage of antigen positive samples in the total group and in morphological subtypes are given in Table 2 and Figure 1. Expression of at least two of the three panmyeloid associated antigens (CD13/CD33/CDw65) was found in 212 of 239 (89%) patients, while 27 patients (11%) disclosed only one or none of these markers. 14 of them were classified as FAB M0 or M7 subtypes. The non-lineage restricted progenitor cell antigen CD34 and HLA-DR were found in 45% and 80% of patients respectively.

The incidence of TdT positivity (≥5%) was 21%.

Table 1. Initial data and overall results of patients with immunological data in Study AML-BFM-87

AML Study-BFM-87	n = 269	
Age (years,median)	7.8	
Sex (m:f)	1.2	
CNS involvement	31/267	(12%)
Extramedullary organ involvement	95/259	(37%)
Liver ≥ 5 cm bcm	55/266	(21%)
Spleen ≥ 5 cm bcm	44/265	(17%)
WBC/mm³ (median)	28.000	
(range)	800–528.000	
Hemoglobin/g/dl (median)	8.2	
Results		
Complete remission	202/269	(75%)
EFS (SE) – 6 years	40%	(3%)

Coexpression of lymphoid associated antigens: 42% of patients tested expressed one or more of the T- or B-lymphoid associated antigens. Coexpression of the T-lymphoid associated antigens, especially CD4, occurred much more frequently than coexpression of the B-lymphoid associated antigens, CD19 (5 patients) and CD10 (3 patients).

T-lymphoid features (CD2, CD4 and CD7 coexpression) were common in all FAB subtypes with the exception of the FAB M6 and M7 types. CD2 was positive in 30% and 23% of the patients with M3 and M4Eo, respectively. CD4 expression was associated with the monoblastic subtypes M4/M5 and was generally negative in M2 with Auer rods. CD7 positivity was found in the immature subtypes M0 and M1 but never in M4Eo.

Correlation of surface antigen expression with FAB subtypes and karyotypes (Table 2 and 3): There was no clear

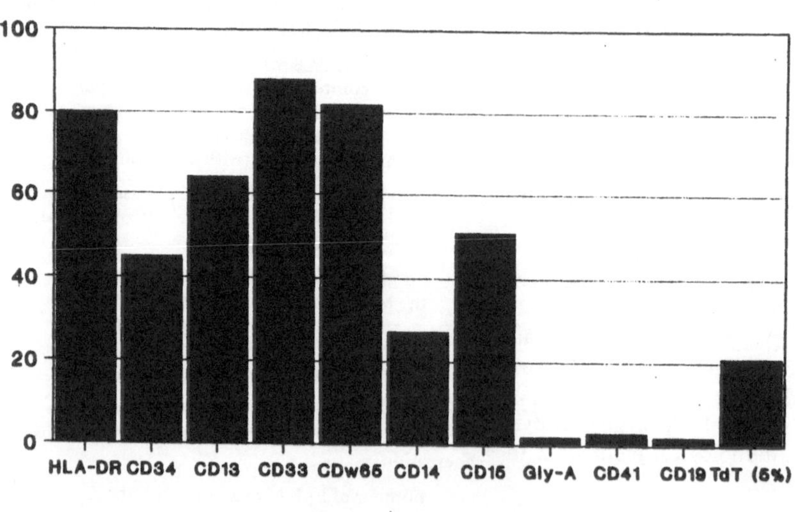

Fig. 1. Percentage of samples expressing the tested surface marker in the total group of patients – Study AML-BFM-87

Table 2. Correlation of surface antigen expression with FAB-subtypes

		Antigen																									
		Progenitor-associated				Panmyeloid						Monocyt./granulocytic-associated				Lineage-specific				Lymphoid-associated							TdT
FAB-Sub-Type	MoAbs (N) pos.	HLA-DR N	%	CD34 N	%	CD13 N	%	CD33 N	%	CDw65 N	%	CD14 N	%	CD15 N	%	GlyA N	%	CD41 N	%	CD2 N	%	CD4 N	%	CD7 N	%	CD19 N	%	TdT N	%
M0	(15)	7	54**	7	64	6	46	8	62**	7	58**	0	0**	4	33	2	20*	0	0	3	25	4	31	4	31*	0	0	5	42*
M1	(10)	5	63	6	75	6	60	9	90	6	60**	0	0**	1	14**	0	0	0	0	1	14	1	14	5	56*	1	13	4	40
M1 Auer	(14)	12	100	10	91*	10	83	10	83	9	75	0	0**	0	0**	1	10	0	0	2	20	2	17	7	58*	0	0	6	55*
M2	(21)	8	38**	5	31	14	67	20	95	17	89	6	32	10	59	0	0	0	0	0	0	6	38	2	10	0	0	2	11
M2 Auer	(51)	48	96*	30	64*	41	82*	47	94	40	82	5	10**	26	53	0	0	0	0	2	4	4	9**	7	14	1	2	15	32*
M3	(14)	0	0**	1	8**	11	79	14	100	10	77	0	0**	3	23**	0	0	0	0	3	30*	2	18	0	0	0	0	2	15
M4	(27)	23	92	7	30	19	76	23	92	20	87	7	30	15	65	0	0	0	0	2	9	13	57*	2	8	0	0	4	16
M4 Eo	(35)	31	89	21	68*	32	94*	31	89	31	91	24	71*	20	59	0	0	1	3	7	23*	15	48	0	0**	0	0	6	18
M5	(59)	55	98*	10	20**	13	25**	50	91	51	98*	23	43*	37	76*	0	0	0	0	3	7	29	64*	3	6	3	6*	2	4**
M6	(7)	5	83	1	20	4	80	4	67	4	67	0	0	0	0**	1	20*	1	25	0	0	0	0	0	0	0	0	2	29
M7	(15)	9	69	5	33	4	31**	8	62**	3	23**	0	0	0	0**	0	0	5	45*	0	0	1	14	0	0	0	0	3	20
Total pos. (%)		203	80	103	45	160	64	224	88	198	81	65	28	116	51	4	2	7	3	23	11	77	36	30	12	5	2	51	21
Total no. of patients tested+		253		229		249		254		243		236		228		215		208		211		215		245		237		247	

Abbreviations: +1 patient with basophilic leukemia excluded
*rate of samples positive higher than in other patients, Fisher's test, $p \leq .10$
**rate of samples positive lower than in other patients, Fisher's test, $p \leq .10$

Table 3. Correlation of surface antigen expression with cytogenetic findings

Karyotype	MoAbs pos. (N)	Progenitor-associated HLA-DR N	HLA-DR %	CD34 N	CD34 %	Panmyeloid- CD13 N	CD13 %	CD33 N	CD33 %	CDw65 N	CDw65 %	Monocytic-/granulocytic-associated CD14 N	CD14 %	CD15 N	CD15 %	Lineage-specific Gly.A N	Gly.A %	CD41 N	CD41 %	Lymphoid-associated CD2 N	CD2 %	CD4 N	CD4 %	CD7 N	CD7 %	CD19 N	CD19 %	TdT N	TdT %
n.d.	(134)	117	83	50	41	91	65	126	91	107	82	36	27	60	47	0	0	3	3	10	8	47	38	16	12	3	2	29	22
normal	(27)	21	78	6	27**	19	73	25	93	24	92	7	28	13	50	1	5	0	0	2	8	7	30	4	15	0	0	2	7**
random	(43)	25	69	26	70*	22	61	28	76**	22	61**	6	19	14	50	2	6	3	10	7	24	8	26	7	18	1	3	13	37*
+8#	(16)	9	75	2	18**	10	91*	10	83	8	73	3	25	3	30	1	10	0	0	1	10	2	20	3	27	0	0	5	42*
t(8;21)#	(23)	16	94*	14	88*	14	78	16	89	17	94	3	18	14	78*	0	0	0	0	1	7	2	13	0	0	1	6	7	39*
t(15;17)#	(5)	0	0**	1	20	4	80	5	100	5	100	0	0	1	25	0	0	0	0	1	33	0	0	0	0	0	0	1	20
inv(16)#	(9)	8	89	8	89*	8	100*	7	78	7	78	6	75*	5	71	0	0	0	0	3	43*	2	29	0	0	0	0	0	0
t(9;11)#	(16)	13	93	1	8**	2	15**	13	93	11	92	3	23	9	75	0	0	0	0	0	0	9	82*	0	0	0	0	0	0**
11q23#	(8)	4	57	2	29	3	43	6	86	7	100	4	67*	4	57	0	0	0	0	1	14	5	71*	2	29	0	0	1	14
- 7 / 7q#	(6)	3	100	3	100	3	100	2	67	2	67	1	33	1	50	0	0	0	0	0	0	0	0	0	0	0	0	1	33
Total positive		203	80	104	45	161	64	225	88	199	82	65	27	116	51	4	2	7	3	23	11	77	36	31	13	5	2	52	21

*the total number of patients for each marker tested varies, mainly due to insufficient cell numbers. Besides, immunological data were not always submitted in patients with existing cytogenetic data.

Abbreviations: n.d. = no cytogenetic data available

+ additional aberrations

*rate of samples positive higher than in other patients, Fisher's test, $p \leq .10$

**rate of samples positive lower than in other patients, Fisher's test, $p \leq .10$

association between any individual surface antigen expression and FAB subtype with the exception of CD41 with FAB type M7 (predictive value 71%). However, the expression of several of the antigens was not distributed equally. Characteristic combinations of higher or lower rates of positive samples could be attributed to certain morphological subtypes and specific karyotypes (Figs. 2a–d).

FAB M0 and random chromosomal abnormalities (Fig. 2A): Negativity of one or two of the three panmyeloid associated antigens, especially CDw65 or CD13 was frequent (9/11 patients), and CD14 was always negative. Expression of the progenitor-associated antigen CD34 (64%) and TdT (42%) as well as coexpression of T-cell antigens (25%–31%) were not uncommon.

Nearly the same was found in random chromosomal abnormalities. Negativity of at least two of the three panmyeloid markers tested was more common than in other karyotypes (11/23 vs. 3/71, $p = .0001$).

FAB M1 (with or without Auer rods): Antigen Expression was similar to that of Mo-subtype with lack of CD14 and CD15 expression and coexpression of T-cell associated antigens, especially CD7 in more than 50% of patients.

FAB M2 (without Auer rods): The rate of samples being HLA-DR negative was higher than in most other subtypes.

FAB M2 with Auer rods and t(8;21) (Fig. 2b): Generally all progenitor associated antigens as well as panmyeloid-associated markers were expressed; contrary to CD14 and CD4 which were usually negative. TdT was relatively often positive.

Although surface antigens expression in *t(8;21)* was similar to that of FAB subtype M2 with Auer rods, expression of CD15 was detected slightly more often ($p = .07$).

FAB M3 and t(15;17) (Fig. 2c): Characteristic for FAB M3 was the absence of HLA-DR (specificity 85%) compared to 15% in non-M3 patients (= sensitivity 28%). In contrast to other subtypes, e.g. M4Eo and M5, expression of CD14 and CD15 was rare. Expression of CD34 was found in 1 patient only. The panmyeloid-associated markers, especially CD33, were generally positive.

As all 5 patients with *t(15;17)* were classified as FAB type M3, surface antigen expression was nearly identical with that of the total group of this subtype.

FAB M4Eo and inv(16) (Fig. 2d): The expression of antigens in FAB M4Eo subtype was similar to that of M2 with Auer rods, however expression of CD14 and CD15 was more common. Of 34 patients 32 expressed CD13 and the incidence of CD34 was significantly higher compared to M3 and M5 subtypes. Coexpression of CD2 was more frequent in M4Eo, and also in M3, compared to other subtypes (Table 4).

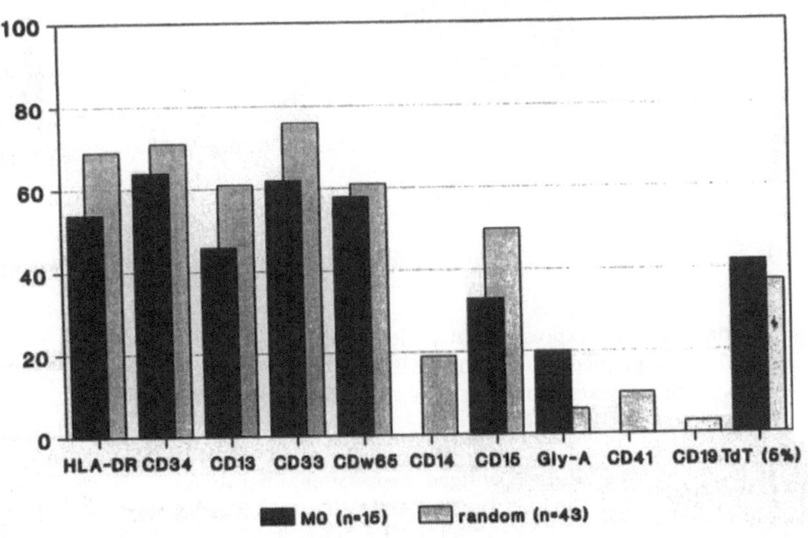

Fig. 2a. Percentage of samples expressing the tested surface marker in patients with FAB Mo and random abnormalities

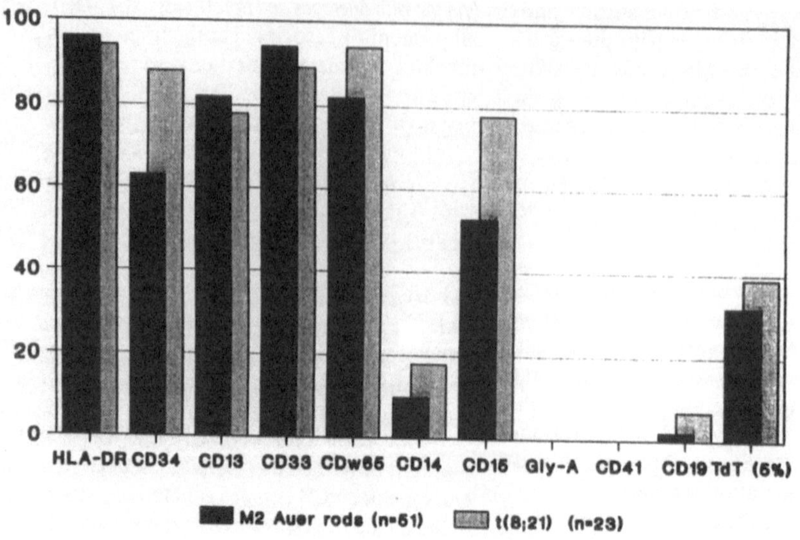

Fig. 2b. Percentage of samples expressing the tested surface marker in patients withFAB M2 Auer rods and t(8;21)

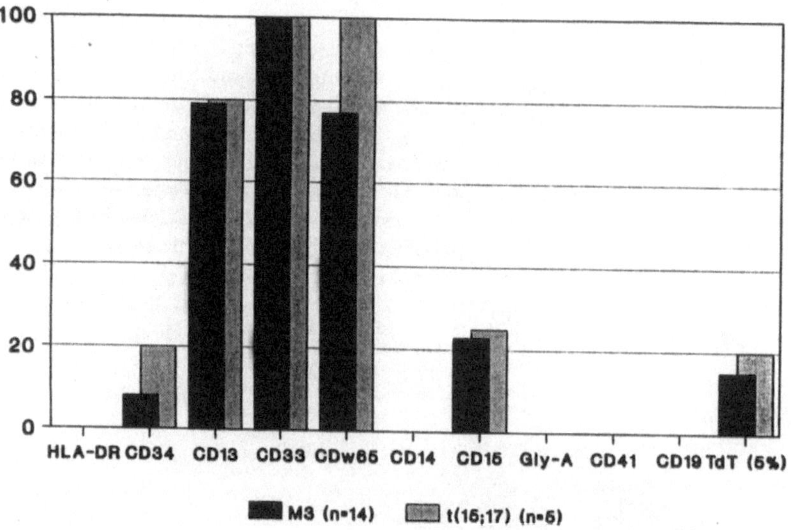

Fig. 2c. Percentage of samples expressing the tested surface marker in patients with FAB M3 and t(15;17)

Surface antigen expression of patients with *inv(16)* corresponded to that of FAB subtype M4Eo. With one exception, blasts of all 9 children expressed CD13 and CD34 .

FAB M4 (Eo negative): Surface antigen expression was uncharacteristic in this subtype, only CD4 coexpression was a frequent finding, but was also found in M5 type.

FAB M5 and t(9;11) (Fig. 2e): CD34 and CD13 were negative in 80% and 75% of M5 samples, CD14 often positive (43%). Moreover, expression of CD15 and CD4 (64%) was found in the majority of patients, whereas in 53 of 55 patients TdT was negative.

Furthermore, the marker combination in *t(9;11)* was similar to that of the FAB M5 subtype, however, CD14 was only occasionally positive.

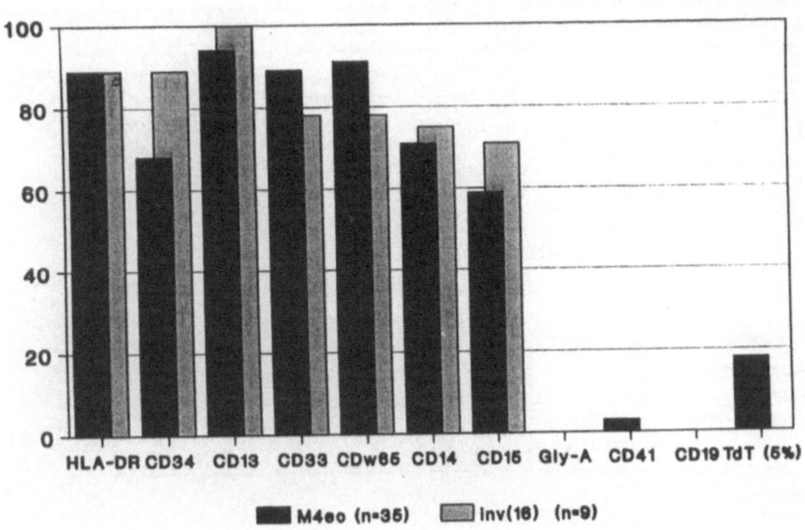

Fig. 2d. Percentage of samples expressing the tested surface marker in patients with FAB M4Eo and inv(16)

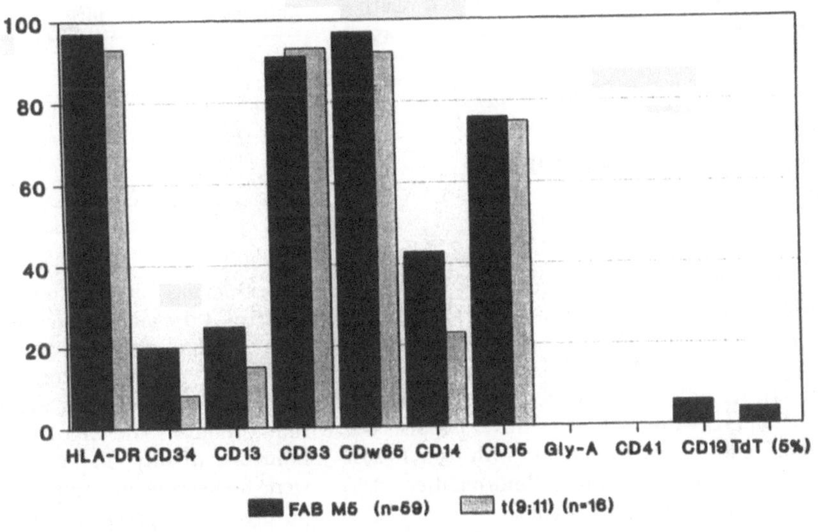

Fig. 2e. Percentage of samples expressing the tested surface marker in patients with FAB M5 and t(9;11)

FAB M7: The lineage specific antigen CD41 was found in 5 patients (CDw42 or CD61 were positive in 6 other patients). All patients showed negativity of all (2 patients) or one or two of the three panmyeloid-associated markers. CD14 and CD15 were always negative.

Association of surface antigen expression with initial white blood count (WBC) and age: With the exception of a higher frequency of HLA-DR negativity in patients with a low WBC (28/101 patients = 28% with WBC $<20000/mm^3$ vs. 23/153 = 15% with WBC $\geq 20000/mm^3$, p=.013) and more CD14 positive patients with higher WBC (17/102 = 17% with WBC $<20000/mm^3$ vs.48/145 = 33% with WBC $\geq 20000/mm^3$, p =.001), there were no remarkable associations between marker expression and WBC (data not shown).

Table 4. Information value regarding morphological subtype diagnosis of finding a given chromosomal abnormality or a given immunophenotype – Data of Study AML-BFM-87

		Sensitivity	Specificity	Predictive Value	Morphologic Type
Aberration	t(8;21)	0.68	0.93	0.74	
Immuno-phenotype	(CD34 or CD13 pos.), and (CD14 or CD4 neg.)	0.90	0.49	0.31	M2 with Auer rods
Aberration	t(15;17)	1.00	1.00	1.00	
Immuno-phenotype	HLA-DR, CD34, CD14 neg., and CD33 pos.	1.00	0.94	0.48	M3
Aberration	inv (16)	0.73	0.99	0.89	
Immuno-phenotype	(CD34 or CD13 pos.) and (CD14 or CD2 pos.)	0.69	0.84	0.41	M4 Eo
Aberration	t(9;11)	0.68	0.97	0.81	
Immuno-phenotype	(CD34 or CD13 neg.) and (CD33 or CDw65 pos.) and (CD15 or CD4 pos.)	0.72	0.72	0.41	M5

The correlation of immunophenotyping and age revealed that children under 2 years of age disclosed CD13 in only 20/54 (37%) vs. 141/196 in over 2-years-old (72%, p< =.001), and relatively more often CD14 (20/52=38% vs. 45/185 =24%, p=.044) and CD15 (33/43=77% vs. 83/186=45%, p< =.001).

Table 5. Prognostic significance of immunological markers

Antigens	low CR rate p(^{2})	low EFS p(Log-rank)
HLA-DR neg.	0.08	0.80
CD34 neg.	0.07	0.40
CDw65 neg.	0.003	0.17
CD14 neg.	0.07	0.13
CD15 neg.	0.56	0.15
All other AG	>0.25	>0.20

Correlation of Other Features with FAB Subtypes

Correlation between morphological subtypes and myeloperoxydase (MPO)-staining: MPO-positivity (>3%) was associated with the FAB types M1, M2, M3 and M4, and was found only rarely in other subtypes (e.g. 26% in FAB M5). Blasts with the karyotypes t(8;21), t(15;17), inv(16) were always MPO positive, whereas the rate of positive samples was significantly lower in patients with t(9;11) (29% positive) and in random abnormalities (57% positive) than in other patients.

Correlation between morphological subtypes and karyotypes: The informative value regarding a specific aberration for a morphological subtype diagnosed was high for the well-known karyotypes t(15;17) for FAB M3 (pv=100%), i.e. all children with this aberration were classified as M3. For the aberration t(8;21) for M2 with Auer rods, inv(16) for M4Eo and t(9;11) for M5, predictive values exceeded 70% (Table 4).

Prognostic significance of surface marker expression (Table 5): A statistically significant correlation for achieving CR was found only for CDw65. Lack of this marker was associated with an unfavourable outcome. When testing the influence of a single marker, none of the other immunological markers was predictive for CR rates. Analysis for EFS showed no significant influence of any marker; differences for EFS were highest when comparing CD14 and CD15 positive vs. negative patients (p-logrank= .13 and .15). Regarding patients disclosing only one or none of the three panmyeloid associated antigens a tendency to a lower CR-rate was found (17/27 patients=63% vs. 166/212=78%, p=.08), but the estimated probability of a 6-year EFS was not significantly different (EFS .36 SE .09 vs. .41 SE .04, p-logrank=.18).

Coexpression of lymphoid associated antigens was not associated with an adverse prognosis, if reactivity of one of these markers was considered. It was also without any prognostic significance if groups of patients expressing at least one B- or T- lymphoid- associated antigen

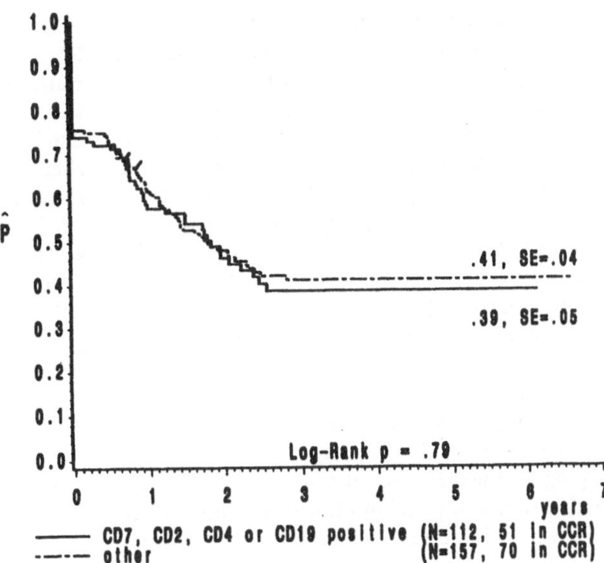

Fig. 3. EFS in patients with coexpression of the lymphoid associated antigens CD2, CD4, CD7 or CD19 vs. others. Slash indicates last patient of the group

were compared with patients expressing no lymphoid- associated antigen (EFS CD7, CD2, CD4 or CD19 positive vs. others = .39, SE .05 vs. .41, SE .04, p-logrank = .79, Fig. 3).

Looking for the possible prognostic relevance of every possible combinations of 2 or 3 antigens for CR rate, no further information was gained, but the small patient numbers in some of these subgroups have to be taken in consideration.

Discussion

The sensitivity for the panmyeloid-associated antigens CD13, CD33 and CDw65 was high for the detection of AML, as leukemic blasts from 236 of 239 (99%) of the patients tested in this study disclosed at least one of these antigens. Expression of lymphoid- (predominantly T-cell) associated antigens in children with AML was common (42%) and in the same range as in recent reports of other pediatric studies [19,26]. CD2 coexpression was relatively frequent in M3 and M4Eo suptypes, CD4 mainly in the monocytic suptypes, and CD7 in the immature subtypes Mo and M1. The latter group was often TdT positive. Expression of the B-lymphoid associated antigen CD19 was rarely seen.

Characteristic immunophenotypic features could be found for some specific entities, which are shown in Figure 2 and Table 4.

In FAB M2 with Auer rods expression of panmyeloid associated antigens as well as HLA-DR was similar to that in t(8;21). In contrast to the report of Hurwitz et al. [12] and Kita et al. [17], CD19 expression was seen in 1 patient only.

For M3 and t(15;17) the lack of HLA-DR was characteristic, and also positivity of CD33 in 100% of patients. As children with M3 usually present with a low WBC, the association of HLA-DR negativity and low WBC was not unexpected.

Children with the karyotype of inv(16) and those with M4Eo presented with the same combination of surface marker expression. All children with inv(16) were positive for CD13, and nearly all patients (33/35) with M4Eo.

Another characteristic group were children with t(9;11) and those with FAB type M5. CD34 and CD13 were mostly negative and a higher rate of CD15 and CD4 positive samples was found compared to other subtypes. In contrast to the total group of children with M5, CD14 was less often positive in those with t(9;11), reflecting the occurrence of more immature monoblastic cells in these children. As the M5 subtype was predominating in children under 2 years (>50%, study AML-BFM-87), the association of CD14 and CD15 with this age group was reasonable.

The FAB type Mo showed less often expression of all three panmyeloid-associated markers compared to other subtypes, the same concerned children with random chromosomal abnormalities.

These results indicate in specific entities an association of morphological, cytogenetic and immunological findings (Table 4).

Our results, that lymphoid-, progenitor- and most myeloid-associated antigens had no influence on prognosis, confirm the findings of the Pediatric Oncology Group [19] and the Children's Cancer Study Group [26], and were in contrast to many other reports concerning the prognostic significance of myeloid antigens in adults with AML [9,11,17,24]. A possible explanation for the discrepancy of these findings and the pediatrics studies may reflect the influence of different treatment regimens or different patient populations (adult vs. children).

In summary, the impact of immunophenotyping for the diagnosis of AML and its subtypes with a standard panel of MoAbs is limited. Only in specific situations, e.g. undifferentiated acute leukemia or M7, immunphenotyping is essential. The discrimination of AML from ALL is usually possible with MoAbs, but coexpression of lymphoid-associated markers is common and without any prognostic relevance in AML. Characteristic subgroups of AML, which are defined by morphological features and karyotypes can be described by low or high expression rates of MoAbs compared to the other patients. This may be helpful if the other diagnostic features are not clear. The contribution of immunophenotyping for prognosis is low in childhood AML and cannot achieve that of morphology and karyotyping.

Participating members: R. Mertens (Aachen); A. Gnekow (Augsburg); R. Dickerhoff (St. Augustin); G.F. Wündisch (Bayreuth); G. Henze (Berlin); U. Bode (Bonn); H.-J. Spaar/Th. Lieber (Bremen); W. Eberl (Braunschweig); W. Andler/ I. Meyer (Datteln); U. Göbel (Düsseldorf); J.D. Beck (Erlangen); W. Havers/B. Stollmann-Gibbels (Essen); B. Kornhuber (Frankfurt); Ch. Niemeyer (Freiburg); M. Lakomek (Göttingen); F. Lampert/R. Blütters-Sawatzki (Gießen); H. Winkler (Hamburg); R. Ludwig, B. Selle (Heidelberg); H. Riehm, P. Weinel, H. Otten (Hannover); N Graf/M. Müller (Homburg/Saar); G. Nessler (Karlsruhe); Th. Wehinger (Kassel); M. Rister (Koblenz); F. Berthold (Köln-Univ.); W. Sternschulte (Köln); R. Schneppenheim (Kiel); P. Bucsky (Lübeck); O. Sauer (Mannheim); P. Gutjahr (Mainz); R. Eschenbach (Marburg); W. Müller (Möchengladbach); R.J. Haas (München); St. Müller-Weihrich (München-Schwabing); Ch. Bender-Götze/R. Köglmeier (München-Univ.); P. Klose (München-Harlaching); H. Jürgens (Münster); A. Jobke (Nürnberg-Cnopf'sche); U. Schwarzer (Nürnberg /Städt.-Kinderklinik); J. Treuner (Stuttgart); D. Niethammer/H. Scheel-Walter (Tübingen); W. Hartmann (Ulm); J. Kühl (Würzburg)

Acknowledgement. Supported by the Deutsche Krebshilfe.

References

1. Ball ED, Davis RB, Griffin JD, Mayer RJ, Davey FR, Arthur DC, Wurster-Hill D, Noll W, Elghetany MT, Allen SL, Rai K, Lee EJ, Schiffer CA, Bloomfield CD (1991) Prognostic value of lymphocyte surface markers in acute myeloid leukemia. Blood 77: 2242–2250
2. Bennett JM, Catovsky D, Daniel MT, Flandrin G, Galton DA, Gralnick HR, Sultan C (1991) Proposal for the recognition of minimally differentiated acute myeloid leukaemia (AML-MO). Br J Haematol 78: 325–329
3. Bennett JM, Catovsky D, Daniel MT, Flandrin G, Galton DAG, Gralnick HR, Sultan C, French-American-British (FAB) Cooperative Group (1976) Proposals for the classification of the acute leukaemias. Br J Haematol 33: 451–458
4. Bennett JM, Catovsky D, Daniel MT, Flandrin G, Galton DAG, Gralnick HR, Sultan C (1985) Proposed revised criteria for the classification of acute myeloid leukemia. Ann Intern Med 103: 626–629
5. Bennett JM, Catovsky D, Daniel MT, Flandrin G, Galton DAG, Gralnick HR, Sultan C (1985) Criteria for the diagnosis of acute leukemia of megakaryocyte lineage (M7). A report of the French-American-British Cooperative Group. Ann Intern Med 103: 460–462
6. Cox DR, Oakes D (1984) Analysis of Survival Data. Chapman and Hall
7. Creutzig U, Ritter J, Schellong for the AML-BFM Study Group G (1993) Does cranial irradiation reduce the risk for bone marrow relapse in acute myelogenous leukemia (AML): unexpected results of the childhood AML Study BFM-87. J Clin Oncol 11: 279–286
8. Creutzig U, Ritter J, Schellong G (1990) Identification of two risk groups in childhood acute myelogenous leukemia after therapy intensification in the study AML-BFM-83 as compared with study AML-BFM-78. Blood 75: 1932–1940
9. Cross AH, Goorha RM, Nuss R, Behm FG, Murphy SB, Kalwinsky DK, Raimondi S, Kitchingman GR, Mirro J (1988) Acute myeloid leukemia with T-lymphoid features: A distinct biological and clinical entity. Blood 72: 579–587
10. Geller R, Zahurak M, Hurwitz CA, Burke PJ, Karp JE, Piantadosi S, Civin CI (1990) Prognostic impor-

tance of immunophenotyping in adults with acute myelocytic leukaemia: the significance of the stem-cell glycoprotein CD34 (My10). Br J Haematol 76: 340–347
11. Griffin JD, Davis R, Nelson DA, Davey FR, Mayer RJ, Schiffer C, McIntrye OR, Bloomfield CD (1986) Use of surface marker analysis to predict outcome of adult myeloblastic leukemia. Blood 68: 1232–1241
12. Hurwitz CA, Raimondi SC, Head D, Krance R, Mirro J,Jr., Kalwinsky DK, Ayers GD, Behm FG (1992) Distinctive immunophenotypic features of t(8;21)(q22;q22) in acute myeloblastic leukemia in children. Blood 80: 3182–3188
13. ISCN (1985) An international system for human cytogenetic nomenclature. In: Harnden DG, Klinger HP (eds). Karger, Basel
14. ISCN (1991) Guidelines for cancer cytogenetics, supplement to an international system for human cytogenetic nomenclature. In: Mitelman F (ed). Karger, Basel
15. Kalbfleisch JD, Prentice RL (1982) The Statistical Analysis of Failure Time Data. John Wiley & Sons, Inc New York
16. Kaplan EL, Meier P (1958) Non-parametric estimation from incomplete observations. J Am Statist Assoc 53: 457–481
17. Kita K, Miwa H, Nakase K, Kawakami K, Kobayashi T, Shirakawa S, Tanaka I, Ohta C, Tsutani H, Oguma S, Kyo T, Dohy H, Kamada N, Nasu K, Uchino H, (The Japan Cooperative Group of Leukemia/Lymphoma) (1993) Clinical importance of CD7 expression in acute myelocytic leukemia. The Japan Cooperative Group of Leukemia/Lymphoma. Blood 81: 2399–2405
18. Kristensen JS, Ellegaard J, Hansen KB, Clausen N, Hokland P (1988) First-line diagnosis based on immunological phenotyping in suspected acute leukemia: a prospective study. Leuk Res 12: 773–778
19. Kuerbitz SJ, Civin CI, Krischer JP, Ravindranath Y, Steuber CP, Weinstein HJ, Winick N, Ragab AH, Gresik MV, Crist WM (1992) Expression of myeloid-associated and lymphoid-associated cell surface antigens in acute myeloid leukemia of childhood: A Pediatric Oncology Group Study. J Clin Oncol 10: 1419–1429
20. Lee EJ, Yang J, Leavitt RD, Testa JR, Civin CI, Forrest A, Schiffer CA (1992) The significance of CD34 and TdT determinations in patients with untreated de novo acute myeloid leukemia. Leukemia 6: 1203–1209
21. Ludwig WD, Bartram CR, Ritter J (1988) Ambiguous phenotypes and genotypes in 16 children with acute leukemia as characterized by multiparameter analysis. Blood 71: 1518–1528
22. Mitelman F, Heim S (1992) Quantitative acute leukemia cytogenetics. Genes Chrom Cancer 5: 57–66
23. Peto R, Pike MC (1973) Conservatism of the approximation $(O\text{-}E)^2/E$ in the logrank-test for survival data or tumor incidence data. Biometrics 29: 579–584
24. Schwarzinger I, Valent P, Köller U, Marosi C, Schneider B, Haas O, Knapp W, Lechner K, Bettelheim P (1990) Prognostic significance of surface marker expression on blasts of patients with de novo acute myeloblastic leukemia. J Clin Oncol 8: 423–430
25. Second MIC Cooperative Study Group (1988) Morphologic, immunologic, and cytogenetic (MIC) working classification of the acute myeloid leukaemias. Br J Haematol 68: 487–494
26. Smith FO, Lampkin BC, Versteeg C, Flowers DA, Dinndorf PA, Buckley JD, Woods WG, Hammond GD, Bernstein ID (1992) Expression of lymphoid-associated cell surface antigens by childhood acute myeloid leukemia cells lacks prognostic significance. Blood 79: 2415–2422
27. Third International Workshop on Chromosomes in Leukemia 1980 (1981) Clinical significance of chromosomal abnormalities in acute lymphoblastic leukemia. Cancer Genet Cytogenet 4: 111–137

Acute Leukemias V
Experimental Approaches
and Management of Refractory Diseases
Hiddemann et al. (Eds.)

Expression of CD7 and CD15 on Leukemic Blasts Are Prognostic Parameters in Patients with Acute Myelocytic Leukemia – Irrelevance of CD34

Klaus Fenchel[1], Christine Heller[1], Eckhart Weidmann[1], Bernhard Wörmann[2], Jürgen Brieger[1], Arnold Ganser[1], Paris S. Mitrou[1], Lothar Bergmann[1], and Dieter Hoelzer[1]

Abstract. In order to investigate the clinical significance of surface markers in correlation to therapeutic outcome of induction therapy in acute myelocytic leukemia (AML), the blasts from 94 adult patients with AML were analyzed prospectively. We used a panel of 32 monoclonal antibodies reactive with normal lymphoid and myeloid cells at various stages of differentiation in a direct immunofluorescence technique. There was no strict correlation of antigen expression with the French-American-British (FAB) classification. All patients were treated with an intensive induction treatment. Staining by two antibodies had a prognostic value. The achievement of complete remission (CR) was significantly correlated with a high ($>50\%$ of cells) expression of CD7 in de novo AML. All patients (8/39) with de novo AML and high expression of CD7 achieved CR, so far ($p<0.03$). The high expression of CD15 was also correlated with the achievement of CR ($p<0.05$). In contrast to recent reports, we found no correlation between CD34 surface expression and the prognosis of the disease. These results confirm earlier reports of antigenic heterogeneity in AML, and indicate that immunologically defined subgroups of AML patients which are of potential clinical significance can be identified.

Introduction

Acute myelocytic leukemia (AML) is the most common form of acute leukemia in adults. Despite considerable improvements in the rate of remission following treatment with chemotherapy, most patients will ultimately die with relapsed leukemia. Although there is clinical, morphological, and laboratory evidence of patient heterogeneity, identification of prognostically important subgroups has proven difficult. Age greater than 60 years has been an adverse feature in most studies [1,2], and some studies have identified other poor prognostic categories including a history of myelodysplastic syndrome [2], specific cytogenetic abnormalities [3] and subgroups within the French-American-British (FAB) classification system [4]. The analysis of surface markers has been particularly useful in acute lymphoblastic leukemia (ALL) [5]. The study of surface markers is far less advanced in AML than in ALL. Preliminary data published so far are controverse, partly demonstrating that prediction of the clinical outcome can not be obtained from the expression patterns of certain surface molecules and partly showing an association of CD34 expression with the prognosis of the disease [6–9].

In a study with a relative small patient population, unfavourable outcome after induction therapy was related to expression of CD54 [10]. This was contradictionary to the results of later findings [11,12] , showing that CD54 was of no evidence for prognosis. Furthermore as a marker of a poor prognosis expression of CD7 and CD13 on myelocytic blasts were reported in a few cases [13]. Because CD13 is known as a myeloid marker and CD7 as a lymphoid marker, coexpression of this two antibodies was explained to characterize a certain "crosslineage" of the leukemia .

[1]Div. of Hematology, Dept. of Internal Medicine, J.W. Goethe-University, Frankfurt/M., Germany
[2]Div. of Hematology, Dept. of Internal Medicine, University-Hospital, Göttingen, Germany

Here, we report the results of a prospective study, investigating the reactivity of 32 MoAbs with blast cells in 94 samples of AML at the time of diagnosis, designed to assess the diagnostic and prognostic value of surface marker expression in AML.

Patients and Methods

Patient selection. Between January 1992 and February 1994, 94 consecutive adult patients with AML were entered into the study. In 58 patients, de novo AML was diagnosed, 21 had a history of an antecedent haematologic disorder (AHD), and 13 patients were in first relapse of AML (FR) (Table 1). Diagnosis was based on Wright-Giemsa-stained bone marrow smears and cytochemistry, according to the FAB Group criteria [14,15]. CR and relapse were defined according to the Cancer and Leukemia Group B criteria [16].

Patients were stratified based upon the disease categories; AHD, FR, and de novo AML. Patients with de novo AML were treated on the European G-CSF-AML protocol. In brief, patients received three courses of intensive therapy, the first course consisted of daunorubicin (DNR), 45 mg/m², given daily on day 1,2 and 3 and ara-C (100mg/m²) as a 24h continous infusion on day 1–7. Additionally, VP-16 was administered in a dosage of 100mg/m² on day 1–5. In the following two cycles, DNR was given only on day 1 and 2, and ara-C was given only on day 1–5. A fourth cycle of consolidation enclosed ara-C 3g/m² (twice a day, day 1–6), and DNR, 30mg/m², on day 7 and 8.

Patients with AHD were treated with ara-C 100mg/m² as a continous infusion on day 1–7, and idarubicin, 10mg/m², on day 1,2,and 3 in the first cycle. In the following two cycles ara-C was administered only on day 1–5 and idarubicin was given only on day 1 and 2. For consolidation patients were treated with m-AMSA 60mg/m² (day 1–5) and ara-C 600mg/m² (twice a day, day 1–5).

Patients in relapse received 3 courses intermediate-high dose (iHD) ara-C 600mg/m² twice a day on day 1–4 and VP-16 100mg/m² on day 1–7.

A complete remission was defined by a marrow normal cellularity with less than 5% blasts and normal-appearing haematopoiesis, and peripheral blood values within normal range. Patients with > 5% blasts were considered non-responders (NR).

Table 1. Patient characteristics

92 total patients included	
58 patients with de novo AML	
21 with antecedent haematologic disorder (AHD)	
13 patients in first relapse of AML	
sex: 48 females, 46 males	
age: median 52,5 (range: 19–78)	
FAB-subtypes (de novo and first relapse, n = 49):	
M0: 3	M4: 9
M1: 11	M5: 2
M2: 20	M6: 1
M3: 2	M7: 1

Immunofluorescence analysis. Mononuclear cells were recovered from heparinized bone marrow aspirated at diagnosis, prior to therapy. After density gradient sedimentation using Ficoll-Hypaque, the cells were washed three times, stained by double color direct immunofluorescence (phycoerythrin- and fluorescein-isothiocyanate labeled) with a series of monoclonal antibodies (MoAbs.) and studied immediately. The mononuclear cell fraction in all evaluable cases contained at least 50% morphologically malignant cells; detection was gated primarily on the subpopulation of malignant cells. Analysis was performed using a FACScan flow cytometer and the Lysys II software (both Becton-Dickinson, Heidelberg, FRG). The MoAbs. used were as follows: CD4 (Leu3), CD8 (Leu2), CD45 (HLE 1), CD14 (LeuM3), CD10 (Calla), CD19 (Leu 12), CD20 (Leu 16), CD22 (Leu 14), CD41a, CD13 (My7), CD71 (ATR), CD45 (KC56), CD34 (HPCA-2), CD2 (Leu 5), CD16 (Leu 11), CD11b (AntiCR 3), DR, CD11c (LeuM5), CD7 (Leu 9), CD15 (LeuM1), CD33 (LeuM9), CD38 (Leu 17), CD25 (Tac), Erymarker, My4, BB10, Tu27, CD11a (LFA-1A), CD18 (LFA-1ß), CD54 (ICAM-1), CD29 (VLA-1), and CD58 (LFA-3). Antibodies were purchased from Becton-Dickinson, Heidelberg, FRG, except: CD45 (Coulter Company, Krefeld, FRG), CD11a, CD18, CD54, CD29, and CD58 (all by Dianova, Hamburg, FRG). Controls were performed with unstained cells and non-reactive antibodies (MsIgG and MsIgM). Double fluorescence analyses were performed with at least 32 combinations of 2 MoAbs each (Fig. 1).

Statistical analysis. Statistical analyses were performed using Statplot and Statgraph softwares.

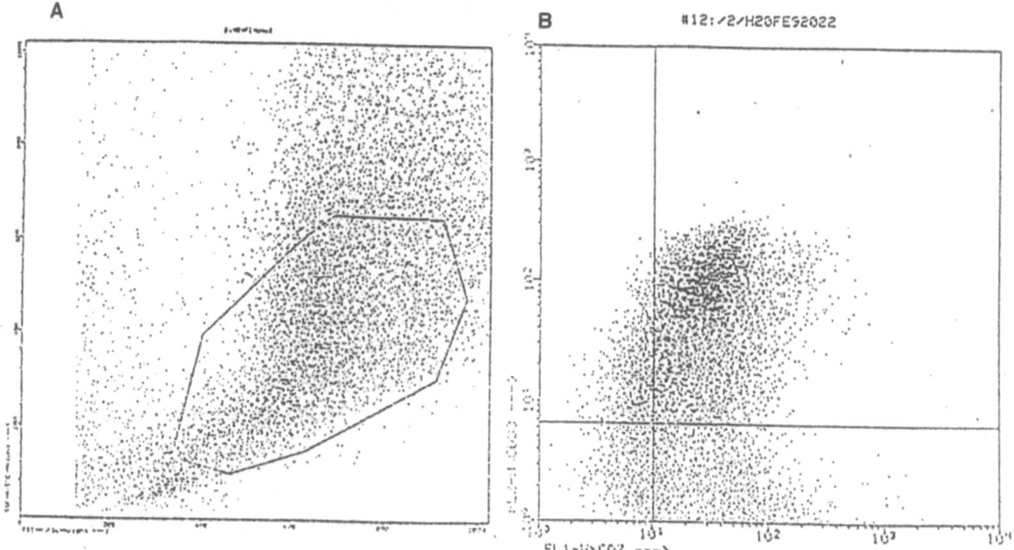

Fig. 1. Flow cytometry of bone marrow cells prior to therapy, cells gated for malignant population in forward (x-axis)/sideward (y-axis) scatter (**A**) and expression of CD7 (x-axis)/CD33 (y-axis) on blast cells (**B**)

The relationships of each surface antigen, single and in combination, to therapeutic outcome were studied by the chi square test and the Fisher's exact test [17].

Results

The relationship of surface marker expression to the outcome of induction treatment was proven for all tested antibodies. Patients were analyzed either in the whole group and in the subgroups de novo, AHD, and FR. Correlation was proved between achievement of CR and different percentages of antibody-expression on the leukemic blasts. When tested only for positive versus negative expression, none of the tested antibodies showed any predictive value, neither alone nor in combination with a second antibody. A positive correlation was found when detection was focussed on leukemias, in which more than 50% of the blast cells expressed a certain antibody. The CR rate was significantly higher in de novo AML with a high expression of CD7 on the leukemic blasts. Out of 39 evaluable patients all eight with high expression achieved CR ($p < 0.03$) (Table 2). This correlation could not been stated in the disease entities FR or AHD (Table 2). There was also a trend to a higher CR rate in CD15 positive group. Analyzed in the whole group of evaluable patients (61, all disease entities together), 15 with high expression of CD15 were in CR after induction therapy ($p < 0.05$). None of the other tested antibodies showed any predictive value. Especially no correlation between CD34 expression and fatal outcome of induction therapy could be stated. None of the studied adhesion molecules, in particular CD54, correlated to achievement of CR.

In this series, age, initial biological parameters (leucocyte and platelet counts, hemoglobin level, bone-marrow blast cell number), extramedullary disease, and expression of other surface markers were not linked to CR rate.

Discussion

This study reflects once again the heterogeneous reactivity of AML cells reported in the literature. The expression of antigens defined as T-lineage-specific is a common observation in AMLs. CD7, highly expressed on normal precursor cells, has been reported in 10 to 26% of cases, especially in M0 and M1 FAB subgroups [6,7,18–22]. The significance of the expression of this lymphoid marker for response to induction therapy and long time survival was discussed controverse:

Table 2. Expression of surface marker on leukemic blasts in correlation to induction therapy response

	de novo AML			AHD / FR		
moAb.	CR (n)	failure (n)	stat. value	CR (n)	failure (n)	stat. value
CD7+	8	0	$p<0.03$	0	2	n.s.
CD7−	15	10		6	13	
CD33+	19	8	n.s.	2	10	n.s.
CD33−	4	1		4	5	
CD7+/CD33+	9	0	$p<0.05$	0	2	n.s.
CD7−/CD33−	9	9		5	6	
CD54+	4	1	n.s.	0	0	n.s.
CD54−	11	4		1	5	
CD34+	8	9	n.s.	4	9	n.s.
CD34−	12	3		2	5	
CD2+	5	0	n.s.	1	1	n.s.
CD2−	20	13		5	15	
CD13+	44	22	n.s.	8	23	n.s.
CD13−	6	6		4	9	
CD15+	14	5	n.s.	1	1	n.s.
CD15−	11	9		5	15	

moAb. = monoclonal antibody, + = expression on >50% of cells, − = expression on <50% of cells

some of the reports indicated it as a marker of bad prognosis [13,23]. This seems convincing, because it represents a certain "bilineage" of the leukemia, which should not respond to a therapy, adapted to a myeloid leukemia. Furthermore, a recent study showed an association of multi drug resistance (MDR1) gene with the expression of CD7 in both acute lymphocytic and nonlymphocytic leukemias, but without any correlation to clinical outcome of this patients [24]. In contrast to these findings, some recent reports failed to find a prognostic value of CD7 [21,25].

Recently we were able to demonstrate in a smaller patient group a positive predictive value of CD7 [26]. This apparent contradiction may be explained by several facts. Even in this study CD7 shows no predictive value, if the correlation to therapeutic response is made just on the base of positive or negative expression. The statistical significant predictive value is given clearly, if the discrimation is done at a limit of 50% of the blast cells positive for CD7. When the limit is reduced down to 30%, the significance vanishes. Another important factor is the difference in the course of the distinct AML disease entities: AMLs in first relapse are in a certain way resistant to standard chemotherapy regimens; from AML after AHD it is known that response rates are smaller than in de novo AML [2]. This was proved to be true in this study, too. The positive correlation of CD7 with response to induction therapy was given only for de novo AML, with no correlation in FR or AHD. This shows the necessarity to differentiate between the subgroups of AMLs included in a study. The difference in results between de novo AMLs and AHD and FR may also be explained by one factor of the induction therapy: in de novo AML induction therapy includes adriamycine, which is not given in FR or AHD. In 1993 a better responsiveness of CD7+ leukemias to this P-gp-related anticancer agent was already observed [27]. In those studies showing a negative correlation of CD7 with therapeutic outcome no differentiation between AHD and de novo AML was done and though the median age of patients was quite ten years higher than in the present study, it seems convincable that a higher frequency of AHD with its poorer prognosis were included [13,23].

The positive correlation of high expression of CD15 with achievement of CR is not as sensational as it is for CD7. Already Griffin et al. found a predictive value for CD15 [28]. In Griffin's study the expression even in lower percentages than 50% of the blasts correlated with a higher rate of CR. This was supported by a study, which found a correlation with a higher rate of continuous CR [26].

This study demonstrates the value of immunophenotyping to identify subsets of patients with different clinical features. It also provides preliminary informations regarding the prognostic value of CD7 and CD15 expression in AML. These markers could be of use for the early identification of patients responding better to chemotherapy induction protocols. Further investigations for pathophysiological explanations such as MDR1 or WT1 gene expression in vitro and in vivo are expected to answer open questions and to help develop therapeutic regimens adapted to the probability of induction response.

Acknowledgements. The authors like to thank S. Christ, S. Fuck, D. Ludwig, C. Seitz, B. Schneider, and B. Würz for skillful technical assistance.

This work was supported by the Deutsche Krebshilfe grant W22/92 and the Dr. Paul and Cilli Weill-Stiftung.

References

1. Peterson BA, Bloomfield CD: Treatment of acute nonlymphocytic leukemia in elderly patients. Am. J. Med. 1982; 72: 963–970
2. Keating MJ: Early identification of potentially cured patients with acute myelogenous leukemia – a recent challenge, in: Bloomfield CD (ed.): Adult Leukemias 1, Boston, Nijhoff, 1982, p 237–241
3. The Fourth International Workshop on Chromosomes in Leukemia: The clinical significance of chromosomal abnormalities in acute nonlymphoblastic leukemia. Cancer Genet. Cytogenet. 1984; 11: 332–340
4. Bennett JM, Begg CB: Eastern Cooperative Oncology Group Study of the cytochemistry of adult acute myeloid leukemia by correlation of subtypes with response and survival. Cancer Res. 1981; 41: 4833–4841
5. Sallan SE, Ritz J, Pesando J, Gelber R, O'Brien C, Hitchcock S, Coral F, Schlossman SF: Cell surface antigens: prognostic implications in childhood acute lymphoblastic leukemia. Blood 1980; 55: 395–402
6. Geller RB, Zahurak M, Hurwitz CA, Burke PJ, Karp JE, Piantadosi S, Civin CI: Prognostic importance of immunophenotyping in adults with acute myelocytic leukaemia: the significance of the stem-cell glycoprotein CD34 (My10). Br. J. Haematol. 1990; 76: 340–347
7. Borowitz MJ, Gockerman JP, Moore JO, Civin CI, Page SO, Robertson J, Bigner SH: Clinicopathology and cytogenetic features of CD34 (My10)-positive acute nonlymphocytic leukemia. Am. J. Clin. Pathol. 1989; 91: 265–270
8. Solary E, Casasnovas RO, Campos L, Bene MC, Faure G, Maingon P, Falkenrodt A, Lenormand B, Genetet N and GEIL: Surface markers in adult acute myeloblastic leukemia: correlation of CD19+, CD34+ and CD14+/DR- phenotypes with shorter survival. Leukemia 1992; 6: 393–399
9. Campos L, Guyotat D, Archimbaud E, Devaux Y, Treille D, Larese A, Maupas J, Gentilhomme O, Ehrsam A, Fiere D: Surface marker expression in adult acute myeloid leukemia: correlations with initial characteristics, morphology and response to therapy. Br. J. Haematol. 1989; 72: 161–166
10. Del Vecchio L, Lo Pardo C, Pane N, Fusco C, Tremiterra E, Selleri C, Notaro R, De Renzo A, Rotoli B: Contribution of DAF and ICAM-1 to the immunological characterization of AML. Haematologica 1991; 76: 82
11. Selleri C, Notaro R, Catalano L, Fontana R, Del Vecchio L, Rotoli B: Prognostic irrelevance of CD34 in acute myeloid leukemia. Br. J. Haematol. 1992; 82: 479–482
12. Archimbaud E, Thomas X, Campos L, Magaud JP, Dore JF, Fiere D: Expression of surface adhesion molecules CD54 (ICAM-1) and CD58 (LFA-3) in adult acute leukemia: relationship with initial characteristics and prognosis. Leukemia 1992; 6: 265–271
13. Bassan R, Biondi A, Benvestito S, Tini ML, Abbate M, Viero P, Barbui T, Rambaldi A: Acute undifferentiated leukemia with CD7+ and CD13+ immunophenotype – lack of molecular lineage commitment and association with poor prognostic features. Cancer 1992; 69: 396–404
14. Bennett JM, Catovsky D, Daniel MT, Flandrin G, Galton DAG, Gralnick HR, Sultan C.: Proposals for the classification of the acute leukemias. Br. J. Haematol. 1976; 33: 451–458
15. Bennett JM, Catovsky D, Daniel MT, Flandrin G, Galton DAG, Gralnick HR, Sultan C.: Proposed revised criteria for the classification of acute myeloid leukemias: a report of the French-American-British Cooperative Group. Ann. Intern. Med. 1985; 103: 626–629.
16. Ellison RR, Holland JF, Weil M, Jacquillat C, Boiron M, Bernard J, Sawitsky A, Rosner F, Gussoff B, Silver RT, Karanas A, Cuttner J, Spurr CL, Hayes DM, Bloom J, Leone LA, Haurani F, Kyle R, Hutchinson JL, Forcier RJ, Moon JH: Arabinosyl cytosine: a useful agent in the treatment of acute leukemia in adults. Blood 1968; 32: 507–523
17. Armitage P: Statistical methods in medical research. John Wiley, New York, 1971.
18. Merle-Beral H, Nguyen Cong Duc L, Leblond V, Boucheix C, Michel A, Chastang C, Debre P: Diagnostic and prognostic significance of myelomonocytic cell surface antigens in acute myeloid leukemia. Br. J. Haematol. 1989; 73: 323–330
19. Cross AH, Goorha RM, Nuss R, Behm FG, Murphy SB, Kalwinsky DK, Raimondi S, Kitchingman GR, Mirro J: Acute myeloid leukemia with T-lymphoid features: a distinct biologic and clinical entity. Blood 1988; 72: 579–587
20. Del Vecchio L, Schiavone EM, Ferrara F, Pace E, Lo Pardo C, Pacetti M, Russo M, Cirillo D, Vacca C: Immunodiagnosis of acute leukemia displaying

ectopic antigens: proposal for a classification of promiscuous phenotypes. Am. J. Haematol. 1989; 31: 173–180

21. Lo Coco F, de Rossi G, Pasqualetti D, Lopez M, Diverio D, Latagliata R, Fenu S, Mandelli F: CD7 positive acute myeloid leukemia: a subtype associated with cell immaturity. Br. J. Haematol. 1989; 73: 480–485

22. Zutter MM, Martin PJ, Hanke D, Kidd PG: CD7+ acute non-lymphocytic leukemia: evidence for an early multipotential progenitor. Leuk. Res. 1990; 14: 23–26

23. Del Poeta G, Stasi R, Venditti A, Simone MD, Masi M, Tribalto M, Papa G: Clinical relevance of CD7 expression in acute myeloid leukemia (AML). Blood 1993; 82(10): 123a

24. Miwa H, Kita K, Nishii K, Morita N, Takakura N, Ohishi K, Mahmud N, Kageyama S, Fukumoto M, Shirakawa S: Expression of MDR1 gene in acute leukemia cells: association with CD7+ acute myeloblastic leukemia/acute lymphoblastic leukemia. Blood 1993; 82[11]: 3445–3451

25. Schwarzinger I, Valent P, Köller U, Marosi C, Schneider B, Haas O, Knapp W, Lechner K, Bettelheim P: Prognostic significance of surface marker expression on blasts of patients with de novo acute myeloblastic leukemia. J. Clin. Oncol. 1990; 8: 423–430

26. Fenchel K., Bergmann L., Heller C., Christ S., Weidmann E., Brieger J,m Mitrou P.S., Hoelzer D.: Prognostic value of simultaneous expression of CD7 and CD33 on leukemic blasts in AML. Blood 82 Suppl. (1993), 122a

27. Kita K, Miwa H, Nakase K, Kawakami K, Kobayashi T, Shirakawa S, Tanaka I, Ohta C, Tsutani H, Oguma S, Kyo T, Dohy H, Kamada N, Nasu K, Uchino H: Clinical importance of CD7 expression in acute myelocytic leukemia. Blood 1993; 81: 2399–2405

28. Griffin JD, Davis R, Nelson DA, Davey FR, Mayer RJ, Schiffer C, McIntyre OR, Bloomfield CD: Use of surface marker analysis to predict outcome of adult myeloblastic leukemia. Blood 1986; 68: 1232–1241

Acute Leukemias V
Experimental Approaches
and Management of Refractory Diseases
Hiddemann et al. (Eds.)

IL-2 Receptor (IL-2R) Alpha, Beta, and Gamma Chains Expressed on Blasts of Acute Myelocytic Leukemia May Not Be Functional

E. Weidmann, J. Brieger, K. Fenchel, D. Hoelzer, L. Bergmann, and P. S. Mitrou

Introduction

Preliminary clinical studies including IL-2 in chemotherapeutic strategies for treatment of acute myelocytic leukemia suggest that IL-2 may improve the overall outcome of the patients [1, 2]. To date, the mechanisms of eradication of blast cells are still unclear. Cytotoxic T and NK cells or secondary cytokines released after administration of IL-2 have been discussed to contribute to the elimination of leukemic cells [3–5]. However, it is important to know, whether IL-2 may directly influence AML blasts [6]. In initial sudies, using flow cytometry, we found expression of considerable levels of the IL-2R alpha chain on blast cells in a low proportion of patients with AML. However, the IL-2R beta chain was more frequently expressed ranging from 0% to 98%. To confirm these results on a transcriptional level, we studied the expression of RNA of the IL-2R α, β, and γ chains by RT PCR in the bone marrow of 39 newly diagnosed patients with AML and in three AML derived cell lines. RNA for all three IL-2R chains was expressed in lines KG1, HEL 92.1.7 and K562. Surface expression of the IL-2R β chain was observed in all three lines, but of the α chain only in KG1 cells. In comparison with unstimulated cell lines incubation of the three lines with various amounts of IL-2 over 3 and 14 days did not influence their growth, measured by cell numbers and 3H-thymidin incorporation. RNA for the α chain was detectable in 12/39 patients, of the β chain in 10/39 patients and the γ chain in 29/39 patients with AML. Altogether the data suggest that the IL-2R expressed on AML blast cells may be incomplete and not functional. In future studies, functional properties of IL-2 R on blast cells obtained from newly diagnosed patients with AML will have to be investigated.

Methods

Blast cells. Heparinized bone marrow was obtained by aspiration from patients with previously untreated patients with AML. Mononuclear cells (MNC) were isolated by Ficoll Hypaque sedimentation.

Cell lines. The myeloid cell lines K562, HEL 92.1.7 and KG1 were obtained from ATCC (Rockville, MD, USA) and maintained in culture according to the provided instructions. For functional analyses, lines were cultured without and in addition of 150 IU/ml, 6000 IU/ml or 60000 IU/ml IL-2 for 3 and 14 days.

Proliferation assay. Blast cell lines were cultured with and without IL-2 as described above. After 3 and 14 days, they were counted and the proliferation was assayed by ^{3}H-thymidine uptake. 5×10^4 cells were plated in 96 well plates and 0.5 uCi ^{3}H-thymidine/well (Amersham, Braunschweig, FRG) was added. After 18 h of incubation in a humified atmosphere cells were harvested and the ^{3}H-thymidine uptake was measured in a β-counter.

Colony assays. Prior to colony assay, cryopreserved blasts from the bone marrow of one AML

Division of Hematology, Department of Internal Medicine, J.W. Goethe University, 60590 Frankfurt/M, FRG

patient were thawn and incubated in RPMI 1640 media (Gibco BRL, Berlin, FRG) supplemented with 10% FCS (Roth, Karlsruhe, FRG), 1% l-glutamine 100 U/ml penicillin and 100 ug/ml streptomycin (Flow Laboratories, Irwine, UK) with addition of 10 ng/ml GM-CSF (Essex-Pharma, Munich, FRG) and 10 ng/ml IL-3 (Amgen, Munich, FRG) for 48 h. Then 1×10^5 cells were transferred into culture dishes containing 1 ml of 1,25% methylcellulose media (Gibco) supplemented with 30% FCS, 1% l-glutamine, 1% 2mM mercapto-ethanol (Gibco), 2,5% IMDM (Gibco), and 10 ng IL-3, 10 ng G-CSF (Amgen) and 10 ng GM-CSF. Cells were incubated for 10–14 days before growing colonies were picked. Then total RNA was extracted from colonies consisting of 20–30 cells, as described below.

RNA purification. RNA was extracted using the RNAzol B method (Biotex, Wak-Chemie, Bad Homburg, FRG). Briefly, cells were washed in PBS and subsequently treated with 0.2 ml RNAzol B solution and 0.02 ml chloroform per 2×10^6 cells. After vigorous shaking and cooling on ice for 5 min, the samples were centrifuged at $12000 \times g$ at 4 °C for 15 min. The aequous RNA-containing phase was removed and the RNA was precipitated with equal volumes of isopropanol for 15 min on ice, and then pelleted and washed with 75% ethanol. For isolation of RNA from small numbers of cells (20–30 cells) obtained from colony assays (see above) 20 ug glycogen were added to the aequous phase prior to precipitation.

cDNA synthesis. Aliquots of 5 ug or less total RNA were reverse transcribed. RNA was incubated for 30 min at 4 °C with a mixture of 200 U of Molononey leukemia virus reverse transcriptase (MMLV-RT), 2 ug oligo-dT, 0.2 ul 100mM dNTP, 0.9 ml DTT 100 mM, 40 U RNAse inhibitor, 6ul $5 \times$ MMLV first-strand buffer: 250 mM Tris-HCl (pH 8.3), 375 mM KCl, 15 mM $MgCl_2$, in a total volume of 30 ul. The reaction was stopped by heating to 99 °C for 5 min. All reagents were purchased from Gibco BRL, Berlin, FRG.

Polymerase chain reaction. The cDNA synthesized as described above was amplified using oligonucleotide primers, which were designed according to published sequencies for IL-2R α, β, and γ chain genes [7–9]:

		primer sequences	size of PCR-product
IL-2Rα:	3′	5′-GGGACTGAG CTGGCATAGAG-3′	544 bp
	5′	5′-GGCTCTACA CAGAGGTCCTG-3′	
IL-2Rβ:	3′	5′-GCTGCAGGC TTTGTCCTGAA-3′	472 bp
	5′	5′-CCCGTGAGT CAAGCATCCTG-3′	
IL-2Rγ:	3′	5′-CCCGTGCTATT CAGTAACAAG-3′	493 bp
	5′	5′-GGCCACACAGA TGCTAAAACT-3′	

The primers were synthesized by Roth, Karlsruhe, FRG. The reaction was performed in solution containing cDNA from 250 ug of total RNA (or less, when RNA from blast colonies was used), 1 U Taq polymerase (Serva, Heidelberg, FRG), 20 pmol of each primer, 10 nmol dNTP, 1.5 mM $MgCl_2$, 50 mM KCl, 10 mM Tris-HCl (pH 9.0) and 0.1% Triton X-100 in a total volume of 50 ul. 35 PCR cycles were performed with 30 sec denaturation at 94 °C, with 30 sec annealing at 60 °C and with 30 sec extending at 72 °C. The amplified products were separated and visualized in ethidium bromide stained 1% agarose gels.

Flow cytometry. Surface expression of the IL-2Rα and β chains was analysed by labeling with monoclonal antibodies [anti IL-2R (CD25), Becton Dickinson, Heidelberg, FRG, and anti IL-2Rβ (p75) Endogen, Boston, MA, USA] and measuring in a FACScan (Becton Dickinson). Gating was set around the blast cell population.

Results

Cell surface expression of IL-2R α and β chains. Blast cells obtained from the bone marrow of 48 patients with previously untreated acute myelocytic leukemia were analyzed for surface expression of IL-2R α and β chains. Blasts from 7/48 patients were shown to express IL-2Rα chains in a frequency higher than 5% ranging between 10% and 42% (Table 1). Cell surface expression of the IL-2R β chain, measured with the monoclonal antibody TU27, was more frequent ranging between 0% and 98% on blast cells from AML patients (Table 1). Also, the three lines of myelopoietic origin expressed the IL-2R β chain

Table 1. Frequency of the patients' blast samples showing expression of the α, β and γ chains on the cell surface or at the mRNA level, and the percentage of cell surface expression and the level of RNA expression by 3 cell lines

	cell surface (>5%)		mRNA		
	α 7/48	β 38/48	α 12/39	β 10/39	γ 29/39
cell lines					
HEL	0%	99%	++	+	++
KG1	37%	97%	++	++	++
K562	0%	98%	++	+	++

+ = moderate expression; ++ = strong expression

(Table 1). However, only the KG1 cell line was demonstrated to express the IL-2Rα chain (Table 1).

IL-2R, α, β and γ chain message expression by bone marrow derived MNC from patients with AML and AML derived cell lines. RT-PCR analysis of IL-2R message expression was performed as described in materials and methods for the α, β and γ chain in 39 patients with newly diagnosed AML. After 35 PCR cycles, signals representing RNA expression of the IL-2R α and β chains occurred only in about 1/3 to 1/4 of the patients' bone marrow samples. Message of the IL-2R γ chain, however, was detectable in 29 out of the 39 patients (Table 1). To study IL-2R expression at a more clonal level, bone marrow derived MNC from 1 patient were cultured in methyl cellulose supplemented with growth factors for the myeloid lineage. After 12 days, 9 colonies were picked and RNA was isolated as described in methods and transferred into RT-PCR. As demonstrated in Table 2, in none of the colonies message for the α chain was detectable. IL-2R β chain RNA was found in at least 3 of the colonies and the γ chain gene was transcribed at a detectable level in 8/9 colonies (Table. 2).

Analysis of the influence of IL-2 on the growth of three AML derived cell lines. The cell lines K562, HEL 92.1.7 and KG1 (for IL-2R surface and gene expression see Table 1) were incubated with various concentrations of IL-2 for 72 h and 14 days. Proliferation was measured by cell numbers and by ^{3}H-thymidine uptake. The results are shown in Table 3. None of the 3 lines, even though they expressed

Table 2. IL-2 R message expression by AML blast colonies

IL-2R	1	2	3	4	5	6	7	8	9
α									
β			+	+		+	+	+	
γ	++	++		++	++	++	++	++	+

Blast colonies were grown, harvested and RT-PCR was performed as described in methods.
+ = moderate expression; ++ = strong expression

IL-2 receptors to a certain level, seemed to respond in growth to IL-2.

Discussion

Interleulin 2 is a low molecular weight (15 kd) glycoprotein involved in growth, differentiation and activation of certain lineages of white blood cells. Receptors for IL-2 (IL-2R) have been shown to be present on T, B and NK cells and on monocytes [10–13]. The IL-2R consists of 3 chains, α, β, and γ and the way they are associated determines the affinity of IL-2 binding [7–9]. Expression of the IL-2R α, chain allows low affinity binding whereas association of the β and γ chains or α, β and γ chains results in intermediate or high affinity of IL-2 binding [9].

More recently, the spectrum of IL-2-binding cells was demonstrated to be wider than originally assumed. IL-2R have been reported to be expressed by leukemic cells [14], certain lymphomas [14], and on solid tumors as malignant melanomas [15] or squamous cell cancers [16]. However, there is a paucity of information regarding the function of IL-2R on tumor cells.

Recently preliminary treatment studies have been reported, demonstrating evidence that administration of IL-2 in patients with acute myelocytic leukemia may prolong remission duration [1, 2]. Since IL-2R were shown to be expressed on myelocytic leukemia blasts, we were interested in the pattern of expression and a possible proliferative response to IL-2. By FACS analysis using monoclonal antibodies against the α and the β chain, low expression of the α chain but more frequent and higher expression of the β chain was found. The results were not exactly reflected by PCR analysis showing less frequent detectable RNA expression for the β chain. Similar findings have been

Table 3. Proliferation of AML derived cell lines in response to IL-2

cell line	time	IL-2 conc. (IU)	thymidine uptake (cpm)	cell number ($\times 10^6$/ml)
K 562	72 h	0	44.038	1.8
		150	34.146	2.8
		6.000	39.287	2.4
		60.000	36.390	2.0
	14 d	0	20.217	6.6
		150	17.666	8.2
		6.000	14.719	6.8
		60.000	15.232	7.6
HEL 92.1.7	72h	0	18.045	6.4
		150	24.181	6.1
		6.000	16.414	6.7
		60.000	17.886	5.2
	14d	0	34.823	7.2
		150	32.987	6.9
		6.000	29.719	7.4
		60.000	30.510	6.7
KG 1	72 h	0	59.032	5.3
		150	58.257	6.8
		6.000	56.363	5.8
		60.000	65.420	7.2

demonstrated in cell lines obtained from squamous cell cancer of the head and neck [16]. The reason for weak β chain message expression remains to be clarified. Message of the IL-2R γ chain was detected in 3/4 of the samples studied. Thus possibly the intermediate IL-2R is expressed on the majority of bone marrow derived blast populations. However, since the γ chain is also a functional component of other cytokine receptors as IL-4 [17, 18], IL-7 [19] and possibly IL-13 [17, 18], strong γ chain message expression may indicate that this part of the receptor expressed on blast cells is associated with other receptors.

To study whether IL-2 may have proliferative activity on AML blasts, 3 AML derived cell lines were cultured with addition of IL-2. According to the data of Foa and coworkers [6] no major changes of cell numbers or ^{3}H-thymidine uptake were observed after 3 and 14 days. Although cell lines do not represent blasts from AML patients, our previous observation that in IL-2 activated bone marrow cultures from AML patients T cells proliferated and blasts disappeared [20] may additionally indicate that IL-2 does not induce proliferation of AML blasts.

In conclusion, our results indicate that IL-2R expressed by AML blast cells may not be functional, possibly by incomplete expression, or mutated genes. However, since IL-2 has been introduced in the treatment of AML, further functional parameters of IL-2R as signal transduction or cytokine production will have to be carried out.

References

1. Foa R: Does interleukin 2 have a role in the management of acute leukemia? J Clin Oncol 11 (1993) 1817–1825.
2. Bergmann L, Heil G, Kolbe K, Lengfelder E, Brücher J, Lohmeyer J, Mitrou PS, Hoelzer D: Interleukin 2 (IL-2) is a feasible consolidation treatment and may prolong second complete remission (CR) of acute myelocytic leukemia. Ann Hematol 67 (1993) A9.
3. Adler A, Chervenik PA, Whiteside TL, Lotzova E, Herberman RB: Interleukin 2 induction of lymphokine-activated killer (LAK) activity in the peripheral blood and bone marrow of acute leukemia patients with active disease and in remission. Blood 71 (1988) 709–716.
4. Archimbaud E, Bailly M, Dore JF: Inducibility of lymphokine-activated killer cells in patients with acute leukemia in complete remission and its clinical relevance. Brit J Haematol 77 (1991) 328–335.
5. Foa R, Guarini A, Tos GA, Cardena S, Fierro MT, Meloni T, Tosto S, Mandelli F, Gavosto F: Peripheral blood and bone marrow immunophenotypic and functional modifications induced in acute leukemia treated with interleukin 2: Evidence for in vivo lymphokine-activated killer cell generation. Cancer Res 51 (1991) 964–968.

6. Foa R, Carretto P, Fierro MT, Bonferroni M, Cardena S, Guarini A, Lista P, Pegoraro L, Mandello F, Forni G, Gavosto F: Interleukin 2 does not promote the in vitro and in vivo proliferation and growth of human acute leukemia cells of myeloid and lymphoid origin. Brit J Haematol 75 (1990) 34–40.
7. Leonard WJ, Depper JM, Crabtree GR, Rudikoft S, Pumphrey J, Robb RJ, Kronke M, Svetlik PB, Peffer NJ, Waldmann TA, Greene WC: Molecular cloning and expression of cDNAs for the human interleukin 2 receptor. Nature 311 (1984) 626–631.
8. Hatakeyama M, Tsudo M, Minamoto S, Kono T, Doi T, Miata T, Miasaka M, Taniguchi T: Interleukin 2 receptor β chain gene: generation of three receptor forms by cloned human α and β chain cDNAs. Science 244 (1989) 551–556.
9. Takeshita T, Asao H, Ohtani K, Isshi N, Kumaki S, Tanaka N, Munakata H, Nakamura M, Sugamura K: Cloning of the γ chain of the human IL-2 receptor. Science 257 (1992) 379–382.
10. Smith KA: Interleukin 2. Annu Rev Immunol 2 (1984) 319–333.
11. Mingari MC, Gerosa F, Carra G, Accolla RS, Moretta A, Zubler RH, Waldmann TA, Moretta L: Human interleukin 2 promotes proliferation of activated B cells via surface receptors similar to those of activated T cells. Nature 312 (1984) 641–643.
12. Siegel JP, Sharon M, Smith PL, Leonard WJ: IL-2 receptor β chain (p70): role in mediating signals for LAK, NK and proliferative activities. Science 238 (1987) 75–78.
13. Herrmann F, Cannistra SA, Levine H, Griffin JD: Expression of interleukin 2 receptors and binding of interleukin 2 by γ IFN induced human leukemic and normal monocytic cells. J Exp Med 162 (1985) 1111–1116.
14. Allouche M, Sahraoui Y, Augery-Bourget Y, Ohashi Y, Sugamura K, Jasmin C, Georgoulias V: Presence of a p70 IL-2 binding peptide on leukemic cells from various hemopoietic lineages. J Immunol 143 (1989) 2223–2229.
15. Aliléche A, Plaisance S, Han DS, Jasmin C, Azzarone B: In human melanoma cells interleukin 2 down modulates the surface expression of histocompatibility antigens class I and class II. Proc Am Assoc Cancer Res 33 (1992) 415.
16. Weidmann E, Sacchi M, Plaisance S, Hoe DS, Yasumura S, Lin W-c, Johnson JT, Herberman RB, Azzarone B, Whiteside TL: Receptors for interleukin 2 on human squamous cell cancer cell lines and tumor in situ. Cancer Res 52 (1992) 5963–5970.
17. Kondo M, Tashekita T, Ishii N, Nakamura M, Watanabe S, Arai K-i, Sugamura S: Sharing of the interleukin 2 receptor γ chain between receptors for IL-2 and IL-4. Science 262 (1993) 1874–1877
18. Russel SM, Keegan AS, Harada N, Nakamura Y, Noguchi M, Leland P, Friedmann C, Miyajiama A, Puri RK, Paul WE, Leonard WJ: IL-2 receptor γ chain: A functional component of the interleukin 4 receptor. Science 262 (1993) 1880–1883.
19. Noguchi M, Nakamura Y, Russel SM, Ziegler SF, Tsang M, Cao X, Leonard WJ: Interleukin 2 receptor γ chain: A functional component of the IL-7 receptor. Science 262 (1993) 1877–1880.
20. Jahn B, Bergmann L, Fenchel K, Weidmann E, Schwulera U, Mitrou PS: CD3+CD4+ T cells as effective cells of autologous blast specific cytotoxicity in acute myelocytic leukemia. Ann Hematol 65, suppl. (1992) A122.

Acute Leukemias V
Experimental Approaches
and Management of Refractory Diseases
Hiddemann et al. (Eds.)

Stromal Function in Long Term Bone Marrow Culture of Patients with Acute Myeloid Leukemia

Michail Ya. Lisovsky and Valeri G. Savchenko

Introduction

Inhibition of normal hemopoiesis-peripheral blood pancytopenia and complete absence of normal colony forming cells in bone marrow [3, 4], is a regular finding in acute (AML) myeloid leukemias [1]. However, this inhibition is reversible. Polyclonal normal hemopoiesis is reestablished in more than two thirds of cases of AML during complete remission, demonstrating the existence of normal stem cells [15]. A few pathogenic mechanisms have been proposed to account for this process: cell crowding, synthesis by leukemic cells of inhibitor substances, cell contact processes and deficiency in the stromal cell microenvironment [2]. Several humoral inhibitors were found to be produced by leukemic cells such as acidic isoferritins, LAI and TNF-alpha [4, 5, 6]. Very little is known about the role of the microenvironment in the inhibition of normal hemopoiesis.

The earlier attempts to study the hemopoietic microenvironment in leukemia have been based on the use of the fibroblast colony forming unit assay (CFU-F) [7] and cultures of passaged bone marrow fibroblasts. It is still unknown which cell population's progenitor represents CFU-F [16]. However suppression of CFU-F in AML demonstrated that leukemia can adversely influence at least some stromal cell types.

Long term bone marrow cultures (LTBMC) as first described by Dexter et al. [8] offer a much more adequate system to study the interaction of hemopoietic cells with stroma because that system reproduces in vitro many of the features of stromal cell mediated regulation of hemopoiesis in vivo.

In order to evaluate the possibility of functional abnormality of stromal microenvironment in AML we studied the effects of adherent stromal cell layer (ASCL) from LTBMCs generated from patients with AML, AML in remission and normal individuals on CFU-GM production by reference normal bone marrow cells. We showed that ASCLs from normal LTBMCs were capable of supporting CFU-GM production in chimeric LTBMC; ASCLs from AML patients had no stimulatory effect and stromal cell layers from AML in remission patients had intermediate effect.

Materials and Methods

Patients. A total of 11 patients and 7 normal controls were included in the study. 6 patients had newly diagnosed AML and they were categorized according to the French-American-British classification as follows: 3 patients with M4 variant (30%, 57%, 67% and 80% of bone marrow blasts), 1 patient with M1 variant (80% of blasts), 1 – with M2 variant (82% of blasts) and 1 patient with M3 variant (80% of blasts). 6 patients were in complete remission of AML, 3 of them had M1 variant, 1 – M2 and 2 – M3 variant. 7 normal controls were donors of allogenic bone marrow transplants.

Establishment of adherent stromal cell layers. LTBMCs from AML and normal marrows were initiated as follows. Bone marrow cells were obtained

Dept. of Hematological Oncology and Bone Marrow Transplantation, Hematological Research Center, Novozykovsky pr. 4A, Moscow, 125167 Russia

from the supernatant after sedimentation in 0.1% methylcellulose (Sigma, St.Lois, MO) for 30 min. 2×10^7 nucleated bone marrow cells were placed in 25 cm^2 tissue culture flasks (Lux, Miles Scientific, Il) containing 10 ml of growth medium, consisting of a-MEM (Flow Labs, UK) with 12.5% preselected fetal calf serum (FCS) (Vector, Russia), 12.5% preselected horse serum (Pansystem, Germany; Vector, Russia), 10^{-4} mol 2-mercaptoethanol, 10^{-6} mol hydrocortisone sodium succinate (Sigma, St.Lois, MO), 2×10^{-4} mol inositol, 20×10^{-6} mol folic acid, 4 mmol glutamine and 1% mixture of the antibiotics penicillin and streptomycin (Flow Labs, UK). The flasks were placed in a 37 °C, 5% CO_2 incubator for 3–5 days and thereafter were maintained at 33 °C. Every week half of the supernatant medium with cells was removed and replaced with fresh growth medium.

The cellularity of ASCLs was counted at 4 and 8 weeks of primary LTBMCs after trypsinisation.

Coculture of Irradiated ASCLs and Reference Bone Marrow Cells. At the time of maximal confluency of ASCLs (3–5 weeks in culture) they were exposed to 40 Gy using a cesium 137 source afterwhat the cultures were overlayed with 5×10^5/ml normal thawed allogenic bone marrow cells. These cells had been previously depleted of adherent cells and cryopreserved. Cells from one donor were used for all LTBMC overlays. All the cocultures were manipulated as conventional LTBMCs.

Adherent cell depletion. For adherent cell depletion the donor bone marrow cells were incubated in 75 cm^2 flasks at a concentration of 2×10^6 cells/ml for 2 hours twice consequently.

To have control cultures without preestablished ASCLs, 5 experiments were performed in which 5×10^6 adherent cell-depleted, thawed reference bone marrow cells were grown in LTBMC. Nonadherent cell counts as well as CFU-GM content in nonadherent cell fraction were monitored weekly.

Culture of CFU-GM. The harvested cells from nonadherent fraction of LTBMCs were counted and assayed weekly for CFU-GM. CFU-GM were assayed in a double agar system. The 0.5% agar underlayer contained 20% of U5637 conditioned medium as a source of colony stimulating activity. Colonies of granulocytes and macrophages numbering 40 cells or more were scored on day 14 using an inverted microscope.

Statistics. Statistical analysis was performed by using the Student t-test.

Results

ASCL formation. On the whole the cellularity of ASCL was significantly decreased in LTBMCs of patients with untreated AML and in patients with AML in remission (Fig. 1).

3 out of 6 patients with untreated AML and all 6 patients with AML in remission formed well-developed ASCLs with moderately decreased cellularity. 3 untreated AML patients with M2, M3 and M4 variants formed atypical poorly developed ASCLs. The cellularity of these ASCLs was greatly decreased (Fig. 1). Fat cells were greatly reduced or absent in cultures from patients with the untreated AML. Cells with fibroblastoid appearance were greatly reduced or absent in the cultures with poor ASCLs.

There was no correlation between ASCL and bone marrow cellularities ($r = 0.13$ for untreated AML).

Hemopoietic supportive capacity of ASCLs. Coculture experiments were performed to determine the possible existense of stromal dysfunction in AML LTBMC... In comparison with normal controls inoculated bone marrow cells demonstrated a defect in CFU-GM production when grown on AML ASCLs. The cumulative production of nonadherent CFU-GM in cocultures of untreated AML patients was 27% and in cocultures of AML in remission patients – 70% of that seen in cocultures with normal ASCLs. The significant difference between the CFU-GM production in normal and untreated AML cocultures became evident beginning from week 3 (Fig. 2). From the same time point – week 3, nonadherent CFU-GM numbers in untreated AML cocultures did not differ from that in the cultures not containing preestablished ASCLs. CFU-GM production did not differ between subgroups of AML cocultures with well developed and poorly developed ASCLs.

In the AML in remission group the pattern of the CFU-GM production curve had much in common with that of normal cocultures apart from insignificantly decreased CFU-GM numbers (Fig. 2).

In order to evaluate the difference in the supportive capacity of well developed and poor ASCLs, CFU-GM production was compared bet-

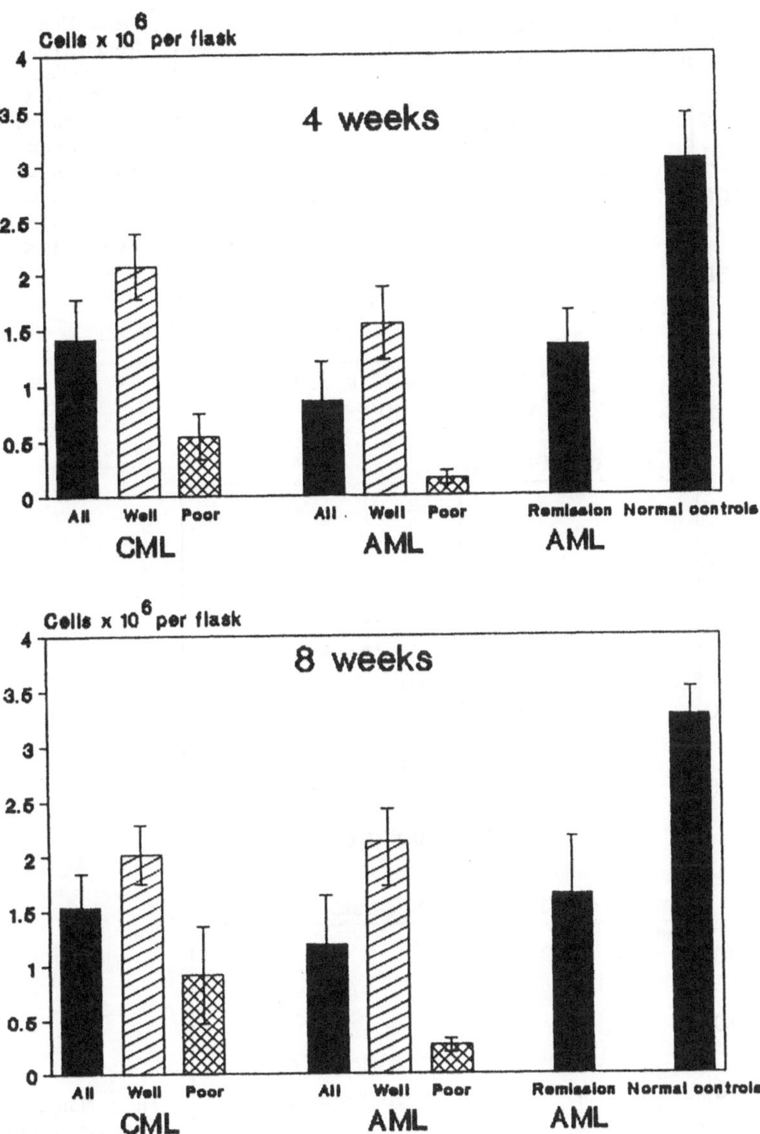

Fig. 1. Cellularity of ASCLs in the normal and AML LTBMCs

ween subgroups with well developed and poorly developed ASCLs (Fig. 3). There was no difference in CFU-GM production between subgroups.

Discussion

In the present study we used the LTBMC system to evaluate in AML the functional integrity of the in vitro hemopoietic microenvironment represented by ASCL.

As a whole ASCL cellularity was decreased in untreated AML by a factor of 2.7 and in AML in remission by a factor 2,1 when compared with the normal controls. 3 out of 6 untreated AML patients did not form well developed ASCL. The general feature of all LTBMCs of untreated AML patients was a greatly decreased amount or absence of fat cells.

The most apparent cause for poor stroma formation in untreated AML – dilution of stromal progenitors – is not likely to be the cause of

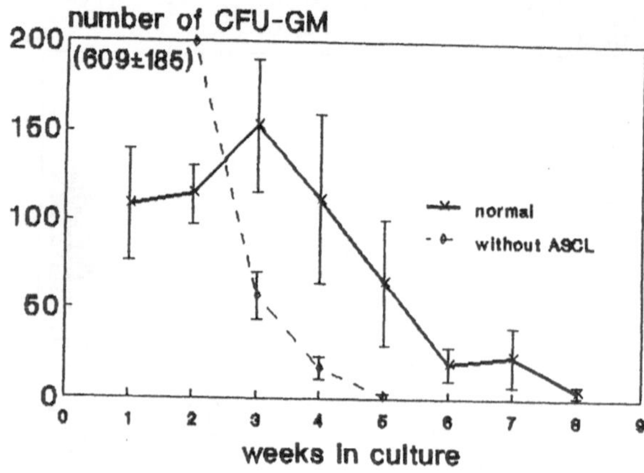

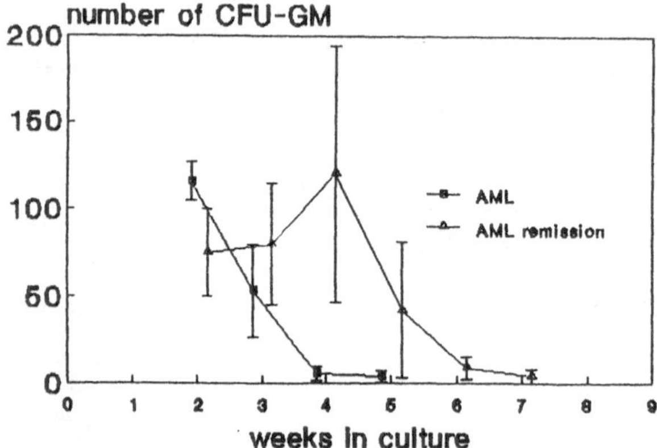

Fig. 2. Nonadherent CFU-GM production from normal bone marrow cells cultured on the irradiated ASCLs of the AML and normal LTBMCs. A – the CFU-GM production on the normal ASCLs and in the flasks without preformed ASCL; B – the CFU-GM production on the, AML and AML in remission ASCLs. In all experiments data of two to three flasks were used per point. The results are expressed as mean ± SD for data of the separate experiments in the groups

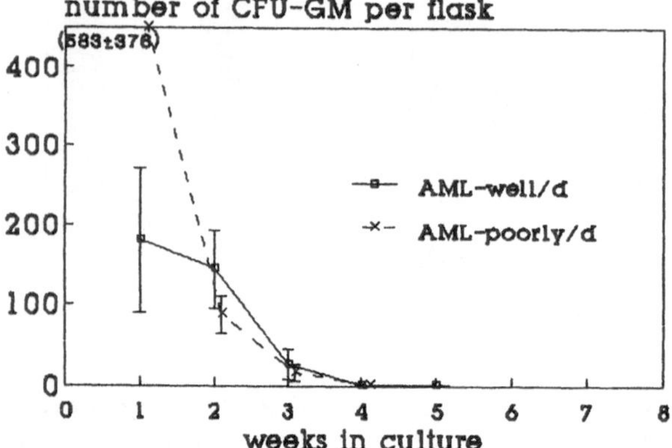

Fig. 3. Nonadherent CFU-GM production from the normal bone marrow cells cocultured with the irradiated well developed (3 patients) and poorly developed (3 patients) ASCLs of the LTBMCs of patients with untreated AML

decreased ASCL cellularity because there is no correlation between ASCL and bone marrow aspirate cellularity. Thus abnormality of obscure origin in stromal cell function represent the most reasonable explanation for decreased stroma formation in untreated AML group. However in the AML in remission group the reduction of ASCL cellularity may be associated with drug treatment [9]. The normal CFU-GM production curve is preserved though at reduced level in AML in this group. This fact indicates that the damage to the stromal population originating from drug treatment is qualitatively different from what is seen in LTBMCs of untreated AML patients.

In the coculture experiments we found a defect in the regenerative capacity of the bone marrow cells reflected in the number of CFU-GM detected weekly in the nonadherent layer of LTBMC and in the shorter period of time during which CFU-GM could be assayed. Our observation is not the only one. The incapacity of stroma in the LTBMCs of 6 untreated AML patients to support generation of granulocyte, erythroid and multipotential progenitors during 5 weeks of cultivation was recently shown by Mayani et al. [10]. Two of those patients developed poor ASCLs as did three of our AML patients.

It was recently shown that division of clonogenic precursors is under the double control of these stimulatory and inhibitory factors produced by stromal cells and it was suggested that the ratio of concentrations of these opposing factors is what is important for the proliferation of hemopoietic progenitor cells [11, 12, 13]. Thus possible explanations for the lack of hemopoietic supportive capacity of stroma in AML LTBMC are underproduction of growth factors or overproduction of inhibitors. Though inhibitor substances were found in supernatants from AML and chronic lymphatic leukemia ASCLs [10, 14] it is still largely unknown what kind of alterations are present in stromal cells of leukemic LTBMC.

In conclusion cellularity, morphology of stromal cell layers and their ability to support hemopoiesis in AML LTBMC is abnormal. This may be indicative of microenvironmental defect in AML in vivo.

References

1. Najman, A., Kobari, L., Khoury, E, Baillou, C.L. Lemoine, F., Guigon, M. (1991) Suppression of normal hematopoiesis during acute leukemias. Annals of New York Academy of Sciences, 628, 140–147.
2. Metcalf, D. (1977) Hemopoietic colonies, p.109. Berlin: Springer Verlag.
3. Bernstein, I.D., Singer, J.W., Smith, F.O., Andrews, R.G., Flowers, D.A., Petersens, J., Steinman, L., Najfeld, V., Savage, D., Frauchtman, S., Arlin, Z., Fialkow, P.J. (1992) Differences in the frequency of normal and clonal precursors of colony forming cells in chronic myelogenous leukemia and acute myelogenous leukemia. Blood, 79, 1811–1816.
4. Broxmeyer, H.E., Bognacki, J., Dorner, M.H., Sousa, M. (1981) Identification of leukemia associated inhibitory activity as acidic isoferritins. Journal of Experimental Medicine, 153, 1426–1444.
5. Olofsson, T., Olsson, I. (1980) Suppression of normal granulopoiesis in vitro by a leukemic associated inhibitor (LAI) of acute and chronic leukemia. Blood, 55, 975–982.
6. Kobari, L., Wail, D., Lemione, F.M., Dubois, C., Thiam, D., Baillon, C.L., Guigon, M., Gorin, N.C., Najman, A. (1990) Secretion of TNF-a by fresh human ANLL cells: Role in the disappearance of normal CFU-GM progenitors. Experimental Hematology, 18, 1187–1192.
7. Castro-Malaspina, H., Gay, R.E., Resnick, G., Kapoor, N., Meyers, P., Chiarieri, D., McKenzie, S., Broxmeyer, H.E., Moore, M.A.S. (1980) Characterisation of human bone marrow fibroblast colony forming cells (CFU-F) and their progeny. Blood, 56, 289–301.
8. Dexter, T.M., Allen, T.D., Lajtha, L.G. (1977) Conditions controlling the proliferation of hemopoietic stem cells in vitro. Journal of Cell Phisiology, 91, 335–344.
9. Rice, A., Reiffers, J., Bernard, Foure, E., Bascans, E., Lacombe, F., Marit, G., Broustet, A. Incomplete stroma formation after allogeneic marrow or autologous blood stem cell transplantation. Nouv.Rev. Fr. Hematol, 34,167–174.
10. Mayani, H., Guilbert, L.J., Clark, J.C., Belch, A.R., Janowska-Wieczorek, A. (1992) Composition and functional integrity of the in vitro hemopoietic microenvironment in acute myelogenous leukemia: Effect of macrophage colony-stimulating factor. Experimental Hematology, 20, 1077–1084.
11. Cashman, J.D., Eaves A.C., Raines, E.W., Ross, R., Eaves, C.J., (1990) Mechanisms that regulate the cell cycle status of very primitive hematopoietic cells in long term human marrow cultures. I. Stimulatory role of a variety of mesenchymal cell activators and inhibitory role of TGF-beta. Blood 75: 96–101.
12. Sutherland, H.J., Eaves, C.J., Lansdorp, P.M., Thacker, J.D., Hogge, D.E. (1991) Differential regulation of primitive human hematopoietic cells in long term cultures maintained on genetically engineered murine stromal cells. Blood 78: 666–672.
13. Eaves, C.J., Cashman, J.D., Kay, R.D., Dougherty, C.J., Otsuka, T., Gaboury, L.A., Hogge, D.E., Lansdorp, P.M., Eaves, A.C., Humphries, R.K. (1991) Mechanisms that regulate the cell cycle status of very primitive hematopoietic cells in long term human marrow cultures. II. Analysis of positive and negative regulators produced by stromal cells within the adherent layer. Blood, 78, 110– 117.
14. Delforge, A., Lagneaux, L., Dorval, C., Bron, D., Bosmans, E., Stryckmans, P. (1993) Excessive production of TGF-beta by bone marrow stromal cells in B-cell chronic lymphocytic leukemia (B- CLLo inhibits growth of hematopoietic precursors and IL-6 production. Experimental Hematology, 21, 1090 (abstr).
15. Fialkow, P.J., Janssen, J.W.G., Bartram, C.R. (1991) Clonal remissions in cutenonlymphocytic leukemia: Evidence for a multistep pathogenesis of the malignancy. Blood, 77, 1415–1417.
16. Lichtman, M.A., (1984) The relationship of stromal cells to hemopoietic cells in marrow. In: Long term bone marrow cultures, edited by D.G.Wright and J.S.Greenberg, pp. 3–29. New York: Alan R.Liss.

Acute Leukemias V
Experimental Approaches
and Management of Refractory Diseases
Hiddemann et al. (Eds.)

Fluorescence In Situ Hybridization for the Diagnosis and Follow-up of BCR-ABL Positive ALL

G. P. Cabot[1], M. Bentz[2], K. Fischer[1], A. Ganser[3], M. Moos[1], C. Scholl[1], P. Lichter[2], and H. Döhner[1]

Introduction

The BCR-ABL fusion, which is the molecular counterpart of the t(9;22), is the most common genetic abnormality in adult acute lymphoblastic leukemia (ALL) [1]. Due to its important diagnostic and prognostic significance a rapid and sensitive detection of this alteration is necessary [2,3]. We recently published a fluorescence in situ hybridization (ISH) protocol that allows the detection of breakpoints within both the major (M-bcr) and the minor (m-bcr) breakpoint cluster regions of the BCR gene on chromosome 22 [4]. In the present study the new protocol was applied to screen a larger number of ALL patients. Furthermore, samples from a few patients in clinical remission were examined.

Patients and Methods

Patients. Five probands and thirteen patients with ALL (age 17–58 years, median 45 years, 6 female and 7 male) were examined by fluorescence ISH at initial diagnosis or relapse. In all patients data from G-banding analysis or/and reverse transcriptase PCR (Rt-PCR) were available. In addition, in two BCR-ABL positive patients hybridizations were performed on immunomagnetic beads sorted cells from autologous bone marrow.

Probes. For fluorescence ISH experiments we used the yeast artificial chromosome (YAC) clone D107F9 (kindly provided by Dr. H. Riethmann, Philadelphia, and Dr. T. Cremer, Heidelberg), amplified by ALU-PCR [5,6]; this clone is splitted by the translocation event; and the cosmid clone cos-abl 8 (kindly provided by Dr. N. Heisterkamp, Los Angeles, USA) recognizing sequences distal to the breakpoint in the ABL protooncogene [7]. In BCR-ABL positive cells one of the cos-abl 8 signals colocalizes with one signal from the BCR-YAC on the Philadelphia chromosome (Ph^1). Both DNA probes were labeled by nick translation with either biotin 16-dUTP or digoxigenin-11-dUTP.

Fluorescence in situ hybridization. Hybridizations were performed as described [4,8]. The hybridization protocol was initially established on methanol/acetic acid fixed cells and extended in a second step on stained and unstained blood or bone marrow smears. For dual colour hybridization 100–200ng of labeled YAC derived probe and 40–100ng of labeled cos-abl 8 were combined with 100–200μg of unlabeled Cot-1 DNA fraction and 2μg herring sperm DNA. After denaturation (76 °C, for 6 min) the probes were preannealed (at 37 °C, for 10 min).

After posthybridization washes the probes were detected with anti-streptavidin Cy3 and/or conjugated fluorescein anti-digoxigenin. The samples were visualized on a conventional fluorescence photomicroscope with a dual band pass filter. Cells were only considered to be BCR-ABL positive, if they exhibited three D107F9 signals and if one of these signals colocalized with one cos-abl 8 signal.

[1]Medizinische Klinik und Poliklinik V, Universität Heidelberg, Germany
[2]Deutsches Krebsforschungszentrum, Heidelberg, Germany
[3]Zentrum der Inneren Medizin, Universität Frankfurt, Germany

Results

We previously reported that for the diagnosis of the BCR-ABL fusion the cut-off level could be reduced from 4.6% in single colour to 1.0% in dual colour hybridization [4]. An unambiguous diagnosis was made retrospectively in cells from a series of ALL (see Fig. 1) and CML patients known to carry the Ph[1]. In this study thirteen ALL patients with unknown BCR-ABL status were screened. In 12 patients the percentage of positive cells was below the cut-off level (range: 0.0%–0.5% mean: 0.16%). In one patient (no. 12) 65.0% of the cells exhibited three YAC-signals and the colocalization of one of these signals with one cos-abl signal (see Fig. 1). In this patient the diagnosis was confirmed by Rt-PCR (break in m-bcr). By G-banding or/and Rt-PCR no Ph[1] or BCR-ABL fusion was detected in any of the other patients. In the BCR-ABL positive patient follow-up samples were analysed following reinduction therapy.

Although the disease was in complete remission, fluorescence ISH (see Fig. 2) showed persistence of the malignant clone: Hybridization on blood and bone marrow smears showed 5.0% and 7.5% BCR-ABL positive cells, respectively. The patient underwent allogeneic bone marrow

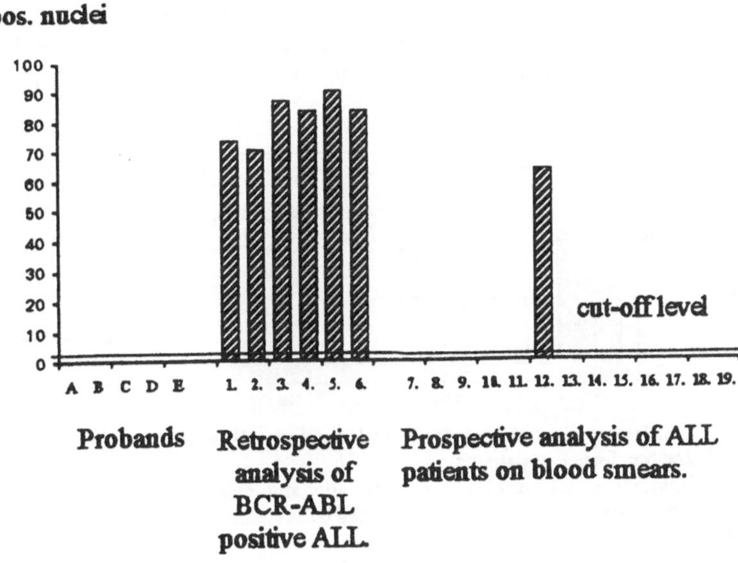

Fig. 1. Screening for BCR-ABL positive ALL using dual colour hybridization

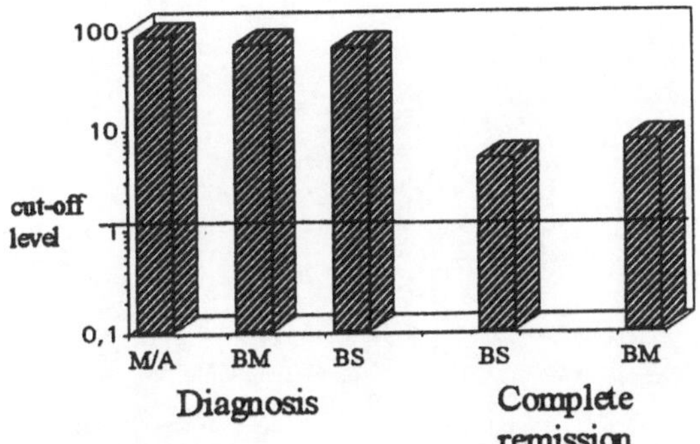

Fig. 2. Detection of BCR-ABL positive cells during remission (note the logarithmic scale)

Hybridization was performed on M/A: methanol / acetic acid fixed cells, BM: bone marrow smears or BS: blood smears

transplantation; so far, an analysis after transplantation has not been performed.

In two BCR-ABL positive patients autologous bone marrow grafts harvested in complete remission were assessed. Analysis was performed on a cell fraction that was enriched for the CD10 – and CD19 – positive cells by immunomagnetic beads purging. In both cases the percentage of BCR-ABL positive cells was above the cut-off level (see Fig. 3: no. 20 8.5% and no. 21 6.0%). Rt-PCR showed amplification signals in both patients (breaks in M-bcr), while the G-banding karyotype remained normal (no. 21). Patient no. 20 died from complication related to bone marrow transplantation. In patient 21 further specimens were available two months after bone marrow transplantation. While morphological evaluation of the bone marrow showed less than 5% blasts, fluorescence ISH exhibited 21% BCR-ABL positive cells. The patient relapsed two months afterwards (Fig. 4).

Discussion

Previously, the applicability of fluorescence ISH for the diagnosis of the BCR-ABL fusion has been shown in only a few studies in CML. Two groups used cosmid clones flanking the breakpoints in the BCR and ABL gene [9,10]. With this probe set only breaks with the M-bcr could be detected. Two other groups used probe pools from microdissected chromosomes or derived from interspecies somatic cell hybrids; these probe sets are suitable for metaphase, but not for interphase cytogenetics [11,12]. However, neither of these probes had been applied to a larger series of patients. In our study we

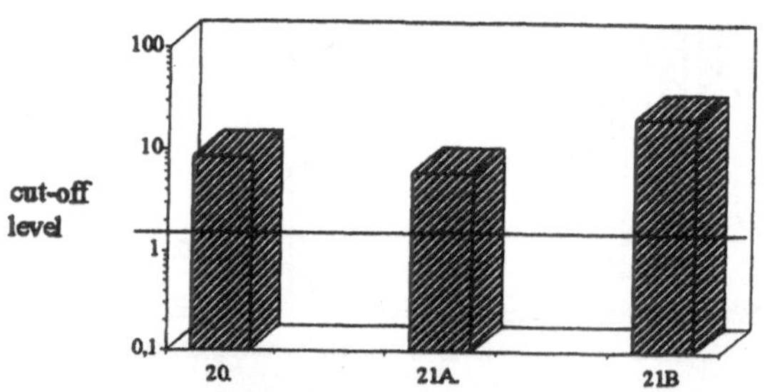

20+21 A: Increased number of BCR-ABL positive cells in the beads fraction from two patients.
21B: Follow-up of patient 21A two months after autologous bone marrow transplantation and two months before clinical relapse.

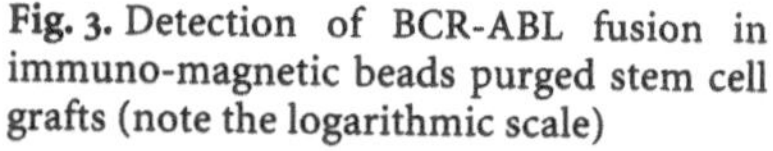

Fig. 3. Detection of BCR-ABL fusion in immuno-magnetic beads purged stem cell grafts (note the logarithmic scale)

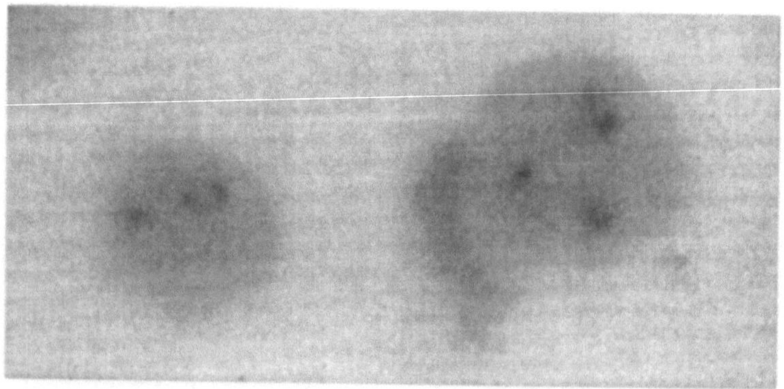

Fig. 4. Hybridization of YAC clone D107F9 to methanol/acetic fixed cells from patient 21. two months after autologous bone marrow transplantation. Although the disease was in complete remission, fluorescence ISH revealed 21.0% BCR-ABL positive cells. Note the three YAC signals in both cells indicating the translocation event

achieved a high sensitivity and specificity by using dual colour hybridization with the YAC-clone D107F9 and the cosmid-clone cos-abl 8. In contrast, in our study breaks both within the M-bcr and m-bcr were detected in interphase cells of ALL patients. The applicability for clinical diagnosis was demonstrated by hybridizing cells on blood smears of 13 consecutive ALL patients. In three patients, we used the probe set for the detection of residual disease.

So far, the use of fluorescence ISH for the monitoring of therapies and the detection of residual tumor cells was only demonstrated on metaphase cells from CML patients after alpha-interferon therapy [12,13]. Using our probe set this analysis can be extended to interphase cells. Using dual colour experiments we could drastically reduce the percentage of false positive nuclei. In comparison to PCR, the detection of minimal residual disease by fluorescence ISH is less sensitive. However, PCR has several drawbacks and any quantification of the malignant clone remains delicate. The sensitivity of fluorescence ISH may further be increased by hybridizing cells enriched for the malignant clone.

Acknowledgement. This work was supported by a grant DO 436/3-1 from the Deutsche Forschungs-gemeinschaft.

References

1. Kurzrock R, Gutterman JU, Talpaz M: The molecular genetics of Philadelphia chromosome-positive leukemias. New Engl J Med 319: 990, 1988.
2. Maurer J, Janssen JWG, Thiel E, van Denderen J, Ludwig WD, Aydemir Ü, Heinze B, Fonatsch C, Harbott J, Reiter A, Riehm H, Hoelzer D, Bartram C: Detection of chimeric BCR-ABL genes in acute lymphoblastic leukemia by the polymerase chain reaction. Lancet 337: 1055, 1991.
3. Westbrook CA, Hooberman AL, Spino C, Dodge RK, Larson RA, Davey F, Wurster-Hill DH, Sobol RE, Schiffer C, Bloomfield CD: Clinical significance of the BCR-ABL fusion gene in adult acute lymphoblastic leukemia: A Cancer and Leukemia Group B Study (8762). Blood 80: 2983, 1993.
4. Bentz M, Cabot G, Moos M, Speicher M, Ganser A, Lichter P, Döhner H: Detection of chimeric BCR-ABL genes on bone marrow samples and blood smears in chronic myeloid and acute lymphoblastic leukemia by in situ hybridization. Blood: (in press), April 1994.
5. Lengauer C, Green ED, Cremer T: Fluorescence in situ hybridization of YAC clones after Alu-PCR amplification. Genomics 13: 826, 1992.
6. Lengauer C, Riethman HC, Speicher MR, Taniwaki M, Konecki D, Green ED, Becher R, Olson MV, Cremer T: Metaphase and interphase cytogenetics with Alu-PCR-amplified yeast artificial chromosome clones containing the BCR gene and the protooncogenes c-raf-1, c-fms and c-erbB2. Cancer Res 52: 2590, 1992.
7. Heisterkamp N, Groffen J, Stephenson JR: The human v-abl cellular homologue. J Mol Appl Genet 2: 57, 1983.
8. Lichter P, Ward DC, in Human Cytogenetics D.E. Rooney, B.H. Czepulkowsky, Eds. (Oxford University Press, New York, 1992), vol. I, pp. 157.
9. Arnoldus EPJ, Wiegant J, Noordermeer IA, Wessels JW, Beverstock GC, Grosveld GC, van der Ploeg M, Raap AK: Detection of the Philadelphia chromosome in interphase nuclei. Cytogenet Cell Genet 54: 108, 1990.
10. Tkachuk DC, Westbrook CA, Andreef M, Donlon TA, Cleary ML, Suryanarayan K, Homge M, Redner A, Gray J, Pinkel D: Detection of bcr-abl fusion in chronic myelogeneous leukemia by in situ hybridization. Science 250: 559, 1990.
11. Zhang J, Meltzer P, Jenkins R, Guan XY, Trent J: Application of chromosome microdissection probes for elucidation of bcr-abl fusion and variant Philadelphia chromosome translocations in chronic myelogenous leukemia. Blood 81: 3365, 1993.
12. Zhao L, Kantarijan HM, von Oort J, Corn A, Trujillo JM, Liang JC: Detection of residual proliferating leukemic cells by fluorescence in situ hybridization in CML patients in complete remission after interferon treatment. Leukemia 7: 168, 1993.
13. Seong DC, Liu P, Siciliano J, Zhao Y, Cork A, Henske E, Warburton D, Yu MT, Champlin R, Trujillo JM, Deisseroth A, Siciliano MJ. Detection of variant Ph-positive chronic myelogenous leukemia involving chromosome 1,9, and 22 by fluorescence in situ hybridization. Cancer Genet. Cytogenet, 1993; 65: 100–103.

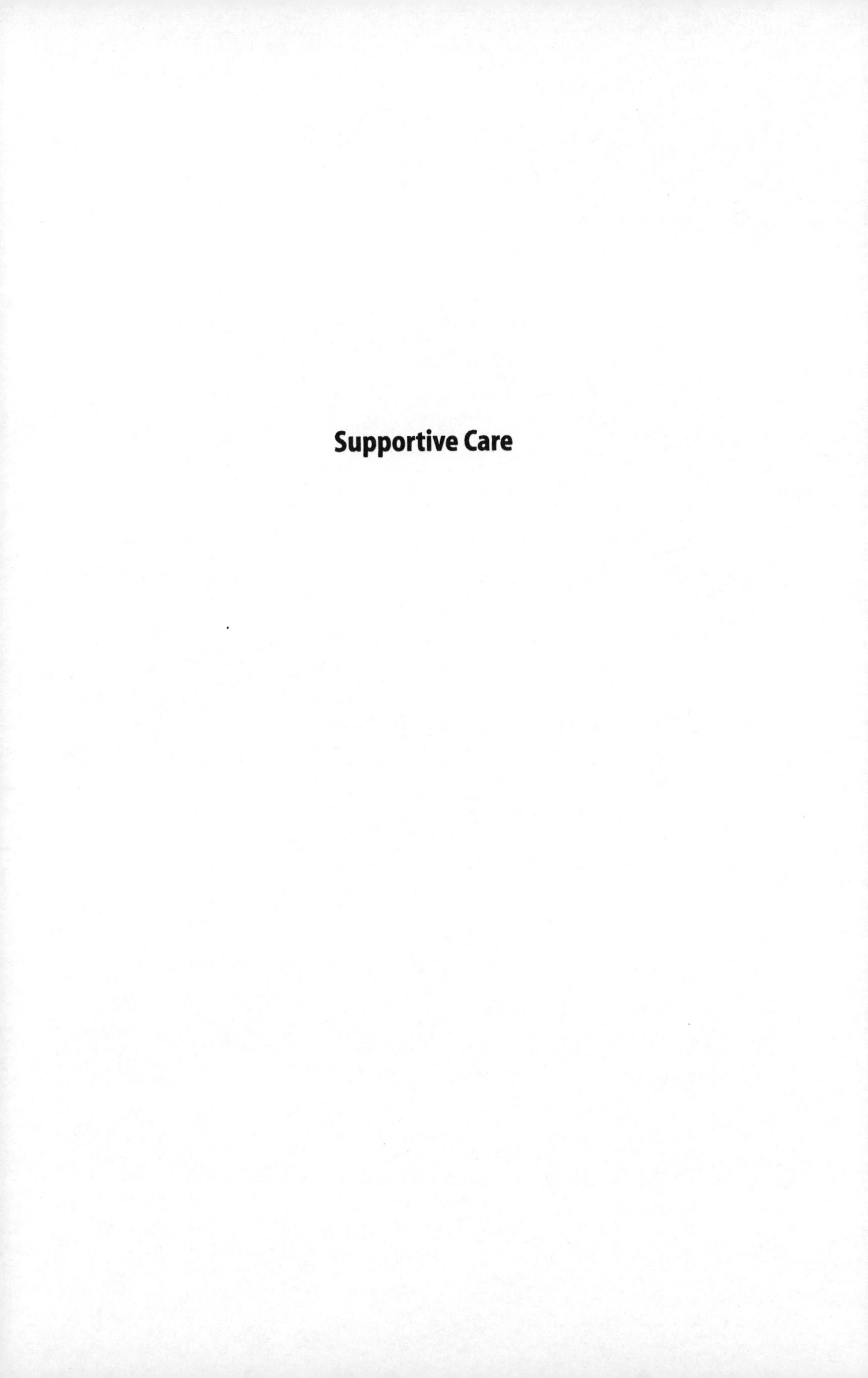

Supportive Care

Acute Leukemias V
Experimental Approaches
and Management of Refractory Diseases
Hiddemann et al. (Eds.)

Incidence and Severity of Amphotericin B-induced Acute Toxicity in Leukemic Patients After Treatment with Three Different Formulations (Amphotericin B, AmBisome and Amphotericin B/Intralipid) – A Pilot Study

M. Arning, K. O. Kliche, A. Wehmeier, A. H. Heer-Sonderhoff, and W. Schneider

Introduction

Intravenous amphotericin B (AmB) is the most potent drug for treatment of systemic fungal infections in leukemic patients. However, use of this drug is often limited by renal side effects and acute toxicity (fever, chills, nausea, vomiting). A far better tolerance has been reported with the use of AmBisome, a liposomal preparation of AmB, but this formulation is extremely expensive. In search of a cheaper AmB preparation with a better tolerance than conventional AmB, french scientists recently reported that AmB mixed in fat emulsion (Intralipid) has a significantly better tolerance profile compared to conventional AmB (Caillot et al., 1992, Chavanet et al., 1992). Our pilot study was performed to get information about the tolerance of the three different AmB preparations in individual patients.

Material and Patients

Patients participating in the study had acute myelogenous or lymphoblastic leukemia and received intravenous antifungal therapy during chemotherapy-induced bone marrow aplasia because of clinically suspected or microbiologically documented systemic fungal infections. For protection of nephrotoxicity, sodium loading with 50 ml NaCl 10% using a central venous catheter was performed in all patients receiving conventional AmB.

Patients were not included if they gave no informed consent, had preexisting renal insufficiency (serum creatinine values > 1,5 mg/dl), or had received an intravenous AmB preparation before start of the study.

AmB Study Protocol

At day 1 of study protocol, patients were given AmB (5 to 30 mg) mixed in 250 ml glucose 5% within 2 hours. On the next day, patients received AmBisome at a dose of 3mg/kg body weight over 1 hour. Therapy on day 3 consisted of 50 mg AmB mixed in 100 or 250 ml Intralipid 10%, given within 2 hours. After each AmB infusion, AmB-related side effects (fever and chills) were documented using modified WHO- and CALGB-expanded common toxicity criteria (Perry, 1992)(Table 1).

Drug-induced fever was assumed when AmB application was followed by the typical, well-known temporal elevation of body temperature within three hours after beginning of AmB infusion, especially when accompanied by chills. To distinguish drug-fever from infectious fever, AmB infusion was started when patients had body temperatures <37,5 degree Celsius at least four hours before start of the study.

No premedication was given.

After application of AmB infusion on day three, patients were asked which AmB preparation they would prefer for further antifungal treatment.

Department of Hematology, Oncology and Clinical Immunology, Heinrich-Heine-University Medical Center, Düsseldorf, Germany

Table 1. Grading for AmB-related side effects

toxicity	grade 0	grade 1	grade 2	grade 3	grade 4
fever	no fever	<38 °C	38 – 40 °C	> 40 °C	fever with hypotension
chills	none	minor chills, without temperature elevation	chills with temperature elevation <40 °C	chills with temperature >40 °C	chills with hypotension

Chi square tests were performed to calculate differences of the tolerance profiles between the three drugs. A p value < 0.05 was considered significant.

Results

18 patients participitated in the study. Fourteen patients received all three AmB preparations, four refused AmB/Intralipid infusions after experiencing acute toxicity with conventional AmB and no side effects after AmBisome infusions. All together 50 AmB infusions were studied.

The incidence and severity of AmB-related side effects is given in Table. 2

Grade 3 toxicity with temperature >40 °C and chills were documented after 6/18 infusions in the AmB group, significantly more often compared to 2/14 infusions in the AmB/Intralipid group and 1/18 infusion in the AmBisome group. The patient who did not tolerate AmBisome also did not tolerate the other two preparations without multi-drug premedication.

Of the six patients who showed grade 3 toxicity after conventional AmB, three later refused AmB/Intralipid infusions. The other three patients with grade 3 toxicity during conventional AmB also experienced toxicity after AmB/Intralipid infusions (2 patients grade 2, 1 patient grade 3).

Table 2. Incidence and severity of AmB-related side effects

	AmB (n = 18)	AmB/Intralipid (n = 14)	AmBisome (n = 18)
grade 0	4	3	10
grade 1	3	2	4
grade 2	5	7	3
grade 3	6	2	1

No grade 4 toxicity was seen after the AmB infusions

Moderate toxicity (grade 2) occurred in 5/18 infusions after conventional AmB, 7/14 in the AmB/Intralipid group and 3/18 in the AmBisome group.

Minor reactions were documented in 3/18 infusions in the AmB group, 2/14 in the AmB/Intralipid group and 4/18 in the AmBisome group.

10/18 AmBisome infusions were tolerated without any adverse reactions, significantly more compared to only 3/14 infusions with AmB/Intralipid.

The questionnaire after all three infusions revealed that 11/18 patients did not find subjective significant differences of the infusion-related adverse reactions. Seven patients clearly stated that AmBisome infusions were much better tolerated than conventional AmB or AmB/Intralipid infusions. Among them were the four patients who refused further participation in the study after experiencing grade 3 and 4 toxicity with conventional AmB infusion and excellent tolerance of AmBisome infusions.

Discussion

Our results confirm that AmBisome is tolerated without acute toxicity in most leukemic patients. The good tolerance of this preparation was especially impressive in five patients who showed grade 3 toxicity after conventional AmB and excellent tolerance of AmBisome.

In contrast, we could not confirm that the AmB/Intralipid formulation has a similar good tolerance profile compared to AmBisome. Major side effects necessitating the administration of antipyretics and/or corticosteroids occurred in 9/14 patients during AmB/Intralipid administration. Although the most severe reactions were observed less frequently compared to conventional AmB, this is only slightly superior to the profile of conventional AmB, where 11/17 patients showed major toxicity (grade 2 and 3).

These results are in contrast to the findings of Caillot et al, 1992, who reported a significantly better tolerance of the lipid formulation as compared to conventional AmB. However, the study of Caillot et al. was a retrospective one and did not compare the tolerance of the different formulations in the same patients. Moreover, they primarily focused on nephrotoxicity and not on acute side effects.

It is well-known that some patients tolerate conventional AmB for weeks without any side effects while other patients do not tolerate even 1mg of the drug without fever and chills. We think that our study design is more adequate to investigate the toxic profile of different AmB preparations.

In this small study, we compared the tolerance profile of a small dosage of conventional AmB with a high dose of AmBisome and a high dose of AmB/Intralipid. Although there are no prospective, controlled studies indicating that incidence and severity of AmB-related acute toxicity increases with AmB dose, we followed current recommendations not to start AmB-treatment with the maintenance dosage of 0,7 to 1 mg/kg body weight.

We made efforts to differentiate drug-induced fever and chills from fever of other causes, but one has to keep in mind that our patients received the AmB formulations because of suspected or documented fungal infections during chemotherapy-induced bone marrow aplasia. We cannot exclude the possibility that in some cases fever due to fungal infection has influenced our study results. However, administration of AmB to normal volunteers must be considered unethical in view of its toxic profile and the administration of the different preparations within three days should minimize any bias of the results due to underlying infection.

This pilot study was performed during the first three days of AmB therapy. Toxic reactions usually decrease with continuation of AmB therapy, and further studies are needed to investigate the toxic profiles of the three formulations during long-term treatment. In this study, we did not focus on nephrotoxicity as we have learned that sodium loading effectively minimizes AmB-induced nephrotoxicity. In our experience, cessation of AmB therapy because of nephrotoxicity has become rare (Arning and Scharf, 1989, Branch, 1988).

At present, we do not know the influence of infusion time and the optimal dose of AmB in lipid emulsions for optimal tolerance of this new drug combination, nor even do we know the equivalent dose of AmB/Intralipid compared to conventional AmB. It may be that changes of these variables may strongly influence our results. Moreover, as it seems that severity of AmB/Intralipid-related side effects tends to be a litte bit lower when compared to the severity after conventional AmB, the routine use of a premedication with paracetamol or similar antiinflammatory drugs may further increase the tolerance of AmB/Intralipid compared to conventional AmB. Further comparative, prospective studies are necessary to answer these questions.

In conclusion, AmBisome was tolerated best of the three AmB preparations. The AmB/-Intralipid emulsion was marginally better tolerated than the conventional preparation with regard to acute toxic reactions.

References

1. Arning M, RE Scharf (1989), Prevention of Amphotericin B-induced nephrotoxicity by loading with sodium chloride: A report of 1291 days of treatment with amphotericin B without renal failure. Klin Wochenschr 67: 1020–9
2. Branch RA (1988), Prevention of amphotericin B-induced renal impairment. A review on the use of sodium supplementation. Arch Intern Med 148: 2389–94
3. Caillot D, P Chavanet, O Casasnovas, E Solary, G Zanetta, M Buisson, O Wagner, B Cuisenier, A Bonnin, P Camerlynck, H Portier, H Guy (1992), Clinical evaluation of a new lipid-based delivery system for intravenous administration of amphotericin B. Eur J Clin Microbiol 11: 722–5
4. Chavanet PY, I Garry, N Charlier, D Caillot, JP Kisterman, M D'Athis, H Portier (1992), Trial of glucose versus fat emulsion in preparation of amphotericin B for use in HIV infected patients with candidiasis. Brit Med J 305: 921–5
5. Perry MC (ed.) (1992), The Chemotherapy Source Book. Williams & Wilkins, 1133–40

Acute Leukemias V
Experimental Approaches
and Management of Refractory Diseases
Hiddemann et al. (Eds.)

Pulmonary Infiltrates in Patients with Hematologic Malignancies: Clinical Usefulness of Non-bioptic Bronchoscopic Techniques

M. von Eiff, N. Roos, M. Zühlsdorf, M. Thomas, and J. van de Loo

Introduction

The increase in the intensity of cancer chemotherapy has created new problems, and has shifted the major obstacles against a successful treatment of neoplastic diseases from tumor-resistance to the management of therapy related myelosuppression. Persistant neutropenia in the course of intensive antineoplastic treatment exposes patients to an increasing risk of infectious, especially pulmonary infections. The highest mortality between 55 and 90% occurred when the source was respiratory (Pizzo et al 82, Singer et al 77, Whimbey et al 87). To lower the high mortality rate in these patients the earliest possible detection of causal pathogens is needed to start specific treatment.

Patients and Methods

A fiberoptic bronchoscope was advanced into a segmental bronchus supplying an area of radiographic abnormality. Microbiology specimen brush-catheter (Microvasive[R], Watertown, USA) was placed through the channel of the bronchoscope and the plug of the catheter was pushed out using visual guidance. For BAL the bronchoscope was wedged into a segmental bronchus. Alveolar lavage was performed by sequential instillation and suctioning of 50 ml volumes of sterile physiologic saline. The procedure was repeated four times, and the fluid returns were pooled. After BAL bronchial secretions were suctioned via the working channel of the bronchoscope.

An aliquot of the BAL fluid was used for culture of aerobic bacteria, Legionella, Mycobacteria, fungi and viruses. Cytopreparation smears were routinely stained with Grocott for detection of Pneumocystis carinii and fungal organisms, with gram stain for bacteria and with auramine-rhodamine for Mycobacteria. They were studied by direct immunofluorescence assay for Legionella and for cytomegalovirus. Papanicolaou stains were examined for the presence of malignant cells, intracytoplasmatic or intranuclear viral inclusion bodies and hemosiderin-loaden macrophages. Bronchial secretions were submitted for bacterial, fungal, mycobacterial, and Legionella culture and stains. Protected specimen brush was done in 71 patients additionally to BAL and bronchial washings and cultured for bacteria and fungi.

Clinical information on each patient was obtained from the physician who followed the patient's course and by review of the patient's chart. Serum samples obtained during the acute and convalescent phases were tested for antibodies against a variety of pathogens. Blood cultures were taken when clinically indicated and were processed for bacteria and fungi.

Results

103 fiberoptic bronchoscopies in 90 episodes of newly diagnosed pulmonary infiltrates were performed in 90 immunocompromised patients with fever above 38.4 °C. 59 patients had acute leukemias, 31 had other hematological

University of Münster, Department of Hematology and Oncology, Germany

malignancies. The study population comprised 52 males and 38 females, ranging from 16 to 83 years of age. 82 patients had received cytostatic treatment and 66 patients had consecutively developed severe neutropenia (<500 neutrophils/mm^3). The median interval between beginning of fever (> 38.4 °C) and/or detection of pulmonary infiltrates and bronchoscopy was 14 days (range 2 to 35 days). Before bronchoscopy all patients with acute leukemias and 27 of 31 patients with other hematological malignancies were already receiving broad spectrum antibacterial agents, and 31 were also receiving Amphotericin B and 5 Fluorocytosine.

The microbiological findings in bronchoscopic specimens are shown in Table 1. In BAL, bronchical secretions and/or protected specimen brush 226 organisms (on the average two different organisms/bronchoscopy) could be identified. Gram-positive bacteria, especially Koagulase-negative staphylococci and Candida species were cultured in BAL, bronchial secretions and/or protected specimen brush most often.

Altogether, the diagnostic yield of non-bioptic bronchoscopic techniques in detecting infectious episodes in patients with hematologic malignancies was 66 %. Sensitivity and specificity differed between lavage fluid, bronchial secretions, and protected specimen brush, and especially between the organisms themselves. The sensitivity of BAL in detecting different organisms is demonstrated in Figure 1. The sensitivity was 100 % for Pneumocystis carinii and herpes viruses and 85 % for gram-positive bacteria. Fungi were detected with a sensitivity of 43% in BAL and 67 % in bronchial secretions. The lowest sensitivity was found in culturing gram-negative rods. In bronchoscopic specimens of patients with acute leukemia only 6 of 15

Table 1. Microbiologic findings in bronchoscopic specimens of 90 patients with acute leukemias and other hematological malignancies (n = number of bronchoscopies, 13 patients had more than 1 bronchoscopy examination)

	Acute leukemia n = 67	Other hematological malignancies n = 36
Pneumocystis carinii	2	3
Aspergillus species	8	–
Candida species	26	26
Herpes viruses (unclassified)	1	–
Cytomegalovirus	7	7
Herpes simplex virus	–	2
Legionella pneumophila	15	8
Escherichia coli	1	2
Proteus species	1	1
Pseudomonas species	2	3
Klebsiella species	1	1
Enterobacter species	1	1
Acinetobacter species	–	1
Staphylococcus Koagulase positive	–	6
Staphylococcus Koagulase negative	39	20
Streptococcus viridans	16	
Streptococcus faecalis/faecium	8	10
Streptococcus pneumoniae	1	1

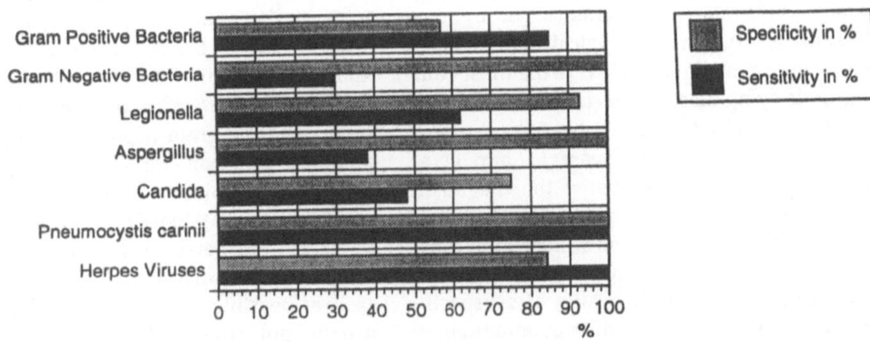

Fig. 1. Sensitivity and specificity of BAL

gram-negative pneumonias could be identified. Legionella pneumophila was cultured only once in bronchoscopic specimens, in the other patients Legionella was detected by direct immunofluorescence assay.

Detection of Pneumocystis carinii, Aspergillus species and gram-negative rods in bronchoscopic specimens was 100% specific. Specificity of detecting herpes viruses was 84%; positive culture of Candida species in lavage fluid and protected brush had a specificity of 75 %, however, in bronchial secretions specificity was only 58%. The cultural detection of gram-positive bacteria had the lowest specificity ranging from 40 to 54% between the three types of bronchoscopic specimens.

Discussion

The expanding number of patients susceptible to opportunistic organisms has increased the need for rapid diagnosis of pulmonary infection. Bioptic techniques such as transbronchial biopsies or perthoracal needle aspiration often cannot be performed because of coagulopathies in this patient population. Lung biopsy – still the gold standard in the differential diagnosis – was of little help in directing medical therapy or influencing clinical outcome (McCabe et al. 85, Potter et al. 85).

In recent years BAL has emerged as a valuable technique to obtain pulmonary specimens for cytologic and microbiologic analysis (Broaddus et al. 85, von Eiff et al. 90, Golden et al. 86, Martin et al. 87, Pisani et al. 92, Saito et al. 88, Stover et al. 84).

Until now little is known about the value of BAL in determining the causative agent of pulmonary infiltrates in patients with acute leukemia or other hematological malignancies. Hematological malignancies were the most common underlying diseases in the study of Stover et al. (1984) and BAL had an overall diagnostic yield of 66% (61 of 92 diseases). Saito et al. (1988) retrospectively evaluated the diagnostic yield of BAL in 22 adults with acute leukemia and compared the results with those at autopsy performed within 3 weeks of BAL. The diagnostic yield of BAL was only 15% (3 of 20 specific diseases); all three were Candida pneumonia.

In our study diagnostic yield of non-bioptic bronchoscopic techniques in detecting infectious pulmonay infiltrates was 66%. As expected BAL was most effective in the diagnosis of Pneumocystis carinii and Cytomegalovirus pneumonia, however, sensitivity and specificity of BAL, bronchial washing and protected brush in detecting fungal or bacterial pneumonia was low.

Candida species often were cultured in bronchoscopic specimens, but in retrospective analysis often were regarded as colonizers and not as etiologic agents of pneumonia.

Staphylococcus epidermidis could be cultured in 38 to 49% and in 33 to 42% of bronchoscopic specimens of patients with acute leukemias, and other hematological malignancies, respectively. The high number of positive cultures of Staphylococcus epidermidis, especially in patients with acute leukemia, may be explained by the intensive cytostatic treatment and secondary destroyment of mucosal barriers. However, in retrospective analysis this bacteria was also seldomly regarded as the etiologic agent of pneumonia because other more likely pathogens were identified.

Legionella infections could be diagnosed with high sensitivity and specificity by monoclonal antibody. Other gram-negative bacteria were rarely cultured in bronchoscopic specimens, particularly in patients with acute leukemia. All patients with acute leukemia had received broad spectrum antibacterial agents before BAL. The low sensitivity was most likely caused by the correct empirical treatment with antibacterial agents.

In conclusion, because of its availability and safety, non-bioptic bronchoscopic techniques remain an important procedure for the evaluation of pulmonary infiltrates in patients with hematological malignancies. BAL was most effective in the diagnosis of Pneumocystis carinii and herpes virus pneumonia, but sensitivity and specificity of BAL, bronchial washing and protected brush in diagnosing bacterial and/or fungal pneumonia was low. Because of the high incidence of pneumonias caused by fungi and/or gram-negative bacteria in this patient population empirical therapy with broad spectrum antibiotics and antimycotics is ur gently indicated when fever and new pulmonary infiltrates are detected. In the course of pneumonia, bronchoscopy should be performed as early as possible to identify organisms which are usually not covered by empiric antimicrobial treatment such as Pneumocystis carinii, Cytomegalovirus or Legionella.

References

1. Broaddus C, Dake MD, Stulbarg MS, Blumenfeld W, Hadley WK, Golden JA, Hopewell PC (1985). Bronchoalveolar lavage and transbronchial biopsy for the diagnosis of pulmonary infections in the acquired immunodeficiency syndrome. Ann Intern Med 102: 747–752
2. von Eiff M, Steimann R, Roos N, van Husen N, Wailger P, Baumgart P, Fegeler W, Junge E, Baumeister H, Wilms B, Heinicke A, van de Loo J (1990). Pneumonien bei abwehrge-schwächten Patienten: Stellenwert nicht-bioptischer bronchoskopischer Untersuchungsverfahren in der Erregerdiagnostik. Klin Wochenschr 68: 372–379
3. Golden JA, Hollander H, Stulbarg MS, Gamsu G (1986). Bronchoalveolar lavage as the exclusive diagnostic modality for pneumocystis carinii pneumonia. A prospective study among patients with acquired immunodeficiency syndrome. Chest 90: 18–22
4. Martin WJ, Smith TF, Brutinel WM, Cockerill III FR, Douglas WW (1987). Role of bronchoalveolar lavage in the assessment of opportunistic pulmonary infections: Utility and complications. Mayo Clin Proc 62: 549–557
5. McCabe RE, Brooks RG, Mark JB, Remington JS (1985). Open lung biopsy in patients with acute leukemia. Am J Med 78: 609–616
6. Pisani RJ, Wright AJ (1992). Clinical Utility of bronchoalveolar lavage in immunocompromised hosts. Mayo Clin Proc 67: 221–227
7. Pizzo PA, Robichaud KJ, Wesley R, Commers JR (1982). Fever in the pediatric and young adult patient with cancer. A prospective study of 1001 episodes. Medicine 61: 153–165
8. Potter D, Pass HJ, Brower S, Macher A, Browne M, Thaler M, Cotton D, Hathorn S, Wesley R, Longo D, Pizzo P, Roth JA (1985). Prospective randomized study of open lung biopsy versus empirical antibiotic therapy for acute pneumonitis in nonneutropenic cancer patients. Am Thorac Surg 40: 422–428
9. Saito H, Anaissie EJ, Morice RC, Dekmezian R, Bodey GP (1988). Bronchoalveolar lavage in the diagnosis of pulmonary infiltrates in patients with acute leukemia. Chest 94: 745–749
10. Singer C, Kaplan MH, Armstrong D (1977). Bacteremia and fungemia complicating neo-plastic disease. A study of 364 cases. Am J Med 62: 731–742
11. Stover DE, Zaman MB, Hajdu SI, Lange M, Gold J, Armstrong D (1984). Bronchoalveolar lavage in the diagnosis of diffuse pulmonary infiltrates in the immunosuppressed host. Ann Int Med 101: 1–7
12. Whimbey E, Kiehn TE, Brannon P, Blevins A, Armstrong D (1987). Bacteremia and fungemia in patients with neoplastic disease. Am J Med 82: 723–730

Fludarabine in Chronic Lymphocytic Leukemia and Malignant Lymphomas

Acute Leukemias V
Experimental Approaches
and Management of Refractory Diseases
Hiddemann et al. (Eds.)

New Aspects in the Treatment of Chronic Lymphocytic Leukemia

J. L. Binet and the French Cooperative Group on CLL

Abstract. For new aspects in the treatment of chronic lymphocytic leukemia are discussed: rationale for selection of patients for treatment, results of new drugs, auto and allogeneic bone marrow transplantation and response criteria to treatment.

Introduction

We analyse here for new aspects in the treatment of chronic lymphocytic leukemia (C.L.L): rationale for selection of patients for treatment, new drugs, auto and allogeneic bone marrow transplantation (B.M.T.) and response criteria to treatment.

Rationale for Selection of Patients for Treatment

In the last decades, the first advance in the treatment of chronic lymphocytic leukemia (C.L.L.) was the advent of clinical staging systems (Raïs classification O, I, II, III, IV and international workshop classification A, B, C) which allowed to identify patients with different risks and to plan therapy accordingly. Results of trial based on these staging system have demonstrated that treatment, in early stage C.L.L. patients (Raï O and A stage), is of no benefit and may even be harmful. By contrast, there is general agreement that patients belonging to advances stages (B, C or III, IV and same I and II of Raï classification) of the disease should be treated.

New Drugs

More than 5000 C.L.L. have received Fludarabine monophosphate IV. M.J. Keating and his co-investigators confirmed the first results of M.D. Grever and reviewed the largest clinical, non randomized experience developed at the M.D. Anderson Cancer Center. Remissions occured in 54 out of 101 (12% of complete remissions, 24% of nodular complete remissions and 19% of partial remissions). One third of patients were resistant to treatment. Clinical stages were strongly predictive for reponse to treatment. In untreated patients, 83% of the patients achieved a complete or partial remission. M. Keating has proved correlation between overall survival or time to progression and complete or partial remission.

In 1990, the French cooperative group on C.L.L. started a randomised clinical trial (C.L.L.-90) in which 262 patients, previously untreated in stage B and C were allocated to receive fludarabine (25 mg/m^2 i.v., daily for 5 days) or CAP regimen -consisting of cyclophosphamide 750 mg/m^2 i.v. day 1, doxorubicin 50 mg/m^2 i.v. day 1 and prednisone 40 mg/m^2 orally on days 1 to 5 – or to the CHOP regimen, consisting of intravenous vincristin 1 mg/m^2 and doxorubicin 25 mg/m^2 on day 1, plus cyclosphosphamide 300 mg/m^2 and prednisone 40 mg/m^2 given orally on days 1 to 5. The first six courses of treatment were given at monthly intervals and the last six at 3-month intervals. In case of disease progression within the first three months after randomization, initial treatment was carried on, but thereafter choice of treatment could be made

Groupe Hospitalier Pitie-Salpetriere, Department of Hematology, Paris, France

according to the following rule. At 3-month, patients allocated to CAP or FDB who were considered as treatment failure (see below) were switched to FDB or CAP, respectively. At the sixth month, patients exhibiting disease progression were administered FDB, except in case of previous failure; doxorubicin dose reduction of 50% was made whenever remission was observed. Finally, all responders (see below) who were administered FDB at the sixth month were discontinuation of FDB. In an early study, we proved a more efficiency of fludarabine in stage B than in stage C.

In stage B, at the sixth month follow-up examination, remission status ("clinical and hematological remission", partial remission, stabilisation and progression), assessed in 158 patients, differed between the three treatment groups [p = 0.05, 6 degrees of freedom (df) chi square test]. "Clinical and hematological remission" was observed for 9 (19%) patients in the FDB group as opposed to 4 (7%) in the CAP group and 5 (10%) in the CHOP group (table II). Moreover, stage at the sixth month differed between the treatment groups (p = 0.02, 6 df chi square test), with 40 (83%) out of the 48 FDB patients in stage A or in remission, as compared to 31 (54%) in the CAP group and 29 (58%) in the CHOP group.

In stage C, remission status at the sixth month was not different between the three groups (p = 0.14, 6 df chi square test), though slight improvement could be observed in the CAP group, with 84% patients exhibiting remission (complete or partial) as compared to 64% in the FDB group and 63% in the CHOP group (table II). In terms of staging at the sixth month follow-up examination, no difference were longer observed between the three groups (p = 0.92, 6 df chi square test), with 55% of CAP patients in stage A or in remission, as compared to 50% in the FDB group and 43% in the CHOP group.

Auto and Allogeneic Bone Marrow Transplantation

A recent study from the European group for Bone Marrow Transplantation (B.M.T.) reported 20 patients with advanced disease who received *allogeneic B.M.T.* Ten patients were alive in complete remission with a mean follow-up of 30 months. S.N. Rabinowe undertook a non randomised study of *autologous* and allogeneic bone marrow transplantation in 20 patients, 8 allogeneic, 12 autologous with a minimal disease state, 13 patients have been staged for remission status (12 in clinical remission). I. Khouri treated patients with advanced stage BCLL who relapsed after fludarabine.

We report 2 cases of International Workshop'stage B C.L.L. with bulky nodal tumor, refractory to conventional therapy and to Fludarabine, who finally responded to a polychemotherapy associating Etoposide, Cytarabine, Cisplatin and Methyl-Prednisolone (ESAP). The bone marrow was harvested after 3 cycles of ESAP for the first patient and 4 cycles for the second one, and purged with anti CD19 and anti-CD20 moabs plus complement. The treatment was then completed with 2 more cycles for both patients. Autologous BMT was performed after TBI (10 grays), Etoposide 50 mg/kg. Both patients are now in clinical remission, for the first time, at 6 and 3 months post BMT respectively, as assessed by clinical and CT scan examinations.

The problem is tolerance and efficiency of these protocol ESAP in bulky nodal forms refractory to Adriamycin and Fludarabine: in 9 patients, 4 deaths by septicemia or hemorragia and refractory or in partial response after 1, 2, 5 and 5 cures, and 3 non response or insufficient responses were observed.

Therefore, we have to better define patients and the timing of autobone marrow group in refractory C.L.L.

Response Criteria to Treatment

With the aim of standardizing the response criteria to treatment, the IWCLL and the National Cancer Institute (NCI) Sponsored Working Group defined complete remission (CR), partial remission (PR), stable disease (SD), and progressive disease (PD) [12]. In fact, all of these criteria define clinical remission rather than CR, which seems very difficult to obtain. Furthermore, assessment of CR is difficult to make with current therapeutic approaches. More sensitive methods are required to detect residual malignant cells. Flow cytometry with the simultaneous use of CD5 and CD19 markers, kλ clonal excess, and analysis of gene rearrangement by the polymerase chain reaction are under study in this setting.

Although it is effective in vitro in C.L.L., Interferon-α (IFN-α) [13] has showed a low response rate in vivo except in early stages of the disease. Its use once response has been achieved after chemotherapy needs to be investigated.

References

1. Rai, K., Sawitsky, A., Cronkite, E., Chanana, A.B., Levy, R.N. and Pasternack, B.S. Clinical staging of chronic lymphocytic leukemia. Blood, 46, 219–234, 1975
2. Binet, J.L., Auquier, A., Dighiero, G., Chastang, C., Piguet, H., Goasguen, J., Vaugier, G., Potron, G., Colona, P., Thomas, M., Tchernia, G., Jacquillat, C., Boivin, P., Lesty, C., Duault, M.T. and Montconduit, M. A new prognostic classification of chronic lymphocytic leukemia derived from a multivariate survival analysis. Cancer, 48, 198–206, 1981
3. Keating, M.J., Kantarjian, M., Redman, J., Koller, C., Barlogie, B., Velasquez, W., Plunkett, W., Freireich, E.J., McCredie, K.B. Fludarabine: a new agent with major activity against chronic lymphocytic leukemia. Blood, 74, 19–25, 1989
4. Keating, M.J. Fludarabine phosphate in the treatment of chronic lymphocytic leukemia. Seminars in Oncology, 17 (suppl 8), 49–55, 1990
5. Grever, M.R., Kopecky, K.J., Coltman, C.A., Files, J.C. Greenberg, B.R., Hutton, J.J., Talley, R., Von Hoff, D.D., Balcerzak, S.P. Fludarabine monophosphate: a potentially useful agent in chronic lymphocytic leukemia. Nouv Rev Fr Hematol, 80, 457–460, 1988
6. Dillman, R.O., Mick, R. and McIntyre, O.K. Pentostatin in chronic lymphocytic leukemia: a phase II trial of cancer and leukemia group. B J Clin Oncol, 7, 433–439, 1989
7. Piro, L.D., Carrera, C.J., Beutler, E. and Carson, D.A. Chlorodeoxyadenosine: an effective new agent for the treatment of chronic lymphocytic leukemia. Blood, 72, 1069–1073, 1988
8. Michallet, M., Corront, B., Grathwohl, A., Milpied, N., Dauriac, C., Brunet, S., Soler, J., Jouet, J.P., Esperou Bourdeau, H., Arcese, W., Witz, F., Moine, A. and Zwaan, F.E. ( ) Allogeneic bone marrow transplantation in chronic lymphocytic leukemia: 17 cases. Bone Marrow Transplantation, (in press)
9. Rabinowe, S.N., Soiffer, R.J., Gribben, J.G., Freedman, A.S., Pesek, K.W., Daley, H.L., Daley, J.F., Spector, N.L., Anderson, K.C., Robertson, M.J., Ritz, J. and Nadler, L.M. Autologous and allogeneic bone marrow transplantation (BMT) for patients with Binet stage B and C B-cell chronic lymphocytic leukemia (B-CLL). Blood, 80, 170a, 1992
10. Khouri, I., Thomas, M., Andersson, B., Deisseroth, A., Keating, M., Champlin, R. Purged autologous bone marrow transplantation for chronic lymphocytic leukemia: preliminary results. Blood, 80, 66a, 1992
11. Sutton, L., Boccaccio, C., Gabarre, J., Maloum, K., Ben-Othman, T., Soussain, C., Cosset, JM., Merle-Béral, H., Binet, JL., Leblond, V. Intensification thérapeutique par chimiothérapie suivie d'autogreffe dans les leucémies lymphoides chroniques réfractaries. Nouv Rev Fr Hématol, 36, 104, 1994
12. International Workshop on chronic lymphocytic leukemia. Chronic lymphocytic leukemia: recommendations for diagnosis, staging and response criteria. Ann Inter Med, 110, 236–237, 1989
13. Pangalis, G.A. and Griva, E. Recombinant alpha-interferon in untreated stages A and B chronic lymphocytic leukemia: a preliminary report. Cancer, 61, 869–872, 1988

Acute Leukemias V
Experimental Approaches
and Management of Refractory Diseases
Hiddemann et al. (Eds.)

The Use of Fludarabine in Chronic Lymphocytic Leukemia and Malignant Lymphomas

Michael J. Keating

Abstract. Fludarabine is a new purine analogue which has demonstrated activity in low grade lymphoproliferative disorders. Initially, fludarabine was noted to have activity against lymphoma in phase I studies. Subsequently, major activity was demonstrated in the treatment of patients with previously treated and refractory chronic lymphocytic leukemia (CLL). The use of fludarabine (Fludara) in previously treated CLL is associated with a response rate of more than 50% with approximately one-third of patients obtaining a complete remission (CR) using NCI Working Group criteria. When Fludara is used in previously untreated patients with CLL, the response rate is 75–80% with the majority of responses being complete remissions. The median time-to-progression of CLL in responders is 18–27 months in previously treated patients and 42 months in previously untreated patients. The impact of Fludara on survival in these patient populations, so far, has not demonstrated in comparative trials. Fludara was noted to have activity against Waldenstrom's macroglobulinemia in previously treated patient populations. More than half of these patients will respond, particularly those with primary refractory disease or disease relapsing off treatment. Refractory relapsed patients who have had multiple attempts at therapy have a lower response rate. The phase I activity of Fludara against malignant lymphoma has been confirmed in subsequent studies with the activity being noted predominantly in low grade lymphomas. Activity is minimal in intermediate and high grade lymphoma. Overall approximately 60% of patients with previously treated low grade lymphoma will respond to Fludara with 20% CRs. More recently Fludara has been combined with mitoxantrone and dexamethasone and is associated with a high CR+PR rate in low grade lymphomas. Fludara has an expanding role in the management of CLL and low grade lymphoma.

Introduction

The 5′ monophosphate of fluoro-arabinosyl adenine, which is known as Fludarabine, fludarabine phosphate, or Fludara IV, is an adenine nucleoside analogue. Initially synthesized by Montgomery, the molecule was improved from arabinosyl adenine by the addition of the fluorine atom to diminish metabolism by adenosine deaminase and by the addition of the phosphate moiety to the sugar to increase solubility [1]. Fludarabine (Fludara) was studied in phase I/II clinical trials and myelosuppression was found to be dose-limiting [2,3]. Clinically significant activity was noted in lymphoid malignancies [2,3]. The major subsequent therapeutic trials have been conducted in the treatment of chronic lymphocytic leukemia (CLL) and low grade lymphoma (LGL) and major clinical activity has been noted in these tumor types. A number of activities of Fludara have been noted relevant to inhibition of DNA synthesis and inhibition of DNA repair as well as inhibition of ribonucleotide reductase, incorporation into DNA and inducing apoptosis [4]. The exact mechanism of action, however, has not been established. This manuscript describes the activity of Fludara in patients with previously treated CLL, previously untreated CLL, and low grade lymphoma alone or in combination.

Department of Hematology, University of Texas M.D. Anderson Cancer Center, Houston, TX 77030, USA

Chronic Lymphocytic Leukemia

Grever and colleagues were the first to demonstrate that Fludara was active in CLL [5]. Subsequently, investigators at the M.D. Anderson Cancer Center (MDACC) have conducted clinical trials with a variety of schedules of Fludara in previously treated patients with CLL [6–9]. In the initial studies, 68 patients were treated with 39 achieving a CR or PR using NCI Working Group criteria [6]. Subsequently, an additional 10 patients were treated with Fludara on that clinical trial (Table 1). Fifteen percent of patients achieved a marrow complete remission documented by biopsy and another 23% of the patients with a CR, using NCI criteria, had persistent interstitial aggregates or nodules in the bone marrow.

The next study utilized the addition of prednisone to Fludara in the five-day schedule every four weeks [7]. The response rate was almost identical to the use of Fludara as a single agent in the same dose and schedule and the only additional feature noted was an increase in the incidence of opportunistic infections with *Pneumocystis carinii* pneumonia and *Listeria* monocytogenes in the group treated with a combination of Fludara and prednisone. There was absolutely no difference in survival of the patients treated. Subsequent clinical trial utilized a once-a-week schedule of 30mg/m² weekly until maximum response or resistance was noted [8]. This schedule had a cumulative dose intensity of 80% compared with the five-day every four weeks schedule. There was a substantial decrease in the response rate with only 24% of patients achieving a complete or partial response. There was no decrease in the early death rate or morbidity associated with this regimen and it was discontinued after accrual of only 47 patients.

A subsequent clinical trials has utilized a three-day schedule of Fludara 30mg/m²/day for three days every four weeks [9]. Eighty patients have been entered on this clinical trial and 46% of the patients have achieved a complete remission (25%) or partial remission (21%) (Table 1). When the survival of these four clinical trials have been compared there is no difference in the survival of any of the four regimens suggesting a biologic predeterminism of survival (Fig. 1).

The three-day regimen is associated with a reduction in incidence of infections to approximately 50% of that noted with the five-day schedules (Table 2). The major morbidity associated with the use of Fludara in previously treated CLL is the development of infectious complications. The majority of the infections are fevers of unknown origin, but as noted in Table 2, a number of patients developed major infections which are usually pneumonias, either unilateral or bilateral. The causative organisms in these pneumonias is variable and is often unknown. Apart from the use of corticosteroids, there is not a high frequency of documented opportunistic infections in patients treated with Fludara regimens.

Fludara has subsequently been administered to previously untreated patients with CLL (Table 3). The initial study reported on 35 previously untreated patients and a response rate of 80% was obtained with three-quarters of the patients achieving a CR using the NCI criteria [10]. The speed of response was rapid and an association of response with Rai and Binet stage was noted.

Subsequently, prednisone has been added to the five-day Fludara regimen and as in the previously treated patient population, no difference was noted in the response rate or the survival (Fig. 2).

When prednisone was added to the five-day schedule, the CR rate was in fact a little lower than when Fludara was used as a single agent [7]. One-half of the patients who achieved a CR by NCI criteria have persistent lymphoid nodules which occurred in the bone marrow. When two parameter flow cytometry is used to

Table 1. Results of fludarabine regimens in previously treated CLL

	FLU × 5	FLU+P × 5	FLU q1w	FLU × 3	TOTAL
Patients	78	169	47	80	374
CR%	39%	37%	15%	25%	32%
PR%	19%	15%	9%	21%	16%
Fail%	33%	35%	66%	45%	41%
Early Death%	9%	12%	11%	9%	11%

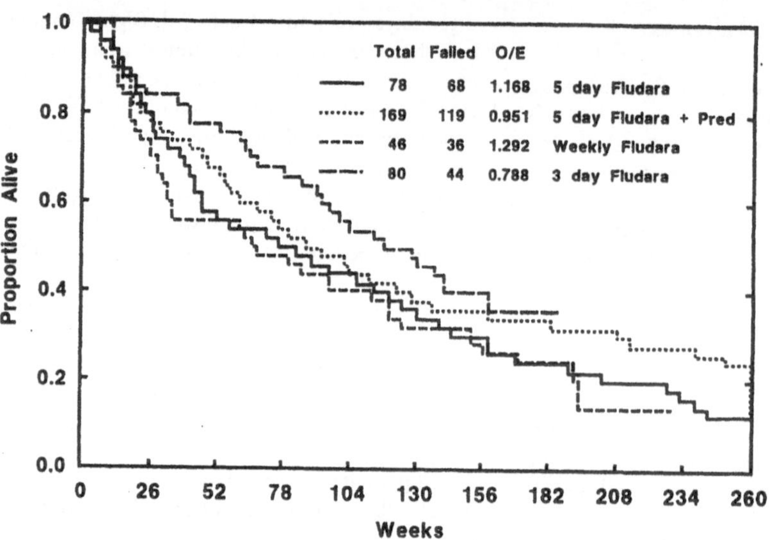

Fig. 1. Survival of previously treated CLL by Fludara regimen

Table 2. Incidence of infections/fever by fludarabine regimen (episodes/100 courses)

Infection	5 Day FLU (437 Courses)	5 Day FLU+P (686 Courses)	3 Day FLU (451 Courses)
Major	44(10)	98(11)	24(5)
Minor	25(6)	34(4)	19(3)
FUO	35(8)	79(9)	13(3)
Atypical	5(1)	14(2)	2(0.4)
Herpes Zoster	5(1)	11 (1)	5(1)
Total	109(25)	254(29)	63(14)

Table 3. Results of fludarabine regimens in untreated CLL

	Fludarabine	Flu+ Prednisone	Total
Patients	35	120	155
CR%	74	61	64
PR%	6	18	15
Fail%	11	20	19
Early Death%	9	1	3

evaluate residual disease or rearrangement of the immunoglobulin heavy and light chains is performed, persistent abnormalities are noted in a substantial number of patients who are said to be in CR [11].

The major concern with the use of Fludara in the management of CLL is a decrease in the T-lymphocyte subsets [12]. Both CD4 and CD8 lymphocyte counts decrease quite promptly in all regimens studied. The median range of lymphocytes which are obtained in patients treated with Fludara with or without corticosteroids is of the order to 150 to 200 CD4 lymphocytes per microliter [7,9].

The starting CD4 and CD8 lymphocytes are usually in the range of 1000–1500/µl. When the number of episodes of infectional fever per patient year-at-risk is analyzed in patients off treatment with persistent low CD4 counts, the incidence of febrile episodes is low with only one febrile episode for every 2.5–3 patient years-at-risk [13]. Thus while the CD4 count is an important parameter to be noted, it does not appear to be associated with a high incidence of opportunistic infections. The incidence of infections is significantly high in patients who have received previous treatment and is much more common in patients with advanced stage disease who start off with low hemoglobin and platelet counts and there is an association with the extent of prior therapy. In addition, patients

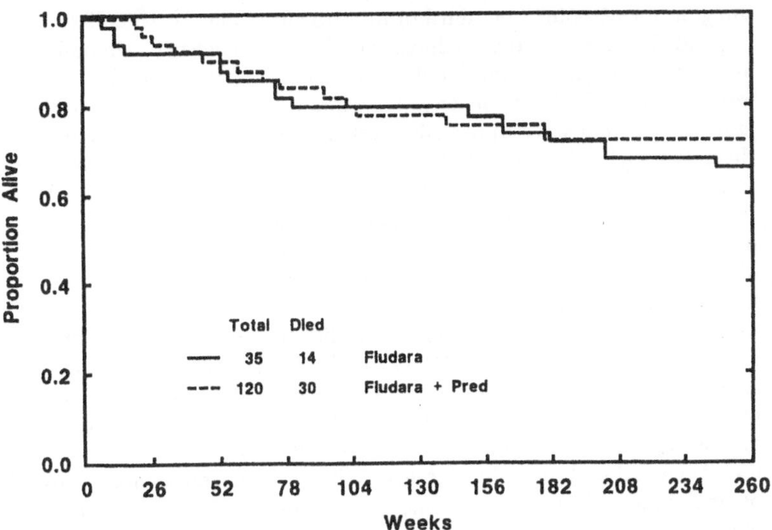

Fig. 2. Survival untreated CLL - Fludara + Prednisone

who are hypoalbuminemic have a high frequency of fevers and infection [6,7].

A number of other investigators have evaluated Fludara in CLL. Fenchel and Hiddemann have both shown response rates of 55% in 11 and 20 patients respectively [14,15]. In the initial study published by Grever et al., 4/20 (20%) of patients achieved a CR or PR. Puccio et al. have published a study of 51 patients with previously treated CLL using a loading dose with a continuous infusion schedule [16]. Forty-two patients were evaluable for response. The criteria for CR were unusually rigorous requiring normalization of bone marrow aspirate and biopsies as well as a conventional criteria and disappearance of all cells that expressed leu-1 (CD5). Correction of hypogammaglobulinemia was also required. Fifty-two percent of the 42 evaluable patients achieved a PR. Improvement in Rai stage was noted in 13/22 responders. As in the MDACC patients, myelosuppression was the most prominent and toxicity, with 40 episodes of infections, 10 of which were fatal. Two mycobacterial infections were seen along with five fungal infections. Only one episode of *Pneumocystis carinii* pneumonia was noted.

Waldenstrom's Macroglobulinemia

Waldenstrom's macroglobulinemia is a low grade lymphoid lymphoma with plasmacytoid lymphocytes which produce a monoclonal immunoglobulin. Traditional therapy has been with alkylating agents and very little information has been published on salvage therapy. Dimopoulos et al. initially reported on the use of Fludara in 11 patients with Waldenstrom's macroglobulinemia (WM) with a 40% response rate in previously treated patients [17]. This study has been increased to 28 patients [18]. Two patients were previously untreated and 26 previously treated. Fourteen patients were considered to be primary refractory, 12 were relapsing receiving salvage therapy. Fludara was given at a dose of 20–30mg/m² daily for five days in 20 patients and 30 mg/m² daily for three days in 8 patients. The response required a sustained decrease of at least 50% in monoclonal IgM synthesis for at least two months with a reduction of more than 50% of tumor infiltrates in liver, spleen, lymph nodes, or bone marrow. Ten of the 28 patients achieved a CR or PR. Seven patients had greater than a 75% cytoreduction. The response rate was higher in the five-day regimen (45%) versus 25% for the three-day schedule. The responses have been sustained with a median duration of response of 38 months. The median survival was 32 months. Both of the previously untreated patients responded with 6/14 of the primary refractory patients and 2/12 for refractory relapse patients.

Fludarabine in LGL

The initial phase I studies noted activity of Fludara in patients with lymphoma [19]. In 26 patients with NHL, who received Fludara 20mg/m² followed by continuous infusion of

30mg/m² for 48 hours, one-third of the patients responded. Subsequently, Redman et al. has used a dose of 25mg/m² for five days every four weeks on 67 evaluable patients with lymphoma [20]. All patients were previously treated with chemotherapy and over 40% had been treated with radiation. Twenty-eight (36%) and 37% of the 76 patients responded. No responses were noted in diffuse small cleaved cell lymphoma, diffuse large cell lymphoma, diffuse lymphoblastic lymphoma, or diffuse unclassified lymphoma. The response rate was 4/12 (33%) for diffuse small lymphocytic lymphoma (DSLL) and 13/21 (62%) for the most common low grade lymphoma namely follicular small cleaved cell lymphoma (FSCCL). Impressively, 4/5 follicular mixed cell and both the follicular large cell lymphoma patients responded. Thus, activity of Fludara was strikingly associated with the low grade lymphomas. Myelosuppression was noted to be the major toxicity and seven patients had treatment discontinued because of prolonged myelosuppression after a median of five courses. While there was no evidence of cumulative granulocytopenia, cumulative thrombocytopenia was noted. Episodes of infection or fever occurred in more than half of the patients. The most common infections were gram-positive coccal infections although one-third of the infections were noted to be associated with gram-negative organisms. As opposed to the CLL patients, most of these patients had indwelling central catheters. Five patients were found to have fungal infections with Candida spp being noted in three, aspergillus in one, and torulopsis glabraba in one. Two patients had *Pneumocystis carinii* pneumonia, one cytomegalovirus, and one a dermatomal herpes zoster. Subsequently, Hochster from the Eastern Cooperative Oncology Group has treated 62 evaluable patients with Fludara 18mg/m² for five days [21]. Cycles were repeated every four weeks. All but one of the patients had been previously treated. The median number of prior treatment regimens was two. More than half the patients [35] had intermediate to high grade histology with low grade histology being noted in 27 patients. The overall response rate was 30%. Hochster confirmed the association of response in low grade lymphomas and the disappointing response in intermediate and high grade histologies. Myelosuppression was noted in that study to be the major morbidity. Subsequently, both Whelan and Zinzani have published the results of their clinical trials in 25 and 21 patients [22,23]. The response rates were above 60% in both studies for previously treated patients and 75% for the previously untreated patients [6/8] in Zinzani's study. Thus, Fludara has been noted to have substantial activity in low grade lymphoma in a broad range of phase I and phase II studies.

Combination Studies

Phase I studies of Fludara have been conducted with Fludara combined with mitoxantrone and dexamethasone (FMD) in low grade lymphoma (the phase I studies found a response rate of 15/21 with the combination FMD) [24]. Recommended dose for phase II studies is Fludara 25mg/m²/day for three days, mitoxantrone 10mg/m² on day one and dexa methasone 20mg per day on days 1–5 [25]. Cycles are repeated every four weeks. Twenty-eight patients are evaluable. Thirty-two percent achieved a CR and 50% a PR with 89% overall response rate. These studies are continuing and have now been inserted as a comparative arm in frontline treatment of low grade lymphoma. The major toxicity which was noted in this study was *Pneumocystis carinii* pneumonia which may be associated with a concomitant use of corticosteroids with the purine analogue.

Future Studies in CLL and LGL

The marked diversity of interactions of Fludara with DNA damaging drugs and radiation gives rise to a number of future possibilities [4]. Fludarabine enhances the formation of ara-C triphosphate in AML and CLL cells and the combination of Fludara/ara-C has activity in refractory patients [26,27]. Fludara also inhibits the repair of DNA damage associated with cisplatinum and a combination of Fludara, ara-C, and cisplatinum has been used in refractory CLL and low grade lymphoma with promising early results [28,29]. The radiation sensitization potential of Fludara should also be considered in the management of lymphoma with radiation [30]. Fludara is the most active single agent in the treatment of CLL and one of the most active single agents noted in low grade lymphoma. Increasing use of this drug should take into consideration its myelosuppressive and immunosuppressive potential.

References

1. Montgomery JA, Hewson K: Nucleosides of 2-fluoroadenine. J Med Chem 12: 498–504, 1969
2. Von Hoff DD: Phase I clinical trials with fluda rabine phosphate. Semin Oncol 17: 33–38, 1990 (suppl 1)
3. Grever MR, Leiby J, Kraut E, et al: A comprehensive phase I and II clinical investigation of fludarabine phosphate. Semin Oncol 17:39–48, 1990 (suppl 8)
4. Plunkett W, Gandhi V, Huang P, et al: Fludarabine: Pharmacokinetics, mechanisms of action, and rationales for combination therapies. Semin Oncol 20: 2–12, 1993
5. Grever MR, Coltman CA, Files JC, et al: Fludarabine monophosphate in chronic lymphocytic leukemia. Blood 68: 223a, 1986 (suppl 1) (abstr)
6. Keating MJ, Kantarjian H, Talpaz M, et al: Fludarabine: A new agent with major activity against chronic lymphocytic leukemia. Blood 74: 19–25, 1989
7. O'Brien S, Kantarjian H, Beran M, et al: Results of fludarabine and prednisone therapy in 264 patients with chronic lymphocytic leukemia with multivariate analysis derived prognostic model for response to treatment. Blood 82: 1695–1700, 1993
8. Kemena A, O'Brien S, Kantarjian H, et al: Phase II clinical trial of fludarabine in chronic lymphocytic leukemia on a weekly low-dose schedule. Leuk Lymphoma 10: 187–193, 1993
9. Robertson LE, O'Brien S, Koller C, et al: A three-day schedule of fludarabine in chronic lymphocytic leukemia. Blood, in press
10. Keating MJ, Kantarjian H, O'Brien S, et al: Fludarabine: A new agent with marked cytoreductive activity in untreated chronic lymphocytic leukemia. J Clin Oncol 9: 44–49, 1991
11. Robertson LE, Huh YO, Butler JJ, et al: Response assessment in chronic lymphocytic leukemia after fludarabine plus prednisone: Clinical, pathologic, immunophenotype, and molecular analysis. Blood 80: 29–36, 1992
12. Keating MJ: Immunosuppression with purine analogues – The flip side of the gold coin. Ann Oncol 4: 347–348, 1993
13. Keating MJ, O'Brien S, Kantarjian H, et al: Long-term follow-up of patients with chronic lymphocytic leukemia treated with fludarabine as a single agent. Blood 81: 2878–2884, 1993
14. Fenchel K, Bergmann L, Jahn B, et al: Fludarabine phosphate in refractory chronic lymphocytic leukemia. Onkologie 14: 190, 1991 (suppl 2)
15. Hiddeman W, Rottman R, Wormann P, et al: Treatment of advanced chronic lymphocytic leukemia by fludarabine: Results of a clinical phase II study. Ann J Hematol 63: 1–4, 1991
16. Puccio CA, Mittelman A, Lichtman SM, et al: A loading dose/continuous infusion schedule of fludarabine phosphate in chronic lymphocytic leukemia. J Clin Oncol 9: 1562–1569, 1991
17. Dimopoulos MA, O'Brien S, Kantarjian H, et al: Fludarabine therapy in Waldenstrom's macroglobulinemia. Am J Med 95: 49–52, 1993
18. Keating MJ, O'Brien S, Plunkett W, et al: Fludarabine phosphate: A new active agent in hematologic malignancies. Semin Hematol 31: 28–39, 1994
19. Leiby JM, Snider KM, Kraut EH, et al: Phase II trial of 9-β-D-arabinofuranosyl-2-fluoroadenine 5′ monophosphate in non-Hodgkin's lymphoma: Prospective comparison of response with deoxycytidine kinase activity. Cancer Res 47: 2719–2722, 1987
20. Redman JR, Cabanillas F, Velasquez WS, et al: Phase II trial of fludarabine phosphate in lymphoma: An effective new agent in low grade lymphoma. J Clin Oncol 10: 790–794, 1992
21. Hochster HS, Kim K, Green MD, et al: Activity of fludarabine in previously treated non-Hodgkin's low grade lymphoma: Results of an Eastern Cooperative Oncology Group study. J Clin Oncol 10: 28–32, 1992
22. Whelan JS, Ganjoo R, Johnson PWM, et al: Treatment of low grade non-Hodgkin's lymphomas with fludarabine. Leuk Lymphoma 10: 35–37, 1993
23. Zinzani PL, Lauria F, Rondelli D, et al: Fludarabine: An active agent in the treatment of previously treated low grade non-Hodgkin's lymphoma. Ann Oncolo 4: 575–578, 1993
24. McLaughlin P, Hagemeister FB, Swan Jr F, et al: Phase I study of the combination of fludarabine, mitoxantrone, and dexamethasone in low grade lymphoma. J Clin Oncol, in press
25. Keating MJ, McLaughlin P, Plunkett W, et al: Fludarabine – Present status and future developments in chronic lymphocytic leukemia and lymphoma. Ann Oncol 5: 79–83, 1994
26. Gandhi V, Plunkett W: Modulation of arabinosyl nucleoside metabolism by arabinosyl nucleotides in human leukemia cells. Cancer Res 48: 329–334, 1988
27. Estey E, Plunkett W, Gandhi V, et al: Fludarabine and arabinosylcytosine therapy of refractory and relapsed acute myelogenous leukemia. Leuk Lymphoma 4: 343–350, 1993
28. Yang LY, Trujillo JM, Keating MJ, et al: Effect of fludarabine on the tumoricidal synergy produced by the combination of arabinosylcytosine and cisplatin in human LoVo colon carcinoma cells. Proc Am Assoc Cancer Res 33: 443, 1992 (abstr)
29. Robertson LE, Kantarjian H, O'Brien S, et al: Cisplatin, fludarabine, and ara-C: A regimen for advanced fludarabine refractory chronic lymphocytic leukemia. Proc Am Soc Clin Oncol 12: 308, 1993 (abstr)
30. Gregoire C, Hunter N, Milas L, et al: Enhancement of radiation response by fludarabine in murine tumor models. Proc Am Assoc Cancer Res 33: 85, 1992 (abstr)

Acute Leukemias V
Experimental Approaches
and Management of Refractory Diseases
Hiddemann et al. (Eds.)

Response to Fludarabine in Patients with Low Grade Lymphoma

A. Pigaditou[1], A. Z. S. Rohatiner[1], J. S. Whelan[1], P. W. M. Johnson[1], R. K. Ganjoo[1], A. Rossi[1], A. J. Norton[2], J. Amess[3], J. Lim[1], and T. A. Lister[1]

Abstract. Eighty-eight adults with low grade lymphoma were treated with Fludarabine phosphate at a dose of 25 mg/m^2 intravenously, daily for five days, every three to four weeks. The response rate was 44% for those who had received prior treatment and 69% for those who had not. The major toxicity was myelosuppression, neutropenia ($< 1.0 \times 10^9$/l) occurring in 55% of previously treated and 31% of previously untreated patients respectively. Further studies will determine the precise role of Fludarabine in the therapy of low grade lymphoma.

Introduction

The clinical course of the low grade lymphomas particularly follicular lymphoma is characterised by repeated regression of lymphadenopathy following relatively innocuous chemotherapy. The regressions are usually incomplete [1–3] and the median survival is between 5 and 10 years, death almost always occurring as a result of the disease [1,2,4,5]. It is therefore heartening that a new class of compounds, the purine analogues is showing promise [6–10]. The results below reflect the experience gained at St. Bartholomew's Hospital in a collaborative trial [11] and a single centre phase II study [12].

Patients and Methods

Patients. Fifty five men and thirty three women, aged 20–82 years commenced therapy with Fludarabine. Thirty nine had 'refractory' and twelve had 'recurrent' (but possibly still responsive to alkylating agent) disease. All of them had received Chlorambucil at least once, and the majority had received an Adriamycin-containing regimen. Twenty one patients were treated with Fludarabine after having been induced into a partial remission with conventional treatment, in the hope that complete remission might be achieved prior to myelo-ablative therapy supported by autologous bone marrow transplantation. Sixteen patients had received no previous treatment (Table 1).

Therapy. Fludarabine was given daily for 5 days, intravenously, at a dose of 25 mg/m^2 over 10 minutes, having been reconstituted in 10 ml of sterile water. This was repeated every three weeks if possible or as dictated by the clinical condition of the patient and the peripheral

Table 1. Clinical characteristics (n:88)

Gender M:F	55:33
Median age (range)	48(20–82 yrs)
Histology (Kiel classification)	
– small lymphocytic (SLL)	1
– lymphoplasmacytoid (LPC)	38
– centroblastic/centrocytic follicular (FL-CB/CC)	29
– centroblastic/centrocytic difuse (DF-CB/CC)	5
– peripheral T-cell (Per-T)	2
– T-zone	3
– low grade unclassified	10

[1] ICRF Dept of Medical Oncology
[2] Department of Histopathology - St. Bartholomew's Hospital
[3] Department of Haematology - St. Bartholomew's Hospital

blood count. The intention was to give two further cycles of therapy after 'maximum response' had been achieved. In practice, therapy was delayed because of cytopenia in 17 patients, with dose reduction in two, because of profound myelosuppression.

Definition. Complete remission was documented when the patient was in normal health, with neither clinical, radiological (computed axial tomography) or morphological (bone marrow) evidence of disease.

Partial remission was defined as having been achieved when there was a greater than 50% reduction in the estimated bulk of tumour in lymph nodes on bone marrow. Lesser responses were considered failure.

Results

Response to therapy. Complete [4] and partial [16] remissions were documented in 20/45 (44%) evaluable 'previously treated patients', there being the same outcome regardless of whether the treatment was given in the recurrent or refractory situation. There were twenty patients in whom therapy failed and five treatment related deaths.

There was an improvement in the degree of response in 9/20 (CR2, PR7) of the patients treated with the intention of proceeding to more intensive therapy.

The response rate was highest in patients who had received no prior therapy, being 11/16 with six complete remissions (Table 2).

Toxicity. The treatment was generally well tolerated although two patients complained of lethargy and one of visual disturbance. There were five potentially treatment related deaths. All occurred in patients who had been previously treated and none were showing evidence of responsiveness to Fludarabine.

The neutrophil count fell below 1.0×10^9/l in 55% of previously treated and 31% of previously untreated patients. Thrombocytopenia was much less common. Infection, including three cases of herpes zoster was documented in 24/49 (49%) of previously treated patients with more than half of them requiring admission to hospital. Five (31%) of the newly diagnosed patients were admitted because of infection.

Discussion

These results confirm the unequivocal activity of Fludarabine against low grade B cell lymphoma. The response rate, exceeding 50% is similar to that achieved with either single agent or combination chemotherapy in patients with recurrent or progressive disease.

The toxicity incurred was 'acceptable' although there is undoubtedly a real risk of infection, probably related to T Cell dysfunction since it may occur when the total peripheral white blood count is normal. In addition, in a subsequent group of patients potential neurological toxicity has been recorded (Johnson personal communication), although it must be emphasised that a causative role for Fludarabine has not been demonstrated.

The critical issue now is how best may Fludarabine be incorporated into the management of patients with follicular lymphoma in 1994. Clinical trials are being conducted to determine how it compares with conventional combination chemotherapy in those with newly diagnosed disease. These will provide valuable information about whether long term freedom from recurrence occurs following Fludabarine alone, in addition to how it compares with 'CVP'. Increasingly it is being used as a second line choice.

Table 2. Response rate according to histology [CR+PR]

Patients	SLL	LPC	FL-CB/CC	DF-CB/CC	PER-T	L-G/unclass	T-zone	Total	(%)
Previously treated	1/1	10/29	5/11	1/2	0/1	3/8	–	20/45	(44)
Partial remission (Pre-ABMT)	–	3/3	6/15	0/1	–	0/1	–	9/20	(45)
Previously untreated	–	6/10/	–	1/1	1/1	1/1	2/3	11/16	(69)

The next decade will reveal the role of Fludarabine in the treatment of follicular lymphoma. Whether this is as a single agent or in combination or sequence with other drugs, as part of palliative or curative therapy, it is a welcome weapon in the therapeutic armamentarium.

Acknowledgements. We are particularly pleased to acknowledge the contribution of the nursing and medical staff of the Bodley Scott Unit for the care of the patients; the expertise of the departments of Pathology and Diagnostic Radiology; the data management staff and secretarial staff of the Medical Oncology Unit for the preparation of the paper.

References

1. Gallagher CJ, Gregory WM, Jones AE, Stansfeld AG, Richards M, Dhaliwal HS, Malpas JS & Lister TA. Follicular lymphoma: prognostic factors for response and survival. J Clin Oncol, 1986; 4: 1470–1480
2. Richards MA, Hall PA, Gregory WM, Dhaliwal HS, Stansfeld AG, Amess JA & Lister TA. Lymphoplasmacytoid and small cell centrocytic non-Hodgkin's lymphoma – a retrospective analysis from St. Bartholomew's Hospital 1972–1986. Haematol Oncol, 1989; 7: 19–35
3. Jones SE, Fuks Z, Bull M et al. Non Hodgkin's lymphoma IV. Clinicopathologic correlation in 405 cases. Cancer, 1973; 31: 806–823
4. Anderson T, De Vita VT, Simon RM et al. Malignant lymphoma II. Prognostic factors and response to treatment of 473 patients at the National Cancer Institute. Cancer, 1982; 50: 2708–2721
5. Brittinger G, Bartels H, Common H et al. Clinical and prognostic relevance of the Kiel Classification of non-Hodgkin's lymphoma. Results of a prospective multi-centre study by the Kiel Lymphoma Group. Haematol Oncol, 1984; 2: 269
6. Hutton JJ, von Hoff DD, Kuhn J, Phillips J, Hersh M & Clark G. Phase I clinical investigation of 9-b-D-arabinofuranosyl-2-fluoroadenine 5′-monophosphate (NSC 312887) a new purine antimetabolite. Cancer Res, 1984; 44: 4183
7. Huang P, Plunkett W. Preferential incorporation of arabinofuranosyl-2-fluoroadenine (F-ara-A) into poly (A+) RNA and its inhibitory effects on transcription and translation. Proc AACR, 1986; 27: 21
8. Leiby JM, Snider KM, Kraut EH et al. Phase II trial of 9-b-D-arabinofuranosyl-2-fluoroadenine 5′-monophosphaate in on-Hodgkin's lymphoma: Prospective comparison of respone with deoxycytidine kinase activity. Cancer Res, 1987; 47: 2719
9. Redman J, Cabanillas F, McLaughlin P & 6 others. Fludarabine phosphate: a new agent with major activity in low grade lymphoma. Proc AACR, 1988; 29: 211
10. Hochster H & Cassileth P. Fludarabine phosphate therapy of non-Hodgkin's lymphoma. Semin Oncol, 1990; 17: 63
11. Whelan JS, Davis CL, Rule S, Ranson M, Smith OP, Mehta AB, Catovsky D, Rohatiner AZ, Lister TA. Fludarabine phosphate for the treatment of low grade lymphoid malignancy. Br J Cancer 1991; 64 (1): 120
12. Whelan JS, Ganjoo RK, Johnson PWM, Rohatiner AZS, Lister TA. Treatment of low grade non-Hodgkin's lymphomas with fludarabine. Leukemia and Lymphoma 1993 10 (Supp) 35–37

Acute Leukemias V
Experimental Approaches
and Management of Refractory Diseases
Hiddemann et al. (Eds.)

Fludarabine in Combination with Mitoxantrone and Dexamethasone in Relapsed and Refractory Low-Grade Non-Hodgkin's Lymphoma

C. Pott, M. Unterhalt, D. S. Sandford, H. Markert, M. Freund, A. Engert, W. Gassmann, W. Holtkamp, M. Seufert, K. Hellriegel, B. Knauf, R. Nieberding, B. Emmerich, P. Koch, B. Wörmann, and W. Hiddemann

Abstract. Fludarabine Phosphate is an active agent in the treatment of patients with low-grade Non-Hodgkin's-Lymphoma. This phase II study was initiated to evaluate the antilymphoma activity and toxicity of a combination therapy of Fludarabine with Mitoxantrone and Dexamethasone (FMD) in the treatment of patients with relapsed or refractory low-grade Non-Hodgkin's-Lymphoma. Up to now, 36 patients from 8 participating centers have been treated with FMD and achieved an over all response rate of 56% with 2 (9%) complete and 11 (47%) partial remissions. All patients were heavily pretreated and had received 2–5 preceeding regimen (median 2). Histologic subtypes included 13 centroblastic-centrocytic NHL, 9 centrocytic NHL, 12 lymphoplasmocytoid immunocytoma, one T-chronic lymphocytic leukemia and one monocytoid B-cell lymphoma, respectively. Treatment associated toxicity was moderate with myelosuppression comprising the major side effect. In contrast to other investigators we did not see an increased risk of infections. Non hematologic toxicity was mild.

Introduction

As we know about the natural history and clinical outcome of chronic lymphocytic leukemia (CLL) and indolent Non-Hodgkin's-Lymphoma (NHL), these diseases follow a continous remitting course and are in general considered to be incurable. Most patients respond to initial therapy but induction of complete remission has shown not to be associated with a prolongation of survival. The overall-survival of patients with low-grade Non-Hodgkin-lymphoma is 6–10 years and no plateau in the survival curve is achieved either with single agent or combination chemotherapy [1–3]. If patients become symptomatic with progressive bone marrow infiltration, lymphadenopathy or organ infiltration, palliative treatment regimen containing alkylating agents, Chlorambucil and Cyclophosphamide alone or in combination with corticosteroids are applied. These agents are able to achieve responses in 60–75% of patients with 10–20% achieving a complete remission [4,5] but all eventually relapse and succumb to progressive disease. The failure to cure low-grade NHL has lead to a variety of therapeutic approaches but there has no standard therapy been identified. Therefore current treatment protocols range from a watch and wait approach to intensive multidrug regimen and even new approaches with myeloablative chemotherapy in selected patient subgroups are under investigation [6–9].

With the development of the structurally related purine analogs Fludarabine Phosphate, 2-Deoxycoformycine and 2-Chlordeoxyadenosine new perspectives in the therapy of low-grade lymphoid malignancies were provided. While 2-Deoxycoformycine and 2-Chlorodeoxyadenosine are mainly effective in the treatment of hairy cell leukemia [10–12], Fludarabine has shown to be effective in the treatment of chronic lymphocytic leukemia (CLL) [13–17] and low-grade NHL, predominantly of the follicular subtype [18–25]. A number of phase I and II

Department of Hematology and Oncology, University of Göttingen, Göttingen, Germany, for the German Low-Grade Non-Hodgkin's-Lymphoma Study Group

studies have shown a significant activity of Fludarabine in the treatment chronic lymphocytic leukemia (CLL) and relapsed or refractory low-grade NHL [8–11]. In five different studies for the treatment of patients with relapsed or refractory low-grade NHL with a Fludarabine monotherapy response rates ranging from 31–38% were seen with complete remissions in 4–18% and partial remissions in 15–30% of the cases (Table 1).

The ability of Fludarabine to inhibit DNA repair makes it a potent partner for other chemotherapeutic agents. It has shown to enhance the crosslinking of Cisplatinum in LoVo cell lines and seems to neutralize Cisplatinum resistence [26–28]. Mitoxantrone, an anthracenedione, has shown significant activity in a broad spectrum of lymphomas particularly in low-grade NHL, inducing response rates of 95% in primarily untreated patients and 30–67 % in patients with relapsed NHL [29,30]. The mechanism of action of Mitoxantrone is induction of DNA strand-breaks, whereas Fludarabine is supposed to inhibit DNA repair by interference with some key enzymes in DNA synthesis. At high concentrations F-Ara-A has additional inhibitory effects on RNA and protein synthesis [31,32]. Basis of a combination therapy of Fludarabine and Mitoxantrone is the assumption, that effects of both substances on DNA damage may act synergistically.

There is only very limited experience with Fludarabine in combination with other myelosuppressive agents. The experimental data of synergistic effects of Fludarabine and Mitoxantrone were basis of a phase I study of a combination therapy conducted by McLaughlin et al. (1992) in 18 relapsed NHL patients which was primarily directed towards defining the optimal drug dosage and schedule [33]. Evaluating five escalation steps a combination of Fludarabine 25 mg/m^2/d day 1–3, Mitoxantrone 10 mg/m^2/d day 1 and Dexamethasone 20 mg/m^2 day 1–5 was found tolerable. The response rate of 72% was significantly higher than comparable results of a Fludarabine monotherapy.

On the basis of these results the German Cooperative NHL Study Group initiated a phase II study for the treatment of relapsed low-grade NHL to investigate the antilymphoma activity and toxicity of Fludarabine in combination with Mitoxantrone and Dexamethasone (FMD) in the treatment of patients with relapsed or refractory low grade NHL.

Patients and Methods

Patient population. Patients were primarily recruited from the multicenter trial of the German Cooperative NHL Study Group with a randomized comparison of two different induction regimen (COP versus PmM) followed by Interferone alpha maintenance or observation only [34]. Criteria for the evaluation of FMD were the rate of complete and partial remission and the duration of a subsequent event free interval as well as the incidence and severity of treatment related side effects.

We included patients with recurrent or refractory NHL who had progressive or bulky disease and required therapy as defined by the presence of B-symptoms and/or signs of impairment of the hematopoetic system. The following histologic subtypes have presently been included into the study: 13 centroblastic-centrocytic NHL, 9 centrocytic NHL, 12 lymphoplasmocytoid immunocytoma, one T-chronic lymphocytic leukemia and one monocytoid B-cell lymphoma.

Table 1. Results of Fludarabine monotherapy in the literature

Reference	No. of Patients	Regimen mg/m^2/d	Clinical response (%)		
			CR	PR	total
Hochster al.(1992)[21]	60	18	9(15)	9(15)	18(30)
Leiby et al.(1987)[19]	25	20+30x	1(4)	7(28)	8(32)
Redman et al.(1992)[20]	60	20–30	5(8)	18(30)	23(38)
Whelan et al.(1991)[22]	34	25	6(18)	7(20)	13(38)
Hiddemann et al.(1993)[23]	38	25	5(13)	7(18)	12(31)
Pigaditou et al. (1994)[24]	45	25	4(9)	16(36)	20(44)
Zinzani et al.(1993)[18]	21	25	3(14)	11(52)	14(67)
Dumontet et al.(1993)[25]	50	25	4(8)	26(52)	30(60)

All patients were required to have adequate marrow function unless caused by lymphoma infiltration of the bone marrow with granulocytes >1500/µl and platelets >100.000/µl liver function (bilirubin <2.0 mg/dl), renal function (creatinine <1.5 mg/dl) as well as a sufficient cardiac function. Dose reduction was assigned in case of treatment associated myelosuppression not related to bone marrow involvement.

Patients were excluded from the study if there was any possibility of primary potentially curative radiotherapy or if they were older than 75 years.

Tumor response and toxicity were evaluated and graded according to WHO criteria. Complete remission (CR) was defined as absence of all signs of disease for more than four weeks including normalization of peripheral blood counts with granulocytes >1500/mm^3, Hb >12 g/dl and platelets >100.000/mm^3. Partial remission (PR) was defined as more than 50% decrease of all measurable lymphoma manifestations for at least 4 weeks and normalization of peripheral blood counts. Remission duration was committed as the time from documentation of remission until relapse. As survival we defined the period from first day of therapy until death.

Treatment plan. Preceding initial therapy, dianostic staging procedures including physical examination, chest X-ray, abdominal sonography, bone marrow aspirate and biopsy and computed tomography scan was performed. Repeated evaluation of involved sites of disease were done after every two cycles. Fludarabine was administered at a dose of 25 mg/m^2/d by a 30 minute infusion on day 1–3 together with Mitoxantrone 10 mg/m^2/d on day 1 as a 30 minute infusion and Dexamethasone 20 mg/d on days 1–5 orally. Cycles were repeated every 28 days for an initial series of 4 courses. Further treatment was adapted to response as follows: Patients achieving a complete remission after 4 cycles received 2 further courses of therapy as consolidation and no further treatment subsequently.

Patients with CR or PR after 6 cycles received also 2 further courses of therapy until a maximum of 8 courses, independent whether a CR or PR was achieved. Patients with minor response or stable disease after 4 cycles were excluded from the study as well as patients with progressive NHL at any stage.

Results

Until now, 36 patients from 8 participating centers have entered the study and 150 cycles of therapy are currently evaluable. Histologic subtypes included 13 centroblastic-centrocytic (CB-CC) NHL, 9 centrocytic (CC) NHL, 12 lymphoplasmocytoid immunocytoma (LP-IC), one T-chronic lymphocytic leukemia and one monocytoid B-cell lymphoma.

All patients were heavily pretreated and had received 2–5 preceeding regimens (median 2). Looking on the temporal course from first diagnosis until start of therapy with FMD an average period of 4 years of disease (range 1/2–15 years) was revealed. (Fig. 1).

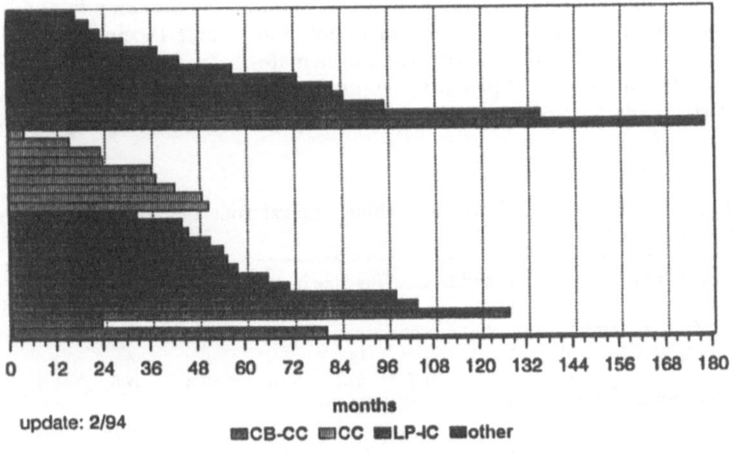

Fig. 1. Time between first diagnosis and start of therapy with Fludarabine

It is apparent that patients with centrocytic NHL have a shorter course of disease due to a more aggressive behaviour of this lymphoma subtype.

According to the normal age distribution observed in patients with low-grade NHL the patient population in our study comprised of mainly elderly patients with the majority being older than 50 years.

Presently we can evaluate 32 patients who have completed at least 2 cycles of therapy. A total of 150 courses have been administered so far. Of 32 evaluable patients 14 (41%) achieved a PR. After 4 cycles 23 patients were evaluable for response. 2 (8.7%) achieved a complete (CR) and 11(47.8%) achieved a partial remission (PR), this is an over all response rate of 56% (Table 2). At present evaluation our results are preliminary yet and the response rate of 56% relates to the evaluation after 4 courses of therapy because the study is still ongoing. 18 patients experienced a minimal response or stable disease after 4 cycles of therapy and 5 patients died during treatment. From these 5 deaths there was 1 patient who died from myocardial infraction apparently not associated to lymphoma therapy and 4 patients died from infections or progressive disease respectively. Presently there seems to be no correlation of probability of response and the number of prior therapies. In contrast to experiences with chronic lymphocytic leukemia response to Fludarabine required a longer time of treatment and remissions did not occur before 3–4 treatment cycles (Table 2).

Analysis of the side effects shows that acute toxicity of FMD was mild. Only a few cases of nausea and vomiting occured as we have seen in previous studies [23]. The main treatment associated side effects of FMD consisted in hematotoxicity. 20–30% of the patients presented with a WHO grade 3–4 toxicity (Table 3). Platelets were mainly affected with 20 % of patients having grade 3–4 toxicity but only a few moderate bleeding complications resulted from that. Almost 30 % of the patients experienced a severe neutropenia (WHO grade 3–4) which did not contribute to a high incidence of grade 3–4 severe infections, which we observed in only 6 % of cases.

Table 3. Toxicity of the combination Fludarabine, Mitoxantrone and Dexamethasone in NHL patients

Toxicity of Fludarabine, Mitoxantrone and Dexamethasone	n	grade 1+2	grade 3+4
hemoglobin	133	28%	8%
leukocytes	134	33%	12%
neutrophils	93	24%	20%
platelets	136	17%	17%
bleeding	114	3%	0%
nausea/vomitting	115	10%	0%
mucositis	114	4%	4%
alopecia	116	9%	1%
infections	118	20%	4%
cardiac dysfunction	117	3%	5%
per. neurotoxicity	118	3%	0%
CNS toxicity	119	7%	0%

There seems to be no cumulative hematotoxicity because almost no dose reduction was necessary due to therapy induced myelosuppression.

Discussion

The current study clearly demonstrates that Fludarabine in combination with Mitoxantrone and Dexamethasone (FMD) is effective in the treatment of heavily pretreated patients with relapsed NHL and has shown an acceptable toxicity. Our group could show in a previous phase

Table 2. Preliminary results of Fludarabine, Mitoxantrone and Dexamethasone (FMD) in combination therapy

Fludarabine, Mitoxantrone and Dexamethasone in relapsed low-grade NHL	n	eval.	CR	PR	MR	SD	PD	EX	AB	
after course 2:	36	34	0	14	3	9	4	2	2	
			0.0	41.2	8.8	26.4	11.8	5.9	5.9	%
after course 4:	26	23	2	11	2	4	2	0	2	
			8.7	47.8	8.7	17.4	8.7	0.0	8.7	%
after course 6:	19	13	1	4	1	0	3	3	1	
			7.7	30.8	7.7	0.0	23.1	23.1	7.7	%

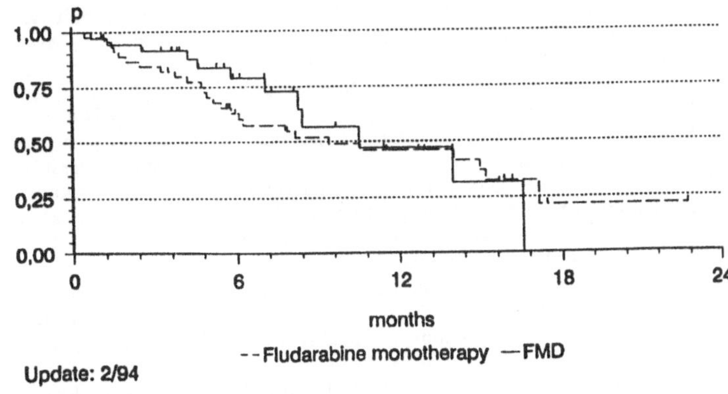

Fig. 2. Survival curves of patients treated with Fludarabine as single agent and in combination (FMD)

II trial for the treatment of relapsed low grade NHL [23] that an over all response rate of 31 % is achieved with Fludarabine as single agent. These results correspond to the response rates found in the literature (Table 1). From 44 evaluable patients treated with Fludarabine as single agent 7 patients achieved a PR after 2 cycles of therapy, none a complete remission. After 4 treatment courses we observed 2 patients with a CR (6.7 %) and 8 patients (26.7 %) with a PR. Although our results for FMD therapy are preliminary yet the combination appears to be more effective with an overall response rate of 56 % after 4 cycles of therapy. These data thus confirm previous reports of McLaughlin [33] who could show remission rates of 72 % in relapsed low-grade NHL patients.

In the treatment of chronic lymphocytic leukemia (CLL) with Fludarabine peripheral lymphocytosis responded rapidly to therapy followed by a regression of lymphnode size and hepatosplenomegaly [35]. In contrast to experiences with chronic lymphocytic leukemia response to FMD required a longer phase of treatment and remissions did not occur before 3–4 treatment cycles.

Analysis of the survival of patients after a treatment with Fludarabine as single agent have been shown in our previous study and patients who achieved a CR or PR after Fludarabine treatment have a significant higher probability of survival compared to patients with minimal or no response [23]. A comparison of the survival curves of all patients in the 2 different studies shows that at present evaluation there seems to be no advantage in survival for the patients treated with FMD compared to Fludarabine alone although patients probably achieve higher response rates with the combination therapy (Fig. 2).

But these results are preliminary and a longer follow up time is needed to finally judge the impact of FMD on remission duration and survival.

Treatment related toxicity was acceptable and comprised predominatly myelosuppression. An increased risk of infection was not observed however different authors report contradictory results [35,36].

Undoubtfully Fludarabine has immunesuppressive effects through a depletion of T-cell subsets. Different investigators found a decrease in the absolute CD4+ and CD8+ counts associated with Fludarabine therapy and an increased incidence of opportunistic infections has been discussed [36,37]. On the other hand long term follow up of patients in remission after single agent therapy with Fludarabine revealed no increased incidence of opportunistic infections despite diminished CD4+ counts [37].

Because low-grade malignancies themselves can lead to decreased numbers of T-cells, effects of Fludarabine on the immune system have to be carefully evaluated and long-term observation of these patients is necessary to evaluate the impact of Fludarabine on long-term immune suppression.

References

1. Horning SJ, Rosenberg SA (1984): The natural history of initially untreated low-grade Non-Hodgkin's Lymphoma. N Engl J Med 311:1471

2. Horning SJ (1994): Low-grade lymphoma 1993: State of the art. Ann Oncol 5 (suppl.2), 23
3. Brittinger G, Meusers P, Engelhard M (1986): Strategien der Behandlung von Non-Hodgkin Lymphomen. Internist 27, 485
4. Knospe WH, Loeb B, Huguley CM(1974): Bi-weekly chlorambucil therapy of CLL. Cancer 33, 555
5. Sawitsky A, Rai KR, Glidewell O, Silver RT (1977): Comparison of daily vs intermittent Chlorambucil and prednisone therapy in the treatment of patients with CLL. Blood 50, 1049
6. Young RC, Longo Dl, Glatstein E et al.(1988): The treatment of indolent lymphomas: Watchful waiting versus aggressive combined modality treatment. Semin Hematol 25 (suppl.2), 11
7. Freedman L, Gorin NC, Laporte JCH et al.(1991): Autologous bone marrow transplantation in 69 patients with a history of low-grade Non-Hodgkin's Lymphoma. Blood 77, 2524
8. Schouten HC, Colombat P, Verdonck LF, Gorin NC, Björkstrand B, Taghipour G, Goldstone AH (1994): Autologous bone marrow transplantation for low-grade Non-Hodgkin's lymphoma: The European Bone Marrow Transplant Group Experience. Ann Oncol 5 (suppl.2), 147
9. Rohatiner AZS, Freedman A, Nadler L, Lim J, Lister TA (1994): Myeloablative therapy with autologous bone marrow transplantation as consolidation therapy for follicular lymphoma. Ann Oncol 5 (suppl.2), 143
10. Spiers A, Moore D, Cassileth P, Harrington D, Cummings F, Neiman R et al. (1987): Remissions in hairy cell leukemia with pentostatin (2'-Deoxycoformycin): N Engl J Med 316, 825
11. Cassileth P, Cheuvart B, SWpiers A, Harrington D, Cummings F, Neimann R et al.(1991): Pentostatin induces durable remissions in hairy cell leukemia. J Clin Oncol 9, 243
12. Tallman MS, Hakimian D, Variakojis D et al. (1992): A single course of 2-Chlorodeoxy adenosine results in complete remission in the majority of patients with hairy cell leukemia. Blood 80, 2203
13. Grever MR, Kopecky KJ, Coltman CA, Files JC, Greenberg BR et al. (1988): Fludarabine monophosphate: a potentially useful agent in CLL. Nouv Rev Fr Hematol 30, 457
14. Keating MR, Kantarjian H, Talpaz M, Redman J, Koller C et al. (1989): Fludarabine: a new agent with major activity against CLL. Blood 74, 19
15. Keating MR, Kantarjian H, O'Brien S et al. (1991): Fludarabine: A new agent with marked cytoreductive activity in untreated CLL: J Clin Oncol 9, 44
16. Cheson BD, Vena DA, Sorenson JM et al. (1991): Current status of US: clinical trials in CLL. Leuk Lymph 5, 119
17. Hiddemann W, Rottmann R, Wörmann B, Theil A, Esink M et al. (1991): Treatment of advanced CLL by fludarabine: results of a clinical Phase II study. Annals Hematol 63, 1
18. Zinzani PL, Lauria F, Rondelli D, Benfenati D, Raspadori D, Bocchia M, Bendandi M, Gozzetti A, Zaja F, Fanin R, Russo D, Galieni P, Tura S (1993): Fludarabine: an active agent in the treatment of previously treated and untreated low-grade NHL. Ann Oncol 4, 575
19. Leiby JM, Snider KM, Kraut EH, Metz EN, Malspeis L (1987): Phase II trial of 9-β-D-arabinofuranosyl-2-fluoroadenine-5'-monophosphate in Non-Hodgkin's lymphoma: prospective comparison of response with deoxycytidine kinase activity. Cancer Res 47, 2719
20. Redman JR, Cabanilas F, Velasques WS, McLaughlin P, Hagemeister FB (1992): Phase II trial of Fludarabine Phosphate in lymphoma: an effective agent in low-grade lymphoma. J Clin Oncol 10, 790
21. Hochster HS, Kim K, Green MD, Mann RB, Neimann RS et al. (1992): Activity of fludarabine in previously treated Non Hodgkin's low-grade lymphoma. Results of an Eastern Cooperative Oncology Group Study. J Clin Oncol 10, 28
22. Whelan JS, Davis CL, Rule S, Ranson M, Smith OP et al. (1991): Fludarabine Phosphate for the treatment of low-grade lymphoid malignancy. Br J Cancer 64, 120
23. Hiddemann W, Unterhalt M, Pott C, Wörmann B, Sandford D, Freund M, Engert A, Gassmann W, Holtkamp W, Seufert M, Hellriegel K, Knauf B, Emmerich B, Kanz L, Koch P (1993): Fludarabine single agent therapy for relapsed low grade non-Hodgkin's lymphomas: a phase II study of the German low-grade non-Hodgkin's lymphoma study group. Sem Oncol 20 (5) (suppl.7), 28
24. Pigaditou A, Rohatiner AZS, Whelan JS, Johnson PWM, Ganjoo RK, Rossi A, Norton AJA, Lim J, Lister TA (1994): Fludarabine in low-grade lymphoma. Sem Oncol, in press
25. Dumontet C, Bastion Y, Bazin M, Salles G, Felman P, Bryon PA, Coiffier B (1993): Fludarabine therapy in low-grade NHL: Results of the Lyon Sud experience. Proceedings of the Fifth International Conference on Malignant Lymphoma, p97, Lugano
26. Yang LY, Trujillo JM, Keating M, Plunkett W (1992): Effect of Fludarabine on the tumoricidal synergie produced by the combination of Arabinosylcytosine and Cisplatin in human LoVo colon carcinoma cells. Proc Am Ass Cancer Res 33, 2647 (abstr.)
27. Yang LY, Li L, Trujillo JM, Liu YZ, Plunkett W, Keating M (1993): Fludarabine synergizes Cisplatin cytotoxicity in human LoVo colon carcinoma cells by inhibiting repair of Cisplatin-induced DNA damage. Proc Am Ass Cancer Res 34, 2070 (abstr.)
28. Gregoire V, Huntering N, Milas L, Brock WA, Plunkett W, Hittelman WN (1992): Enhancement of radiation response by Fludarabine in murine tumor models. Proc Am Ass Cancer Res 33, 511 (abstr.)
29. Hansen SW, Nissen NI, Hanssen MM et al.(1988): High activity of Mitoxantrone in previously untreated low-grade lymphoma. Chemother Pharmacol 22: 27
30. Gams RA, Bryan S, Dukart G et al.(1985): Mitoxantrone in malignant lymphoma. Invest New Drugs 3, 219

31. Huang P, Plunkett W (1991): Action of 9-β-D-arabinofuranosyl-2-fluoroadenine on RNA metabolism. Molec Pharmacol 39, 449
32. Ghandi V, Plunkett W (1988): Modulation of arabinosylnucleoside metabolism by arabinosylnucleotides in human leukemia cells. Cancer Res 48, 329
33. McLaughlin P, Swan F, Hagemeister F, Pate O, Romaguera J, Rodriguez M, Redman J, Keating M, Cabanillas F (1992): Phase I study of the combination Fludarabine, Mitoxantrone and Dexamethasone in low-grade lymphoma (LGL). Proc Am Ass Cancer Res 33, 1363 (abstr.)
34. Hiddemann W, Unterhalt M, Koch P, Nahler M, Herrmann R (1994): New aspects in the treatment of advanced low-grade Non-Hodgkin's Lymphomas: Prednimustine/Mitoxantrone (PmM) vs. Cyclophosphamide/ Vincristine/ Prednisone (COP) followed by Interferone – alpha vs. observation only – A preliminary update of the German Low-Grade Lymphoma Study Group. Sem Oncol, in press
35. Bergmann L, Fenchel K, Jahn B, Mitrou PS, Hölzer D (1993): Immunosuppressive effects and clinical response of fludarabine in refractory CLL. Ann Oncol 4, 371
36. O'Brien S, Kantarjian H, Beran M, Smith F, Koller C, Estey E, Robertson LE, Lerner S, Keating M (1993): Results of Fludarabine and Prednisone therapy in 264 patients with chronic lymphocytic leukemia with multivariate analysis-derived prognostic model for response to treatment. Blood 82, 1695
37. Keating M, O'Brien S, Kantarjian H, Plunkett W, Estey E, Koller C, Beran N. Freireich E, (1993): Longterm follow up of patients with CLL treated with fludarabine as a single agent. Blood 81 (11), 2878

Novantrones – Current Status and Future Perspectives

Acute Leukemias V
Experimental Approaches
and Management of Refractory Diseases
Hiddemann et al. (Eds.)

New Anthracyclines – A Comparative Analysis of Efficacy and Toxicity

Anthony D. Ho

Introduction

The anthracyclines doxorubicin and daunorubicin have been a mainstay for the treatment of hematologic and solid tumors for approximately twenty-five years. While daunorubicin has played a major role in the treatment of acute myelogenous leukemias (AML), doxorubicin has been a key component in the chemotherapy of Hodgkin's disease, non-Hodgkin's lymphomas (NHL), breast cancer, small cell lung cancer, as well as a series of other solid tumors. Other than myelotoxicity, one of the major dose limiting side effects of the anthracyclines is cardiotoxicity. Since the mid-1970s, structurally similar compounds such as the anthracene-diones, and analogues of both daunorubicin and doxorubicin have been synthesized and a few of these compounds have been demonstrated to have improved therapeutic index and have been incorporated into primary and salvage therapy regimens for leukemias, lymphomas and solid tumors. This presentation gives a brief overview on the relative merits of the most commonly used new anthracyclines, idarubicin and epirubicin, as well as mitoxantrone, an anthracene-dione.

4-Demethoxydaunorubicin (Idarubicin)

The daunorubicin analogue idarubicin lacks the methoxyl group in position 4 of the aglycone of the parent compound. It has been tested extensively in experimental leukemias. Early on in the development, several features have indicated that idarubicin is an important agent for acute leukemias. It was shown from phase I and II trials that the drug was active over a broad dose range without significantly increasing extramedullary toxicity, especially cardiotoxicity (Carella et al, 1990). Remission was induced with doses as low as 24 mg/m^2 but escalation to a total dose of 45 mg/m^2 was performed without unacceptable non-hematologic toxicity. This relatively broad therapeutic index has identified idarubicin as an important agent for acute leukemia. Efficacy was found both in acute myeloid (AML) as well as acute lymphoblastic leukemia (ALL) (Petti and Mandelli, 1989; Carella et al, 1990). Subsequently the drug was combined with other agents and encouraging results for relapsed AML and ALL have been developed. Finally three independent randomized trials have demonstrated the superiority of idarubicin over daunorubicin in the treatment of AML, both in inducing complete remission (CR) rates as well as in prolonging the CR-duration and survival (Berman et al, 1991; Vogler et al, 1989; Wiernik et al, 1992).

Another special feature of this drug is that it can be administered orally, even though few data is available on its relative efficacy as compared to the intravenous route of administration. Some early clinical trials have suggested that the oral route of administration might offer some advantage for the treatment of myelodysplasias and elderly patients with AML (Lowenthal, 1987).

Few data has been reported on the activity of idarubicin in lymphomas, multiple myeloma

---

Stem Cell Transplant and Malignant Hematology Program, University of California, San Diego Cancer Center, 8421, San Diego, California 92103-8421 U.S.A.

and in other solid tumors and the role of this drug in these diseases has not yet been defined.

4-Epidoxorubicin (Epirubicin)

Epirubicin is a semisynthetic analogue of doxorubicin that differs from the parent molecule in an epimerization of the 4-OH group of doxorubicin. In advanced breast cancer, monotherapy with epirubicin shows an antitumor effect comparable to that of doxorubicin but better subjective tolerance and less cardiac toxicity (Hayat et al, 1989). In randomized trials comparing the relative efficacy and toxicity of 5FU, doxorubicin and cyclophosphamide (CAF) versus CEF (epirubicin instead of doxorubicin), similar antitumor activity has been demonstrated as regards response rate, duration of response, time to progression (TTP) and survival (Hayat et al, 1989; Armand et al, 1984). However, patients treated with the FEC regimen experienced overall better tolerance and cardiac toxicity was reduced. Based on these encouraging results, the use of weekly doses versus every-4-week administration (Blomqvist et al, 1993) and intensified schedule of epirubicin to 50mg/m^2 on days 1 and 8 have recently been explored (Focan et al, 1993). In the latter study, a significant improvement in response rate, response duration and time to progression was observed for the epirubicin-intensified group. Except for myelotoxicity and stomatitis, which are more frequent in the group receiving the double dose of epirubicin, no significant difference in other extramedullary side effects were observed. These studies all indicate that myelotoxicity instead of cardiotoxicity is the limiting factor for dose escalation with epirubicin. The use of hematopoietic growth factors might then offset this side effect and facilitate delivery of intensified epirubicin dosage in a safe manner to accomplish a maximum tumor reduction in breast cancer.

The experience with epirubicin in other solid tumors or malignant lymphomas is less extensive than in breast cancer. A recent report on patients with diffuse large-cell lymphoma showed that a higher proportion of patients could receive 100% of the planned anthracycline dose by replacing epirubicin for doxorubicin in an 8-week short combination regimen P/DOCE (consisting of epirubicin, vincristine, cyclophosphamide, etoposide and prednisone) for patients aged 65 to 85 (O'Reilly et al, 1993). The rate of grade 3 and 4 mucositis is 18% in patients who received doxorubicin versus 7% in those who received epirubicin. Overall, the regimen is equal in efficacy and similar in toxicity to 3 months of chemotherapy administered on a weekly basis and, for that matter, similar to the results reported in the literature for longer, anthracycline-based chemotherapy treatment. Thus a regimen with a very brief course of administration is attractive for elderly patients and causes minimization of the duration of toxicity.

Mitoxantrone

Since its introduction into clinical trials in 1979, mitoxantrone, an anthracene-dione, has been studied extensively. As a single agent, it has demonstrated promising activity in relapsed and refractory AML or ALL, Hodgkin's disease and NHL, breast cancer as well as other solid tumors (Prentice et al, 1985; Coams et al, 1985; Ho et al 1990; Neidhart et al, 1983). It seems to possess similar activity spectrums as both daunorubicin and doxorubicin but with less cardiac toxicity, less subjective side effects as nausea and vomitting, and less rate of alopecia. Mitoxantrone in combination with high dose or standard dose cytarabine, or in combination with etoposide has shown significant activity against relapsed or primary refractory AML (Paciucci et al, 1987; Hiddemann et al, 1987; Ho et al, 1988).

Moreover, these phase I and II studies provided evidence that there was no absolute cross-resistance between mitoxantrone and the anthracyclines. Patients with AML or ALL who were refractory to anthracyclines can still achieve a CR to mitoxantrone (Hiddemann et al, 1987; Ho et al, 1988). In the mean time this drug plays an important role in the primary treatment for leukemia, NHL, and breast cancer. Replacement of daunorubicin or doxorubicin in standard regimens for AML, ALL or metastatic breast cancer with an equivalent dose of mitoxantrone has produced similar response rates but induced less side effects such as nausea/vomiting, stomatitis, alopecia, or cardiac toxicity (Arlin et al, 1990; Ho et al, 1990; Haas et al, 1994; Bezwoda et al, 1994). Arlin et al (1990) compared daunorubicin combined with cytarabine versus mitoxantrone 12 mg/m^2/d substituted for daunorubicin in the regimen for

3 days and showed that patients treated with mitoxantrone were more likely to achieve CR with one induction course. Therapy with mitoxantrone also reduced the need for antibiotics and transfusions. A greater number of patients also failed daunorubicin plus cytarabine due to persistent leukemia, thus suggesting that equitoxic mitoxantrone containing regimens are better therapy than daunorubicin regimens for patients with newly diagnosed AML.

Similar observations of at least equivalent efficacy but significantly better tolerence and less toxicity have been reported in randomized trials comparing CAF (cyclophosphamide, doxorubicin and 5FU) versus CNF (replacing doxorubicin with mitoxantrone) in metastatic breast cancer (Neidhart et al, 1985; and recently also in a randomized trial comparing CHOP versus CNOP in malignat NHL (Bezwoda et al, 1994).

In all clinical trials, the extramedullary toxicity profile of mitoxantrone has been favorable when compared with the first generation anthracyclines administered in equivalent myelosuppressive dose. This observation, in conjunction with in vitro studies demonstrating a steep dose-response relationship for mitoxantrone in human tumor clonogenic assays (Grant et al, 1991), has made mitoxantrone an ideal drug for dose intensification. It has recently been reported that escalation of mitoxantrone far beyond the conventional dose range is possible without undue toxicity in acute leukemia. Feldman et al (1993) showed that mitoxantrone pharmacokinetics remained relatively linear with doses of up to 80 mg/m^2 and that dose ranges between 40mg to 80mg/m^2 combined with high-dose cytarabine can be administered safely in treatment of patients with AML. Dose levels of 80mg/m^2 administered over 15 minutes as a single intravenous infusion have led to a CR rate of 85% in untreated and relapsed patients with AML or ALL.

Future Directions

As mitoxantrone and the new anthracyclines idarubicin and epirubicin are associated with less cardiotoxicity, less distressful side effects such as nausea/vomitting or mucositis, myelotoxicity has become the major dose limiting toxicity. This special feature render them ideal targets for dose intensification with hematopoietic growth factor support. Recently, we have exploited a dose intensified regimen CEF (cyclophosphamide and 5FU both at 750mg/m^2, and epirubicin at 100mg/m^2) as induction regimen for patients with metastatic breast cancer and simultaneously as mobilization regimen for hematopoietic stem cells (Ho et al, 1993). Two to three cycles were administered to achieve a maximum response and the stem cells collected were used for a mega-dose regimen containing mitoxantrone. This pilot study showed very encouraging preliminary results in terms of safety and efficacy. Further regimens using double transplants have in the mean time been developed to maximize the effects of mitoxantrone, epirubicin and alkylating agents to improve the long-term outcome of patients with metastatic breast cancer, especially those with poor-risk factors.

Furthermore, mitoxantrone has demonstrated no absolute cross-resistance to the anthracyclines. The Goldie-Coldman hypothesis suggests that clones of malignant cells resistant to individual cytotoxic agents might be present primarily. Treatment with a combination of cytotoxic drugs that are non cross-resistant and applied sequentially might circumvent the growth advantage of such clones. Based on the premise that higher remission rates could be achieved if alternating regimens with non cross-resistant drugs are administered as soon as no adequate response to first line treatment is observed, we have initiated a pilot study using flexible numbers of courses of idarubicin/cytarabine (IDAC) or mitoxantrone/etoposide (NOVE) for the primary treatment of AML (Haas et al, 1993). Patients were all treated initially with IDAC and those achieving CR or PR received a second cycle of IDAC. Those failing to respond to IDAC received NOVE as the second course. Patients achieving CR or PR after two cycles of IDAC or one cycle each or IDAC and NOVE received a subsequent cycle of NOVE as early consolidation therapy. Of 54 patients evaluable for response, 46 (85%) achieved a CR, 32 did so after one course of IDAC, 10 after the second cycle of IDAC and 4 further patients after treatment with NOVE. This strategy has now been modified slightly to switch the primary treatment to NOVE if no CR is achieved with the initial attempt with IDAC, and has become a collaborative multicenter protocol for patients with de novo AML.

References

1. Arlin Z, Case DC Jr, Moore J, et al: Randomized multicenter trial of cytosine arabinoside with mitoxantrone or daunorubicin in previously untreated adult patients with acute nonlymphocytic leukemia (ANLL). Leukemia 4: 177–183, 1990
2. Armand JP: Phase II and phase III studies with epirubicin in breast cancer in France, in Bonnadonna G (ed.): Advances in Anthracycline Chemotherapy: Epirubicin, Milan, Italy, Masson, 1984, pp75–82
3. Berman E, Geller G, Santorsa J, et al: Results of a randomized trial comparing idarubicin and cytosine arabinoside with daunorubicin and cytosine arabinoside in adults patients with newly diagnosed acute myelogenous leukemia. Blood 77: 1666–1674, 1991
4. Bezwoda W, Rastogi R, Richards, E, et al: A multicenter randomized, comparative phase III trial of CHOP vs. CNOP regimens in patients with intermediate and high-grade lymphoma. J Clin Oncol (in press, 1994)
5. Blomqvist C, Elomaa I, Rissanen P, et al: Influence of treatment schedule on toxicity and efficacy of cyclophosphamide, epirubicin and fluorouracil in metastatic breast cancer: A randomized trial comparing weekly and every-4-week administration. J Clin Oncol 11: 467–473, 1993
6. Carella AM, Berman E, Maraone MP, et al: Idarubicin in the treatment of acute leukemias. An overview of preclinical and clinical studies. Haematologica 75: 1–7, 1990
7. Coams RA, Ryan S, Dukart G, et al: Mitoxantrone in malignant lymphoma. Invest New Drugs 3: 219–222,1985
8. Feldman EJ, Alberts DS, Ahmed T, et al: Phase I clinical and pharmacokinetic evaluation of high-dose mitoxantrone in combination with cytarabine in patients with acute leukemia. J Clin Oncol 11: 2002–2009, 1993
9. Focan C, Andrien JM, Closon MTh, et al: Dose-response relationship of epirubicin-based first-line chemotherapy for advanced breast cancer: A prospective randomized trial. J Clin Oncol 11: 1253–1263, 1993
10. Grant S, Arlin Z, Gewitz D, et al: Effect of pharmacologically relevant concentrations of mitoxantrone on the in vitro growth of leukemic blast progenitors. Leukemia 5: 336–339, 1991
11. Hayat M, Ostronoff A, Ibrahim A: Epirubicin in breast cancer. Adv Oncol 2: 49–63, 1989
12. Haas R, Ho AD, Del Valle F, et al: Idarubicin/cytosine arabinoside and mitoxantrone/etoposide for the treatment of de novo acute myelogenous leukemia. Semin Oncol 20(Supp 8): 20–26, 1993
13. Ho AD, Lipp T, Ehninger G, et al: Combination of mitoxantrone and etoposide in refractory acute leukemia – an active and well-tolerated regimen. J Clin Oncol 6: 213–217, 1988
14. Ho AD, Del Valle F, Engelhard M, et al: Mitoxantrone/high-dose Ara-C and recombinant human GM-CSF in the treatment of refractory non-Hodgkin's lymphoma. Cancer 66: 423–420, 1990
15. Ho AD, Glück, Germond C, et al: Optimal timing for collections of blood progenitor cells following induction chemotherapy and granulocyte-macrophage colony-stimulating factor for autologous transplantation in advanced breast cancer. Leukemia 7: 1738–1746, 1993
16. Lowenthal RM: A possible special role for oral idarubicin in the treatment of leukemia following myelodysplastic syndrome, in Mandelli F (ed): Idarubicin in the Treatment of Acute Leukemia. Amsterdam, the Netherlands, Excerpta Medica, 1987, pp 50–55
17. Neidhart JA, Gochnour D, Roach RW, et al: Mitoxantrone versus doxorubicin in advanced breast cancer: a randomized cross-over trial. Cancer Treat Rev 10(Supp B): 41–46, 1983
18. O'Reilly SE, Connors JM, Howdle S, et al: In search of an optimal regimen for elderly patients with advanced-stage diffuse large-cell lymphoma: Results of a phase II study of P/DOCE chemotherapy. J Clin Oncol 11: 2250–2257, 1993
19. Petti MC, Mandelli F: Idarubicin in acute leukemias: Experience of the Italian cooperative group GIMEMA. Semin Oncol 16: 10–15, 1989 (Supp2)
20. Prentice HG, Robbins G, Ma DD, Ho AD: Sequential studies on the role of mitoxantrone in the treatment of acute leukemia. Cancer Treatment Rev (Supp B) 10: 57–63, 1983
21. Stiff PJ, McKenzie RS, Alberts DS, et al: Phase I clinical and pharmacokinetic study of high-dose mitoxantrone combined with carboplatin, cyclophosphamide, and autologous bone marrow rescue: High response rate for refractory ovarian carcinoma. J Clin Oncol 12: 176–183, 1994
22. Vogler WR, Velez-Garcia E, Omura G et al: A phase III trial comparing daunorubicin combined with cytosine arabinoside in acute myelogenous leukemia. Seminars Oncol 17: 21–24, 1989
23. Wiernik PH, Banks PLC, Case DC Jr, et al: Cytarabine plus idarubicin or daunorubicin as induction and consolidation therapy for previously untreated adult patient with acute myeloid leukemia. Blood 79: 313–319, 1992

Acute Leukemias V
Experimental Approaches
and Management of Refractory Diseases
Hiddemann et al. (Eds.)

Hematologic and Therapeutic Effects of High-Dose AraC/Mitoxantrone (HAM) in the Induction Treatment of Patients with Newly Diagnosed AML. A Trial by AML Cooperative Group

T. Büchner, W. Hiddemann, B. Wörmann, A. Boeckmann, H. Löffler, W. Gaßmann, G. Maschmeyer, W.-D. Ludwig, E. Lengfelder, A. Heyll, B. Lathan, G. Innig, E. Augion Freire-Innig, K. Buntkirchen, M. C. Sauerland, and A. Heinecke

Abstract. In a multicenter randomised trial in newly diagnosed AML under age 60 double induction using TAD-HAM was more effective than TAD-TAD by more remissions in slow responders ($p = .03$) and a trend to higher overall remission and 5 year remission rates. In the TAD-HAM arm a progressive delay of blood cell recovery times from course to course suggests an impairment of normal and possibly also of leukemic stem cells which can explain the 40% continuous remissions in unselected patients.

Introduction

The combination of high dose AraC with mitoxantrone (HAM) has been introduced into first line treatment of AML as an approach to very early intensification and as a part of the double induction strategy [1]. HAM emerged from promising results with high dose AraC in refractory AML [2,3], intensified consolidation [4,5] and from recent preliminary data also in remission induction [6]. In combination with mitoxantrone high dose AraC was first administered in patients with refractory AML where it proved highly effective [7]. Both partner drugs of HAM exhibit differential non-hematologic toxicities with cerebellar dysfunction being typically observed in some patients after high dose AraC [8] and congestive heart failure resulting from treatment with mitoxantrone, mainly when acumulating with previously applied anthracyclines [9,10]. 10 fold overdosage of mitoxantrone in 5 patients resulted in 3 severe and 1 moderate cardiotoxicities while 2 patients died early due to tumor progression (11,12,one own observation). In all 5 patients three of whom treated for acute leukemias severe neutropenia and thrombocytopenia occurred but was reversible after 18–35 days from the overdosage.

In the 1986 trial of the AML Cooperative Group HAM was used as second induction course starting routinely on day 21 even in aplasia with no residual bone marrow blasts (double induction), and was randomly compared with conventional dose 6-thioguanine/ AraC/ daunorubicin (TAD).

Patients and Methods

Patients under age 60 with newly diagnosed AML were initially randomized to receive double induction by the sequence of TAD-TAD or TAD-HAM before responders received TAD consolidation and 3 year maintenance by monthly reduced TAD courses as published before [13]. HAM was AraC 3 g/m^2 q 12 h day 1–3 and mitoxantrone 10 mg/m^2 day 3–5.

Results

665 patients 16–59 years of age were randomised, entered treatment and were evaluated. As hematological effects we compared the recovery times of neutrophils and platelets after the two induction courses and the consolidation

Department of Medicine, Hematology/ Oncology, University Münster, Germany

course both sequentially and between the two randomised arms. Recovery times after the second courses (TAD vs HAM) were documented by all participating centers whereas data for the first courses and consolidations restrict to one center (Münster). Results are shown in Figure 1.

Table 1 shows data of response to induction treatment.

Among the responders 12 (6%) in the TAD-TAD arm and 20 (8%) in the TAD-HAM arm died while in remission, most of them in hypoplasia after consolidation. The event free survival (events are non-achievement of remission, death or relapse) of all patients shows a median of 10 months with 25% continuing event

Table 1. Response to double induction treatment

Double induction	TAD-TAD	TAD-HAM	p
Patients	329	336	
Complete remissions (CR)	216 (66%)	244 (73%)	
Hypoplastic deaths	53 (16%)	42 (12%)	
Persistent leukemia	60 (18%)	50 (15%)	
CR if day 16 blasts > 40%	12/48 (25%)	27/60(45%)	.03

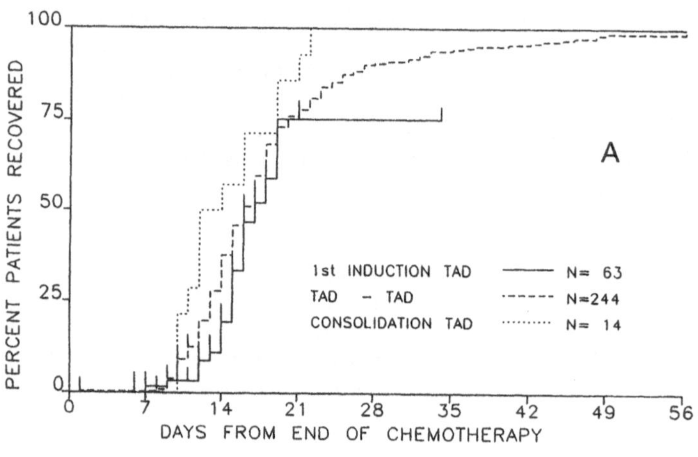

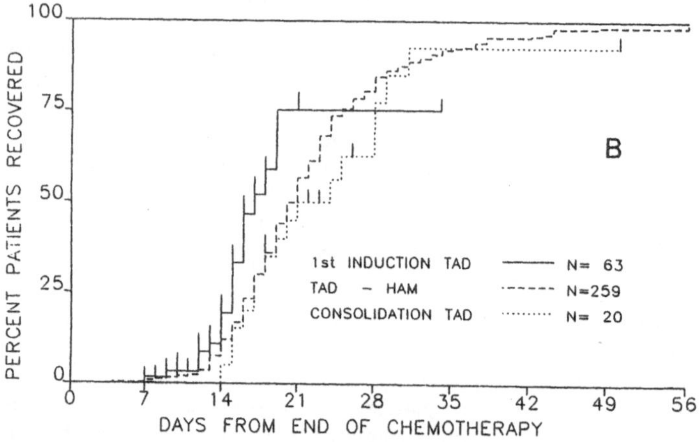

Fig. 1. Kaplan-Meier plots of recovery time of peripheral blood neutrophils to 500/cmm and platelets to 20.000/cmm after chemotherapy for the first induction, the second induction and the consolidation course. Tic marks indicate patients not recovered at this time. **A** = second induction with TAD, **B** = second induction with HAM. Differences between **A** and **B** are significant for second induction (p = .0001) and for consolidation (p = .0001)

free survival in the TAD-HAM arm vs 9 months and 17% in the TAD-TAD arm (p = 0.13).

Figure 2 shows remission duration for the two double inductions compared. Once randomised and entered induction treatment no exclusions were done during the further course. Patients receiving bone marrow transplantation in first remission were censored at the time of transplant.

Discussion

After high dose AraC/mitoxantrone (HAM) was found to induce more than 50% CR in patients with refractory AML [7] its introduction into the double induction strategy was equally successful. When compared with TAD as second induction course HAM exhibits a higher antileukemic activity with significantly more remissions in patients with > 40% residual blasts in their day 16 bone marrow and also with a trend to a higher overall response rate and longer remission duration. Since the 40% 5 year remission rate in the TAD-HAM arm was obtained in unselected patients with no exclusions after achievement of remission this cure rate compares favourably to all published results. The hematologic effects of the two randomised double inductions show a prolonged recovery time of neutrophils and platelets after HAM even more expressed after the subsequent consolidation in this arm. This progressive delay of hematopoietic reconstitution in the TAD-HAM arm not seen in the TAD-TAD arm suggests an impairment of hematopoiesis at an early progenitor or stem cell level. As from the hypoplastic death rates and event free survival the hematopoietic impairment does not increase the therapeutic risk. The progressive delay of blood cell recovery, however, suggests that a compartment of leukemic progenitor or stem cells may also be impaired more effectively by the TAD-HAM than the TAD-TAD sequence thus explaining a positive trend in the therapeutic results.

References

1. Büchner Th, Hiddemann W, Löffler G et al. (1991) Improved cure rate by very early intensification combined with prolonged maintenance chemotherapy in patients with acute myeloid leukemia: Data from the AML Cooperative Group. Sem Hematol 28 (Suppl. 4): 76–79
2. Willemze R, Zwaan FE, Colpin G et al. (1982) High dose cytosine arabinoside in the management of refractory acute leukaemia. Scand J Haematol 29: 141–146
3. Herzig RH, Wolff SN, Lazarus HM et al. (1983) High-dose cytosine arabinoside therapy for refractory leukemia. Blood 62: 361–369
4. Wolff SN, Marion J, Steins RS et al. (1985) High-dose cytosine arabinoside and daunorubicin as consolidation therapy for acute nonlymphocytic leukemia in first remission: A pilot study. Blood 65: 1407–1411
5. Mayer RI, Davis RB, Schiffer CA et al. (1992) Comparative evaluation of intensive post-

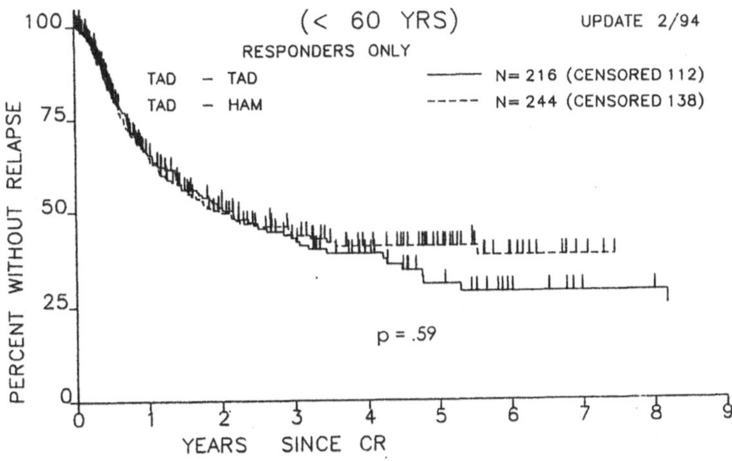

Fig. 2. Kaplan-Meier plots of remission duration for patients receiving double induction in the TAD-TAD arm and in the TAD-HAM arm. Censored are patients without relapse, also indicated by tic marks

remission therapy with different dose schedules of Ara-C in adults with acute myeloid leukemia (AML): initial results of a CALGB phase III study. Proc ASCO 11: 853
6. Bishop JF, Young GA, Szer J et al. (1992) Randomized trial of high dose cytosine arabinoside (Ara-C) combination in induction in acute myeloid leukemia (AML). Proc ASCO 11: 849
7. Hiddemann W, Kreutzmann H, Straif K et al. (1987) High-dose cytosine arabinoside and mitoxantrone: a highly effective regimen in refractory acute myeloid leukemia. Blood 69: 744–749
8. Herzig RH et al. (1987) Cerebellar toxicity with high-dose cytosine arabinoside. J Clin Oncol 5: 927–932
9. Janmohammed R, Milligan DW (1989) Mitoxantrone induced congestive heart failure in patients previously treated with anthracyclines. Br J Hematol 71: 292–293
10. Pratt CB, Crom DB, Wallenberg J et al. (1983) Fatal congestive heart failure following mitoxantrone treatment in two children previously treated with doxorubicin and cisplatin. Cancer Treat Rep 67: 85–87
11. Siegert W, Hiddemann W, Koppensteiner R et al. (1989) Accidental overdose of mitoxantrone in three patients. Med Oncol & Tumor Pharmacother 6: 275–278
12. Hachimi-Idrissi S, Schots R, DeWolf D et al. (1993) Reversible cardiopathy after accidental overdose of mitoxantrone. Ped Hemat and Oncol 10: 35–40
13. Büchner Th, Urbanitz D, Hiddemann W et al. (1985) Intensified induction and consolidation with or without maintenance chemotherapy for acute myeloid leukemia (AML): Two multicenter studies of the German AML Cooperative Group. J Clin Oncol 3: 1583–1589

Acute Leukemias V
Experimental Approaches
and Management of Refractory Diseases
Hiddemann et al. (Eds.)

Comparison of Front-Line Chemotherapy for Intermediate Grade and Follicular Non-Hodgkin's Lymphoma Using the CAP-BOP Regimens

Julie M. Vose, James R. Anderson, Philip J. Bierman, and James O. Armitage for the Nebraska Lymphoma Study Group

Abstract. The CAP-BOP series of induction regimens (cyclophosphamide, doxorubicin, mitoxantrone, procarbazine, bleomycin, vincristine, and prednisone) was administered to 389 patients with advanced aggressive non-Hodgkin's lymphoma as primary therapy. The overall complete response rates were not different between the three regimens: CB-A (64%), CB-AI (66%), and CB-M (65%). In addition, the 3-year failure-free survivals did not differ by regimen: CB-A (42%), CB-AI (45%), and CB-M (40%). 158 patients with follicular lymphoma were treated with the identical regimens during the same time period. The complete response rates were also similar in the follicular lymphoma patients with CB-A (71%), CB-AI (67%), and CB-M (68%).

Toxicity was regimen specific with CB-AI having a 22% incidence of neurotoxicity, compared to 7% for CB-A and 13% for CB-M ($p = 0.01$). Complete alopecia was seen in 100% of the patients receiving CB-A or CB-AI, compared to 38% of those patients receiving CB-M ($p < 0.01$). Although all three regimens had similar efficacy in the treatment of aggressive and follicular non-Hodgkin's lymphoma, the toxicity profiles were regimen dependent.

Introduction

The development of combination chemotherapy for the treatment of advanced aggressive non-Hodgkin's lymphomas (NHL) has been one of the most successful oncologic strategies developed over the past two decades. The first generation regimens, such as the CHOP regimen (cyclophosphamide, doxorubicin, vincristine, and prednisone) were first developed in the 1970's and were reported to produce a long-term disease-free survival of approximately 30% – 35% of patients [1]. Over the ensuing 15–20 years, additional agents shown to have activity against NHL were added to cyclophosphamide and doxorubicin to form the second and third generation strategies.

Initial reports of these more dose intensive regimens were hopeful, with the complete response rates increase up to 60–80% [2–5]. However, long-term follow-up of these original trials, and the diffusion of the third-generation regimens to a more generalized patient population has demonstrated the lack of a significant difference between the major regimens when compared to the original CHOP regimen [6].

With the realization that many regimens could produce the same results when used as induction therapy for aggressive NHL, toxicity issues and the identification of prognostic factors which could predict for patients with a poor outcome have become important issues. This article will outline a series of trials performed through the Nebraska Lymphoma Study Group evaluating the substitution of bolus or infusional agents and different anthracyclines in an attempt to modify the toxicity profile of the CAP-BOP regimen. In addition, identification of poor prognosis patients within these trials will allow alternative therapies to be offered when appropriate for this patient population.

Department of Internal Medicine, University of Nebraska Medical Center, Omaha, Nebraska, USA

Patients and Methods

Patients. Patients were entered at the time of diagnosis to one of three sequential treatment protocols and registered through the Nebraska Lymphoma Study Group. Between 9/82 and 1/92, 389 patients with advanced aggressive NHL were treated on one of these three protocols. In addition, 158 patients with follicular lymphoma were entered on the same protocols.

The criteria for inclusion in this analysis were a histologic diagnosis of diffuse mixed large and small cell NHL, diffuse large cell NHL, or immnoblastic NHL in the aggressive categories or follicular mixed cell, or follicular large cell NHL according to the Working Formulation [7]. The patients ranged in age from 15 to 92 years (median 66 years) and were bulky stage I or II (mass ≥10 cm), stage III or IV according to the Ann Arbor staging criteria [8].

Staging included physical examination, blood cell counts, routine blood chemistries, lactic dehydrogenase (LDH), computed tomography (CT) of chest, abdomen, and pelvis, and bone marrow aspirate and biopsy. Other tests such as gastrointestinal series, lumbar puncture with spinal fluid examination, magnetic resonance images (MRI), or SPECT gallium scans were done if clinically indicated. Restaging was done with repeat CT scans of chest, abdomen and pelvis, and repeat of any other previously positive tests after three cycles of therapy. Patients were given two cycles of therapy past complete remission, or to a maximum of seven cycles of therapy.

Complete remission (CR) was defined as normalization of physical examination, laboratory values, and radiologic abnormalities for a minimum of 4 weeks. A partial response (PR) was defined as ≥50% reduction in the bidimensional sum of the perpendicular area of any abnormalities for a minimum of 4 weeks. No response (NR) was defined as a <50% reduction in any abnormalities. An early death (ED) was considered any death while the patient was still on therapy.

Regimens. Of the patients with aggressive NHL, one hundred fifteen patients were treated with CB-A (cyclophosphamide, doxorubicin, procarbazine, bleomycin, vincristine, and prednisone). One hundred thirty eight patients received CB-AI (cyclophosphamide, doxorubicin, procarbazine, infusional bleomycin and vincristine, and dexamethasone). And one hundred thirty six patients received CB-M (cyclophosphamide, mitoxantrone, procarbazine, bleomycin, vincristine, and prednisone). In addition of the follicular lymphoma patients, 28 received CM-A, 43 CB-AI, and 87 CB-M (Table 1). There was a 1/3 dose reduction of the myelosuppressive drugs for age ≥70 years.

Statistical methods. All patients started on treatment were considered assessable. Survival duration was measured from the beginning of treatment to date of death from any cause or last follow-up alive. Failure-free survival (FFS) was defined as the time from the beginning of treatment to progression, relapse or death from any cause. Survival and FFs were plotted according to the method of Kaplan and Meier [9]. Comparisons of time to event distributions were made using the long-rank test [10].

Table 1. CAP-BOP Regimens

CB-A Regimen:	Cyclophosphamide 650 mg/M² Day 1
	Doxorubicin 50 mg/M² Day 1
	Procarbazine 100 mg/M²/day Days 1–7
	Bleomycin 10 mg/M² (max 15 mg) Day 15
	Vincristine 1.4 mg/M² (max 2.0 mg)Day 15
	Prednisone 100 mg/day Days 15–21
CB-AI Regimen:	Cyclophosphamide 500 mg/M² Day 1
	Doxorubicin 50 mg/M² Day 1
	Procarbazine 100 mg/M²/day Days 1–5
	Bleomycin 4 mg/M²/day CI Days 1–5
	Vincristine 1.0 mg/M²/day (max 2.0 mg) Days 1,2 CI
	Dexamethasone 10 mg/M²/day Days 1–5
CB-M Regimen:	Cyclophosphamide 650 mg/ M² Day 1
	Mitoxantrone 12 mg/M² Day 1
	Procarbazine 100 mg/M²/day Days 1–7
	Bleomycin 10 mg/M² Day 15
	Vincristine 1.4 mg/M² (max 2.0 mg) Day 15
	Prednisone 100 mg/day Days 15–21

CI = Continuous infusion
*1/3 dose reduction for age ≥70 with all regimens

Results

Clinical characteristics. The clincal characteristics of the patients with aggressive NHL on the three protocols are listed in Table 2. The median age of the entire patient population was 66 years, with 68% of the patients being ≥60 years of age at the time of diagnosis.

Response to treatment. The overall response rates were as follows: CB-A (69%), CB-AI (73%), CB-M (71%). Seventy-four of 115 (64%) patients treated with CB-A achieved a complete response (CR). This compares to a CR rate of 66% with CB-AI, and 65% with CB-M (p=NS). For the patients with follicular lymphoma complete response rates included: CB-A (71%), CB-AI (67%), and CB-M (68%) (p=NS).

Survival and failure-free survival. With a median follow-up of 75 months (CB-A), 47 months (CB-AI), and 15 months (CB-M), the predicted 3-year survivals were 50%, 56%, and 47% respectively (p=NS). The 3-year failure-free survivals for the regimens were 42% (CB-A), 45% (CB-AI), and 40% (CB-M) (p=NS). There was no difference by treatment regimen with respect to the failure-free survival in patients less than 60 years of age (Fig. 1). In addition, the failure-free survival in patients treated for follicular NHL was not different based on the extent of follicularity. Patients ≥age 70 years who received a 1/3 dose reduction of the myelosuppressive agents had a significantly decreased FFS when compared to patients aged 60–70. This was seen in the results of all three regimens.

The 6-year failure-free survival for the patients treated for follicular lymphoma were as follows: follicular small cleaved (42%), follicular mixed cell (48%), and follicular large cell (39%), (p=NS) (Fig. 2). No differences were seen between the patients treated with the different CAP-BOP regimens.

Table 2. Patient Characteristics: Histologies

Characteristics	CB-A (N=115)	CB-AI (N=138)	CB-M (N=136)
Age (median)	18–90 (65)	18–89 (66)	15–92 (67)
Male : Female	52% : 48%	54% : 46%	47% : 53%
Stage I/II	38%	46%	54%
III/IV	62%	54%	47%
Histology			
Diffuse Mixed	12%	13%	8%
Diffuse Large	43%	48%	67%
Immunoblastic	45%	40%	25%
LDH > Normal	56%	49%	47%
Mass ≥ 10 cm	21%	14%	19%
Immunophenotype			
B-cell	88%	87%	90%
T-cell	12%	13%	10%

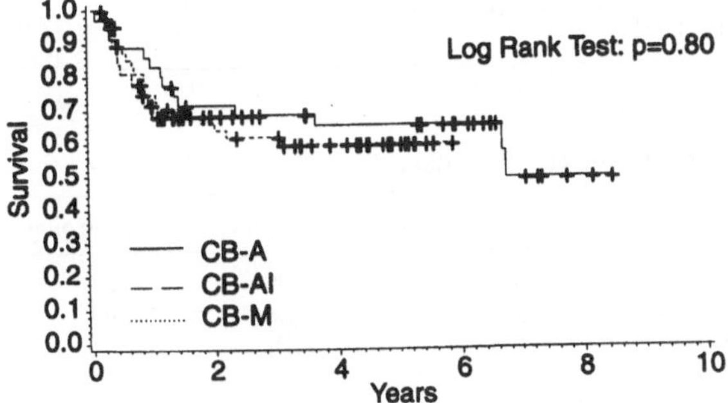

Fig. 1. Failure-free survival (age < 60) for patients with aggressive NHL treated with CB-A, CB-AI, or CB-M

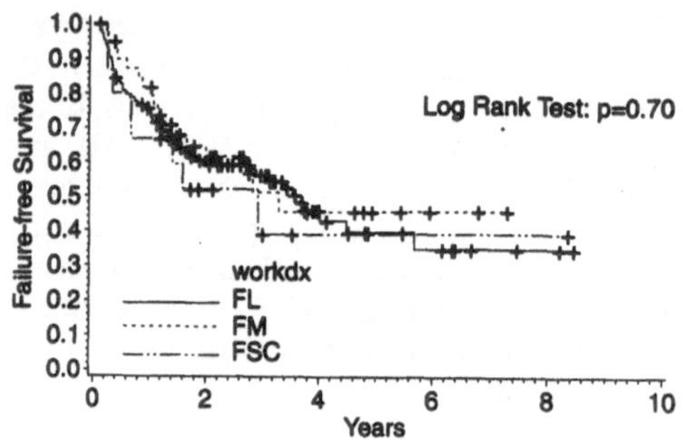

Fig. 2. Failure-free survival for patients with follicular NHL treated with CB-A, CB-AI, or CB-M

Prognostic index analysis. The International Prognostic Index was applied to the prognostic variables identified in this analysis. Since the overall age of the patient population treated in the CAP-BOP series was significantly higher than that in the International Prognostic Index, a comparison of only those patients less than age 60 was evaluated. For patients less than age 60, the three characteristics identified in the International Prognostic Index were Ann Arbor Stage III or IV, lactic dehydrogenase (LDH) > normal, or ECOG performance status ⩾2 at the time of diagnosis [11]. These characteristics divide the patient population into four distinct risk groups with patients having 0, 1, 2, or 3 of the risk indicators. Table 3 compares the 5-year survivals for patients in the CAP-BOP series with aggressive NHL to those obtained in the International Prognostic Index analysis. The FFS for both risk categories 2 and 3 were ⩽20% at 5 years following diagnosis.

Table 3. Patients ⩽ Age 60: 5-Year Survival

Prognostic Category	International Index	CAP-BOP Regimens
Low [0]	83%	85%
Low-Intermediate [1]	70%	62%
High-Intermediate [2]	46%	48%
High [3]	32%	33%

Toxicity analysis. Toxicity assessments were defined as follows: pulmonary toxicity was defined as any interstitial infiltrate on a chest radiograph for which no infectious etiology was found and the bleomycin was discontinued. Cardiac toxicity was defined as the development of symptomatic congestive heart failure for which no other etiology or anatomic abnormality was identified. Neurologic toxicity was defined as symptomatic peripheral neuropathy for which the vincristine was discontinued. Complete alopecia was defined as estimated hair loss ⩾80% of normal.

The pattern of toxicities differed slightly by regimen. Patients treated on the three regimens had pulmonary and cardiac toxicities that were not statistically different. However, patients treated on the CB-AI regimen with infusional bleomycin and vincristine had a significantly higher incidence of neurologic toxicity (22%) compared with the CB-A regimen (7%) and the CB-M regimen (13%) ($p = 0.01$). Also, patients treated with the CB-M regimen had significantly less comple alopecia (38%) compared with the two doxorubicin containing regimens (100%) ($p < 0.01$) (Table 4).

Discussion

Over the past 20 years, many different combination chemotherapy regimens have been developed for the treatment of aggressive non-Hodgkin's lymphoma. Although the third-generation regimens appeared to produce a higher complete remission rate, the overall long term disease-free survival appears to be equivalent in a large prospective randomized trial [6]. Explanations for this discrepancy include the equivalent follow-up available for the patients in the prospective randomized trial and the application of these regimens to a more generalized patient population.

Table 4. Toxicity Evaluation

Regimen	Pulmonary	Cardiac	Neurologic	Alopecia
CB-A	13%	1.5%	7%	100%
CB-AI	13%	1.5%	22%	100%
CB-M	10%	1.0%	13%	38%
p-value	NS	NS	0.01	<0.01

The use of chemotherapeutic agents given by a different route or length of administration has also been evaluated with renewed interest over the past few years. The half-life of many chemotherapeutic agents is quite short, and infusional administration has been evaluated by some groups in an attempt to increase the bioavailability of these agents [12, 13]. Some studies have demonstrated responses with the infusional approach following failure of regimens with the same agent given by bolus [14].

The regimens described in this article (CB-A, CB-AI, and CB-M) have no major differences with respect to survival or failure-free survival. As the gradual realization that the newer third generation regimens would not greatly increase the long term disease-free survival of patients diagnosed with NHL, other priorities such as decrease in the toxicities associated with the therapy and additional treatment strategies have been the focus of studies within the last few years. In elderly patients with NHL, diminished toxicity is extremely important as quality of life issues become foremost when the probability of cure is otherwise similar.

In the younger patient population age ⩽60, toxicity is also an important consideration. However, a priority that has been identified from various trials is the selection of high-risk patients by utilization of the International Prognostic Index which has allowed the direction of these patients into dose intensity trials such as the use of high-dose chemotherapy and autologous bone marrow transplantation in first partial or complete remission [15–17]. Future prospective randomized trials using this approach will perhaps demonstrate the improved disease-free survival in the dose-identification group which was hoped to be seen in the patients receiving the third-generation regimens.

References

1. Coltman CA, Dahlberg S; Jones SE et al: CHOP is curative in thirty per cent of patients with large cell lymphoma: A twelve year South West Oncology Group (SWOG) follow-up. In Skarin AT (ed): Advances in cancer chemotherapy update treatment for diffuse large cell lymphoma. New York, NY Wiley, p71–82, 986.
2. Connors JM, Klimo P: MACOP-B chemotherapy for malignant lymphomas and related conditions: 1987 update and additional observations. Semin Hematol 25: 41–46, 1988.
3. Shipp MA, Harrington DP, Klatt MM et al.: Identification of major prognostic subgroups of patients with large-cell lymphoma treated with m-BACOD or M-BACOD. Ann Intern Med 104: 757–765, 1986.
4. Fisher RI, DeVita VT Jr, Hubbard SM et al.: Randomized trial of ProMACE-MOPP vs. ProMACE-CytaBOM in previously untreated, advanced stage, diffuse aggressive lymphomas. Proc Am Soc Clin Oncol 3: 242a, 1984
5. Weick JK, Dahlberg S. Fisher RI et al.: Combination chemotherapy of intermediate-grade and high-grade non-Hodgkin's lymphoma with MACOP-B: a Southwest Oncology Group Study. J Clin Oncol 9: 748–753, 1991
6. Fisher RI, Gaynor ER, Dahlberg S et al.: Comparison of a standard regimen (CHOP) with three intensive chemotherapy regimens for advanced non-Hodgkin's lymphoma. N Engl J Med 328: 1002–1006, 1993
7. The Non-Hodgkin's Lymphoma Pathologic Classification Project. National Cancer Institute sponsored study of classifications of Non-Hodgkin's lymphomas: summary and description of a working formulation for clinical usage. Cancer 49: 2112–2135, 1982
8. Carbone PP, Kaplan MS, Musshoff K et al.: Report of the Committee on Hodgkin's Disease staging classification. Cancer Res. 31: 1860–1861, 1971
9. Kaplan E, Meier P: Nonparametric estimation from incomplete observations. J Am Stat Asso 53: 457–481, 1958
10. Idem. Regression models and life-tables. J R Stat Soc 34: 187–220, 1972
11. Shipp MA, Harrington D, Anderson J et al.: Development of a predictive model for aggressive lymphomas: the International NHL Prognostic Factors Project. Proc Am Soc Clin Oncol 11: 319a, 1992
12. Jackson DV, Paschold EH, Spurr CL et al.: Treatment of advanced non-Hodgkin's lymphoma with vincristine infusion. Cancer 53: 2601–2606, 1984
13. Banavali SK, Advani SH, Gopal R et al: Continuous cyclophosphamide, doxorubicin, vincristine, and prednisolone. Cancer 65: 1704–1710, 1990
14. Hollister D, Silver RT, Gordon B et al.: Continuous infusion vincristine and bleomycin with high dose methotrexate for resistant non-Hodgkin's lymphoma. Cancer 50: 690–1694, 1982.
15. Gulati SC, Shank B, Black P et al.: Autologous bone marrow transplantation for patients with poor-prognosis lymphoma. Clin Oncol 6: 1303–1313, 1988
16. Philip T, Hartmann O, Biron P et al.: High-dose therapy and autologous bone marrow transplantation in partial remission after first-line induction therapy for diffuse non-Hodgkin's lymphoma. J Clin Oncol 6: 1118–1124, 1988
17. Nademanee A, Schmidt GM, O'Donnell MR et al.: High-dose chemoradiotherapy followed by autologous bone marrow transplantation as consolidation therapy during first complete remission in adult patients with poor-risk aggressive lymphoma: a pilot study. Blood 80: 1130–1135, 1992.

Acute Leukemias V
Experimental Approaches
and Management of Refractory Diseases
Hiddemann et al. (Eds.)

Prednimustine and Mitoxantrone in the Treatment of Low-Grade Non-Hodgkin Lymphomas

M. Unterhalt[1], P. Koch[2], C. Pott-Hoeck[1], R. Herrmann[3], and W. Hiddemann[1] for the German Low-Grade Lymphoma Study Group

Abstract. In 1988, Landys et al. reported a high anti-lymphoma activity of the combination of prednimustine and mitoxantrone (PmM). These data were confirmed by a phase II study of our group in 19 pretreated patients with advanced low malignant non-Hodgkin lymphomas using PmM (prednimustine 100 mg/m²/day orally days 1–5 and mitoxantrone 8 mg/m²/day i.v. days 1 and 2) with a response rate of 68%. Based on these data a randomized multicenter comparison of PmM with standard COP (cyclophosphamide 400 mg/m²/day i.v. days 1–5, vincristine 1,4 mg/m² (max. 2 mg) i.v. day 1 and prednisone 100mg/m²/day orally days 1–5) was initiated in untreated patients with advanced centrocytic or advanced centroblastic-centrocytic lymphomas. Patients with no progression during treatment, received six or eight courses of PmM or COP depending on the response to therapy. Patients who had at least a reduction of the lymphoma mass of more than 50% during the first six courses, were considered as responders and were subsequently randomized for IFN-α maintenance versus observation only. The study was monitored by a onesided sequential test with a working significance level of 0.05. Based on an estimated rate of 65% remissions after COP the test was designed to detect an improvement of 20% by PmM with a probability of 90%. In October of 1993 a decision was stated by this sequential procedure. At that time 140 randomized patients, 74 treated with COP and 66 treated with PmM, were evaluable. Both regimens achieved comparable response rates of 84.8% with PmM and 82.4% with COP. So there was no significant improvement by PmM compared with COP. Granulocytopenia was the most important side effect after both protocols and was observed after 235 (42%) of 554 PmM treatment cycles and after 181 (32%) of 564 COP treatment courses ($p < 0{,}0001$). Severe infections were very rare however under both regimens. (2.2% after COP and 1.0% after PmM) These data indicate a high efficiency of PmM and COP in advanced low-grade lymphomas. Further data are needed to assess their impact on disease free and overall survival as well as to evaluate the impact of IFN-α maintenance on these parameters.

Introduction

The prognosis of patients with low-grade malignant non-Hodgkin lymphomas in advanced stages III and IV has not significantly changed within the past decades[6,10]. The median survival after diagnosis is 6 to 10 years. While patients in stages I and II, in isolated cases also in stage III, may be cured by radiotherapy[11], only palliative treatment concepts are available for patients with advanced disease. New aspects recently emerged from a report by Karl Landys et al.[9], who reported on a high anti-lymphoma activity of the combination of prednimustine and mitoxantrone with a low incidence of therapy associated side effects.

Based on these data we initiated a phase II study in 1987 for patients with advanced

[1]Dept. of Internal Medicine, University of Göttingen, Germany
[2]Dept. of Internal Medicine, University of Münster, Germany
[3]Dept. of Internal Medicine, Kantonsspital Basel, Switzerland

low-grade non-Hodgkin lymphomas who had failed on standard therapy using Prednimustin and Mitoxantron for a initial cytoreductive therapy and Interferon-alpha for maintenance[4,5,6]. 19 patients were enrolled in this study and 13 achieved a complete or partial remission. These data were the basis for a randomized multicenter study to compare the efficency of the standard COP therapy with the new PmM regimen in patients with advanced centroblastic-centrocytic and centrocytic lymphomas.

Patients and Protocols

The PmM therapy consisted of 8mg/m² mitoxantrone on days 1 and 2 and 100mg/m² prednimustine for days 1–5. For the COP treatment a dose of 400mg/m² cyclophosphamide on days 1 –5, a single dose vincristin of 1.4mg/m² up to a maximum of 2mg on day 1 and a prednisone dose of 100mg/m² on days 1–5 was applied. The therapy was repeated every four weeks for the PmM regimen and every three weeks for COP. Only untreated patients with centroblastic/centrocytic or centrocytic lymphoma at advanced stages III and IV were enroled into this study. Treatment was stated in all patients with centrocytic lymphoma and in CB/CC NHL upon the presence of B symptoms, hematopoietic insufficiency, bulky disease, or objective progression of the lymphoma. All patients, that did not show progression of the lymphoma under therapy received a minimum of 6 therapy cycles and a maximum of 8 cycles, depending on the therapy results after 4 cycles of therapy. Patients who achieved at least a partial remission, defined as at least 50% reduction of the initial lymphoma mass, were randomized for maintenance therapy with interferon-α versus no therapy, in order to determine the effect of an IFN-maintenance on the event-free survival.

Results

Recruitment. As of February 1994 407 patients from 108 centers have entered the study. The histological diagnoses were centroblastic-centrocytic lymphoma in 314 patients and centrocytic lymphoma in 80 patients. 13 patients with different histological diagnoses had to be excluded. Patient recruitment has increased steadily after start of the study in May 1988. 344 patients of the 407 patients entered the study after June 1989 and have been randomized between COP and PmM. Before this date each center treated with either PmM or COP. Only the randomized patients formed the basis for the statistical evaluation of chemotherapy arms.

Patient characteristics. There were 185 male patients and 159 female patients. For centroblastic-centrocytic lymphomas there were 48% male patients and 52% female cases, while a preponderance of males (74%) was found in centrocytic lymphomas. The distribution of age shows a median age of 54 years for all randomized patients. For the patients with centroblastic-centrocytic lymphoma the median age is 53 years while for the patients with centrocytic lymphomas it is significantly higher with a median of 60 years.

Statistics and evaluation of response. The first aim of this study was to show whether PmM was superior to COP in initial response to therapy. Patients were classified as responders if they achieved at least a partial remission after 6 cycles and were still in remission one month after the end of the consolidation therapy. Patients that had progressive disease or less than a partial remission after 6 cycles or patients who died during therapy were classified as treatment failures. Patients who did not adhere to the protocol were classified as abort of treatment and were not evaluated for the statistical decision. The study was monitored by a onesided sequential test with a working significance level of 0.05. Thus the probability of a wrong decision in favour of PmM would be smaller than 5%. To determine the power of the test it was stated that based on an estimated rate of 65% remissions after COP an improvement of 20% by PmM shoud be detected with a probability of 90%. The test statistic was calculated after each evaluable patient and in October 1993 the procedure decided, that no statistical significant improvement by PmM for the response-rate could be stated. At that time 74 COP patients and 66 PmM patients were evaluable. There were 61 responders and 13 treatment failures after COP indicating a response rate of 82.4%. For the PmM regimen there were 56 responders and 10 failures, meaning a response rate of 84.8%. As of February 1994 99 patients are evaluable for COP and 93 patients for PmM. For both therapies 15 patients have to be classified as abort of treatment. A complete remission after only 4 courses of therapy (CR 4) was achieved by 10 patients after COP and by 19 patients after PmM. Another 8 patients by COP and 9 by PmM reached a complete remission after 6 courses (CR 6). A partial remission (PR) after 6 courses was seen in 53 patients with COP and in 39 patients with PmM therapy (Fig. 1.) So the overall response rate for COP is 84.5% and 85.9% for the PmM regimen; PmM, however, induced more complete remissions (35.9% vs. 21.4%).

For the subgroup of patients with centrocytic lymphomas (Fig. 2.) results are preliminary because of small numbers. After treatment of 18 patients with COP we observed in this group 13 partial remissions and 1 complete remission after course 6. Four patients showed progressive disease under therapy. Fifteen patients with centrocytic lymphoma were treated with PmM. Three patients did not show a response to therapy. There was one patient who achieved a complete remission after course 4 and 3 others after course 6. Eight patients responded with a partial remission to the PmM therapy.

For patients older than 60 years at randomization the response rate for COP was 88.9% while it was 91.6% for PmM (Fig. 3). Even in this group the tendency for more complete remissions after PmM was observed. The rate of death was not significantly higher than in the whole group of randomized patients.

The actual Kaplan-Meier estimates (Fig. 4) for all patients who were randomized for PmM versus COP and for IFN-maintenance versus no therapy show a tendency for a longer event-free interval in the group of PmM treated patients. Further data and analyses are needed to substantiate this findings and to assess wether PmM might have a long term beneficial effect on disease free survival.

Side effects. Analysis of therapy related toxicity revealed myelosuppression, most notably leukocytopenia as the predominant side effect (Table 1). For leukocytes and granulocytes

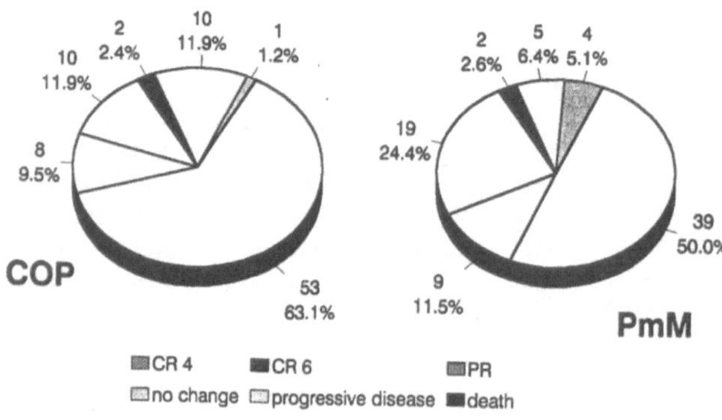

Fig. 1. Response of all randomized patients

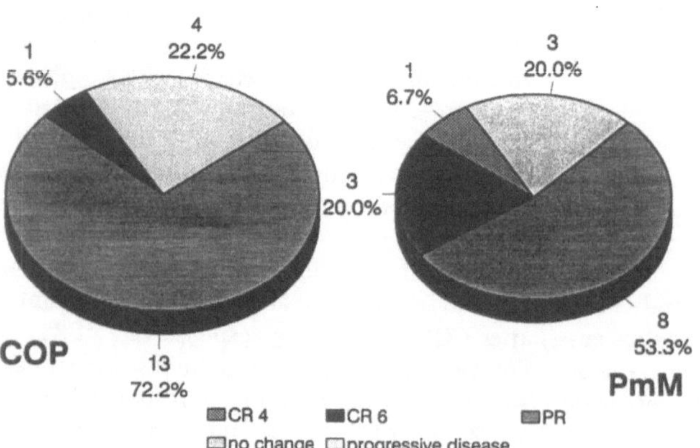

Fig. 2. Response of all randomized patients with centrocytic lymphoma

Fig. 3. Response of patients older than 60 years at randomization

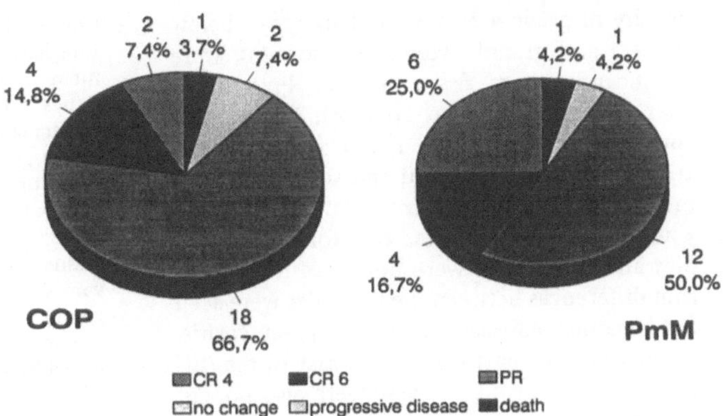

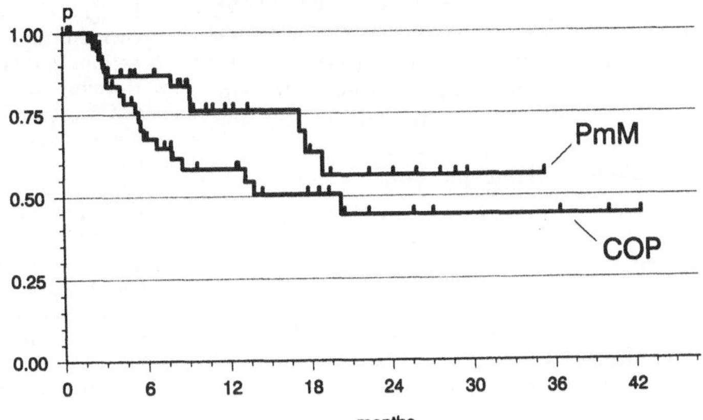

Fig. 4. Event-free interval. All patients randomized for PmM vs. COP and interferon vs. no maintenance therapy

Table 1. COP vs. PmM – Side Effects

	COP			PmM		
	n	Gr. 1+2	Gr. 3+4	n	Gr. 1+2	Gr. 3+4
Hemoglobin	694	17.4%	1.3%	671	18.6%	0.6%
Leukocytes	**687**	**33.2%**	**37.3%**	**672**	**32.3%**	**47.9%**
Granulocytes	**564**	**26.6%**	**32.1%**	**554**	**28.0%**	**42.4%**
Thrombocytes	**688**	**7.4%**	**1.9%**	**673**	**19.8%**	**2.4%**
Bleeding	723	0.1%	0.1%	687	1.5%	0.0%
Nausea/Vomiting	719	25.6%	1.3%	691	27.8%	2.5%
Mucositis	718	4.7%	0.4%	688	6.5%	0.4%
Obstipation	719	4.6%	0.4%	687	2.5%	0.1%
Diarrhea	719	6.1%	0.4%	688	3.3%	0.3%
Fever	720	6.8%	0.8%	688	4.9%	0.3%
Alopecia	**722**	**44.0%**	**32.4%**	**685**	**33.1%**	**1.0%**
Infection	720	7.9%	2.2%	688	9.2%	1.0%
Cardiac dysfunction	721	1.2%	1.5%	687	3.3%	0.4%
Neurotoxicity	**719**	**21.7%**	**1.4%**	**689**	**1.6%**	**0.0%**

toxicity of grade 3 and 4, i.e. leukocytes below 2000/μl and granulocytes below 1000/μl, were significantly more frequent after PmM than after COP treatment ($p < 0.0001$). For platelet counts toxicity of grade 1 and 2, i.e. platelet counts between 100 000/μl and 50 000/μl, were more often seen in PmM treated patients. Grade 3 and grade 4 toxicity was rare for both therapies and differences were not seen. No significant differences between the therapies were seen for bleeding, nausea and vomiting, mucositis, obstipation, or diarrhea. In contrast to the differences in neutropenia there were also no significant differences in fever and infections. A significant difference in cardiac dysfunction was also not found. A very impressive difference was seen for alopecia. After 32% of the therapy cycles with COP a complete alopecia was observed, complete alopecia was very rare after PmM therapy. Neurotoxicity caused by vincristin was more often seen after COP therapy. Because of this in 15 patients the therapy had to be continued without vincristin.

Conclusions

The randomized comparison of COP versus PmM did not indicate a significant advantage of PmM for the overall response to therapy mainly because of a substantially higher efficiency of COP than expected. Still a substantially higher rate of complete remissions and a tendency towards a longer event free interval emerged. These data need to be substantiated by further follow-up. This is also necessary to judge the impact of IFN-α on the long-term perspectives of patients with advanced low-grade NHL entered into this trial.

References

1. Balkwill FR: Antitumor effects of interferons in animals, in Finter NB, Oldham RK (eds): Interferon, in vivo and Clinical Studies, vol 4. Amsterdam, Elsevier, 1985, pp 23–45
2. Brittinger G; Meusers P; Engelhard M: Strategien der Behandlung von Non-Hodgkin-Lymphomen.(Strategies in the treatment of non-Hodgkin's lymphomas) Internist (Berl), 27 [8] 485–97, 1986 Aug
3. Chisesi T; Capnist G; Vespignani M; Cetto G: Interferon alfa-2b and chlorambucil in the treatment of non-Hodgkin's lymphoma. Invest New Drugs, 5 Suppl S35–40, 1987
4. Hiddemann W, Koch P, Essink M, et al: Treatment of low-grade non-Hodgkin's lymphoma with prednimustine/mitoxantrone followed by interferon alpha-2b. A clinical phase II study. Contrib Oncol 37: 287–291, 1989
5. Hiddemann W, Unterhalt M, Koch P, Nahler M, van de Loo J: Treatment of low-grade non-Hodgkin's lymphoma by cytoreductive chemotherapy with prednimustine/mitoxantrone followed by interferon alpha-2b maintenance: results of a clinical phase II study. Semin Oncol, 17 (6 Suppl 10) 20–3, 1990
6. Hiddemann W, Unterhalt M, Koch P, Nahler M, Herrmann R, van de Loo J: alpha Interferon maintenance therapy in patients with low-grade non-Hodgkin's lymphomas after cytoreductive chemotherapy with prednimustine and mitoxantrone. Eur J Cancer, 27 Suppl 4: 37–9, 1991
7. Horning SJ; Nademanee AP; Chao NJ; Schmidt GM; Hoppe RT; Lipsett JA; Negrin RS; Forman SJ; Blume KG: Regimen-related toxicity and early post-transplant survival in patients undergoing autologous bone marrow transplantation (ABMT) for lymphoma: Combined experience of Stanford University and the City of Hope National Medical Center (meeting abstract): Proc Am Soc Clin Oncol; 9: 271, 1990
8. Horning SJ; Rosenberg SA: The natural history of initially untreated low-grade non-Hodgkin's lymphomas. N Engl J Med, 311 (23) 1471–5, 1984 Dec 6
9. Landys KE: Mitoxantrone in combination with prednimustine in treatment of unfavorable non-Hodgkin lymphoma: Invest New Drugs; 6(2); 105–13, 1988
10. Ozer H; Anderson JR; Peterson BA; Budman DR; Henderson ES; Bloomfield CD; Gottlieb A: Combination trial of subcutaneous interferon alfa-2b and oral cyclophosphamide in favorable histology, non-Hodgkin's lymphoma. Invest New Drugs, 5 Suppl S27–33, 1987
11. Portlock CS: "Good risk" Non-Hodgkin's lymphomas: Approaches to management. Semin Hematol 20: 25–36, 1983
12. Portlock CS: Non-Hodgkin's lymphomas. Advances in diagnosis, staging, and management. Cancer, 65 (3 Suppl) 718–22, 1990 Feb 1
13. Rohatiner AZ; Richards MA; Barnett MJ; Stansfeld AG; Lister TA: Chlorambucil and interferon for low grade non-Hodgkin's lymphoma. Br J Cancer, 55 (2) 225–6, 1987 Feb
14. Young RC; Longo DL; Glatstein E; Ihde DC; Jaffe ES; DeVita VT Jr: The treatment of indolent lymphomas: watchful waiting v aggressive combined modality treatment. Semin Hematol, 25 (2 Suppl 2) 11–6, 1988 Apr

Acute Leukemias V
Experimental Approaches
and Management of Refractory Diseases
Hiddemann et al. (Eds.)

Mono- Versus Combination-Chemotherapy in Metastatic Breast Cancer

Else Heidemann

The conventional concept to deliver combination chemotherapy to patients with metastatic breast cancer has been questioned in the last years. The rationale for using a polydrug regimen was the assumption of a higher probability to achieve a remission (Falkson et al. 1991, Zinser et al. 1987). Besides others our prospectively-randomized multicenter trial comparing the treatments with 40 mg/m² of epirubicin or with 40 mg/m² of adriamycin or with 12 mg/m² of mitoxantrone each in combination with 600 mg/m² of cyclophosphamide shows that prognostic factors are more important than the chosen treatments for the outcome in metastatic breast cancer patients (Table 1, Fig. 1 and 2) (Heidemann et al. 1993).

Therefore we have to ask, whether in the palliative setting of metastatic breast cancer combination chemotherapy is justified at all when monotherapy can optimize quality of life. Another question is whether any prognostic subgroups do draw survival benefit from combination treatment.

Some scientists quote studies having been performed in the seventies (Table 2). Those studies show either no survival difference when using a sequence of monotherapies instead of giving the same drugs altogether or better survival in the group having liver involvement and receiving polychemotherapy (Chlebowski et al. 1989, Tormey et al 1977).

It has however to be remembered that in the 1970s the diagnosis of liver metastases was possible only in late stages of the disease, and the WHO criteria were not strictly applied to clinical trials. Therefore the quoted results don't have to mean anything for the patients nowadays.

With the aims of palliation, quality of life, and prolongation of survival in mind we started another prospectively-randomized multicenter trial adressing the following questions:

1. Is there a survival benefit for *low risk* patients (Fig. 3) when treatment starts with

Table 1. Outcome of treatment in metastatic breast cancer dependent on subgroup characteristics

subgroup	median survival	multivariate analysis
AC	17 months	no difference
EC	16 months	
NC	18 months	
bone only	27 months	
lung only	25 months	
liver only	19 months	$p<0{,}05$
liver and other	13 months	
one organ only	22 months	
more than one organ involved	13 months	$p<0{,}05$
disease free interval ≤18 month	12 months	
disease free interval > 18 month	22 months	$p<0{,}05$
age <40 J.	12 months	
age 46–50 J.	21 months	$p<0{,}05$
previous adjuv. chemother.	14 months	
no previous adjuv. chemother.	18 months	$p<0{,}05$

Medical Department, Deaconess Hospital, D 70176 Stuttgart, Germany

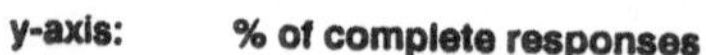

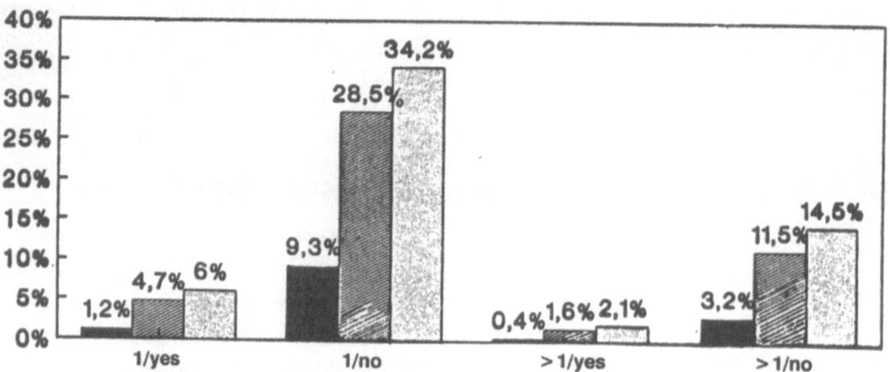

Fig. 1. Chance of achieving a complete response-dependent on a combination of prognostic factors

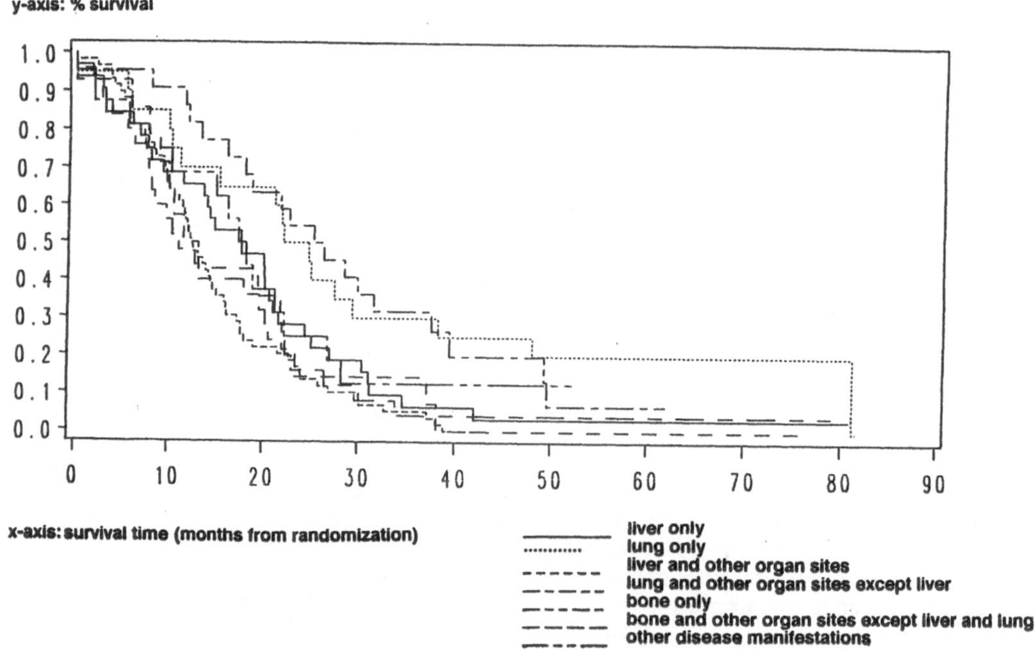

Fig. 2. Projected (Kaplan-Meier) survival for 188 patients with different sites of metastases in breast cancer

cyclophosphamide, methotrexate and fluoro-uracil and is crossed over to mitoxantrone monotherapy in the case of progressive disease in comparison to the reverse sequence?

2. Is there a survival benefit for *high risk* patients (Fig. 3) when treatment starts with fluoro-uracil, epirubicin and cyclophosphamide and is crossed over to vindesine,

Table 2. Monotherapy vs polychemtherapy. Literature review

		over all survival
Mouridsen 1977	Cys vs. CMFVP	↑
Rubens 1975	HD Cyc vs CMF+VLB	=
Smalley 1967	F-M-C-V-P-vs CMFVP	=
Carmo-1980 Pereira	FU vs CMFVP	↑
Chlebowski 1989 (collection of data 1971–1973)	C-M-F-P vs CMFP	=
	without liver involvement	=
	with liver involvement	↑
Hoogstraten 1976	Adm vs. CMFVP with crossover	=
Ahmann 1987 (collection of data 1972–1975)	CFP (V) -Adm -Ifo -MeCCNU	=
Canellos 1976	L-PAM vs CMF	↑
French Group 1991	Epi vs. FEC (50) vs. FEC (75)	=

= no difference
↑ combination better than monotherapy

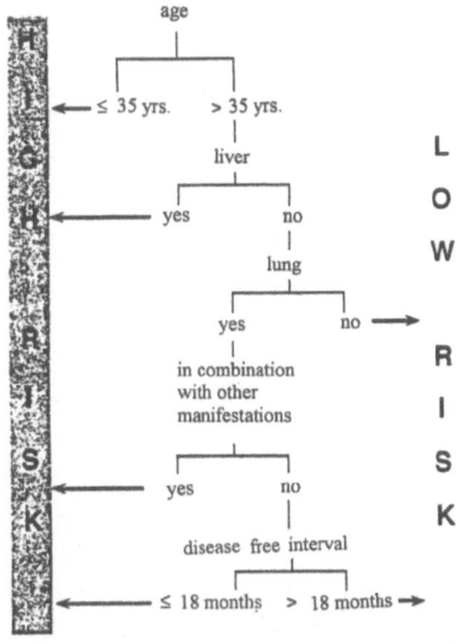

Fig. 3. Advanced Breast Cancer Risk Flow Sheet

mitomycin and prednisolone in the case of progressive disease in comparison to starting with mitoxantrone monochemotherapy and crossing over to vindesine, mitomycin, prednisolone in the case of progressive disease?

Today combination chemotherapy still must be considered standard for hormone-resistant metastatic breast cancer. After having completed our ongoing study we will probably know better whether there is a subgroup of patients that does draw survival benefit from combination chemotherapy. If there is no such group, then monotherapy may become the treatment of choice for patients with hormone-resistant metastatic breast cancer.

References

1. Ahmann, L., Schaid, D. J., Bisel, H. F., Hahn, R. G., Edmonson, J. H., Ingle, J. N. (1987) The effect on survival of initial chemotherapy in advanced breast cancer: polychemotherapy versus single drug. J. Clin. Oncol. 5, 1928–1932.
2. Canellos, G. P., Pocock, S. J. , Taylor, S. G., Sears, M. E., Klaasen, D. J., Band, P. R. (1976). Combination chemotherapy for metastatic breast carcinoma. Prospective comparison of multiple drug therapy with L-phenylalanine mustard. Cancer 38, 1882–1886.
3. Carmo-Pereira, J., Costa, F. O. Henriques, E. (1980) Single drug vs combination cytotoxic chemotherapy in advanced breast cancer: a randomized study. Europ. J. Cancer 16, 1621–1625.
4. Chlebowski R. T., Smalley, R. V., Weiner J. M., Irwin, L. E., Bartolucci, A. A., Bateman, J. R. (1989) Combination versus sequential single agent chemotherapy in advanced breast cancer: associations with metastatic sites and long-term survival. Br. J. Cancer 59, 227–230.
5. Falkson, G., Gelman, R. S., Leone L., Falkson C. I. (1990) Survival of premenopausal women with metastatic breast cancer. Cancer 66, 1621–1629.
6. French Epirubicin Study group (1991) A prospective randomized trial comparing epirubicin monotherapy to two fluorouracil, cyclophosphamide, and epirubicin regimens differing in epirubicin dose in advanced breast cancer patients. J. Clin. Oncol. 9, 305–312.
7. Heidemann, E., Steinke, B., Hartlapp, J., Schumacher, K., Possinger, K., Kunz, S., Neeser, E., v. Ingersleben, G., Hossfeld, D., Caffier, H., Souchon, R., Waldmann, R., Blümner, E., Clark, J. (1993) Prognostic subgroups: the key factor for treatment outcome in metastic breast cancer. Onkologie 16, 344–353.
8. Hoogstraten, B., George, S. L., Samal, B. (1979) Combination chemotherapy and adriamycin in patients with advanced breast cancer. Cancer 38, 13.
9. Mouridsen, H. T. , Palshof, T., Brahm, M. (1976) Evaluation of single-drug vs. multiple-drug chemotherapy in metastatic carcinoma of the breast. Cancer Res. 36, 3911

10. Rubens, R. D., Knight, R., Hayward, J. L. (1975) Chemotherapy of advanced breast cancer: a controlled randomized trial of cyclophosphamide versus a four-drug combination. Br. J. Cancer 32, 739.
11. Smalley, R. V. , Murphy, S., Huguley, C. M., Bartolucci, A. (1976) Combination vs. sequential five-drug chemotherapy in metastatic carcinoma of the breast. Cancer Res. 36, 3911–3916.
12. Tormey D., Carbone, P., Band, P. (1977) Breast cancer survival in single and combination chemotherapy trials since 1968. Proc. Am. Assoc. Cancer Res. 18, 64
13. Zinser, J. W., Hortobagyi, G. N. , Buzdar, A. U., Smith, T. L., Fraschini, G. (1987) Clinical course of breast cancer patients with liver metastasis. J. Clin. Oncol. 5, 773–782.

Springer-Verlag and the Environment

We at Springer-Verlag firmly believe that an international science publisher has a special obligation to the environment, and our corporate policies consistently reflect this conviction.

We also expect our business partners – paper mills, printers, packaging manufacturers, etc. – to commit themselves to using environmentally friendly materials and production processes.

The paper in this book is made from low- or no-chlorine pulp and is acid free, in conformance with international standards for paper permanency.